The Great Ormond Street Hospital Manual of Children's Nursing Practices

The Great Ormond Street Hospital Manual of Children's Nursing Practices

Edited by

Susan Macqueen OBE
Previous Lead Nurse and Director of Infection Prevention and Control
Great Ormond Street Hospital for Children
London, UK

Elizabeth Anne Bruce
Clinical Nurse Specialist, Pain Control Service
Great Ormond Street Hospital for Children
London, UK

Faith Gibson
Clinical Professor of Children and Young People's Cancer Care
Great Ormond Street Hospital for Children and
London South Bank University London, UK

WILEY-BLACKWELL
A John Wiley & Sons, Ltd., Publication

Blackwell Publishing was acquired by John Wiley & Sons in February 2007. Blackwell's publishing program has been merged with Wiley's global Scientific, Technical and Medical business to form Wiley-Blackwell.

Registered office: John Wiley & Sons, Ltd, The Atrium, Southern Gate, Chichester, West Sussex, PO19 8SQ, UK

Editorial offices: 9600 Garsington Road, Oxford, OX4 2DQ, UK
The Atrium, Southern Gate, Chichester, West Sussex, PO19 8SQ, UK
350 Main Street, Malden, MA 02148-5020, USA

For details of our global editorial offices, for customer services and for information about how to apply for permission to reuse the copyright material in this book please see our website at www.wiley.com/wiley-blackwell

Library of Congress Cataloging-in-Publication Data
The Great Ormond Street Hospital manual of children's nursing practices / edited by Susan Macqueen, Elizabeth Anne Bruce, Faith Gibson.
    p. ; cm.
  Manual of children's nursing practices
  Includes bibliographical references and index.
  Summary: 'Clinical skills are a fundamental aspect of nursing care of children and young people. The Great Ormond Street Hospital Manual of Children's Nursing Practices is an evidenced-based manual of practical skills in children's nursing, which builds on the extensive expertise developed at Great Ormond Street Hospital. It encompasses all aspects of children's nursing from the most basic aspects of everyday practice to advanced practice in high dependency and intensive care to provide a comprehensive resource for all qualified nurses, students, and other health-care professionals involved in caring for children, both in the hospital and the community setting'–Provided by publisher.
  ISBN 978-1-4051-0932-1 (pbk. : alk. paper) – ISBN 978-1-4443-6118-6 (e-book)
  I. Macqueen, Susan. II. Bruce, Elizabeth (Elizabeth A.) III. Gibson, Faith, 1960– IV. Hospital for Sick Children (London, England) V. Title: Manual of children's nursing practices.
  [DNLM: 1. Pediatric Nursing–methods. 2. Adolescent. 3. Child. 4. Infant. WY 159]
  618.92′00231–dc23
                          2012009759

A catalogue record for this book is available from the British Library.

Wiley also publishes its books in a variety of electronic formats. Some content that appears in print may not be available in electronic books.

Also available in other electronic formats
• e-book, ISBN 978-1-4443-6118-6
• Kindle, see www.amazon.co.uk
• Wiley Desktop Edition, see http://eu.wiley.com/WileyCDA/WileyTitle/productCd-1118307798,descCd-ebook.html

Set in 9.5/11 pt Minion by Toppan Best-set Premedia Limited
Printed and bound in Singapore by Markono Print Media Pte Ltd

1   2012

Contents

Foreword

It is a great pleasure to be able to introduce the first edition of *The Great Ormond Street Hospital Manual of Children's Nursing Practices*. Great Ormond Street Hospital for Children has an international reputation in the care and treatment of sick children. The underpinning nursing practice principles can be adopted by nurses working across all settings. We hope this manual will be viewed by children's nurses across the world as a comprehensive evidence base which they can draw upon to support their day-to-day practice.

Healthcare for children and young people has changed beyond all recognition over the last thirty years. These developments have been in response to a number of factors including advances in medical science, technology and pharmacology, and more and more children are surviving long-term, life-limiting and life-threatening conditions.

Excellent nursing practice makes a significant contribution to the work of the healthcare team and the overall care of the child and family. As a result clinical colleagues, children, families and the public expect nurses to deliver high-quality patient care with exemplary nursing skill in a highly complex and emotionally charged environment. To maximise this contribution requires the development of sound clinical skills: an ability to critically analyse a particular situation; to gather comprehensive and relevant information to make an accurate clinical assessment ensuring early detection and recognition of deterioration; decision-making and taking appropriate action.

This requires a nurse to be well informed, knowledgeable and keep up-to-date. This can be challenging – to meet these many priorities, and balance the demands of practice in a wide range of busy clinical environments. It is hoped this manual will help children's nurses to ensure their practice is evidence-based and up-to-date.

Predominantly written by nurses from Great Ormond Street Hospital there are a number of highly respected contributors to this long-awaited book from several organisations and clinical settings representing the breadth and complexity of children's services. The coordination required to produce this manual has been no mean feat for the editors, Susan Macqueen, Elizabeth Bruce and Faith Gibson, whose tenacity is to be admired. The importance of collaboration across the wider healthcare team outweighs the challenges to produce this text which emphasises the delivery of seamless care across a range of settings and professional groups.

Liz Morgan
Chief Nurse
Great Ormond Street Hospital for Children NHS
Foundation Trust

Fiona Smith
Advisor for Children & Young People's Nursing
Royal College of Nursing

Acknowledgements

The Editors and Wiley-Blackwell would like to thank the many reviewers who provided welcome feedback and recommendations on individual chapters within the Manual.

They would also like to thank other staff at Great Ormond Street Hospital who contributed to the development of the Manual, including Sarah Allen (Chapter 14), Jennifer Grehan (Chapter 14), Jane Stevens (Chapter 3) and Crispin Walklin-Lee (Chapter 13).

Every effort has been made to acknowledge by name the many staff at the Great Ormond Street Hospital for Children NHS Foundation Trust who have contributed to earlier drafts of the Manual. The Editors and Publisher are very grateful for their assistance and would like to apologise for any inadvertent omissions.

List of contributors

Editorial Panel

Breidge Boyle MSc, BSc (Hons), RN (Child), RN (Adult), ANNP
Advanced Neonatal Nurse Practitioner
Great Ormond Street Hospital for Children NHS Foundation Trust
London, UK

Chris Caldwell RN (Adult), RN (Child), RNT, BSc (Hons), MSc, PGDip Ed
Assistant Director of Education and Organisational Development (Assistant Chief Nurse)
Great Ormond Street Hospital for Children NHS Foundation Trust
London, UK

Kathryn Halford RN (Adult), RN (Child), BSc
Assistant Chief Nurse
Great Ormond Street Hospital for Children NHS Foundation Trust
London, UK

Joy Hayes RN (Child), BSc (Hons), MSc, Dip Nurse Ed
Matron for Paediatrics
Whittington Health NHS Trust
London, UK

Kate Khair RN (Adult), RN (Child), MSc, MCGI
Nurse Consultant, Haemophilia
Great Ormond Street Hospital for Children NHS Foundation Trust
London, UK

Lindy May RN (Adult), RN (Child), MSc (Neuroscience), Diploma in Counselling
Nurse Consultant, Neurosurgery
Great Ormond Street Hospital for Children NHS Foundation Trust
London, UK

Liane Pilgrim RN (Child), BSc (Hons)
Sister
Haemodialysis Unit
Great Ormond Street Hospital for Children NHS Foundation Trust
London, UK

Vanessa Shaw MBE, MA, RD, FBDA
Head of Dietetics, Honorary Associate Professor University of Plymouth
Great Ormond Street Hospital for Children NHS Foundation Trust
London, UK

Elisabeth Smith RN (Adult), RN (Child), Advanced Diploma in Child Development, MSc Child Development
Lead Advanced Nurse Practitioner & ECMO Coordinator
Cardiorespiratory Services, Paediatric Cardiology and Cardiac Surgery
Great Ormond Street Hospital for Children NHS Foundation Trust
London, UK

Mark Whiting PhD, MSc, BNursing, RGN, RSCN, HV Cert, DN Cert, PGDip (Ed), RNT
Consultant Nurse, Children's Community and Specialist Nursing
Hertfordshire Community NHS Trust
Peace Children's Centre, Watford, Hertfordshire, UK

List of Contributors

Katie J. Allen RN (Adult), RN (Child), Bsc (Hons) Professional Practice
Children's Neuroscience Unit
Great Ormond Street Hospital for Children NHS Foundation Trust
London, UK
(Chapter 18)

Katrina Anthony RN (Adult), DipHE (child)
Pre-Admission Nurse Specialist, Urology
Great Ormond Street Hospital for Children NHS Foundation Trust
London, UK
(Chapter 29)

Tina Banks DCR (R)
Former CT Superintendent Radiographer, MRI research radiographer
Great Ormond Street Hospital for Children NHS Foundation Trust
London, UK
(Chapter 14)

Helen Bedford BSc, MSc, PhD, RN (Adult), RHV, FFPH, FRCPCH
Senior Lecturer in Children's Health
Centre for Epidemiology and Biostatistics
UCL Institute of Child Health
London, UK
(Chapter 11)

Fiona Bell BSc (Hons) Children's Nursing, ENB 147
Lecturer Practitioner, Nephro-urology
Great Ormond Street Hospital for Children NHS Foundation Trust
London, UK
(Chapter 29)

Nikki Bennett-Rees RN (Child), RN (Adult), Diploma advanced nursing
Clinical Nurse Specialist, Bone Marrow Transplant
Great Ormond Street Hospital for Children NHS Foundation Trust
London, UK
(Chapter 3)

Margaret Bird RN (Adult), RN (Child), BSc Hons, MSc
Clinical Lead Nurse
Children's Community Nursing Team, Children's Centre
Norwich, UK
(Chapter 23)

Fiona Blackwell RN (Child), RN (Adult), Dip Child Development
Matron for Children's Services
Wye Valley Trust, Hereford County Hospital, Hereford
(Chapter 14)

Breidge Boyle MSc, BSc (Hons), RN (Child), RN (Adult), ANNP
Advanced Neonatal Nurse Practitioner
Great Ormond Street Hospital for Children NHS Foundation Trust
London, UK
(Chapter 17)

Emma Brady BSc (Hons) Physiotherapy
Physiotherapist
Physiotherapy Department
Great Ormond Street Hospital for Children NHS Foundation Trust
London, UK
(Chapter 20)

Eileen Brennan RN (Adult), RN (Child), ENB 147, MSc
Nurse Consultant in Paediatric Nephrology
Great Ormond Street Hospital for Children NHS Foundation Trust
London, UK
(Chapters 1, 9)

Kathryn Bridgwater RN (Child), BSc (Hons) Child Health, Advanced Diploma in Child Development
Nurse Practice Educator, Orthopaedics
Great Ormond Street Hospital for Children NHS Foundation Trust
London, UK
(Chapter 20)

Joanne Brind RN (Adult), RN (Child), MSc, Dipl (IPresc)
Clinical Nurse Specialist
Great Ormond Street Hospital for Children NHS Foundation Trust
London, UK
(Chapter 19)

Elizabeth Bruce MSc, BSc (Hons), RN (Adult), RN (Child)
Clinical Nurse Specialist, Pain Control Service
Great Ormond Street Hospital for Children NHS Foundation Trust
London, UK
(Chapters 15, 21, Editor)

Sue Chapman RN (Adult), RN (Child), Advanced Diploma (child development), MSc Paediatric Critical Care (advanced nursing practice), ENB100
Nurse Consultant, Acute and High Dependency Care and Associate for Safer Care (Paediatrics)
NHS Institute for Innovation and Improvement
Great Ormond Street Hospital for Children NHS Foundation Trust
London, UK
(Chapters 1, 16)

Robert Cole RN (Child), RN (Adult), MA Ed, PGDip Ed, BSc (Hons)with ENB Higher Award, ENB 199, ENB998, ENB A53. APLS Instructor
Nurse Lecturer/ Practitioner
King's College London
Florence Nightingale School of Nursing and Midwifery
London, UK
(Chapter 25)

Sue Cole RN (Adult), RN (Child), DipHE Children's Oncology Nursing
Paediatric Oncology CNS, Paediatric Ward
South London Healthcare NHS Trust
Kent, UK
(Chapter 13)

Amber Conley Bachelor of Health Science Nursing, BSc Nursing Studies (Child), MSc Nursing
Matron and Lead Principal Treatment Centre Nurse for Children and Young People
The Royal Marsden NHS Foundation Trust and St George's Healthcare NHS Trust
Sutton, Surrey
(Chapter 8)

Joanne Cooke TD, MSc, BSc (Hons), RN (Adult), RN (Child)
Nurse Practitioner, Tracheostomy Care
Great Ormond Street Hospital for Children NHS Foundation
Trust
London, UK
(Chapter 28)

Catherine Dunne Dip PT, MSc Physiology
Clinical Specialist Physiotherapist
Cardiorespiratory Physiotherapy
Great Ormond Street Hospital for Children NHS Foundation
Trust
London, UK
(Chapter 26)

Teresa Durack RN (Adult), RM, DipN, PGDip, MSc
Modern Matron, Corporate Facilities
Great Ormond Street Hospital for Children NHS Foundation
Trust
London, UK
(Chapters 2, 23)

Netty Fabian RN (Child)
Formerly Senior Staff Nurse, Transitional Care Unit
Great Ormond Street Hospital for Children NHS Foundation
Trust
London, UK
(Chapter 19)

Róisín Fitzsimons RN (Child), BSc (Hons), Dip HE
Clinical Nurse Specialist
The Children's Allergy Service
St Thomas' Hospital
London, UK
(Chapter 2)

Sheryl Gettings MSc, BSc (Hons), RN (Child)
Senior Lecturer
London South Bank University
London, UK
(Chapter 19)

Faith Gibson PhD, MSc, RN (Child), RN (Adult), ONC Cert,
Cert Ed, RNT, FRCN
Clinical Professor of Children and Young People's Cancer Care,
Great Ormond Street Hospital for Children NHS Foundation
Trust and London South Bank University
London, UK
(Chapters 10, 15, Editor)

Claire Gilbert BSc (Hons) (Children's Nursing), Diploma
(Child Health), RN (Adult), RN (Child)
Clinical Nurse Specialist, Hypoglycaemia
Great Ormond Street Hospital for Children NHS Foundation
Trust
London, UK
(Chapter 14)

Ambrose Gullet RN (Adult), RN (Child), BSc
Clinical Research Nurse, Nephro-urology
Institute of Child Health
University College London
London, UK
(Chapter 29)

Julia Hannan RN (Adult), RN (Child), Adv Dip Child
Development, BSc Child Health, MA Death and Society
Clinical Nurse Specialist, Paediatric Oncology Outreach and
Palliative Care Team
Great Ormond Street Hospital for Children NHS Foundation
Trust
London, UK
(Chapter 22)

Juanita Harrison RN (Adult), RN (Child), BA Hons
Specialist Practitioner Children's Nursing
Alder Hey Children's NHS Foundation Trust
West Derby, Liverpool, UK
(Chapter 6)

Joy Hayes RN (Child) BSc (Hons), MSc, Dip Nurse Ed,
Matron for Paediatrics
Whittington Health NHS Trust
London, UK
(Chapters 13, 14)

June Hemsley RN (Child), BSc Children's Nursing
Clinical Nurse Specialist, Paediatric Oncology Outreach and
Palliative Care Team
Great Ormond Street Hospital for Children NHS Foundation
Trust
London, UK
(Chapter 22)

Sylvia J. Hennem MSc, CSci, FIBMS
Specialist Practitioner of Transfusion
Great Ormond Street Hospital for Children NHS Foundation
Trust
London, UK
(Chapter 4)

Melanie Hiorns MBBS, MRCP, FRCR
Consultant Paediatric Radiologist
Great Ormond Street Hospital for Children NHS Foundation
Trust
London, UK
(Chapter 14)

Penny Howard RN (Adult), RN (Child)
Clinical Nurse Specialist, Orthopaedics
Great Ormond Street Hospital for Children NHS Foundation
Trust
London, UK
(Chapter 20)

Helen Ingall Dip HE Child Health, BSc (Hons)
Sister, Urology and General Surgery
Great Ormond Street Hospital for Children NHS Foundation
Trust
London, UK
(Chapter 29)

Carole Irwin BSc (Hons), PGCE, ENB 219
Practice Educator, Surgery
Great Ormond Street Hospital for Children NHS Foundation
Trust
London, UK
(Chapter 20)

Helen Johnson BSc (Hons) RN (Adult), RN (Child), ENB 216
Clinical Nurse Specialist Stoma Care
Great Ormond Street Hospital for Children NHS Foundation
Trust
London, UK
(Chapter 5)

Julie Sharon Jones RN (Child), Dip Nursing Studies
Senior Staff Nurse
Great Ormond Street Hospital for Children NHS Foundation
Trust
London, UK
(Chapter 15)

Monica King RN, SCM, HVCert, PG Cert (Child Protection
and Family Support)
Sessional Lecturer for post-graduate module 'Protecting and
Safeguarding Children'
Department of Children's Nursing
Faculty of Health and Social Care
London South Bank University
London, UK
(Chapter 7)

Trisha Kleidon Bachelor of Health Science (Nursing), Grad
dip Paediatrics, Child and Young Health Nursing
Nurse Practitioner Candidate
Royal Children's Hospital, Brisbane, Australia
(Chapter 14)

Lorraine Laccohee RN (Child), BA (Hons), PG Diploma
Children's Community Nurse
Croydon Health Services
Surrey, UK
(Chapter 6)

Susan Macqueen OBE, RN (Adult), RN (Child), MSc (Medical
Anthropology), ENB 910
Formerly Lead Nurse and Director of Infection Prevention and
Control
Department of Microbiology, Virology and Infection
Prevention and Control
Great Ormond Street Hospital for Children NHS Foundation
Trust
London, UK
(Chapters 12, 14, Editor)

Pippa Mashford DCR(R)
Senior Radiographer
Great Ormond Street Hospital for Children NHS Foundation
Trust
London, UK
(Chapter 14)

Jan E. Maxwell RN (Child), SCM, MPH
Clinical Nurse Specialist – Plastic Surgery
Great Ormond Street Hospital for Children NHS Foundation
Trust
London, UK
(Chapter 10)

Nicola McAdam RN (Child)
Senior Staff Nurse
Paediatric Intensive Care Unit
Great Ormond Street Hospital for Children NHS Foundation
Trust
London, UK
(Chapter 20)

Beth McCann RN (Child)
Clinical Nurse Specialist, Children & Young People's Cancer
Unit
University College Hospital
London, UK
(Chapter 13)

Rachel McCann RN (Child), BSc (Hons) Critical Care
Nursing, ENB405
Practice Educator, Surgery
Great Ormond Street Hospital for Children NHS Foundation
Trust
London, UK
(Chapter 10)

Brian McGowan MSc, RN
Lecturer, Institute of Nursing Research
School of Nursing
University of Ulster
Newtownabbey
Co. Antrim
(Chapter 6)

Clare McLaren DCR (R)
Clinical Specialist Radiographer
Interventional Radiology
Great Ormond Street Hospital for Children NHS Foundation
Trust
London, UK
(Chapter 14)

Nikki Mumford RN (Child), EN
Metabolic Clinical Nurse Specialist
Metabolic Medicine
Great Ormond Street Hospital for Children NHS Foundation
Trust
London, UK
(Chapter 14)

Nikki Nabney RN (Child)
Transitional Care Unit
Ward Manager / Sister
Great Ormond Street Hospital for Children NHS Foundation
Trust
London, UK
(Chapter 26)

Helen Nulty FIBMS
Chief Biomedical Scientist, Blood Transfusion – Haematology /
Oncology
Great Ormond Street Hospital for Children NHS Foundation
Trust
London, UK
(Chapter 4)

Nic O'Brien BHSc (Physiotherapy), MCSP
Senior Occupational Health Physiotherapist
Great Ormond Street Hospital for Children NHS Foundation
Trust
London, UK
(Chapter 16)

Maura O'Callaghan RN (Child)
Lead Nurse, ECMO
Cardiorespiratory Unit
Great Ormond Street Hospital for Children NHS Foundation
Trust
London, UK
(Chapter 26)

Julia Petty BSc, MSc, PGDipEd, RN (Adult), RN (Child)
Senior Lecturer in Neonatal Lecturer
City Community and Health Sciences
City University
London, UK
(Chapter 10)

Liane Pilgrim RN (Adult), RN (Child)
Sister
Haemodialysis Unit
Great Ormond Street Hospital for Children NHS Foundation
Trust
London, UK
(Chapter 29)

Paula Pollock RN (Child)
Senior Staff Nurse
Demelza House
Eltham, UK
(Chapter 26)

Zoe Pullar RN (Child)
Sister
Paediatric Unit
Watford General Hospital
Watford, Herts, UK
(Chapter 26)

Claire Richardson BSc (Hons), ENB 147, RN (Child)
Senior Staff Nurse, Nephrology
Great Ormond Street Hospital for Children NHS Foundation
Trust
London, UK
(Chapter 13)

June Rogers MBE, RN, RN (Child), BSc (Hons), MSc
Continence Advisor with special interest in Paediatrics
Team Director, PromoCon
Burrows House, Worsley
Manchester, UK
(Chapter 5)

Jacqueline Rouse-Robinson RN (Child), BSc (Hons) in
Child Health
Modern Matron – Neurosciences
Great Ormond Street Hospital for Children NHS Foundation
Trust
London, UK
(Chapter 15)

Stephen Rowley RN (Adult), RN (Child), BSc (Hons), MSc
Lead Cancer Nurse and Clinical Director ANTT (www.antt.
org.uk), Haematology Unit
University College London Hospitals
London, UK
(Chapter 12)

Karen Ryan RN (Adult), RN (Child)
Clinical Nurse Specialist, Bladder Exstrophy
Urodynamics
Great Ormond Street Hospital for Children NHS Foundation
Trust
London, UK
(Chapter 29)

Paul Sacher BSc (Med) Hons RD
Childhood Nutrition Research Centre
Institute of Child Health
London, UK
(Chapter 19)

Rebecca Saul RN (Child)
Lecturer Practitioner, Paediatric Pain
Great Ormond Street Hospital for Children NHS Foundation
Trust
London, UK
(Chapter 30)

Katie Self RN (Child), DipHe, BSc, Paediatric Nephro-urology
Nursing
Paediatric Urology, Clinical Nurse Specialist
Portland Hospital for Women and Children
London, UK
(Chapter 10)

Vanessa Shaw MBE, MA, RD, FBDA
Head of Dietetics, Honorary Associate Professor University of Plymouth
Great Ormond Street Hospital for Children NHS Foundation Trust
London, UK
(Chapters 10, 19)

Sheila Simpson BA (Hons), DPSN, RN (Child), RN (Adult)
Resuscitation Services Manager
Great Ormond Street Hospital for Children NHS Foundation Trust
London, UK
(Chapters 26, 27)

Lynn Speedwell BSc, MSc (Health Psych), DCLP, FAAO, FBCLA
Head of Optometry, NHS Trust
The Clinical and Academic Department of Ophthalmology
Great Ormond Street Hospital for Children NHS Foundation Trust
London, UK
(Chapter 10)

Deborah St Louis RN (Child)
Gastro Day Care
Great Ormond Street Hospital for Children NHS Foundation Trust
London, UK
(Chapter 14)

Maggie Stewart
Formerly Clinical Nurse Specialist
Nutrition, Gastroenterology
Great Ormond Street Hospital for Children NHS Foundation Trust
London, UK
(Chapter 19)

Mary Wallis SRN, SCM, RN (Child)
Neonatal Nurse Advisor
Great Ormond Street Hospital for Children NHS Foundation Trust
London, UK
(Chapter 17)

Cynthia Wenden RN (Adult), RN (Child), BSc (Hons)
Clinical Nurse Specialist, Symptom Care team
Great Ormond Street Hospital for Children NHS Foundation Trust (now Marie Curie)
London, UK
(Chapter 22)

Zoe Wilks BSc (Hons) Child health, Adj Dip Cu Dev, RN (Child), RN
Modern Matron, Outpatients
Great Ormond Street Hospital for Children NHS Foundation Trust
London, UK
(Chapter 3)

Lesley Wilson NNEB, HPSEB, Certificate in Education
Formerly Play Services Manager
Great Ormond Street Hospital for Children NHS Foundation Trust
London, UK
(Chapter 24)

Elizabeth Wright BSc (Hons), DipAppSS, RN (Adult), RN (Child), V300, ENB 136 and 870
Clinical Nurse Specialist Dialysis, Dialysis Unit
Great Ormond Street Hospital for Children NHS Foundation Trust
London, UK
(Chapter 9)

Introduction

We made the decision to write this introductory chapter last. We wanted to set the scene for what was to follow and therefore needed to know what followed before we put finger to keyboard. Our intention here is to highlight a number of principles that should underpin all clinical care given in the community and hospital setting, and which are the cornerstone of the content of chapters in this textbook. All the guidelines contained herein are not intended to replace individual assessment and personalised treatment of the child and family. Our intention for presenting this information is to bring to nurses delivering child healthcare the latest evidence that underpins clinical care, the 'how to' and 'why' of many clinical procedures. Our first principle that guides us in our work is that of individualised care.

Individualised care

The motto for Great Ormond Street Hospital for Children NHS Foundation Trust is 'The child first and always'. Each child or young person needs to be seen as a 'whole', in the context of their family, carers, school, friends and local community. This perspective should involve an understanding that as children and young people grow up, and develop, their needs change. Knowledge of child development, family structures, communication patterns and the wider social networks children live within is important for us to understand how we approach care delivery. Using a family systems approach to nursing is not new, but we, like other authors and practitioners, would recommend its use to focus on the care of the whole family (Hemphill and Dearmun 2010).

Children also have rights as human beings and need special care and attention (United Nations International Children's Emergency Fund – UNICEF Convention on the Rights of the Child 1989). This Convention is the first legally binding international instrument to incorporate the full range of human rights for children – civil, cultural, economic, political and social rights. Each child has the right:

- for survival – to be given food and water and grow healthily
- to develop to the fullest – to achieve and enjoy through education
- to protection from harmful influences, abuse and exploitation – to stay safe
- to participate fully in family, cultural and social life – to make a positive contribution and achieve economic well-being.

Our role in healthcare is to ensure children reach their fullest potential, and thus limit where we can the short- and long-term effects that result from health changes. Most children will experience the healthcare system in some way during their life; vaccinations, school health checks, dental checks, sexual health, maternity services or if they become unwell a visit to their local doctor, or a hospital referral. It is important that within each of these different contexts the child is seen as an individual within the family. Throughout this textbook there are many examples of approaches to ensure this aim will be achieved in your approaches to care.

Family-centred care

Our second principle is the need to fully understand the principles of, and work always using, a family-centred approach to care. This takes the notion of individualised care further with family-centred care viewed as a central tenet of children's nursing (Coleman 2002). A 'family-centred care' (FCC) model is widely used in the care of children and young people in hospital. This encompasses the holistic psychosocial-economic need to always see children within a family concept. Hutchfield (1999) analysed the concepts of FCC and found that partnership with parents/carers, parent's participation and care by parent were the most common systems applied in practice. These systems were meant to help clarify for parents/carers their caring roles, and make explicit how professionals and parents/carers would work together. 'The social construct of family-centred care has been refined again and again and within this construct parents/carers have moved from a passive presence to being allowed to take on a more active role in their child's care in hospital' (Coleman 2002, page 9). It is even more evident that family presence in healthcare settings is important, from the perspective of the parents/carers and the child (Soderback et al 2011).

The effectiveness of family-centred care, however, has not been measured sufficiently, and many argue that although nurses would support the principles of it very few can really define it and say what works best in what situation. Corlett and Twycross (2006) in their review on FCC commented on the relevance to clinical practice 'for family-centred care to be a reality nurses need to negotiate and communicate with children and their families effectively'. Parents/carers need to be able to negotiate with health staff what this participation will involve and to negotiate new roles for themselves in sharing care of their sick child. Parents/carers should be involved in the decision-making process. However, research suggests that a lack of effective communication, professional expectations and issues of power and control often inhibit open and mutual negotiation between families and nurses.

A Cochrane Database of Systematic Reviews (Shields 2008) concluded that there is a 'dearth of high quality qualitative research about family-centred care. A much more stringent examination of the use of FCC as a model for care delivery to children and families in health services is needed.' Despite this need for better definition and evaluation we would support the notion of family involvement in care, where nurses work within family structures to care for children and young people effectively and support family members in their roles, whether they be nursing or family roles. We recommend the family-centred practice continuum described by Smith *et al* (2010) to practitioners; this will help you help parents to decide on the degree to which they may be active participants in their child's care, including planning, delivery, and management.

Legislation

Our third principle stresses the need for clinical professionals working with children and young people to be conversant with legislation and general guidance for the welfare of children and young people. This knowledge will always be timely, and it falls to the professional to keep this up to date. Access to computers at clinical level makes this task much easier than it ever was, with access to professional data bases and Pubmed. We draw the reader's attention to some of the legislation relevant today:

1. The Human Rights Act (1998), which came into force in October 2000, giving further effect in the UK to the rights enshrined in the European Convention on Human Rights.
2. The Children Act (2004), which is the legal framework for England. In Scotland the legislative provisions for protecting children and promoting their welfare are contained in the Protection of Vulnerable Groups (Scotland) Act 2007 and the Children (Scotland) Act 2003. The principles of co-operation and information sharing between agencies in the safeguarding of children are, however, important themes in the legislative framework and guidance governing the delivery of children's services in Northern Ireland, where the legislative provisions are the Children (Northern Ireland) Order 1995, and the Safeguarding Vulnerable Groups (Northern Ireland) Order 2007. In both jurisdictions Area Child Protection Committees are the means of providing local procedures and processes for agencies to comply with the legislation to safeguard children and to co-operate together, and for anyone working with children. The Welsh Assembly Government has produced its own version of *Safeguarding Children: Working together Under the Children Act 2004* (2006).
3. The government's document on *Every Child Matters* (2003) which was the beginning of the 10-year plan to further improve the lives of children, young people and their families.
4. *The National Service Framework for Children, Young People and Maternity Services* (2007), which establishes clear standards for promoting the health and well-being of children and young people.
5. *Every Child Matters – change for children* (Home Office UK Border Agency 2009). This is a statutory guidance to the UK Border Agency on making arrangements to safeguard and promote the welfare of children.
6. *Healthy Lives, Brighter Futures* (2009) – a joint strategy between the Department of Health and the Department for Children, Schools and Families for children and young people's health and well-being.

Code of conduct

The need to be conversant with the code of conduct is our fourth principle. Nurses and other healthcare staff must act as advocates for the child when necessary (NMC 2008). The people in your care must be able to trust you with their health and well-being. To justify that trust, you must:

1. make the care of people your first concern, treating them as individuals and respecting their dignity
2. work with others to protect and promote the health and well-being of those in your care, their families and carers, and the wider community
3. provide a high standard of practice and care at all times
4. be open and honest, act with integrity and uphold the reputation of your profession.

As a professional, you are personally accountable for actions and omissions in your practice and must always be able to justify your decisions. The code should be considered together with the Nursing and Midwifery Council's rules, standards, guidance and advice available from www.nmc-uk.org. The NMC web site is kept up to date and should be able to guide you in aspects of the codes and guidance: your role as a practitioner is to keep up to date with this.

Ethnicity

As nurses, we need to be confident in our role to deliver culturally sensitive care to families, and this is our fifth principle. Family ethnicity includes race, culture, religion and nationality, which impact on a family or person's identity and how they are seen by others. Health is shaped by many different factors, such as lifestyle, material wealth, educational attainment, job security, housing conditions, psycho-social stress, discrimination and health services. We know that health inequalities exist for different ethnic minority groups and represent the cumulative effect of these factors over the life-course; they can be passed on from one generation to the next through maternal influences on baby and child development. Initiatives aiming to reduce poverty, social exclusion and difficulty in accessing health services have the potential to tackle the root causes of health inequalities. Some community initiatives which are aiming to reduce health inequalities and social exclusion by targeting deprived areas are: Health Action Zones (www.haznet.org.uk), Neighbourhood Renewal (www.neighbourhood.statistics.org.uk), the New Deal for Communities (www.communities.gov.uk), Sure Start (www.direct.gov.uk/en/Parents/Preschooldevelopmentandlearning/NurseriesPlaygroupsReceptionClasses) and most recently, the Spearhead Area initiatives (www.dh.gov.uk). An understanding of such schemes can help nurses to be aware of support networks available to families in our care.

The concept of 'culture' is not homogeneous and one should avoid using generalisations in explaining a family's beliefs or behaviours. One should differentiate between the rules of a culture, which governs how one *should* think and behave, and how people actually behave in real life. Generalisations can be dangerous as they often lead to misunderstanding, prejudices and discrimination. There may be conflict within a family who has certain beliefs when their child has been influenced by different outside social forces. Cultural background has an important influence on many aspects of a child's life, including their beliefs, behaviours, perceptions, emotions, language, religion, rituals, family structure, diet, dress, body image, concepts of space and time. It also plays a part in attitudes to illness, pain and other misfortunes (Helman 2007). It is important to interpret behaviour or beliefs within their particular context, which is made up of historical, economic, social, political and geographical elements. This may, for example, have an influence on children or parents who are non adherent with their medical/nursing care and are seen as 'difficult'.

In most cultures boys and girls are socialised in different ways and this varies throughout the world. For example, men may play a more predominate part in public life in some cultures but the 'grandmother' of the family (who is seen as being wiser) may be the decision maker on the way the child is brought up.

Artificial changes of the body such as in body piercing, tattooing or artificial fattening in some cultures are often deemed as notions of beauty. Extreme cases such as female circumcision or severe obesity may affect health and should be dealt with accordingly. Different religious beliefs may include ritual immersions, fasts, food taboos, circumcision, communal feasts or mass pilgrimages. Some of these may be associated with incidences of certain diseases such as malnutrition with food taboos.

Health professionals should not assume that everyone knows how their body works. Many people see it as a 'plumbing system' or machine and that body parts and cavities are connected by pipes (Helman 2007). It is important to ensure that families and children understand their particular health problem and that this is communicated by both oral and written information in their native language, using props that might best help us explain what is happening. An interpreting service should be available to families and children whose first language is not English. Healthcare workers must be sensitive to the world that children and their families live in and ensure that cultural differences or even different views on health are taken into consideration, recorded where necessary and communicated appropriately to the clinical team.

Consent and involving children in decisions

Throughout this book there is an emphasis on ensuring direct communication with children and involving them in all decisions about them. This might include small decisions such as which arm they want to use for their blood pressure to be taken, to bigger decisions such as what kind of central line they want inserted. In all relevant sections authors have provided supporting literature on the issue of consent relevant to the clinical procedure. We thought this an important sixth principle, and want to highlight in particular Department of Health guidance that should be fully understood by all nurses delivering child healthcare. The following information is taken from the Department of Health's *Reference Guide to Consent for Examination or Treatment* (2009). It provides an update on legislation relating to obtaining valid consent: the Human Tissue Act 2004 (see www.hta.org.uk), the Mental Capacity Act 2005 (see www.publicguardian.gov.uk/mca/code-of-practice.htm) and recent legal cases. It is based on English law and therefore healthcare practitioners must follow professional and local guidelines and ensure they are kept up to date, as further legal developments may occur and the law may differ in other countries. It should be read in conjunction with the issues highlighted in each section of this textbook.

Paragraph 1 states:

> It is a general legal and ethical principle that valid consent must be obtained before starting treatment or physical investigation, or providing personal care, for a person. This principle reflects the right of patients to determine what happens to their own bodies, and is a fundamental part of good practice. A healthcare professional (or other healthcare staff) who does not respect this principle may be liable both to legal action by the patient and to action by their professional body. Employing bodies may also be liable for the actions of their staff.

The guidance states 'that case law ("common law") has established that touching a patient without valid consent may constitute the civil or criminal offence of battery'.

Consent may be expressed verbally or non-verbally: an example of non-verbal consent would be where a person, after receiving appropriate information, holds out an arm for their blood pressure to be taken. However, the person must have understood what examination or treatment is intended, and why, for such consent to be valid. If your work involves healthcare of any kind for children – in the healthcare context this includes anything from helping a child get dressed to carrying out major surgery, whether in hospital or in the child's own home – you need to make sure that you have consent to do what you propose to do.

Most consent is obtained by medical staff for operations and specific medical treatments. Information given including risks (both orally and written) must be written in the medical/nursing notes. However, nurses must ensure that children and parents understand the risks. If nurses are giving specific treatments as part of the expanded role of the nurse, where written consent is required they must follow the same procedure. Any care or treatment and alternatives must be discussed with parents and the child as appropriate. If students are to give care, an explanation that they are learning, under whose supervision, should be given and for any extra care, such as examining a child, permission should be sought. The trained nurse is responsible for ensuring the student is competent in the relevant activity. Written consent should be obtained for any visual or audio recording, including photographs or other visual images and also participation in any kind of research. Consent must be seen as a continuum and can be withdrawn at any time.

Paragraph 4 states:

> Legal advice should always be sought if there is any doubt about the legal validity of a proposed intervention. While much of the case law refers specifically to doctors, the same principles will apply to other healthcare practitioners involved in examining or treating patients.

It is important that nurses do not obtain consent for operation or treatment (unless specifically indicated in the expanded role of the nurse). For example, nurses may give cytotoxic drugs but the consent for the overall treatment regimen is obtained currently by doctors.

Paragraph 12 states:

> The standards expected of healthcare professionals by their regulatory bodies may at times be higher than the minimum required

by the law. Although this guidance focuses primarily on the legal position, it will also indicate relevant guidance from regulatory bodies. It should be noted that the legal requirements in negligence cases have historically been based on the standards set by the professions for their members; therefore where the standards required by professional bodies are rising, it is likely that the legal standards will rise accordingly.

This is known as the 'Bolan test' (1957).

Section 3 of the reference guide outlines the law for consent for children and young people. The legal position concerning consent and refusal of treatment by those under the age of 18 is different from the position for adults. The guidance states 'For the purposes of the guidance 'children' refers to people aged below 16 and 'young people' refers to people aged 16–17.'

Section 3 paragraph 22 sets out persons who may have parental responsibility:

- the child's mother
- the child's father, if he was married to the mother at the time of birth
- unmarried fathers, who can acquire parental responsibility in several different ways:
  1) For children born before 1 December 2003, unmarried fathers will have parental responsibility if they:
     - marry the mother of their child or obtain a parental responsibility order from the court
     - register a parental responsibility agreement with the court or by an application to court.
  2) For children born after 1 December 2003, unmarried fathers will have parental responsibility if they:
     - register the child's birth jointly with the mother at the time of birth
     - re-register the birth if they are the natural father
     - marry the mother of their child or obtain a parental responsibility order from the court
     - register with the court for parental responsibility
     - the child's legally appointed guardian.
- a person in whose favour the court has made a residence order concerning the child
- a local authority designated in a care order in respect of the child.

For consent to be valid, it must be given voluntarily by an appropriately informed person who has the capacity to consent to the intervention in question (this will be the patient or someone with parental responsibility for a patient under the age of 18, someone authorised to do so under a Lasting Power of Attorney (LPA) or someone who has the authority to make treatment decisions as a court appointed deputy. If the 16/17-year-old is capable of giving valid consent then it is not legally necessary to obtain consent from a person with parental responsibility for the young person. For children under 16 years the concept of 'Gillick competence'(1986), where the child has sufficient understanding and intelligence to enable them to understand fully what is involved in a proposed intervention, will also have the capacity to consent to that intervention. This legal concept is said to reflect a child's increasing development and maturity. A child under 16 years of age may be 'Gillick competent' to consent to medical treatment, research, donation or any other activity that requires their consent.

Although parental consent does not have to be obtained for competent young people or those who are 'Gillick competent', it is good practice to involve the parents in the decision making providing the young person or child agrees. Although a child or young person may have the capacity to give consent, this is only valid if it is given voluntarily. This requirement must be considered carefully. Children and young people may be subject to undue influence by their parent(s), other carers or a sexual partner (current or potential), and it is important to establish that the decision is that of the individual him or herself.

Further information can be obtained from the Department of Health guidelines (2009), and knowledge about the consent process must be kept up to date, as nurses need to be able to refer families to guidance that might help them.

Communication and handover

Communication, and the ability to communicate complex information to children, young people and family members features in all our stated principles so far. We encourage practitioners to learn effective communication strategies to ensure that children, young people and their parents/carers have the information they need in the appropriate format (Matthews 2010). In our seventh and final principle we want to turn to the importance of communication between professionals. Nurses have always had a 'ritual' for handing over patient information from one another when changing shifts, but the quality and accuracy of the information has often been called into question. One of the greatest sources of frustration for children, young people and their families is the lack of integration and communication between different services within an organisation or between organisations.

Handover is the system by which the responsibility for immediate and ongoing care is transferred between healthcare professionals. Children, young people and their families expect, and should have, a designated consultant and nurse to coordinate the multidisciplinary team. However, at times (e.g. at night, weekends or during an emergency admission) the responsibility for care must pass from one team, or consultant, to another (Royal College of Physicians 2011). Poor handover between doctors, nurses and multidisciplinary teams is a common cause of error in hospitals, and is a major preventable cause of patient harm. It can lead to inefficiencies, repetitions, delayed decisions, repeated investigations, incorrect diagnoses, incorrect treatment, and poor communication with the patient. Some hospitals do not even have a handover protocol in place (RCP 2011). The handover should be written or recorded and each professional involved in the child's care should have access to it at all times. There is no reason why children, young people or their parents should not listen to their own handover unless this is felt to be medically inappropriate.

Various examples of a handover template can be found at www.rcplondon.ac.uk/resources/clinical-resources/standards-medical-record-keeping/hospital-admission-handover-and-disc-0. At Great Ormond Street, a template which is an adaptation of SBAR and ABCD (see Chapter 1) has been introduced to improve all forms of communication and handover (see Table I.1) (Beckell and Kipnis 2009, Dunsford 2009, Resuscitation Council 2011).

Table I.1 Example of a high-dependency cardiac ward handover sheet

SBARD and ABCD Assessment Tool – Paediatric Cardiac Ward GOSH		
Situation	Name	Introduce parents/carers if present, name band with date of birth, hospital number
	Age	
	Diagnosis	
	Weight	Height, head circumference
	Allergies	
	Surgery, intervention, **Expected discharge date**	Days post operative
	Infection Precautions	Standard precautions, isolation, PPE requirements
Background	Any past or present information of relevance	Comment on parental concerns, previous day's care, developments, or changes
Assessment (CEWS Score)	Airway	Airway patency, airway obstruction, tracheostomy
	Breathing	Mode of Ventilation (SV, CPAP, BIPAP inc. Settings)
		Saturations
		Respiratory rate, rhythm, depth
		Work of breathing, recession, use of accessory muscles, auscultation of chest.
		Oxygen requirement (Delivery method, NC, HB,FM)
		Colour, pale, cyanosis
	Circulation	Heart Rate, rhythm, volume
		Pacing (Mode, rate, last pacing check)
		Blood pressure
		Temperature
		Capillary refill, peripheral pulses, mottled appearance
	Neurological assessment	AVPU, pupils, posture (Blood glucose if altered)
		Sedation, pain management
	Drugs	Infusions – Morphine, Inotropes, Heparin
		Antibiotics, EP up to date, drug levels required
	Elimination / Fluids	Current Fluid Allowance ml/kg/day
		Balance mls (Comment on Diuretics)
		Urine ml/kg/hr
		Diuretics
		Weight Today's (Comment +/– gms)
		Feeding Method (SALT, dietician)
		Bowels (Time since last stool)
	Healthy Skin/Skin Integrity	Surgical Wound (Date dressing due)
		Pressure ulcer prevention score
	Invasive Devices **(Also see patient body map for locations)**	Chest drains, pacing wires, sutures
		IV access (Peripheral, central, arterial)
		NG, NJ, NO, PEG, PEJ (Safety log complete, parent training)
		Tracheostomy, Berlin heart
	Investigation and Pathology Results	Pathology Results, ECG, ECHO, CXR, EEG
Recommendations	Investigations and pathology requests	
	Referrals	
Decision	Discharge checklist, transfer, **EDD**	Discharge Letter – Nurses/Doctors
	Medication	TTA ordered
	Parent Teaching, information for parents	
	Transport	Outpatient appointment booked

Developed for the Paediatric Cardiac Ward by Ashley Hurford, Practice Educator, Cardiac Services, with thanks to Sue Chapman, Nurse Consultant Acute and High Dependency Care, and Fiona Horrox, Senior Lecturer, Children's Nursing, London South Bank University.
Based on SBARD and ABCD assessment.

Communication during verbal handover should also be standardised to improve accuracy and safety. A communication aid developed by the US Navy and adapted for healthcare (Hohenhaus *et al* 2006) has been further adapted by clinical teams at GOSH. Where a 'D' for decisions has been added to the acronym SBAR, this is to 'round off' each conversation and improve clarity. Over one-third of wards at GOSH have improved the efficiency and effectiveness of their handover using the SBARD (Situation, Background, Assessment, Recommendation, Decision) communication aid. On average, wards using SBARD have reduced the length of time spent in handover by 30–50% – that is 10–20 minutes twice each day. Nurses who now use SBARD also report that their handovers feel safer and more effective, as everyone involved focuses on patient care needs for the next shift and beyond, rather than reviewing what has happened in the past. This method is also being used to communicate the needs of the deteriorating child. Although yet to be formally evaluated within the context of healthcare, we are recommending its use to readers of this textbook.

These seven principles, outlined here briefly, are, we suggest, important to all the chapters that follow. Delivering safe care, managing procedures effectively and working with all family members sensitively are important to ensure we as nurses can be confident of delivering high-quality care. Nurses have a central role in helping children, young people and their family members to manage the demands of clinical procedures as part of a unique illness experience. Even when the procedure has been undertaken many times before, and we are caring for 'expert patients', our attention to individualised patient assessment will enable us to work effectively alongside family members.

Susan Macqueen OBE
Elizabeth Anne Bruce
Faith Gibson

References

Beckell C, Kipnis G. (2009) Collaborative Communication: Integrating SBAR to Improve Quality/Patient Safety Outcomes. Available at http://onlinelibrary.wiley.com/doi/10.1111/j.1945-1474.2009.00043.x/pdf (last accessed 31st January 2012)

Bolam v Friern Hospital Management Committee (1957) 2 All ER 118 Available at http://oxcheps.new.ox.ac.uk/casebook/Resources/BOLAMV_1%20DOC.pdf (last accessed 20th June 2011)

Coleman V. (2002) The evolving concept of family-centred care. In Smith L, Coleman V, Bradshaw M. (eds) Family-centred Care: concept, theory and practice. Basingstoke, Palgrave, pp 3–18

Corlett J, Twycross A. (2006) Negotiation of parental roles within family-centred care: a review of the research. Journal of Clinical Nursing, 15(10), 1308–1316

Department of Health (2009) Reference Guide to Consent for Examination or Treatment, 2nd edition. Available at www.doh.gov.uk/consent (last accessed 12th June 2011)

Dunsford J. (2009) Structured communication – improving patient safety with SBAR. Nursing for Women's Health, 13(5), 385–390

Every Child Matters (2003) Available at https://www.education.gov.uk/publications/eOrderingDownload/CM5860.pdf (last accessed 13th June 2011)

Gillick v West Norfolk and Wisbech AHA (1986) AC 112 Available at http://www.hrcr.org/safrica/childrens_rights/Gillick_WestNorfolk.htm (last accessed 20th June 2011)

Healthy Lives, Brighter Future (2009) Available at http://www.dh.gov.uk/en/Publicationsandstatistics/Publications/PublicationsPolicyAndGuidance/DH_094400 (last accessed October 2011)

Helman C. (2007) Culture, Health and Illness, 5th edition. London, Hodder Arnold Publications

Hemphill AL, Dearmun AK. (2010) Working with children and families. In Glasper A, Richardson J. (eds) A Textbook of Children's and Young People's Nursing. Churchill Livingstone, Edinburgh, pp 17–29

Hohenhaus S, Powell S, Hohenhaus JT. (2006) Enhancing patient safety during hands-off: standardized communication and teamwork using the SBAR method. American Journal of Nursing, 106(8), 72A–72B

Home Office UK Border Agency (2009) Section 55 Borders, Citizenship and Immigration Act – Every Child Matters – change for children. Available at http://www.ukba.homeoffice.gov.uk/sitecontent/documents/policyandlaw/legislation/bci-act1/change-for-children.pdf?view=Binary (last accessed 11th June 2011)

Hutchfield K. (1999) Family-centred care: a concept analysis. Journal of Advanced Nursing, 29(5), 1178–1187

Matthews J. (2010) Communicating with children and their families. In Glasper A, Richardson J. (eds) A Textbook of Children's and Young People's Nursing. London, Churchill Livingstone Elsevier, pp 121–136

Nursing and Midwifery Council (2008) The Code: Standards of Conduct, Performance and Ethics for Nurses and Midwives. Available at http://www.nmc-uk.org/Nurses-and-midwives/The-code/The-code-in-full/ (last accessed 11th December 2011)

Protection of Vulnerable Groups (Scotland) Act 2007 Available at http://www.legislation.gov.uk/asp/2007/14/contents (last accessed 11th June 2011)

Resuscitation Council (2011) Medical Emergencies and Resuscitation. Available at http://www.resus.org.uk/pages/MEdental.pdf (last accessed 31st January 2012)

Royal College of Physicians (2011) Acute Care Toolkit 1 – Handover. Available at http://www.rcplondon.ac.uk/sites/default/files/acute-medicine-toolkit-may-2011.pdf (last accessed 12th July 2011)

Safeguarding Children: Working Together Under the Children Act 2004 (2006) Available at http://cymru.gov.uk/pubs/circulars/2007/nafw-c1207en.pdf?lang=en (last accessed 11th June 2011)

Shields L, Pratt J, Davis L, Hunter J (2008) Family-centred care for children in hospital. DO1: 10.1002/14651858.CD004811.pub2

Smith L, Coleman V, Bradshaw M. (2010) Family-centred care. In Glasper A, Richardson J. (eds) A Textbook of Children's and Young People's Nursing. Churchill Livingstone, Edinburgh, pp 73–86

Soderback M, Coyne I, Harder M. (2011) The importance of including both a child perspective and the child's perspective within health care settings to provide truly child-centred care. Journal of Child Health Care, 15(2), 99–106

The Children Act (2004) Available at http://www.legislation.gov.uk/ukpga/2004/31/notes/division/2/2/1/2 (last accessed 11th June 2011)

The National Service Framework for Children, Young People and Maternity Services (2007) Available at http://www.dh.gov.uk/en/Publicationsandstatistics/Publications/PublicationsPolicyAndGuidance/Browsable/DH_4094329 (last accessed 12th June 2011)

The Protection of Children (Scotland) Act (2003).Available at http://www.scotland.gov.uk/Resource/Doc/232370/0063586.pdf (last accessed 11th June 2011)

UNICEF Convention on the Rights of the Child (1989) Available at http://www.unicef.org/crc/index_30160.html (last accessed 11th June 2011)

The GOSH website http://www.gosh.nhs.uk contains helpful information for parents, children, teenagers and healthcare professionals. Under 'Healthcare Professionals' further clinical guidelines and integrated care pathways can be accessed.

Chapter 1

Assessment

Chapter contents

Procedure guidelines

The Great Ormond Street Hospital Manual of Children's Nursing Practices, First Edition. Edited by Susan Macqueen, Elizabeth Anne Bruce, Faith Gibson.
© 2012 Great Ormond Street Hospital for Children NHS Foundation Trust. Published 2012 by Blackwell Publishing Ltd.

2

Introduction

Assessment forms the first part of any nursing activity and is the first step in the nursing process. Without a comprehensive assessment of the child and family's needs, care cannot be planned, delivered or evaluated effectively. For most children and their families, the performing of the nursing assessment is often the first contact that they have with the nursing team and it is important that this is seen as a positive, helpful and informative process.

Each child and their family should be approached as an individual. Much about the child's illness or problem can be discovered through observing the child at play or interacting with their family, without the nurse needing to touch or examine the child.

To aid ease of use, this chapter is organised into five distinct sections. (1) The first section outlines the general principles that should run throughout the assessment process, which should support the nurse's assessment role. (2) Issues surrounding the child's 'present illness' are then explored and this includes examining the current issues that have brought the child into the healthcare setting. (3) For many children, their current problems may be related to previous illnesses and/or injuries and this forms an important part of the assessment process. (4) Likewise, many conditions may be hereditary or have a tendency to run in families, so the health history of other family members may provide important information on actual or potential health problems for the child. (5) The measuring of vital signs including blood pressure is a core nursing role, which allows the child's condition or response to treatment to be monitored. Vital sign measurements provide information about the child's state of health and can identify signs of illness, disease or deterioration, allowing early intervention and treatment. Other routine measurements, such as height and weight, provide essential information about the child's growth and development, which is especially important in cases of chronic illness. These are adapted from the clinical practice guidelines at Great Ormond Street Hospital with the kind permission of the lead authors (Godwin *et al* 2005, Wilks *et al* 2001la, 2011b).

Together, these five sections form an important part of the health assessment and information is gained through effective communication with the child and/or their parents/carers.

The subsequent physical examination is broken down into nine 'systems' based on the approach used throughout the 'admission assessment' documentation currently in use at Great Ormond Street Hospital. The information gained thus far should be utilised to guide the nurse on the structure and depth of the physical examination of each system. The process is not designed to be fragmented but to encourage the nurse to structure the examination around the child and family's individual needs, while providing a comprehensive healthcare assessment. Not every system will need to be examined to the same depth, but if actual or potential problems are identified within a certain system, special attention should be paid to examining that area in detail. The 'systems review' section is designed to be read in conjunction with other relevant chapters of this book.

The last section briefly discusses the need for full and accurate documentation of the assessment, which should be completed during or shortly after the assessment.

Finally, assessment is an ongoing, dynamic process. Although this chapter provides a structured approach to performing a full nursing assessment, it is not designed to be prescriptive and the nurse should remain responsive to the child and family's needs at all times.

Procedure guideline 1.1 General principles of assessment

Statement	Rationale
1. Before undertaking the assessment, the nurse should consider the child's gender, cultural and religious beliefs.	**1.** The child's gender and their cultural and religious beliefs should influence how the nurse approaches the assessment process.
2. Throughout the assessment process, the nurse should refer any serious concerns about any aspect of the child's well-being to a senior nursing or medical colleague.	**2.** To ensure that, if help is immediately required, it is sought quickly and from the appropriate source.
3. Familiarise yourself with the parent-held child health record (commonly known as the 'red book'), previous healthcare records and referral letter if appropriate.	**3.** To guide the assessment process, avoid unnecessary repetition and highlight priorities for assessment.
4. Establish who has parental responsibility (PR) for the child.	**4.** Only a person with PR can consent to any form of care or treatment (including the assessment process) of a child under 16 years of age (unless the child is considered competent to consent for themselves). Fathers do not automatically acquire PR and either parent can have this revoked by the Court.

Procedure guideline 1.1 (*Continued*)

Statement	Rationale
5. Establish a rapport with the child and family by: • Introducing yourself by name and role • Establish what the child would like to be called • Be welcoming in a warm, friendly fashion • Maintaining good eye contact throughout the assessment process.	**5.** To reduce any anxiety the child and family may have and promote effective assessment (Ford and Munro 2000).
6. Ensure all explanations are described in language appropriate for the child's age and development.	**6.** To ensure understanding.
7. Use jargon-free, non-technical terms throughout the assessment process. If jargon is unavoidable, ensure this is clearly explained and documented.	**7.** To ensure understanding.
8. Explain to the child and family the purpose and format of the assessment process.	**8.** To reduce any anxiety that the child and family may have. Cooperation and open communication is more likely if they understand what is happening and why.
9. Select an environment where the assessment is to be conducted. Ensure it is warm and private and if possible is decorated in an age appropriate manner (Engel 1997).	**9.** To promote comfort for the child and maintain confidentiality. The needs of an adolescent are different to those of an infant.
10. When recording the child's health assessment, use the child and family's own words wherever possible.	**10.** To ensure accuracy of information.
11. Encourage the child and family to ask questions and voice any concerns.	**11.** To ensure effective communication and reduce anxiety. Parents/carers who state that they have serious concerns about their child may be an important clue about the child's overall condition (Stawser 1997).

12. What is the child and family's first language?
   Are there any other language needs such as British Sign Language or Makaton?
   If it is not spoken English, do they need an interpreter or 'signer' to be present?
	12. Effective communication is essential to the assessment process.

13. Use a mixture of open and closed questions.	**13.** Open questions elicit broader, more general information. Closed questions can be used to gain more specific information and clarify information.
14. Clarify your understanding of the issues by reflecting back the child's and family's statements, such as 'When you said that you had a headache in your tummy, did you mean that your tummy was hurting?'.	**14.** To ensure correct interpretation of the child's and family's information.
15. Are the child and family aware of why they are at the hospital or clinic today?	**15.** To ensure the child and family are fully informed about their treatment.

4

Procedure guideline 1.2 **Present illness**

Statement	Rationale
1. Find out what the child and family's reason for attending the hospital or clinic is.	**1.** This will provide important information about their perception of their needs and healthcare problems.
2. Ascertain what they consider to be the main health problem or need.	**2.** The major needs of the child and family may not be the same as those perceived by the healthcare professionals. This will also help the nurse to structure the assessment process.
3. Ask the child and family to describe the symptoms of the illness or problem in their own words.	**3.** To ensure effective assessment and communication. To help the nurse to structure the assessment process.

4. If they have symptoms of pain, what words or sounds does the child use to describe their pain?
    Establish with the child and family the exact location, duration and frequency of the pain. Does anything trigger the pain to start? What helps to relieve the pain (including over-the-counter medicines used)?
    Severity may be assessed using pain assessment tools appropriate for the children age (Royal College of Nursing 2009). For further information, see Chapter 21 on Pain management.
	4. To ensure effective communication and assessment of pain.
	    Establishing factors that aggravate or relieve the pain may help with the diagnosis as well as aiding the planning of nursing care.
	    Pain assessment tools will help to monitor the child's pain and response to treatment more accurately.

5. Does the child have any known infections?	**5.** If so, the child may need to be isolated to prevent the spread of infection. For further information, see Chapter 12 on Infection Prevention and Control.

Principles table 1.1 **Past history**

Principle	Rationale
1. Taking details of the child's past history and illnesses is an important part of the assessment process.	**1.** The child's past history may glean important information about their current healthcare issues.
2. Children who are experiencing developmental or neurological problems and all those under 2 years of age should have their prenatal, birth and neonatal history assessed (Engel 1997).	**2.** The prenatal, birth and neonatal history is especially important for these children as developmental and neurological problems may be related to their prenatal and birth history.
3. The pre-natal history should include details about maternal health, any infections or medications taken, abnormal maternal bleeding, weight gain, the duration and any other difficulties encountered during the pregnancy.	**3.** To provide a comprehensive assessment.
4. The birth history should include the duration of labour, type of delivery and any maternal complications.	**4.** To provide a comprehensive assessment.
5. The neonatal history should include the child's weight and condition at birth, as well as details of any admission to special care or neonatal intensive care. Any other complications or difficulties, such as respiratory distress, jaundice or feeding problems should also be noted. The results of an infant's Guthrie test should be established.	**5.** To provide a comprehensive assessment.

Principles table 1.1 (*Continued*)

Principle	Rationale
6. Has the child been in hospital before? If so, when was this and what was wrong with them? More detailed information may be found within the child's healthcare records.	**6.** The child's current illness may be related to previous illness or past surgery.
7. How has the child responded to previous illnesses, procedures and hospitalisations?	**7.** A child who is chronically ill or who has been in hospital numerous times may need different support from a child who has never been in hospital before. Identification of procedures that are known to distress the child (such as venepuncture) may allow practitioners to adopt strategies to lessen the distress (Duff 2003).
8. What medicines is the child currently taking? Note the dosage and frequency of all medications, including 'over-he-counter' medicines. Establish the child and parents'/carers' understanding of the drugs and the reasons for their use.	**8.** To allow a review of the current medications and ensure that the current regimen is continued. The assessment also provides an opportunity for education surrounding their medications.

9. Is the child allergic to anything? If so, what are the medicines or products that they are allergic to?
    What type of reaction did they have to the medicine/product? Who told you that it was an allergic reaction?
    Has your child taken this or similar drugs/productions after this reaction occurred? If yes, did they experience similar problems?
	9. Failure to document a serious allergy places the child at risk of anaphylaxis if the medicine/product is subsequently given (Henderson 1998).
	    The child and family may mistake a medication's side-effects for an allergy (e.g. GI disturbance during antibiotic therapy).
	    Misdiagnosing a reaction can lead to the child being deprived of effective treatment (Campbell and Glasper 1995).

10. Have they had any of the common communicable diseases such as chickenpox, mumps or measles? Have they been in recent contact with anyone else who has these illnesses?	**10.** It is important to establish if they have acquired immunity to any of these common illnesses as well as establishing that they are not currently an infection risk to other children.

11. Has the child been immunised? Is so, take details of which vaccinations they have received and when. Check this against the current recommended immunisation schedule (Department of Health 2011).
    Make a note of any vaccinations they have not received and the reason why.
	11. The child may be at risk of illness if they have not received their vaccinations.
	    The assessment may also provide an opportunity for education and health promotion. For further information see Chapter 11 on Immunisations.

Principles table 1.2 **Family history**

Principle	Rationale
1. What is the family composition? Who lives at home with the child? Do they have siblings? If so what are their names and ages.	**1.** To develop an understanding of the child as an individual and member of a family.
2. Are the parents/carers employed in work? If so, what is their occupation? If both parents work, who cares for the child?	**2.** Parental occupation can have an impact on the health and well-being of the child and family. Financial difficulties may adversely affect the health and well-being of the family and the individual.

(Continued)

Principles table 1.2 (*Continued*)

Principle	Rationale
3. Where do the child and family live? Do they own their own house or rent? How long have they lived at that address?	**3.** Problems with housing can have a significant effect on the child's physical, emotional and psychological well-being (Chaudhuri 2004, Emond *et al* 1997). Hospitalisation that is a significant distance from the family home may affect the ability of other family members to visit and lead to isolation and stress.
4. Are both parents and grandparents still alive? Have they had any significant health problems?	**4.** The health of the parents and grandparents may give clues as to the nature of the child's illness.
5. Do any family members have a history of serious or inherited illness?	**5.** To aid with the diagnosis and planning of nursing care.
6. Does the child attend school? Which one? Overall, how are they progressing? Are there any problems that the parents/carers or child are aware of?	**6.** Problems at school may negatively impact on the child's health. Problems may be related to current health problems (e.g. difficulties with hearing or eyesight may affect the ability to learn) or can be the cause of health problems (e.g. bullying at school may lead to anxiety causing behavioural problems, weight loss, sleeping difficulties, etc.) (Oliver and Candappa 2003).
7. Do the family see any other medical or allied health professionals on a regular basis?	**7.** Other professionals may provide important information about the child and family. Communication and liaison with other healthcare teams is equally important.
8. Do the child and/or family have any other concerns regarding the child's general health and social needs?	**8.** To allow the child and family to voice concerns about issues that may not have been covered within the assessment.

Measuring vital signs, height and weight

Procedure guideline 1.3 Monitoring plan and early warning score

Statement	Rationale
1. All Children admitted to hospital should have a documented monitoring plan.	**1.** To facilitate communication between the multi-professional team.
2. The monitoring plan should be reviewed at least daily by the multi-professional team.	**2.** To ensure the plan is appropriate for the child's needs.
3. All children should also be assessed using an Early Warning Score or similar 'track and trigger' tool (Pearson 2008).	**3.** To detect early signs of deterioration and ensure appropriate escalation to a senior healthcare professional if needed (Chapman *et al* 2010).

Procedure guideline 1.4 Assessing the temperature

Statement	Rationale
1. Core temperature varies in childhood and is dependent on a number of factors including age, environmental factors and illness (Hockenberry and Wilson 2007).	**1.** It is important to assess temperature against age appropriate values, taking into account environmental factors and current state of health.
2. Peripheral temperature monitoring is useful for children where there are concerns about fluid balance status or peripheral perfusion.	**2.** A significant difference between the core and peripheral temperature may indicate poor perfusion to the skin from dehydration or shock (Advanced Life Support Group 2005).

3. All children should have a temperature recorded on admission.
    The ongoing frequency of temperature monitoring should reflect the child's clinical condition.
	3. To establish a baseline.
	    To provide child centred, individualised care.

4. If the temperature reading falls outside the normal range, measurements should be taken more frequently until the temperature normalises.	**4.** To assess temperature instability and severity, to monitor disease progression and to monitor temperature control techniques (NICE 2007).
5. The site and equipment selected for temperature measurement should take into account the child's age, local policy guidance and the preferences of the child and family (Carr *et al* 2011, Royal College of Nursing 2011). Infants under the age of 4 weeks should have their temperature measured with an electronic thermometer in the axilla. Infants and children from 4 weeks to 5 years should have their temperature measured with an electronic/chemical dot thermometer in the axilla or an infra-red tympanic thermometer (NICE 2007, Royal College of Nursing 2011). **a)** The equipment should be appropriate for the site of measurement and the staff should be trained in its use. Equipment must be cleaned, serviced and calibrated in accordance with manufacturer's guidelines and local policies (Royal College of Nursing 2011). **b)** The rectal route is not recommended unless other routes and methods are impossible or impractical [(Royal College of Nursing 2011).	**5.** To ensure the child's safety and improve adherence. **a)** To ensure the measuring device is used safely and accurately. **b)** There is a risk of bowel perforation, discomfort and distress to the child and the invasive nature of this route (Casey 2000).

6. Axillary temperature measurement:
    To measure the axillary temperature in a younger child, it may be helpful to position them on the parent's/carer's lap.
    Measurements via this route may be inaccurate in the early stages of a fever (Carr *et al* 2011, Engel 1997).
	6. To ensure the child's safety and improve adherence.

7. Oral temperature measurement To measure the oral temperature, ensure the child is sitting or lying. Do not measure the temperature via this route if the child has had a hot or cold drink in the previous 20 minutes. **a)** Also avoid this route if the child is uncooperative, comatosed, seizure prone or had recent oral surgery (Engel 1997, Carr *et al* 2011).	**7.** To prevent inaccurate readings. **a)** To prevent complications.

(Continued)

8 **Procedure guideline 1.4** (*Continued*)

Statement	Rationale
8. Tympanic temperature measurement: Tympanic thermometer measurements may be unreliable due to the large number of variables which may influence the readings (Dunleavy 2010, Rush and Wetherall 2003). Do not use this route if the child has acute otitis media, sinusitis or had recent surgery to the ear. It may also be difficult in children with very small external ear canals. **a)** Ensure the child is sitting or lying. **b)** Perform an ear tug: For children under 1 year – pull the ear straight back. For children aged 1 to adult – pull the ear up and back. **c)** While tugging the ear, fit the probe snugly into the ear canal (with a firm seal around the external auditory meatus) orientating tip towards tympanic membrane (Casey 2000).	**8.** To ensure the child's safety and improve adherence. **b)** To straighten the ear canal in order to allow a clear view of the eardrum. **c)** To allow the sensor to measure the heat from drum and not the sides of the ear canal.
9. Rectal temperature measurement: If the rectal route must be used, younger infants may be placed in the supine position with knees flexed towards the abdomen. For older children, place prone or lying on their side. **a)** Do not use if the child has had anal or rectal surgery, chemotherapy, has diarrhoea or rectal irritation (Engel 1997).	**9.** To ensure the child's safety and improve adherence. **a)** To prevent secondary complications.
10. Assess the temperature against age appropriate values. **a)** The measurement should be documented according to local policy and the method and device from which the temperature was recorded should be noted (Rush and Wetherall 2003).	**10.** Normal temperature varies slightly with age. **a)** To ensure accuracy, consistency and comparability.

Procedure guideline 1.5 **Assessing the heart rate**

Statement	Rationale
1. In older children, the heart rate can be assessed by palpating the radial artery (Rawling-Anderson *et al* 2008, Royal College of Nursing 2011). In infants and children under 2 years of age, it is more reliable to listen to the apical beat with a stethoscope (Royal College of Nursing 2011).	**1.** To obtain an accurate recording.
2. If the child is crying or very distressed, you may have to wait until they are calmer (Engel 1997).	**2.** Crying and distress may increase the pulse rate.
3. Count the pulse for a full minute.	**3.** To ensure an accurate reading as the pulse may be irregular (Rawling-Anderson *et al* 2008, Royal College of Nursing 2011).
4. Assess the heart rate against age-appropriate values (Advanced Life Support Group 2005, Rawling-Anderson *et al* 2008).	**4.** Normal pulse rate varies with age. To identify abnormal values.
5. Document the heart rate on the appropriate chart, noting the child's activity at the time.	**5.** To ensure accuracy, consistency and comparability.

Procedure guideline 1.6 Assessing the respiratory rate

Statement	Rationale
1. Avoid letting the child know that respirations are being counted.	**1.** Self-consciousness may alter the respiratory rate and depth.
2. If the child is crying or very distressed, you may have to wait until they are calmer.	**2.** To gain an accurate recording as crying and distress may increase the respiratory rate (Aylott 2006b, Simoes et al 1991).
3. In infants and young children, place a hand just below the child's xiphoid process. Observation alone is adequate in the older child.	**3.** To feel the child's breathing.
4. Count the child's breaths for 1 full minute.	**4.** To ensure an accurate reading as the respirations of infants and young children may be irregular (Simoes et al 1991).
5. Assess respiratory rate against age-appropriate values.	**5.** Normal respiratory rate varies with age (Advanced Life Support Group 2005). Rapid respiratory rates (tachypnoea) may indicate fever, anxiety, pain or respiratory distress. Low respiratory rates (bradypnoea) may indicate overdosage with opiates. Bradypnoea following a period of respiratory distress may indicate exhaustion. This is a clinical emergency and appropriate action must be taken (Advanced Life Support Group 2005).
a) Document the respiratory rate on the appropriate chart.	**a)** To ensure accuracy, consistency and comparability.

Procedure guideline 1.7 Height

Statement	Rationale
1. Assessment of growth is vital and provides a sensitive guide to: • health • development • nutritional status • the response to treatment. (Freeman et al 1995, Hall 2000, Voss 2000).	**1.** A healthy adequately nourished and emotionally secure child grows at an optimal rate (Stanhope et al 1994). A slow rate of growth could suggest a pathological disorder requiring diagnosis and possible treatment, e.g. malabsorption, an eating disorder, hypertension, pyschosocial problems, craniopharyngioma (Sherwood et al 1986, Skuse 1989). Regular measurement of children in primary care can allow early diagnosis of these problems (Stern et al 1985).
2. Whenever a child is admitted to hospital, their height or length must be measured and must be: • recorded in the child's healthcare record • recorded in the admission assessment record • recorded in the child's parent held record plotted on a centile chart. The date, time and the name of the measurer must also be recorded (Voss 2000).	**2.** Many diseases do not cause obvious symptoms and poor growth may be the first or only indicator of a problem (Voss 2000). To maintain accurate documentation and communication.
3. All children in hospital should have their height measured and plotted on a centile chart every 3 months. A single measurement does not reflect the rate of growth.	**3.** Hospitalised children are at nutritional risk. Serial measurements allow for a more accurate assessment of a child's growth rate.

(Continued)

Procedure guideline 1.7 (*Continued*)

Statement	Rationale
4. Standard equipment for measuring height in children of varying ages should be available in all areas where children are to be assessed.	**4.** To facilitate monitoring of the child's height.
5. All equipment should be checked, calibrated and cleaned prior to use.	**5.** To ensure the accuracy of measurement. To minimise the risk of cross-infection.
6. The appropriate equipment to height of the child should be selected. This is dependant on the child's age and developmental and physical ability.	**6.** To obtain an accurate measurement. To maintain the safety of the child and staff.
7. Children under 2 years of age and those who are unable to stand (or find standing difficult) should be measured supine. All others should be measured standing.	**7.** To obtain an accurate measurement (Voss 1990).
8. A child who has one leg shorter than the other should be measured standing on the longest leg. They should always be measured on the same leg.	**8.** To obtain an accurate measurement (Voss 1990).

9. In some forms of short stature body proportions may also be clinically relevant, e.g. achondroplasia, or after spinal irradiation.
    The most useful body proportion is the relationship between trunk length and leg length.
    This is obtained by measuring a sitting height and subtracting this from the total height.
    Children who need to be measured lying down should have their crown–rump length measured, i.e. head to bottom. This measurement is then subtracted from the child's total length.
	9. To determine body proportions (Voss 1990).

10. The positioning of the child is crucial.	**10.** Poor positioning results in inaccurate measurement.

11. The child should normally have the following removed:
  • nappy
  • their socks and shoes
  • any bulky clothing
  • hairclips
  • braids, i.e. undo hair
  • orthopaedic braces.
The child's healthcare records must indicate if any of these items are not removed (Voss 1990).
	11. To avoid inconsistencies of measurements.
	To enable visualisation of the child's feet.
	To enable an accurate measurement to be taken.
	To maintain an accurate record.

12. When measuring a child standing, the child's body must be positioned with their:
  • feet together
  • feet flat on the ground
  • heels touching the back plate of the measuring instrument
  • legs must be straight
  • buttocks against the backboard
  • scapula, wherever possible, against the backboard
  • arms loosely at their side.	

13. When measuring a child in the supine position, two people are required.	**13.** One to ensure contact of the feet and other contact of the head with the measuring board.

Procedure guideline 1.7 (Continued)

Statement	Rationale
14. Place the measuring board on a firm surface and lay the child on the board. One person should ensure the head is held in contact with the headboard. The other person should position the child with their: • feet together • feet flat against the foot board • heels touching the back plate of the measuring instrument • legs straight and in alignment with the body • buttocks against the backboard • scapula, wherever possible, against the backboard. The ankles should be held to ensure this position is maintained and firm pressure may need to be applied to keep the child's legs in position. The child should be completely aligned and flat on the board.	**14.** To ensure stability of the measuring device and obtain an accurate measurement. To ensure the head and body are in complete alignment.
15. In both measurement methods, the child's head should be positioned with the lower margins of the orbit in the same horizontal plane as the external auditory meati, i.e. the corner of the eyes horizontal to the middle of the ear.	**15.** This position is referred to as the Frankfort plane and ensures accuracy of measurement (Voss 1990).
16. The measuring instrument should then be read (ensuring it is at eye level for the standing method) when the child has fully exhaled. Record the measurement to the last complete millimetre and do not round up the measurement (Schling and Hulse 1997).	**16.** To obtain an accurate height of child.
17. Record the child's height in their healthcare records as appropriate. Documentation should include the date and time of the measurement as well as the name of the person who performed the procedure.	**17.** To maintain accurate documentation.
18. The child's height should also be plotted on a centile chart. The 'Four in One Growth Chart' is the centile chart that is recommended for general use (Cole 1994, Fry 1994).	**18.** To compare the child's growth against evidence based data.
19. Any abnormality or deviation from the expected centile should be reported to the child's doctor.	**19.** To facilitate appropriate management.

Procedure guideline 1.8 Weight

Statement	Rationale

1. All children should be weighed on admission to hospital and at least weekly thereafter.	**1.** Hospitalised children are at nutritional risk.
	    To establish a baseline for future assessment.
	    To monitor the child's growth.

2. Inform the child and family of the procedure and the reason.	
3. Before undertaking the procedure, consider the child's gender, culture and religious beliefs.	

12

Procedure guideline 1.8 (*Continued*)

Statement	Rationale
4. Children under 2 years of age should be weighed naked. Children over 2 years of age should be weighed in minimal clothing or light underwear. If worn, nappies should be removed. Shoes and slippers should not be worn during the measurement.	**4.** To ensure accurate measurement. To avoid inconsistencies in measurement.
5. If clothing has not been removed or the child is weighed with additional equipment, such as a splint or cast, this must be recorded in the child's healthcare records.	**5.** To maintain an accurate record.
6. Standard equipment for weighing children of varying ages should be available in all areas where children are to be assessed.	
7. All weighing equipment should be checked, calibrated and cleaned prior to use.	**7.** To ensure the accuracy of measurement. To minimise the risk of cross-infection.
8. The appropriate equipment to weigh the child should be selected. This is dependant on the child's age and developmental and physical ability.	**8.** To obtain an accurate measurement. To maintain the safety of the child and staff.
9. If the child is very sick or unable to sit unaided, the child should be supported by a carer and weighed together on the scales. The carer should then be weighed alone and their weight subtracted from the combined weight of the child and carer.	**9.** To obtain an accurate measurement. To maintain the safety of the child.
10. The child must be completely on the scales and their weight fully borne.	**10.** To ensure an accurate measurement.
11. Record the figure shown on the scales to the last complete gram for infants under 4 kg and to the last 100 grams for older children above 4 kg. Do not round up the measurement.	**11.** To ensure an accurate measurement.
12. Help the child and family to redress the child.	**12.** To maintain safety, comfort and dignity.
13. Record the child's weight in their healthcare records as appropriate. Documentation should include the date and time of the measurement as well as the name of the person who performed the procedure.	**13.** To maintain accurate documentation.
14. The child's weight should also be plotted on a centile chart. The 'Four in One Growth Chart' is the centile chart that is recommended for general use (Cole 1994, Fry 1994).	**14.** To compare the child's growth against evidence based data.
15. Any abnormality or deviation from the expected centile should be reported to the child's doctor.	**15.** To facilitate appropriate management.

Review of systems

Procedure guideline 1.9 Respiratory and cardiovascular system review

Statement	Rationale

1. Observe and note the child's activity level. Are they calm and behaving appropriately? Are they restless or agitated? Listless and drowsy?	1. A child's activity is a valuable indicator of their overall state of health.
	   Agitation and restlessness may indicate shock or hypoxia.
	   Drowsiness and listlessness may indicate serious problems such as late shock or a neurological problem (Advanced Life Support Group 2005, Bowler 1998).

2. Observe the child's body posture.	2. A child may alter their body position to alleviate symptoms:
	   A child with severe airway obstruction or respiratory distress may sit upright in a 'tripod' position to ease their breathing (Advanced Life Support Group 2005, Kline 2003).
	   'Squatting' may indicate a diagnosis of tetralogy of Fallot (Engel 1997).

3. Note the child's general colour. Is this normal for the child?	3. Skin colour varies between and within different ethnic groups.
	   Parents/carers will generally have noticed if the child's colour has altered from the baseline.
	   Skin colour may indicate underlying disease problems.
	   Pallor (especially when combined with drowsiness and fever in infants) may indicate serious problems such as shock or hypoxia (Hewson *et al* 2000).
	   A yellow tinge (jaundice) may indicate liver problems.

4. Observe for peripheral and central cyanosis (blue/purple discolouration).
   a) Check the colour of the child's tongue.
	4. Peripheral cyanosis may be due to vasoconstriction and can be a healthy response to a cold environment.
	   a) Central cyanosis is a blue or purple discolouration of the tongue and indicates severe hypoxaemia or polycythaemia (Gill and O'Brien 1998, McGrath and Cox 1998)

5. Observe the child for mottling and oedema.
 	
   a) Look at the child's hands and nails for colour, shape and condition.
	5. Pallor and mottling may indicate heart disease or shock. Oedema may be present in congestive heart failure or renal failure.
	   a) Finger clubbing is due to chronic hypoxia and may indicate a chronic heart or lung condition (Gill and O'Brien 1998).
	   Splinter haemorrhages (small red or black lines in the fingernail beds) may be present in infective endocarditis (Ford and Munro 2000).

6. Look at the shape of the child's chest. Are there any deformities of the chest wall?	6. Prominence of the sternum and costal cartilages may indicate respiratory or cardiac problems. In older children a round chest is often indicative of a chronic lung disorder.
7. Does the chest move symmetrically on breathing?	7. In health, the chest should move symmetrically. Decreased movement on one side may indicate pneumonia, pneumothorax or inhalation of a foreign body.

(Continued)

14 ## Procedure guideline 1.9 (*Continued*)

Statement	Rationale
8. Are there signs of recession (indrawing of the chest wall)?	**8.** Recession is more commonly seen in younger children as their ribs and chest wall are more compliant (Hazinski 1992). 　　Recession generally indicates increased work of breathing and respiratory distress (Aylott 2006b). Recession in an older child suggests severe respiratory distress (Advanced Life Support Group 2005).
a) If so, where is it located and how marked is it (mild, moderate or severe)?	**a)** The degree of recession generally correlates to the severity of the condition. Severe recession, especially if accompanied by other signs of respiratory distress, is a sign of severe illness and should be referred to a doctor immediately (Carter and Laird 2005, Hewson *et al* 2000)
9. Are there visible pulsations or scars? Where are they located?	**9.** A visible pulsation in the left chest may indicate left ventricular enlargement or other cardiac problems. 　　Scars may indicate previous surgery for respiratory or cardiac problems.
10. Does the child make any noises when they are breathing? 　　If so, what do they sound like and when do they occur (on inspiration, expiration or both).	**10.** Stridor (a high pitched sound generally worse on inspiration) indicates severe upper airway obstruction and may be due to infection (such as croup or epiglottis), post-traumatic injury, neoplasia or developmental problems such as subglottic haemangioma or laryngomalacia (Carter and Laird 2005, La Buda *et al* 2005). 　　Wheeziness may indicate asthma, an acute respiratory tract infection or foreign body inhalation. 　　Grunting is a sign of severe respiratory distress (Advanced Life Support Group 2005, Aylott 2006b.
11. Does the child have a cough? If so, what does it sound like and when does it occur? 　　Is the cough productive? If so, describe the nature of the expectorant.	**11.** A severe barking cough, especially with stridor, may indicate croup. 　　A paroxysmal prolonged bout of coughing (sometimes ending in a sharp intake of breath) may indicate pertussis (whooping cough). 　　A productive cough is rare in children and may indicate cystic fibrosis.
12. Do the child and/or family have any other concerns regarding the child's respiratory or cardiovascular needs?	**12.** To allow the child and family to voice concerns about issues that may not have been covered within the assessment.

Procedure guideline 1.10 Neurological system review

Statement	Rationale
1. Ask the parent/carer the age at which the child first rolled over, sat unaided, crawled, walked, spoke their first words, spoke their first sentence and dressed without help (Engel 1997). Assess these against developmental guidelines.	**1.** A through history of the child's development is important in order to plan nursing care appropriate for the child's developmental age. The assessment can also identify neurological and developmental abnormalities.

Procedure guideline 1.10 *(Continued)*

Statement	Rationale
2. Check the child's head circumference against age-appropriate values.	**2.** A large head (especially within the frontal area) may indicate hydrocephalus. A small head (microcephaly) may be linked to abnormality during the prenatal period (maternal infection, drug use), chromosomal abnormality or perinatal trauma.
3. Observe the child for any abnormalities of movement.	**3.** Abnormal movement may result from neurological problems or local injury to the affected limb.
4. Assess the strength and symmetry of the child's muscles by asking them to squeeze your fingers, and push away the examiner's hands from the soles of their feet. Test the arms and legs by asking the child to push against gentle pressure applied by the examiner's hands. Note any weakness or asymmetry.	**4.** Weakness or asymmetry should be considered abnormal and may result from the current or previous illness, local injury to the affected limb or trauma.
5. Check the child's ability to move all their limbs. Ask them to walk up and down to assess the movement of their lower limbs. Note any areas of flaccidity or spasticity.	**5.** Abnormal limb movement may be seen while observing the child at play. Abnormal movement may be related to neurological problems, trauma, previous illness or congenital disorder.
6. Ask the child to hop, skip or walk heel-to-toe.	**6.** Inability or difficulty to perform any of these may indicate cerebellar dysfunction (Orfanelli 2001).
7. Does the child have any problems with their vision? Can they see objects that are close by and further away?	**7.** Visual difficulties may be related to problems with the eye itself, cranial nerve II or the brain (particulary the pituitary, hypothalamic and chiasmatic region). Double vision may indicate problems with cranial nerve IV or the midbrain.
8. Do the child's pupils constrict in response to a bright light? Is the response equal in both pupils?	**8.** Unreactive or unequal pupil responses to light may indicate problems with cranial nerve II or III or within the brainstem (Marcoux 2005).
9. Can the child follow an object through the full range of movement (ask the child to follow an object moved in an 'H' shape without moving their head)? Do they have a droopy eyelid?	**9.** Normally you can see the child's pupil fully. Problems moving the eyeball (up, down or inwards) or droopy eyelids (ptosis) may indicate problems with cranial nerve III, IV, the midbrain or brainstem (Orfanelli 2001).
10. Does the child blink if a wisp of cotton touches the eye?	**10.** Abnormal corneal reflexes may indicate an abnormality of cranial nerve V or the brainstem.
11. Can the child see objects in their field of vision? Are they able to move the eyeball laterally (sideways)? Are there signs of nystagmus (rapid eye movement back to the midline)? Is the child able to direct both eyes at one object (inability to do this is termed strabismus)?	**11.** Inability to move the eyeball laterally may indicate damage to cranial nerve VI or abnormality of the pons, cavernous sinus or result from a basal skull fracture. Strabismus may also indicate problems with cranial nerve VI, the extraocular muscle of the eye or may be due to mal-alignment of the eyes (squint) (Rudolf and Levene 1999). Nystagmus (repetitive to-and-fro movement of the eyes) may be related to cranial nerve VI abnormality or may be idiopathic.
12. Ask the child to clench their teeth. Feel the jaw and temple area for symmetry and strength. Can the child feel light touch on their forehead, checks and jaw?	**12.** Inability or weakness may indicate problems with cranial nerve V or the brain, particularly the pons or may result from previous surgery or illness (such as trigeminal neuralgia or neuropathy) (Orfanelli 2001).

(Continued)

16 Procedure guideline 1.10 (*Continued*)

Statement	Rationale
13. Ask the child to make a 'scary face', to smile, show their teeth and puff out their cheeks. Observe for abnormal expressions, movement or weaknesses.	**13.** Abnormal expressions, movements or facial weaknesses may indicate problems with cranial nerve VII, the pons region of the brain, infection, inflammation or trauma (Riordan 2001).

14. Does the child have any hearing problems? The ability to hear can be checked by snapping the fingers behind each ear or gently rubbing together a lock of the child's hair.
    Is there any discharge from the ear itself?
	14. Hearing problems may result from problems with the ear itself (such as infection or damage related to prematurity or previous injury) or abnormality of cranial nerve VIII.
	    The presence of soft yellow brown wax is normal. Foul-smelling yellow or green discharge may indicate rupture of the tympanic membrane or infection (Engel 1997). Blood may indicate the presence of a foreign body, scratching from irritation or a fracture of the base of the skull.

15. Ask the child to swallow. Check if the uvula is in the mid-line by asking the child to stick out their tongue.	**15.** Inability to swallow or a poor gag reflex may result from brain stem problems or abnormality of cranial nerve X or XII (Orfanelli 2001). Further assessment may be needed to ensure the child is able to protect their airway to prevent subsequent airway and breathing problems. Abnormal position of the uvula may indicate problems with cranial nerve IX, X or the brain stem.
16. Can the child shrug their shoulders and turn their head from side to side? Check the symmetry and strength of this by asking the child to perform this against the resistance of the assessor's hand.	**16.** Abnormality or weakness of the sternomastoid and trapezius muscles may result from damage to cranial nerve XI or local injury to the neck and shoulder.
17. Does the child have any difficulties pronouncing words or sounds? Ask the child to stick out their tongue and check if it is in the midline.	**17.** Difficulty with pronunciation or movement of the tongue may indicate abnormality of cranial nerve XII as a result of lesions of the basal skull, posterior fossa or fourth ventricle.
18. Does the child and/or family have any other concerns regarding the child's neurological needs?	**18.** To allow the child and family to voice concerns about issues that may not have been covered within the assessment.

Procedure guideline 1.11 **Nutrition system review**

Statement	Rationale
1. Weigh and measure the height of the child and check these against age-appropriate values and previous records.	**1.** To establish if the child is growing and developing normally.
2. Is the child gaining weight and growing? Are the parents/carers concerned about any aspect of the child's development?	**2.** Parents/carers are generally the first person to detect poor nutrition or weight gain. Failure to thrive may indicate a number of chronic illnesses such as gastro-oesophageal reflux, cardiac, respiratory, liver, renal, endocrine and metabolic disorders (Shah 2002).
3. What is the child's normal feeding regimen? Do they need help with eating or drinking? Do they use a knife and fork or fingers to feed themselves? Do they drink from a cup/beaker/bottle?	**3.** Continuing the child's normal regimen will help to decrease anxiety and stress.

Procedure guideline 1.11 (*Continued*)

Statement	Rationale
4. For infants, are they breast or bottle-fed and if so, which milk do the parents/carers use?	**4.** To maintain the child's current regimen.
5. What are the child's likes and dislikes? Are there any foods to which the child is allergic or cannot tolerate?	**5.** To establish the child's current regimen and aid the planning of nursing care.
6. Does the child require a special diet or food supplements?	**6.** Wherever possible, these should be continued while the child is in hospital.
7. Does the child require any additional nutritional support such as overnight feeding or total parenteral nutrition?	**7.** To establish the child's current regimen and aid the planning of nursing care.
8. Is the child seeing any other professional, such as a dietician or nurse specialist?	**8.** To ensure effective communication between professionals, that may offer additional information about the child.
9. Do the child and/or family have any other concerns regarding the child's nutritional needs?	**9.** To allow the child and family to voice concerns about issues that may not have been covered within the assessment.

Procedure guideline 1.12 Elimination and sexual development review

Statement	Rationale
1. What is the child's normal toilet regimen? Can they use the toilet unaided? For younger children are they potty trained?	**1.** To plan the child's individual care and maintain the child and family's normal routine wherever possible.
2. What is the colour and consistency of the child's urine? Does it have an odour? Does it hurt when they pass urine?	**2.** Dark, concentrated urine may indicate dehydration. Cloudy urine and/or smelly may indicate infection. Red or brown urine suggests haematuria.
3. What is the colour and consistency of the child's faeces? Does it have an odour? Does it hurt when they have their bowels opened?	**3.** Black stools may indicate melaena from gastrointestinal bleeding. Grey or clay coloured stools may indicate biliary atresia. Pale loose, bulky offensive stools may indicate coeliac disease (Chand and Mihas 2006) Liquid or watery green stools may indicate diarrhoea due to infection, inflammation, chemotherapy or laxative use. Ribbon-like stools may indicate Hirschsprung's disease (Engel 1997).
4. Does the child need aperients, such as laxatives, suppositories or enemas? If so, how often are they required?	**4.** To maintain current therapy and promote normal bowel actions.
5. Is there any abnormal discharge from the genital area?	**5.** Abnormal discharge may result from the presence of a foreign body or infection. Sexually transmitted diseases may result from consensual sex or sexual abuse.
6. In older boys, have they reached puberty? If so, at what age did this occur?	**6.** Puberty in boys usually starts between 11 and 14 years and is considered delayed if there are no signs by age 14 years (Rudolf and Levene 1999).

(*Continued*)

Procedure guideline 1.12 (*Continued*)

Statement	Rationale
7. In older girls, have they developed secondary sexual characteristics (breasts, pubic hair)? If so, at what age did this occur?	**7.** Breast development before 8 years of age may be normal, but needs further assessment. Delayed breast development (none by age 13) should also be further assessed (Engel 1997).
8. In older females, have they started menstruating? If so, what was the date of their last period?	**8.** The possibility that the child could be pregnant should be examined. Children may not declare this in front of their parents/carers.
9. Do they have painful periods? If so, what relieves the pain?	**9.** To maintain the child's comfort and assess development.
10. For older children and adolescents, are they sexually active (remembering that they may not disclose this if their parents/carers are present)? If so, are they practising safe sex and using contraception?	**10.** Adolescents may be sexually active and not disclose this to their parents/carers. The health assessment may be an appropriate opportunity for health promotion and discussion about sexual health.
11. Do the child and/or family have any other concerns regarding the child's elimination needs or sexual development?	**11.** To allow the child and family to voice concerns about issues that may not have been covered within the assessment.

Procedure guideline 1.13 Skin hygiene review

Statement	Rationale
1. Observe the general colour and pigmentation of the skin.	**1.** Overall skin colour varies between individuals and across ethnic groups. A yellow discolouration may indicate jaundice or liver disease; redness may indicate inflammation or bruising, and paleness may indicate anaemia, or shock.
2. Observe the general condition of the child's hair. What is the texture and colour? Is it normally distributed?	**2.** To establish a baseline for future assessment.
3. Observe the general condition of the child's nails. What are their shape and colour?	**3.** To establish a baseline for future assessment.
4. Observe the general condition of the child's mouth. Ask about their normal dental routine. When did they last visit the dentist?	**4.** To establish a baseline for future assessment.
5. Is there any abnormal odour?	**5.** This may indicate a fungal infection or poor personal hygiene.
6. Are there any abnormal areas of skin? If so, describe their location and appearance.	**6.** To establish a baseline for future assessment and help to plan nursing care.
7. Is there a rash? If so, describe its duration, site of onset, how it has developed and if it has spread.	**7.** Rashes may indicate an infection, infestation, allergy or systemic illness.

Procedure guideline 1.13 (*Continued*)

Statement	Rationale
8. Does the rash 'come and go' or is it consistent?	**8.** Urticaria is a transient itchy rash that appears rapidly but then fades. Causes can include a food or drug allergy, infection (particularly viral infection) or contact allergy (Budd and Gardiner 1999).
9. Does the rash blanch when pressure is applied?	**9.** Haemorrhagic rashes do not fade under pressure and may be associated with meningococcal septicaemia, acute leukaemia or Henoch-Schonlein purpura (Bowler 1998). More experienced advice should be sought immediately.
10. Does the rash itch?	**10.** Not all rashes itch and this may aid the diagnosis. Allergic reactions, eczema, chickenpox (varicella zoster) and bacterial infections such as impetigo may be very pruritic (itchy).
11. Is anyone else in the family affected?	**11.** Infestations (such as scabies) or infectious disease may affect other children or adults in the same household.
12. Does anyone else in the family have a history of skin disorders?	**12.** Diseases such as eczema or psoriasis can run in families.
13. What is the child's normal hygiene routine? Do they prefer a bath or shower? Are there any soaps or products they or their parents/carers would not use?	**13.** Maintaining the child's normal regimen will help to reduce anxiety and promote continuity. For further information see Chapter 10 on Personal Hygiene and Pressure Ulcer Prevention.
14. Does the child need any assistance with hygiene needs?	**14.** To plan the child's nursing care.
15. Establish with the child and carer their level of involvement and participation in meeting their hygiene needs.	**15.** To plan the child's nursing care.
16. Are there any bruises? If so, where are they located, what is the size and colour and how did they happen?	**16.** Bruises may frequently be found on the legs of toddlers as they learn to walk. Multiple bruises or unusual patterns/locations may be indicative of non-accidental injury and should be referred to a senior colleague for assessment. Suspicions of abuse should be documented and referred to the appropriate social worker. For further information see Chapter 7 on Child Protection.
17. Does the child have any wounds? If so, describe their reason, location, size and appearance. **a)** Does the wound need any form of dressings? If so, describe when and how this is changed.	**17.** Wounds may indicate previous surgery or illness. **a)** To maintain the child's care.
18. Do the child and/or family have any other concerns regarding the child's skin or hygiene needs?	**18.** To allow the child and family to voice concerns about issues that may not have been covered within the assessment.

Procedure guideline 1.14 Mobility review

Statement	Rationale
1. Ask the parent/carer the age at which the child first rolled over, sat unaided, crawled, walked and dressed without help (Engel 1997). Assess these against normal developmental criteria.	1. A through history of the child's development is important in order to plan nursing care appropriate for the child's developmental age. The assessment can also identify mobility and developmental abnormalities.
2. How does the child normally mobilise? How far can they walk independently?	2. To plan appropriate and individualised nursing care.
3. Observe the child for any abnormalities of movement and assess against 'age-appropriate' development.	3. Abnormal movement may result from neurological problems or local injury to the affected limb.
4. If the child can walk, observe the gait and note any abnormalities.	4. Infants and toddlers tend to walk bow-legged with a wide-based gait. Limping may indicate a variety of abnormalities including trauma, septic arthritis/osteomyelitis, transient synovitis, slipped femoral capital epiphysis, congenital dislocation of the hip, irritable hip, scoliosis or cerebral palsy (Fischer and Beattie 1999).
5. Does the child need any mobility aids such as crutches or a wheelchair?	5. To plan appropriate and individualised nursing care.
6. Do the child and/or family have any other concerns regarding the child's mobility?	6. To allow the child and family to voice concerns about issues that may not have been covered within the assessment.

Procedure guideline 1.15 Psychological review

Statement	Rationale
1. How does the child address his parents/carers (e.g Mummy, Daddy, Mamma, etc)?	1. To ensure effective communication and promote the child's sense of security.
2. Does the child have any special toys or comforters? Have they brought them with them?	2. To promote the child's normal regimen and sense of security.
3. What is the child's normal daily routine? What time do they wake, eat meals, go to sleep? a) How has the child reacted to their illness?	3. To plan the child's individual care and maintain the child and family's normal routine wherever possible. a) To plan appropriate nursing care as individual children react differently to illness.

4. Is the diagnosis and prognosis of the child's illness known to the child and/or family? What exactly do they understand about their current condition?	4. To maintain confidentiality.
	   To plan appropriate and individualised nursing care.
	   To ensure adequate psychological and emotional support.

5. Does the child have any emotional, developmental or mental health problems?	5. To plan appropriate and individualised nursing care.
6. Do the child and/or family have any other concerns regarding the child's emotional, or psychological needs?	6. To allow the child and family to voice concerns about issues that may not have been covered within the assessment.

Procedure guideline 1.16 Communication review

Statement	Rationale
1. Do the family have a health visitor? If so, what is their name and contact details?	1. To maintain inter-professional communication and continuity.
2. Do the family see any other medical or allied health professionals on a regular basis?	2. Other professionals may provide important information about the child and family. Communication and liaison with other healthcare teams is equally important.
3. Does the child or family have any other specific needs or difficulties?	3. To plan appropriate and individualised nursing care. The child's parents/carers may also have specific health needs or disabilities which impact on their ability to care for the child at home and/or in hospital.
4. Does the child have any problems with their hearing, speech or eyesight? If so, what specifically are the problems and when was this last assessed?	4. In order to plan the child's nursing care and ensure effective communication.
5. Do the child and family have any other questions about any aspect of their care?	5. To ensure that all concerns have been addressed and all aspects of the child's care recorded.

Assessment: documentation

Document the assessment as soon as possible. This will ensure that accurate records are kept (Ayott 2006a) and allows re-assessment in the event of a change of condition.

Blood pressure

Accurate blood pressure (BP) measurement in children has been the subject of an intense debate for many years; the first issue is around cuff size and the second is the methods of measurement. Recommendations to start to address these difficulties were published by European experts managing children and adolescence with hypertension (Lurbe et al 2009).

Many well-known textbooks endorse a number of different criteria for choosing the correct cuff size for measuring BP of children based on cuff width; many do not include the most important measurement, which is the length of the cuff. Manufactures have added to this inconsistency of choice by using 'range finder' which differs depending on the brand used. Interestingly, the 'range finder' measurement on most cuffs does not correlate with the recommendations for adult and children, which recommends that the internal cuff length covers a minimal of 80% of the circumference of the upper arm. This in practice often resulted in falsely high blood pressure readings resulting in a phenomenon known as 'under cuffing' or 'cuff hypertension' (Update on the 1987 Task Force Report on High Blood Pressure in Children and Adolescents 1996).

'Under cuffing' is when the blood pressure cuff is too small, resulting in falsely high BP readings. The recommendations for children and adults are that the internal bladder of the cuff covers 80–100% of the circumference of the upper arm, the centre of the bladder of the cuff (marked artery) should be placed in line with the radial artery with the bladder encircling the upper arm (Lurbe et al 2009); this will ensure that the arterial blood flow is completely occluded during the measurement procedure, ensuring accurate measuring and less variability of readings. In paediatrics, the correct cuff bladder size to arm circumference rather than arm width of cuff is more important for consistent and valid measurements (Vyse 1987) (Figure 1.1).

The recommendations for cuff size, for all ages of children, are often much larger that most healthcare professionals realise. Very few areas actually measure the cuff bladder against the child's arm, often opting for the cuff that 'looks about right' for the size of child, its label (infant, small child, small adult, etc) or the 'range finder' (Arafat 1999). This practice has contributed to some children being over treated for high blood pressure during periods of acute illness and an increased numbers of referrals of babies and young children to specialist units for suspected hypertension.

The cuff should be measured against the child's upper arm. The cuff is the correct size if the bladder encircles 80-100% of the circumference of the upper arm, as mentioned above (NIH 2005, Lurbe et al 2009), if not, use the next cuff size up. A small bladder overlap is considered preferable to a cuff that covers less than 80% of the circumference of the arm (Dillon 1991). Many specialists recommend a cuff that is as much as 90–100% the circumference of the upper arm in children with hypertension (Morgenstern and Butani 2004). When measuring the BP manually, and if the cuff covers the area of the brachial artery where auscultation is usually detected, the radial arterial pulse can be used and a Doppler ultrasound is recommended in this situation (Dillon 1991).

The second ongoing debate is about automated blood pressure monitors. Since the turn of the century, automated

(a)

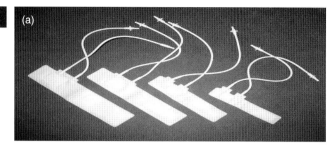

(b)

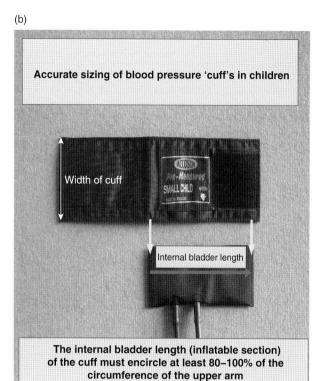

Accurate sizing of blood pressure 'cuff's in children

Width of cuff

Internal bladder length

The internal bladder length (inflatable section) of the cuff must encircle at least 80–100% of the circumference of the upper arm

Figure 1.1 Blood pressure cuffs. (a) Integrated bladder; (b) cuff with internal bladder.

monitors have flooded the market place; they are found in all GP practices, hospitals and many homes throughout the UK. Automated blood pressure reading has been found to be highly variable in a number of areas and in general they read higher than traditional methods of measurement (Chino 2011). Unfortunately these monitors have largely replaced the traditional technique of using a stethoscope and sphygmomanometer. Paediatrics had been identified as one of the high-risk areas of high variability especially in the younger age groups and children with hypertension (www.bhsoc.org). It must be recognised that the accuracy on BP measuring devices should not be solely on claims from manufacturers (O'Brien *et al* 2003). Of note to date there are no automated monitors on the market that have been validated by the British Hypertension Society (BHS), for use in children with hypertension. For the above reasons, European experts responsible for the management of children with hypertension recommend that children's BP is measured manually using auscultatory methods (Doppler in the under 5s and a stethoscope in older children) (Lurbe *et al* 2009). Unfortunately, this standard is rarely achieved outside specialist units. Importantly, since most epidemiologic data are based on auscultation (manual) blood pressure measurements, healthcare professionals working in paediatric should recognise that the current BP centiles used by most paediatricians are not transferable to automated monitors (Dinamap, Critikon, Philips, Hewlett Packard).

In practice measuring manual BP in babies and young children is technically challenging and requires additional skills and equipment. However, in this technological age the skill of BP measurement has largely been lost. Specialists in this area recommend that all paediatric nurses and clinicians are taught the theory and practice of measuring a BP using auscultation, as the alternative methods of measurement (automated) are not consistent or accurate enough to diagnose hypertension in babies and young children (Lurbe *et al* 2009). A lack of knowledge in this area leads to an increase in the number of children being referred to specialist units for investigations into hypertension or, worse, high automated readings being dismissed as machine error (Brennan 2008). This presents a significant risk to children as an elevated BP is often the only early sign of renal disease and aortic coarctation. If a child's BP is found to be continually elevated following a period of BP monitoring using the correct sized cuff, the BP should be measured manually by auscultation to confirm hypertension (Lurbe *et al* 2009). This section will cover techniques for measuring manual BP and best practice when using automated monitors.

Blood pressure (BP) is defined as 'the pressure exerted by blood on the wall of a blood vessel' (Tortora 1992).

There are two main phases of a BP, the systolic phase and the diastolic phase: the systolic represents the pressure when the heart is beating and the diastolic the pressure when the heart is at rest (Edwards 1997).

A BP is made up of five Korotkoff sounds, which are defined as follows:

- Phase 1 – The first appearance of faint, repetitive, clear tapping sounds that gradually increase in intensity for at least two consecutive beats: this is the systolic BP.
- Phase 2 – A brief period may follow during which the sounds soften and acquire a swishing quality.

An auscultatory gap may occur here in some patients (usually elderly and hypertensive patients) – this is where sounds may disappear altogether for a short time.

- Phase 3 – The return of sharper sounds, which become crisper to regain, or even exceed, the intensity of Phase 1 sounds.

  The clinical significance, if any, of phases 2 and 3 has not been established.

- Phase 4 – The distinct, abrupt muffling sounds, which become soft and blowing in quality.

- Phase 5 – The point at which all sounds finally disappear completely: this (in adults) is the diastolic pressure, and current recommendations suggest Phase 5 should be recorded (Lurbe *et al* 2009).

It is widely recognized, that a Korotkoff 5 phase is not always present in children under the age of 13 (Korotkoff 5 can be 0); in this situation Korotkoff 4 is taken as the diastolic reading (but this is subject to many measurement difficulties and is therefore inconsistent). It is reasonable to measure only a systolic BP in most children being treated for hypertension (Brennan 2002, O'Sullivan 2001).

A normal BP is age, height and gender related, and there is a range of acceptable limits for each age and group. Figure 1.2 shows BP centiles modified from the Task Force on High Blood Pressure in children and adolescents (O'Brien *et al* 2003) for age and height defined blood pressure levels for the 50th and 95th percentile, for boys and girls.

Blood Pressure Levels for Boys by Age and Height Percentile

Age (Year)	BP Percentile ↓	Systolic BP (mmHg) ← Percentile of Height →							Diastolic BP (mmHg) ← Percentile of Height →						
		5th	10th	25th	50th	75th	90th	95th	5th	10th	25th	50th	75th	90th	95th
1	50th	80	81	83	85	87	88	89	34	35	36	37	38	39	39
	90th	94	95	97	99	100	102	103	49	50	51	52	53	53	54
	95th	98	99	101	103	104	106	106	54	54	55	56	57	58	58
	99th	105	106	108	110	112	113	114	61	62	63	64	65	66	66
2	50th	84	85	87	88	90	92	92	39	40	41	42	43	44	44
	90th	97	99	100	102	104	105	106	54	55	56	57	58	58	59
	95th	101	102	104	106	108	109	110	59	59	60	61	62	63	63
	99th	109	110	111	113	115	117	117	66	67	68	69	70	71	71
3	50th	86	87	89	91	93	94	95	44	44	45	46	47	48	48
	90th	100	101	103	105	107	108	109	59	59	60	61	62	63	63
	95th	104	105	107	109	110	112	113	63	63	64	65	66	67	67
	99th	111	112	114	116	118	119	120	71	71	72	73	74	75	75
4	50th	88	89	91	93	95	96	97	47	48	49	50	51	51	52
	90th	102	103	105	107	109	110	111	62	63	64	65	66	66	67
	95th	106	107	109	111	112	114	115	66	67	68	69	70	71	71
	99th	113	114	116	118	120	121	122	74	75	76	77	78	78	79
5	50th	90	91	93	95	96	98	98	50	51	52	53	54	55	55
	90th	104	105	106	108	110	111	112	65	66	67	68	69	69	70
	95th	108	109	110	112	114	115	116	69	70	71	72	73	74	74
	99th	115	116	118	120	121	123	123	77	78	79	80	81	81	82
6	50th	91	92	94	96	98	99	100	53	53	54	55	56	57	57
	90th	105	106	108	110	111	113	113	68	68	69	70	71	72	72
	95th	109	110	112	114	115	117	117	72	72	73	74	75	76	76
	99th	116	117	119	121	123	124	125	80	80	81	82	83	84	84
7	50th	92	94	95	97	99	100	101	55	55	56	57	58	59	59
	90th	106	107	109	111	113	114	115	70	70	71	72	73	74	74
	95th	110	111	113	115	117	118	119	74	74	75	76	77	78	78
	99th	117	118	120	122	124	125	126	82	82	83	84	85	86	86
8	50th	94	95	97	99	100	102	102	56	57	58	59	60	60	61
	90th	107	109	110	112	114	115	116	71	72	72	73	74	75	76
	95th	111	112	114	116	118	119	120	75	76	77	78	79	79	80
	99th	119	120	122	123	125	127	127	83	84	85	86	87	87	88
9	50th	95	96	98	100	102	103	104	57	58	59	60	61	61	62
	90th	109	110	112	114	115	117	118	72	73	74	75	76	76	77
	95th	113	114	116	118	119	121	121	76	77	78	79	80	81	81
	99th	120	121	123	125	127	128	129	84	85	86	87	88	88	89

Figure 1.2 Blood pressure levels for boys and girls by age and height percentiles.

Age (Year)	BP Percentile ↓	Systolic BP (mmHg)							Diastolic BP (mmHg)						
		← Percentile of Height →							← Percentile of Height →						
		5th	10th	25th	50th	75th	90th	95th	5th	10th	25th	50th	75th	90th	95th
10	50th	97	98	100	102	103	105	106	58	59	60	61	61	62	63
	90th	111	112	114	115	117	119	119	73	73	74	75	76	77	78
	95th	115	116	117	119	121	122	123	77	78	79	80	81	81	82
	99th	122	123	125	127	128	130	130	85	86	86	88	88	89	90
11	50th	99	100	102	104	105	107	107	59	59	60	61	62	63	63
	90th	113	114	115	117	119	120	121	74	74	75	76	77	78	78
	95th	117	118	119	121	123	124	125	78	78	79	80	81	82	82
	99th	124	125	127	129	130	132	132	86	86	87	88	89	90	90
12	50th	101	102	104	106	108	109	110	59	60	61	62	63	63	64
	90th	115	116	118	120	121	123	123	74	75	75	76	77	78	79
	95th	119	120	122	123	125	127	127	78	79	80	81	82	82	83
	99th	126	127	129	131	133	134	135	86	87	88	89	90	90	91
13	50th	104	105	106	108	110	111	112	60	60	61	62	63	64	64
	90th	117	118	120	122	124	125	126	75	75	76	77	78	79	79
	95th	121	122	124	126	128	129	130	79	79	80	81	82	83	83
	99th	128	130	131	133	135	136	137	87	87	88	89	90	91	91
14	50th	106	107	109	111	113	114	115	60	61	62	63	64	65	65
	90th	120	121	123	125	126	128	128	75	76	77	78	79	79	80
	95th	124	125	127	128	130	132	132	80	80	81	82	83	84	84
	99th	131	132	134	136	138	139	140	87	88	89	90	91	92	92
15	50th	109	110	112	113	115	117	117	61	62	63	64	65	66	66
	90th	122	124	125	127	129	130	131	76	77	78	79	80	80	81
	95th	126	127	129	131	133	134	135	81	81	82	83	84	85	85
	99th	134	135	136	138	140	142	142	88	89	90	91	92	93	93
16	50th	111	112	114	116	118	119	120	63	63	64	65	66	67	67
	90th	125	126	128	130	131	133	134	78	78	79	80	81	82	82
	95th	129	130	132	134	135	137	137	82	83	83	84	85	86	87
	99th	136	137	139	141	143	144	145	90	90	91	92	93	94	94
17	50th	114	115	116	118	120	121	122	65	66	66	67	68	69	70
	90th	127	128	130	132	134	135	136	80	80	81	82	83	84	84
	95th	131	132	134	136	138	139	140	84	85	86	87	87	88	89
	99th	139	140	141	143	145	146	147	92	93	93	94	95	96	97

BP, blood pressure.

*The 90th percentile is 1.28 SD, 95th percentile is 1.645 SD, and the 99th percentile is 2.326 SD over the mean.

Figure 1.2 (*Continued*)

Blood Pressure Levels for Girls by Age and Height Percentile

Age (Year)	BP Percentile ↓	Systolic BP (mmHg) ← Percentile of Height →							Diastolic BP (mmHg) ← Percentile of Height →						
		5th	10th	25th	50th	75th	90th	95th	5th	10th	25th	50th	75th	90th	95th
1	50th	83	84	85	86	88	89	90	38	39	39	40	41	41	42
	90th	97	97	98	100	101	102	103	52	53	53	54	55	55	56
	95th	100	101	102	104	105	106	107	56	57	57	58	59	59	60
	99th	108	108	109	111	112	113	114	64	64	65	65	66	67	67
2	50th	85	85	87	88	89	91	91	43	44	44	45	46	46	47
	90th	98	99	100	101	103	104	105	57	58	58	59	60	61	61
	95th	102	103	104	105	107	108	109	61	62	62	63	64	65	65
	99th	109	110	111	112	114	115	116	69	69	70	70	71	72	72
3	50th	86	87	88	89	91	92	93	47	48	48	49	50	50	51
	90th	100	100	102	103	104	106	106	61	62	62	63	64	64	65
	95th	104	104	105	107	108	109	110	65	66	66	67	68	68	69
	99th	111	111	113	114	115	116	117	73	73	74	74	75	76	76
4	50th	88	88	90	91	92	94	94	50	50	51	52	52	53	54
	90th	101	102	103	104	106	107	108	64	64	65	66	67	67	68
	95th	105	106	107	108	110	111	112	68	68	69	70	71	71	72
	99th	112	113	114	115	117	118	119	76	76	76	77	78	79	79
5	50th	89	90	91	93	94	95	96	52	53	53	54	55	55	56
	90th	103	103	105	106	107	109	109	66	67	67	68	69	69	70
	95th	107	107	108	110	111	112	113	70	71	71	72	73	73	74
	99th	114	114	116	117	118	120	120	78	78	79	79	80	81	81
6	50th	91	92	93	94	96	97	98	54	54	55	56	56	57	58
	90th	104	105	106	108	109	110	111	68	68	69	70	70	71	72
	95th	108	109	110	111	113	114	115	72	72	73	74	74	75	76
	99th	115	116	117	119	120	121	122	80	80	80	81	82	83	83
7	50th	93	93	95	96	97	99	99	55	56	56	57	58	58	59
	90th	106	107	108	109	111	112	113	69	70	70	71	72	72	73
	95th	110	111	112	113	115	116	116	73	74	74	75	76	76	77
	99th	117	118	119	120	122	123	124	81	81	82	82	83	84	84
8	50th	95	95	96	98	99	100	101	57	57	57	58	59	60	60
	90th	108	109	110	111	113	114	114	71	71	71	72	73	74	74
	95th	112	112	114	115	116	118	118	75	75	75	76	77	78	78
	99th	119	120	121	122	123	125	125	82	82	83	83	84	85	86
9	50th	96	97	98	100	101	102	103	58	58	58	59	60	61	61
	90th	110	110	112	113	114	116	116	72	72	72	73	74	75	75
	95th	114	114	115	117	118	119	120	76	76	76	77	78	79	79
	99th	121	121	123	124	125	127	127	83	83	84	84	85	86	87
10	50th	98	99	100	102	103	104	105	59	59	59	60	61	62	62
	90th	112	112	114	115	116	118	118	73	73	73	74	75	76	76
	95th	116	116	117	119	120	121	122	77	77	77	78	79	80	80
	99th	123	123	125	126	127	129	129	84	84	85	86	86	87	88
11	50th	100	101	102	103	105	106	107	60	60	60	61	62	63	63
	90th	114	114	116	117	118	119	120	74	74	74	75	76	77	77
	95th	118	118	119	121	122	123	124	78	78	78	79	80	81	81
	99th	125	125	126	128	129	130	131	85	85	86	87	87	88	89

Figure 1.2 (*Continued*)

Age (Year)	BP Percentile ↓	Systolic BP (mmHg) ← Percentile of Height →							Diastolic BP (mmHg) ← Percentile of Height →						
		5th	10th	25th	50th	75th	90th	95th	5th	10th	25th	50th	75th	90th	95th
12	50th	102	103	104	105	107	108	109	61	61	61	62	63	64	64
	90th	116	116	117	119	120	121	122	75	75	75	76	77	78	78
	95th	119	120	121	123	124	125	126	79	79	79	80	81	82	82
	99th	127	127	128	130	131	132	133	86	86	87	88	88	89	90
13	50th	104	105	106	107	109	110	110	62	62	62	63	64	65	65
	90th	117	118	119	121	122	123	124	76	76	76	77	78	79	79
	95th	121	122	123	124	126	127	128	80	80	80	81	82	83	83
	99th	128	129	130	132	133	134	135	87	87	88	89	89	90	91
14	50th	106	106	107	109	110	111	112	63	63	63	64	65	66	66
	90th	119	120	121	122	124	125	125	77	77	77	78	79	80	80
	95th	123	123	125	126	127	129	129	81	81	81	82	83	84	84
	99th	130	131	132	133	135	136	136	88	88	89	90	90	91	92
15	50th	107	108	109	110	111	113	113	64	64	64	65	66	67	67
	90th	120	121	122	123	125	126	127	78	78	78	79	80	81	81
	95th	124	125	126	127	129	130	131	82	82	82	83	84	85	85
	99th	131	132	133	134	136	137	138	89	89	90	91	91	92	93
16	50th	108	108	110	111	112	114	114	64	64	65	66	66	67	68
	90th	121	122	123	124	126	127	128	78	78	79	80	81	81	82
	95th	125	126	127	128	130	131	132	82	82	83	84	85	85	86
	99th	132	133	134	135	137	138	139	90	90	90	91	92	93	93
17	50th	108	109	110	111	113	114	115	64	65	65	66	67	67	68
	90th	122	122	123	125	126	127	128	78	79	79	80	81	81	82
	95th	125	126	127	129	130	131	132	82	83	83	84	85	85	86
	99th	133	133	134	136	137	138	139	90	90	91	91	92	93	93

BP, blood pressure.
*The 90th percentile is 1.28 SD, 95th percentile is 1.645 SD, and the 99th percentile is 2.326 SD over the mean.
Reproduced with permission from Pediatrics Vol. (4), pp. 649–658, Copyright 1998 by the AAP.

Figure 1.2 (*Continued*)

Principles table 1.3 Measuring blood pressure

Principle	Rationale
1. A BP should be measured on all children admitted to hospital (de Swiet *et al* 1989), if the measurement is considered within the normal ranges for the child and there are no other indications for a BP to be performed this may be the only BP necessary (Edwards 1997).	1. Research suggests that some children can have a high BP without any signs or symptoms of hypertension, if a high blood pressure is recorded at the initial assessment, the BP measurement should be repeated until the readings are within normal limits. If the blood pressure continues to be high make sure the cuff size is correctly measured (Figure 1.1). If a sphygmomanometer is available measure the BP manually. This episode of high BP must be noted in the child's records and followed up (de Swiet *et al* 1989).

Principles table 1.3 (*Continued*)

Principle	Rationale

2. A BP should be measured regularly and/or monitored:
 	
a) If the initial reading is shown to be outside normal ranges (de Swiet 1986) (see Figure 1.2).
b) If the child has a previous history of hypertension (de Swiet *et al* 1989).
c) If there is a strong family history of hypertension
d) On all children with conditions that may affect their BP:
• Low birth weight
• Renal (Rascher 1997)
• Urological (Dillon 1991)
• Cardiac (Edwards 1997)
• Diabetes (Adler 2000)
• Neurology
• Neurofibromatosis
• Pregnant (Dillon 1988)
• Obesity
• Before antihypertensive medication is administered
• Oncology
• According to specific protocols, such as during albumin infusion or blood transfusion
• Pre and post surgery (Wong 2001)
• During anaesthetic
• During critical illness.
e) Children with:
• Headaches
• Facial palsy
• Visual symptoms
• With syndromes associated to hypertension.
	2. Measuring BP is an essential component of a child's physical assessment. A base line BP is a very important observation for all children requiring admission to a hospital.
	
	d) Low birth weight babies seem to be a particular risk factor (Strufaldi, 2009, Uiterwaal *et al* 1997).
	   In children with renal conditions hypertension is common and will always need to be treated. About 70–80% of hypertension in children is due to renal parenchymal abnormality (Luma and Spiotta 2006).
	   Childhood obesity increases the risk of childhood hypertension. Several studies found that the odds ratios in obese children were 2.4 for raised diastolic blood pressure and 4.5 for raised systolic blood pressure (Freedman 1999)
	• An adequate blood pressure is essential to maintain the blood supply and function of vital organs. Measurement of blood pressure is therefore a key part of the monitoring of the child during anaesthesia and critical care.
	• High BP is often seen in sick children secondary to medical treatment or post surgery. This is usually transient and will resolve over time.

3. The first BP measurement should be taken on the child's right arm. If the BP measurement is consistently high and there are no other contributing factors, a measurement should be performed on both arms and legs (Beevers *et al* 2001a, Perloff *et al* 1993) and the **arm** with the highest reading should then be used regularly (McAlister and Strauss 2001, Perloff *et al* 1993).	**3.** The right arm is generally the preferred arm for blood pressure measurement for consistency and comparison with the reference tables. The pressure differences between arms can be >10 mmHg in some hypertensive children (McAlister and Strauss 2001). A high reading on the right arm BP and a low reading on the leg BP can be a sign of coarctation of the aorta. This can be confirmed by bilateral weak femoral pulses and echocardiogram.

Procedure guideline 1.17 Methods of blood pressure monitoring

Statement	Rationale
1. There are two main methods of BP monitoring, direct and indirect. **a)** Direct A direct BP can only be performed when the child has an arterial line in situ. It is regarded as the 'gold standard' or 'true' BP (Derrico 1993). This is obviously, not always practical to perform, and is rarely performed outside of intensive care units, high dependency care units and renal transplant centres (Clarke 1999). **b)** Indirect The indirect methods are more commonly performed, but there are several different ways to achieve a measurement of indirect BP:	1. The two methods can be used together or interchangeably. **a)** Arterial lines are usually only used in critical care settings because of the associated risks with use, e.g. haemorrhage, thrombosis and infection (Roberts 2002). **b)** There are now two types of manual manometers freely available: Aneroid and more recently the Accoson green light 300 (Graves *et al* 2004). Aneroid manometers are commonly used in practice; they need to be checked for calibration yearly. Recalibration is only done by the manufactures; this is seldom done in practice. The Accoson Greenlight 300 is a manual manometer that has been validated by the BHS (www.bhsoc.org). The advantage of this particular monitor is its proven accuracy and reproducibility, self-calibration and ease of maintenance (Graves *et al* 2004).
2. Palpation (using a sphygmomanometer with examination using gentle pressure of the fingers to detect the pulse).	2. This is a very effective way of achieving a quick and approximate BP.
3. Doppler (sphygmomanometer with doppler ultrasound).	3. The doppler and sphygmomanometer are the most accurate method of gaining a systolic reading in children under five (Dillon 1988). Recording of systolic BP is preferred to diastolic pressure (Beevers *et al* 2001a). The systolic reading is the preferred reading to use in the treatment of children with hypertension because of its greater accuracy and reproducibility (Brennan 2008).
4. Auscultation (sphygmomanometer with stethoscope).	4. Due to the limitations of automated monitors, auscultation and sphygmomanometers/doppler are still the most accurate method of measuring BP in children with hypertension (Brennan 2008, Lurbe *et al* 2009).

Procedure guideline 1.17 (*Continued*)

Statement	Rationale
5. Oscillometry (Dinamap or similar)	**5.** Oscillometry (automated) methods of BP measurement in children can be problematic (Update on the 1987 Task Force on High blood pressure in children and adolescence, 1996), the accuracy of several models used by many paediatric areas has known limitations (Lurbe *et al* 2009). Oscillometric devices calculate BP from the oscillations detected in the cuff, this determines the mean BP directly from the maximum point of oscillation, the systolic and diastolic are then calculated using an algorithm (Lurbe *et al* 2009). The problem with this method is that the oscillation in children is often short so the potential for erroneous measurements is increased significantly (Lurbe *et al* 2009), leading to an increased variability in measurements. It has been well documented that these devices do not function well in patients with arrhythmias, the elderly, dialysis patients and patients with reduced vascular elasticity such as diabetics (O'Brien *et al* 2003), in practice children with hypertension appear to be a group at risk. Many of the above problems found in adults also apply to children with hypertension and critical illness. Very few monitors have been validated for paediatrics and those that have, are not validated for children with high BP (www.bhsoc.org). For this reason they cannot be recommended in younger children with high blood pressures. Care should be taken if an oscillometric device inflates and deflates repeatedly 'hunting' without displaying the BP; this can indicate the BP is either too low or high for the automated monitor to register (Lunn *et al* 2009). If this occurs, a manual BP should be measured (Figure 1.3). Automated devices tend to under-read at low BP and over-read very high BP.

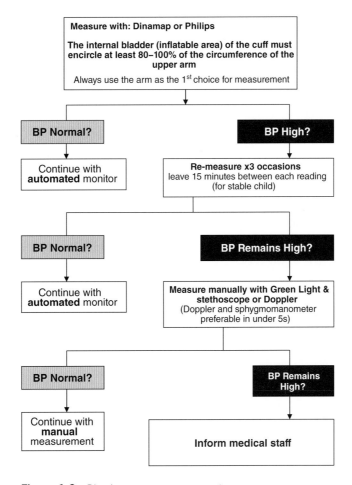

Figure 1.3 Blood pressure measurement.

Procedure guideline 1.18 Equipment for blood pressure monitoring

Statement	Rationale
1. The equipment required should be gathered and checked prior to performing the BP (Petrie *et al* 1986).	**1.** To prevent additional distress to the child by delayed procedure.
2. Equipment for manual BP measurement	**2.** To ensure that it will provide an acceptably accurate measurement and meets recommendations. Literature has demonstrated that up to 50% of BP measuring equipment is thought to be inaccurate and in need of repair (Nolan and Nolan 1993) and can result in the recording of an inaccurate BP (Petrie *et al* 1986).

a) Sphygmomanometer light is on zero
   • Pointer on zero.

b) Maintenance/recalibration
   • They should be serviced yearly by biomedical engineering department to confirm accuracy
   • The date of calibration should be clearly stated on the manometer.

c) Cuff
   • Bladder, tubing, connections, inflation bulb and valves are sound
   • Nylon cuffs should be wiped with disinfectant wipes between use
   • Fabric cuffs should be washed regularly.

d) A variety of cuff sizes should be available (Figure 1.1).

e) Inflation/deflation device
   • Control valves, leaks, vents
   • Tubing should be clean and not perished
   • The system must be able to inflate rapidly
   • Deflation should be smooth and able to be reduced at 2 mmHg/second (Beevers *et al* 2001b)
   • Stethoscope or doppler and water-soluble jelly or palpation by hand.

f) Stethoscope
   • Good condition, with clean well fitting earpieces (Petrie *et al* 1986).

g) Doppler
   • Clean (using water not alcohol) (Parks 2002)
   • Used according to manufacturer's guidelines.
   OR

h) An automated blood pressure monitor
   • Refer to manufacturer's guidelines. The BP upper and lower limits are usually set automatically, this should be confirmed before attempting to measure a BP
   • Choose the cuff size according to guidelines (Figure 1.1)
   • If any of the equipment is defective or unsuitable alternative equipment should be used.

e) The green light 300 is a non-automated mercury-free device for auscultatory BP measurement. This device has an additional benefit of displaying a light that shows you are reducing the pressure at the correct speed. If you are measuring the BP according to the recommendations, the green light illuminates confirming the correct reduction of pressure. This reduces observer-related error and inappropriately rapid deflation rates are reduced significantly.
   • The upper and lower limits for inflation needs to be set before measuring a BP as a higher inflation than necessary can cause considerable discomfort and will cause the BP to be artificially elevated. This is especially important in small children who may move during the measurement.
   • Two cuff types are usually available for most automated monitors, disposable and non-disposable. Both usually have an internal and external range finder. These do not always fulfil the recommendations of a bladder 80–100% of the circumference of the upper arm, measurement of the inflatable cuff against the arm using the 80–100% coverage is more accurate, i.e. the largest cuff size that will fit the arm (Figure 1.1).

Procedure guideline 1.18 (*Continued*)

Statement	Rationale
3. Ensure that the examiner • Has washed hands • Is appropriately trained and familiar with the equipment.	**3.** To minimise spread of infection. To minimise any potential error in BP recording (Nolan and Nolan 1993).

4. The examiner should be aware that a child's BP can increased or decreased by a number of factors:
• Defence reaction
• Time of day
• Meals
• Smoking
• Anxiety
• Temperature
• Season of year
• Sleeping
• Medication
• Urinary retention
• Pain
• Exercise
• Age
• Upper and lower limbs.
	4. 'White coat' hypertension
	   High BP can occur as a result of anxiety during a clinical examination.
	   This tends to subside when the child becomes accustomed to the procedure and the observer. In these children readings are likely to be lower when taken in the home by the community nurse.
	   The examiner should ask the child and family about their history, circumstances that may have affected the BP (Beevers *et al* 2001a). It is important to remember that a child's BP while asleep tends to be lower. Care must be taken if the measurement is on the higher side of normal while sleeping as this could be masking mild hypertension. In this circumstances it is important to measure a waking BP if possible.

5. Explain procedure to the child and family • Outline procedure briefly • Warn of minor discomfort that may be caused • Explain that the procedure may be repeated. The child should be informed of the need for BP measurement (Update of the 1987 Task Force report on high blood pressure in children and adolescents 1996). If the child is anxious or distressed the play specialist should be involved.	**5.** To minimise the risk of anxiety which may result in a temporarily elevated BP (Brennan 2008).
6. The environment that the child is in should be calm and relaxed. The child should be asked to sit and relax/play quietly before measuring the BP.	**6.** These variables can alter a BP (Ramsey *et al* 1999).
7. Posture of the child. **a)** The child should be in a seated position for 3–5 minute, if possible their feet should be on the ground (Beevers *et al* 2001a). **b)** The child's or young adult's legs should be uncrossed (Foster-Fitzpatrick 1999).	**7.** **a)** If the child is lying down, the BP may read slightly lower (Beevers *et al* 2001a). With the exception of acute illness, the blood pressure should be measured with the child in the seated position with the antecubital fossa supported at heart level. It is preferable that the child's feet are on the floor while the blood pressure is measured, if this is not possible the legs should be well supported, not dangling in the air. **b)** BP can be significantly increased by the child's leg being crossed (Foster-Fitzpatrick 1999).

(*Continued*)

Procedure guideline 1.18 (*Continued*)

Statement	Rationale
8. Position the child's arm. The arm should be horizontal at the level of mid-sternum well supported. If the BP is measured on the leg, the child should be lying flat on the bed.	**8.** If the child's arm is below heart level BP can be overestimated by 10 mmHg and if above it can be underestimated by same amount (Petrie *et al* 1986). BP centiles are calculated on arm BP only. For treatment purposes the arm BP is the measurement of choice. If it is not possible to measure the BP on the child's arm a leg BP can be measured, however this must be documented as a leg BP and a larger cuff size should be used. Normally in healthy children the systolic blood pressure is lower in the arms than in the legs due to peripheral amplification of the pulse pressure (Lurbe *et al* 2009).
9. The process of BP measurement should be quick and effective and cause minimal disruption to the child.	**9.** A true BP measurement can only be achieved if the child is calm, relaxed and stress free. It is important to avoid over inflation of the cuff because this causes discomfort, particularly in younger children. If the person measuring the BP is having difficulties, take a break and come back with another person who can distract the young child while you try and measure the BP. If the child is distressed by the procedure you will get an artificially high reading. A play specialist is particularly helpful in these circumstances with distraction therapy. For further information see Chapter 24 on Play as a Therapeutic Tool.

Procedure guideline 1.19 **Manual blood pressure with doppler**

Statement	Rationale
1. Ensure the child is comfortable.	**1.** To ensure accuracy.
2. The child should be in a warm environment, tight or restrictive clothing should be removed from the arm/leg (Thompson 1981).	**2.** To minimise the effect of extraneous influences which may temporarily alter the BP (Perloff *et al* 1993).
3. Apply cuff, ensure that the inflatable bladder length is long enough to encircle at least 80–100% of the upper arm circumference (Figure 1.1), this should fit firmly and be well secured (Perloff *et al* 1993).	**3.** To prevent recording an inaccurate BP (Lurbe *et al* 2009, Morgenstern and Butani 2004, National high BP education program 2004, Vyse 1987).
4. Position the manometer It should be: • Vertical at eye level • Not more than 1 m from the observer (Perloff *et al* 1993).	**4.** To prevent observer error (Beevers *et al* 2001b).
5. The observer should be comfortably positioned in order to be able to inflate and deflate the cuff gradually with ease (Perloff *et al* 1993).	**5.** To prevent injury to the staff performing the BP measurement and to ensure that the procedure is performed accurately on the first attempt, this will prevent unnecessary repeating of the procedure and reduce the risk of further distressing the child (Perloff *et al* 1993).

Procedure guideline 1.19 (*Continued*)

Statement	Rationale
6. The centre of the cuff bladder (usually labelled artery) should be placed over the brachial artery. The tubing from the blood pressure cuff should not cross the auscultatory area, the tubing may lie inferiorly (going down) or superiorly (going up).	**6.** To ensure that the most accurate BP reading can be measured and avoid 'cuff hypertension' (National Heart, Lung and Blood Institute Task Force on Blood Pressure Control in Children 1987).
7. The first BP should be estimated by: **a)** Placing a doppler over the position of maximal pulsation of the brachial artery in the arm or radial pulse in the wrist, pumping up the cuff, when the pulse sound disappears, this is the estimated BP, now deflate the cuff.	**7.** Prevents underestimation of systolic pressure by misreading the Korotkoff sound, this will ensure that the auscultatory gap is not missed (Perloff *et al* 1993). Contact of the stethoscope with the cuff or tubing may produce artefactual sounds; if the cuff is long, use the radial pulse instead.
8. Place stethoscope (or doppler or fingers to palpate) gently over artery, do not press too firmly or touch the cuff, inflate the bladder rapidly and steadily to a pressure of 30 mmHg above the previously estimated systolic BP (McAlister and Straus 2001).	**8.** To maximise the accuracy and reproducibility of the measurement (Perloff, *et al* 1993), avoid pressing down too firmly on the artery, which could occlude it. Do not move the doppler too quickly or you may hear false pulse sounds (artefact).
9. Reduce the pressure at 2–3 mmHg per second.	**9.** To avoid inaccuracies in BP measurement. A rapid deflation can result in recording errors (Nolan and Nolan 1993) and a slow inflation can cause venous congestion and increases the likelihood of an inaccurate measurement. Using the Accoson green light reduces this risk as it displays a green light when the reduction of pressure is at the recommended speed (Graves *et al* 2004).
10. The point at which repetitive, clear tapping sounds (Phase 1) first appear for consecutive beats gives the systolic BP (McAlister and Straus 2001).	**10.** Both measurements should be taken to the nearest 2 mmHg (Beevers *et al* 2001b).

11. The point at which repetitive sounds disappear (Phase 5) gives the diastolic BP (McAlister and Straus 2001). This is only achievable using a stethoscope.	**11.** A doppler will not pick up the diastolic BP because it only detects the acoustic waves moving towards the transducer only.
	  A diastolic BP can only be measured manually with a stethoscope and may be difficult to detect in some children. The diastolic pressure should be recorded at the point where muffling of the repetitive sounds is taken (Phase 4). It should be clearly documented as Phase 4.
	  When using a stethoscope there may be a 'silent' or 'auscultatory gap' where sounds disappear shortly after the systolic phase is heard, this should be documented if it is noted.

12. Continue to completely deflate the cuff rapidly (McAlister and Straus 2001).	**12.** Prevent discomfort.
13. If the reading is difficult to ascertain (common in small, unsettled children) stop, take a rest and retry when the child is settled.	**13.** To enable an accurate reading to be taken, BP will be elevated in unsettled children.
14. Number of measurements: If it is necessary to repeat the BP, the cuff should be allowed to fully deflate, and then a minute should elapse before the next measurement is taken (Ramsey *et al* 1999).	**14.** To prevent venous congestion, which would give an inaccurate BP on the second reading (Nolan and Nolan 1993). Only repeat the measurement if the child is settled to prevent falsely high readings.

Procedure guideline 1.20 Automated measurement of blood pressure

Statement	Rationale
1. Be aware of the limitations of automated monitoring in young children.	1. The manufacturers warn that clinical judgement should be used in the appropriateness of using an automated monitor on patients who are moving, shivering or convulsing, with cardiac arrhythmias, if the patient's BP is changing rapidly over a period of time (renal replacement therapy or fluid shifts), severe shock or hypothermia where blood flow to the peripheries is reduced, heart rate extremes (<40 bpm–>300 bpm). Care must also be taken with obese children as a thick layer of fat surrounding the arm dampens the oscillations coming from the artery, and accuracy is reduced (User Guide to M3046A 2001).
Posture of the child: 1. The child should be in a seated position for 3 minutes before performing BP (Beevers *et al* 2001a).	If the child is lying down, the BP may read slightly lower (Beevers *et al* 2001a). With the exception of acute illness, the blood pressure should be measured with the child in the seated position with the antecubital fossa supported at heart level. It is preferable that the child's feet are on the floor while the blood pressure is measured.
2. The child/young adult's legs should be uncrossed (Foster-Fitzpatrick 1999).	2. BP can be significantly increased by the child's legs being crossed (Foster-Fitzpatrick 1999).
3. Position the child's arm horizontal at the level of mid-sternum well supported. If the BP is measured on the leg the child should be lying flat on the bed for 5 minutes.	3. If the child's arm is below heart level BP can be overestimated by 10 mmHg and if above it can be underestimated by same amount (Petrie *et al* 1986). BP centiles are calculated on arm BP only. For treatment purposes the arm BP is the measurement of choice. If it is not possible to measure the BP on the child's arm a leg BP can be measured, however this must be documented as a leg BP and a larger cuff size should be used. Normally, in healthy children, the systolic blood pressure is lower in the arms than in the legs due to peripheral amplification of the pulse pressure.
4. Cuff (size chosen Figure 1.1) should fit firmly and be well secured (Perloff *et al* 1993). Do not measure a BP on an arm that has an intravenous infusion or cannula in place (User Guide to M3046A 2001).	4. To ensure that the most accurate BP reading can be made and avoid 'cuff hypertension' (National Heart, Lung and Blood Institute Task Force on Blood Pressure Control in Children 1987). The manufacturer's recommendations are not to measure BP on arms with infusions or cannula as there is an increased risk of tissue damage and extravasation (User Guide to M3046A 2001).
5. The centre of the cuff bladder (usually labelled artery) should be placed over the brachial artery.	5. For greater accuracy and reproducibility.
6. Make sure the correct patient size setting is set on the monitor and press the start button as recommended by the manufacturers. Set the monitor for a single measurement or automatic measurement for the frequency required as recommended in the manufacturer's guide. The cuff should be reapplied frequently for regular BP monitoring is required.	6. If the monitor inflation settings are too high this may cause considerable discomfort to the child and cause the BP to increase due to a pain response. Frequent repeated measurement can cause purpura, ischaemia and neuropathy (User Guide to M3046A 2001), for this reason the BP cuff should be reapplied hourly and the skin observed for colour, warmth and sensitivity.
7. The arm should remain still during the measurement.	7. Movement artefact is often responsible for falsely high readings or an inability for the monitor to register a reading, but this is not always the case. In this situation a manual BP should be taken.

Procedure guideline 1.20 (*Continued*)

Statement	Rationale
8. Record the measurement. If the BP readings are above the expected level for age and height and the child is calm and not in any discomfort during the procedure the BP measurement should be repeated three times, leaving at least 1 minute between readings. Make sure the cuff bladder size is correct and continue to monitor. If the readings obtained are consistently high; a 4 limb BP should be measured. If the problem continues manual BP measurement should be obtained (Figure 1.3).	**8.** The BP readings on automated monitors do tend to be slightly higher than manual readings on normotensive children. On hypertensive children the variability seems to be significant. To date there are no automated monometers that have be successfully validated for use in hypertensive children in the UK. Lunn *et al* (2009) published a case study of a 3-year-old child with a BP of 210 systolic, which was unrecordable on an automated monitor.
9. If the child's BP is to be monitored continually make sure the cuff is not wrapped too tightly around the limb, remove regularly.	**9.** This may cause discolouration and even ischaemia.

Procedure guideline 1.21 **Recording the blood pressure**

Statement	Rationale
Record the BP	
1. The BP should be written down as soon as it is recorded.	**1.** To prevent the measurement being forgotten.
2. The BP should be recorded with arrow tops pointing up, e.g. ∧ or as a ∨, with the arrows pointing down – but the tip of the point should be at the number.	**2.** For consistency of documentation.
3. The arm in which the pressure is being recorded and the position of the subject should be noted, for example: left arm, sitting.	**3.** The same limb and cuff size should be used for repeated measurements to ensure consistency (Brennan 2008).
4. In children the arm circumference and bladder size should be indicated.	**4.** It is important to consistently use the same arm and cuff size to ensure reproducibility of results (Update on the 1987 Taskforce Report. National High Blood pressure education Program Working group on hypertension control in Children and adolescents 1996).
5. If the child/young adult is anxious, restless or distressed, a note should be made with the BP (Beevers *et al* 2001b).	**5.** There are many factors that can cause a spuriously high reading to be taken and, if not indicated as such, this reading could be considered as a true BP, which may lead to instigation of inappropriate treatment (Beevers *et al* 2001b).

References

Adler A, Stratton I, Neil H, Yudkin J, Matthews D, Cull C, Wright A, Turner R, Holman R. (2000) Association of systolic blood pressure with macrovascular and microvascular complications of type 2 diabetes (UKPDS 36): prospective observational study. British Medical Journal, 321, 412–419

Advanced Life Support Group (2005). Advanced Paediatric Life Support: The Practical Approach, 4th edition. London, BMJ Books

Arafat M, Mattoo TK. (1999) Measurement of blood pressure in children: Recommendations and perceptions on cuff selection. Paediatrics, 104(3), e30

Aylott M. (2006a) Developing rigour in the observation of the sick child: Part 1. Paediatric Nursing, 18(8), 38–44

Aylott M. (2006b) Observing the sick child: Part 2a Respiratory Assessment. Paediatric Nursing, 18(9), 38–44

Beevers G, Lip G, O'Brien E. (2001a) ABC of Hypertension: Blood Pressure Measurement. Part I – Sphygmomanometry: factors common to all techniques. British Medical Journal, 322, 981–985

Beevers G, Lip G, O'Brien E. (2001b) ABC of Hypertension: Blood Pressure Measurement. Part II – Conventional sphygmomanometry: technique of auscultatory blood pressure measurement. British Medical Journal, 322, 1043–1114

Bowler S, (1998) Meningococcal disease. Nursing Standard, 13(5), 49–52, 55–56

Brennan E. (2002) Care of Infants with Renal Disorders. In Crawford D. (ed.) Neonatal Nursing, 2nd edition. London, Chapman and Hall, pp 204–225

Brennan E. (2008) Assessment of blood pressure. In: Kelsey J, McEwing G. (eds) Clinical Skills in Child Health Practice. Edinburgh, Churchill Livingstone, pp 88–95

Budd C, Gardiner RM. (1999) Paediatrics (Crash Course series). St Louis, Mosby

Campbell S, Glasper EA. (1995) Whaley and Wong's Children's Nursing (UK edition). St Louis, Mosby

Carter S, Laird C. (2005) Assessment and care of ENT problems. Emergency Medicine Journal, 22(2), 128–139

Carr EA, Wilmoth ML, Beoglos Eliades A, Baker PJ, Shelestak D, Heisroth KL, Stoner KH. (2011) Comparison of temporal artery to rectal temperature measurements in children up to 24 months. Journal of Pediatric Nursing, 26, 179–185

Casey G. (2000) Fever management in children. Paediatric Nursing, 12(3), 38–43

Chand N, Mihas A. (2006) Celiac disease: Current concepts in diagnosis and treatment. Journal of Clinical Gastroenterology, 40(1), 3–14

Chapman SM, Grocott MPW, Franck LS. (2010) Systematic review of Paediatric Alert Criteria for identifying children at risk of critical deterioration. Intensive Care Medicine, 36, 600–611]

Chaudhuri N. (2004) Interventions to improve children's health by improving the housing environment. Reviews on Environmental Health, 19(3–4), 197–222

Chino S, Urbina E, LaPointe J, Tsai J, Berenson G. (2011) Korotkoff sound versus Oscillometric cuff sphygmomanometers comparison between auscultatory and DynaPulse blood pressure measurements. Journal of the American Society of Hypertension, 5(1), 12–20

Clarke S. (1999) Arterial Lines: an analysis of good practice. Journal of Child Health Care, 3(1), 23–27

Cole TJ. (1994) Do growth chart centiles need a face lift? British Medical Journal, 308(6929), 641–642

Department of Health (2011) http://www.dh.gov.uk/en/Publichealth/Immunisation/index.htm (last accessed 11th November 2011)

Derrico D. (1993) Comparison of blood pressure measurement methods in critically ill children. Dimensions of Critical Care Nursing, 12(1), 31–33

de Swiet M. (1986) The epidemiology of hypertension in children. British Medical Bulletin, 42(2), 172–175

de Swiet M, Dillon MJ, Littler W, O'Brien E, Padfield PL, Petrie JC. (1989) Measurement of blood pressure in children. British Medical Journal, 289, 497

Dillon MJ. (1988) Blood pressure. Archives of Disease in Childhood, 63, 347–349

Dillon MJ. (1991) Blood pressure measurement in childhood. In: O'Brien E, O'Malley K. (eds) Handbook of Hypertension. Amsterdam, Elsevier, pp126–138

Duff AJ. (2003) Incorporating psychological approaches into routine paediatric venepuncture. Archives of Disease in Childhood, 88(10), 931–937

Dunleavy KJ. (2010) Which core body termperature measurement is most accurate? Nursing, December, 18–19

Edwards S. (1997) Recording blood pressure. Professional Nurse Study Supplement, 13(2), S8–S11

Emond AM, Howat P, Evans JA, Hunt L. (1997) The effects of housing on the health of preterm infants. Pediatric and Perinatal Epidemiology, 11(2), 228–239

Engel J. (1997) Pediatric Assessment, 3rd edition. St Louis, Mosby

Fischer SU, Beattie TF. (1999) The limping child: epidemiology, assessment and outcome. Journal of Bone and Joint Surgery (British edition), 81-B(6), 1029–1034

Ford MJ, Munro JF. (2000) Introduction to Clinical Examination, 7th edition. Edinburgh, Churchill Livingstone

Foster-Fitzpatrick L, Ortiz A, Sibilano H, Marcantonio R, Braun L. (1999) The effects of crossed leg on Blood Pressure Measurement. Nursing Research, 48(2), 105–108

Freedman DS, Dietz WH, Srinivasan SR, et al (1999) The relation of overweight to cardiovascular risk factors among children and adolescents: the Bogalusa Heart Study. Paediatrics, 103(6 Pt 1), 1175–1182

Fry T. (1994) Introducing the new Child Growth Standards. Professional Care of Mother and Child, 4(8), 231–233

Godwin H, Thomas L, Richardson C. (2005) Clinical Practice Guideline: Temperature Measurement and management of pyrexia. London, Great Ormond Street Hospital

Gill D, O'Brien N. (1998) Paediatric Clinical Examination, 3rd edition. Edinburgh, Churchill Livingstone

Graves J, Tibor M, Murtage B, Klein L, Sheps SG. (2004) The Accoson Greenlight300 the first non-automated mercury-free blood pressure measurement device to pass the international protocol for blood pressure measurement devices in adults. blood Pressure Monitoring, (9)1, 13–17

Hall DM. (2000) Growth monitoring. Archives of Diseases in Childhood, 82(1), 10–15

Hazinski MF. (1992) Nursing Care of the Critically Ill Child, 2nd edition. St Louis, Mosby

Henderson N. (1998) Anaphylaxis. Nursing Standard, 12(47), 49–55

Hewson PH, Poulakis Z, Jarman F, Kerr JF, McMaster D, Goodge J, Silk G. (2000) Clinical markers of serious illness in young infants: A multicentre follow-up study. Journal of Paediatrics and Child Health, 36(3), 221–225

Hockenberry MJ, Wilson D. (2007) Wong's Nursing Care of Infants and Children, 7th edition. St Louis, Mosby

Kline A. (2003) Pinpointing the cause of pediatric respiratory distress. Nursing, 33(9), 58–64

La Buda CS, Ruess L, Rooks VJ. (2005) Stridor in children: Imaging and etiologies. Contemporary Diagnostic Radiology, 28(25), 1–5

Luma GB, Spiotta RT. (2006) Hypertension in children and adolescents. American Family Physician, May 1, 73(9), 1558–1568

Lunn A, Blyton D, Watson AR. (2009) Blood pressure measurement in children: Declining standard. Archives of Diseases in Childhood, 94, 995

Lurbe E, Cifkova J, Cruickshank K, Dillon MJ, Ferreira I, Invetti C, Kuznetsova T, Laurent S, Mancia G, Morales-Olivas F, Rascher W, Redon J, Schaefer F, Seeman T, Stergiou G, Wuhl E, Zanchetti A. (2009) Management of high blood pressure in children and Adolescence: Recommendations of the European society of hypertension. Journal of Hypertension, 27, 1719–1742

Marcoux KK. (2005) Management of increased intracranial pressure in the critically ill child with an acute neurological injury. American Association of Critical-Care Nurses Journal (Clinical Issues: Advanced Practice in Acute and Critical Care), 16(2), 212–231

McAlister F, Straus S. (2001) Evidence based treatment of hypertension: Measurement of blood pressure: an evidence based review. British Medical Journal, 322, 908–911

McGrath A, Cox C. (1998) Cardiac and circulatory assessment in Intensive Care Units. Intensive and Critical Care Nursing, 14(16), 283–287

Morgenstern B, Butani L. (2004). Casual blood pressure measurements methodology. In Portman RJ, Sorof JM, Ingelfinger JR. (eds) Pediatric Hypertension, pp 77–96. Humana Press, Totowa, NJ, USA

National Heart, Lung and Blood Institute Task Force on Blood Pressure Control in Children (1987) Report of the Second Task Force on Blood Pressure Control in Children. Paediatrics, 79(1), 1–25

National Institutes of Health (NIH) (2005) The fourth report on the diagnosis, evaluation, and treatment of high blood pressure in children and adolescents. NIH Bethesda, MD, USA

National Institute for Health and Clinical Excellence (2007) Feverish illness in children: NICE guideline. Available at http://www.nice.org.uk/nicemedia/pdf/CG47NICEGuideline.pdf (last accessed 14th November 2011)

Nolan J., Nolan M. (1993) Can nurses take an accurate blood pressure? British Journal of Nursing 2 (14) pp. 724–729

O'Brien E, Asmar R, Beilin L, Imai Y, Mallion JM, Mancia G, Mengden T, Myers M, Padfield P, Palatini P, Parati G, Pickering T, Redon J, Staessen J, Stergiou G, Verdecchia P. (2003) On behalf of the European Society of Hypertension Working Group on Blood Pressure Monitoring. European Society of Hypertension recommendations for conventional, ambulatory and home blood pressure measurement. Journal of Hypertension, (21), 821–848

Oliver C. Candappa M. (2003) Tackling bullying: listening to the views of children and young people. London, DfES publications

Orfanelli L (2001) Neurologic Examination of the Toddler: How to assess for increased intracranial pressure following head trauma. American Journal of Nursing, 101(12), 24CC–24FF

O'Sullivan J, Allen J, Murray A. (2001) A clinical study of the korotkoff phases of blood pressure in children. Journal of Human Hypertension, 15, 197–201

Parks Medical Electronics (2002) Pocket Doppler Operating Manual. Aloha, Parks Medical Electronics

Pearson G. (ed.) (2008) Why Children Die: A pilot study. Available at http://www.cemach.org.uk/ (accesssed 14ᵗʰ November 2011

Perloff D, Grim C, Flack J, Frohlich E, Hill M, McDonald M, Morgenstern B. AHA (1993) Medical/Scientific Statement: Special report. Human Blood Pressure Determination by Sphygmomanometry. Circulation, 88(5), 2460–2467

Petrie JC, O'Brien ET, Littler WA, de Swiet M. (1986) British Hypertension Society: Recommendations on Blood Pressure Measurement. British Medical Journal, 293, 611–615

Ramsey LE, Williams B, Johnston GD, Macgregor GA, Poston L, Potter JF, Poulter NR, Russell G. (1999) British Hypertension Society Guidelines: Guidelines for management of hypertension: report of the third working party of the British Hypertension Society. Journal of Human Hypertension, 13, 569–592

Rawling-Anderson K, Hunter J (2008) Monitoring pulse rate. Nursing Standard, 22(31), 41–43

Rascher W. (1997) Blood Pressure Measurement and Standards in Children. Nephrology Dialysis and Transplantation, 12(5), 868–870

Riordan M. (2001) Investigation and treatment of facial paralysis. Archives of Disease in Childhood, 84(4), 286–287

Roberts C. (2002) Arterial Line Sampling. ICU Online: CRACC Protocols. London, Great Ormond Street Hospital for Children NHS Foundation Trust

Royal College of Nursing (2009) The recognition and assessment of acute pain in children. Available at http://www.rcn.org.uk/__data/assets/pdf_file/0004/269185/003542.pdf (last accessed 14ᵗʰ November 2011)

Royal College of Nursing (2011) Standards for assessing, measuring and monitoring vital signs in infants, children and young people – RCN guidance for children's nurses and nurses working with children and young people. Available at http://www.rcn.org.uk/__data/assets/pdf_file/0004/114484/003196.pdf (last accessed 11ᵗʰ September 2011)

Rudolf MCJ, Levene MI. (1999) Paediatrics and Child Health. Oxford, Blackwell Science

Rush M, Wetherall A. (2003) Temperature measurement: practice guidelines. Paediatric Nursing, 15(9), 25–28

Schling S, Hulse T. (1997) Growth monitoring and assessment in the commmunity. A guide to good practice. London, Child Growth Foundation

Shah MD. (2002) Failure to Thrive in Children. Journal of Clinical Gastroenterology, 35(5), 371–374

Sherwood MC, Stanhope R, Preece MA, Grant DB. (1986) Diabetes insipidus and occult intracranial tumours. Archives of Diseases of Childhood, 61(12), 1222–1224

Simoes EA, Roark R, Berman S, Esler LL, Murphy J. (1991) Respiratory rate: measurement of variability over time and accuracy at different counting periods. Archives of Diseases in Childhood, 66(10), 1199–1203

Skuse D. (1989) ABC of child abuse. Emotional abuse and delay in growth. British Medical Journal, 299, 113–115

Stanhope R, Wilks Z, Hamill G. (1994) Failure to grow: lack of food or lack of love? Prof Care of Mother and Child, 4(8), 234–237

Stern M. (1985) Assessing the child with short stature. Archives of Diseases in Childhood, 11, 106

Strawser D. (1997) Pediatric bacterial meningitis in the emergency department. Journal of Emergency Nursing, 23(4), 310–315

Strufaldi MW, Silva EM, Franco MC, et al (2009) Blood pressure levels in childhood: probing the relative importance of birth weight and current size. European Journal of Pediatrics, 168(5), 619–624

Thompson DR. (1981) Recording patient's blood pressure: a review. Journal of Advanced Nursing, 6, 283–290

Tortora GJ, Grabowski SR. (1992) Principles of Anatomy and Physiology, 7ᵗʰ edition. New York, Harper Collins

Update on the 1987 Task Force Report on High Blood Pressure in Children and Adolescents (1996) A Working Group from the National High Blood Pressure Education Program. National High Blood Pressure Education Program Working Group on Hypertension Control in Children and Adolescents. Pediatrics, 98, 649–658

Uiterwaal CS, Anthony S, Launer LJ, et al (1997) Birth weight, growth, and blood pressure: an annual follow-up study of children aged 5 through 21 years. Hypertension, 30(2 Pt 1), 267–271

Voss LD. (2000) Growth Monitoring. Archives of Disease in Childhood, 82, 14–15

Voss LD, Bailey BJ, Cumming K, Wilkin TJ, Betts PR. (1990) The reliability of height measurement (the Wessex Growth Study). Archives of Disease in Childhood, 65(12), 1340–1344

Vyse TJ. (1987) Sphygmomanometer bladder length and measurements of blood pressure in children. Lancet, 1, 561–562

Wilks Z, Bryan S, Mead V. (2011a) Clinical Guideline: Measuring a child: Height. Available at http://www.gosh.nhs.uk/health-professionals/clinical-guidelines/weight-measuring-a-child/ (last accessed 14ᵗʰ November 2011)

Wilks Z, Bryan S, Mead V, Davies EH, Shaw V, Peters C. (2011b) Clinical Guideline: Measuring a child: Height. Available at http://www.gosh.nhs.uk/health-professionals/clinical-guidelines/height-measuring-a-child/?locale=en (last accessed 14ᵗʰ November 2011)

Wong D. (2001) Wong's Essentials of Pediatric Nursing. St Louis, Mosby

Chapter 2

Allergy and anaphylaxis

Chapter contents

Introduction

Allergic conditions or hypersensitivity reactions are common and their prevalence is increasing. They cause a range of symptoms from mild reactions, such as rashes and sneezing, to severe, life-threatening reactions such as anaphylaxis. Food is the most common cause of allergic reactions in children, with most children who have a food allergy showing sensitisation to specific foods by the age of 2 years. Other allergic diseases such as eczema, asthma and allergic rhinitis are increasing in prevalence across the world. Approximately 40% of children in the UK have a diagnosed condition, such as asthma, eczema, allergic rhinitis or food allergy. With increasing awareness of allergic disease, many more parents/carers believe their child has an allergy. Unfortunately there is a need for greater knowledge regarding the management of allergic disease by healthcare professionals in the UK and more adequate allergy care for children. Consequences of the lack of understanding and provision includes heightened anxiety, risk taking, inappropriate food exclusion with nutritional consequences and unneccesary omission of vaccination because of fear of an allergic reaction. National Institute for Clinical Excellence (NICE) guidelines are now available for the diagnosis and assessment of food allergy in children in primary care (NICE 2011).

The range of allergic diseases is wide and outside the realms of this chapter but the following aspects will be explored:

1. Allergy and the immune response
2. Diagnosis and management of allergy
3. Management of anaphylaxis
4. Food allergy
5. Respiratory allergy
6. Allergens in the healthcare setting.

Further reading is recommended and a number of key texts are suggested at the end of the chapter.

Allergy and the immune response

The word allergy is derived from the Greek, meaning altered reactivity. The immune system is responsible for allergic responses, Gell and Coombes (Johansson *et al* 2001) proposed a classification for allergic responses in the 1960s which has been used widely for many years:

Type I   IgE mediated (immediate) hypersensitivity
Type II   Antibody mediated hypersensitivity
Type III Immune complex interactions
Type IV   Cell mediated (delayed) hypersensitivity.

A revised nomenclature for allergy was devised by the European Academy of Allergy and Clinical Immunology (EAACI) taskforce in 2001 (Figure 2.1) (Johansson *et al* 2001). This has helped to simplify and define 'allergic responses' to reactions being either IgE or non-IgE mediated and it is more common now for clinicians to use this new definition, which aids diagnosis and management of reactions (Johansson *et al* 2004).

Allergic reactions are inappropriate immune responses by an atopic individual to a protein within a substance, which is usually harmless. The production of immunoglobulin E (IgE) and subsequent allergic reactions are responses of the immune system to an allergen (antigen). The first part of this process is the uptake of the allergen by an antigen presenting cell. The allergen passes through the body's barriers, such as the skin, nasal mucosa, respiratory or gastrointestinal tract and is captured and internalised by an antigen presenting cell, the most efficient of which are dendritic cells. The antigen is broken down by the dendritic cell and through a series of complex immune processes immunoglobulin E (IgE) is produced. IgE binds with high affinity receptors known as FcεR1 on the outside of mast cells, an effector cell in the allergic response found in all tissues of the body.

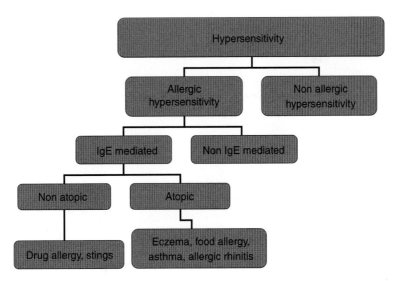

Figure 2.1   EAACI 2001 Nomenclature for hypersensitivity reactions. Reproduced with the kind permission of the Resuscitation Council (UK).

When IgE on the mast cell subsequently comes into contact with the specific allergen it triggers the mast cell to degranulate and release its contents; histamine, tryptase, heparin and leukocytes, mediators of an allergic response.

As histamine is released by mast cells it acts on surrounding blood vessels, causing them to dilate. This initial vasodilatation causes redness (erythema) in the skin, which occurs rapidly after the release of histamine. As the blood vessels dilate, their walls become permeable and plasma leaks out, causing swelling (oedema). Histamine also stimulates the nerves to cause further vasodilatation and the sensation of feeling itchy. The release of mediators also sends signals via cytokines to recruit the effector cells in the allergic response, T helper cells and eosinophils, which cause inflammation, the late phase of the allergic response, and can lead to a systemic reaction.

Atopy is the predisposition to produce immunoglobulin E (IgE) on encountering a potential allergen. How atopy manifests itself is known as allergic disease and can include: asthma, eczema, allergic rhinitis and conjunctivitis, food allergy and, in severe cases, anaphylaxis. An atopic individual may have one or all of these conditions. A phenomenon known as 'the allergic march' has been recognised, where children follow an atopic pattern. Many children present as young babies with eczema, develop food allergies within the first few years of life, and then in their mid-childhood to teenage years develop asthma and allergic rhinitis.

Diagnosis and management of allergy

Accurate history is the cornerstone of allergy diagnosis and should underpin a decision to perform testing. Diagnosis of allergy should begin with a careful allergy focused history of symptoms and their relation to foods eaten, the home environment, pets, seasons of the year and medicines. Family history is important, as it gives an indication as to whether the child is at increased risk of being atopic. Children who have either one or both parents with an atopic disease are at increased risk of being atopic themselves. This may manifest as eczema or food allergy as a baby, or allergic rhinitis in adulthood, as the parent passes on a genetic predisposition to develop an allergic disease rather than a specific allergy itself. Hence, a child whose parent has peanut allergy may not have peanut allergy themselves.

History alone is not enough to confirm allergy. Firm diagnosis requires confirmatory testing. Two common tests used to assess atopic children are skin prick tests (SPT) and specific IgE (SpIgE) testing (formerly known as RAST testing). Skin prick tests are simple and inexpensive to perform and they give immediate results.

Skin prick testing

SPT introduces the allergen into the top layer of skin. If the child is allergic to the allergen a wheal and flare (hive) will appear at the site within 15–20 minutes. The skin is marked to identify each allergen, a small droplet of the allergen is placed on the skin, with at least 2cm between each droplet and the skin is pricked gently, with a metal lancet at 90° angle, through the allergen, which is then carefully removed with tissue. To avoid contamination the child should remain as still as possible to prevent the droplets running into one another and a new lancet should be used for each allergen and care taken when wiping the droplets away. After 15 minutes, the wheal is measured in millimetres at the widest point and recorded. The size of wheal relates to the likelihood of clinical allergy but not to severity of reaction. A negative (saline) and positive (histamine) control should be performed to ensure the child reacts appropriately and validates the test (Høst et al 2003).

There are a number of things to be aware of with regard to SPT. There is a small theoretical risk that a severe systemic reaction could occur when SPT is performed and therefore SPT should be carried out in a clinical area where facilities are available for resuscitation. The clinician performing SPT should ensure the child is well and if they have asthma, this is well controlled and the child is not requiring a bronchodilator or is wheezy on the day of testing. There are some situations when SPT is not appropriate, for example if the child has severe eczema, as a clear patch of skin may not be available and itching as a response to SPT may cause the child more discomfort. Some children have a condition called dermatographism where their skin may mark quite easily and SPT may return false positive results to all allergens tested. If the child has taken an antihistamine or medicine containing a sedative (e.g. cough medicine), the SPT may give a false negative response, which could lead to an unsafe diagnosis. Proper use of positive and negative control tests ensures this is detected and thus prevented. Immediate diagnosis of an allergy with SPT enables us to give patients the information regarding allergen avoidance and a management plan, detailing how to treat an allergic reaction at their clinic visit (see Figure 2.2).

Blood tests

SpIgE testing is not as instantaneous as SPT (see Table 2.1), as blood must be taken from the patient and sent to a laboratory where it undergoes a process to measure the amount of IgE (in Ku/l) present to a specific allergen. The results may take a long time to return depending on local laboratory facilities and this may lead to a delay in diagnosis and risk of subsequent allergic reactions.

As mentioned earlier, there is an underprovision of allergy services within the UK, which may cause a delay in the child receiving appropriate assessment, diagnosis and management of their allergic disease. This delay may lead the family to turn to alternative and unreliable forms of diagnostic techniques, such as VEGA (bioelectrical) testing and kinesiology, to confirm and treat any suspected allergy. The family may exclude foods unnecessarily from their child's diet, which could have a detrimental effect on their nutritional intake and impair their growth and development. Alternatively, if there is no confirmation of an allergy, the patient may not avoid a food they are allergic to, putting themselves at risk of an allergic reaction.

Managing allergy

Avoidance of the allergen is essential to ensuring the child does not have an allergic reaction and this will be discussed in the individual sections relating to specific disease processes. In

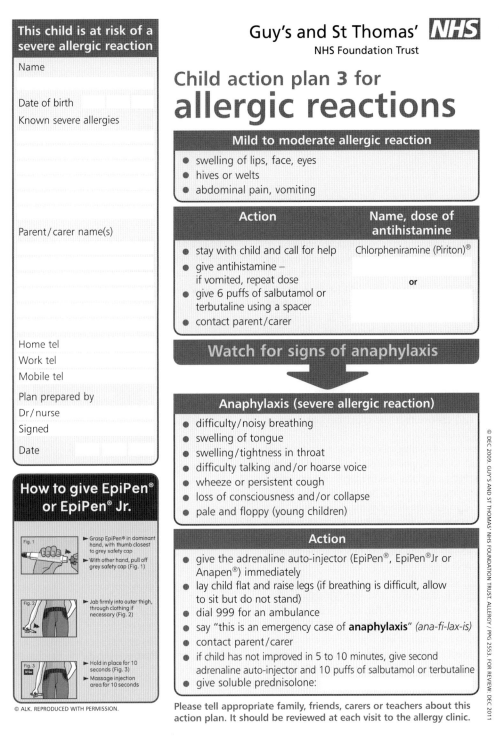

This child is at risk of a severe allergic reaction

Name

Date of birth

Known severe allergies

Parent/carer name(s)

Home tel

Work tel

Mobile tel

Plan prepared by

Dr/nurse

Signed

Date

Guy's and St Thomas' **NHS**
NHS Foundation Trust

Child action plan **3** for
allergic reactions

Mild to moderate allergic reaction
- swelling of lips, face, eyes
- hives or welts
- abdominal pain, vomiting

Action	Name, dose of antihistamine

• stay with child and call for help
• give antihistamine –
  if vomited, repeat dose
• give 6 puffs of salbutamol or
  terbutaline using a spacer
• contact parent/carer
	Chlorpheniramine (Piriton)®
	
	or

Watch for signs of anaphylaxis

Anaphylaxis (severe allergic reaction)
- difficulty/noisy breathing
- swelling of tongue
- swelling/tightness in throat
- difficulty talking and/or hoarse voice
- wheeze or persistent cough
- loss of consciousness and/or collapse
- pale and floppy (young children)

Action
- give the adrenaline auto-injector (EpiPen®, EpiPen®Jr or Anapen®) immediately
- lay child flat and raise legs (if breathing is difficult, allow to sit but do not stand)
- dial 999 for an ambulance
- say "this is an emergency case of **anaphylaxis**" (ana-fi-lax-is)
- contact parent/carer
- if child has not improved in 5 to 10 minutes, give second adrenaline auto-injector and 10 puffs of salbutamol or terbutaline
- give soluble prednisolone:

**How to give EpiPen®
or EpiPen® Jr.**

Fig. 1
► Grasp EpiPen® in dominant hand, with thumb closest to grey safety cap
► With other hand, pull off grey safety cap (Fig. 1)

Fig. 2
► Jab firmly into outer thigh, through clothing if necessary (Fig. 2)

Fig. 3
► Hold in place for 10 seconds (Fig. 3)
► Massage injection area for 10 seconds

© ALK. REPRODUCED WITH PERMISSION.

Please tell appropriate family, friends, carers or teachers about this action plan. It should be reviewed at each visit to the allergy clinic.

© DEC 2009. GUY'S AND ST THOMAS' NHS FOUNDATION TRUST. ALLERGY / PPG 2553. FOR REVIEW: DEC 2011

Figure 2.2 Child action plan. Reproduced with permission from Guy's and St Thomas' NHS Foundation Trust.

addition, the child and family should be given strategies to manage an allergic reaction. In the case of potentially severe allergies such as food allergy, this should include a written treatment plan, prescription of emergency and rescue medication and training in how to use an adrenaline auto-injector device, if appropriate. This shall be discussed in detail below. Regular medical review and assessment is important, particularly during childhood, as the course of allergic conditions may change as the child grows.

Management of anaphylaxis

Anaphylaxis is an increasing problem in the UK, with food allergy being the most common cause in UK children. While

Table 2.1 A comparison of SPT and SpIgE testing

Test	Advantages	Disadvantages
Skin prick testing	• Convenient • Quick • Visual • Cheap • High sensitivity	• Must stop taking antihistamines at least prior to testing • Close monitoring, oxygen, suction and rescue medication required • May elicit false negative and positive results • Requires trained person
Specific IgE	• Patient does not have to stop taking antihistamines • No risk of systemic reaction	• Long wait for results • Expensive • Blood test can be distressing

allergen avoidance is the cornerstone of management, it is vital that when accidental reactions occur they are quickly recognised and managed appropriately. If there are features of anaphylaxis, first line management is with intramuscular adrenaline; a safe drug that is rapidly effective in most cases, although a second dose may be required. Early administration of adrenaline is associated with better outcomes and where there is uncertainty regarding the severity of a reaction, it is best to err on the side of caution and administer the adrenaline. In milder reactions, a quick acting antihistamine is sufficient. Children at risk of allergic reactions should have an individualised treatment plan in place at school (see Figure 2.2). An accidental reaction should be used as an opportunity to consider how to reduce the chance of a repeat occurrence and ensure that the child has appropriate ongoing medical care in place.

Anaphylaxis is a serious systemic allergic reaction, rapid in onset, which may lead to death and differs from other allergic reactions due to its severity and the involvement of respiratory and/or cardiovascular symptoms. While hypotension and shock are more commonly seen as part of anaphylaxis in adults, it is respiratory features that are most commonly implicated in severe reactions in childhood (Muraro *et al* 2007). The Resuscitation Council (2008) provide an algorithm for the management of anaphylaxis (see Figure 2.3).

The most common cause of allergic reactions in children is food. Common allergens include milk and egg (which are often outgrown), as well as peanuts, tree nuts, fish and shellfish (which are seldom outgrown). It is peanuts and tree nuts that most commonly cause severe reactions. Other, less common causes of anaphylaxis include insect stings, latex and medications such as penicillin (see Table 2.2).

The fundamental principle of managing allergy is to avoid the allergen. Unfortunately, in severe food allergies, even small exposures (particularly by mouth) may cause severe reactions. However, most reactions to food are mild, self limiting and respond well to antihistamines such as chlorphenamine. Severe reactions are more common in children who have had a history of severe reactions or who also have asthma. This is because children, who have poorly controlled asthma, may already have airways that are inflamed and narrowed. If an allergic reaction were to occur, any additional airway narrowing due to the systemic release of allergic inflammatory mediators, would cause respiratory distress and anaphylaxis.

Severity of a reaction cannot be predicted and may depend on factors such as the amount and state of the allergen ingested

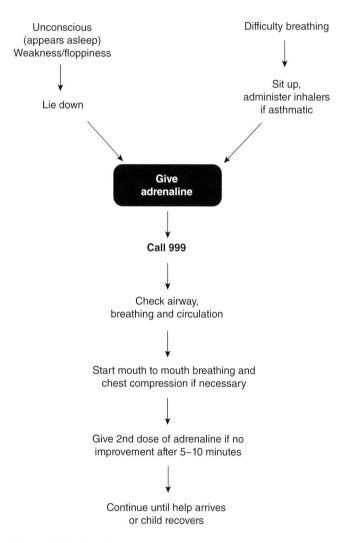

Figure 2.3 Anaphylaxis algorithm (Resuscitation Council 2008).

(e.g. cooked/uncooked), alcohol consumption, exercise and intercurrent illness. Therefore, the European Academy of Allergy and Clinical Immunology (EAACI) taskforce for anaphylaxis in children have identified criteria that assist clinicians in categorising children who may be at higher risk of anaphylaxis and who should be prescribed an adrenaline auto-injector device (AAD).

Table 2.2 Children at increased risk of anaphylaxis (Muraro *et al* 2007)

Absolute risk of anaphylaxis, i.e. should be prescribed an adrenaline auto-injector device	Relative risk of anaphylaxis
Co-existent asthma	Reacted to trace quantities of allergen, i.e. vapour or topical contact
Previous anaphylaxis to food, drug or insect sting	Peanut or tree nut allergy
Food dependent exercised induced anaphylaxis (FDEIA)	Teenager with a food allergy
Idiopathic anaphylaxis	Living in a remote area, far from medical services

Table 2.3 Doses of adrenaline auto-injector devices

Weight of child	Dose of adrenaline auto device
10–30 kg	Epipen junior 0.15 mg Anapen 0.15 mg JEXT 0.15 mg
>30 kg	Epipen 0.3 mg Anapen 0.3 mg JEXT 0.3 mg
>60 kg	Anapen 0.5 mg (this was new to the market in Autumn 2009 and is more likely to be prescribed for adults)

Adrenaline

Adrenaline, the optimal drug for treating an allergic reaction, increases vasoconstriction, reduces oedema, causes bronchodilation and inhibits the release of inflammatory mediators, such as histamine and tryptase. In the event of a severe allergic reaction, the priority is to administer intramuscular adrenaline. Adrenaline is a safe drug which is rapidly effective, although a further dose may be required if there is no improvement in the symptoms and an ambulance has not arrived within 5 minutes of administration. Of individuals who have required a dose of adrenaline, 20% have required a further dose (Muraro *et al* 2007).

Adrenaline auto-injector devices (Epipen, JEXT and Anapen) are syringes and needles pre loaded with adrenaline. Anyone who carries an AAD should have two with them at all times as they are single use only. For children it is advisable they should be prescribed four, two to keep at home and two at school. Families should be encouraged to check and make a note of the expiry date of the AAD, as most last for approximately 12–18 months and should be renewed before they expire. Table 2.3 provides the dose of an adrenaline auto device for a child's weight.

An individual with a diagnosed food allergy should have a formal emergency treatment plan in place, with which all carers should be familiar. The emergency plan is unique to each child, identifies what the individual is allergic to, and clearly outlines how to treat an allergic reaction should one occur. Families are strongly advised to keep this emergency management plan with the emergency medications (antihistamines, adrenaline auto-injector, and inhalers if a child is asthmatic), which should be available to the child at all times.

Training regarding how and when to administer an adrenaline auto-injector device should be provided at diagnosis, and should be re-iterated at subsequent meetings with relevant healthcare professionals. Early use of adrenaline during an anaphylactic reaction results in rapid recovery and a better outcome (Muraro *et al* 2007). Carers are encouraged to use the auto-injector as soon as signs of anaphylaxis have been identified and before calling an ambulance. Features of an anaphylaxis manifest as increased work of breathing, wheeze, stridor, persistent cough, hoarse voice, the child may become pale, floppy or unresponsive. Some young people and adults have described a 'feeling of impending doom'. Good advice for carers is that if they are unsure whether the reaction warrants use of an AAD it is best to err on the side of caution and administer adrenaline immediately.

Following this, many children's emergency plans will advise to call for help and to give an antihistamine, if the child is able to swallow, to reduce symptoms of a pruritic urticarial rash. The child's Salbutamol inhaler can be given via a spacer device, following administration of adrenaline, to act locally to reduce the symptoms of respiratory distress. Following an anaphylaxis and administration of the AAD, the person should be placed in a lying position and exercise should be avoided. If an ambulance has not arrived within 5 minutes of administration of adrenaline and the child is still exhibiting signs of an anaphylaxis a second AAD should be administered (Muraro *et al* 2007).

In order to minimise the risk of accidental exposure of the food the child is allergic to, communication with schools and nurseries is vital. All carers involved in the care of the child with a food allergy should be aware of allergens they need to avoid, as well as their treatment plan. Emergency medication should be readily available, and all staff should be able to identify the child and be confident in identifying and managing an allergic reaction. School nurses or community nurses who have been trained to provide teaching and support to nurseries/schools regarding management of allergies in schools and administration of AADs, should provide regular updates (Muraro *et al* 2010).

Allergen avoidance is the cornerstone of management of an allergy. However, it is paramount that when allergic reactions do occur they are recognised and managed promptly. Early administration of adrenaline is associated with better outcomes. Knowledge should be passed to carers so that in the event of anaphylaxis, they are well equipped and confident to deal with the emergency.

Food allergy

As mentioned above, common food allergens among the paediatric population include milk and egg (which are often outgrown) as well as peanuts, tree nuts, fish and shellfish (which are seldom outgrown). Around 6–8% of children in the UK suffer from a food allergy and there has been a particular increase in peanut and tree nut allergies, with almost 1 in 50 children affected. Most British classrooms now contain at least one child with a food allergy. This has implications for families, carers, schools and primary care.

Allergic reactions to food may present in a variety of ways, due to different underlying mechanisms. Food allergy falls under the umbrella of food hypersensitivity, and includes both IgE and non IgE mediated food allergy. IgE mediated allergic reactions to food often occur on the second or subsequent exposure to the allergen. Sensitisation (and subsequent allergy) may occur without ingestion of the allergen. It is now thought that cutaneous exposure to peanut for example may lead to sensitisation in atopic infants with eczema. In the past, delayed allergies were referred to as intolerances (e.g cow's milk intolerance), which imply a non-immune mediated process. However, our improved understanding means that while exact details of the underlying mechanisms are unclear, they do have an immunological basis involving T cells (Fox and Thompson 2007).

Most food allergies are diagnosed in the first few years of life, when new foods are introduced into the child's diet. Cow's milk is the most common food allergy in childhood, followed closely by hen's egg, soya, peanuts, tree nuts, fin fish, shell fish, sesame and wheat, although these vary across the world. For most children who are cow's milk, hen's egg, wheat or soya allergic, these are often outgrown by school age, whereas other allergies are less frequently outgrown.

Diagnosis

Any child who is believed to have a food allergy would benefit from being seen at a specialist children's allergy clinic, where medical history, examination and allergy testing can be performed. History is the cornerstone of accurate diagnosis of a food allergy and will guide the clinician as to which allergens should be tested for.

Timing of the allergic reaction is important in establishing if this was an IgE or non IgE mediated allergic reaction, or indeed an allergic reaction at all. How long after the food was consumed did the child react? An IgE mediated reaction typically occurs within 30 minutes of ingesting the food but can occur up to 2 hours after ingestion. This close relationship between ingestion and reaction aids the diagnosis of IgE mediated allergies. Reproducibility of symptoms is also key to uncovering an allergic response; it is unlikely that a child would suddenly become allergic to a food if they have eaten it without adverse effect on numerous previous occasions (NICE 2011).

Some children can tolerate small amounts of the allergen, i.e. egg as a baked ingredient in cakes, but refuse plain egg. For some food allergens (e.g. egg) the state of the allergen (cooked or raw) can affect the protein structure. In the case of egg, when it is heated up the protein is broken down and it becomes less allergenic, therefore it is common that children may tolerate small amounts of the allergen in a highly processed form but may not tolerate it in a more raw form. Young children may not be able to vocalise that they are having an allergic reaction and may feel a strange sensation in their mouths complaining their mouth feels 'itchy, spicy or tickly'. These children may be deemed a 'fussy eater', therefore it should be ascertained, whether the child can eat a whole portion of the suspected food, as refusal may be a sign of an allergic response, the local release of histamine in the mouth, causing a strange sensation.

Sometimes, food allergies can be more subtle, causing delayed symptoms often related to ongoing exposure to the food due to

Table 2.4 Presentation of IgE and non-IgE mediated allergic responses to food

IgE mediated allergic reactions	Non IgE mediated allergic reactions
Skin	Skin
• Urticaria	• Eczema
• Oedema	Gastrointestinal
• Itching	• Gastro-oesophageal reflux
Gastrointestinal	• Food protein induced enterocolitis syndrome
• Vomiting	• Enteropathy
• Diarrhoea	• Proctocolitis
Respiratory	• Failure to thrive
• Wheezing	• Constipation
• Anaphylaxis	
Circulatory	
• Anaphylaxis	
• Decreased blood pressure	

its inclusion in the diet (see Table 2.4). Delayed reactions are not so obvious and a child may continue to eat or be offered a particular food and suffer from persistent symptoms such as eczema, reflux or they may start to refuse to eat. These delayed, or non-IgE mediated allergies tend to be more of a problem in infancy and are most commonly due to milk although soya, wheat and egg are also common culprits.

Family and past medical history also help when establishing the child's allergic status. Babies who suffer from eczema are at risk of having food allergies. The more severe the eczema and the earlier in life that it begins, the more likely there is to be a food allergy. A baby with severe eczema before 3 months of age is very likely to suffer from food allergies.

Testing

SPT and SpIgE are the only validated confirmatory tests used in the diagnosis of IgE mediated food allergy. Measurement of the size of the SPT wheal or level of SpIgE in the blood helps to ascertain the likelihood of a child being allergic to a suspect food. It is a common misconception among parents/carers that the larger the size of the wheal or higher the level of SpIgE, the more severe an allergic reaction will be. This is not the case; there are no tests which can give an indication of severity of an allergic reaction. For some common food allergens, validated studies have demonstrated that a wheal above a certain size or SpIgE above a certain level has a 95% predictive value that the child is clinically allergic, although results vary between populations (Table 2.5). The size of the SPT wheal or level of SpIgE may vary over time and may indicate when a child has outgrown their allergy. Therefore, children are reviewed and retested regularly to see if they have developed tolerance. This is helpful when deciding which children should have an oral food challenge (OFC) to explore the possibility they may be able to tolerate the allergen (Eigenmann and Sampson 1998, Roberts and Lack 2000, Sampson 1999, Sporik et al 2000).

Results of SPT and SpIgE tests must be treated with caution; an incorrect diagnosis may prove fatal if the child was still

Table 2.5 95% specificity in predicting the outcome of food challenges

Allergen	Size of wheal in children >2 years	Size of wheal in children <2 years	Level of SpIgE in children >2 years	Level of SpIgE in children <2 years
Cow's milk	8 mm	6 mm	15 kU/l	5 kU/l
Hen's egg	7 mm	5 mm	7 kU/l	2 kU/l
Peanut	8 mm	4 mm	14 kU/l	14 kU/l

Table 2.6 Examples of food challenge doses

Dose	Cow's milk	Hen's egg
Lip	Lip	Lip
1	5 ml	0.5 g
2	10 ml	4 g
3	30 ml	10 g
4	200 ml	30 g

allergic to a food and they were to consume the allergen based on a false negative result. This highlights the importance of accurate history taking. If a child had a good history of reacting to a food but had a negative SPT or specific IgE result, they fall into a 'grey area' and the only safe way to know if that food can be eaten is to perform an oral food challenge (OFC) in a supervised, safe clinical environment.

Oral food challenge

The OFC is an inpatient procedure that involves feeding the child the suspected allergen in increasing portions until the child has consumed 8–10g of dried weight of protein of the allergen or an appropriate portion size of the allergen. The OFC must be performed on a children's ward, so the child can be observed for any sign of an allergic reaction, all rescue medications should be to hand and the OFC is supervised by a specialised nurse, trained in recognition and treatment of signs of an allergic reaction.

The OFC is the gold standard test as it can objectively demonstrate tolerance or allergy. The OFC begins with the allergen being rubbed on the child's lip and then increasing amounts of the food is consumed over a period of approximately 2 hours, with 15–30 minutes between each dose. Table 2.6 shows examples of OFC doses. If the child shows any sign of an allergic reaction the OFC should be discontinued immediately and the reaction treated appropriately. The allergen can be disguised in any vehicle that will facilitate the child eating the food. This can be anything from cow's milk mixed with soya milk, which the child may be used to drinking, to cod in jam sandwiches, to disguise the taste. As long as the vehicle is something the child has eaten before, is not allergic to and helps the child eat the challenge allergen, anything goes!

If at any point during the OFC the child exhibits any sign of an allergic reaction, the OFC will be stopped and the child will

be treated for an allergic reaction according to its severity. The child is then observed for a period of at least 2 hours once they have finished consuming the food, regardless of whether they tolerate the top dose or if the OFC is discontinued at an earlier portion because they have reacted (Sicherer 1999).

Preparation

There are a number of factors which need to be considered when performing an OFC. Preparation is essential to ensure the OFC is performed safely and runs smoothly. The family should be fully informed of the procedure before the appointment, this includes providing them with written information and discussing the procedure with the family either at their outpatient appointment or on the telephone before the OFC. This will help the family prepare their child for the OFC, which will hopefully ensure the day goes well. The family should also be aware that if the child has a negative OFC and consumes the required amount of allergen, they must incorporate the food into their diet at home at least twice a week.

To ensure the safety of the OFC there are a number of measures that need to be taken. The child should be well on the day of the OFC and should have stopped taking antihistamines as they can mask the early signs of an allergic reaction. Long-acting antihistamines, such as cetirizine and loratidine, should be stopped five days before the OFC, short-acting, such as chlorphenamine, should be stopped 48 hours before the OFC. The child should not have had a viral illness, exacerbation of asthma, eczema or allergic rhinitis in the week preceding the OFC. If the child is unwell in any way they could have a much more severe allergic reaction if they were to react to the allergen. If there are any exacerbations of atopic disease it is difficult to know if the child is reacting during the OFC; for example, if their eczema is very troublesome and they are itchy it is often difficult to gauge during the OFC if the child is having a reaction or if this amount of itch is normal for them. Similarly, it is often best to challenge someone with allergic rhinitis out of the pollen season, as it may be difficult for them to come off of their antihistamines, or if they develop rhinorrhea during the course of the OFC, it may be difficult to ascertain if this is a response to the challenge allergen.

Troubleshooting

The child or family may be very anxious as the child is being exposed to something they are possibly allergic to and have previously been warned could prove life-threatening if accidentally consumed. The role of the nurse is to explain to the family why the OFC is being performed and build up their confidence. For some families, just coming into hospital is progress. The child may be anxious due to previous experience, so having the opportunity to speak to the specialist nurse or dietician is a positive experience, which helps them to build their confidence to either continue with the OFC, or develop strategies to manage their allergy with confidence at home.

Some children may get mid-way through the OFC and decide they no longer want to eat the food. This is a difficult situation, because, if the child has not consumed enough of the allergen, the findings will not be reliable. To give the child a diagnosis of allergy at this point could mean that the child will continue to avoid a food to which they are not allergic. This has a huge impact on the family's quality of life and may have implications on the child's nutritional requirements. Alternatively, if the child was allergic to the food and they were told they could consume it, this could have disastrous consequences as they could have an allergic reaction. This is where bringing in food the child commonly eats, i.e. soya milk or a favourite sandwich filling helps to disguise the challenge allergen. The skills of a play specialist, or rewards such as stickers may help to encourage the child to continue eating.

Often the child may report subjective symptoms of an allergic reaction such as itchy throat or abdominal pain, or a younger child may become very quiet and withdrawn. These must be taken seriously as they may herald a more severe allergic reaction. However, many children are very anxious about consuming the challenge food and these symptoms may be due to fear rather than a genuine reaction. This is a difficult situation to manage; it would be unwise to stop the challenge without a definitive diagnosis, yet you do not want to elicit an anaphylaxis. There are a number of approaches which may be utilised in this situation; in the first instance, preparing the child and gaining their trust, by explaining the procedure so they feel reassured, should help avoid this scenario. Distraction is very useful (e.g. engaging the child in an activity such as a computer game) to see if the symptoms disappear. If the symptoms persist and the child cannot be distracted, a discussion with the family should then ensue, to make a decision as whether or not to stop the OFC. If it is felt this is not an allergic response, the OFC should proceed with caution; it may be wise to repeat the previous dose and see if the symptoms persist. If the symptoms do persist or get worse, the OFC should be stopped and the child confirmed allergic. If they do not, hopefully the OFC will continue and the allergen can be safely reintroduced into the child's diet.

Following a negative OFC, where the child tolerated the food, the allergen can be reintroduced into the child's diet. If the OFC was positive and the child reacted, the family should be advised to strictly avoid that allergen, at this point a dietician is essential either to guide reintroduction or to give assistance with avoidance strategies.

Unfortunately there are no reliable tests available for delayed non IgE mediated food allergies. A food exclusion diet under the guidance of a paediatric dietician and subsequent reintroduction of the suspected allergen is the recommended method to confirm a delayed allergy. The symptoms should disappear when the food is removed from the diet and return when the food is reintroduced.

Respiratory allergy

Increase in atopy is not limited to food allergy. It is estimated that 80% of asthma in children is driven by aeroallergens and there is an increase in children presenting at a younger age with symptoms of allergic rhinitis. This disease now affects between 10 and 40% of children across the world. The link between asthma and allergic rhinitis is now much better understood. The nasal cavity is the beginning of the respiratory tract and the epithelium has similarities to that of the lower airway. The nose acts as a gatekeeper, warming, humidifying and filtering air before it passes through into the lungs. If the nasal passage becomes blocked the nose cannot do its job, the child will begin to breathe through their mouth. Cold, dry air will pass into the respiratory tract and can cause bronchospasm. In addition, the air is not filtered, which allows small airborne particles to enter the lower airways, introducing infection and causing inflammation, which can lead to coughing, constriction of the airways and symptoms of asthma.

The inextricable link between asthma and allergic rhinitis is well established. In the 1990s an international group of clinicians got together to look at allergic rhinitis and its impact on asthma (ARIA). The group have produced guidelines and regular updates on the management of patients with allergic rhinitis and asthma. Upper airway symptoms of allergic rhinitis include rhinorrhea, sneezing, blocked nose, nose bleeds, headaches and ocular symptoms; red, watery, itchy eyes, which often become swollen and painful (Brozek *et al* 2010).

Diagnosis

Clinical history is again the cornerstone of diagnosis of a respiratory allergy and this should include symptoms, whether these are persistent, time of year of onset and how troublesome these symptoms are. This is important as different aeroallergens are prevalent in the atmosphere at different times of year. For example, children who notice exacerbation of asthma in the autumn months may well be sensitised to moulds such as cladosporium, alternaria and aspergillus, which are commonly found on decaying leaves, fruit and vegetables. Children who have symptoms of allergic rhinoconjunctivitis such as runny nose, runny eyes, itchy nose and sneezing during spring (February to April) are more likely to be sensitised to tree pollen as this is in abundance in the atmosphere at these times. Children who have these symptoms later on in the year (May, June and July) are likely to be grass pollen allergic as this is the height of the grass pollen season. Other children may have symptoms of allergic rhinitis all year round and these are caused by indoor aeroallergens such as house dust mite, cats and dogs.

To fully assess the impact of the disease on an individual, severity must also be considered. The impact on respiratory allergy is often underestimated but for children who suffer with allergic rhinitis their quality of life is significantly affected. Those who are affected in the height of the pollen season report a huge impact on outdoor activities. They are unable to join in with their friends when playing sports, or enjoy trips to the park. Children with allergic rhinitis are woken at night frequently due to a runny nose or blocked nose, which causes them to be very tired during the day. In addition, children with allergic rhinitis may take daily sedating antihistamines to combat the symptoms. These sedating antihistamines have an effect on their school lives and they frequently underperform at school. Public exams are taken at the height of the grass pollen season when children with allergic rhinitis are most affected. It has been seen that children with allergic rhinitis are more likely perform better in their mock exams which are held in the winter months, than exams which are held in the summer time, when compared with children without hayfever (Walker *et al* 2007).

There are a number of presenting features of the child with allergic rhinitis; they may have dark circles under their eyes, due

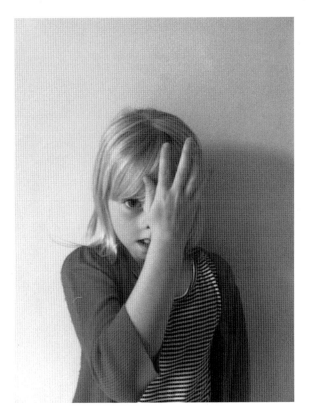

Figure 2.4 The 'allergic salute' in a child with allergic rhinitis.

to vasodilation and inflammation in the blood vessels around the sinuses, which impinges on blood drainage. The child often has a nasal crease which results from rubbing their nose frequently. This is often called the 'allergic salute' and a child may do this continuously during the consultation (Figure 2.4). They frequently mouth breathe because their nose is blocked and they are unable to breath adequately through their nose. This causes dry lips and some children, may persistently lip lick and develop a perioral rash.

The nasal mucosa of children with allergic rhinitis often appear very red and inflamed, with visible inferior nasal turbinates and a clear, watery nasal discharge. This clinical picture and history is, therefore, suggestive of allergic rhinitis. The onset of symptoms and time of year when the child is affected can indicate to which aeroallergens they are likely to be sensitised. Skin prick testing to a panel of aeroallergens, as previously described, would confirm the suspected allergens driving the child's allergic rhinitis.

Management

Avoidance is usually the cornerstone of management of allergy, but is harder to achieve in children who are sensitised to aeroallergens, as they are found in abundance in the environment. Parents/carers may wish to try bed covers, mattress encasings and removing soft toys from the child's bed, to reduce the exposure to house dust mite. However, these are costly and no proven benefit has been shown to avoidance of aeroallergens. The main-

stay of management of children with allergic rhinitis is pharmacotherapy. The first line treatment is an intranasal corticosteroid, which reduces the inflammation in the nasal mucosa. Correct administration technique is essential to ensure the nasal spray is effective (Figure 2.5). The child should sit or stand with their head bent forward and the hand that is administering the nasal spray should be on the opposite side to the nostril into which the nasal spray is administered. The child must not sniff following administration, as this would cause the medication to be swallowed, rather than remaining in the area of inflammation (Scadding *et al* 2008).

Pre-emptive administration of the intranasal corticosteroid should commence pre seasonally to ensure that there is minimal inflammation of the nasal mucosa before being exposed to the allergen. In addition, if the child continues to have symptoms of allergic rhinitis, a once daily, non-sedating antihistamine should be administered regularly. A sedating antihistamine will only add to drowsiness and contribute to poor performance at school. In addition to the nasal spray and antihistamines, eye drops are useful for those who suffer with troublesome ocular symptoms. A recent advance in the treatment of allergic rhinitis is the addition of a leukotriene receptor antagonist (montelukast), which was previously an add-on therapy for asthma, but the benefits of this drug for allergic rhinitis have been demonstrated (Brozek *et al* 2010).

Despite maximal pharmacotherapy, some children still have severe symptoms of allergic rhinitis and for these children specific immunotherapy may be considered. This is the administration of the allergen in small but increasing doses until maintenance dose has been reached. This can either be given sublingually or subcutaneously. Immunotherapy has been in existence for over a 100 years, however, it went out of vogue in the UK during the 1980s and 1990s, due to a number of fatalities. It is much more widely used now, although only in specialised clinics where the clinicians have the knowledge and expertise to safely administer this treatment to a highly selected population. There is some suggestion that by treating the cause of allergic rhinitis with immunotherapy this may halt the progression to asthma in children and there are studies underway to assess the plausibility of this (Penagos *et al* 2006).

It is important to be aware of the association between allergic rhinitis and asthma, as evidence of a blocked and inflamed nasal mucosa may be suggestive of lower airway inflammation. Children may be asymptomatic most of the year but develop symptoms during the pollen season. Therefore questioning and treatment should also include symptoms of asthma, such as nocturnal cough, wheeze and difficulty in breathing or coughing following exertion (exercise, playing, laughing). Any reports of such symptoms must be investigated. Spirometery, is a reliable method of assessing lung function in children who are symptomatic. It entails the child blowing into a machine to measure the amount of air that can be expelled from the lungs in one second. A baseline reading is measured following which salbutamol is administered to the child and 15–20 minutes later, a second test is performed if the difference is more than 15% and there is a clinical history suggestive of lower airway inflammation. The child should be followed up to monitor their progress and managed in accordance with the British Thoracic Society (2011) guidelines, which are reviewed regularly and

(a)

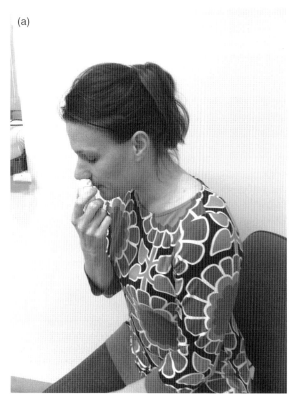

(b)

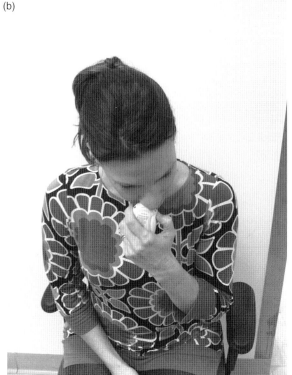

Figure 2.5 Correct administration of an intranasal corticosteroid.

encourage a stepwise approach to the management of children with asthma.

Allergens in the healthcare setting

This section will focus on an area of allergy that causes much concern for healthcare professionals and can have far reaching consequences for children who may be allergic to certain medication or latex.

Drug allergy

There are only a small number of studies that have looked at the prevalence of drug allergy in children and these have shown that approximately 2% of hospital admissions are due to an adverse reaction to a drug. With regards to hospitalised children, approximately 9.5% have had a drug reaction that has prolonged their visit during their inpatient stay and in the outpatient setting, approximately 1.5% of children prescribed drugs have had adverse reaction to them, 12.3% of which were classified as a severe reaction (Impicciatore *et al* 2001, cited by Mirakian *et al* 2009).

While adverse reactions to drugs are a real concern, a large number of parents/carers believe their children have a drug allergy. Incorrect diagnosis of a drug allergy has far-reaching implications; if the child is indeed allergic to a particular drug, subsequent exposure could cause an allergic reaction, potentially severe in nature and could even cause death. Therefore, if the

child is allergic to a particular drug, they should be aware of the importance of informing all healthcare professionals of this at every encounter. However, if the child is not allergic to the suspected drug and has not had any confirmatory testing they may well avoid a particular drug unnecessarily and as a result, be treated with more expensive, less effective medication. Penicillin is commonly used to treat childhood infections and many parents/carers believe their children to be allergic to it. This is either based on a family history of drug allergy, or a rash that occurred at time of administration. Frequently a rash that develops at this time may be part of the infection process, rather than a response to the medication.

Presentation

The drugs most commonly implicated in allergic reactions are beta-lactams such as penicillin and cephalosporin. Non-steroidal anti-inflammatory drugs (NSAIDs), insulin, anticonvulsants and drugs used in anaesthesia, most commonly neuromuscular blocking agents (NMBAs) such as rocuronium and suxamethonium are also common allergens. The Gell and Coombes classification of allergic response describes four types of responses to allergic reactions to drugs (Mirakian *et al* 2009). Most commonly it is Type 1, IgE mediated allergic reactions that occur, usually caused by penicillin. The Type 4, non IgE mediated delayed hypersensitivity reactions are usually T-cell mediated and are commonly driven by antibiotics, anticonvulsants and non-steroidal anti-inflammatory drugs (Mirakian *et al* 2009).

Diagnosis

If the child is an inpatient at the time of a suspected adverse reaction the suspected drug should be stopped immediately and the child treated appropriately. Antihistamines should be administered to reduce urticaria and puritus if the child exhibits symptoms of a mild allergic reaction. If the child has had anaphylaxis, adrenaline should be administered as early as possible and local resuscitation guidelines for management of an anaphylaxis should be followed. Following this, the child should be referred to a specialist allergy service, where clinicians are experienced in the investigation of a suspected drug allergy in children.

History is essential to establish accurate diagnosis and this should include timing of administration of a drug and subsequent allergic reaction. If the child was an inpatient, their drug chart and notes are essential to help build up a clinical picture. Included in the history should be any history of the child previously taking the drug and either reacting to it or tolerating it. If the suspected drugs were administered during anaesthesia it is essential that the anaesthetic records are forwarded to the allergy clinic and used as part of the diagnostic procedure. Parents/carers often have taken photos of rashes that have developed after taking a drug, and these maybe helpful to establish the type of reaction. A history of all drugs taken at the time of the reaction is essential, including 'over the counter medication' and homeopathic remedies that may have been administered by carers (Ewan et al 2009).

There are a number of risk factors that may predispose a child to be at increased risk of an allergic reaction to medication, including recurrent administration of the drug either orally or topically. Children with chronic conditions such as cystic fibrosis may be at increased risk, due to prolonged use of antibiotics. Atopy is not a risk factor, but children who are atopic may have a more severe reaction if they do react to a drug.

Testing

If a child is hospitalised at the time of an allergic reaction, blood should be taken immediately after the reaction to measure tryptase levels. Tryptase is released by mast cells at the time of an allergic reaction and is elevated in the blood up to 2 hours after the allergic reaction begins. It may remain elevated up to 7 hours after a reaction; hence blood should be taken again at 6 hours, then at 24 hours, to record the child's baseline level of tryptase, which will help in diagnosing an allergic reaction to a drug.

Skin prick testing and intradermal testing can be helpful in the diagnosis of drug allergy, although studies have concentrated on their use in penicillin allergy and suspected allergy to drugs used in general anaesthesia. Neat concentrations of the drugs can cause an irritation reaction and therefore the drugs are diluted and skin testing is performed as described earlier in the chapter. Intradermal testing can also be performed, which involves injecting a small amount of the drug (0.03 ml of the solution) into the top layer of the skin to raise a bleb of approximately 3 mm in diameter. After 15–20 minutes it can be measured to see if the size of the bleb has increased. If the bleb increases by 3 mm it may be considered a positive reaction. Skin testing and intradermal testing should be carried out by clinicians who are experienced in this procedure, as expertise is needed to interpret the results and differentiate a true positive result from an irritant reaction. A negative skin test should not automatically indicate tolerance to the drug, especially if the history is suggestive of an allergic reaction. The child may need an oral drug challenge, if appropriate, to confirm diagnosis or tolerance to the suspected drug. In the case of many drugs, such as NMBAs, other drugs used during general anaesthesia, insulins and drugs which are not available as oral preparations, a challenge is not appropriate and the only definitive way to test for allergy or tolerance is intradermal testing, which is why it is essential this is carried out by clinicians who are experts in this area (Ewan et al 2009, Mirakian et al 2009).

An oral drug challenge should be performed in an inpatient setting equipped to manage a severe allergic reaction. The suspected drug is administered to the child in increasing doses, starting with a 100th of the dose and increasing in four steps until a cumulative therapeutic dose has been administered. The doses are given in 30 minute intervals and the child observed between doses. As with OFC, the child will be kept for 2 hours following the final administration of the dose. If the child reacts at any point the challenge will be stopped immediately and the reaction treated appropriately. If the child does not exhibit signs of an adverse reaction to the suspected drug, they will be discharged home on a course of that particular drug for three to five days. The duration of the course will depend on the history of onset of the suspected allergic reaction.

Management of drug allergy

If drug allergy has been diagnosed, management is strict avoidance of the allergen. The child and family should alert all healthcare professionals of their allergic status. If the child is admitted to hospital, a red allergy name band should be worn and the allergy documented in the child's notes and on their prescription chart. The child should be encouraged to wear an item that identifies they have an allergy, such as a 'Medic Alert' bracelet, which carries an internationally known symbol identifying the child and the drug to which the child is allergic. A suitable alternative drug should be found so that they have a safe treatment option in the future. If there are no suitable alternatives and the child needs a particular drug that they are allergic to, desensitisation can be carried out so that the child can use that drug. This is not a common procedure and should only be carried out under the guidance of an allergist, in a setting where full resuscitation facilities are available.

Vaccination

Many parents/carers who have a child with a food allergy have concerns regarding immunisation of their child. This has come to the forefront in recent years with the drive to immunise all high-risk groups of children, including those with asthma, with the Swine Flu and seasonal flu vaccine and there has always been a query over the MMR for children with an egg allergy. A common misconception is that the MMR vaccines and some others contain egg and may cause an allergic reaction in those children allergic to egg, and alongside unfounded concerns relating to autism was partly to blame for the dip in the immunisation rate for MMR in the UK in the late 1990s to less than 80%.

The British Society of Allergy and Clinical Immunology have recently examined the suitability of MMR immunisation in egg allergic children. It was concluded that any hen's egg protein content is negligible, and it is safe for use in those children who are allergic to hen's egg in the Primary Care setting. The only caution would be for those children who have had anaphylaxis to a vaccine previously and they should be referred to a specialist allergy service. Vaccination should be postponed in children who are unwell or who have poorly controlled asthma on the day scheduled for administration (Baxter 2003, BSACI–PAG 2007, Demicheli *et al* 2005, Fox and Lack 2003, World Health Organization 2004).

Anyone, irrespective of whether they have an egg allergy or not may be at risk of an allergic reaction to any vaccine, caused by one of the excipients, such as gelatine or neomycin contained in the vaccine. However, the concern of parents/carers who have a child with an egg allergy is not unfounded as some vaccines are grown on egg (Table 2.7). These children may be at higher risk of an allergic reaction when egg-containing vaccine is administered and should have the vaccine administered as a day case in hospital, where emergency medication and equipment is available.

Severe allergic reactions or anaphylaxis to vaccines are extremely rare; however, there are many common vaccine related adverse events or side effects. WHO acknowledges this and classifies adverse events following immunisations (AEFIs) according to four main categories, which are outlined below, examples given are not exhaustive and the Department of Health's *Green Book* provides further explanation of AEFIs (Department of Health 2011):

1. Programme-related – this relates to incorrect practice of administering vaccines, such as, not allowing enough time between vaccinations, incorrect reconstitution or administration of the vaccine.
2. Vaccine induced – these are events which are directly related to the administration of the vaccine, for example, redness and swelling at the site of administration, a fever or rash following DTaP/HiB/IPV or MMR. These reactions are common and self-limiting; however, there have been reports of anaphylaxis following administration of vaccines and anyone administering a vaccine should remain vigilant.
3. Coincidental – many children may develop a cold following administration of a vaccine, such as the influenza vaccine. This cold may have developed irrespective of the vaccination being administered and commonly the influenza vaccine is administered in the winter months when cold viruses are prevalent.
4. Unknown – an adverse event which does not fit into any of the first three criteria.

AEFIs can be managed in a number of ways; in the first instance, preparation and managing parental/carers' expectations is essential. Vaccinations should be administered in settings equipped to provide resuscitation, by healthcare professionals who are trained in administering vaccinations and managing emergency situations. The child's past medical history should be established, including previous responses to vaccination and any existing allergies. Carers should be advised that some events are normal following immunisation, such as fever within 48 hours following DTaP/HiB/IPV and a rash or fever one week following the MMR vaccine. Advice regarding management of fever and signs to observe for should be given.

An anaphylaxis commonly occurs within 30 minutes of exposure to the allergen and in the case of vaccines, other than previous anaphylaxis to a vaccine, there are no known predisposing factors, which put children at an increased risk of having an anaphylaxis to a vaccine. Therefore, children should remain in the setting where the vaccine was administered for a period of time after administration; this will vary according to local guidelines. Any child who is suspected of having an anaphylaxis or allergic reaction to a vaccination should be referred to a high-risk vaccine service, within an allergy department, for investigation and subsequent administration of vaccines in an inpatient setting.

Latex allergy

Latex use is now commonplace in industrialised societies, from tyres and dummies, to surgical gloves and sundry medical products. Latex gloves were introduced for medical use more than 100 years ago. Other than three isolated incidents (two in Germany and one in the United States of America in 1927), there were no reports of systemic latex allergy until the late 1980s (Slater 1994). It is now recognised that there is a risk associated with the wearing of latex gloves, particularly those with a powder lining.

Latex allergy is now known to affect an increasing number of the population and many healthcare providers now have a latex free policy. There are some children who have an increased risk of being allergic to latex; those who have had multiple surgical procedures, i.e. children with spina bifida, are at higher risk of

Table 2.7 Vaccines grown on hen's egg

Vaccinations containing egg	Alternatives to egg-containing vaccine
Yellow fever vaccine	No vaccine alternative, patient should check area they are travelling to and if possible they should obtain an exemption certificate. However, they should be aware some countries will not allow travel without vaccination. Yellow fever vaccination can only be performed in a setting with a certificate to administer the vaccine, by staff with the appropriate knowledge and training.
Seasonal influenza vaccine	This vaccine is developed each year according to the strain of influenza, some companies manufacture vaccines with very low egg content and may be suitable for those children who are tolerating egg in a highly processed form, i.e. baked in cakes. The manufacturers should be consulted for information regarding egg content.
Rabies vaccine	Some Rabies vaccines are not grown on egg and are therefore suitable for children with an egg allergy. If there is any uncertainty the child should be referred to a specialised high-risk vaccine service, where the vaccine can be administered.

developing a latex allergy as numerous exposures to latex perioperatively can lead to sensitization (Alenius *et al* 1993). Proteins in certain fruits (i.e. banana and avocado) cross-react with latex and some children who are allergic to these fruits may also be allergic to latex. Latex allergy should be suspected in children who report an allergic reaction to balloons or sports equipment or who have had an allergic reaction in a healthcare setting, such as the dentist, when no other allergens are present. However, children may also have come into contact with latex in the community, e.g. balloons, sports equipment, such as racquet handles. Therefore history should include questioning regarding tolerance of these items. If there is no reliable history of tolerance to latex and the child falls into a high-risk group, SPT or SpIgE testing could be performed. An equivocal result would warrant an inpatient challenge to latex.

Management of children with a latex allergy

As with all allergens, avoidance is the mainstay of management to reduce the risk of allergic reaction. As there is an increased awareness of latex allergy, many trusts now have a 'Latex free' policy, written in conjunction with the procurement department, to ensure products containing latex can not be ordered, or it is brought to the requisitioner's attention that the product contains latex and an alternative is suggested. In addition all children who are allergic to latex need to be identified, for example, they should wear red 'allergy' wristbands, ensuring everyone caring for that child is aware of their allergy. In some instances, such as in theatre, where some products still contain latex, there are a number of measures that can be taken to minimise the child's risk of exposure. Where possible latex products should be removed from the environment, the number of people in theatre at the time of the child's procedure should be kept to a minimum and if possible the child who has a latex allergy should be first on the list for surgery.

Not all dentists have moved to latex free products, therefore parents/carers should be advised to tell all medical professionals if their child has a latex allergy and may like their child to wear a bracelet identifying their allergic status to all, just in case the child is ever in a position where they are unable to speak for themselves.

Any allergic reaction to latex should be treated in the same way as any other allergic reaction and for an anaphylaxis, adrenaline should be administered at the earliest opportunity and help sought immediately. In a hospital setting, this would involve putting out a 'crash call' as per hospital policy; in the community, an ambulance should be called.

Conclusion

The incidence of atopy is increasing across the world and disease manifests in a variety of ways, from food allergy in the young child to asthma, allergic rhinitis in older children, or drug allergy, which can affect children regardless of their atopic status. Unfortunately the rapid increase in atopy is not mirrored by the provision of allergy services in the UK. However, with a better understanding and recognition of allergic presentations and the knowledge of how to treat and manage children with allergic

disease, these children are being referred to the appropriate specialist. In specialist clinics children with an allergic condition can be managed in a safe way and receive the appropriate education and empowerment they need to manage their condition and achieve optimal quality of life.

Key texts

British Thoracic Society and Scottish Intercollegiate Guidelines Network (2011) British Guideline on the Management of Asthma. Available at www.brit-thoracic.org.uk

Høst A, Andrae S, Charkin S, *et al* (2003) Allergy testing in children: why, who, when and how? Allergy, 58(7), 559–569

Mirakian R, Ewan PW, Durham SR, *et al* (2009) BSACI guidelines for the management of drug allergy. Clinical and Experimental Allergy, 39, 43–46

Muraro A, Roberts G, Clark A, *et al* (2007) The management of anaphylaxis in childhood: position paper of EAACI. Allergy, 62, 857–871

Muraro A, Clark A, Beyer K, *et al* (2010) The management of the allergic child at school: EAACI/GA2LEN Task Force on the allergic child at school. Allergy DOI: 10.1111/j.1398-9995.2010.02343.x

Resuscitation Council (UK) (2008) Emergency treatment of anaphylactic reactions. Guidelines for healthcare providers. Available a: www.resus.org.uk/pages/reaction.pdf (last accessed 1st August 2011)

National Institute for Health and Clinical Excellence (2011) Diagnosis and assessment of food allergy in children and young people in primary care and community settings. London, National Institute for Health and Clinical Excellence

Scadding GK, Durham SR, Mirakian R, *et al* (2008) BSACI guidelines for the management of allergic and non-allergic rhinitis. Clinical and Experimental Allergy, 38, 19–42

References

Alenius H, Palosuo T, Kelly K, Kurup V, Reunala T, Makinen-Kiljunen S, Turjanmaa K, Fink J. (1993) IgE reactivity to 14-kD and 27-kD natural rubber proteins in latex-allergic children with spina bifida and other congenital anomalies. International Archives of Allergy and Immunology, 102(1), 61–66

Baxter DN. (2003) Measles immunization in children with a history of egg allergy. Vaccine 14(2), 131–134

British Society of Allergy and Clinical Immunology–Paediatric Allergy Group (BSACI) (2007) Recommendations for Combined Measles, Mumps and Rubella (MMR) Vaccination in Egg-Allergic Children. Available at www.BSACI.org (last accessed 21st October 2011)

British Thoracic Society and Scottish Intercollegiate Guidelines Network (2011) British Guideline on the Management of Asthma. Available at www.brit-thoracic.org.uk (last accessed September 2011)

Brożek JL, Bousquet J, Baena-Cagnani CE, Bonini S, Canonica GW, Casale TB, van Wijk RG, Ohta K, Zuberbier T, Schünemann HJ. (2010) Allergic Rhinitis and its Impact on Asthma (ARIA) Guidelines 2010. Available at http://www.whiar.org/docs/ARIAReport_2010.pdf (last accessed May 2011)

Demicheli V, Jefferson T, Rivetti A, Price D. (2005) Vaccines for measles, mumps and rubella in children. Cochrane Database of Systematic Reviews, 4. CD004407. DOI: 10.1002/14651858.CD004407.pub2.

Department of Health (2011) Department of Health Green Book. Available at http://www.dh.gov.uk/en/Publicationsandstatistics/Publications/PublicationsPolicyAndGuidance/DH_079917 (last accessed September 2011)

Eigenmann PA, Sampson HA. (1998) Interpreting skin prick tests in the evaluation of food allergy in children. Pediatric Allergy and Immunology, 9, 186–191

Ewan, PW, Dugué, P, Mirakian, R, Dixon, TA, Harper, JN, Nasser SM. (2009) BSACI guidelines for the investigation of suspected anaphylaxis during general anaesthesia. Clinical and Experimental Allergy, 40, 15–31

Fox A, Lack G. (2003) Egg allergy and MMR vaccination. British Journal of General Practice, 53, 801–802

Fox AT, Thompson M. (2007) Adverse reactions to cows' milk. Paediatrics and Child Health, 17(7), 288–294

Høst A, Andrae S, Charkin S, Diaz-Vázquez C, Dreborg S, Eigenmann PA, Friedrichs F, Grinsted P, Lack G, Meylan G, Miglioranzi P, Muraro A, Nieto A, Niggemann B, Pascual C, Pouech MG, Rancé F, Rietschel E, Wickman M. (2003) Allergy testing in children: why, who, when and how? Allergy, 58(7), 559–569

Impicciatore P, Choonara I, Clarkson A, Provasi D, Pandolfini C, Bonati M. (2001) Incidence of adverse drug reactions in paediatric in/out-patients: a systematic review and meta-analysis of prospective studies. Br J Clin Pharmacol, 52, 77–83

Johansson SGO, O'B Hourihane J, Bousquet J, Bruijnzeel-Koomen C, Dreborg S, Haahtela T, Kowalski ML, Mygind N, Ring J, van Cauwenberge P, van Hage-Hamsten M, Wüthrich B. (2001) A revised nomenclature for allergy. An EAACI position statement from the EAACI nomenclature task force. Allergy, 56, 813–824

Johansson SGO, Bieber T, Dahl R, Friedmann PS, Lanier B, Lockey R et al (2004) A revised nomenclature for allergy for global use: Report of the Nomenclature Review Committee of World Allergy Organization. J Allergy Clin Immunol, 113, 832–836

Mirakian R, Ewan PW, Durham SR, Youlten LJF, Dugue' P, Friedmann PS, English JS, Huber PAJ, Nasser SM. (2009) BSACI guidelines for the management of drug allergy. Clinical and Experimental Allergy, 39, 43–46

Muraro A, Roberts G, Clark A, Eigenmann P A, Halken S, Lack G, Moneret-Vautrin , Niggemann B, Rance F, EAACI Task Force on Anaphylaxis in Children (2007) The management of anaphylaxis in childhood: position paper of EAACI. Allergy, 62, 857–871

Penagos M, Compalati E, Tarantini F, Baena-Cagnani R, Huerta J, Passalacqua G, Canonica GC. (2006) Efficacy of sublingual immunotherapy in the treatment of allergic rhinitis in pediatric patients 3 to 18 years of age: a meta-analysis of randomized, placebo-controlled, double-blind trials. Annals of Allergy Asthma Immunology, 97, 141–148

National Institute for Health and Clinical Excellence (2011) Diagnosis and assessment of food allergy in children and young people in primary care and community settings. London: National Institute for Health and Clinical Excellence. Available at www.nice.org.uk/guidance/CG116. (last accessed 21st October 2011)

Resuscitation Council (UK) (2008) Emergency treatment of anaphylactic reactions. Guidelines for healthcare providers. Available at www.resus.org.uk/pages/reaction.pdf (last accessed 1st August 2011)

Roberts G, Lack G. (2000) Food allergy-getting more out of your skin prick tests. Clinical and Experimental Allergy, 30, 1495–1498

Sampson HA (1999) Food Allergy. Part 2: Diagnosis and management. The Journal of Allergy and Clinical Immunology, 103(6), 981–989

Scadding GK, Durham SR, Mirakian R, Jones NS, Leech SC, Farooque S, Ryan D, Walker SM, Clark AT, Dixon TA, Jolles SRA, Siddique N, Cullinan P, Howarth PH, Nasser SM. (2008) BSACI guidelines for the management of allergic and non-allergic rhinitis. Clinical and Experimental Allergy, 38, 19–42.

Sicherer SH. (1999) Food Allergy: When and how to perform oral food challenges. Pediatric Allergy and Immunology, 10, 226–234

Slater JE. (1994) Latex allergy. Journal of Allergy and Clinical Immunology, 94(2)(Part 1), 139–149

Sporik R, Hill DJ, Hosking CS. (2000) Specificity of allergen skin testing in predicting positive open food challenges to milk, egg and peanut in children. Clinical and Experimental Allergy, 30, 1540–1546

Walker S, Khan-Wasti S, Fletcher M, Cullinan P, Harris J, Sheikh A. (2007) Seasonal allergic rhinitis is associated with a detrimental effect on examination performance in United Kingdom teenagers: case-control study. Journal of Allergy and Clinical Immunology, 120, 381–387

World Health Organization (2004) Measles vaccines; WHO position paper. Weekly Epidemiological Record, 14, 130–142

Useful websites

The Allergy Academy – www.allergyacademy.org
American Academy of Allergy Asthma and Immunology – www.aaaai.org
The Anaphylaxis Campaign – www.anaphylaxis.org.uk
The Association of Anaesthetists of Great Britain and Ireland – www.aagbi.org
British Society of Allergy & Clinical Immunology – www.bsaci.org
The Cochrane collaboration – www.cochrane.org
The European Academy of Allergology and Clinical Immunology – www.eaaci.net
European Resuscitation Council – www.erc.edu
Health protection agency – www.hpa.org.uk
Resuscitation Council UK – www.resus.org.uk
World Allergy Organisation – www.worldallergy.org
http://www.food.gov.uk/multimedia/pdfs/allergyfactsheet1.pdf
http://www.food.gov.uk/multimedia/pdfs/allergyfactsheettwo.pdf

Chapter 3

Biopsies

Chapter contents

Procedure guidelines

The Great Ormond Street Hospital Manual of Children's Nursing Practices, First Edition. Edited by Susan Macqueen, Elizabeth Anne Bruce, Faith Gibson.
© 2012 Great Ormond Street Hospital for Children NHS Foundation Trust. Published 2012 by Blackwell Publishing Ltd.

Introduction

This chapter includes sections on liver biopsy, punch skin biopsy, renal biopsy, and bone marrow aspirate and trephine (BMT). Each of these topics is dealt with under separate headings, in which rationale, the procedure is detailed here. Care of the child undergoing general anaesthesia can be found in other chapters in this book, including pre- and post-operative care.

Liver biopsy

Introduction

The liver (Figure 3.1 and 3.2) is located in the upper right quadrant of the abdomen, just behind the lower portion of the ribs (which protect it from injury) and is the largest and most metabolically complex organ in the body. It carries out hundreds of different functions designed to maintain a favourable internal environment in the body (metabolic homeostasis), and helps to protect against infection. This anatomical knowledge is an essential part of preparation.

Liver biopsy is sometimes used in the investigation of patients with suspected liver disease, e.g. enlargement of liver and/or

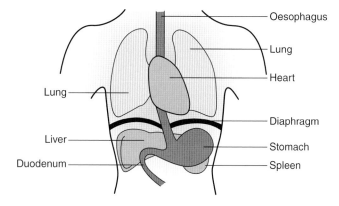

Figure 3.1 The position of the liver within the body.

spleen, abnormal liver enzymes, an abnormal appearance of the liver on a scan, low blood sugar, raised blood ammonia, etc. The benefits and risks of a liver biopsy must be assessed carefully for each child and the results of other routine investigations taken into account.

Liver biopsy samples can be obtained by different methods, such as percutaneous core needle biopsy sampling, using a trans-jugular core needle approach, or by laparoscopic or open surgical techniques.

Percutaneous liver biopsy is associated with small but definite risks to the child, even in the most experienced hands, and therefore it should only be performed when the potential benefits of the test outweigh the risks. The potential benefit of knowing what the liver looks like under the microscope (or how it functions biochemically, or whether it is the site of infection) is that this will lead to specific, effective treatment or at least define the likely disease outcome. This benefit should be continually re-evaluated as alternative diagnostic tests (e.g. DNA analysis) and new treatment options become available, such as has occurred with the new antiviral therapies in viral hepatitis and in liver transplantation.

In the majority of cases, percutaneous core needle sampling is the modality of choice, due to the relative technical ease of the procedure and its high diagnostic accuracy (Cohen *et al* 1992, Hoffer FA 2000, Lachaux *et al* 1995, Litchtman *et al* 1987, Nobili *et al* 2003, Rivera-Sanfeliz *et al* 2005).

Indications for liver biopsy

Liver biopsy (in combination with the child's clinical history, physical examination, data from imaging and laboratory tests) is a powerful clinical tool for diagnosing, treating and monitoring liver disease. At GOSH, all liver biopsies are performed by the Interventional Radiology (IR) department, usually under general anaesthetic. It is assumed that all children referred to IR for a liver biopsy will have had previous imaging of the liver and biliary tree. This imaging will be reviewed by IR and discussed with the referring team prior to accepting the biopsy request.

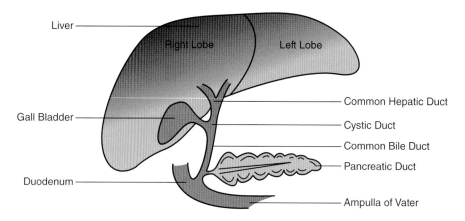

Figure 3.2 Liver anatomy.

Indications for a liver biopsy include:

- Investigation of suspected diffuse liver disease, such as infective, autoimmune, cholestatic and congenital forms of hepatitis, Langerhans' cell histiocytosis (LCH), metabolic liver disease such as Wilson's disease and glycogen-storage disorders, and some types of neuroblastoma (diffuse forms of stage 4 and stage 4S)
- Investigation of focal liver disease, such as mesenchymal hamartoma, teratoma, hepatoblastoma, rhabdoid tumour, sarcoma, non-Hodgkin lymphoma, hepatocellular carcinoma and hepatic adenoma (Roebuck 2008)
- Management of liver transplant
- Management of drug therapies that affect the liver parenchyma.

Contraindications to liver biopsy

Contraindications to liver biopsy include:

- A patient who is too unstable or critically unwell to undergo this procedure. There is an increased risk of mortality for an acutely sick child.
- Significant coagulopathy, significant thrombocytopenia (usually taken to be less than 80,000/mm^3). There is no published safe lower limit for platelet count, though studies usually consider levels below 50–100,000/mm^3 to be unsafe for a percutaneous approach (Gonzalez-Vallina *et al* 1993, Hatfield *et al* 2008, Hoffer 2000, Lindor *et al* 1996, Little *et al* 1996, Nobili *et al* 2003, Rivera-Sanfeliz *et al* 2005, Schiemann *et al* 2000, Sharma *et al* 1982). Sharma *et al* (1982) have shown that the risk of bleeding increases if the platelet count is below 60,000/mm^3. It makes sense that the risk of haemorrhage increases in the presence of abnormal clotting parameters (Lachaux *et al* 1995), but Cohen *et al* (1992) have noted that pre-biopsy coagulation parameters were not predictive of subsequent complications. Importantly, operators should be wary of temporary correction of significant coagulopathies, as the abnormality may recur in the hours or days following the procedure, leading to delayed bleeding. In such circumstances, there should be a low threshold for considering a transjugular approach.
- Significant ascites. A small volume of ascites can probably be tolerated by most operators, particularly if the percutaneous biopsy track is to be plugged, though significant volumes of ascites should prompt consideration of a transjugular approach. Published studies vary in their definition of the volume of ascites, making interpretation of the data difficult. It may be that image-guided percutaneous procedures are less risky in cases of mild–moderate ascites than previously thought (Little *et al* 1996).

A patient in whom any of these factors are present should be discussed with the IR team on a consultant-to-consultant basis, in order to decide whether the potential benefits of biopsy outweigh the risks; some of these factors may be only relative contraindications. In some cases, transjugular biopsy route may be appropriate, as the risks of bleeding are greatly reduced using this technique.

Clotting abnormalities must be discussed with a consultant haematologist, and corrected, as far as possible, prior to the procedure.

Patients on anticoagulant medication or a non-steroidal should have their medication discussed with their clinical team and the haematology team prior to a decision to proceed with the biopsy.

A complete patient assessment is required to assess patient suitability and subsequent complications.

Equipment

The following equipment is required:

- An ultrasound machine with a standard 13–6 MHz linear transducer. Occasionally a small parts 13–6 MHz linear probe is useful in infants.
- Co-axial core needle biopsy system. Semi-automated systems are available from various manufacturers (examples include Coaxial Temno: Allegiance Healthcare). Older series describe the use of aspiration needles, but more recent series have shown that automated devices are safe and accurate (Hoffer 2000, Rivera-Sanfeliz *et al* 2005). There is no strong evidence to recommend a particular biopsy needle size; although the literature suggests that an 18G core needle sample is adequate for a diagnostic sample in the majority of cases (Hoffer 2000, Nobili *et al* 2003).
- The appropriate medium for the biopsy should be obtained from the relevant laboratory prior to the procedure to ensure optimal condition of the biopsy when it arrives in the laboratory for analysis. The medium is usually a very small amount of sterile normal saline in a sterile specimen pot. If saline is used, the sample must be transported immediately to the laboratory so that it can be processed correctly, e.g. some are fixed in formalin, some in glutaraldehyde, or frozen.
- Some investigations require that the liver is snap frozen immediately and this will require solid carbon dioxide (Card ice) or liquid nitrogen at the venue of the procedure.

Complications of liver biopsy

Paediatric studies suggest an overall complication rate for percutaneous biopsy of 0–6.83% (2.4–4.5% major complications) (Cohen *et al* 1992, Gonzalez-Vallina *et al* 1993, Lachaux *et al* 1995, Nobili *et al* 2003, Schiemann *et al* 2000). Mortality rates are quoted at 0–0.6% (Cohen *et al* 1992, Lichtman *et al* 1987, Lachaux *et al* 1995). The data is difficult to compare between series as authors vary in their definition of major and minor complications, and in the exclusion criteria they employ.

Complications include intraperitoneal haemorrhage, biliary peritonitis, haemobilia and injury to the duodenum, colon or lung. The risk of significant bleeding after an image-guided percutaneous liver biopsy, as measured by a decrease in haematocrit, is reported to be 1.2–2%. Lachaux *et al* (1995), McGill *et al* (1990) and Rivera-Sanfeliz *et al* (2005) showed that the risk of significant bleeding is increased in malignant versus non-malignant liver disease. Paediatric studies have shown that the risk of complications is greater in children with malignant disease, cirrhosis or recent bone marrow transplant (Cohen *et al*

Procedure guideline 3.1 Pre-operative preparation (liver biopsy)

Statement	Rationale
Percutaneous core needle biopsy technique	
1. Careful child preparation prior to undertaking a liver biopsy is essential. Ideally, child and parent/carer education should begin at an outpatient visit, prior to the biopsy. Explain the procedure in sufficient detail, with careful attention to anxiety and pain management issues. Explain the potential benefits and (at least to the parent/carer) the risks involved.	**1.** To ensure safety through the procedure.
2. The child will usually be asked to complete a 6 hour fast. Some children (those at risk of a low blood sugar) will require an intravenous infusion during this time.	**2.** An empty stomach may decrease the likelihood of post-procedure nausea and vomiting, which reduces the risk of inadvertent peri-operative aspiration of stomach contents.
3. In most instances, the biopsy procedure is undertaken on an inpatient basis, following the recommendations outlined below.	
4. On the day before the biopsy, the clinical team review recent laboratory evaluation of prothrombin time activated, partial thromboplastin time and complete blood count, including platelets.	**4.** To check the child's clotting status and to minimise the risk of haemorrhage.
5. Normal coagulation parameters and platelets >80,000 (sampled within the last month) are acceptable if the child's clinical condition is stable and they do not have cholestatic jaundice.	**5.** If the patient is unwell, the results should be from a sample collected within 24 hours of the biopsy. In an emergency situation the biopsy may proceed with fresh frozen plasma (FFP) cover to minimise the risk of haemorrhage, but this should be agreed by all parties prior to commencing the procedure. If there is abnormal coagulation or thrombocytopenia that cannot be corrected, a transjugular biopsy may be more appropriate.
6. Explain the procedure to the parents/carers and child as appropriate. The consent should include adequate understanding of the risks and benefits of the procedure, complications, post-procedural care and home care.	**6.** To obtain informed and written consent (see Department of Health Consent Web Pages, DoH 2009, Patient information 2011).
7. A pre-medication can be administered to the child prior to attending theatre, to make the experience less frightening or stressful. This decision will be made by the anaesthetist in charge of the case.	**7.** A play specialist may be able to assist in preparing the child for the procedure.
8. An intravenous cannulae may need to be inserted prior to the procedure.	**8.** To facilitate the anaesthetic induction and to manage fluid balance. The decision to place the cannulae in prior to induction should be made by the anaesthetist in charge of the case.

9. Children with an underlying metabolic disorder or a history of hypoglycaemia should commence an intravenous infusion of glucose at the commencement of fasting:
 	
5% Glucose   **5–10 mg/kg/min**
                    0.1–0.2 ml/kg/min
10% Glucose   **5–10 mg/kg/min**
                    0.05–0.1 ml/kg/min
	9. To prevent hypoglycaemia and minimise the risk of metabolic acidosis.

10. Record the child's blood glucose 1–2 hourly depending on the child's underlying condition. The blood glucose should be maintained at 5–8 mmol/l. Medical staff should provide clear, written instructions of action to be taken in the event of hypoglycaemia during fasting.	**10.** To ensure child's safety.

Procedure guideline 3.2 Peri-operative procedure (liver biopsy)

Statement	Rationale
1. Universal precautions and personal protective equipment (PPE) is standard practice within an intra-operative theatre environment.	**1.** To safeguard the practitioner and patient.

Patient positioning

2. The child should be placed in a supine position.	**2.** To allow ultrasound examination of the abdomen.
3. Consider moving and handling risks when positioning and moving the child.	**3.** To ensure staff safety.

Procedure

4. A suitable biopsy site is identified by the radiologist, using ultrasound.	**4.** To ensure the safest approach to the liver parenchyma is used.
5. Prepare the field with alcohol-based solution (povidone–iodine) and place sterile drapes over the child.	**5.** To sterilise the operative field.
6. Administer local anaesthetic with 0.25% levobupivacaine 2.5mg/ml in both superficial and deep planes.	**6.** Local anaesthetic minimises post-procedural pain. Levobupivacaine has a long duration of action and ensures the child's comfort post-operatively. Lidocaine 1% buffered with sodium bicarbonate may be used for non-GA (general anaesthetic) cases, as it is less painful, but most children have this procedure performed under general anaesthetic.
7. A small nick in the skin is made with a surgical blade, usually using a subcostal approach, to allow introduction of the biopsy needle.	**7.** For ease of access.
8. The radiologist will then advance the co-axial biopsy needle through the skin and into the liver, under direct ultrasound guidance. While this is done, the anaesthetist usually ensures that the child is breath-holding, so that the passage of the needle through the liver capsule is accurate.	**8.** This allows the time spent in the liver to be kept to a minimum.
9. If the biopsy is non-targeted (for investigation of diffuse liver disease), the semi-automated inner needle of the co-axial system is fired twice, in slightly different areas of the liver, to ensure two good cores are obtained. This is done under real time ultrasound guidance. The number of cores may vary depending on the clinical situation.	**9.** This technique allows collection of many cores with only one hole in the liver capsule.
10. In targeted biopsies (for focal liver lesions) the outer needle is usually advanced through normal liver parenchyma into the abnormal liver lesion and then the inner needle is used to sample from the area of abnormality; again, this is performed using real time ultrasound guidance. The number of cores obtained may be as many as 15, so that the pathologist has enough tissue to ensure a diagnosis can be made.	

(Continued)

Procedure guideline 3.2 (Continued)

Procedure	Procedure
11. Once the biopsy samples have been taken, the inner needle of the system is removed and the track is filled with several plugs of a haemostatic substance such as gelatine foam sheets (Gel foam, Pharmacia and Upjohn), as the outer needle is withdrawn.	**11.** The gelatine plugs act to minimise the risks of both tumour spill and of bleeding (Smith *et al* 1996). In one paediatric series, detectable bleeding occurred in three children (14%) despite biopsy track embolisation, two with focal disease and one with diffuse disease (Hoffer 2000); in another series, there was no statistical difference in complication rates between patients who did or did not undergo track embolisation (Hatfield *et al* 2008).
12. The biopsy sample is obtained and placed in the correct medium. The medium is usually a very small amount of sterile normal saline in a sterile specimen container.	**12.** To ensure optimal condition of the biopsy arriving in the laboratory for analysis.
13. The biopsy site may be closed with a wound closure strip, e.g. Steri-strip and an adhesive dressing is then applied (Autio *et al* 2002).	**13.** To close the wound and prevent infection.
14. The child is rolled onto the right side and postoperative instructions are given for them to remain in this position for 1 hour to help prevent bleeding or bile leakage complications.	**14.** When the child is positioned with their right side down, pressure is being applied to the liver to encourage haemostasis.
15. The practitioner undertaking the procedure must ensure that the sample is clearly labelled with the patient's details, sample type, date and time, prior to sending it to the appropriate laboratory. A request form must accompany the sample and include accurate patient details and clear instructions for the analysis of the sample.	**15.** To ensure that the sample is analysed appropriately.
16. The operator performing the biopsy should record the procedure in the child's healthcare record including: • How many passes were made? • Any medication administered • Any apparent complications • Specific post-operative care requirements.	**16.** To maintain an accurate record and documentation.

Procedure guideline 3.3 Post-operative care (liver biopsy)

Statement	Rationale
1. Measure and record vital signs: • Every 15 minutes for the first 2 hours • Every 30 minutes for 2 hours thereafter • Hourly thereafter until 8 hours post biopsy. At 8 hours post biopsy, the child should be reviewed by a member of the clinical team (doctor) to ensure the child is well enough to be discharged or to discontinue specialist nursing care, where appropriate (see discharge section). 　　Any rise in pulse rate, fall in blood pressure or respiratory distress should be notified immediately to the clinical team looking after the child. They will assess and determine the possible need for blood transfusion, clotting factors, platelets, etc. If significant bleeding is suspected they will need to inform the person who undertook the procedure and the consultant in overall charge of the child. A surgeon should be informed at this early stage. Urgent imaging, embolisation or surgery may be required.	**1.** To monitor vital signs and to act promptly to restore circulating blood volume and stop bleeding.

Procedure guideline 3.3 (*Continued*)

Statement	Rationale
2. Observe the actual site of the biopsy for any signs of bleeding, at the same time as vital signs are recorded, for the first 12-hour period after the procedure. An intravenous cannula must remain in situ for the 24-hour period post biopsy.	**2.** Complications usually occur within the first 3 hours of liver biopsy as the blood pressure returns to normal parameters for the child. (Grant and Neuberger 1999). **Note that most children who bleed post liver biopsy do so into the peritoneal cavity and therefore there is often no external sign of bleeding**.
3. It is important to remember that sick children deteriorate for reasons unrelated to the liver biopsy. For example, a child with mitochondrial disease who appears slow to recover from anaesthesia or regained consciousness may have undetected severe hypoglycaemia.	**3.** Junior staff must inform a more senior nurse/doctor should this occur for advice/appropriate medical intervention.
4. Assess the child's need for analgesics post-operatively and administer as appropriate.	**4.** To ensure the child's pain free and comfortable to help minimise the risk of complications.
5. The child may eat and drink 2 hours post procedure, once awake and orientated.	**5.** To prevent aspiration and vomiting.
6. The child should remain on bed rest for 8 hours post procedure. However, the child can be allowed brief toilet visits under supervision by a nurse or a responsible family member during this period, provided their vital signs are stable. The position in which the child should be nursed following liver biopsy is not significant. There is no consensus in the literature and no controlled trials have been carried out to assess the various possible positions. The child should be encouraged to adopt a position that is comfortable and reassuring (Grant and Neuberger 1999, Perraul *et al* 1978).	**6.** It can be difficult to ensure that children remain on bed rest for this period and creative thinking may need to be used. The family and play specialist could be involved in keeping the child occupied while on bed rest.
7. Ensure that the child has passed urine post anaesthetic.	**7.** To ensure they are not dehydrated or showing signs of post-operative urine retention.
8. Most children will remain in hospital for 24 hours post biopsy. Children who are otherwise well, with no clotting abnormalities, may be discharged 8 hours post procedure, if the biopsy was performed early on the morning theatre list, but this decision must be discussed and agreed with all clinical teams prior to biopsy. **The child must then be reviewed by a senior doctor on the clinical team prior to discharge**. The child should have a responsible person to stay with them on the first post-biopsy night at home and should be able to return to hospital in a timely manner should the need arise.	**8.** To observe for late signs of complications.

1992, Lachaux *et al* 1995). It may be that these children should always be considered for a transjugular biopsy approach.

Tumour seeding along the biopsy track remains a significant concern but, unlike in hepatocellular carcinoma in the adult population, it is rare in the commoner paediatric lesions such as hepatoblastoma.

Smaller risks include lack of an adequate sample (see earlier). With good operative technique, post-operative pain should be minimal and post-operative infection rare.

The majority of complications occur in the first 3 hours after liver biopsy (Grant and Neuberger 1999).

Discharge planning

Post discharge, the parents/carers should be supplied with a liver biopsy advice leaflet, if they do not already have one, so that they can be supported with advice when at home. They should be advised that the histology results are usually available no earlier than 2 days after the procedure being performed. This may be due to the complexity of the analysis being performed on the biopsy specimen. For microbiology and metabolic analysis, for example, these results will take longer. The family must also be made aware of how they will receive the results. Usually, results will be available at the next outpatient appointment for discussion with the child's consultant.

When children go home they can resume a degree of normal activity. There should be an interval of somewhere between 2 weeks and 3 months where the child may have restrictions. Children may have to avoid contact sports and swimming for 6–8 weeks. This is to allow the internal organ to heal following the biopsy and to minimise the risk of internal haemorrhage post-operatively. Advice from their clinician will be given as relevant to the child's age and lifestyle. However, parents/carers should be aware of siblings and other children indulging in rough and tumble play that might inadvertently knock the liver area.

If the dressing and wound closure strip, e.g. Steri-strip, is in place it may be removed after 3 days or soaked off in the bath (Autio *et al* 2002). If the skin looks red and angry and/or the child develops pyrexia, parents/carers should seek medical advice from their GP. This may be due to infection and the child will need to visit their GP who will contact the hospital to advise whether they need to return to the hospital for blood test analysis and appropriate treatment.

It has been shown that delayed haemorrhage can occur up to 15 days after percutaneous liver biopsy in patients who develop a post-biopsy coagulopathy. The parents/carers need to look out for signs of a high temperature, unexpected lethargy and generally being unwell or irritable.

The occurrence of delayed haemorrhage is also documented after the reinstatement of warfarin therapy several days after percutaneous liver biopsy. The child's consultant must give the family clear advice regarding re-commencing a child's anti-coagulant drugs (see Contraindications section earlier).

Punch skin biopsy

Introduction

The skin is complex with an array of functions. It is the largest body organ, undertaking the major physiological functions of regulation of the body temperature, protection, sensation, excretion, immunity and synthesis of vitamin D (Tortora 1994). Children can present with a wide range of skin anomalies. Some of these can prove to be relatively normal, while, in the extreme, others can be life threatening. Accurate and timely assessment and diagnosis is therefore crucial. Many skin disorders can be diagnosed through direct observation and palpation. Others may require referral to a dermatology specialist or expert. Children with a persistent skin problem or an unusual presentation may be referred to a dermatologist for further investigations in order to achieve differential diagnosis prior to initiating a clinically effective treatment regimen. This may involve a microscopic or histo-pathological examination of the area of skin involved, or radiological imaging. When a sample of the skin is required for the purpose of aiding accurate diagnosis or further investigation, a minor surgical procedure is undertaken in order to obtain a biopsy sample.

To identify disease processes in the deeper dermis and to confirm diagnosis (Godsell 1998), a biopsy can be performed by a punch biopsy, shave biopsy or surgical excision of part of a lesion. When the full thickness of the skin (deeper dermis) needs to be assessed and analysed, a punch skin biopsy is performed. Pigmented and oily skins tend to have more scar formation than pale, dry skins. Children with anaemia may have impaired healing due to reduced oxygen transportation in the blood (McClaren 1992).

Rare metabolic disorders and chromosomal abnormalities may sometimes be confirmed by examination of the fibroblasts and chondrocytes, which are cultured from skin.

Although this procedure may be performed on the ward or theatre, only a Health Care Professional (HCP) who has been trained in this skill should undertake the punch skin biopsy. Any training should acknowledge the physical act part of the procedure, as well as the psychological aspects and the sequence of events.

To ensure that their knowledge remains valid and up to date, and that their practice is safe and efficient, the HCP who undertakes this role should be responsible for ensuring that they work within their Code of Professional Practice and competency. The newly trained HCP should continue to make themselves aware of developments in practice, research and available products.

Preparation of equipment and environment

The child should be assessed for their sedation requirements to facilitate adherence and minimise anxiety. Avoid using the child's own bed space or room; rather use a clinical room if possible, where all equipment is close at hand. This also ensures that the child's own bed space remains a safe haven and provides greater privacy for the child and family (Frederick 1991). The clinical area should be clean and an adjustable magnifying lamp should be available to allow good visualisation of the biopsy area.

The medium for a skin biopsy should be obtained from the appropriate laboratory. Ensure the laboratory request form has the correct clinical information for analysis.

The following special arrangements need to be made for specific mediums:

- Formalin is used for routine histology and is obtainable from Histology.
- Liquid nitrogen is used for immunofluoresent investigations (Harper 1990). Special guidelines for the handling of liquid nitrogen, covering the Control of Substances Hazardous to Health Regulations (COSHH), may be obtained from the bone marrow laboratory.
- A 'special fixative' for electron microscopy investigation (Harper 1990) may be obtained from the Virology department.

If a pneumatic tube is available in a Trust to deliver specimens to a laboratory this cannot be used in this instance. The mediums must be collected by porters or delivered to the appropriate ward or clinical area.

Equipment should be prepared as outlined in the following procedure guideline.

Procedure guideline 3.4 **Punch skin biopsy**

Statement	Rationale
1. a) A local anaesthetic is used when carrying out the procedure. **b)** Oral sedation may also be required. **c)** An aseptic non-touch technique (ANTT) should be employed throughout the procedure.	**1. a)** To minimise pain, stress and anxiety. **b)** In giving sedation the child is better able to tolerate the overall procedure. **c)** To minimise the risk of infection.
2. The site to be biopsied must be identified by the relevant multidisciplinary team. The site chosen for the purpose of investigating metabolic disorders is under the arm or axilla.	**2.** To aid the diagnosis for the child and family. To minimise visible scarring and provide a good cosmetic outcome.
3. Cytogenetics and chromosomes specimens are sent via Biochemistry to a Cytogenetics department. Fibroblast culture specimens are sent to an Enzymology Laboratory.	
4. Universal precautions, personal protective equipment (PPE) must be adopted according to hospital policy.	**4.** To prevent contamination and safeguard the person performing the procedure.

Procedure guideline 3.5 **Preparation of the child and family (skin biopsy)**

Statement	Rationale
1. Obtain verbal and written consent from the child and family for the procedure (DoH 2001 a,b, UN General Assembly 1989, Orr 1999). **a)** Allow enough time between giving information to the family and child and performing the procedure.	**1.** To ensure that informed consent is obtained and to allow the family to develop coping strategies. **a)** Too much or too little time the child will become anxious. The better informed the child the better able they would be to develop coping strategies (Sclare and Waring 1995).
2. The child and family should be given Trust specific information and directed to relevant websites, in particular direct to the GOSH website where written information and some podcasts are available that help when preparing children for procedures.	**2.** To address any information requirements and to empower the child and family alleviating any worries or concerns.
3. Inform the child and family of the following: **a)** That a punch skin biopsy is necessary. **b)** The reason for the biopsy. **c)** What it entails. **d)** The potential risks of a punch skin biopsy. **e)** Are there any alternatives? **f)** The duration of the procedure. **g)** The expected cosmetic outcome. **h)** What happens afterwards? **i)** When to expect results.	**3.** To obtain informed written consent according to the Trust Hospital Policy. **b)** To minimise anxiety. **d)** To empower the family.
4. A play specialist and the child's named nurse can help the child to be adequately prepared for the procedure (Heiney 1991). **a)** Discuss with the family and child the appropriate method of distracting the child that will be used during the procedure itself. Attempt to discover what techniques are most likely to consume their attention, e.g. pop-up books, musical books, blowing bubbles and guided imagery where the child is encouraged to imagine something pleasant, e.g. a favourite holiday.	**4.** To prepare the child according to their age and cognitive development in language they can understand: avoiding jargon and complex words. **a)** To prevent the child's whole attention being centred on the invasive procedure. These techniques can help to distract and relax the child (Heiney 1991, Langley 1999).

Procedure guideline 3.6 **Preparation of equipment (skin biopsy)**

Statement	Rationale
1. Clean dressing trolley or appropriate clean surface or tray.	
2. Skin Biopsy Pack (obtainable from a HSDU department) or a sterile dressing pack containing sterile non-woven swabs and a sterile towel.	**2.** Some literature suggests that fibres shed from cotton wool swabs can become entwined in tissue and a focus for infection (Briggs 1996).
3. Alcohol based antiseptic cleaning solution, e.g. chlorhexidine gluconate 0.5%.	**3.** Active against a wide range of Gram-positive and negative organisms. Routine use of povidone–iodine solution should be avoided in small babies and children. Iodine absorption may cause hypothyroidism during a critical period of neurological development and stains the skin cells (Smerdely et al 1989).
4. Local anaesthetic, e.g. lidocaine 1%. Lidocaine with adrenaline (epinephrine) is a powerful vasoconstrictor, therefore decreasing the bleeding in wounds. However, this may be contraindicated in areas of end artery flow, i.e. fingers and toes. This can cause palpitations and tremors, so is therefore used with caution.	
5. Disposable scalpel.	
6. Sterile gloves.	
7. Disposable plastic apron.	
8. Prescription chart.	
9. 2 ml syringe.	
10. Blue needle (23 G).	
11. Orange needle (25 G).	
12. Correctly labelled specimen pot containing the appropriate medium. This is decided by the type of investigation required.	
13. A sterile occlusive latex free dressing, e.g. Cutiplast size 7.2 cm × 5 cm or Opsite size 6.5 cm × 5 cm.	**13.** A wound dressing serves several functions. It protects the wound from further insult, keeps the wound clean, and provides a moist environment that promotes healing (Autio et al 2002). It also minimises the risk of scarring. Choosing an appropriate dressing is difficult especially with the wide and confusing range that is available for use today. For children dressings must be easy to apply and remove; be able to withstand the rigors of children's activities; and be secure enough to prevent the child from interfering with the wound (Teare 1997).
14. Conforming bandage.	
15. Steri-strips.	
16. Tape.	
17. Disposable punch biopsy needle size 0.3 mm or 0.4 mm.	
18. Hypoallergenic dressing, e.g. Mepitel.	**18.** To prevent further breakdown of fragile skin.

Parental/carer role

In order to minimise anxiety to the child and to empower the family/care giver, it is important to identify with the parent/carer their role throughout the procedure. This role includes adopting the appropriate method of distraction with the child to use during the procedure itself. The child's parent/carer may remain with their child if they wish to do so. Throughout the procedure the child and parent/carer should be reassured and the procedure explained to them.

Procedure guideline 3.7 **Punch skin biopsy procedure**

Statement	Rationale
1. A topical local anaesthetic should be applied to the biopsy site prior to the procedure. Consult the child and family on the use of Ametop® cream. Check for previous allergic reactions to the cream and use Emla® if necessary. If Emla® is used, ensure that it remains in situ for the appropriate time. Special precautions may need to be taken with known atopic children with eczema.	**1.** The minimal time for Ametop® is 30 minutes. The optimal application time for Emla® to achieve 95% anaesthesia to the area is 90 minutes. This is due to the nerve fibre size and is particularly relevant in the age group 1–5 years. Application of local anaesthetic will reduce the pain of the procedure (Clark and Radford 1986, Lawson *et al* 1995, Smith & Nephew Ltd 2003).
2. The local anaesthetic used should be prescribed and checked according to the Administration of Medicines Policy.	**2.** To meet hospital policy requirements.
3. While maintaining the dignity of the child, place the child in a comfortable position with the potential biopsy area exposed. Positioning of the child would depend on the site of the skin biopsy. The position should be the most comfortable and reassuring for the child. Small children/infants can lie or sit on an adult's lap. Ensure a young child has their favourite cuddly toy or comforter with them throughout (Robinson and Collier 1997, RCN 2003). Consider moving and handling risks issues.	**3.** To facilitate biopsy taking and to maintain safety, security and dignity. To minimise the stress to the child.
4. Having performed a surgical ward hand wash and wearing the appropriate protective clothing, remove the local anaesthetic cream and wipe dry with a tissue or gauze. Confirm with the child, if appropriate, that the cream has caused numbness of the skin effectively. The biopsy area should be cleaned for 30 seconds with an alcohol based cleansing solution and allowed to dry for another 30 seconds (DoH 2003, Franklin 1998, Macqueen 2008, Niffeneger 1997).	**4.** To reassure the child and help reduce the pain.
5. Check the child's name, date of birth, hospital number and allergies against the prescription charts.	**5.** To prevent a medication error.
6. The local anaesthetic should be prepared using an aseptic non-touch technique. Draw up in a 2 ml syringe with a blue needle (23 G) and change to an orange needle (25 G). **a)** The HCP should warn the child that it will sting or have a burning sensation with subcutaneous infiltration of the local anaesthetic. It should be injected subcutaneously using the 'spider technique' lifting a skin fold to assure that the subcutaneous injection is accomplished. This forms a 'belb' or small bump. **b)** Time must be allowed for the anaesthetic to take effect. Wait 2–3 minutes before proceeding.	**6.** To minimise the risk of infection. **a)** Less adipose tissue leads to greater risk of intra-muscular injection (King 2003, Winslow *et al* 1997). **b)** To gain maximum benefit from anaesthesia and to ensure effectiveness of the anaesthetic.

(Continued)

Procedure guideline 3.7 (*Continued*)

Statement	Rationale
7. To perform the procedure: **a)** Pull the skin around the biopsy area tight. **b)** Introduce a disposable punch biopsy firmly at a perpendicular angle to the anaesthetised area of the skin surface. **c)** The needle should be rotated back and forth with the cutting edge carrying the punch down onto the tissue. **d)** The guard on the sterile punch biopsy will prevent too deep a penetration into the skin. **e)** Withdraw the disposable biopsy punch needle while applying pressure on the puncture site. This should release the skin specimen. **f)** Remove the specimen using the plastic forceps or sterile scissors. **g)** Specimens taken for rare metabolic disorders should be removed using a disposable scalpel blade. **h)** Place the specimen in the appropriate biopsy medium and ensure the container is correctly and clearly labelled. **i)** Apply continuous pressure to biopsy site until bleeding stops. **j)** Apply Steri-strips in a 'star' pattern.	**a)** To immobilise the skin. **b)** To facilitate effective biopsy taking. **c)** To ensure that the full thickness of the deeper dermis is obtained. **d)** To avoid damage to underlying tissue and to minimise pain and bleeding. **f)** To obtain sample and prevent damage to the fibroblasts and skin tissue. **h)** To prepare for laboratory analysis to enable correct analysis. **i)** To achieve haemostasis. **j)** To ensure the edges of the wound are drawn carefully together so as to promote effective healing and improve cosmetic outcome. Steri-strips work best in superficial low-tension wounds. It is inexpensive, easy and painless to apply (Autio *et al* 2002).
k) Once bleeding has stopped apply some Bactroban ointment to the site for immunocompromised children. **l)** Once haemostasis has been achieved apply either: • A dry dressing, e.g. Cutiplast or Op-site or • A low-adherent dressing, e.g. Mepitel, if the surrounding skin is fragile (Harper 1990). **m)** Cover the dressing with a pressure dressing. When tape cannot be applied due to fragile skin use a bandage to secure the dressing. **n)** Dispose of used equipment and sharps according to the Waste Policy. Remove protective clothing and perform a clinical hand wash. **o)** Document the type of specimen the time, date and site where the biopsy was taken. **p)** Place the sample in a polythene specimen bag and send to the appropriate laboratory. **q)** Record the procedure in the child's healthcare records. **r)** Time should be taken to give positive feedback to the child for tolerating the invasive procedure, and to the parent/carer for their valuable contribution.	**l)** To protect the site and minimise infection, in order to maintain comfort and prevent further irritation. **m)** To maintain skin integrity and comfort. **n)** To meet hospital policy and to prevent an inoculation injury reducing the risk of cross-infection. **o)** To enable analysis to take place. **q)** To maintain an accurate record **r)** Concluding the procedure with a positive outcome and to acknowledge the value of the involvement of parent/carer.

Procedure guideline 3.8 **Post-procedural care (skin biopsy)**

Statement	Rationale
1. Once the procedure has been completed the child may return to their bed or the playroom, or they may go straight home. **a)** If sedation has been given, their level of consciousness and their vital signs must be monitored pre discharge.	**1.** To facilitate safety and comfort. **a)** To ensure the child is awake and orientated prior to discharge.

Procedure guideline 3.8 *(Continued)*

Statement	Rationale
2. Assess the child's need for analgesia. Oral analgesia may be required if the child experiences pain or discomfort. The analgesia must be prescribed and administered according to hospital Administration of Medicines Policy.	**2.** To relieve pain and to promote comfort.
3. The dressing should be observed intermittently within the first 24 hours for any signs of bleeding. The pressure dressing should be removed after this point. **a)** The child's doctor should be informed if bleeding is observed. The family/child's carer should be given clear instructions to contact their GP or healthcare professional if a problem occurs.	**3.** To detect early signs of biopsy site complications.
4. A clean wound should be left untouched, leaving the exudates to nourish the natural healing process (Briggs 1996, Dealey 1994). **a)** The site should be left untouched and kept dry for 48 hours. **b)** The dressing may be removed after 48 hours. **c)** The Steri-strips may begin to fall off. Allow this to happen. If still intact they may be removed on the third day. Many children prefer to remove their own dressings by soaking them off in the bath or shower (Bale 1996). **d)** Once skin edges have sealed bathing or showering is not likely to cause any further risk (Briggs 1997).	**4.** To minimise the risk of infection. Children in good health have a vigorous healing reaction. Increased metabolism and good circulation contribute to increased rates of healing (Dealey 1994). **a)** Consider wound healing within the context of the child's childhood disorder. **c)** To minimise the risk of scarring. **d)** To enable normal hygiene practices to resume.
5. Healing in immune-compromised children may be delayed because of reduced efficiency of the immune system. Secondary to this is a decreased resistance to infection, which in turn will delay healing (Morrison 1992).	
6. Immune-compromised children may be prescribed a prophylactic topical antibiotic. Those with an uncomplicated biopsy do not usually develop an infection. The first application is applied after haemostasis has occurred. **a)** The second application should be made 48 hours after the procedure when the dressing is removed.	**6.** To prevent infection. Use of adhesive tapes is also associated with decreased infection rates (Trott 1997). **a)** Antibiotics are often an over-used prophylactic.
7. The topical antibiotics must be prescribed and given according to the Administration of Medicines Policy.	**7.** To meet Hospital Policy.
8. A written instruction sheet on the care of the biopsy site must be given to the main parent/carer on discharge. It should also include parent/carer education about the wound healing process, which should include a discussion of the return to normal activities. **a)** An outpatient's appointment must be given to the family.	**8.** To empower child and family and to ensure that the child does not pick at the tape and remove it. **a)** To inform parents/carers of results and to recommend future action/treatment.
9. The child and family must be informed of the results of the procedure as soon as possible, although they should be advised that some biopsy results take 6–8 weeks depending on the nature of analysis of the biopsy. **a)** This discussion must be recorded in the child's healthcare records.	**9.** To keep the child and family informed. This may be due to time taken for the growing of skin cells. **a)** To provide an accurate record and documentation.

Renal biopsy

Introduction

A renal biopsy is a specialised, minimally invasive procedure with some significant and serious, but rare, complications (Simckes *et al* 2000). It accomplishes an important role in determining, confirming or monitoring a diagnosis or treatment regimen within nephrology (Caione *et al* 2000, Postlethwaite 1994, Simckes *et al* 2000, Tomson 2003, Wallace 1998). The procedure essentially involves the removal of a very small amount of kidney tissue (cortical and medullary) for microscopic analysis and there are several different techniques that can be used to obtain this tissue sample, including open, laparoscopic and percutaneous techniques (Bauer *et al* 2000, Coburn and Mitchell 2002). At Great Ormond Street Hospital the percutaneous method is the most commonly performed technique, unless the child has contraindications to this method. It is usually undertaken in theatre or interventional radiology with ultrasound guidance while the child receives either local or general anaesthesia depending on their age and level of adherence with the procedure.

While specialist medical practitioners perform the biopsy, the nursing role in caring for a child undergoing a renal biopsy is a very important one. The responsibility of the ward nurse is principally to ensure appropriate preparation and safe recovery of the child (Price *et al* 2000, Tomsett and Watson 1996, Wallace 1998). There are several indications for a renal biopsy, a number of contraindications to the biopsy going ahead, as well as various complications that can occur after the biopsy has been performed – all of which it serves the nurse well to understand. A competent and knowledgeable nurse can fulfil a vital role within the specialist expert team, as that knowledge may enable early recognition of potential complications, and therefore swift investigation and correction. A specialist expert team is felt to be an important, if not fundamental, factor in the success and safety of the renal biopsy, and as such, children should be referred to specialist centres with experience if a kidney biopsy is considered necessary (Postlethwaite 1994).

Indications

Renal biopsies, as previously mentioned, are performed for numerous and diverse reasons, but the most prevailing reasons include: to assess steroid resistant nephrotic syndrome, persistent blood or protein in the urine; or to assess the severity of potential transplant rejection (Bauer *et al* 2000, Date 1994, Postlethwaite 1994, Vidhun *et al* 2003. It is important that the biopsy is only performed if it will direct and advance the child's treatment regimen; it should not be used for diagnostic or research purposes alone due to the various associated complications of the process (Bauer *et al* 2000).

Contraindications

To try to reduce the risk of complications occurring there are a number of risk factors that need to be corrected or further investigated prior to a kidney biopsy going ahead. These include uncontrolled hypertension, severe anaemia and having a solitary kidney (Caione *et al* 2000, Webb and Postlethwaite 2003). As bleeding is the most common and potentially serious complication of a biopsy (Whittier and Korbett 2004), children with severe anaemia should not undergo a biopsy as the risk of reducing the haemoglobin level further may be hazardous. Equally, children with hypertension should not experience the procedure as the risk of bleeding is amplified (Whittier and Korbett 2004), so this condition should receive investigation and further management. To prevent the significant risk of bleeding, clotting screens (and bleeding times if the child has severe uraemia) should be checked and corrected if necessary prior to the procedure and any anticoagulation and antiplatelet therapy should be discussed with regard to the pre-emptive discontinuation of treatment (Bauer *et al* 2000, Postlethwaite 1994). The child should have blood taken for group and save, in order that blood can be cross-matched if required or, if at high risk of bleeding, blood should be cross matched ready for use if necessary (Webb and Postlethwaite 2003).

A biopsy must always be preceded by an ultrasound of the kidneys to ensure that the child has two kidneys, in the usual position, to reduce any risk to the child's renal function (Bauer *et al* 2000). In children with transplanted kidneys, it is already known that there is only one functioning kidney, but the need for the biopsy outweighs the risks of the biopsy itself (Bauer *et al* 2000). However, the biopsy is usually still performed under ultrasound guidance to ensure accurate localisation of the kidney (Webb and Postlethwaite 2003).

Complications

As previously mentioned, bleeding is the most commonly witnessed complication after a biopsy; most often exhibited as haematuria, which is almost unavoidable as the kidney is such a vascular organ (Postlethwaite 1994, Simckes *et al* 2000, Whittier and Korbett 2004). Microscopic haematuria is virtually always present and should not cause any anxiety (Postlethwaite 1994), but macroscopic haematuria may occasionally be witnessed; both usually settle quickly with encouragement of fluids, which also has the benefit of reducing the risks of clots forming in the bladder (Postlethwaite 1994). Persistent macroscopic haematuria may indicate bleeding at the site of the biopsy; possibly resulting in the need for a blood transfusion and very occasionally there may be a need for another operation or radiological procedure to stop the bleeding (Postlethwaite 1994). Bed rest is generally thought to prevent the likelihood of haematomas and haematuria, although the optimal length of bed rest is heavily debated (Simckes *et al* 2000, Whittier and Korbett 2004).

Further complications that may occur include haematomas; small insignificant haematomas may never be noticed and are probably quite common, but there are a very small number of children who suffer from larger more noteworthy haematomas. These may cause significant loin pain and warrant further investigation. Minor discomfort and pain are also common after a biopsy over the site, caused by insertion of the needle (Postlethwaite 1994, Simckes *et al* 2000); it is usually easily controlled with mild analgesia (such as paracetamol), but stronger pain relief, such as codeine may be required (Bauer *et al* 2000, Tomsett and Watson 1996).

Other potential, but rare, complications include infection, hypotension, arterio-venous fistula and renal capsular tear (Bauer *et al* 2000, Postlethwaite 1994). A nephrectomy may be required in extreme circumstances if the bleeding from a renal capsular tear is uncontrollable and all other procedures have failed (Bauer *et al* 2000, Postlethwaite 1994). There is also a very small mortality risk, which, on examining the research, usually occurs only as a result of substantial haemorrhage, which is rare (Whittier and Korbett 2004). The final potential problem, which requires a mention, is that of technical failure where insignificant tissue is collected for analysis and a repeat biopsy is required (Postlethwaite 1994). It is important the child and family understand all these potential risks before consenting to the procedure (Bauer *et al* 2000).

Renal biopsy complications have been reported as uncommon after 6 hours and as a result several units that are performing biopsies currently perform them as a day case (Hussain *et al* 2003). The policy at Great Ormond Street Hospital, if the child has undergone a uncomplicated percutaneous biopsy, is to place the child on bed rest and monitor the child for 4 hours post biopsy. However, if the child is considered to be at high risk of complications, with co-morbid conditions (hypertension, bleeding disorders, etc), or is displaying signs of any complications, bed rest and monitoring continues for longer.

Discharge from Great Ormond Street Hospital occurs no sooner than 6 hours after biopsy; the child may need to stay overnight if the biopsy occurred late in the day. If the child's observations are normal, their biopsy site looks satisfactory, the child is pain free, is tolerating food and drink, and has passed urine twice with no evidence of persistent macroscopic haematuria they can be discharged. The child must also live within reasonable travelling distance of the hospital and on discharge it is important that the child and family fully understand all the potential complications. The child should be given advice to rest for a further 12–24 hours, observe urine for signs of bleeding and also be advised to stay off school for 2–3 days. In addition, they should avoid strenuous exercise (for example bike riding and horse-riding) and contact sports for 4 weeks, as this provides time for maximum healing and minimises the likelihood of any further complications (Tomsett and Watson 1996). The child should have an outpatient clinic appointment booked, to receive the results when available, or sooner if the child needs attention for other clinical concerns.

Procedure guideline 3.9 **Pre-operative procedure (renal biopsy)**

Statement	Rationale
1. Ensure that informed consent is gained and a consent form is completed. a) Ensure that the child has a correctly labelled name band in place.	1. To ensure the child and family are fully aware of any potential complications. a) To ensure that the correct child will receive the procedure.
2. A pre-operative set of baseline observations should be performed: a) Temperature. b) Pulse rate. c) Respiratory rate. d) Blood pressure. e) Oxygen saturations.	2. To enable an accurate comparison to be made post-operatively. To assess for any contraindications (such as hypertension).
3. Ensure the following bloods are performed: a) Full blood count. b) Urea and electrolytes (U&Es). c) Clotting screen. d) Group and save. e) Bleeding time if urea >40 mmol/l.	3. To ensure that the child is safely prepared for theatre.
4. Child may need to have any coagulation abnormalities corrected prior to procedure.	4. To reduce the risk of bleeding post-operatively.
5. Discuss anticoagulant or antiplatelet therapy with medical staff (usually discontinued for 1 week before and after the procedure).	5. To reduce the risk of bleeding post-operatively.
6. The child should be nil by mouth appropriately for the type of anaesthetic they will receive.	6. To ensure that the child is safely prepared for theatre.

(Continued)

Procedure guideline 3.9 (*Continued*)

Statement	Rationale
7. Transplant patients and those with good renal function may need to be given IV fluids pre-theatre for hydration.	**7.** To avoid the risk of dehydration.
8. A urinalysis ward dipstick should be performed before the child goes to theatre.	**8.** To assess the level of haematuria pre-theatre (baseline), to enable an accurate comparison to be made post-operatively.
9. Ensure that an ultrasound is performed.	**9.** To ensure that the child has two kidneys to minimise the risk of subsequent renal failure if complications were to occur (unless they are a transplant patient where the benefits should outweigh the risks).
10. The child should receive age-appropriate preparation either by nursing staff or the play specialist.	**10.** To reduce any anxiety.

Procedure guideline 3.10 Post-operative procedure (renal biopsy)

Statement	Rationale

1. Monitor the child's oxygen saturations on return, until stable.
    Record the child's:
a) Temperature.
b) Pulse rate.
c) Respiratory rate.
d) Blood pressure
    i. ¼ hourly for 1 hour
    ii. ½ hourly for 2 hours
    iii. Hourly until discharge.
Reducing or increasing frequency as condition dictates.
	1. To assess/detect:
	• Respiratory distress (recovery from anaesthesia)
	• Haemorrhage
	• Pain
	• Infection.

2. Liberal fluids should be commenced post-biopsy (unless the child is fluid restricted when input should be closely monitored). IV fluids should be started if the child is unable to take fluid orally.	**2.** To promote good urine output in order to reduce and determine haematuria and the risk of clot formation.
3. Monitor the child's input and output.	**3.** To assess fluid status and kidney function.
4. Small urine samples from each void should be collected, labelled with time and date, and saved for duration of stay. **a)** These should be tested with a ward dipstick. **b)** Macroscopic haematuria and passing of clots should be reported to medical staff.	**4.** Microscopic haematuria is normal for 72 hours post-biopsy, but should be decreasing throughout this period. **a)** To observe for diminishing haematuria. **b)** To ensure that any persistent bleeding can be treated promptly (post-operative bloods, an ultrasound and overnight stay may be required).
5. The biopsy site must be observed: • 1/4 hourly for 1 hour • 1/2 hourly for 2 hours • Hourly until discharge.	**5.** To check for bleeding, haematoma and infection, which can be potential complications of a biopsy.
6. Keep the dressing dry and in place for 36–48 hours. **a)** Steri-strips will fall off.	**6.** To promote healing and reduce the risk of scarring.

Procedure guideline 3.10 (*Continued*)

Statement	Rationale
7. The child should receive pain assessment and management according to the pain chapter.	**7.** To assess, manage and treat the child in pain appropriately although site tenderness is normal post-biopsy. Excessive flank/abdominal pain may indicate haemorrhage. Loin pain may indicate a large haematoma.
8. Commence diet when tolerating fluids. **a)** Assess child for nausea and vomiting.	**8.** To ensure child is able to be discharged. **a)** Refer to medical practitioner for anti-emetics as required.
9. The child should be on bed-rest for 4 hours after biopsy. **a)** Distressed toddlers may sit on carers' laps. **b)** A play specialist referral should be made.	**9.** Reduces risk of haemorrhage, haematuria and haematomas. **a)** To encourage the child to stay on bed-rest, and to reduce any distress and subsequent potential damage of any distress. **b)** To occupy the child while on bed rest.
10. The child should start to very gently mobilise prior to discharge.	**10.** To ensure the child is safe to be discharged.
11. Child and family should receive an 'Kidney Biopsy – information for families' booklet.	**11.** Informed parents/carers may recognise complications more promptly.
12. Child and family should be aware that they should contact the ward if they have blood in the urine or pain around site.	**12.** To ensure prompt treatment of any complications.
13. Child should be advised to avoid lifting, strenuous activity (e.g. bike riding, horse riding) and contact sports for 4 weeks.	**13.** Provides time for maximum healing and minimises the likelihood of any further complications.
14. The child's GP and Community Team should be informed that the child has had a biopsy. **a)** School Nurse should be informed that the child has had a biopsy.	**14.** To ensure that appropriate and fully informed assistance can be provided if required when the child is at home. **a)** To ensure that the school is aware that the child will be absent from school for 2–3 days and should not perform school sports for 4 weeks.

Bone marrow aspirate and trephine

Introduction

Healthy bone marrow is a complex tissue which is a fundamental requirement for normal living. The bone marrow contains stem cells for haemopoietic cells and stem cells that are precursors for non-haemopoietic tissues, which are responsible for:

- Maintaining homeostasis
- Maintaining the body's defence system
- Transporting oxygen and carbon dioxide around the body.

It was not until the late 1940s that bone marrow aspiration became a reliable and widely used diagnostic technique (Diamond 1989). A bone marrow aspiration is the removal of adequate amounts of bone marrow to confirm the diagnosis of a malfunctioning marrow. Furthermore, it can be repeated to monitor the child's response to treatment.

Bone marrow can be aspirated from a variety of sites which are rich in marrow. These sites are the sternum, tibia (in small infants only), and the most usual site being the anterior and posterior iliac crests. Cells from the marrow are analysed for their characteristics such as shape, size, number, and are used to aid diagnosis in children with haematological, oncological, immunological, metabolic and infectious problems.

A bone marrow aspirate can be performed either under general anaesthetic, or more usually under local anaesthetic, and usually as a day case in the clinic setting.

Bone marrow trephine/biopsy is a procedure where a small core of both bone and marrow are removed. If this is required it is usually performed at the same time as an aspirate. A bone marrow trephine is used to establish further staging of a child's solid tumour by confirming the presence of metastatic disease.

Complications

These are extremely rare, the more common being:

1. Haemorrhage – this is most likely to occur in children who are thrombocytopenic. Therefore, for children undergoing:
   - A bone marrow aspirate – the platelet count must be greater than 10×10^9/l
   - A bone marrow trephine – the platelet count must be greater than 30×10^9/l.

2. Bleeding/bruising – this can be avoided by applying pressure to the site and, if necessary, a pressure bandage.
3. Infection – if a pressure bandage or plaster has been applied, these must be removed by 24 hours post procedure, as leaving them on will expose the immune-compromised child to infection. The gentlest way to remove the dressing is to soak it off in a warm bath.

Preparation of equipment

The following equipment should be prepared:

- Alcohol-based antiseptic, e.g. chlorhexidene in alcohol
- Sterile dressing pack
- Sterile gloves
- Selection of syringes – including 20 ml syringes and needles
- Bone marrow aspiration needle
- Bone marrow trephine needle (if required)
- Microscope glass slides and container
- Specimen bottles – plain and with heparin
- Specimen pot with formalin for trephine, if required
- Local anaesthetic, if required
- Plaster.

To prepare the equipment and perform the aspiration/trephine, staff must perform a surgical hand wash and use an aseptic technique. By applying these two rules the risk of infection will be minimised.

Procedure guideline 3.11 Preparation of child and family (aspiration/trephine)

Statement	Rationale
1. Inform and prepare the child and family for the following procedure: a) A bone marrow aspirate +/– trephine if required. b) The need for the aspirate +/– trephine. c) What the test involves. d) The potential risks of the aspirate/trephine. e) The approximate duration of the procedure.	To obtain informed consent. To minimise anxiety (Pinkerton *et al* 1993).
2. Contact a play specialist or experienced nurse to work with the child.	2. To help prepare the child.
3. Ensure the appropriate hospital information leaflets are given to the family in a format which they can read.	3. To enable the family to have a full understanding of the procedure.
4. If a general anaesthetic is to be used, ensure a doctor obtains written consent.	4. To comply with hospital policy.
5. If an anaesthetic is to be used the child must be Nil By Mouth as per hospital policy.	5. To minimise the risk of aspiration of stomach contents while under anaesthesia.
6. Blood test results, i.e. full blood count +/– clotting, available prior to performing the procedure.	6. To reduce the risk of haemorrhage.

Procedure guideline 3.12 Aspiration/trephine procedure

Statement	Rationale
1. During the procedure under anaesthetic, monitor the child's: a) Oxygen saturations. b) Respiratory and pulse rate and pattern. c) Colour. d) Airway. e) Secretions. f) Consciousness level.	1. To monitor the child's cardio-pulmonary systems. c) To observe if the child needs suction or atropine if excessive secretions. f) To observe if the child needs further anaesthetic.

Procedure guideline 3.12 (*Continued*)

Statement	Rationale
2. During the procedure under local anaesthetic the parents/carers may wish to remain with their child.	2. To offer comfort and support.
3. The local anaesthetic must be checked as prescribed. a) The doctor will administer the local anaesthetic into the prepared puncture site and must wait for it to take effect.	3. To comply with hospital policy. a) To ensure effectiveness of the anaesthetic.
4. Once the child is ready, position them on the side where the aspirate will be performed, uppermost. This position must be maintained throughout the procedure ensuring an adequate airway is maintained.	4. To facilitate effective aspiration. To maintain safety of the child.
5. The doctor performing the procedure will comply with universal precautions and clean the site of the aspiration with an alcohol-based antiseptic and allow site to dry.	5. To minimise the risk of infection.
6. The marrow needle is inserted into the anaesthetised area and a 20 ml syringe is applied to the hub of the needle. If the marrow is hypercellular and difficult to aspirate, continue repeating the above procedure through the **same** skin puncture site until an adequate specimen is obtained.	6. To obtain an adequate sample for diagnosis.
7. Place the aspirate on the microscope slide and in the specimen pots.	7. To prepare sample for laboratory analysis.
8. Label slides and pots. Once dry place the slides in the slide container.	8. To ensure slides have the correct child's details on.
9. Withdraw the aspirate needle while applying pressure on the puncture site.	
10. Apply continuous pressure until the bleeding stops.	10. To minimise haematoma formation and pain.
11. Apply a dressing to the puncture site (i.e. plaster).	11. To minimise infection.
12. Dispose of used equipment as per hospital policy.	12. To comply with hospital policy.
13. Ensure specimens are sent to the appropriate laboratories.	13. To enable analysis to occur.
14. Record necessary information in appropriate healthcare records.	14. To ensure accurate data collection.

Procedure guideline 3.13 Post-procedure care (aspiration/trephine)

Statement	Rationale
1. Continue to monitor vital signs until the child is fully awake.	1. To ensure a safe recovery from anaesthetic.
2. Keep noise levels to a minimum while child is regaining consciousness.	2. To minimise distress.
3. If the procedure was under general anaesthetic, ask the parents/carers to return once their child is rousable.	3. To minimise the distress for the child and anxiety for the parents/carers (Sepion 1990).
4. Ensure oxygen and suction are available by the child's bed, and are functioning.	4. To maintain a safe environment.

(*Continued*)

Procedure guideline 3.13 (*Continued*)

Statement	Rationale
5. The child can return to their bed once rousable and may sleep in a semi-prone position. If awake the child can be cared for in whichever position is most comfortable.	**5.** To maintain a clear airway.
6. Prescribed analgesia given if needed and repeated as often as necessary.	**6.** To maintain a pain-free state.
7. Resume oral fluids and diet once the child is fully awake.	
8. Observe the puncture site for signs of bleeding. Contact the doctor if there are any problems.	**8.** To detect complications.
9. Inform the parents/carers: **a)** To repeat analgesia as prescribed. **b)** Their child may bathe/shower the following day. **c)** To remove the plaster/dressing within 24 hours.	**9.** **a)** To minimise pain. **b)** To continue normal hygiene practice. **c)** To minimise the risk of infection.
10. They will be informed of results as soon as possible.	**10.** To keep the family informed.

References

Autio L, Koozer K, Olson (2002). The four S's of wound management: Staples, sutures, steri-strips and sticky stuff. Holistic Nurse Practice, 16(2), 80–88

Bale S, Jones V. (1996) Caring for children with wounds. Journal of Wound Care, 5(4), 177–180

Bauer L, Hurst M, Rudge C, Sobeh M. (2000) Practical Procedures in Nephrology. London, Arnold

Briggs SM. (1996) The principles of a specific technique in wound care. Professional Nurse, 11(12), 805–810

Briggs M. (1997) The principles of a closed surgical wound care. Journal of Wound Care, 6(6), 288–292

Caione P, Micali S, Rinaldi S, Capozza N, Lais A, Matarazzo E, Maturo G, Micali F. (2000) Retroperitoneal laparoscopy for renal biopsy in children. Journal of Urology, 164, 1080–1083

Clark S, Radford M. (1986) Topical anaesthesia for venepuncture. Archives of Disease in Childhood, 61, 1132–1134

Coburn S, Mitchell S. (2002) Acute renal failure, early detection and prompt intervention can improve outcomes. American Journal of Nursing, 102(Supp 6–12) 1132–1134

Cohen MB, A-Kader HH, Lambers D, Heubi JE. (1992) Complications of percutaneous liver biopsy in children. Gastroenterology, 102, 629–632

Date A. (1994) The value of the graft biopsy in the care of renal transplant patients. Journal of Postgraduate Medicine, 40(3), 165–167

Dealey C. (1994). The Care of Wounds. Cambridge, Blackwell Science

Department of Health (2001a) Reference Guide to Consent for Examination or Treatment. DoH www.dh.gov.uk/assetRoot/04/01/90/79/040197079.pdf.

Department of Health (2001b) Consent – What you have a Right to Expect. A Guide for Children and Young People. DoH www.dh.gov.uk/assetRoot/04/01/90/21/04019021.pdf

Department of Health (2003) Winning Ways: Working Together to Reduce Healthcare Associated Infection in England. www.dh.gov.uk/assetRoot/04/06/46/89/04064689.pdf

Department of Health (2009) Reference guide to consent for examination or treatment, 2nd edition. Available at http://www.patient.co.uk/doctor/Consent-to-Treatment-in-Children.htm, http://www.dh.gov.uk/en/Publicationsandstatistics/Publications/PublicationsPolicyAndGuidance/DH_4008977 (children and young people), http://www.dh.gov.uk/en/Publicationsandstatistics/Publications/PublicationsPolicyAndGuidance/DH_4005202 (parents)]

Diamond LK. (1989) Forward. In: Miller DR, Baehnerk R, Miller LP (eds) Blood Diseases of Infancy and Childhood. St Louis, CV Mosby

Franklin L. (1998) Skin Cleansing and Infection Control in Peripheral Cannulation and Venepuncture. Paediatric Nursing, 10(9), 33–34

Frederick V. (1991) Paediatric IV Therapy: Soothing the patient. Registered Nurse, 54(12), 43–47

Godsell G. (1998) Performing diagnostic skin biopsies. Professional Nurse, 13(6), 368–371

Gonzalez-Vallina R, Alonso EA, Rand E, Black DB, Whitington PF. (1993) Outpatient percutaneous liver biopsy in children. Journal of Pediatric Gastroenterology and Nutrition, 17, 370–375

Grant A, Neuberger J. (1999) Guidelines on the use of liver biopsy in clinical practice. International Journal of Gastroenterology and Hepatology, 45(suppl IV), IV1–IV11

Harper J. (1990) Handbook of Paediatric Dermatology, 2nd edition. London, Butterworth Heinmann

Hatfield MK, Beres RA, Sane SS, Zaleski GX. (2008) Percutaneous image-guided solid organ core needle biopsy: Coaxial versus noncoaxial method. American Journal of Radiology, 190, 413–417

Heiney P. (1991) Helping children through painful procedures. American Journal of Nursing, 91, 20–24

Hoffer FA. (2000) Liver biopsy methods for paediatric oncology patients. Paediatric Radiology, 30(7),481–488

Hussain F, Watson A, Hayes J, Evans J. (2003) Standards for renal biopsies. A comparison of inpatient and day care procedures. Pediatric Nephrology, 18, 53–56

King L. (2003) Subcutaneous insulin injection technique. Nursing Standard, 17(34), 45–52, quiz 54–55

Lachaux A, Le Gall C, Chambon M, Regnier F, Loras-Duclaux L et al. (1995) Complications of percutaneous liver biopsy in infants and children. European Journal of Pediatrics, 154, 621–623

Langley P (1999) Guided Imagery: a review of the effectiveness in the care of children. Paediatric Nursing, 11(3), 18–21

Lawson RA, Smart NG, Gudgeon AC, Morton NS. (1995) Evaluaton of an amethocaine gel preparation for percutaneous analgesia before venous cannulation in children. British Journal of Anaesthesia, 75(3), 282–285

Litchtman S, Guzman C, Moore D, Weber JL, Roberts EA. (1987) Morbidity after percutaneous liver biopsy. Archives of Disease in Childhood, 62(9), 901–904

Lindor KD, Jorgensen RA, Rakela J, Bordas JM, Gros JB et al. (1996) The role of ultrasonography and automated-needle biopsy in outpatient percutaneous liver biopsy. Hepatology, 23, 1079–1083

Little AF, Ferris JV, Dodd GD, Baron RL. (1996) Image-guided percutaneous hepatic biopsy: Effect of ascites on the complication rate. Radiology, 199, 79–83

Macqueen S. (2008) Clinical Practice Guidelines. Hand Washing. London, Great Ormond Street Hospital for Children NHS Foundation Trust

McClaren S. (1992) Nutrition and wound healing. Journal of Wound Care, 1 (3), 45–55

McGill DB, Rakela J, Zinsmeister AR, Ott BJ. (1990) A 21-year experience with major haemorrhage after percutaneous liver biopsy. Gastroenterology, 99, 1396–1400

Morrison M. (1992) A Colour Guide to Nursing Management of Wounds. London, Wolfe

Niffeneger JP. (1997) Proper hand washing promotes wellness in childcare. Journal of Paediatric Health Care, Jan/Feb, 26–31

Nobili V, Comparcla D, Sartorelli MR, Natali G, Monti L et al. (2003) Biopsy and ultrasound-guided percutaneous liver biopsy in children. Pediatric Radiology, 33, 772–775

Orr FE. (1999) The role of the paediatric nurse in promoting paediatric right to consent. Journal of Clinical Nursing, 8(3), 291–298

Patient information: consent in children http://www.patient.co.uk/doctor/Consent-to-Treatment-in-Children.htm accessed October 6th 2011

Perraul J, McGill DB, Ott BJ, Taylor WF. (1978) Liver biopsy; Complications in 1,000 in-patients and outpatients. Gastroenterology, 74, 103–106

Pinkerton CR, Cushing P, Sepion B. (1993) Impact of diagnosis on the family. In: Pinkerton CR, Cushing P, Sepion B (eds). Childhood Cancer Management. London, Chapman and Hall, p 2

Postlethwaite RJ. (1994) Clinical Paediatric Nephrology, 2nd edition, pp. 465–471. Oxford, Oxford University Press

Price D, Tomsett A, Gartland C. (2000) Preparation for renal biopsy: a play package. Paediatric Nursing, 12(2), 38–39

RCN London Publication (number 001 999) (2003) Restraining, holding still and containing children and young people: Guidance for nursing staff. www.rcn.org.uk/members/downloads/restraining-holding-still-cyp.pdf

Rivera-Sanfeliz G, Kinney TB, Rose SC, Agha AK, Valji K et al (2005) Single pass percutaneous liver biopsy for diffuse liver disease using an automated device: experience in 154 procedures. Cardiovascular and Interventional Radiology, 28(5), 584–588

Robinson S, Collier J. (1997) Holding children still for procedures. Paediatric Nursing, (9)4, 12–14

Roebuck D. (2008) Focal liver lesion in children. Paediatric Radiology, 38 (Suppl 3), S518–522.

Schiemann AO, Barrios JM, Al-Tawil YS, Gray KM, Gilger MA. J (2000) Percutaneous liver biopsy in children: impact of ultrasonography and spring-loaded biopsy needles. Pediatric Gastroenterology Nutrition, 31(5), 536–539

Sclare I, Waring M. (1995) Routine venepuncture: improving services. Paediatric Nursing, 7(4), 23–27

Sepion B. (1990) Investigations, staging and diagnosis – Implications for nurses. In: Thanson J (ed.). The Child with Cancer – Nursing Care. London, Scutari Press

Simckes A, Blowey D, Gyves K, Alon U. (2000) Success and safety of same-day kidney biopsy in children and adolescents. Pediatric Nephrology, 14, 946–952

Sharma P, McDonald GB, Banaji MJ. (1982) The risk of bleeding after percutaneous liver biopsy: relation to platelet count. Clinical Gastroenterology, 4, 451–453

Smerdely P, Boyages S, We D. (1989) Topical iodine containing antiseptics for neonatal hypothyroidism in very low birth weight babies. Lancet, 2, 661–664

Smith & Nephew Ltd. (2003) Ametop product information. http://www.snwmd.co.uk

Smith TP, McDermott VG, Ayoub DM, Suhocki PV, Stackhouse DJ (1996) Percutaneous transhepatic liver biopsy with tract embolization. Radiology, 198, 769–774

Teare J. (1997) A home care team in paediatric wound care. Journal of Wound Care, 6(6), 295–296

Tomsett A, Watson A. (1996) Renal biopsy as a day case procedure. Paediatric Nursing, 8, (5), 14–15

Tomson C. (2003) Indications for renal biopsy in chronic renal disease. Clinical Medicine, 3(6), 513–517

Tortora G. (1994) Introduction to the Human Body: Essentials of Anatomy and Physiology. New York, Harper Collins

Trott A. (1997) Wound and Lacerations: Emergency Care and Closure, 2nd edition. St Louis, Mosby

United Nations General Assembly (1989) Convention on the Rights of the Child. http://www.nrweb.ord/legal/child.html

Vidhun J, Masciandro J, Varch L, Salvatierra O, Sarwal M. (2003) Safety and risk stratification of percutaneous biopsies of adult-sized renal allografts in infants and older pediatric recipients. Transplantation, 76(3), 552–557

Wallace M. (1998) Anatomy and physiology of the kidney. ORN Journal, 68(5), 799–790, 803–804, 806, 808, 810–811, 813–816, 819–824, 827–828

Webb N, Postlethwaite R. (2003) Clinical Paediatric Nephrology, 3rd edition, pp. 131–132. Oxford, Oxford University Press

Whittier W, Korbet S. (2004) Timing and complications in percutaneous renal biopsy. Journal of the American Society of Nephrology, 15(1), 142–147

Winslow EH, Jacobson A, Peragallo-Dittko V. (1997) Rethinking subcutaneous injection technique. American Journal of Nursing, 97(5), 71–72

Chapter 4

Administration of blood components and products

Chapter contents

Procedure guidelines

The Great Ormond Street Hospital Manual of Children's Nursing Practices, First Edition. Edited by Susan Macqueen, Elizabeth Anne Bruce, Faith Gibson.
© 2012 Great Ormond Street Hospital for Children NHS Foundation Trust. Published 2012 by Blackwell Publishing Ltd.

Introduction

Children experience a wide range of chronic diseases, such as haemophilia, sickle cell disease or thalassaemia, leukaemia, or immune deficiency, as well as acute life-threatening episodes such as burns (see Chapter 6), or road traffic accidents, which require treatment with blood components. These may be red cells, platelets, plasma or derivatives of plasma such as coagulation factors, immunoglobulin or albumin. The administration of these components is in itself simple; however, potential hazards such as human error, transfusion reaction, infection, antibody development, and anaphylaxis (see Chapter 2) may be severe (Serious Hazards of Transfusion 2008). For some families, the use of blood components is considered to be unacceptable, due to religious and/or cultural beliefs or and concerns over transmission of infectious diseases. These will be addressed later in this chapter.

Administration of any blood component should form part of a care-plan, involving a trained practitioner, the child and the family/carer. Children with inherited abnormalities such as haemophilia or immune deficiency may require life-long therapy, for these children their parents/carers may administer blood components to them at home, or they may even self-infuse. It is therefore imperative that they, their family/carers and primary/community nurses are involved in the care planning process.

This chapter describes:

- An overview of the history of transfusion
- Nursing practice guidelines relating to:
  - Administration of red blood cells, platelets, plasma and cryoprecipitate
  - Administration of albumin
  - Administration of immunoglobulin
  - Administration of coagulation factors.

An overview of blood transfusion

It is surprising that this relatively simple and yet life-saving procedure has only become part of routine clinical care within the past 100 years. While venesection (blood letting) has been common practice since the times of Hippocrates (approx. 420 BC), evidence of blood transfusion did not appear until after the discovery of the blood circulation by William Harvey in 1628, with written evidence of transfusion in 1666 when, in Oxford, blood was transfused from one dog to another (Giangrande 2000).

Blundell, an obstetrician at Guys Hospital in London, performed the first recorded human blood transfusion in 1828. He recognised that women often died from post-partum haemorrhage and having seen the results of transfusion of blood in animals applied this technique to humans, but realised that only human blood should be used in humans following the death of a dog from transfused human blood (Blundell 1828).

Initially blood transfusion was carried out without knowledge of blood groups, and not surprisingly many recipients died. In 1900, in Vienna, Karl Landsteiner identified four distinct blood groups (now known as A, B, AB, and O). By the 1920s, blood grouping became universal practice and in 1921, Percy Oliver at King's College Hospital London, established the world's first blood donor service. Sister Linstead, a nurse at King's, gave blood for this patient and the first British Red Cross Transfusion Service was established (Giangrande 2000). In 1922 this service was used 13 times, in 2009 National Health Service Blood and Transplant (NHSBT) collected 2.1 million donations (NHSBT 2010).

Despite this vast number of collections, the demand for blood remains high. Whole blood is rarely used, as most recipients only require part of the donation. Almost all donations are separated into their components (red cells, platelets, fresh frozen plasma ([FFP]), cryoprecipitate [Cryo]), coagulation factors, immunoglobulin and albumin). These are used singly or in combination as necessary to treat children; for example, a child with liver disease may receive individual coagulation factors as well as platelet and red cell transfusions.

Since the 1980s, the viruses that cause hepatitis A, B and C, cytomegalovirus (CMV), human T-cell leukaemia viruses (HTLV) I and II and human immunodeficiency virus (HIV) have been identified. In each case tests have been developed to detect virally positive donors who are then excluded from donor panels. The risk of being infected with these viruses from UK donated blood components is now extremely low. However, blood components should still be considered to be potentially infectious and their administration should be avoided unless there is no other option. Viral inactivation processes, such as treatment with methylene blue or solvent detergent are utilised for plasma components. There are concerns regarding the spread of variant Creutzfeldt-Jakob disease (vCJD) by transfusion of infected blood components. The prion protein responsible for vCJD is detectable in white cells, platelets and plasma (Wallington 2000) suggesting that transmission via transfusion is possible (Peden et al 2004). However, although over 2 million blood components are transfused annually, only a small number of recipients have become infected. Several steps have been introduced in the UK to prevent the spread of vCJD.

Since 1999, all NHSBT components are white cell depleted. Since 2004 potential donors who have themselves been transfused are no longer able to donate and also since 2004 FFP for use by children has been sourced from the United States of America. US sourced cryoprecipitate has been used since it became readily available in the UK in 2009.

It is good practice to screen children who receive repeated blood transfusions, for known blood-borne pathogens and to vaccinate them against hepatitis B.

In 1996, the Serious Hazards of Transfusion (SHOT) committee was established to monitor blood transfusion safety. The 2008 SHOT report contains a chapter relating to paediatric cases and summarises reported incidents involving children, these are most commonly incidents of incorrect blood component transfusion and are due to:

- Failure to meet special requirements such as irradiated or CMV negative products
- Miscalculated prescriptions (over/under transfusion)
- Failure of correct patient identification process.

The most important role that nurses have is ensuring that the blood component they are giving is for the right child – by following hospital procedure, checking the blood component against the prescription AND the child's wrist band, which MUST be attached to the child and not to their cot or bed. The wristband is the final identifying protector of a child who cannot identify themselves. In the community or in exceptional cases, where children are not wearing hospital

identity bracelets, local policy for checking the child's identity must be in place.

Cultural and religious belief may affect treatment with blood components. The most numerous group who fall into this category are Jehovah's Witnesses who refuse to accept blood transfusion based on literal interpretation of a number of passages in The Bible (Genesis 9:4, Leviticus 17:14 and Acts 15:20, 15:29 and 21:25). Some may accept fractionated blood products (albumin, immunoglobulin, coagulation factors) and these with careful surgical techniques may avoid the need for blood transfusion. In children with life-threatening bleeding or diseases where blood or platelet transfusion is unavoidable it might be necessary to apply for a court order (see Chapter 1).

Recent advances in the use of cell salvage and pre-operative haemoglobin elevation by the use of iron and/or erythropoetin supplementation (Spahn and Casutt 2000) have reduced the need for transfusion in elective surgery. Children and adults with haemophilia are now treated with genetically engineered factor VIII and IX. Recombinant technology will continue to affect 'blood' component therapy in the future.

Administration of red cells

The term 'red cells' describes several components, which are available for transfusion and which are used in different circumstances. Whole blood is rarely used and available by special order only. Red cells in additive solution (SAG-M, saline adenine glucose mannitol)) are used for children with blood loss, anaemia or leukaemia, where transfusion of 4ml/kg will raise the haemoglobin by 1g/dl.

Administration of platelets

Platelets are produced by two processes: single donor (apheresis) or pooled from four donors. Single donor platelets are used in children to reduce donor exposure; these can be divided into neonatal packs for use in neonates and small children. Human leukocyte antigen (HLA) matched platelets are available on a named patient basis for children who have either developed or are at risk of developing HLA antibodies. Platelets in PAS (platelet additive solution) are platelets where most of the plasma has been removed; these are used for children who react to plasma components, e.g. those who have allergic reactions to HLA matched platelets or those with some immune deficiencies.

Administration of fresh frozen plasma (FFP)

FFP for children is manufactured from single donations, from untransfused, American male donors. All donations are virally inactivated by methylene blue treatment. The decision to source this plasma from the US was taken to further minimise the risk of vCJD. FFP is used to correct abnormal clotting, disseminated intravascular coagulation, in liver disease and cardiac surgery or when there is a known single coagulation factor deficiency for which a coagulation factor concentrate is unavailable, e.g. factor V deficiency.

Administration of cryoprecipitate

Cryoprecipitate is produced by freezing and thawing FFP, the precipitate contains significant quantities of factor VIII and fibrinogen which is used to treat abnormal clotting and low fibrinogen levels.

The general principles for IV administration are covered in **Chapter 13**. The following additional procedures and information are related to the specifics of administration of blood products.

Procedure guideline 4.1 Preparation – child and family (transfusion)

Statement	Rationale
1. Inform the child and family of the following: • That a blood component transfusion is necessary • The reason for the transfusion • What it entails • The likely duration of the process • Obtain and document consent.	1. To inform the child/parent/carer and address any issues or concerns they may have. To obtain 'informed consent'.
2. Ensure the child is wearing an identity wristband.	2. To enable positive patient identification.
3. Ensure pre-transfusion vital signs are recorded (no more than 60 minutes before commencement of transfusion): • Temperature • Respiration rate • Pulse • Blood pressure.	3. To establish baseline parameters for the child; these may alter if a reaction occurs.
4. Ensure venous access has been established.	4. To enable infusion to commence.

Procedure guideline 4.2 Preparation – prescription (transfusion)

Statement	Rationale
1. Blood products must only be administered if prescribed on a prescription chart. Blood components must be prescribed by an appropriately trained, competent and locally authorised, practitioner.	1. To ensure the correct treatment of the child. To comply with the Guideline on the Administration of Blood Components (BSCH 2012)

2. The prescription should include:
• Patient demographics:
  ○ First name and family name
  ○ Hospital number
  ○ Date of birth
• Date and time infusion required
• Type of blood component to be administered
• Any special requirements, e.g. gamma-irradiation, CMV-seronegative
• Volume in **ml** to be transfused
• A suitable infusion rate for the child
• An infusion time of 4 hours or less.
	2. To ensure the correct volume of product is administered to the correct child.
	   To ensure transfusion completed within 4 hours of product removal from storage to reduce risk of infection.

3. Ensure there is sufficient blood component supplied to meet the prescription requirements.	3. To enable Blood Bank and clinical area to plan adequately.
4. If administering an intravenous pre-medication of an anti-histamine and steroid do so prior to commencing transfusion.	4. To prevent reactions in children who have reacted previously.
5. Ensure there are instructions for what should happen after the transfusion.	5. To ensure planning takes place.

Procedure guideline 4.3 Preparation – transfusion

Statement	Rationale
1. Arrange for the collection of the blood component from storage.	1. To ensure blood component is in optimum condition for use.
2. The person collecting the component must have documentation containing the child's: • First name and family name • NHS/Hospital number • Date of birth. The details on the documentation must match the details on the blood component label.	2. To ensure the correct component is collected for the child.
3. When a blood component is collected it must be checked out, stating date and time of removal from storage, according to local systems in use. Documentation of receipt of component on the ward should be returned to Blood Bank.	3. To enable blood component traceability and documentation of 'cold chain' in order to comply with the UK Blood Safety and Quality Regulations (2005).

(Continued)

Procedure guideline 4.3 (*Continued*)

Statement	Rationale
4. Check the child's details are the same on the blood component label, prescription and report form, i.e. • First name and family name • NHS/Hospital number • Date of birth.	**4.** To ensure correct component is given to the correct child.
5. An appropriate blood component administration set, which has an integral 170–200μm micro-aggregate filter, should be used. Paediatric blood administration sets, with a smaller priming volume, are appropriate for small volume transfusions Infusion pumps and syringe drivers can be used, **provided** they are verified as safe for this purpose. Blood components administered using a syringe driver require an administration system that should incorporate an integral three-way system. However, care should be taken as this system carries an inherent risk. When using an administration set of this type: • The component bag **must** remain attached throughout the procedure • The transfer of patient and blood component details to the syringe is not advised • The three-way system must be checked prior to transfusion • A new syringe and administration set should be used when administering different components • Blood components from more than one donation should not be mixed in the syringe, but given sequentially using a new syringe.	**5.** To remove particulate matter, e.g. fibrin and to prevent cell damage to blood products. To reduce wastage in the administration set. To ensure Positive Patient Identification. Due to risk of transcription errors. To ensure the component is administered from the syringe and **not** allowed to flow freely from the component bag. In order to be able to identify the relevant donation in case of a reaction.

6. When preparing the transfusion:
• Check the child's details are the same on the component bag and prescription:
  ○ First name and family name
  ○ NHS/Hospital number
  ○ Date of birth
• Check unit number on label and component bag are the same and match the details on the report form
• Check the blood group on the component is compatible with that of the child
• Check the expiry date of the component
• Check any special requirements are met, e.g. CMV negative, irradiated components
• Check the bag is intact.
	6. To ensure the correct component is given to the correct child, preventing incompatibility, administration of out-of-date components, preventing infection.

7. Prime the administration set using universal precautions and aseptic non-touch technique.	**7.** To minimise the risk of infection, prevent air embolism and ensure the set is patent.
8. If the transfusion is cancelled at this point inform the Blood Transfusion Laboratory.	**8.** To ensure the Blood Transfusion Laboratory records are accurate.

Procedure guideline 4.4 Infuse component – identity check and administration

Statement	Rationale
1. Check the child's identity wristband and prescription chart.	1. To ensure the components are being administered to the correct child.
2. Check the child's details on the component label and prescription chart match for: • First name and family name • NHS/Hospital number • Date of birth.	2. To ensure the component is being administered to the correct child.
3. Recheck the child's identity using the wristband.	3. To ensure correct patient identification.
4. Connect the prepared blood component to the child according to the relevant intravenous therapy guidelines using the general principles of IV administration.	4. To reduce risk of infection.
5. Set the infusion rate according to the prescription **but** ensure the infusion is completed within 4 hours of removal of blood component from appropriate storage.	5. To ensure it is administered within 4 hours.

Procedure guideline 4.5 Infuse product – observations, recordings and traceability

Statement	Rationale
1. Closely monitor the child for the first 30 minutes of transfusion. This should be negotiated with any family members in attendance. Regular visual observations should continue throughout the transfusion.	1. This is when reactions are most likely to occur.
2. Record the date and time of starting infusion in the child's medical records and sign that you are responsible for its administration.	2. To ensure accuracy of records and determine accountability for infusion.
3. Ensure positive traceability for each blood component transfusion is recorded by sending details of the transfusion to the Blood Transfusion Laboratory.	3. To comply with current legislation.

4. Observations should be undertaken and clearly documented for every unit transfused. Minimum monitoring must include:
• Pulse rate, blood pressure, temperature and respiration rate:
  ○ No more than 60 minutes prior to the start of the transfusion
  ○ 15 minutes after the start of the transfusion
  ○ No more than 60 minutes after the completion of the transfusion.
• If the child becomes unwell or shows signs or symptoms of a transfusion reaction further observations should be undertaken, recorded and appropriate action taken
• Routine patient observations, as defined by the clinical area, should be continued throughout the transfusion period.
	4. To monitor for any potential complications and comply with the BCSH guidelines (2009).

(Continued)

79

Procedure guideline 4.5 (Continued)

Statement	Rationale
5. Check cannula site half hourly for: • Redness, swelling/inflammation • Pallor • Leakage/oozing • Skin temperature change • Tenderness. If ANY appear **STOP** the transfusion.	**5.** To monitor for extravasation and phlebitis.
6. Record the following hourly: • Transfusion rate • Volume infused • Total volume infused.	**6.** To ensure the rate remains correct, prevent over-transfusion and ensure the pump or syringe driver (if used) is working correctly.
7. Observe the child throughout the transfusion for signs of transfusion reactions: • Sweating/fever • Rash/mottled appearance • Dizziness • Flushing • Tachycardia • Nausea • Chills/rigors • Laboured breathing/wheezing • Chest or loin pain • Loss of consciousness • Sudden collapse.	**7.** To ensure the safety of the child.

Administration of albumin

Albumin is available in two strengths: 4.5% is used to increase the serum albumin levels and to expand plasma; 20% is used when there are problems of fluid overload and when sodium levels are either high or low. The stronger 20% albumin is available in 10–100 ml doses while doses of 4.5% are in 100–500 ml. Albumin is most commonly used in hypovolaemia to restore volume, in hypoproteinaemia and in hypoalbuminaemia to replace protein and to maintain blood pressure. It is most commonly used in children with renal and liver disease.

Albumin is administered as an intravenous infusion follow the guidelines in Chapter 13, and administration of red cells and platelets in this chapter. Additionally follow procedure 4.7 below.

Administration of immunoglobulin

Immunoglobulin is a blood product prepared from pooled human plasma, which carries a degree of risk from viral transmission. To minimise the risk of transmitting infections such as hepatitis, all plasma is obtained from selected screened donors, and then undergoes validated, virus inactivation processes during the manufacturing designed to inactivate most common viruses, including HIV, hepatitis B and hepatitis C.

Immunoglobulin is used in the treatment of children with inherited primary antibody deficiency or other complex immunodeficiency disorders to prevent life-threatening infections. In addition, it can be used as supportive therapy for secondary immunodeficiencies where intensive treatments, such as chemotherapy have caused temporary damage to the immune system, e.g. during stem cell transplantation. The aim of treatment is prevention of infection by providing passive immunity through antibody replacement from plasma; therefore children have some degree of protection from common infections such as measles and chickenpox and many other viral and bacterial infections. Children on immunoglobulin replacement therefore do not need the routine childhood immunisations.

Immunoglobulin therapy has also been shown to be effective in a wide range of other diseases, for example Kawasaki's disease and idiopathic thrombocytopenic purpura where 'modulation' of the immune system is required, although the exact mechanism of action is not understood.

Before commencing immunoglobulin therapy a risk assessment should be undertaken. Parents/carers and children should have the opportunity to discuss the implications of treatment, including practical aspects, patient friendly information leaflets should be provided and consent/assent should be obtained and recorded in the case notes.

Procedure guideline 4.6 Reaction management (transfusion)

Statement	Rationale
1. If the child shows signs of a reaction: • Stop the transfusion • Maintain IV access • Inform doctor • Record vital signs • Give prescribed steroid and anti-histamine • Record incident in child's healthcare records • Continue transfusion when child has recovered, if appropriate • Inform Blood Transfusion Laboratory • **Remember the 4-hour rule** • Report incident according to local trust protocol.	1. To stop/reduce the reaction, maintain accurate records, and maintain patency of IV line.

2. If a severe reaction occurs:
• Stop transfusion **immediately**
• Maintain IV access
• Seek **urgent** medical assistance
• Give prescribed steroid and anti-histamine if prescribed
• Record vital signs
• Record incident in child's healthcare records
• **Do not recommence transfusion**
• Inform Blood Transfusion Laboratory and:
  ○ Return blood component and administration set to the laboratory
  ○ Send a full blood count
  ○ Send a sample to Blood Transfusion (for transfusion reaction assessment)
  ○ Obtain a urine sample collected after the reaction
• Report incident according to local trust protocol.
	2. To stop the reaction and minimise the impact, maintain accurate records, maintain patency of IV line and assist in investigation of the incident.

Procedure guideline 4.7 Infuse component (albumin)

Statement	Rationale
1. Set infusion rate according to prescription BUT ensure infusion is completed within **3 hours** following the manufacturer's instructions.	1. To maintain the effectiveness of the component, to meet the manufacturer's recommendations and to minimise the risk of infection.
2. **Remember albumin may need to be changed during the infusion if the prescribed rate means that the above recommendation will be exceeded.**	
3. Intravenous administration set should be flushed with 20 ml normal saline to ensure the total amount of albumin prescribed is infused.	3. The administration set may retain up to 20 ml of albumin.
4. Give diuretic **if** prescribed at required time according to the Drug Policy.	4. To prevent fluid overload especially if fluids are being restricted.

Procedure guideline 4.8 Observations and recordings (albumin)

Statement	Rationale
1. Record date and time of starting the infusion.	1. To ensure accuracy of records.
2. Sign that you are administering the albumin.	2. To determine who is accountable for the infusion.
3. Record the batch of the albumin in the child's notes.	3. To assist component and child tracing.
4. Establish the frequency and type of observations that the child may require during the infusion according to their clinical condition.	
5. Do not leave the child unattended for the first 30 minutes of the infusion.	5. This is when reactions are most likely to occur.
6. This should be negotiated with any family members in attendance.	
7. If a reaction occurs inform Pharmacy and seek advice.	7. To assist investigation of incident.
8. If more than one bottle is required the same administration set can be used.	
9. If large volumes of albumin are required this should be planned with the department supplying the albumin.	9. To ensure adequate stock is available.

Immunoglobulin is usually given as an intravenous infusion (IVIG) but it can also be given by rapid subcutaneous infusion (SCIG). With new products being licensed specifically for this purpose, SCIG is becomingly increasingly popular as a safe and effective treatment, particularly in small children where venous access is difficult. It is also easy to administer at home, with parents/carers being taught how to administer this treatment.

It is considered poor practice to change products once a child is established on one particular product, because the components are not identical, and children who tolerate one product may not tolerate another. In addition, switching components exposes the child to another plasma pool and increases the risk of exposure to blood borne viruses.

Minor adverse reactions occur relatively frequently during and after the first few infusions, while more severe reactions are uncommon when the infusions are administered appropriately. Most systemic adverse reactions are associated with the intravenous route and occur when infusions are given too quickly or if there is a concurrent febrile illness.

Immunoglobulin is administered either as a subcutaneous or an intravenous infusion. The general principles for IV therapy are covered in Chapter 13 and administration of blood are given previously in this chapter. The following additional procedures and information are related to the specifics of administration of intravenous immunoglobulin and subcutaneous immunoglobulin infusions.

Procedure guideline 4.9 Preparation – child and family (immunoglobulin)

Statement	Rationale
1. Carry out a risk assessment to ensure the family understand the need for treatment and how it is administered: • **Intravenous** • **Subcutaneous** – use with caution if the child has low platelets.	1. To inform the family and gain consent. • To reduce the risk of severe bruising.
2. Explain the procedure to the child and family and include: a) The reason for treatment. b) The risks and benefits. c) The options for on-going treatment.	2. To prepare them for treatment and obtain consent. c) To plan ahead and liaise with local services.

Procedure guideline 4.9 (*Continued*)

Statement	Rationale
3. Assess that the child is fit for treatment and perform baseline observation of temperature, respiration rate, heart rate.	3. To establish the normal for the child, ruling out pre-existing disease processes.
4. Weigh the child.	4. To calculate the dose.
5. Complete pre-treatment blood tests and investigations: • Immunoglobulin trough levels (IgGAM) • Serum and plasma for long-term storage (store Ig) • Liver function tests • Hepatitis C screen.	5. • To monitor treatment efficacy • To enable look back in the event of an infectious outbreak • To monitor the effectiveness of treatment.

Procedure guideline 4.10 Preparation – prescription (immunoglobulin)

Statement	Rationale
1. Immunoglobulin is a blood product and **MUST NOT** be administered unless prescribed on the child's prescription chart.	1. To ensure treatment is necessary and given as prescribed.
2. Calculate the dose: a) Replacement therapy – 300–500 mg/kg/3 weeks. b) Modulation – 1–2 g/kg (single dose). c) Round the dose to the nearest whole bottle.	a) To give appropriate dose. c) To prevent wastage.
3. Prescribe the **named product** to be used. Calculate the infusion rate in ml/hr (rate is product specific and should be calculated in ml/kg/hr).	3. To avoid product switching. For intravenous infusion rates the product insert should be read.
4. Prescribe pre-medication if required. a) Check the product dose, batch number and expiry date. b) Record in the child's medical and nursing records and blood product register. c) Ensure immunoglobulin is at room temperature. d) Check the child's identity band and prescription according to the Drug Policy before starting the infusion.	4. Pre-medication is usually only given if there has been a recent infusion reaction. a) To avoid medication errors. b) This enables accurate recording of infusion details. c) This is more comfortable and avoids chilling the child. d) To ensure the immunoglobulin is being administered to the correct child.

Procedure guideline 4.11 Preparation – equipment for intravenous or subcutaneous infusion of immunoglobulin

Statement	Rationale
1. Gather equipment for **intravenous** infusion (see Chapter 13).	1. To ensure safe infusion.
2. Topical local anesthetic creams may be used.	2. To minimise discomfort of procedure.
1. Gather equipment for **subcutaneous** infusion.	1. To ensure safe infusion.
2. Apply local anaesthetic cream to sites 1–2 hours prior to infusion.	2. To minimise discomfort.
3. Ensure pumps are available and working.	3. For safe subcutaneous infusion.

Procedure guideline 4.12 Procedure – intravenous infusion (immunoglobulin)

Statement	Rationale
1. If using powder/diluent read mixing instructions carefully.	1. To reconstitute as per manufacturer's instructions.
2. Prime administration set with immunoglobulin using universal precautions and an aseptic non-touch technique.	2. To minimise the risk of infection.
3. Check the child's identity band and prescription according to the Drug Policy.	3. To ensure the immunoglobulin is being connected to the right child.
4. Infuse immunoglobulin a the prescribed rate, starting slowly, and increasing to maximum rate over 30–60 minutes.	4. To minimise the risk of, and promptly detect adverse reactions.
5. Do not leave the child unattended during the infusion as there is risk of adverse reactions.	5. To monitor for potential adverse reactions (see adverse reactions).
6. **This should be negotiated with any family members in attendance.** Check peripheral infusion access site half hourly for: • Inflammation (tenderness, swelling, redness) • Leakage.	6. To detect for signs of extravasation (see additional information in IV infusion guidelines).
7. Check the site and the infusion system is intact and record the infusion rate and pressures, hourly volume infused and total volume infused.	7. To ensure rate remains correct, to detect signs of extravasation and to ensure infusion pump is working correctly.
8. The intravenous solution administration set will need flushing with 0.9% sodium chloride **if the total amount of immunoglobulin infused is less that 100 ml.**	8. The administration set may retain up to 20 ml of the product.

Procedure guideline 4.13 Procedure – subcutaneous infusion (immunoglobulin)

Statement	Rationale
1. Select suitable infusion sites, abdomen, thighs or buttocks: a) Thighs are preferred in children under 2 years. b) Abdomen is preferred in older children as the thighs become more muscular.	1. a) To minimise discomfort and swelling. b) To promote steady absorption.
2. Remove local anaesthetic cream (if used) 5 minutes before needles are inserted.	2. To allow the skin to dry and maximise its effect.
3. Draw up the drug for the infusion in the syringe and prime the administration line using a no touch technique.	3. To prevent infection.
4. Lift a skin fold and insert the needle into the subcutaneous tissue. The angle of insertion will depend on the needle type, length and the amount of subcutaneous tissue the child has.	4. To prevent the needle going into the muscle underneath.
5. Secure the needle with tape or occlusive dressing as appropriate.	5. To prevent the infusion being dislodged.

Procedure guideline 4.13 (*Continued*)

Statement	Rationale
6. Assess the child's subcutaneous tissue to decide on infusion rate: • 5–10 ml can be infused in babies 1–6 months over 1 hr • <10 ml can be infused in 40–60 mins in children under 7 years • 10–25 ml can be infused in 60–90 mins in older children • >30 ml may need to be split between two sites. NB Initial discomfort at the site is normal.	**6.** To maximise the child's comfort and mobility.
7. Set the pump at the appropriate rate for the syringe size: **a)** Observe the child. **b)** Record details of the infusion, site, rate. **c)** Check the infusion site. NB Swelling and redness at the site is normal, but will disappear 24hrs after the infusion.	**7.** To observe for leakage.
8. Do not leave the child unattended during the infusion as there is risk of adverse reactions. This may be negotiated with any family members in attendance.	**8.** To monitor for potential adverse reactions (see adverse reactions).

Procedure guideline 4.14 Reaction management (immunoglobulin)

Statement	Rationale
1. If the reaction is mild: • Headache • Fever, chills, sweating • Flushing • Nausea. Reduce the infusion rate, administer paracetamol/ibuprofen.	**1.** To minimise reaction and to make the child comfortable.
2. If the reaction is moderate: • Vomiting • Severe headache, dizziness • Urticarial rash, wheals • Mild wheezing • Chest pain. **a)** Stop the infusion. **b)** Call medical assistance.	**a)** To stop reaction. **b)** To make the child comfortable while assessing them and treating with anti-histamine.
3. If the reaction is severe: • Tightness of throat or chest • Difficulty breathing or wheezing • Back or loin pain/darkened urine • Loss of consciousness • Sudden collapse. **a) Stop the infusion** and infuse 0.9% sodium chloride. **b)** Call urgent medical assistance. **c)** Record incident in child's healthcare records. **d)** Complete an incident report form. **e)** Continue the infusion when possible.	**a)** To minimise impact from reaction. **b)** To make the child comfortable while assess them and treating with anti-histamine and steroids. **c)** To maintain accurate records. **d)** To promote accurate recording of incidents. **e)** To fully treat the child.

Procedure guideline 4.15 Completing the infusion (immunoglobulin)

Statement	Rationale
1. Dispose of equipment in a sharps bin in accordance with the Trust Waste policy.	1. To reduce risk of infection by safe disposal.
2. Document in the child's medical and nursing healthcare records and blood products register: • The batch of the immunoglobulin • Date and time of starting infusion • Sign that you are responsible for its administration.	2. To ensure accuracy of records, assist product and child tracing and determine accountability for the infusion.

Administration of coagulation factors

Single, plasma derived or recombinant, coagulation factors (factors VII, VIII, IX, XI, XIII, fibrinogen, von-Willebrand factor, antithrombin and protein C concentrates) are generally available in 250 iu, 500 iu and 1000 iu vials and occasionally in vials of 1500 iu, 2000 iu or 3000 iu. These are mainly used by children with congenital bleeding disorders such as haemophilia. They can also be used in combination for children with acquired coagulation disorders such as those with liver or cardiac disease. Genetically engineered factor VII, VIII, IX and XIII are available and pose minimal risk of transfusion of human blood-borne viruses and are generally considered 'safe' for use in any child.

Many children with bleeding disorders have life-long replacement therapy, administered at home by their parents/carers, themselves and their community nurses. This is done in partnership between the hospital, community team and family. All aspects of discharge planning, procedures for undertaking this care as a community nurse etc are covered in Chapter 1.

With the exception of fibrinogen concentrate all coagulation factors are administered by bolus intravenous injection, through a 23 G butterfly (unless a cannula or central venous access is in situ). The guidelines for administration of IV injection (see Chapter 13) should be followed. Fibrinogen concentrate is given as an intravenous infusion following the guidelines in (Chapter 13). Coagulation factors **MUST NOT** be filtered as this will lead to the coagulation factors being removed by the filters, leading to the administration of a sub-optimal dose and resulting in bleeding.

Conclusion

Administration of blood and its components is both a life-saving and potentially life-threatening procedure. It is imperative that the administration of these products, in hospitals and the community, is undertaken following rigorous training and procedure. For many children administration of these products is part of their everyday lives and parental/self-administration in the community facilitates good quality of life outcomes for them and their families (Khair 2002).

References

Blundell J. (1828) Observations on transfused blood by Dr Blundell with a description of his gravitor. Lancet, ii, 321–324

British Committee for Standards in Haematology (BCSH) (2012) Guidelines on the Administration of Blood Components. Available at www.bcshguidelines.com (last accessed 4th January 2012)

Giangrande P. (2000) Historical review – the history of blood transfusion. British Journal of Haematology, 110, 758–767

Khair K. (2002) Pilot testing of the 'Haemo-QoL' quality of life questionnaire for haemophiliac children in six European countries. Haemophilia, 8, 47–54

National Health Service Blood and Transplant Annual Review 2010/11 www.nhsbt.nhs.uk/annual review (last accessed January 2012)

Peden AH, Head MW, et al. (2004) Preclinical vCJD after blood transfusion in a PRNP codon 129 heterozygous patient. Lancet, 364(9433), 527–529

Serious Hazards of Transfusion (2008) Annual Report. Available at http://www.shotuk.org/wp-content/uploads/2010/03/SHOT-Report-2008.pdf (last accessed 21st October 2011)

Spahn D, Casutt M (2000) Eliminating blood transfusions new aspects and perspectives. Anaesthesiology, 93, 242–249

DoH (2005) The Blood Safety and Quality Regulations (2005) (Available at http://www.legislation.gov.uk/uksi/2005/50/resources (last accessed 21st October 2011)

Wallington TB (2000) CJD/vCJD research within the NBS and its Partners Blood Matters (3). Available at http://www.blood.co.uk/pdf/publications/blood_matters_3.pdf (last accessed 21st October 2011)

Bowel care

Chapter contents

Procedure guidelines

Introduction

Elimination has been cited by Roper *et al* (1990) as one of the activities of daily living. As nurses it is important to understand the elimination routines of the children and young people in the hospital's care and cater for any variations. Although elimination is a natural body function, there is a lot of taboo surrounding the subject and discussion can cause embarrassment and discomfort. Consideration must be given to religious and cultural beliefs, particularly in relation to acceptance of an altered body image following stoma formation (Black 2009a).

Various methods can be used to empty or clean the bowel. Different approaches are used in different circumstances. In the majority of cases it is preferable to use laxatives. However, if the child has a mechanical obstruction of the bowel, laxative use may be contra-indicated. Stimulating peristalsis in an obstructed bowel will cause increased discomfort and possibly perforation. Emptying or cleansing the bowel is necessary to: treat constipation; prepare the bowel for investigation or surgery; or to control faecal incontinence.

This chapter includes guidelines on the following practices:

- Management of constipation
- Management of diarrhoea
- Administering a suppository
- Administering an enema
- Rectal washout (infant)
- Rectal washout (older child)
- Colonic irrigation (ACE washout)
- Stoma care.

For further information, the reader is directed to the National Institute for Clinical Excellence (NICE) guideline on the management of constipation in children and young people (NICE 2010).

Constipation

Constipation is a common childhood condition and is responsible for 90–95% of all bowel problems in children. In most cases the constipation develops as a result of a number of factors, which is then often made worse by the passage of a large painful stool, which perpetuates the problem when the child begins to associate pain with having their bowels opened (Loening-Baucke 1998).

There have been a number of definitions of constipation but it is now generally accepted that for a diagnosis of constipation to be made it must include two or more of the following in a child with a developmental age of at least 4 years with insufficient criteria for diagnosis of irritable bowel syndrome (IBS):

1. Two or fewer defecations in the toilet per week.
2. At least one episode of faecal incontinence per week.
3. History of retentive posturing or excessive volitional stool retention.
4. History of painful or hard bowel movements.
5. Presence of a large faecal mass in the rectum.
6. History of large diameter stools that may obstruct the toilet.

Criteria must be fulfilled at least once per week for at least 2 months before diagnosis (Rasquin *et al* 2006).

It is expected that most children will open their bowels at least three times per week, however it has been shown that the consistency, as well as frequency of the stool is of equal importance. The awareness of stools that are difficult or painful to pass is important, as it has been identified that a high number of children develop constipation as a result of experiencing pain with defecation (Loening-Baucke 2007). This is obviously an important trigger factor for the development of constipation and questions regarding stool consistency and presence of pain or discomfort should always be included in any paediatric continence assessment.

Constipation can be divided into two types:

1. Idiopathic(functional) constipation – the majority of children will present with this type of constipation where there is no underlying cause.
2. Constipation associated with an underlying disorder – either with the bowel – such as Hirschsprung's disease, neurological – such as spina bifida or systemic – such as hypothyroidism.

Idiopathic constipation

For the majority of children with constipation the problem is functional or 'idiopathic'. Constipation is referred to as 'idiopathic' if it cannot be explained by anatomical or physiological abnormalities. The exact cause of constipation is not fully understood but factors that may contribute include pain, fever, dehydration, dietary and fluid intake, psychological issues, toilet training, medicines, such as anticholinergics, and familial history of constipation.

Non-idiopathic constipation

There are a number of conditions, both congenital and acquired that can result in constipation. These include anorectal anomalies, such as imperforate anus and Hirschsprung's disease, neurological conditions such as spina bifida, sacral agenesis and spinal cord injuries and endocrine conditions such as hypothyroidism.

Investigations

The first and most important investigation in constipation is a detailed history of the problem, to determine cause and treatment. Areas to be questioned include:

- What is the normal bowel habit, how has it changed and over what period of time?
- What is the normal diet and how has it changed recently?
- What medication is the child receiving?
- Are there any other medical conditions?
- Have there been any changes in the child's normal routines; changing schools or attending for the first time can disrupt toileting habits?
- Has the child suffered previous bowel problems or abdominal surgery?

NICE (2010) produce a number of supportive documents alongside their guidance and currently there are two history-taking questionnaires (one for children aged under 1 year and one for children older than 1 year) available to download from their website (http://guidance.nice.org.uk/CG99/Questionnaire).

It is important to recognise that children may perceive rectal examinations as abuse particularly when force or coercion is used and therefore the routine carrying out of a digital rectal examination (DRE) is not recommended by NICE in those children over the age of 1 year. NICE (2010) also make clear recommendations regarding other investigations that are not to be carried out routinely as part of the initial assessment. As well as DRE these include, amongst others, abdominal X-ray, transit studies and ultrasound. It is important, however, particularly if the symptoms have been noted from birth and if the child's symptoms do not improve with the recommended treatment, that the perianal area is inspected and the position of the anus is noted. As many of the children who present in this group are of the younger age and still in nappies this can be done quite easily by asking the mum to change the child's nappy and the area inspected while their bottom is exposed.

By taking a careful detailed history the diagnosis of idiopathic constipation can be confirmed and any 'red flags' easily identified. The 'red flags' findings and clues that may indicate an underlying disorder include:

- Constipation reported from birth with delayed passage of meconium
- Abnormal appearance or position of anus
- Gross abdominal distension
- Unexplained abnormal gait.

If any 'red flags' are identified then the child should be referred urgently to a healthcare professional experienced in the specific aspect of the child's health that is causing concern. It is at this stage that a more detailed examination, including a digital rectal examination, would be carried out if necessary. If any 'amber flags', including faltering growth and possible maltreatment, are identified then the constipation should be treated but the child referred on for further investigation as per local guidelines and policies.

Plain abdominal X-ray, to show any faecal loading or obstruction, should not be performed purely to establish a diagnosis of constipation. NICE make the following recommendation: 'Consider using a plain abdominal radiograph only if requested by specialist services in the ongoing management of intractable idiopathic constipation' (NICE 2010).

Further investigations, when underlying conditions are present/suspected, are:

- Sigmoidoscopy – allows a detailed examination of the rectum and sigmoid colon
- Colonoscopy – allows a detailed examination of the bowel as far as the caecum
- Barium enema – allows a clear picture of the structure of the colon
- Rectal biopsy, suction biopsy or full thickness biopsy to examine the presence of ganglion nerve cells, to exclude Hirschsprung's disease
- Colonic transit studies – the child will be given radio-opaque markers, made up of different shapes, to swallow at intervals. Abdominal X-rays note how long it takes for the different markers to be evacuated.
- Ano-rectal manometry – measurements are taken of the pressures within the anal canal. A small tube placed in the rectum records the pressure created by contraction and relaxation of anal muscles.

Treatment of constipation

For successful treatment of constipation there needs to be a clear understanding of the various factors involved for each individual child, which in some cases necessitates a multi-disciplinary approach to ensure all the child's needs are met. The general principles in managing constipation in children and young people are to soften and clear any faecal impaction, establish a regular pain-free pattern of defecation and prevent relapse by supportive management including demystification and education for the child and family.

Laxatives

NICE recommend laxatives as first line treatment, with Movicol being the laxative of choice.

Disimpaction

It is important to clear out the bowel first if the child is impacted and NICE (2010) make the following treatment regimen recommendations for disimpaction:

- Polyethylene glycol 3350 + electrolytes, i.e. Movicol Paediatric Plain (Movicol PP) using an escalating dose regimen as the first-line treatment
- Movicol PP may be mixed with any cold drink
- Add a stimulant laxative, such as sodium picosulfate, if Movicol PP does not lead to disimpaction after 2 weeks
- Substitute a stimulant laxative singly or in combination with an osmotic laxative such as lactulose if Movicol PP is not tolerated
- Inform families that disimpaction treatment can increase symptoms of soiling and abdominal pain initially
- It is important that children undergoing disimpaction are reviewed within a week to check progress and adjust dosage regime if necessary.

NICE also advise that rectal medications, including sodium citrate enemas, should not be used unless all oral medication has failed and that phosphate enemas should only be used under specialist supervision in hospital.

Maintenance

As a rough guide the suggested starting maintenance dose for children following disimpaction is roughly half the dose required for disimpaction. However, the correct dose is whatever produces the optimum results of at least three soft, easily passed stools per week with the consistency of the stool and the ease of passage being the important factors. Clinical experience has shown that the best way to reach the optimum maintenance dose is to slowly titrate the dose of Movicol down from the disimpaction dose until the optimum dose is reached.

NICE recommend the following regimen for maintenance:

- Movicol PP (Polyethylene glycol 3350 + electrolyte) as the first-line treatment

- Adjust the dose of Movicol PP according to symptoms and response
- Add a stimulant laxative if Movicol PP does not work
- Substitute a stimulant laxative, such as sodium picosulfate, if Movicol PP is not tolerated by the child or young person. Add another laxative such as lactulose or docusate if stools are hard
- Continue medication at maintenance dose for several weeks after regular bowel habit is established – this may take several months
- Children who are toilet training should remain on laxatives until toilet training is well established
- Do not stop medication abruptly: gradually reduce the dose over a period of months in response to stool consistency and frequency
- Some children and young people may require laxative therapy for several years with a small minority requiring continued ongoing laxative therapy.

Diet

Encourage a well-balanced, high-fibre diet along with increased fluid intake. Excessive milk drinking in later infancy should be avoided. It is generally accepted that once a child is fully weaned milk intake should not exceed 1 pint per day.

Toileting

Children should be encouraged to sit on the toilet after meals. Enough time should be allowed for the bowel to empty.

Suppositories and enemas

When oral laxatives have failed, particularly if the child has an underlying disorder, suppository or enema may be prescribed. It must be remembered, however, that some children may find rectal administration distressful so it is important that these procedures are only undertaken with the child's full cooperation.

Children should be followed up regularly to assess progress and re-evaluate laxative use. The families should also be given the contact details of a healthcare professional they can contact for advice if problems develop between appointments.

Biofeedback

This is a treatment to retrain the nerves and muscles used in evacuation. The treatment can be lengthy and needs full commitment from the child and family (Brazzelli and Griffiths 2006, Cox et al 1998). The evidence base, however, for the use of biofeedback is poor and it is not currently recommended by NICE (2010) as a standard treatment intervention for idiopathic constipation.

Invasive treatments

For children with intractable constipation and for those whose constipation is related to an underlying disorder further invasive treatments may be indicated and include:

- Rectal washouts such as Peristeen® (Ausili et al 2010, Bohr 2009)
- The ACE procedure (Malone 2004, Sinha et al 2008, Yardley et al 2009) (see later in this chapter)
- Bowel resection would be the last resort but subtotal colectomy with ileorectal anastomosis or ileosigmoid anastomosis may be performed.

Preparation for investigations or surgery

All centres will have protocols for preparation of the bowel for investigation or surgery. These can vary in use of certain laxatives or enemas. It is important, therefore, to identify and follow local guidelines and protocols regarding bowel preparations for specific investigations/surgical interventions. However, no child with inflammatory bowel disease should have rectal washouts or enemas except for foam enemas which are used for ulcerative colitis.

Treatment of faecal soiling/incontinence

Children can suffer faecal soiling/incontinence for a number reasons including:

- Constipation with overflow
- Anorectal anomalies, spina bifida
- Resection of bowel leading to a shortened gut
- Emotional difficulties (encopresis).

Nurses need to be aware of the psychological effects faecal incontinence has on the child and the family (Ludman 2003). These effects can be minimised more easily the earlier the problem is addressed.

Whatever the cause, faecal soiling/ incontinence needs to be treated. It would be hoped before the child begins school that some programme of management will have started.

For those children with overflow soiling associated with constipation, once the constipation has been resolved the soiling should stop. For children with faecal incontinence related to an underlying condition, treatment options for these children could include:

- Timed evacuations using a combination of oral/rectal preparations and a toileting programme
- Rectal washouts
- Colonic irrigation
- ACE washouts.

Sometimes further surgery, such as repeat pull through, colonic resection, levatorplasty, colostomy or stimulated graciloplasty, will be performed.

Products to help with the management of faecal incontinence/soiling

There are a range of containment products available, both disposable and reusable to help manage faecal incontinence. The degree of soiling will dictate the most appropriate product to be used.

Further information regarding the full range of products and resources available can be obtained via PromoCon (part of the charity Disabled Living) which provides national advice and information via its web site and helpline (www.promocon.co.uk, helpline: 0161 607 8219).

Diarrhoea

There are a number of causes of diarrhoea in childhood including infection, food allergy, disaccharide malabsorption, general malabsorption (coeliac disease and cystic fibrosis), inflammatory bowel disease, and toddler diarrhoea, which is by far the commonest cause. A careful history with an understanding of associated symptoms will give a clue as to the underlying cause and help direct the most appropriate treatment.

Toddler diarrhoea

Toddler's diarrhoea is also known as chronic nonspecific diarrhoea. Affected children develop 3–10 watery loose stools per day. The stools are often more smelly and pale than usual and parents/carers may report bits of undigested vegetable food in the stools (such as bits of carrot, sweetcorn, etc). Mild abdominal pain sometimes occurs, but apart from the loose stools the child is usually symptom free.

A child with just toddler's diarrhoea is otherwise well, grows normally, plays normally and is usually not bothered about the diarrhoea. No detailed tests are usually needed if the child is otherwise well. Symptoms usually go, with or without treatment, by the age of 5–6 years.

The cause of the diarrhoea is not clear but it is **not** due to malabsorption of food or to a serious bowel problem. It is also not due to an intolerance of a type of food.

Often, no treatment is needed, particularly if symptoms are mild. Reassurance that it will ease in time may be all that is

required. However, in many cases slight changes to the child's diet may be all that is needed. They are the 4 Fs – fat, fluid, fruit juices and fibre and include the following:

1. Increase fat in the diet.
2. Decrease fluid in the diet.
3. Avoid fructose and sorbitol – decrease fruit juices.
4. Increase dietary fibre.
5. Normal diet for age.
6. Reassurance.
7. There is no role for medications.
8. The parents/carers should be told that there is no serious sequelea and this is not a precursor to inflammatory bowel disease.
9. Most children are better by 4 years of age, and are better by the time they become potty trained.

Suppositories

NICE does not recommend suppositories as a treatment for idiopathic constipation. Suppositories can be used as a method of evacuating faeces or as a means of administering medication. Whatever the use the administration is the same. The route of administration is normally into the rectum, but they can be inserted into a colostomy using the same principles.

Ensure the environment where the procedure is to take place is private, and has a toilet, commode or bed pan available if the suppository being used is to evacuate the rectum.

Explanation of the procedure to child and parents/carers will alleviate anxiety. Some families regard the rectal route for medication to be the least acceptable (Seth *et al* 2000). Suppositories may be contra-indicated in some children, e.g. post rectal surgery, or children who are neutrapoenic.

Procedure guideline 5.1 Administering a suppository

Statement	Rationale
1. Gather equipment: • Suppository • Lubricating jelly • Gloves.	1. To allow the procedure to be carried out promptly without interruption.
2. Take off nappy or underwear. Ask child to lie on left side with knees bent up to abdomen. Infants can lie on their back with feet and legs held up.	2. Insertion of suppository will be easier in this position. This position is easier to maintain in an infant.
3. Put on gloves.	3. To adhere to universal precautions.
4. Open suppository, lubricate the end. Holding the suppository between index finger and thumb, locate the anus and gently insert the suppository with the index finger. The suppository should be fully inserted into the rectum next to the rectal wall.	4. Lubrication will make insertion easier. Fully inserting the suppository against the wall of the rectum will allow it to be retained longer and therefore be more effective.

(Continued)

91

Procedure guideline 5.1 (*Continued*)

Statement	Rationale
5. Ask the child to try and retain the suppository as long as possible.	**5.** The longer the suppository is retained the better the result.
6. If the suppository is used to evacuate the rectum, sit the child on the toilet or commode to empty the bowel.	**6.** Allow enough time sitting on the toilet/commode for the rectum to empty.
7. If the suppository is for medication purposes, e.g. analgesia, wipe excess lubricating jelly off perineum and replace nappy or underwear.	**7.** The suppository will dissolve and medication absorbed through bowel mucosa.

Enemas

NICE does not recommend the administration of enemas for treatment of idiopathic constipation. This can be seen as an unpleasant and embarrassing procedure for some children. Therefore, consideration must be given to certain aspects that can lessen anxiety. Ensure the environment where the procedure is to be carried out is private and has a toilet, bedpan or commode available. Children who are bed-bound will need to remain on the bed and will need incontinence sheets or a nappy.

Allow enough time for the procedure to be undisturbed. Generally 30–40 minutes is needed to ensure the enema and stools are evacuated. Explain the procedure to the child and parents/carers. While the enema is given, due to the child's position they will not be able to see what you are doing. If only a part of the enema is prescribed, the amount should be measured prior to the procedure starting.

Procedure guideline 5.2 **Administering an enema**

Statement	Rationale

1. Gather equipment:
  • Enema
  • Gloves
  • Lubricating jelly
  • Rectal catheter if needed
  • Incontinence sheet.
	1. To allow the procedure to be carried out promptly with no interruption.

2. Take off nappy or underwear. Ask the child to lie on their left side with knees bent up to abdomen.
  Infants can lie on their back with feet and legs held up.
	2. Insertion of the enema nozzle or rectal catheter is easier.
	
	  • This position is easier to maintain with an infant.

3. Put on gloves.	**3.** To adhere to universal precautions.

4. Lubricate the end of the enema nozzle.
  If a rectal catheter is to be used, attach it to the enema nozzle and lubricate the end.
	4. Lubrication ensures easier insertion.
	  Using a catheter allows the enema to be instilled high up in the colon. If the rectum is loaded with faeces the tube will be able to bypass it and produce a better result.

5. Gently squeeze the enema bottle to allow the solution to prime the nozzle or rectal catheter.	**5.** Air needs to be expelled from the nozzle or catheter.
6. Identify the anus and gently insert the nozzle or catheter into anus. Squeeze the enema bottle until all the solution has entered the rectum. Continue squeezing the enema bottle as the nozzle or catheter is gently removed.	**6.** The catheter or nozzle should be inserted far enough into the rectum to stop the enema solution from running out of the anus. Squeezing the bottle while taking out the catheter or nozzle stops fluid running back into the bottle.

Procedure guideline 5.2 (*Continued*)

Statement	Rationale
7. Older children should be asked to try and keep the enema solution in their bowel for as long as they can.	**7.** This allows the enema solution to be as effective as possible. If the solution is pushed out immediately the result will not be as effective.
8. Sit the child on the toilet, commode or bedpan, allowing time to empty the bowel.	**8.** Sitting on the toilet or commode offers the best position for emptying the bowel. The child needs to sit on the toilet/commode long enough for the bowel to empty fully.
9. Continually reassure the child if abdominal cramps occur.	**9.** The enema causes peristalsis, which can be uncomfortable. As the bowel empties the cramps lessen.

Procedure guideline 5.3 **Rectal washout on an infant**

Statement	Rationale

1. Gather equipment and ensure the room is warm and private.
 	
  a) Apron.
  b) Disposable gloves.
  c) Incontinence sheets.
  d) Disposable bowls.
  e) Rectal/nasogastric tube (10 or 12 Fr).
  f) Syringe (50 ml).
  g) Warm saline.
  h) Lubricating jelly.
	1. Having equipment ready ensures the procedure can be uninterrupted. The baby will be stripped or partially stripped; therefore, the room needs to be warm.
	  a–d) To adhere to universal precautions and minimise the risk of infection.

2. Explain procedure fully to parents/carers and undress infant feet to waist.	**2.** Can be seen as a distressing procedure; if all questions and fears are answered parents/carers will feel more comfortable.
3. Pour warm saline into bowl, draw up about 20 ml into syringe and attach rectal tube. Prime the tube with saline.	**3.** Tube needs to be primed to prevent the introduction of air into the rectum, which could cause extra distension. Saline is used as it will not be absorbed by the gut.
4. Infants are generally more content to lie on their backs during the procedure, but any position they want to assume can be accommodated. Ask parents/assistant to lift up the infant's feet and hold.	**4.** It is easier to control all equipment during the procedure if legs are supported and not kicking out. Parents/carers are closer to the infant to provide comfort.
5. Put on disposable gloves. Lubricate the end of the tube. Locate the anus and gently insert the tube about 1–2 inches.	**5.** 1–2 inches is far enough to begin with, the rectum can be emptied and the tube can then be advanced more easily if necessary.
6. Slowly inject the saline into the rectum, once it has entered gently draw back on the syringe. If any pressure is felt stop drawing back. If no saline can be drawn back, disconnect syringe from tube gently moving the tube back and forth can stimulate evacuation by gravity.	**6.** Drawing back on the syringe makes the procedure quicker and will cause no problem as long as there is no pressure felt.
7. Evacuated stool and saline should be collected in a disposable bowl.	**7.** It is important to check that the amount of saline being instilled is returned, to avoid abdominal distension.

(*Continued*)

Procedure guideline 5.3 (*Continued*)

Statement	Rationale
8. No more than 20 ml of saline should be instilled at one time in small infants.	**8.** Overfilling the rectum/sigmoid colon could cause distension and possible perforation.
9. Repeat the above steps until the abdomen is deflated or the saline is running clean.	**9.** It depends on why the washout has been prescribed. If the baby has Hirschsprung's disease or is constipated the washout stops when the infant's abdomen is deflated. If the washout is prescribed to clean the colon for surgery it will need to be repeated until saline is running clean.
10. Medical staff may have prescribed how much saline to be used in total. If not, the infant's warmth dictates. When the washout has been completed gently remove the catheter, clean the infant then dress.	**10.** Attempts should be made to keep the infant warm at all times. If this is unsuccessful the washout should be stopped and if required repeated later.

Procedure guideline 5.4 Rectal washout (older child)

Statement	Rationale
1. Gather equipment: • Disposable gloves • Incontinence sheets • Rectal washout kit (funnel with tubing and connector attached) • Rectal tube (sizes of catheter that accommodate funnel are 10–18 Fr) • Lubricating jelly • Warm saline • Bucket.	**1.** Having equipment ready ensures procedure can be uninterrupted.
2. a) Ensure room is warm and private. **b)** Explain procedure fully to child and parents/carers.	**2. a)** To ensure that the child is as comfortable as possible during the procedure. **b)** This can be a distressing procedure. Allaying fears by explaining what will happen can help the child cope with the washout.
3. Lower garments must be removed and the child should lie on a couch on top of the incontinence sheets. Lying on the left side with knees bent up to the abdomen is the preferred position.	**3.** This ensures easy insertion of the rectal tube. Tell the child what happens at each stage, as in this position they will not be able to see what you are doing.
4. Put on disposable gloves; attach rectal tube to washout kit. Place bucket on floor beside couch.	**4.** The saline and stools from the washout will flow into the bucket.
5. Pour some saline into the funnel to prime the tube. Pinch the rectal tubing.	**5.** Pinching the rectal tubing is the only means of controlling the flow of saline.
6. Lubricate the end of the rectal tube, locate the anus and gently insert the tube. About 3–4 inches is enough to start the washout.	**6.** The tube can be introduced further when the rectum is empty. If the tube is not inserted far enough the saline will run straight back out of the anus.
7. Lift up the funnel to allow the saline to enter the rectum by gravity. When the saline in the funnel has entered the rectum, lower the funnel and allow saline and stool to run into the bucket.	**7.** Ensure that the saline instilled comes back out of the rectum. Moving the rectal tube gently may help to evacuate the stool and saline – some may be evacuated around the tube.

94

Procedure guideline 5.4 (*Continued*)

Statement	Rationale
8. Leaving the rectal tube in the rectum, refill the funnel with saline and repeat the last step. Do not overfill the funnel.	**8.** Overfilling the rectum with saline could cause abdominal pain. Reassure the child that the saline will empty back quickly.
9. The process can continue until the saline runs clear and/or the rectum has emptied.	**9.** If the washout is as a preparation for surgery the bowel needs to be clean. For constipation, the evacuation of stool from the rectum may be all that is needed.
10. At the end of the washout gently remove the catheter. It is useful to ask the child to sit on the toilet and try to evacuate any stool or saline that may still be in the bowel.	**10.** Sometimes the movement from the couch to the toilet will allow any saline or stool to move down the bowel. This will then evacuate into the toilet.

Transanal colonic irrigation

Colonic irrigation is a means of emptying the transverse and descending colon. This can be performed either by using a colostomy irrigation kit (a bag for holding saline with a long tube attached that has a soft plastic cone at the end) or a Peristeen® trans anal washout kit or the Shandling catheter. The Shandling catheter is a rectal catheter that has a retaining balloon; it is useful for children who have a patulous (wider opening) anus (Fitzpatrick 1996). The balloon will stop the washout from running straight back out of the anus. The catheter is rather cumbersome and children will need help to perform the irrigation and as a result it is generally no longer used in practice.

New developments such as the Peristeen® system for transanal irrigation have superseded the older systems such as the Shandling catheter and can be used from the age of 3 years. The majority of children can learn to carry out the procedure themselves, which facilitates independence (Ausili *et al* 2010, Bohr 2009, Christensen *et al* 2006).

Anal irrigation (Peristeen®)

Trans anal irrigation is performed to evacuate stools from the rectum and lower colon in the management of faecal incontinence and chronic constipation. It involves introducing water into the rectum and colon via the anus. The water and contents of the rectum and descending sigmoid colon are subsequently evacuated into the toilet. Although initially performed by a parent/carer it is a procedure that the child can be taught to carryout independently.

This section is based on using the Peristeen® anal irrigation system as that is the only device currently available that is licensed for use in children. The reader will need to check local policy to determine what systems are available for use in their own area.

As this procedure is designed to take place over the toilet or commode, appropriate toileting aids (such as a seat reducer/

step) should be in place if necessary to enable the child to sit comfortably. Distraction techniques may be useful for some children to help them relax during the insertion of the rectal catheter. If the child is able; encourage them to operate the control unit – this will not only act as a distraction technique but also help facilitate the child's later independence. Some children may experience abdominal cramps during the procedure – try to pump the water more slowly and check the temperature. Adjust the volume of air in the balloon if there is leakage of fluid or the catheter is expelled prematurely.

The following precautions should be noted:

- The Peristeen® anal irrigation is designed to be used in children over the age of 3 years, special caution must be used in children under 3 years
- Special caution must also be taken in children with recent abdominal or anal surgery, anal fissure or inflammatory bowel disease
- Rectal irrigation should not be used when there is a known obstruction of the large bowel or acute stage of inflammatory bowel disease or diverticulitis.

Antegrade colonic enema – ACE

The use of the ACE procedure is now considered to be the follow on option if a trial of transanal irrigation (Peristeen®) does not prove to be either acceptable or effective for the child.

The appendix is brought out onto the abdominal wall as a small opening. This allows a catheter to be inserted directly into the caecum, through which a washout can be performed while the child is sitting on the toilet. The whole of the colon can be evacuated and the child can be clean for up to 48 hours.

If the child has had an appendicectomy, a caecal flap can create this channel.

Washout solutions for the ACE vary from centre to centre so it is important to always follow local policies and guidelines, but generally include an enema solution and saline. It is usual to mix equal measures of enema and saline; this is given and then followed by a saline flush.

Procedure guideline 5.5 **Anal irrigation**

Statement	Rationale
1. Gather the following equipment: • Anal irrigation kit (Peristeen®) • Irrigation bag and tubing • Control unit • Rectal catheter (two sizes, small/large) • Lukewarm (body temperature) water (approx 20 ml per kg – but local policy/guidelines will dictate) • Apron and gloves (non latex) – if procedure carried out by carer.	**1.** Having equipment ready ensures procedure can be uninterrupted.
2. Undertake a comprehensive nursing and medical assessment.	**2.** To identify any contraindications.
3. Performing rectal irrigation is not without risk and the decision to undertake it should be made in consultation with senior medical personnel and the child's GP if the procedure is to be continued in the community.	**3.** To ensure the procedure is suitable and appropriate for the child.
4. Explain the procedure to the child.	**4.** To enlist the child's cooperation and gain consent.
5. Fill the irrigation bag with lukewarm water and run it through the system until there is sufficient water in the catheter packaging.	**5.** To enable the catheter to become lubricated.
6. Position the child as appropriate. If the child is able to stand unsupported insertion of the catheter is best carried out with the child standing next to the toilet. This can involve standing directly in front of the toilet facing away and leaning slightly forwards or standing to the side of the toilet depending on the space available. If the child is unable to stand, the child should be positioned on a bed or changing mat for insertion of the catheter and inflation of the balloon. The child can then be lifted onto the toilet or commode using a hoist and toileting sling if necessary. If the child is confident to sit on the toilet and has good sitting balance then the catheter can be inserted while the child is sitting on the toilet. With time this is a procedure that some children can be taught to do independently.	**6.** To ensure the child is comfortable and to enable the procedure to be carried out as easily as possible. To help promote independence.
7. Once the catheter has been inserted into the rectum (approx 2.5 cm past the balloon section, but this will differ depending on the size of the child) the catheter balloon is inflated by turning the dial to the appropriate symbol and using sufficient pumps of the balloon (usually 2–3 for the large catheter, 1–2 for the small catheter).	**7.** To retain the catheter and instilled fluid.
8. The dial is then turned to the water symbol and water is pumped slowly into the rectum – the exact quantity instilled will depend on each individual child but is usually 350–500 ml.	**8.** To commence the washout.
9. When the appropriate volume of water has been instilled the dial is turned to the air symbol and the balloon is deflated. The water and contents of the rectum and descending colon are subsequently evacuated into the toilet.	**9.** To allow the rectal catheter to slide out.
10. Once the evacuation is complete the child should be assisted to wipe their bottom if able, otherwise this should be carried out by their carer.	**10.** To make the child comfortable.
11. The rectal catheter should be disposed of as per local policy and the remaining equipment cleaned and stored away.	**11.** To minimise the risk of infection.
12. The results of the rectal irrigation should be documented in the child's healthcare records.	

Procedure guideline 5.6 ACE washout

Statement	Rationale
1. Ensure bathroom is private.	**1.** The child will be more relaxed in privacy.
2. Gather equipment: • Washout solutions • Size 10 FR catheter • Lubricating jelly • Gloves • 60 ml bladder syringe.	**2.** To ensure procedure is uninterrupted.
3. Put on gloves, lubricate the end of the catheter and gently introduce into the ACE stoma. It needs to be inserted about 3–4 inches. It is easier to insert the catheter with the child standing up or lying down.	**3.** To adhere to universal precautions. The catheter needs to go through the appendix and into the caecum. If it is not introduced far enough the washout solution will not enter the colon. Sitting down may make passing the catheter more difficult.
4. Draw up the half-strength enema solution into the bladder syringe. Attach the syringe into the catheter and slowly inject the solution. Continue until all the enema solution has been instilled. Keep the empty syringe attached to the catheter for a few minutes.	**4.** Injecting the enema solution too quickly may not produce enough stimulation for the colon to empty fully. This gives time for the enema solution to move through the colon before the saline is instilled. Otherwise it will be diluted more.
5. Bend back the catheter and remove syringe. Refill the syringe with saline and reattach to the bent catheter. Slowly inject the saline flush until all prescribed saline is given.	**5.** Bending back the catheter will stop the already instilled enema solution returning through the catheter. The volume of saline flush will help flush out faeces.
6. When all solution has been instilled gently remove catheter.	**6.** The tube needs to be removed otherwise the fluid will run back out into the syringe.
7. The child needs to sit on the toilet for up to about 45 minutes or until all fluid and stool has been evacuated. The child should try to push out the washout solution and stool.	**7.** Evacuation of the bowel can take at least 30–45 minutes. The bowel will empty more quickly if the child tries to evacuate their bowel.

Stoma care

The word stoma comes from the Greek meaning mouth or opening. The majority of stomas raised in childhood are formed in the neonatal period, and are usually a temporary measure in the surgical correction of congenital abnormalities. Conditions that may require stoma surgery include: imperforate anus, Hirschsprung's disease, cloacal extrophy, necrotising enterocolitis, ulcerative colitis, Crohn's disease, familial adenomatous polyposis, tumours and trauma (Fitzpatrick 1996).

There are four main types of output stomas:

1. Colostomy – a portion of the colon is brought out through the abdominal wall and is normally sited in the left iliac fossa. (In children the transverse, descending or sigmoid colon may be used.)
2. Ileostomy – a portion of ileum is brought out through the abdominal wall and is normally sited in the right iliac fossa.
3. Jejunostomy – a portion of the jejunem is brought through the abdominal wall. (This stoma has a high output and these children generally require total parental nutrition.)
4. Urinary diversions – these include:

a) Ileal conduit – a section of the ileum is isolated to act as a reservoir and the ureters implanted into it. This stoma can be sited in the left or right iliac fossa.
b) Ureterostomy – one or two of the ureters can be brought out onto the abdominal wall, either side by side or at either side of the abdomen.
c) Vesicostomy – the neck of the bladder is brought through the abdominal wall low down at the pelvis.

The success of any surgery is generally related to the level of understanding and the support given to the child and family. Families need to know what is happening, what the surgery involves and how they will cope afterwards. It is vitally important to be honest when preparing children for surgery. Meeting another family whose child has had stoma surgery can be an excellent support. They can answer questions from a personal perspective and share experiences such as what support is needed at school.

Factors to note

A number of infants who have undergone surgery on the small intestine can have a temporary intolerance to lactose. Their ileostomy output will be very loose, and test positive to sugar. These babies will need special lactose-free formula milk. It is important that when these infants start weaning they are given a milk-free diet. When all corrective surgery is completed the child will probably be able to take a normal diet. This decision will be taken on an individual basis, with the support of a dietician.

Children and their parents/carers need to understand that some foodstuffs will affect stoma function. Some foods can produce more odorous stools, e.g. eggs, onions, fish and cheese. Green vegetables, onions, beans and fizzy drinks will increase flatus. Foods such as nuts, popcorn or dried fruits can swell in the gastrointestinal tract and cause bowel obstructions if eaten in large amounts. However, children should eat a well balanced diet and most things can be eaten in moderation.

Eating foods that contain a high vitamin C content may be of benefit to a child with a urinary diversion: by increasing the acidity of the urine and drinking plenty of fluids, urine is prevented from becoming concentrated and hence urinary infections are reduced (Reid 2002).

Infants and children with ileostomies are susceptible to sodium depletion. Older children may complain of cramps in their legs if sodium is low. Regular urinary sodium levels need to be taken and, if low, sodium supplements should be given. Older children may just be told to use extra salt on their food. Foods such as marmite, cheese or crisps are a good source of salt.

Dehydration is a potential problem for infants and children with ileostomies. Maintaining fluid balance can be difficult in small babies. Parents/carers should be advised on signs of dehydration, i.e. sunken fontanel, decrease in urinary output, increase in stoma output, dark shadows under eyes, dry skin and lethargy. Medical advice should be sought if the family are concerned. Intravenous fluids may be necessary.

Some older children may want to try colostomy irrigation as a means of managing their colostomy. However, many of them will have tried rectal or ACE washouts in the past and want to be free of washouts. Using a colostomy plug may provide the older child with an alternative to wearing a pouch, especially for sporting activities.

There is no doubt that surgery resulting in an altered body image is difficult to come to terms with. For some, after many years of soiling and washouts, a stoma is a means of having control over one's bowel with less attention needed than washouts. Ongoing support is needed as the child goes through different stages of their life. Meeting other youngsters who have had similar surgery can be a valuable support; often children feel they are the only one to have such problems. Some children may need extra psychological support in coming to terms with the surgery.

Parents/carers of children undergoing stoma surgery should have discussion with the school about their child's condition. In some areas a child will have the support of a welfare assistant, in other areas the parents/carers have to attend to the child's care if necessary. Older children may prefer to utilise the privacy of the school nurses room to perform stoma care, as communal toilets in school are notorious for lack of privacy. Starting these discussions early will ensure as little disruption as possible to the child's education.

All stoma appliances are available on prescription. Prior to discharge it is usual to give the family a supply that will last until the GP prescribes more. Chemists may take a day or two ordering stock, therefore the family should not wait until they are using their last pouch before ordering more. Some companies offer a home delivery service but a prescription is still required from the GP. Children who have a permanent stoma after the age of 16 will be exempt from prescription charges.

Procedure guideline 5.7 **Stoma siting**

Statement	Rationale
1. It is generally not necessary to mark the site of the stoma in a newborn infant.	**1.** The stoma will usually be of a temporary nature and will be closed before the child is out of nappies.
2. If the child is older and out of nappies, or if the child will have a stoma as a more permanent treatment, the stoma should be sited prior to surgery. When marking a stoma site the following points should be considered:	**2.** If the stoma is placed in the optimal position the child should have no problems with stoma management. Thus making acceptance of the stoma a little easier.
3. The child should be able to see the stoma site.	**3.** It is important to be able to see the stoma when lying down, sitting up and standing. Changing a pouch is extremely difficult if the stoma cannot be seen.
4. The stoma should be brought through the rectus abdominis sheath.	**4.** This muscle grips the bowel and will help to prevent prolapse or retraction of the stoma.
5. Any bony prominences must be avoided.	**5.** If the stoma is too near the hip, movement will loosen the adhesive of the pouch.
6. Any previous scars must be avoided.	**6.** Skin creases; folds and scars make the skin surface uneven. Loose stools will leak along these tracts.

Procedure guideline 5.7 (*Continued*)

Statement	Rationale
7. The waistline of clothes should be avoided.	**7.** Stomas should be under the waistline both for discretion and pouch security.
8. Ensure that any prostheses or braces do not cover the site.	**8.** Any appliances worn can usually be adapted so as not to interfere with the pouch.
9. If the child is wheelchair bound, the stoma must be sited while they are in the wheelchair.	**9.** Children confined to wheelchairs usually have their stomas sited higher on the abdomen, as they will be easier to see and manage.

Stoma pouch selection

Many nurses ask which is the right pouch to use. There are various things to consider when selecting the most appropriate pouch (Black 2009b). Using an inappropriate pouch is time-consuming and can cause needless discomfort for the child.

Principles table 5.1 **Stoma pouch selection**

Principle	Rationale
1. There are many different pouches produced by a number of manufacturers. However, there are basically two designs of pouch: **a)** A one-piece pouch has an adhesive flange with a pouch bonded onto it. **b)** A two-piece pouch has an adhesive flange and a separate pouch, which attaches to the flange.	**1.** **a)** This pouch is designed to stay in place for 1–3 days. It also has a flat profile. **b)** This allows the opportunity to keep the flange on for a few days but change the pouch more frequently.
2. Both the one-piece and the two-piece pouches have either a closed end (for formed stool) or an open, drainable end (for loose stool).	**2.** Closed pouches need to be taken off and discarded when roughly two-thirds full. Ileostomy pouches need to be emptied roughly 3–6 times per day.
3. Urinary pouches have a tap at the end to which an overnight drainage bag can be attached; they also have a non- return valve in the pouch.	**3.** Overnight drainage bags are important for the child to have an uninterrupted sleep. Non-return valves stop urine from splashing back up the ureters.
4. Older children with colostomies that produce formed stools have the opportunity to use a colostomy plug. A flange is placed around the colostomy, a plug with a filter and a cap on the top is inserted into the colostomy, and then the cap snaps over the flange. The plug needs to be taken out at least 12 hourly and a pouch attached to the flange.	**4.** Plugs cannot be used if the stool is loose as the loose stool would probably leak out or the bowel would push out the plug. The bowel needs time to empty at least once a day.
5. The choice of pouch to be used is affected by factors such as manual dexterity, vision and size.	**5.** One-piece appliances may be easier to manage for children with poor vision or dexterity problems. Two-piece pouches are not ideal for use with small infants.
6. In the early postoperative period it is advisable to use a one-piece, clear, drainable pouch.	**6.** The colour of a newly formed stoma needs to be observed following surgery. A two-piece pouch is going to be painful to apply in the early postoperative period.

Changing a pouch

When changing a pouch, especially for the first time, ensure you have enough time to perform the procedure. Children may be very frightened about the procedure, they need explanations of what you are doing and parents/carers will be trying to assimilate what they will need to learn.

100

Procedure guideline 5.8 Changing a pouch

Statement	Rationale
1. Gather appropriate equipment: • Receptacle to empty pouch into • Disposable gloves (for hospital staff) • Bowl of warm water • Gauze squares or cleansing wipes • New pouch • Bag to dispose of used pouch and cleansing materials • Scissors • Template or measuring device.	1. To be prepared to carry out procedure without interruption.
2. Position the child/baby lying down. Older children can lie down or stand up.	2. The child needs to be comfortable. When lying down or standing up the abdomen is smooth. When sitting upright the abdominal skin becomes wrinkled, this will compromise pouch adhesion.
3. Wash hands and put on disposable gloves.	3. To adhere to universal precautions.
4. If a drainable pouch is being used it needs to be emptied before removing it.	4. Unless emptied first the pouch contents will spill. Also, when parents/carers are at home they should not put full pouches in their refuse.
5. Remove old pouch by carefully peeling off the pouch from top to bottom with one hand, whilst supporting the skin with the other. Adhesive removers should not be used on small babies.	5. Supporting the skin makes the procedure less uncomfortable and helps prevent the skin from tearing. Adhesive removers can dry out the skin causing soreness.
6. The pouch can then be put into a disposable bag and discarded as per local policy for disposal of clinical waste.	6. To minimise the risk of contamination/cross-infection.
7. Clean the peristomal skin with warm water and gauze. If some residue is left on the skin from the old pouch, use a dry piece of gauze to remove it before washing. Do not use cotton wool. Ensure the skin is dried thoroughly.	7. The residue will spread over the skin if wet. Any residue left on the skin may interfere with the adhesion of the new pouch. Cotton wool will deposit strands, which may interfere with pouch adhesion.
8. Prepare the new pouch. The aperture should be cut to fit snugly around the stoma with no peristomal skin exposed.	8. It is easier to prepare the new pouch before hand. If any skin is exposed to effluent it will become excoriated.
9. Put on the new pouch. a) If a one-piece pouch is being used, fold the adhesive backwards in half, placing the pouch on the underside of the stoma first, then flip the adhesive over the stoma and secure all around. b) If a two-piece pouch is being used. secure the flange first and then attach the pouch. c) Pull the pouch gently. d) If a drainable pouch is being used ensure the clip is secured correctly at the bottom of the pouch.	9. b) Two-piece pouches usually leak because the pouch has not been attached properly to the flange. c) To ensure it is attached completely. d) If the clip is not secure the pouch will fill up and subsequently leak.

Potential problems with stomas

There can be problems with stoma management in paediatric patients. One of the main problems will be the size of the baby. The majority will be neonates and some will be premature. In this age group complications can be high (Patwardhan *et al* 2001).

Principles table 5.2 Potential problems with stomas

Principle	Rationale
1. A healthy stoma is red/pink in colour. It is very important especially in the postoperative period to check the colour of the stoma regularly. If the stoma appears darker in colour, medical advice should be sought.	1. If the blood supply is compromised the bowel will become necrosed. The stoma will become purple/black. Surgical refashioning of the stoma may be necessary.
2. In the early postoperative period all stomas will be oedematous. At 6 weeks the stoma should have shrunk to its actual size. This is important, as the parent/child needs to cut the pouch or flange to the exact size of the stoma. They have to be aware that the stoma will change shape and size.	2. Only one or two spare pouches should be prepared at a time. This will ensure no abdominal skin is exposed to stoma output as the stoma shrinks. Families are advised to wait 6 weeks before arranging pre-cut pouches or having pouches/flanges cut by prescription companies.
3. Prolapse of loop stomas in infants and children is common. Parents/carers and children need to be told of the possibility, given a description of what a prolapse looks like, and when to seek medical advice. Older children should be discouraged from lifting heavy weights.	3. If the prolapsed bowel remains red/ pink and soft there is usually no cause for concern. If the colour changes, i.e. becomes darker or the bowel is tense to the touch medical advice should be sought. Some prolapses require reducing under sedation or general anaesthetic. Lifting heavy weights puts strain on the abdomen and can cause prolapse.
4. Some stomas can become retracted. This will cause more problems with an ileostomy as the output is much looser, and the stool will leak under the adhesive of the pouch. Parents/carers can seek the advice of the stoma nurse or the doctor if the stoma appears sunken.	4. Retracted stomas can be managed by using a pouch with a convex adhesive flange. This will push out the stoma. If this fails the stoma may need surgical refashioning.
5. Stenosis of the stoma can also occur. Often the narrowing of the bowel cannot be seen at the surface, but there may be a reduction in the amount of stool passed or stools may become ribbon-like.	5. Simple dilation of the stoma can solve the problem. If this does not work surgical revision of the stoma can be undertaken.
6. Overgranulation can occur if the pouch fits too tightly. Continuous rubbing on the bowel mucosa can cause a granuloma to form.	6. Granulomas can bleed easily and can be distressing. Silver nitrate can be used to treat them; if this doesn't work they can be surgically removed.

References

Ausili E, Focarelli B, Tabacco F, Murolo D, Sigismondi M, Gasbarrini A, Rendeli C. (2010) Transanal irrigation in myelomeningocele children: an alternative, safe and valid approach for neurogenic constipation. Spinal Cord, 48(7), 560–565

Black P. (2009a) Managing physical postoperative stoma complications. British Journal of Nursing, 18(7), S4–10

Black P. (2009b) Choosing the correct stoma appliance. British Journal of Nursing, 18(4), 510, 512–514

Bohr C. (2009) Using rectal irrigation for faecal incontinence in children. Nursing Times, 105(7), 42–44

Brazzelli M, Griffiths P. (2006) Behavioural and cognitive interventions with or without other treatments for defaecation disorders in children. Cochrane Review, 4, CD002240

Christensen P, Bazzocchi G, Coggrave M, Abel R, Hultling C, Krogh K, Media S, Laurberg S. (2006) A randomised, controlled trial of transanal irrigation versus conservative bowel management in spinal cord injured patients. Gastroenterology, 131, 738–747

Cox DJ, Sutphen J, Borowitz Kovatch B, Ling W. (1998) Contribution of behaviour therapy and biofeedback to laxative therapy in the treatment of paediatric encoporesis. Annals of Behavioural Medicine, 20(2), 70–76

Fitzpatrick G. (1996) The child with a stoma. In: Myers C. (ed.) Stoma Care Nursing. London, Arnold

Loening-Baucke V. (1998) Constipation in children. New England Journal of Medicine, 339, 1155–1156

Loening-Baucke V. (2007) Constipation as cause of acute abdominal pain in children. Journal Pediatrics, 151(6), 666–669

Ludman L. (2003) Gut Feelings: a psychologists 20 year journey with paediatric surgeons. Journal of the Royal Society of Medicine, 6, 87–91

Malone PSJ. (2004) The antegrade continence enema procedure. British Journal of Urology International, 93(3), 248

National Institute for Clinical Excellence (NICE) (2010) Constipation in children and young people (CG99) Diagnosis and management of idiopathic childhood constipation in primary and secondary care. Available at http://www.nice.org.uk/guidance/CG99 (last accessed 14th June 2011)

Patwardhan N, Keily EM, Drake DP, Spitz L, Pierro A. (2001) Colostomy for anorectal anomalies: high incidence of complications. Journal of Paediatric Surgery, 36(5), 795–798

Rasquin A, Di Lorenzo C, Forbes D, Guiraldes E, Hyams JS, Staiano A, Walker LS. (2006) Childhood functional gastrointestinal disorders: Child/adolescent. Gastroenterology 130, 1527–1537

Reid G. (2002) Critical Reviews in Food Science and Nutrition, 42, 293–300

Roper N, Logan WW, Tierney AJ. (1990) The Elements of Nursing: A model for nursing based on a model of living, 3rd Edition. Edinburgh, Churchill Livingstone

Seth N, Llewelyn NE, Howard RF. (2000) Parental opinions regarding the route of administration of analgesic medication in children. Paediatric Anaesthesia, 10(5), 537

Sinha Ck, Grewal A, Ward HC. (2008) Antegrade continence enema (ACE): current practice. Pediatric Surgery International, 24(6), 685–688

Yardley IE, Pauniaho SL, Baille CT, Turnock RR, Cauldicott P, Lamont GL, Kenny SE. (2009) After the honeymoon comes divorce: long term use of the Antegrade continence enema procedure. Journal of Paediatric Surgery, 44(6), 1274–1276

102

Chapter 6

Burns and scalds

Chapter contents

Procedure guidelines

The Great Ormond Street Hospital Manual of Children's Nursing Practices, First Edition. Edited by Susan Macqueen, Elizabeth Anne Bruce, Faith Gibson.
© 2012 Great Ormond Street Hospital for Children NHS Foundation Trust. Published 2012 by Blackwell Publishing Ltd.

Introduction

A burn is a traumatic multisystem life-changing event and the long-term care of the child who has been burned can extend over several years. Nursing care following a burn injury can be the most significant contribution to a child's well-being (Fowler 1994). It is important to remember that a burn injury can cause extreme stress for all family members. Therefore, children's nurses must ensure that the well-being of parents/carers and siblings is considered, as well as that of the child. Using a family-centred model of nursing and giving consideration to the five outcomes identified within the white paper *Every Child Matters: Change for Children* (Department of Health 2004) the children's nurse should continually assess and evaluate nursing care. According to the National Burn Care Review (NBCR 2001), the goal of burn care is the restoration of form, function and feeling and that treatment should consist of seven phases (see Figure 6.1). With this in mind, this chapter will look at the process of burn management from injury through to healing and will cover the topics listed below:

- Common causes of burns in children
- Overview of anatomy of the skin
- Classification of burns
- First aid following a burn
- Assessment
- Fluid resuscitation for major burns
- Wound healing and wound care
- Dressing changes
- Nutrition
- Psychological care following a burn
- Referral to the Community Children's Nursing Team
- Ongoing care of the child
- Health promotion and education following a burn.

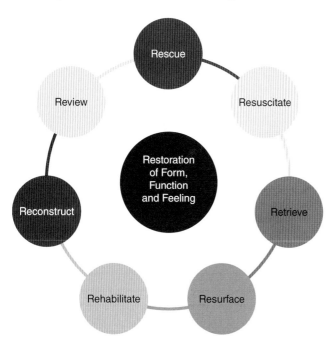

Figure 6.1 Seven phases of burn management (NBCR: National Burn Care Review 2001).

Common causes of burns in children

Burns are a relatively common form of injury in childhood and can be simply defined as the death/necrosis of tissues due to exposure to or contact with a heat source. Burn injuries can usually be attributed to the following sources:

- **Scalds:** Exposure to a hot liquid or gas is the most common cause of burns in children under 5 years old and is responsible for 60% of burns suffered by children less than 3 years of age.
- **Fire:** Exposure to a naked flame will result in a burn.
- **Contact burns:** For example, children coming into contact with an unattended iron or a radiator that is too hot.
- **Electrical burns:** These include contact with a live electrical source or lightning.
- **Radiation:** Children who have been inadequately protected from the sun can suffer from extensive sun burn.
- **Chemical burns:** Chemical (acid and alkali) burns differ from other kinds of burns as the damage caused may be attributed to chemical changes as opposed to heat. However, many chemicals undergo exothermic reactions on contact with the skin and this will also contribute to the severity of the burn. Knowledge of the specific chemical agent involved will direct subsequent intervention.

Overview of anatomy of the skin

The skin is the largest organ of the human body (Taylor 2001). Whilst acting as a cover for the body, the skin provides protection from bacteria as well as maintaining temperature and preventing water loss. In children under 2 years of age, the skin is one-fifth thinner than adult skin (Peters 2001).

The skin is comprised of two main layers, the epidermis and dermis. The epidermis is made up of epithelial cells, split into four layers, and acts as the outermost protective shield of the body. Below this layer lies the dermis, which makes up the bulk of the skin. The dermis has two major layers comprised of connective tissue. Connective tissue is made up of three fibres; the most abundant of which are collagen fibres. The connective tissue gives the skin its strength. Only the dermis is vascularised and nutrients reach the epidermis by diffusing through tissue fluid from blood vessels in the dermis. The dermis is rich in nerve fibres, blood vessels and lymphatic vessels. Below the dermis lays the hypodermis or subcutaneous layer, which is made up of adipose and connective tissue. The subcutaneous layer thus anchors the skin to underlying organs in the body. Approximately half of the body's fat stores are located in the subcutaneous layer and therefore acts as an effective shock absorber as well as an insulator to prevent heat loss (Marieb 2004).

Classification of burns

Classification of a burn relies on clinical observation and this remains the 'standard for diagnosis' (Heimbach *et al* 2002). The following list has been adapted from Appleby (2005).

- **Superficial burns:** Limited to the superficial epidermal layer of the skin. The appearance will be red, caused by erythema and possibly blistered. The skin will blanch on pressure and sensation will be extremely painful, as no nerve endings will have been damaged. The sun and minor scalds mainly cause superficial burns. These burns do not tend to scar.

- **Superficial partial thickness burns:** The entire epidermis will have been burnt causing a pink surface with both open and closed blisters. The skin will blanch less quickly on pressure and will be painful for the child. Scalding to the skin mainly causes this depth of burn.
- **Deep partial thickness burns:** The epidermis and dermis will have been destroyed here leaving some skin appendages. The burn appearance will be a cream base with blisters. The area will not blanch and will be less painful for the child as some nerve endings have been destroyed.
- **Deep or full thickness burns:** This type of burn involves the dermis and underlying fat. The appearance of the skin will be white, brown, black, leathery and waxy as a result of all layers of the skin being penetrated. These burns will not blister and are painless and numb for the child, as all nerve endings will have been destroyed.

First aid following a burn

The course of action taken following a burn injury is dependent on a number of variables, including age, percentage of body surface area affected, depth of burn and any associated injuries. In children, a burn involving more than 10% of the total body surface area requires resuscitation and once this is commenced the child should be referred to a specialist centre. However, smaller burns may also be problematic and require treatment in specialist centres to minimise the risk of complication. The following types of burns should be referred to a specialist unit (NBCR 2001):

- Burns greater than 10% in children
- Infants under 1 year of age
- Burns of special areas – face, hands feet, genitals, perineum and over major joints
- Circumferential burns to limbs or chest
- Full thickness burns greater than 5% total body surface area
- Electrical burns
- Chemical burns
- Burns with associated inhalation injury
- Burns indicative of non-accidental injury.

As with all trauma, children who have been burned should be assessed according to trauma management guidelines beginning with airway (A), breathing (B) and circulation (C). Basic trauma management appropriately performed at this stage can offset the development of complications at a later stage and will have a profound effect on eventual outcomes. The child's condition should be stabilised before treatment of the burn (see Chapter 27 for resuscitation).

Procedure guideline 6.1 First aid following a burn

Statement	Rationale

1. Assess the child's:
  a) Airway:
    • Has the child been in a house fire?
    • Are there burns around the nose, mouth and neck?
    • Is there soot around the nose and mouth?
  b) Breathing:
    • Rate
    • Rhythm
    • Noise
    • Work.
  c) Circulation:
    • Check pulse
    • Are there any circumferential burns or full thickness burns that may restrict blood flow to periphery?
	1.
	  a–b) A child's airway is naturally smaller in diameter than an adult airway. A burn involving the child's airway may result in tracheal oedema and may obstruct breathing.
	
	  c) Swelling from a full thickness or circumferential burn may compromise a child's circulation. In this situation an emergency escharotomy may be performed allowing the tissue to expand and restore blood flow to the burned area of the body.

2. Administer first aid:
  a) Immerse affected area in or place under running cold water promptly.
    NB. Do not use ice as a cooling fluid as this will constrict capillaries.
  b) Limit application of cold water to 10 minutes or 20 minutes in the case of extensive burns or alkali burns.
	2.
	  a) To reduce/remove heat energy from the area. Cold water rapidly cools residual heat, which will relieve pain, reduce tissue damage and reassure the child.
	
	  b) Excessive use of water can cause hypothermia (Fowler 1999). When the skin has been burned it is unable to prevent the loss of body fluid or keep the body at its normal temperature.

(Continued)

Procedure guideline 6.1 (*Continued*)

Statement	Rationale
c) Elevate any limbs involved if possible and sit the child up if the burn is above the navel.	**c)** Elevation of the burnt limb decreases oedema to the affected area.
d) Do not attempt to remove clothing unless the burn is chemical.	**d)** Removal of clothing may de-roof blisters or take off skin thus increasing distress. However, a chemical burn will continue while the material is next to the skin.
e) Topical applications should be confined to wet compresses or sterile dressings, while medical advice is being sought.	**e)** A wet dressing will continue cooling and thus relieve pain. Any other substance used could hinder subsequent examination and assessment.
f) Apply cling film as a temporary dressing or to retain a cold compress while awaiting medical intervention.	**f)** To help relieve pain, as the burn and thus the nerve endings are not exposed to the air so readily. Applying cling film will reduce the risk of bacterial contamination in the first instance. Clingfilm and a compress will also prevent the child from seeing the wound, therefore helping to reduce distress.
g) Cling film should be applied in small, overlapping sections.	**g)** To avoid constrictions to blood flow (Fowler 1998).

Procedure guideline 6.2 Assessment of a burn

Statement	Rationale
1a) Take a detailed chronology of how the burn occurred.	**1a)** To ensure that treatment given is appropriate to the extent of the burn.
b) If there is any suspicion of non-accidental injury then local child protection guidelines must be followed.	**b)** To ensure consistency and identify any discrepancies that might be indicative of a non-accidental injury.
2a) Establish the timescale of when the burn happened and the length of time the child was in contact with the source of the burn.	**2a)** To aid with the classification and depth of the burn. Fluid resuscitation begins from the time of injury NOT the time of admission to hospital. On admission fluid resuscitation may already be in arrears.
b) Establish what first aid measures, if any, were taken.	**b)** To enable more accurate classification of the burn and aid health education once the wound is healing.
3. Assess the depth of the burn:	**3.**
a) Observe and record the colour of the skin, presence of blisters and the texture of the skin (Fowler 1998).	**a)** To determine the severity and extent of the burn.
b) Assess the skin for capillary refill by applying pressure to affected areas.	**b)** Poor capillary refill indicates a deeper burn.
c) Assess the child's level of pain.	**c)** A burn is intensely painful. Deeper burns will have destroyed nerve endings but a burn is usually of mixed depth. Do not assume that a full thickness burn is painless for a child.
d) The percentage of burns on the child's body must also be assessed. This can be carried out using a Lund and Browder chart (1944).	**d)** The Lund and Browder chart accounts for both age and size differences in children. For example, the head will be proportionately larger than the limbs. The child's surface area is therefore accounted for (see Figure 6.2).
e) Alternatively the extent of the burn can be assessed by using the child's own palm size. The rule of nines may also be used (modified for use in children) to calculate the percentage body surface area burned.	**e)** The child's own palm size represents 1% of a burn. This can be a more difficult method unless the child is co-operative and the burn is in one small area.

106

Procedure guideline 6.2 (*Continued*)

Statement	Rationale
f) The assessment of the size of the burn should be checked by two staff.	**f)** Inaccurate estimation of burn size can occur, with small burns being overestimated and large burns being underestimated (Collis *et al* 1998). This has knock-on effects for the calculation of resuscitation fluid.
5. If the child has sustained injuries to the face or neck they should be encouraged to sit up.	**5.** To reduce any oedema that is forming and thus reduce the potential for respiratory distress. NB. Children who have received burns to these areas should be treated at a regional burns unit and may require assessment by an anaesthetist prior to transfer.

107

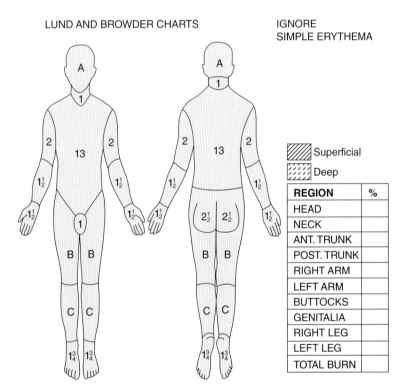

LUND AND BROWDER CHARTS

IGNORE SIMPLE ERYTHEMA

REGION	%
HEAD	
NECK	
ANT. TRUNK	
POST. TRUNK	
RIGHT ARM	
LEFT ARM	
BUTTOCKS	
GENITALIA	
RIGHT LEG	
LEFT LEG	
TOTAL BURN	

RELATIVE PERCENTAGE OF BODY SURFACE AREA AFFECTED BY GROWTH

AREA	AGE 0	1	5	10	15	ADULT
A = ½ OF HEAD	9½	8½	6½	8½	4½	3½
B = ½ OF ONE THIGH	2¾	3¼	4	4½	4½	4¾
C = ½ OF ONE LEG	2½	2½	2¾	3	3¼	3½

Figure 6.2 The Lund and Browder chart (1944) (Bosworth 1997).

Fluid resuscitation for major burns

The first 24 hours following the burn is known as the shock phase. If a child's injuries are over 10% of their body surface area then the child will have lost a large amount of body fluid, which will result in a reduction in the circulating blood volume (Clarke 1992, Fowler 1998). Fluid resuscitation will therefore be needed.

Box 6.1 Parkland formula

Parkland formula for fluid replacement (Pape *et al* 2001)
3–4 ml Hartmann's solution × body weight (kg) × % burn
= Total amount of resuscitation fluid to be infused in 24 hrs.

Principles table 6.1 **Fluid resuscitation**

Principle	Rationale
1. The majority of burns units recommend the use of crystalloids for fluid replacement (Pape *et al* 2001) although colloids are also used.	1. A recent Cochrane review concluded that colloids are more expensive than crystalloids and have not been shown to be any more effective in fluid resuscitation (Perel *et al* 2009).
2. The Parkland formula (Pape *et al* 2001) is used to replace lost fluid over 24 hours (see Box 6.1). a) Half of the calculated total is given over the first 8 hours; the second half is given over the remaining 16 hours. b) Fluid resuscitation begins from the time of the injury and NOT the time of admission.	2. To maintain blood supply to all vital organs, particularly the viscera (organs within the body cavities) (Muir *et al* 1987). To detect and ameliorate the effects of hypovolaemic shock.
3. The child also has a metabolic water requirement. This should be given at 1.5 ml per kg per hour. Infants should receive a minimum of 30 ml per hour (Clarke 1992).	
4. Regular monitoring of urea and electrolytes, packed cell volume and urine output during the resuscitation phase is essential.	4. To replace electrolytes lost through the burn injury. Young children may be particularly prone to hypoglycaemia.
5. Oral consumption of liquids should be encouraged if possible, **unless specifically contra-indicated**. Clarke (1992) recommends the use of Dioralyte.	5, 6. There is a significant risk of paralytic ileus developing and early feeding offsets its development (Davies and Ward 1993).
6. If the burn is >10% total body surface area (TBSA) a nasogastric tube should be passed and enteral feeding started immediately.	
7. Fluid intake and output should be closely monitored. Following fluid resuscitation a child should be able to maintain an adequate urine output while fluid maintenance is decreased.	7. Urine output is the most important indicator of response to fluid resuscitation (Fowler *et al* 1996). If this is not achieved, there is the potential of acute renal failure.

Wound healing and wound care

Wound healing

As with any wound, the healing of a burn goes through several stages: the inflammatory phase, destructive phase, proliferative phase and maturation. The healing of a burn will depend largely on the depth. The following is an approximate guideline:

• Superficial burns; generally heal within 3–7 days
• Superficial dermal burns; up to 14 days. Skin grafting may be required if over a joint

• Deep dermal burn; 28 days/months. Skin grafting is likely to be needed unless area is particularly small
• Full thickness burn; this burn will not heal without surgical intervention. Skin grafting will be needed.

Wound care

Much debate exists over whether blisters from the burn should be de-roofed or remain intact before applying a dressing. Burn blisters are formed as a result of damaged capillaries leaking plasma. This leads to heat damaged epidermis lifting and separating from the dermis and the accumulated fluid thus causing the blister. It has been argued that burn fluid provides an ideal environment for bacteria to grow and multiply. In addition it has also been suggested that the burn fluid actually hinders lymphocyte and neutrophil function (Rockwell and Ehrlich 1990, cited in Flanagan and Graham 2001). However, it has also been argued that leaving the blister intact can promote healing and possibly increase re-epithelialisation by up to 40%. Understandably pain levels are greatly decreased for the child by leaving the blister intact. Flanagan and Graham (2001) recommend leaving blisters intact where possible, particularly for smaller areas of burns. This is an area that needs further research.

Burns dressings are carried out in order to reduce the risk of bacteria colonisation and thus infection of the wound (Fowler 1994). Cleansing of the wound should allow removal of excess exudate and previous dressing product debris (Madsen *et al* 2000). Dressings should be generous in covering the whole of the wound and should not slip. Ideally dressing changes should then be left for the maximum amount of time possible as repeated changes increase the risk of infection by potentially introducing bacteria to the wound surface (Clarke 1992, Holt 1998). In addition, research suggests that antibiotics should not be used as prophylactic treatment, as they may increase the risk

of resistant bacteria developing (Lawrence 1992). The wound contact layer should be chosen to best suit the needs of the wound. A partnership approach to wound management is recommended with the dressing of choice chosen in consultation with colleagues from the multidisciplinary team.

For any child undergoing a dressing change, the scenario should be as stress free as possible. Dressing changes and wound cleansing have been identified as the most painful wound-care interventions for a child (Kammerlander and Eberlein 2002). Appropriate and sufficient pain relief is therefore essential prior to carrying out the dressing change. Following consultation with medical colleagues, appropriate prescription oral morphine may be offered 30 minutes before a dressing change is due to start. This may also be supplemented with an anxiolytic such as Midazolam (Byers *et al* 2001, Hansen *et al* 2001). For children who are more anxious, the use of Entonox may well be more appropriate as it provides both analgesia and anxiolysis. Entonox can also provide distraction and requires the child to take control of their own pain relief and regulate their breathing. For more information on the use of Entonox and other pain guidelines see Chapter 21. The role of the family in this scenario is pivotal and their participation should be discussed in advance to ascertain what role they wish to play.

Procedure guideline 6.3 **Dressing changes**

For any dressing change the following equipment will be needed:

1. Clean dressing trolley or suitable large clean surface
2. Sterile dressing pack and spare galley pot
3. Sterile gloves
4. Appropriate dressings to place over the wound bed – follow local guidelines
5. Gauze/foam dressings appropriate to the size that will be needed for the limb – follow local guidelines
6. Appropriate creams prescribed for the child. In many cases this may be antimicrobial cream
7. Bandages and tape to secure dressing
8. Spatulas to decant any cream into a separate container
9. Plastic disposable apron
10. Disposable plastic bag for soiled dressings, etc
11. Wound swabs.

Statement	Rationale
1. If possible, two nurses should be available to perform the dressing change.	1. This enables one to remain 'clean'.
2. The room should be warmed prior to commencing the dressing change depending on the extent of the injury.	2. Extensive skin loss can result in a rapid reduction in body heat due to convection, conduction and radiation.
3. Explain the procedure in full to the child and the parent/carer using appropriate language that is easily understood. Give the parent/carer the option to remain in the room while the dressing change is carried out. Explanation should include how the dressing change will be done, how long the change might take and what the child might expect from the dressing change.	3. To ensure the child and parent/carer understand the procedure fully. NB Information and explanation should continue throughout the dressing change for the same reason.

(Continued)

109

Procedure guideline 6.3 (*Continued*)

Statement	Rationale
4. If the parents/carers are staying, ensure that their role has been discussed before the procedure begins.	**4.** To help relieve any feelings of anxiety and promote compliance from the child by involving the parent/carer.
5. Involve the skills of a play specialist where appropriate in order to distract and occupy the child while the procedure is being carried out.	**5.** Distraction will capture the child's attention and hopefully imagination and help to reduce distress. Examples include the use of bubbles or water toys if in the bath (Webster 2000).
6. Assess the child's current level of pain and administer pain relief in anticipation of pain during the procedure.	**6.** As well as background pain a dressing change will induce significant breakthrough pain. Administration of pain relief in advance will offset the intensity and or duration of the pain and make the procedure more bearable for the child, family and nurses.
7. Thoroughly wash and dry hands using soap and water (follow local hand washing policies).	**7.** To minimise the risk of infection.
8. Use an aseptic technique to set up the dressing trolley with the appropriate dressings, creams and bandages prior to commencing the dressing change.	**8.** To prevent infection. For more information on the aseptic non-touch technique (ANTT) see Chapter 12 on Infection Prevention and Control.
9. For large areas, by preparing gauze already rolled, the burnt limb can be quickly and easily covered without too much distress to the child.	**9.** Being organised and prepared will cause less anxiety for the child and parent/carer.
10. The number of dressings needed must be estimated and opened before starting the dressing change.	**10.** To ensure a smooth process. Estimation of the number of dressings required will prevent disruption to the nursing task and save money by preventing unnecessary waste.
11. If creams are being used then use a spatula to remove cream from the pots into a separate sterile container. Ensure pots are then labelled with child's name in order that they are not used for any other child.	**11.** The use of a spatula and separate pots of cream for each individual child will avoid cross-infection.
12. For dressing changes being carried out in the bath ensure the bathroom is above 27°C in temperature. Run the bath to an appropriate depth, ensuring that all limbs are covered with tepid water.	**12.** A burn alters the thermo-regulation of the body and wound cleansing causes a significant drop in temperature. After cleansing it takes 40 minutes for the burn to return to temperature and 3 hours for the body to adjust back to an optimum temperature for wound healing (Miller and Dyson 1996). Good technique will minimise this effect.
13. Remove old dressings from the wound. For children having a bath the majority should be removed before they enter the bath.	**13.** Removal of dressings allows reassessment of the burn area and any change of treatment can then be decided. Removal also allows the skin to be cleaned in order that any infection can be identified and swabbed.
14. Do not remove a dressing with force. Stubborn dressings should be soaked off in the bath or soaked off using saline or tepid water.	**14.** Forcing a dressing is extremely traumatic and can destroy new epithelial tissue and delay the healing process further. Bale (1996) states that many children may cope better with the procedure of they are able to soak their own dressings off in the bath.
15. Gently pat skin dry once the burnt area has been cleansed. Clean towels will need to be used if the child has been bathed.	**15.** To avoid destroying new epithelial tissue. To avoid infection of the wound area.

Procedure guideline 6.3 *(Continued)*

Statement	Rationale
16. If carrying out a dressing change without bathing use sodium chloride to cleanse the area.	**16.** Sodium chloride is preferred as it is a simple non-irritant solution that is non-toxic to human tissues. Evidence surrounding the use of tap water as an alternative has been inconclusive (Patel and Beldon 2003).
17. Following cleansing, apply appropriate cream or dressing to the affected area (adhere to local guidelines). The wound contact layer chosen should be determined in partnership with members of the multidisciplinary team following wound assessment.	**17.** All dressings act as a protective layer before application of gauze and should promote wound healing and allow skin to heal without sticking to the new dermal layer.
18. Apply generous layers of gauze or foam dressing over initial dressing ensuring all affected areas are covered.	**18.** Gauze or foam dressing will provide comfort through padding and also soaks up any exudate from blisters as well. This will enable the wound dressing to remain intact for some time.
19. Apply layers of crepe bandage and secure with tape ensuring that the tape does not contract and squeeze the affected area.	**19.** To provide support and fix the dressing in place without affecting circulation.

Table 6.1 Examples of dressing and creams

Dressing type	Rationale
1. Occlusive or low adherent dressings: These are laid directly over the wound surface.	1. Allow exudate through from the wound bed and minimise pain on removal.
2. Foam dressings: If blisters are present, these can be used as a secondary dressing over an occlusive or paraffin gauze dressing.	2. To soak up excess exudates and provide a comfortable cushioned layer to the wound. Foam dressings come in different depths and can be cut to shape without affecting the function of the dressing.
3. Soft gauze: Use over the occlusive dressing if the area is dry with no blistering and secure with a crepe bandage.	3. To provide extra cushioning protection and keep the area clean and dry.
4. Hydrocolloid dressings: Can be laid directly over the wound surface.	4. These dressings soak up exudates and form a gel that keeps the burn moist and warm. The healing wound would need to be reassessed to ensure that exudate does not leak through once its capacity has been reached.
5. Antimicrobial creams may be prescribed and used with dressings.	5. These have good hydrating properties and antimicrobial factors, thus reducing the risk of bacterial infection and promoting child comfort (McKirdy 2001).

Which dressing?

The aim of a burn dressing is to keep the area clean and dry and prevent the wound from becoming infected. However, in addition to this, the dressing used will play a key role by providing the right environment to support and promote wound healing (Baranoski 2005).

No one dressing is suitable for all types of wounds.

Benbow (2004) identifies the following issues that will influence choice of dressing:

- The action of the dressing i.e. what you want the dressing to do
- What the limitations of that dressing are
- How the dressing should be applied and removed.

Consideration of these points will enhance evidence-based practice. Specifically for burns, the depth, surface area and moistness need to be considered when selecting an appropriate dressing. Evidence shows that moisture plays an important part in wound healing. However, there needs to be the correct balance that will draw away excess exudates while maintaining moisture in the wound bed (Baranoski 2005). The nurse must also consider which dressings to combine together in order to promote optimum healing and be cost effective within their own clinical practice.

Table 6.1 gives a few examples of how a burn wound can be dressed. However, choice of dressings will largely depend on local hospital or primary care trust guidelines for wound management and local policy should always be followed.

Nutrition

All children require a balanced diet of vitamins, minerals and nutrients as they grow. Where the skin has been damaged nutrition plays an important role in the promotion of wound healing. Additionally, a burn injury is a major cause of catabolism and is associated with an accelerated metabolic rate and abnormalities in lipid and carbohydrate metabolism. Casey (1998) stated that children who are deficient in nutrients can be susceptible to impaired healing by the following:

- Deficiency in vitamin C inhibits collagen synthesis and capillary development. This is due to the unique structure of this group of proteins, which require vitamin C to form stable bonds between the collagen fibres.
- Protein is also essential for wound healing. Granulation and tissue repair rely greatly on the presence of amino acids and thus a protein deficiency will inhibit these mechanisms (Wallace 1994).
- A deficiency in zinc will inhibit epithelialisation. Zinc is essential for protein synthesis and therefore will be needed wherever cell division is taking place.

A deficiency in iron is not regarded to have a direct impact on wound healing. Casey (1998) argues though that oxygen delivery to the wound site will be directly proportional to the concentration of oxygen circulating the body and that this will be reflected at the wound site, with metabolic activity of the cells in the wound bed decreasing.

In the days following a burn injury involving more than 10% of the total body surface area caloric need of the body is greatly increased (Wilson 2000). For this reason it is recommended that a qualified dietician should carry out an assessment of the child's nutritional state. Appropriate nutritional supplements can then be provided in order to promote wound healing for the child. If a child is unwilling or unable to manage food orally appropriate steps will need to be taken to ensure that the child is receiving adequate nutrition. In the initial stages the child might benefit from having a nasogastric tube inserted. The nutritional need can then be met with reduced problems.

Psychological care following a burn

The psychological recovery from a burn injury is a long process. The child may display signs of extreme anxiety through the initial trauma, repeated exposure to painful procedures and possible separation from parents/carers during procedures. In addition, long-term hospitalisation can also lead to emotional problems for the child. Parents/carers, as well, may require emotional support. Feelings of guilt over the accident or incident are common. Assessment from a psychologist may be indicated to guide care interventions. A compassionate approach to psychological care is recommended from admission to discharge and requires empathy and a non-judgemental attitude. The following information can be used as guidelines when managing psychological aspects of care:

- Ensure information is clear for both the parent/carer and child and that any questions are answered to avoid misunderstandings and decrease anxiety.
- Involve the parent/carer and child in decisions surrounding their care to promote empowerment and control of the situation.
- Encourage adaptive coping behaviours on a daily basis. Maintain a positive attitude towards the child's body. Both the parent/carer and child should be encouraged to explore their feelings about the changes to the skin and its function.
- Focus on the child's personality as a positive aspect of themselves rather than the physical burn/scarring.
- Reintegration to school or college can be daunting and may require input from professionals to prepare the way.
- Children and families have individual needs. An adolescent may require more expert care to meet their emotional needs than a young child would. Care should therefore be delivered on an individual basis. Females show a lower self-esteem following altered body image than males when social support is not prevalent. Acceptance from peers and family is inextricably related to self-esteem, which in turn decreased emotional distress (Orr *et al* 1989).

Procedure guideline 6.4 Referral to the community children's nursing team

Most hospitals will have access to a community children's nursing (CCN) team within the primary care setting who will be able to manage care of the burn once the child is well enough to be discharged from the hospital setting.

Statement	Rationale
1. Check the address and contact telephone numbers for the family before contacting the CCN team.	1. The family may not be returning to their own home and discrepancies often occur with telephone numbers.
2. Telephone the CCN team.	2. To ensure that the referral can be accepted by the CCN team.
3. Fill out the appropriate referral form, including the child's name, date of birth, address, telephone number, name of person with parental responsibility, GP details, diagnosis, nursing care required and any other relevant information about the child's care.	3. To ensure smooth transition from hospital to home for the child and family. To ensure that nursing care is consistent with that given in hospital.

Procedure guideline 6.4 (*Continued*)

Statement	Rationale
4. Clearly explain to the CCN team how the burn occurred.	**4.** The CCN team will carry out their own assessment and may identify discrepancies that need to be investigated further. Good communication and collaborative working is essential for the well-being and safety of the child. The need for open working and safeguarding children is highlighted within government reports such as the National Service Framework for Children (DoH 2004a) and the Children Act (DoH 2004b).
5. Negotiate directly with the CCN about what dressings need to be sent home with the child.	**5.** Usually 2–3 days is needed for the General Practitioner or Nurse Prescriber to prescribe the appropriate dressings and therefore supplies are needed in the meantime.
6. Discharge the child home with appropriate analgesia for dressing changes and ensure that parents/carers know how long before the procedure to administer analgesia.	**6.** Parents/carers can be empowered to administer pain relief before the CCN arrives at the home.
7. Document all liaison and communication.	**7.** Accurate record keeping is essential (NMC 2009).

Procedure guideline 6.5 **Ongoing care of the child**

Scar formation following a burn injury will depend on the depth of the burn. A superficial burn will usually leave minimal scarring, while deeper burns may leave more obvious scars. Redness will be evident for months following healing as the skin has formed new epithelial tissue that needs time to mature fully. At this time the new skin will be hypersensitive to both heat and cold.

Statement	Rationale
1. Educate the child and parent/carer to use total sun block on the new area of skin for at least 12 months (McKirdy 2001).	**1.** New skin needs time to mature and will be extremely sensitive to heat (Howell 1998).
2. Educate the family to gently massage the new area of skin using a skin sensitive moisturiser several times every day.	**2.** Moisturisers will help to restore the skin's normal texture; minimise scar tissue; and prevent flaking and dryness that can occur in freshly healed burns (McKirdy 2001). These symptoms are due to the newly epithelialised tissue producing less skin oils.
3. Encourage the child and family to comply with programmes of occupational therapy and physiotherapy.	**3.** Ongoing adherence will reduce the incidence/effect of contracture formation and will help in the restoration of function. Superficial and partial thickness burns will eventually return to normal function, but full thickness burns will not recover this ability (Fowler 1998).
4. Any burn will alter the skin's make up and has the potential to scar. Pressure garments are extremely effective in the control of scar management and should be applied immediately following wound healing (Robson *et al* 1998). Silicone gels may also help in the control and management of hypertrophic scarring, reducing discomfort and irritation (Colom Majan 2006).	**4.** Application of pressure to the scar area will prevent further shortening of collagen within the new skin area and thus help prevent excessive scarring until the scar is mature. This has been achieved when the scar is avascular, flat and soft (Wilson 2000).

(Continued)

Procedure guideline 6.5 (*Continued*)

Statement	Rationale
5. Encourage the wearing of pressure garments. The garment should be worn for 23 hours per day for 1–2 years until the scar is mature (Wilson 2000). Children may find the garments hot and sometimes confining, so positive reinforcement of the benefits needs to be provided. Garments should be washed regularly to maintain hygiene and may need to be altered as the child grows. Children may find the garments comforting as they cover up marking/scarring and thus draw attention away from the burn injury.	5. Daily adherence will ensure the best results for the child's scarring. Pressure garments work to minimise the appearance of scars but will not prevent scar formation. However, they do help to protect the newly healed skin.

Procedure guideline 6.6 **Health promotion and education following a burn**

For the nurse caring for a child following a burn injury, health promotion becomes an integral part of their nursing care. Health promotion refers to skin care and scar care following the child's discharge home. The newly healed burn will be sensitive to sunlight and must be protected at all times by avoiding contact with direct sunlight and through use of high factor or total block sun creams. Health promotion is also critical for follow-up care in order to avoid further injuries occurring. The parents or carer should be educated as to why the burn might have happened. The following guidelines can be used as a basis for re-educating parents/carers in order that further accidents can be prevented. The guidelines consider how to prevent burns in children.

Statement	Rationale
Hot water/liquids	
1. Keep a hot liquid drink out of reach of a child.	1. If a hot drink is on the floor or low table, the child is more likely to knock or kick the cup over potentially casing a burning scald. Boiling water causes superficial skin loss in just 0.1 seconds and a full thickness burn in 1 second (Clarke 1992).
2. Always check the temperature of bath water before allowing your child to get in. Teach your children not to touch the taps. Never leave the child unsupervised in the bathtub. If possible run the cold water first and then add hot water until a suitable temperature is reached. Alternatively thermostats can be fixed in order that the water temperature doesn't exceed a certain limit, for example, 40°C.	2. Scalding can occur in a matter of seconds. A fall into bath water at 42°C results in partial thickness skin loss in just one second and full thickness loss within 10 seconds (Clarke 1992).
3. Turn saucepan handles towards the back of the stove when cooking. Never leave a child unsupervised in the kitchen.	3. Small children will naturally be tempted to pull a handle that is above them. This could potentially cause burns to the face and body as well and arms and legs.
Electricity	
1. Place plastic childproof plugs into all unused electrical sockets. Always unplug equipment with a heat output when not in use (e.g. electrical heaters, hairdryers, etc).	1. Little fingers fit very easily into plug sockets and thus potentially are at risk of an electrical burn.
2. Always keep irons out of reach even when cooling and never leave unattended.	2. Equipment like this can be easy to operate and may lead to a thermal burn if used by young children unsupervised. Irons remain hot for a period of time after switching off.

Procedure guideline 6.6 (*Continued*)

Statement	Rationale
3. Keep extension cords used out of sight and to a minimum.	**3.** Young children may be easily able to unplug from the extension cord, leaving a potential once again for an electrical burn.

Matches and candles

1. Keep matches in a container that a child cannot open and keep them out of the reach of a child. Remember that children can stand on chairs and climb up to shelves to obtain things.	**1.** To avoid accidental injury.
2. When smoking, avoid having a child on your lap.	**2.** A cigarette tip is a potential burn hazard for the child.
3. Ensure a child is supervised near burning candles or incense. Never leave burning candles unattended.	**3.** A child can easily put their hand into the flame or knock the candle over onto them, potentially causing a burn injury.

Fire safety

1. Keep a small fire extinguisher handy in the kitchen. Ensure older children know how the extinguisher works.	**1.** For a small fire this might be adequate to extinguish the blaze.
2. Educate your children in how to alert the emergency services.	**2.** The parent or adult may not be able to access the telephone and may need to rely on someone else.
3. Educate your children to leave the house quickly and safely if there is a fire and to avoid any smoke filled areas.	**3.** It may not be possible for a person to ensure everyone else is safely outside if the house is filling with smoke.

References

Appleby T. (2005) Burns. In Morton PG, Fontaine DK, Hudak CM, Gallo BM. (eds) Critical Care Nursing; A Holistic Approach, 8th edition. Philadelphia, Lippincott Williams & Wilkins

Ayliffe GAJ, Fraise AP, Geddes AM, Mitchell K. (2000) Control of Hospital Infection, A Practical Handbook, 4th edition. London, Arnold

Bale S. (1996) Caring for children with wounds. Journal of Wound Care, 5(4), 177–180

Baranoski S. (2005) Wound dressings, a myriad of challenging decisions. Home Healthcare Nurse, 23(5), 305–315

Benbow M. (2004) Mixing dressings – a clinical governance issue? Journal of Community Nursing, 18(3), 26–32

Bosworth C. (1997) Burns Trauma: Management and Nursing Care. London, Ballière Tindall

Byers JF, Bridges S, Kijek J, LaBorde P. (2001) Burn Childs' Pain and Anxiety Experiences. Journal of Burn Care Rehabilitation. 22, 144–149

Casey G. (1998) The importance of nutrition in wound healing. Nursing Standard, 13(3), 51–54

Clarke J. (1992) A Colour atlas of Burn Injury. London, Chapman and Hall

Collis N, Smith G, Fenton OM. (1998) Accuracy of burn size estimation and subsequent fluid resuscitation prior to arrival at the Yorkshire Regional Burns Unit. A three-year retrospective study. Burns, 25, 345–351

Colom Majan JI. (2006) Evaluation of a self-adherent soft silicone dressing for the treatment of hypertrophic post operative scars. Journal of Wound Care, 15(5), 193–196

Davies MP, Ward DJ. (1993) Long-term gastrointestinal problems in burns patients. Burns, 19(5), 423–425

DoH (Department of Health), DfE (Department for Education and Skills) (2004) National Service Framework for Children, Young People and Maternity Services. London, HMSO

DoH (Department of Health) (2004b) The Children Act 2004 – available online at: http://www.legislation.gov.uk/ukpga/2004/31/introduction (last accessed 18th April 2011)

Flanagan M, Graham J. (2001) Should burn blisters be left intact or debrided? Journal of Wound Care, 10(1), 41–45

Fowler A. (1994) Nursing management of a child with burns. British Journal of Nursing, 3(21), 1105–1112

Fowler A. (1998) Nursing management of minor burn injuries. Emergency Nurse, 6(6), 31–37

Fowler A. (1999) Nursing care of minor burns. Community Nurse, 5(4), 39–40

Fowler A, Byers J, Flynn MB. (1996) Acute burn injury: A trauma case report. Critical Care Nurse, 16(4), 55–65

Hansen SL, Voigt DW, Paul CN. (2001) A retrospective study on the effectiveness of intranasal Midazolam in pediatric burn childs. Journal of Burn Care Rehabilitation, 22, 6–8

Heimbach D, Mann R, Engrav L. (2002) Evaluation of the burn wound management decisions. In: Herndon D. (ed). Total Burn Care, 2nd edition. London, Saunders

Holt L. (1998) Assessing and managing minor burns. Emergency Nurse, 6(2), 14–16

Howell F. (1998) Management of minor burn injuries. Practice Nurse, 15(4), 208–212

Kammerlander G, Eberlein T. (2002) Nurses views about pain and trauma at dressing changes: a central European perspective. Journal of Wound Care, 11(2), 76–79

Lawrence J. (1992) Infective complications of burns. Care of the Critically Ill, 8(6), 234–236

Lund C, Browder N. (1944) Estimation of areas of burns. In: Bosworth C. (1997) Burns Trauma: Management and Nursing Care. London, Ballière Tindall

Madsen W, Reid-Searl M, Jones J. (2000) Minor burn management: an Australian regional perspective. Journal of Wound Care, 9(9), 431–434

Marieb EN. (2004) The integumentary system. In Marieb EN, Mallatt JB, Hutchings RT. (eds), Human Anatomy and Physiology, 6th edition. New York, Pearson/Benjamin Cummings

McKirdy L. (2001) Management of minor burns. Journal of Community Nursing, 15(10), 28–33

Miller M, Dyson M. (1996) Principles of Wound Care. London, Macmillan

Muir IFK, Barclay TL, Settle JAD. (1987) Burns and Their Treatment, 3rd edition. London, Butterworth's

NBCR (2001) Standards and Strategy for Burn Care – A Review of Burn Care in the British Isles. Manchester, British Burn Association. Available at: http://www.ibidb.org/index.php?option=com_docman&task=cat_view&gid=14&Itemid=28 (last accessed 18th April 2011)

Nursing and Midwifery Council (2009) Record Keeping: Guidance for Nurses and Midwives. Available online at: http://www.nmc-uk.org/Documents/Guidance/nmcGuidanceRecordKeepingGuidanceforNursesandMidwives.pdf (last accessed 18th April 2011)

Orr DA, Reznikoff M, Smith GM. (1989) Body image, self-esteem and depression in burn-injured adolescents and young adults. Journal of Burn Care and Rehabilitation, 10(5), 444–461

Pape S, Judkins K, Settle JAD. (2001) Burns. The First Five Days, 2nd edition. London, Smith & Nephew

Patel S, Beldon P. (2003) Examining the literature on using tap water in wound cleansing. Nursing Times, 99(43), 22–24

Perel P, Roberts I, Pearson M. (2009) Colloids versus crystalloids for fluid resuscitation in critically ill patients (Review). Cochrane Database of Systematic Reviews. issue 3. Available online at: http://www.thecochranelibrary.com/userfiles/ccoch/file/CD000567.pdf (last accessed 8th January 2012)

Peters J. (2001) Caring for dry and damaged skin in the community. British Journal Of Nursing, 6(12), 645–651

Robson MC, et al (1998) Clinical aspects of healing in specialized tissue. In Leaper DJ, Harding KG. (1998) Wounds: Biology and Management. Oxford, Oxford University Press

Rockwell WB, Ehrlich HP. (1990) cited in Flanagan M, Graham J. (2001) Should burn blisters be left intact or debrided? Journal of Wound Care, 10(1), 41–45

Taylor K. (2001) The management of minor burns and scalds in children. Nursing Standard, 16(11), 45–51

Wallace E. (1994) Feeding the wound: nutrition and wound care. British Journal of Nursing, 3(13), 662–667.

Webster A. (2000) The facilitating role of the play specialist. Paediatric Nursing, 12(7), 24–27

Wilson R. (2000) Massive tissue loss: Burns. In Bryant R. (ed.), Acute and Chronic Wounds: Nursing Management, 2nd edition. London, Mosby

116

Child protection

Chapter contents

The Great Ormond Street Hospital Manual of Children's Nursing Practices, First Edition. Edited by Susan Macqueen, Elizabeth Anne Bruce, Faith Gibson.
© 2012 Great Ormond Street Hospital for Children NHS Foundation Trust. Published 2012 by Blackwell Publishing Ltd.

Introduction

Child protection is everybody's responsibility and a key governance issue for the National Health Service. The identification of vulnerable children and young people and those at risk of abuse and neglect is a priority for national action, requiring strategies that support families and promote the health and well-being of children and young people. Child abuse and neglect are forms of maltreatment that can occur across all social classes and within all cultures, and may be caused by an adult or adults, or another child or children (DCSF 2010).

Child abuse and neglect is a complex area for children's nurses. There are many uncertainties, professionals often ask themselves if they have done the right thing, are they over-reacting, how can they possibly think the unthinkable? Public perceptions of professional roles are influenced through media reports of horrific child abuse and neglect. In other cases medical evidence appears to be in doubt and parents/carers are found innocent in the court. Personal sensitivity and awareness of the impact of the nurse's own personal experience of childhood, family life and parenting can evoke strong emotions. Nurses must feel well supported by managers and child protection specialists in their responsibilities. There are often no clear answers and difficult decisions have to be made jointly with partner professional agencies.

Within this chapter, brief summaries are given of important aspects, to aid understanding and to give meaning to the nurses' responsibilities.

The hospital setting

This chapter focuses on child protection in a hospital setting, and the responsibilities of the children's nurse. Children's nurses have an absolute duty to safeguard and protect children and young people from harm under the Nursing and Midwifery Council (NMC) code of professional conduct (NMC 2004), revised in 2008 (NMC 2008). This can mean breaking confidences by sharing information in order to protect (NMC 2006). Their prime responsibility is to the child, to whom they have a crucial, assertive and professional role in upholding their welfare. All children's nurses should be familiar with their local Child Protection Policy and procedures that set out the processes to be followed in safeguarding and promoting the welfare of children, including responding to concerns and taking action to protect a child who has been harmed.

Abused children can present in many ways in almost any department of a hospital. The importance of listening to children and providing them with opportunities to feel safe enough to disclose distress and confusion about what may be happening in their lives cannot be over-emphasised. This may be the one opportunity they have to do so. Children's nurses need to develop working relationships with families so that parents or carers feel confident about providing information about their children, themselves and their circumstances. The challenge is to work in a trusting, supportive partnership with a child's parents or carers but utilise the knowledge from parents or carers as one component of an assessment. The children's nurse can contribute a great deal to communication as well as other aspects that take place between professionals when abuse is suspected.

An individual and corporate responsibility

Safeguarding and protecting the welfare of children is defined as:

1. Protecting children from maltreatment.
2. Preventing impairment of children's health or development.
3. Ensuring that children are growing up in circumstances consistent with the provision of safe and effective care.
4. Undertaking that role as to enable those children to have optimum life chances and to enter adulthood successfully.

(*Working Together to Safeguard Children*, DCSF 2010 p. 34, para 1.20)

The National Society for the Prevention of Cruelty to Children (NSPCC) estimates that on average between one and two children are killed by their parents or carers every week, and infants under 1 year are more at risk of being killed than any other age group in England and Wales (NSPCC 2007). Many more children will suffer harmful effects to their health and well-being for the rest of their lives. Child protection cannot be separated from policies to improve children's lives as a whole, and must be part of a spectrum of services to safeguard children.

Childhood is defined as from birth to 18 years in the Children Act 1989 (England and Wales), the Children (Scotland) Act 1995 and the Children (Northern Ireland) Order 1995. Young people with special needs cared for by Great Ormond Street Hospital (GOSH) up to 19 years old are regarded as children and subject to the same rights for protection from abuse and neglect.

The government in June 2010 commissioned Eileen Munro, Professor of Social Work, to review child protection practice and front line services. Essentially a review of social work practice, Munro calls for the focus to be shifted towards more proactive early interventions that benefit families as a whole and a system that keeps a focus on whether children are being effectively helped and protected (Munro 2010, 2011a, 2011b).

The overwhelming majority of children referred to children's social care are living in families that are likely to be struggling (Munro 2010). In 2008/09, 547,000 children were referred to social services; this increased to 603,700 in 2009/10 (DfE 2010). A small percentage in both years became or continued to be the subject of child protection plans as they were assessed as suffering, or likely to suffer significant harm, but the vast majority were assessed as in need of some support and help (Munro 2010). As of 31 March 2010, a total of 39,100 children were the subject of a Child Protection Plan in England, because of concerns about abuse and neglect (DfE 2010).

Understanding what daily life is like for a child is crucial in order to identify and meet their needs (Horwath 2010). Nurses in their duty of care to children and young people need to be thoughtful and reflective and ask themselves; what is it like for the child to live in this family, today, tomorrow and at weekends?

Concerns about unborn children arise when thinking about safeguarding and protecting children. Maternal health and welfare play a crucial part in the development of the unborn child; the mother and child relationship at birth; and the ability of the mother to safely care for her baby after birth. Action has to be taken to protect unborn babies in some circumstances.

Defining child abuse and neglect

Four categories of child abuse and neglect are defined for the purposes of clarifying the predominant type of abuse to which a child is subject. There is often overlap between them:

Physical abuse

Physical abuse may involve hitting, shaking, throwing, poisoning, burning, scalding, drowning, suffocating, or otherwise causing physical harm to a child. Physical harm may also be caused when a parent or carer fabricates the symptoms of, or deliberately induces illness in a child. (DCSF 2010 p. 38)

Alerting factors may include:

- Unexplained bruising, marks, injuries or burns
- Multiple injuries of different ages/site
- History incompatible with injury/illness, i.e. fractures in a non-mobile baby.

Recent research (Kolko 2002, cited in DCSF 2007 p.15) has shown that children who have been physically abused have higher rates of psychiatric problems, violence and anti-social behaviour in later life.

Fabricated and induced illness (FII) is a complex form of abuse that many children's nurses will meet, especially in specialist and tertiary children's hospitals. The effects to the child are significant, affecting them physically, emotionally, developmentally and socially (DCSF 2008). It is associated with significant mortality, physical illness and disability (RCPCH 2009 Ch 4, 4.1). This is an illness in which the history or the investigations have been falsified, or induced, by the parent or carer. The children will already have undergone a series of investigations and treatment in their district general hospital or other settings before being referred to a tertiary or specialist hospital for further diagnostic tests. They may already have an underlying health disorder that is organic in nature.

There are three main ways of a parent or carer fabricating or inducing illness in a child. These are not mutually exclusive:

1. Fabrication (false reporting) of signs and symptoms, which may include significant exaggeration, and fabrication of past medical history.
2. Falsification of hospital charts and records and falsification of letters and documents. It also includes interference with specimens of body fluids.
3. Induction of illness in the child by a variety of means, including interfering with IV lines.

The early sharing of concerns with senior staff with expertise in the management and diagnosis of this type of abuse are crucial. Children must be kept safe during periods of investigation and observation. Staff, especially children's nurses who spend long periods of time with the parents and carers, must feel well supported. The management of suspected or actual fabricated or induced illness follows the same path as other forms of child abuse and Trust procedures have guidance on the management of perplexing presentations that must be followed.

Neglect

Neglect is the persistent failure to meet a child's basic physical and/or psychological needs, likely to result in the serious impairment of the child's health or development. Neglect may occur during pregnancy as a result of maternal substance abuse. Once a child is born, neglect may involve a parent or carer failing to provide adequate food, clothing and shelter (including exclusion from home or abandonment); failing to protect a child from physical and emotional harm or danger; failure to ensure adequate supervision including the use of inadequate care-takers, or the failure to ensure access to appropriate medical care or treatment. It may also include neglect of, or unresponsiveness to, a child's basic emotional needs. (DCSF 2010 p.39)

Neglect accounted for 45% of children and young people subject to a child protection plan as on 31 March 2009 (DCSF 2009a). A recent small-scale descriptive study (Lewin and Heron 2007) of health visitors' experiences of working with families, ranked the most important characteristics of neglect to include parental behaviour related to violence in the home; a domestic environment of high criticism and low warmth; and the lack of care of children. Stevenson (2007) emphasises the serious effects of neglect and expresses major concern at the persistent high proportion of children registered under this category. Crittenden's evidence (1996 cited in DCSF 2007 p.16) that neglect can result in damage to the overall health, emotional or behavioural development and identity in children demonstrates the catastrophic effects of this type of abuse.

Alerting factors presenting in hospital may include:

- Poor hygiene
- Delay in seeking medical attention
- Underweight with no medical cause.

Sexual abuse

Sexual abuse involves forcing or enticing a child or young person to take part in sexual activities, including prostitution, whether or not the child is aware of what is happening. The activities may involve physical contact, including penetrative (e.g. rape or buggery or oral sex) or non-penetrative acts. They may include non-contact activities, such as involving children in looking at, or in the production of, pornographic material or watching sexual activities or encouraging children to behave in sexually inappropriate ways. (DCSF 2010 p.38)

Much of this type of abuse is hidden and a significant proportion of perpetrators of child sexual abuse are other children and young people, some of whom will have been sexually abused themselves (DfES 2006a). *Staying Safe* (DCSF 2007) cites Home Office statistics from 2003, showing that approximately 25% of people convicted for sexual offences were aged between 10 and 24. Sexual abuse is associated with multiple problems related to social disadvantage, domestic violence and also chronic ill-health (Jones and Ramchandani 1999), but occurs in all social classes. The Sexual Offences Act 2003 introduced new offences to deal with perpetrators who abuse or exploit children and young people through prostitution.

Alerting factors related to sexual abuse may include:

- Sexually transmitted disease
- Pregnancy in a minor
- Bruising or bleeding in the genital area

• Children showing inappropriate sexualised behaviour, e.g. verbally, or through play.

There is very clear guidance for professionals who work with young people who are sexually active, both in the London Child Protection Procedures (2010) and *Working Together* (DCSF 2010). A sexual relationship can present a risk of significant harm to a child. A child under the age of 13 years is not legally capable of consenting to sexual activity, and such a case should always be discussed with a social worker. Any decisions for professionals not to share information with Children's Social Care regarding sexual activity involving children under 13 should be exceptional and made with the documented approval of a senior manager. Sexual activity with a child under 16 is also an offence and in these cases the nurse must consult with the Named Nurse or Children's Social worker. Children who are sexually exploited are a group that have clearly identified risks of running away from home, gang activity, child trafficking and substance misuse (DCSF 2010). The risk of significant harm to children and vulnerable young people who are caught up in any form of sexual activity cannot be underestimated, and the referral of young people to children's social care is for their safety and protection.

Emotional abuse

Emotional abuse is the persistent emotional ill treatment of a child such as to cause severe and persistent adverse effects on the child's emotional development. It may involve conveying to children that they are worthless or unloved, inadequate, or valued insofar as they meet the needs of another person. It may feature age or developmentally inappropriate expectations being imposed on children. These may include interactions that are beyond the child's developmental capability, as well as overprotection and limitation of exploration and learning, or preventing the child participating in normal social interaction. It may involve seeing or hearing the ill-treatment of another. It may involve serious bullying causing children frequently to feel frightened or in danger, or the exploitation or corruption of children. Some level of emotional abuse is involved in all types of ill treatment of a child, though it may occur alone. (DCSF 2010 p. 38)

Emotional abuse may be hard to identify, and the effects of this form of abuse may become recognised over time through observation of a child and interaction with their caregivers.

Alerting factors may include:

• Excessive attention seeking
• Low self-esteem, low self-confidence
• Depressed, withdrawn
• Witnessing harm to another.

The effects of abuse and neglect

Research (Advisory Council 2003, Amiel and Heath 2003, Cleaver *et al* 1999, for example) demonstrate that there are poor outcomes for children's health and welfare when they are affected by parental problems such as domestic violence, drug and alcohol misuse, mental health problems and learning difficulties. These are sources of stress for families. Abuse and neglect occurs as a result of a complex interaction between these different factors, which impair parenting. Impaired and harmful parent-

ing behaviour occurs within all social classes, there is no stereotypical association with social class.

The sustained abuse or neglect of children physically, emotionally or sexually can have major long-term effects on all aspects of a child's health, development and well-being (DCSF 2010). There is much literature on the traumatic impact of child abuse and neglect (for example, Bentovim 1992, Briere 1992, Reder and Duncan 1999, Reder *et al* 1993). Recent research (Glaser 2003) illustrates actual changes in the physically developing brain of maltreated infants, suggesting a wider and perhaps long-term damaging effect of neurological atrophy. Gerhardt (2004) interprets the findings in neuroscience, psychology, psychoanalysis and biochemistry and explains why love is essential to brain development in the early years of life. She describes how early interactions between babies and their parents/carers have lasting and serious consequences. Negative factors can occur in the context of how children and young people are cared for and nurtured by their parents and carers, how their developmental needs are responded to. Howe (2005), using modern attachment theory to explain children's social and emotional development, scientifically explores the formation of children's minds in the context of these early interactions or care-giving relationships and analyses the risks and consequences of child abuse, neglect, rejection and trauma.

Children are affected differently by negative impacts in their life; but not all children are abused. There will be strengths within some families and environments that help to offset negative effects, creating a protective resilience in the child. Examples of strengths are the presence of one nurturing and responsible parent/carer, positive friendships with peers, other supportive adult role models, educational achievement and success (Cleaver *et al* 1999).

Sources of stress for families

Working Together (DCSF 2010 pp. 261–283) reviews and summarises key research findings identified as sources of stress for children and families.

Social exclusion may be caused by factors such as chronic poverty and often multiple disadvantage. Poor housing; poverty and social isolation as a result of racism and ethnic difference; living in economically disadvantaged areas; homelessness and living in temporary accommodation, all have a detrimental effect on the development of children. Children of young parents with little or no support may experience stresses in this category.

Domestic violence, including the threat to an unborn child, is a serious issue and occurs across the social classes. Approximately 75% of children subject to a child protection plan live in homes where domestic violence occurs (DoH 2005) and mothers who are victims may be unable to protect their children from either witnessing the violence or becoming directly involved. Children may be greatly distressed by witnessing the physical and emotional suffering of a parent/carer and prolonged and/or regular exposure to domestic violence can have a serious impact on a child's development and emotional well-being, leading to serious anxiety and distress, despite the best efforts of the victim parent/carer to protect the child (DCSF 2010, LSCB 2007, 2008). Over 30% of domestic violence starts during pregnancy (DoH

2005). Assaults on pregnant women frequently involve kicks and punches directed to the mother's abdomen.

Under the Adoption and Children Act 2002, living with or witnessing domestic violence is identified as a source of 'significant harm' for children. The *London Child Protection Procedures 2nd edition* (LSCB 2003) states that:

> where there is domestic violence the implications for the children . . . must be considered because research evidence indicates a strong link between domestic violence and all types of abuse and neglect. (LSCB 2003 p. 158. 9.4.3)

The 3rd edition (LSCB 2007) elaborates on this earlier guidance making it clear the impact domestic violence can have on children. Furthermore, London Safeguarding Children Board supplementary guidance *Safeguarding Children Abused through Domestic Violence* (LSCB 2008) states that where there is a child under the age of 1 year, or a history of domestic violence in pregnancy, the child protection process must be initiated.

Nurses must follow normal child protection procedures if they know that a child is being exposed to domestic violence, and refer to the hospital social worker. Similarly the nurse must know how to access services to support a mother to protect herself. It is very hard for women in some cultures to talk about domestic violence and the children's nurse will be in situations, caring for a child, where a mother may feel safe to disclose such abuse. A comprehensive toolkit that details the relevant legislation and inter-relationship between domestic violence and the abuse and neglect of children, has been developed for staff to support work with children and young people (DoH 2009).

Staying Safe (DCSF 2007 p. 22) reports evidence that children who grow up in violent households can show a lack of interest in their environment and poorer intellectual development. Serious behavioural problems were shown to be 17 times higher for boys and 10 times higher for girls who had witnessed the abuse of their mother; and one study found that 26% of homeless 16–25 year olds had left home because of domestic violence.

Mental illness in the parent or carer may impact on a child's developmental needs. There should always be an assessment of the parenting capacity and the implication for the child; many parents/carers with a mental illness care very well for their children, and are aware and seek help for times when they are not. Some parents/carers with mental illness may be unable to provide for their child's physical needs, or be emotionally unavailable for the child, leading to neglect and emotional harm. Post-natal depression can also be linked to behavioural and physiological problems in the infants of such mothers.

Drug and alcohol misuse in a parent/carer has complex effects on children, relating to the parents/carers lifestyle and capacity to parent safely and responsibly. As with mental illness in a parent/carer, it is important not to generalise, and a thorough assessment is required. The effect to the child is what is important. The effects include harm caused by maternal transmission of substances during pregnancy and the reduced parenting capacity of those under the influence of drugs and/or alcohol. Children will also be physically affected and distressed by a parent/carer who may show bizarre, unpredictable and dangerous behaviour when using some substances.

It must be remembered that there is often overlap between these known key risk factors; one can lead to another and the effects to the child compounded.

Staying Safe (DCSF 2007) cites research showing that:

> Children of parents/carers with alcohol or drug problems, mental illness or domestic violence issues can have an inability to concentrate at school, perform below expected ability and miss school often to look after parents/carers or siblings . . . alcohol is involved in 33% of child abuse cases, and 40% of domestic violence incidents. In at least 40% of domestic violence cases, there is also childhood physical and sexual abuse, involving the same perpetrator; and, parental substance misuse or domestic violence issues made parents/carers reluctant to own up to their problems because they are fearful their children may be removed from their care. (DCSF 2007 p. 22)

Parent/carer or parents/carers with a learning disability may experience stress and difficulty in bringing up their children. Again it is important not to generalise, and a thorough assessment is required. The effect to the child is what is important. A parent/carer may not have the capacity to respond safely or appropriately to a child's developmental needs, or anticipate what these may be. This is compounded when there are additional stressors such as social exclusion and other health and social issues as already discussed in the above points.

Children with disabilities

Children and young people with disabilities are more likely to use hospital based services than their non-disabled counterparts. 'Disability' used as a term in this chapter also includes the group of children with chronic health needs. The National Service Framework for Children, Young People and Maternity Services (DoH 2004a) includes clear standards for practice when working with this group of children and their families.

Disabled children and young people were found to be over three times more likely to be abused or neglected than their non-disabled peers in the largest and most recent study to examine the prevalence of abuse among disabled children and young people, undertaken in the US (National Working Group on Child Protection and Disability 2003). Smaller scale research in the UK indicates similar levels of abuse or neglect. There is a growing body of evidence that disabled children, especially those with complex needs, are at increased risks of abuse (DCSF 2010 p. 202, 6.43). Evidence suggests that the presence of multiple disabilities increase the risk of both abuse and neglect.

A child with a disability is a child first and safeguards for disabled children are the same as for non-disabled children (DfES 2006a). The presence of a disability is just one issue which may affect the way that assessment is conducted.

The basic rights of the disabled child are as for any other child; that is:

- The right to express one's feelings and have these taken into account
- The right to safety
- The right to communication – by appropriate means of communication as necessary for children who cannot verbally communicate.

Practice Guidance was published in 2009 (DCSF 2009c) to ensure that agencies working at local and strategic level ensure that disabled children are kept safe; their increased vulnerability and risks of abuse are prioritised and they receive the same levels of protection as other children.

Difference and culture

All children have a right to grow up safe from harm. While in England and Wales, children of all nationalities are entitled to protection under the Children Act 1989. Nurses must have awareness and knowledge of culture-specific child rearing practices within the context of child abuse and neglect; differences do not justify harm and all children have the right to be protected. Child abuse and neglect exists within all cultures, but the child's needs must come first.

Certain practices, such as female circumcision, are against the law in the UK and many other countries.

The legal framework, national and political influences

The Children Act 1989 set out the law and guidance for the care and protection of children and young people, emphasising the need for shared responsibilities to safeguard children and young people from abuse and neglect, and to promote their well-being.

The two key principles of the Children Act 1989 are:

1. The child's welfare must always come first (the child's welfare is paramount). This means that a child's needs and best interests must be put above all else. Due consideration must be given to the child's religious beliefs, racial origin and cultural and linguistic background.
2. Parental responsibility replaces the former concept of parental rights. Parental responsibility is defined as the duty of the parents/carers to care for their child physically, emotionally and morally.

Legislation does not clearly define abuse and neglect but the Children Act 1989 describes Harm. Harm is defined under Section 31(9) (s31(9)) of the Children Act 1989, amended by the Adoption and Children Act 2002, as follows:

'harm' means ill-treatment or the impairment of health or development, including, for example impairment suffered from seeing or hearing the ill-treatment of another;
'Development' means physical or mental health; and
'Ill-treatment' includes sexual abuse and forms of ill-treatment which are not physical.

The concept of Significant Harm was introduced as the threshold by which compulsory intervention in family life, in the best interests of the child, was justified. Section 47 (s47) of the Children Act 1989 provides the Local Authority with a duty to investigate any report that a child is suffering, or likely to suffer, significant harm. Significant Harm is defined as: 'injury, ill treatment or avoidable impairment of health and development that is due to a standard of care below that of a reasonable parent'. It also includes the impairment of a child's health or development as a result of witnessing the ill-treatment of another person (as amended by the Adoption and Children Act 2002).

There are no absolute criteria on which to rely when judging what constitutes 'significant harm' and different factors are taken into account, including the duration and frequency of the abuse and neglect and the degree of threat and coercion (DCSF 2010).

Under Section 31(10) (s31(10)) of the Children Act 1989:

Where the question of whether harm suffered by a child is significant turns on the child's health and development, his health or development shall be compared with that which could be reasonably be expected of a similar child.

Children's social care services have a statutory duty to investigate possible or suspected cases of abuse and neglect under the Children Act 1989. Two other agencies have that statutory function, the police and the National Society for the Prevention of Cruelty to Children (NSPCC). Health services have a duty to refer concerns and identified cases to children's social care services and to cooperate in an investigation.

The local authority has a duty to provide services necessary to safeguard and promote the welfare of children 'in need' in their areas under Section 17 (s17) of the Children Act 1989. A child is defined as 'in need' when:

He (or she) is unlikely to achieve or maintain, or to have the opportunity of achieving or maintaining, a reasonable standard of health or development without the provision for him of services by a local authority;

or

His health or development is likely to be significantly impaired, or further impaired, without the provision of such services;

or

He is disabled

Since the Children Act 1989 the 21st century has seen significant development in policy and practice in children's services, aimed at improving safeguards for children and young people.

The National Services Framework for Children, Young people and Maternity Services (NSF) (DoH 2004a) is a 10-year, developing strategy, setting standards to improve delivery and quality of care in the health services, to ensure that services are equitable nationally, accessible, needs led and centred on the child. Standard 5 focuses on safeguarding and promoting the welfare of children and young people, and is further developed in the Standard for Hospital Services (DoH 2004b):

All agencies work to prevent children suffering harm and to promote their welfare, provide them with the services they require to address their identified needs and safeguard children who are being or who are likely to be harmed. (Standard 5)

The *Every Child Matters* (DfES 2003b) agenda, part of the Change for Children programme shapes child care policy and practice in England and Wales. The emphasis is on all children, focusing on universal services which every child uses, with early intervention for children and families who have needs.

It sets out to reform children and young people's services; to protect children from neglect and harm as well as to ensure that each child is able to fulfil their potential, by reducing levels of educational failure, ill health, substance misuse, teenage pregnancy, crime and anti-social behaviour. Wide-ranging proposals lead to services to improve the quality, accessibility and coherence of services to children and their families.

While the NSF focuses on children's health in the broadest sense, the NSF standards will help the National Health Service to achieve the 'five outcomes' for children's services in the Change for Children programme, which is at the heart of the government agenda. All individuals and organisations are working towards shared positive outcomes. The five outcomes, identified in consultation with children, young people and families as priority areas for their well-being, are:

1. To be healthy – including improved physical and mental health and emotional well-being.
2. To stay safe – including protection from harm and neglect, from bullying and discrimination.
3. To enjoy and achieve – in education, training and recreation, with parents or carers to share in their child's learning and support them throughout their school years.
4. To make a positive contribution – the contribution made by them (children and young people) to society, enabling them to enjoy living in a richly diverse culture.
5. To achieve economic well-being – social and economic well-being includes encouragement to engage in further and higher education, training or employment and to be free from the disadvantage of poverty.

The Children Act 2004 provides the legislative foundation to support the wide process of change in the Every Child Matters agenda; focusing and reorganising the provision of services; to ensure that all agencies work together to achieve the five outcomes.

The principle aims of the Children Act 2004 include the establishment of the Children's Commissioner, to promote awareness of the 'views and interests' of children in England and the establishment of Local Safeguarding Children Boards. These Boards are made up of members from public, voluntary and private bodies that have responsibilities to provide services for children and young people. The Boards have a statutory responsibility in their respective children's services authorities to ensure the effectiveness of each agency's capacity, including Hospital Trusts, to safeguard children (Waterman and Fowler 2004).

Section 11 (s11) of the Children Act 2004 reinforces the duty of all organisations (public, voluntary and private bodies) to safeguard and promote the welfare of children and young people, and reinforces the need to ascertain the child's wishes and feelings regarding the provision of services (DfES 2007a).

The Children's Plan (DfES 2007b) was the broad strategy of the government of the time, to strengthen support for families and children during the early years of their children's lives with a focus on their learning and enjoyment, of which staying safe and keeping healthy is an integral part. Since a change of government in 2010, the essence of The Children and Young People's Plan becomes embodied in a principle: local strategic partners have a duty to identify children's welfare as a priority in their 'business' or 'service' plans (London CP procedures 2011, April 4th edition, Sec 1.1–1.4)

Statutory guidance from government on making arrangements under the Children Act 2004 informs a strong and robust safeguarding culture within an organisation that is accountable to inspection by the Care Quality Commission and Joint Area

Reviews (Waterman and Fowler 2004). Internal governance arrangements within the hospital include rigorous review of policies and procedures and audit activity to measure safeguarding capacity. Good nursing practice must reflect evidence based practice in child protection, including documentation; the keeping of records, and referral to appropriate Named and Designated professionals for advice and guidance.

The Children Act 2004 makes separate provision in Wales where there is devolved administration. In Wales there has been a Children's Commissioner since 2001 and whilst the duty to safeguard and promote welfare is the same, local leadership structures are not.

In Scotland a major child abuse inquiry led to a national audit of child protection practice. Policy developments and guidance led to the production of Standards for Practice that applied to all agencies (Scottish Executive 2004).

Learning from serious case reviews

Formal reviews and enquiries following the death or very serious harm to a child through abuse and neglect identify recurring issues, such as poor communication and information sharing between professionals and agencies, and a failure to listen to children (DoH 2002). The Statutory Inquiry into the events surrounding the death of Victoria Climbie (Laming 2003) analysed the role and responsibilities of the professionals involved in the statutory framework for child protection in this country. Both the Inquiry and the first joint Chief Inspectors' Report (DfES 2003a) on safeguarding children highlighted the lack of priority status given to safeguarding. The themes included; a failure to share information, poor coordination of services, the absence of anyone with a strong sense of accountability, frontline workers coping with staff vacancies, poor management and a lack of effective training.

Lord Laming concluded in his Inquiry Report that none of the professionals who had come into contact with Victoria understood what a day in her life was like (Horwath 2010). Of the 108 recommendations that were made, a number applied specifically to health services, and hospital. The Summary and Recommendations should be read by all children's nurses and can be found on-line www.victoria-climbie-inquiry.org.uk. One of the recommendations for hospitals focuses on the critical assessment and management of children whom, there is reasonable cause to suspect, may have been abused or neglected:

> The investigation and management of a case of possible deliberate harm to a child must be approached in the same systematic and rigorous manner as would be appropriate to the investigation and management of any other potentially fatal disease. (Recommendation 83)

The Government publishes biennial reports of serious case reviews so that themes and trends can be identified and lessons can be learned that will inform policy and professional practice. The 2003–2005 study (Brandon et al 2008) gave emphasis to the uncertainly and risk that is at the core of work with children and families. In most reviews there were numerous childhood adversities that had a negative effect on their health and well-being. The impact of domestic violence, parental substance misuse, parental mental illness and neglect cannot be understated and the authors highlight that it is a combination of these factors that is particularly toxic. The 2005–2007 study (Brandon *et al* 2009) and the most recent analysis of 2007–2009 (Brandon *et al* 2010) identified recurring findings that have significant implications for nurses, midwives and health visitors who work predominantly with children under the age of 5, and their families. Drawing on a dataset of over 600 serious case reviews, just under half of the children at the centre of the review were not known to children's social care at the time of death or injury, and secondly almost half of all reviews are in relation to babies under 1 year of age; two-thirds of the reviews are of children under 5. This emphasises the importance of effective universal services but in particular it reinforces that it is everybody's responsibility to safeguard and protect children. Information between the many agencies that have involvement with children this age, including children's nurses in A&E departments and minor injury 'urgent care' centres, must be shared.

Bullying is a growing concern for many children and young people; it can be very damaging and causes considerable stress. Bullying takes many forms and is the most common reason for calls to ChildLine. (NSPCC 2003). Children and young people may disclose to their nurse that they are being bullied, by their peers, or sometimes siblings in the home. The nurse must listen and ensure that the child can discuss the issues with an appropriate person (such as the psychologist, social worker or child advocacy service) to get the right help. Similarly, the hospital setting must have anti-bullying strategies in place to protect the children and young people in their care.

From 1 April 2008 the collecting and analysing of deaths of all children became a compulsory function of each Local Safeguarding Children Board (DCSF 2010). Lessons can be learned from this review process about the health, well-being and safety of children that can lead to appropriate policy for the future; influencing preventive or early intervention strategies at a local or national level (Sidebotham and Fleming 2007). A large proportion of child deaths will be as a result of chronic illness, disability and life limiting conditions, others will be from accidents, and a minority as a consequence of abuse and neglect. In the former, children's nurses should be familiar with their Trust's policy for End of Life plans. In the latter, any suspicious death will be managed as directed in the Trust's child protection policy.

An important factor of safeguarding was highlighted in a report *Why Children Die* (CEMACH 2008). It was found that some of the children who had later died had not been taken to hospital follow-up appointments. Hospitals must have a clear published policy on the process for following up children who miss out-patient appointments (Care Quality Commission (CQC) 2009). Nurses may be the best placed professionals to contact and inform the health visitor or school nurse, as well as the normal process of notification of the family GP of a child's non-attendance.

Following the death of baby Peter Connolly in Haringey in August 2007 and subsequent investigations of serious harm or deaths of children in other areas, Lord Laming published *The Protection of Children in England: A Progress Report* in March 2009 (Laming 2009). Recommendations to further improve the quality of good practice that had been implemented following the Victoria Climbie Inquiry were made. Lord Laming argued for the focus to be on outcomes for the child, keeping the child at the centre of practice, listening to the child and understanding the perspective of the child. The government responded with an action plan (DCSF 2009b) that addressed the requirement for a 'step change in the arrangements to protect children from harm' and for leaders of local services to 'translate policy, legislation and guidance into day-to-day practice on the frontline of every service' (p. 3).

Peter was 17 months old when he died of horrific inflicted injuries. At the time of his death he was the subject of a child protection plan. Peter's life and involvement with professionals reminds us of the need to focus on authoritative practice and authoritative intervention by all professionals and agencies involved with children. Authoritative practice challenges parents/carers with expectations of their responsibilities to parent/carer safely, it challenges other professionals in the expectations of their services, and it assesses a child's experience thoroughly with a low threshold of concern, and keeps the focus on the child.

Within his report Lord Laming made recommendations for hospital Accident and Emergency departments. (Recommendation p. 28, Laming 2009). In many of the cases where a child has experienced significant harm or died as a result of abuse, the child has at some point been taken to an Accident and Emergency department of a hospital. It is vital that children's nurses working in that department are able to recognise abuse and be familiar with local procedures for making enquiries to find out whether a child is subject to a child protection plan. They need knowledge too of whether a child has recently been seen in another hospital Accident and Emergency department, ambulatory care unit, walk-in centre or minor injury unit. This requires appropriate IT systems, but, in the absence of such, telephone enquiries of other Units can be made as appropriate. Where an injury is thought to be non-accidental Children's Social Care Service and the Child's General practitioner (GP) must be notified as soon as possible.

Standards for Hospital Services (DoH 2004b) take into account those recommendations in the Victoria Climbie Inquiry report, which apply to children in hospital. As laid out in *Keeping Children Safe* (DfES 2003a) the challenges for corporate and individual action include:

- Changing cultural attitudes, so that staff consider whether a child's injury or illness might be a result of abuse or neglect
- Having interpreting services that support staff in recognising the particular needs of a child who may be at risk of harm
- Reinforcing the duty of the local authority to safeguard and promote the welfare of children in their area, including those who are in hospital and working with other local authorities and agencies to provide services for the child or family
- Agreeing and recording a multi-agency action plan before the child leaves hospital and emphasising that the need to safeguard a child should always inform the timing of discharge from hospital
- Having records of hospital care that are contemporaneous, clear, accurate, comprehensive, attributable to and signed by the healthcare professional providing the service and the responsible consultant where appropriate, and which detail any prior attendance at that hospital or another.

The government's key guidance for all professionals, *Working Together under the Children Act 1989*, was revised (DCSF 2010).

Key changes include the importance of keeping the child in focus, to ensure that where there are concerns about a child's welfare there is direct contact and observation of them, and assessment is underpinned by rigorous analysis. The definition of children at risk is widened to include young people at risk of harm from community based violence, which includes gang, group and knife crime. Children missing from school may require proactive multi-agency work, as may children affected by parental mental ill-health, who may need protection. The London Safeguarding Board Procedures (LSCB 2007) has been fully updated in line with recent changes to statutory guidance, and will be followed by a fuller revision once the government has responded to the Munro Review of Child Protection. With this upcoming revision in mind, version 4 is available online only (LSCB 2011).

A safeguarding culture

Skilled and competent staff, adequate managerial support and professional supervision are crucial elements in protecting children. Within an organisation there must be senior executive commitment to the importance of safeguarding and promoting welfare, and a clear line of accountability so that nurses know with whom they can discuss their concerns about children and to whom they can make a referral. There must be an environment that supports the sharing of appropriate information, valuing the expertise and skills of individual colleagues and professionals across disciplines who work together in the best interests of the child. Children must be protected from staff who would wish to harm them. Organisations have safe recruitment and selection procedures in place to prevent the employment, paid or otherwise, of any unsuitable person with children. As well as references prior to employment, all staff are subject to a Disclosure from the Independent Safeguarding Authority (ISA). New legislation in the Safeguarding Vulnerable Groups Act 2006 is establishing a more robust and secure vetting and barring protocol.

Health and Social Care Standards and Planning Framework for 2005–2008 sets out core standards that health, social and educational services have to meet by 2014 (DfES 2007a). Core standard C2 is relevant to safeguarding and promoting welfare and requires that:

> Health care organisations protect children by following national child protection guidance within their own activities and in their dealings with other organisations. (DfES 2007a p. 43)

Great Ormond Street Hospital has a child protection policy (Great Ormond Street Hospital for Children NHS Foundation Trust 2010) to ensure all staff are aware of the procedures for dealing with suspicions or actual concerns about a child's welfare or safety. This is compatible with the principles and requirements of the *London Child Protection Procedures* (3rd edition 2007, 4th edition April 2011). Nurses must have knowledge of these and any additional Local Safeguarding Children Board procedures.

Arrangements for 'out of hours' concerns are in place, with a key professional identified with child protection expertise to give advice and guidance, available on a 24-hour basis.

Education and training

Nurses having contact with children or their families need appropriate education and training to enable them to recognise abuse; to keep excellent records and clear documentation of concerns and communications with the child, the family, and professionals involved; and to know when to refer to Children's Social Care.

Competencies for healthcare staff have been developed in the form of a generic knowledge and skills framework (RCPCH 2006, updated 2010). This assists organisations to identify, plan and deliver the training and education needs across the range of their employees, enabling individuals working in any healthcare environment to receive appropriate initial and on-going training in relation to their specific role and responsibilities.

Children's nurses should receive level 3 training as a minimum and progress to level 4 and above depending on their level of responsibility and experience. The hospital must have a training strategy that is dynamic to respond to the needs of its staff. Single agency training (such as within the Hospital Trust) may be delivered through different mediums, which include e-learning as well as face-to-face group training.

Inter-agency training, available through the Local Safeguarding Children Board, helps to build trust and effective communication across professional boundaries by developing a shared understanding of each agency's roles and responsibilities, all of whom have a commitment to safeguarding and protecting children (DCSF 2010).

Child protection supervision

All nurses involved in child protection work should have access to high-quality child protection supervision, stated by Morrison as the 'cornerstone of effective safeguarding of children and young people' that 'should . . . operate effectively at all levels within the organisation' (Morrison 2005 p. 18 cited in *National Service Framework* (DOH 2004a)). Child protection supervision is a formal process, the primary purpose of which is to safeguard the child by undertaking an assessment of risk and formulating a child-centred action plan. It provides a framework, which is used to facilitate a development or problem-solving process with individuals or groups (Morrison 2005). When an individual child is receiving hospital based care over a long period of time there is opportunity to monitor the progress of the plan with the nurse, review and evaluate it.

Individual and group supervision must be available to all children's nurses and integral to a Trust clinical supervision strategy. The supervisor is identified as having some expertise of safeguarding knowledge to support and enable learning; ensuring practitioners develop knowledge and competence in the safety and protection of children in complex clinical situations.

The Chief Nursing Officer for England reviewed the contribution of nursing, midwifery and health visiting to vulnerable children and young people (DfES 2004). **Key skills for nurses** are identified and are underpinned by the *Common Core of Knowledge and Skills for the Children's Workforce* (DfES 2005), central to the Every Child Matters programme. They include:

- A need for all nurses in the acute health sector to have a focus on child protection, with Child Protection training as a core part of nurse education (**Training and Education**)
- Children's nurses to be confident and assertive to act on behalf of children and young people (**Communication skills to engage with children and families**)
- All nurses, including those in neonatal units to work proactively with children and parents/carers in areas such as parenting support and attachment (**Promoting Positive Parenting**)
- Nurses to establish trusting relationships with older children and young people; involving them in their healthcare decisions (**Positive therapeutic relationship to influence choices in health**)
- Children's nurses to be knowledgeable in mental health issues and specialist services to benefit children and young people (**Awareness of Mental health issues**)
- *Nurses to feel confident* in liaison with key professionals that must take place as part of discharge planning (**Inter-professional communication**)
- Nurses in Accident & Emergency departments (A&E) need to assess a family situation and take steps if they think a child is at risk in situations such as domestic violence or aggressive behaviour (**Pro-active intervention in risk situations**)
- Community Children's Nurses work alongside other child and family providers in children's services, in keeping with the principle of following the child and being alert to vulnerability factors and sharing information (**Collaboration with agencies in the interest of the child**).

Children's nurses should have knowledge and understanding of risks to children, how to recognise them, to know how to seek help; and have an understanding of other professional roles in the provision of services. They need to be aware of risks posed by adult behaviours that affect parenting and share concerns with named professionals early.

Implications for nursing practice

The importance of information sharing

Safeguarding and promoting the welfare of children – and in particular protecting them from significant harm – depends on effective joint working between agencies and professionals that have different roles and expertise. Individual children, especially some of the most vulnerable children and those at greatest risk of suffering harm and social exclusion, will need co-ordinated help from health, education, early years, children's social care, the voluntary sector and other agencies, including youth justice services. (DCSF 2010 p. 31 para 1.12)

Effective information sharing by professionals makes an important contribution to safeguarding. If children's needs are identified at an early stage and information shared, appropriate services and support can be provided for families, and more serious problems can be prevented. Children's nurses have a crucial responsibility to share information in their role as advocate for the child. Information that supports the safeguarding and protection of a child cannot be confidential, and must be shared (NMC 2006, NMC 2008, DfES 2006a). The decision to share information is always based on a professional judgement. Helpful guidance (DfES 2006a) gives clarity about confidentiality and consent, issues that cause anxiety for agencies.

The Common Assessment Framework (CAF)

Multi-agency working is supported through tools and processes such as the **Common Assessment Framework (CAF),** and the **lead professional role** (key worker to co-ordinate services for the child) (Figure 7.1). Nurses contribute to the universal CAF for children with health and development needs (DfES 2006b). The CAF is a simple and practical assessment tool that has been developed to enable frontline staff, who first meet the child in an 'ordinary' setting (such as in hospital) to complete an initial assessment, which forms the basis for a discussion and referral to Children's Social Care for services.

The CAF provides the foundation for a systematic and structured assessment of the child's developmental needs; the parent's/carer's capacity to respond to those needs; and wider family and environmental factors (that contribute to the child's health and welfare). Undertaken with the child, with parental permission, and their parents/carers it looks at the strengths as well as the full range of the family's needs, covering aspects that affect a child's development, from health, education and social

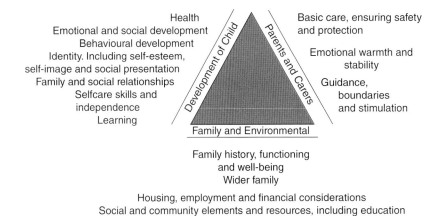

Figure 7.1 The three common assessment framework domains and their elements.

development, through to housing and family relationships. The focus is on early intervention and improved cooperation and communication between agencies that can provide services to meet the needs. It supports the sharing of information and working in partnership with families.

Parents/carers carry a copy of their child's assessment and plan, like the parent-held child record, and practitioners will add information and changes as they arise. In this way parents/carers will not have to keep repeating themselves in different settings. Although primarily a tool to identify a child's needs it can also be used to inform a wider assessment that is undertaken by children's social care where a child protection investigation is required.

Practice guidance for the children's nurse

Children's nurses should be familiar with their own local child protection procedures. They must know when it is appropriate to undertake a Common Assessment (CAF) and refer a child to children's social care for help as a 'child in need', and how to act on concerns that a child may be at risk of significant harm through abuse or neglect.

Procedures in Working Together (DCSF 2010) and *What to do if you're worried a child is being abused* (DfES 2006c) also clearly summarise what action has to be taken. The National Institute of Health and Clinical Excellence (NICE) has published clear and helpful clinical guidelines (NICE July 2009, re-issued December 2009) that cover the alerting features of child maltreatment in children and young people, in an easy-to-read format.

The nurse should inform her Senior Nurse Manager on the ward and the child's consultant of her concerns. All anxieties and concerns about a child's safety and welfare must be discussed with the Named Nurse, Named Doctor, or Social Worker from the hospital's Social Care Department as soon as possible on the same day, without delay. If there are disagreements between nursing, medical or therapy members of staff about making a referral, discussion with a Named professional must take place. All observations, discussions and communications must be recorded in the child's nursing notes. Where a child is presented with possible injury/injuries the Named Doctor will be

called to undertake a detailed medical examination as part of the assessment.

The following guidelines are adapted from Great Ormond Street Hospital Child Protection Policy, Procedures and Guidance November 2010. They reflect nursing procedures that are integral within the policy, and are not published separately. They may be used as a framework onto which specific organisations can incorporate their own policy requirements. They form the basis of statutory responsibilities of the children's nurse, and incorporate Lord Laming's recommendations from the Victoria Climbie Inquiry (Laming 2003) and subsequent law and best practice guidance as emerging from serious case reviews. They reflect the safeguarding standard as laid down in the NSF for children and young people (DoH 2004b)

Aim

1. To ensure that children in whom there are concerns are appropriately referred to the Children's Social Care department or police.
2. To enable professional practice to be audited as part of a quality improvement process in the recognition and management of safeguarding and protecting children.
3. To support adherence to the 'safeguarding' standards in the NSF.
4. To support the philosophy of 'Change for Children' programme and the Children Act 2004 by defining best professional practice, interdisciplinary working and focus on outcomes for the child.

Professional responsibilities of staff at Great Ormond Street Hospital

All staff, (clinical, non-clinical, clinical support and administrative) on joining the Trust Organisation will receive information on the signs and indicators of child abuse and neglect, and how to make a referral or discuss concerns about a child in whom child abuse and neglect is a possibility. This is in line with Level 3 training as defined by the intercollegiate document (RCPCH 2009), which is the minimum level for all staff who work within a children's hospital.

Principles table 7.1 Responsibilities of staff

Principle	Rationale
1. All staff, including children's nurses must be equipped, through training and support, with the knowledge, skills and confidence to make decisions and take appropriate action when queries and concerns are raised about a child in hospital.	1. Every member of staff has access to the Child Protection Policy (procedures and guidance), which is accessible on the Trust intranet.
2. All staff should familiarise themselves with the hospital procedures to safeguard and protect children and know who to contact for advice and consultation, and how to refer to the children's social care department.	2. An aide-memoire for staff, must be visible in all clinic areas.

(Continued)

Principles table 7.1 (*Continued*)

Principle	Rationale
3. Clear information in the form of a flowchart, giving details of how to contact Named Nurse/Doctor for consultation/advice and how to make a referral to Children's Social Care Services must be visible in all clinic areas.	**3.** The flowchart of **IMMEDIATE RESPONSES TO SUSPICIONS AND CONCERNS** must be followed by all staff involved (GOSH 2010 p. 10).
4. Prompt referral to children's social care services must take place where child abuse is suspected, who will decide what process needs to be followed and what the child's immediate safeguarding needs are.	**4.** There must be clear procedures to follow when children are 'in care' – in the care of a local authority, or on any type of 'Care Order'. Communication with the child's social worker must be frequent and documented. Formal written information must be in the child's notes confirming their legal status, who has parental responsibility, who has visiting rights and the plans for the child's safeguarding.
5. Children who are in the care of the local authority in any legal status, be it as an emergency protection order or another, have safeguarding rights that may include restrictions on who can visit them, who can consent to procedures, who has parental responsibility, and measures to ensure their safeguarding that must be communicated and documented to ensure their continuing safety. Nurses must ask on admission and document who has parental responsibility for the child.	

128

Procedures for children attending A&E

Great Ormond Street Hospital does not have an accident and emergency (A&E) department but children's nurses have important roles in A&E departments in other hospitals, therefore this chapter is included. Also, children may be transferred to Great Ormond Street Hospital directly from other A&E departments of other hospitals and it is important that the receiving nurse knows the processes that have taken place and when a referral to Children's Social Care has been made when a child is seriously injured, or abuse or neglect is a possibility.

Nurses in A&E departments must be trained to recognise signs of abuse and neglect, have clear procedures and know who to contact both routinely and in emergency, internally and externally on a 24 hour basis.

Each year, one child in six attends an emergency department because of injury. The true incidence of intentional injury remains uncertain, reported frequencies are between 1% and 10% (Benger and Pearce 2002). To put this into context, in 2007 in England there were around three million attendances in A&E departments of children up to 16 (CQC 2009). Children suffering from abuse and neglect can be brought to any A&E department in the country for treatment and assessment, and staff must be aware of the risk and indicators of intentional injury.

The following questions must be considered and answered:

1. Has there been a delay in seeking medical help for which there is no satisfactory explanation?
2. Is the history consistent?
3. Are there unexplained injuries?
4. Is the child's behaviour and interaction with the adult appropriate?
5. Has the child attended another A&E department or health service provision recently?

If the answer to question 1 and 3 is 'Yes', and 2 and 4 is 'No', this must be treated as suspicious; requiring further history taking, expert medical examination and action taken to safeguard the child, according to the local procedures. This will involve close liaison with social services and it may involve the police immediately, if a Police Protection Order is required to keep the child in hospital while further plans for safety are made and investigations are carried out.

The following indicators must raise concern and the rationale as for the above statement is applicable:

1. Frequent attendee.
2. Any bruising or injury in a young baby.
3. Unexplained bruising or a fracture or head injury in a child under 1 year or in a child who is not physically mobile.
4. Parents, especially young parent(s), presenting with crying or unsettled babies, or babies who are not feeding well.

Parent(s) who are very stressed and anxious with an unsettled baby may be actively seeking help because they cannot cope. Liaison with the Health Visitor, General Practitioner and other professionals involved is important, to request early follow-up in the community. Admission to hospital should be considered for a period of observation.

Principles table 7.2 Children attending A&E

Principle	Rationale
1. Make sure the child's full details are recorded: name (and others used) DOB, full address and telephone number, next of kin details, name and details of adult escorting the child, GP's name and address, name of school, language spoken at home. The accompanying adult or the young person themselves should always be asked if they have a social worker, and the name and contact detail recorded.	**1.** Nurses must have electronic access to an updated and maintained register(s) of the children subject to a child protection plan for the local authorities in their geographical area, to check every child's name against the register.
2. Accurate data on attendance to an A&E department must be collected on all children who attend so that there can be tracking of previous attendances and retrieval of those notes, and there can be checks against the local register of children subject to a child protection plan.	**2.** There must be clear protocols to follow if a child is subject to a child protection plan, which include communicating with the child's key social worker in the community.
3. Ensure history taking from the adult and child is recorded in detail, noting behaviour of both; recording these observations, and documenting injuries as seen and told about, prior to examination by the doctor.	**3.** Documentation and record keeping of what was observed, heard or witnessed at the point of admission in the first interview with the nurse is very important. This is in relation to the conversation with the child and the parent/carer, between child and parent/carer, and observation of the relationship between the child and parent/carer.

Good record keeping is highlighted as an essential part of professional accountability and good practice and a key factor where there is suspicion of abuse and neglect. If there is no record there is no evidence for action to be taken. Record keeping, including detailed documentation of all communications with both family and professionals should be very clear, with the rationale for action take.

Procedures for children admitted to hospital

When any child is seen as a patient for an investigation or examination in an outpatient setting, or is admitted to the ward as an in-patient, the following questions should be asked, or clarified with the parent/carer if they are already recorded:

1. Does the child have a Health Visitor/School Nurse (or school)/Community Nurse?
2. Does the child have a Family Worker or a Social Worker?
3. Is the child's 'Parent held record' book available?
4. Is there an electronic patient alert that states that the child is subject to a child protection plan?
5. Is the language spoken at home recorded? (In consideration for interpreters, information that is given to parents/carers verbally or written will be given in their preferred language where appropriate.)
6. Who has parental responsibility?

History taking should, on admission or attendance as an outpatient, in a walk-in centre or in an ambulatory care setting, record an accurate profile of the child's psychosocial background, as well as their health and developmental history. This facilitates seamless care and liaisons with other professionals as required. It also supports a 'needs assessment' when appropriate to aid the health and welfare of the child.

The following information should be written in the child's admission record:

1. Tick box marked or evidence that the question has been asked for each of the above statements, in admission data in child's medical records. Yes/No/Refuse.
2. Name of Health Visitor/School Nurse or name of School/Community Nurse recorded as appropriate.
3. Name of Social Worker/Family worker recorded if there is one.
4. All records entries signed with date and times recorded.

At Great Ormond Street Hospital (GOSH) a dedicated records section for child protection is included in a child's medical records once the threshold for a child protection referral has been met (except for concerns about fabricated or induced illness – see below) and in all cases of head injuries to children under the age of 2 years, unless that injury has been sustained in a car accident.

The purpose of the separate section is to support effective information sharing, assisting staff to maintain an overview of the welfare of the child and refer as appropriate. It ensures that both a coherent account of the situation and the plans to protect the child are easily available to staff. It is imperative that all staff involved with the child record any aspect of their care that concerns the child protection issue; all relevant contacts from parents/carers and both internal and external agencies involved.

A Lead Consultant for the child protection concerns is identified and their name documented.

Fabricated or induced illness: concerns or suspicion

If there are concerns and suspicions that illness in a child *may be* fabricated or induced, information must be frequently and regularly shared between all professionals concerned, including the Named Doctor for Child Protection. The fact that concerns or 'uncertainty' about the cause of the child's signs and symptoms have been raised must be documented in the child's medical records, nursing records and 'confidential' records (not immediately accessible to the parents/carers) where used.

In cases of suspected or actual fabricated or induced illness information must be frequently and regularly shared between all professionals concerned so that fabrication or induction can be identified. The child protection section should not be inserted into the records until the diagnosis of a natural illness is excluded.

To ensure that a child in whom there are child protection concerns is discharged safely there must be:

1. Documentation in the medical records that the Lead Consultant has notified the Named Doctor for Child Protection of the concerns.
2. Clear documentation in the medical, nursing records and 'confidential' records indicating with whom the concerns have been shared.
3. Conversations between nursing, medical and allied health professionals both internally and externally are documented in the medical records.
4. Conversations between professionals (nursing, medical and allied health) and the family are documented in the medical, nursing records and 'confidential' records where used.
5. All observations documented in the medical and nursing records.
6. Recommendations or investigations, interventions and treatment are documented in the medical records.
7. All notes entries signed with date and times recorded.

Pre-discharge planning procedure

There should be evidence, when child protection concerns have been raised, that plans for discharge are documented in the medical records by the lead consultant. This plan should be summarised in the Child Protection section of the child's records (GOSH) indicating that there is full cooperation and agreement with the social worker, medical, nursing and allied health professionals involved. This will include details of any strategy meeting held and the outcome of that (see The Strategy Discussion/ Meeting later in this chapter).

In keeping with the Laming Report (recommendations 70 and 71), no child about whom there are child protection concerns may be discharged from hospital either to another hospital or to home without a documented plan for their future, including follow-up arrangements.

To ensure that a child in whom there are child protection concerns is discharged safely there must be:

1. A clear plan for discharge in the child's medical record that includes a summary of the issues and future plan for protecting the child, including out-patient follow-up.

2. A clear plan for discharge with respect to child protection concerns, documented in the Child Protection section in the child's medical record, signed by the lead consultant and the children's social care worker.
3. A record in the nursing record that child protection concerns have been passed verbally prior to transfer of the child, between the nurse in charge of the ward and the receiving hospital or community nursing team as appropriate.
4. A record in the medical notes that the lead consultant or the registrar has verbally notified the receiving consultant or the GP as appropriate (if discharging to home).
5. Discharge plan (medical summary) to include names of professionals to whom this information has been conveyed, both internally and externally, e.g. child's social worker, consultant at the receiving hospital, GP and health visitor/community nurse/school nurse as appropriate. A written copy to be faxed to the GP/receiving hospital as per hospital policy.
6. If child protection concerns have been raised and on investigation not substantiated this should be indicated in the discharge plan as 'child protection concerns not founded, case closed with respect to this issue'.
7. All record entries signed with date and times recorded.

The strategy discussion/meeting

Where there is a risk of significant harm and a referral has been made to Children's Social Care, a strategy discussion (which may be an initial telephone discussion between a police officer from the child abuse investigation team, and a social worker) or a meeting will be called; the purpose of which is to share information gathered, and decide whether there are child protection concerns. The strategy discussion will ensure that there are plans in place to protect the child. Specific roles and tasks of each professional and agency are identified and the nurse's role is to participate in the discussions and considerations about the child and a plan of safety, and know the services that their organisation can offer. The nurse should be supported by the Named professional for Safeguarding and Child Protection or a senior colleague with experience. A decision will be made about what and how information will be shared with the parents/carers and the child.

Police specially trained in working with families in the child protection process are involved in the strategy meeting. Their role is to exclude criminal activity, they may need to undertake a criminal investigation and interview both parents/carers and the child.

A Child Protection Conference will be called by Children's Social Care, within 15 working days, if concerns about a child's welfare are substantiated. A Core Assessment must take place to inform the Conference, as part of the profile of the child and indicator of strengths and needs of the family. Authorised by section 47 of the Children Act 1989, this is an in-depth assessment that builds on the information obtained in the CAF, and is undertaken by the social worker (DoH 2000). Nurses may be asked to contribute to the wider Core Assessment and the analysis of the findings as required by Children's Social Care. The nurse will be involved in supporting a child through these procedures, and in turn will be supported by the hospital legal team and Named professionals. They may be required to attend the Case Conference, with the medical Consultant involved.

Where abuse or neglect is substantial or continuing, children and young people become subject to a child protection plan, which means they receive intensive support from children's social care and other services, as children who are judged to be at continuing risk of significant harm and in need of active safeguarding (DCSF 2010).

A child protection plan will be in place, to which all agencies contribute and it identifies what the role of each agency will be in keeping the child safe. The plan will set out the actions to be taken to protect the child. A central register of names of children subject to a plan is maintained by the children's social care department in which the child lives. This list of names is shared, using secure electronic systems; for example, when a child's name is entered into the database in their local Accident and Emergency department the staff will be aware of whether or not the child is subject to a child protection plan. The registers in each local authority are accessible on a 24 hour basis so that agencies and professionals who have concerns about a child are able to make enquiries of the locally held register.

Hospitals make internal arrangements for appropriate senior nursing staff to access the local Children's Social Care service 'out of hours' or when hospital social workers are not available.

When a nurse is alerted to the fact that a child is subject to a child protection plan, the hospital social worker should be notified immediately and the child's consultant and other professionals involved directly with the child's care informed. (This should not influence any decisions they make about a possible referral though.) At Great Ormond Street Hospital this would activate the insertion of a separate Child Protection Section into the child's main set of notes. The social worker informs the child's key worker in the local Children's Social Care team of the reason for admission (or attendance at the accident and emergency department, or as an out-patient in a department). The nurse will be informed of the relevant details of the Child Protection Plan for the child, who and what services are involved and who the key worker co-ordinating the plan is. Information is shared on a 'need to know' basis; the nurse should not expect further details about the child's protection plan to be given to them, other than what is necessary in relation to the nature of the child's presentation.

A final word – communication with other agencies

> The responsibility of both the message initiator and the message receiver to ensure that their communication is being understood.
> (Reder and Duncan 2003)

Problems of communication are frequently identified between professionals in reviews of fatal child abuse. Reder and Duncan (2003) explore the psychology of communication and the complexities involved. Meanings are attributed to messages both given and received, and the contexts in which these communications occur also influence the understanding of the message given. This is indeed a very important issue for children's nurses that can have a major impact on the safety of a child as a classic example below, cited by Reder and Duncan

(2003) from the Victoria Climbie Inquiry Report (Laming 2003), illustrates:

> Victoria was prematurely discharged from one hospital, having been admitted with suspected non-accidental injuries. Sources of the confusion were multiple, but included a nurse's fax that Victoria was 'fit for discharge' being interpreted by the social worker as meaning the ward staff had no concerns at all. It was intended to convey that, although she was medically fit, social services still had their assessment to undertake' (page 148). Then a paediatrician's entry '? Discharge' in the medical notes was understood by a nurse to indicate a definite discharge plan (page 274)

It is crucial that when discussing a child with another professional, in the same or another discipline, where there are suspected non-accidental injuries and/or in whom there are concerns about their welfare the **language used is clear and straightforward**, thinking holistically and clarifying that the person receiving the message has understood what the giver has meant to relay. In addition all communication must be recorded, dated and signed as per the hospital policy. In the same way any record written about the child or involving the child should be **unambiguous and clearly understood** by anybody else.

Acknowledgements

I wish to acknowledge Jane Collins, Chief Executive of Great Ormond Street Hospital for her contribution to the draft of the Introduction to this chapter and the members of the Quality Standards group (2004/5), in particular Sue Constable, lead Clinical Site Practitioner. These guidelines are not published separately but are reflected in nursing admission and procedural documentation.

References

Advisory Council on the Misuse of Drugs (2003) Hidden Harm. Responding to the needs of children of problem drug users. The report of an Inquiry. London, HMSO

Amiel S, Heath I. (eds) (2003) Family Violence in Primary Care. Oxford, Oxford University Press

Benger R, Pearce A. (2002) Simple Intervention to improve detection of child abuse in emergency departments. British Medical Journal, 324, 780–782

Bentovim A (1992) Trauma Organised Systems. London, Karnac Books

Brandon M, Belderson P, Warren C, Howe D, Gardner R, Dodsworth J, Black J. (2008) Analysing Child Deaths and Serious Injury Through Abuse and Neglect: What can we learn? A biennial analysis of serious case reviews 2003–2005. London, DFES. Available at www.dcsf.gov.uk

Brandon M, Bailey S, Belderson P, Gardner R, Sidebotham P, Dodsworth J, Warren C, Black J. (2009) Understanding Serious Case Reviews and Their Impact. A biennial analysis of serious case reviews 2005–2007. London, DFES. Available at www.dcsf.gov.uk

Brandon M, Bailey S, Belderson P. (2010) Building on the Learning from Serious Case Reviews: A two-year analysis of child protection database notifications 2007–2009. London, DFE. Available at www.dfe.gov.uk

Briere JN. (1992) Child Abuse Trauma. Newbury Park, Sage Publications

Care Quality Commission (CQC) (2009) Safeguarding Children: A review of arrangements in the NHS for safeguarding children. London, Care Quality Commission

132

Cleaver H, Unell I, Aldgate J. (1999) Children's Needs – Parenting Capacity: The impact of parental mental illness, problem alcohol and drug use, and domestic violence on children's development. London, HMSO

Confidential Enquiry Into Maternal and Child Health (CEMACH) (2008) Why Children Die. London, RCOG Press

Crittenden P. (1996) Research on maltreating families: Implications for intervention. In Briere J, Berliner L, Bulkley J. (eds), APSAC Handbook of Child Maltreatment. Thousand Oaks, Sage

Department for Children, Schools and Families (DCSF) (2007) Staying Safe: A Consultation Document. Available at www.education.gov.uk

Department for Children, Schools and Families (DCSF) (2008) Safeguarding Children in Whom Illness is Fabricated or Induced. Available at www.education.gov.uk

Department for Children, Schools and Families (DCSF) (2009a) Statistical First Release: Referrals, Assessments and Children and Young People who are the subject of a Child Protection Plan: Year Ending 31 March 2009. Available at www.education.gov.uk

Department for Children, Schools and Families (2009b) The Protection of Children in England: Action Plan. London, The Stationary Office

Department for Children, Schools and Families (DCSF) (2009c) Safeguarding Disabled Children: Practice Guidance. London, The Stationary Office. Available at www.dcsf.gov.uk

Department for Children, Schools and Families (DCSF) (2010) Working Together to Safeguard Children: A guide to inter-agency working to safeguard and promote the welfare of children. London, DCSF Publications. Available at www.education.gov.uk

Department for Education (DfE) (2010) Children in Need in England, including their characteristics and further information on children who were the subject of a child protection plan (2009–10 Children in Need census, Final). Available at www.dfe.gov.uk

Department for Education and Skills (DfES) (2003a) Keeping Children Safe. The Government's response to the Victoria Climbie Inquiry Report and Joint Chief Inspectors' Report Safeguarding Children (paragraph 11). London, HMSO. Available www.dh.gov.uk

Department for Education and Skills (DfES) (2003b) Every Child Matters. London, HMSO. Available at www.everychildmatters.gov.uk

Department for Education and Skills (DfES) (2004) The Chief Nursing Officer's Review of the Nursing, Midwifery and Health Visiting Contribution to Vulnerable Children and Young People. London, HMSO. Available at www.dh.gov.uk

Department for Education and Skills (DfES) (2005) Common Core of Skills and Knowledge for the Children's Workforce. DfES Publications. Available at www.everychildmatters.gov.uk

Department for Education and Skills (DfES) (2006a) Working Together to Safeguard Children: a guide to inter-agency working. Available at www.dfes.gov.uk

Department for Education and Skills (DfES) (2006b) Information Sharing: Practitioner's Guide. Available at www.dfes.gov.uk

Department for Education and Skills (DfES) (2006c) What to Do if You're Worried a Child is Being Abused, 2nd edition. Available at www.everychildmatters.gov.uk

Department for Education and Skills (DfES) (2007a) Statutory Guidance on making arrangements to safeguard and promote the welfare of children under s11 of the Children Act 2004. Available at www.dfes.gov.uk

Department for Education and Skills (DfES) (2007b) The Children's Plan. Building Brighter Futures – Summary. Available (archives) at www.dfes.gov.uk

Department of Health (DH) (2000) Framework for Assessment of Children in Need and their Families. London, HMSO

Department of Health (DH) (2002) Learning from Past Experience – A Review of Serious Case Reviews. Available at www.doh.gov.uk/qualityprotects

Department of Health (DH) (2004a) The National Service Framework for Children, Young People and Maternity Services. London, HMSO. Available at www.dh.gov.uk

Department of Health (DH) (2004b) Core Document, National Service Framework for Children, Young People and Maternity Services (Standard 5. Safeguarding and Promoting the Welfare of Children and Young People). London, HMSO. Available at www.dh.gov.uk

Department of Health (DH) (2005) Responding to domestic abuse: A handbook for Health Professionals. London, HMSO. Available at http://www.dh.gov/publications&statistics

Department of Health (DH) (2009) Improving safety, Reducing harm: Children, young people and domestic violence. A practical toolkit for frontline practitioners. London, HMSO. Available at http://www.dh.gov/publications&statistics

Gerhardt S. (2004) Why Love Matters: how affection shapes a baby's brain. Sussex, Hove, Routledge

Glaser D. (2003) Early experience, attachment and the brain. In: Corrigall J, Wilkinson H. (eds) Revolutionary Connections: Psychotherapy & Neuroscience. London, Karnac, pp 117–133

Great Ormond Street Hospital for Children NHS Foundation Trust (2010) Child Protection Policy, Procedures and Guidance 2010. London, GOSH

Horwath J. (2010) Assessing children in need: Background and context. In: Horwath J. (ed.) The Child's World. The Comprehensive Guide to Assessing Children in Need, 2nd edition. London, Jessica Kingsley

Howe D. (2005) Child Abuse and Neglect: Attachment, Development and Intervention. Basingstoke, Palgrave Macmillan

Jones D. Ramchandani P. (1999) Child Sexual Abuse: Informing Practice from Research. Abingdon, Radcliffe Medical Press

Kolko DJ. (2002) Child physical abuse. In Myers JEB, Berliner L, Briere J, Hendrix CT, Jenny C, Reid T. (eds), APSAC Handbook of Child Maltreatment, 2nd edition, Thousand Oaks, Sage

Laming, Lord (2003) The Victoria Climbie Inquiry: Report of an Inquiry by Lord Laming. London, The Stationary Office. Available at www.victoria-climbie-inquiry.org.uk

Laming, Lord (2009) The Protection of Children in England: A Progress Report. London, The Stationary Office

Lewin D, Heron H. (2007) Signs, symptoms and risk factors: Health Visitors' perspectives of child neglect. Child Abuse Review, 16(2), 93–107

London Child Protection Procedures (2010) 4th edition, Chapter 5.42/43, p. 238. Available at www.londonscb.gov.uk/procedures (last accessed 2nd January 2012)

London Safeguarding Children Board (LSCB) (2003) London Child Protection Procedures, 2nd edition. London, London Safeguarding Children Board. Available at www.londoncpc.gov.uk

London Safeguarding Children Board (LSCB) (2007) London Child Protection Procedures, 3rd edition. London, London Safeguarding Children Board. Available at www.londoncpc.gov.uk

London Safeguarding Children Board (LSCB) (2008) Safeguarding Children Abused through Domestic Violence. London, London Safeguarding Children Board. Available at www.londoncpc.gov.uk

London Safeguarding Children Board (LSCB) (2011) London Child Protection Procedures 4th edition. London, London Safeguarding Children Board. Available at www.londoncpc.gov.uk

Morrison T. (2005) Staff Supervision in Social Care, 3rd edition. Brighton, Pavilion Publishing

Munro E. (2010) The Munro Review of Child Protection Part One: A System's Analysis. London, Department for Education. Available at www.education.gov.uk/munroreview

Munro E. (2011a) The Munro Review of Child Protection Interim Report: The Child's Journey. London, Department for Education. Available at www.education.gov.uk/munroreview

Munro E. (2011b) The Munro Review of Child Protection: Final Report – A child-centred system. Available at www.education.gov.uk/munroreview

National Institute of Health and Clinical Excellence (2009) When to Suspect Child Maltreatment: NICE Clinical Guideline 89. London, NICE Publications. Available at www.nice.org.uk

National Society for the prevention of Cruelty to Children (NSPCC) (2003) Bullying: Policies and best practice. Available at www.nspcc.org.uk/inform

National Society for the Prevention of Cruelty to Children (NSPCC) (2007) Child Deaths/Journalist briefing July 2007. Available at www.nspcc.org.uk

National Working Group on Child Protection and Disability (2003) It Doesn't Happen to Disabled Children. London, NSPCC Publications. Available at www.nspcc.org.uk/inform

Nursing and Midwifery Council (NMC) (2004) The NMC Code of Professional Conduct: Standards for Conduct, Performance and Ethics. London, NMC

Nursing and Midwifery Council (NMC) (2006) Advice on How to Apply the NMC Code of Conduct Rewrite 2006. London, NMC

Nursing and Midwifery Council (NMC) (2008) The Code: Standards of Conduct, Performance and Ethics for Nurses and Midwives. London, NMC

Reder P, Duncan S. (1999) Lost Innocents. A follow-up study of fatal child abuse. London, Routledge

Reder P, Duncan S. (2003) Understanding Communication in Child Protection Networks. Child Abuse Review, 12, 82–100

Reder P, Duncan S, Gray M. (1993) Beyond Blame. Childhood abuse tragedies revisited. London, Routledge

Royal College of Paediatrics and Child Health (RCPCH) *et al* (2006) Safeguarding Children and Young People: Roles and Competencies for Health Care Staff. Intercollegiate Document. Supported by the Department of Health. Available at www.rcpch.ac.uk

Royal College of Paediatrics and Child Health (RCPCH) *et al* (2010) Safeguarding Children and Young People: Roles and Competencies for Health Care Staff. Intercollegiate Document. Supported by the Department of Health. Available at www.rcpch.ac.uk

Royal College of Paediatrics and Child Health (RCPCH) (2009) Fabricated or Induced Illness by Carers (FII): A Practical Guide for Paediatricians. London, RCPCH. Available at www.rcpch.ac.uk

Scottish Executive (2004) Framework for Standards for the Protection of Children and Young People. Edinburgh, The Stationary Office

Sidebotham P, Fleming P. (2007) Unexpected Death in Childhood. A handbook for practitioners. Chichester, John Wiley & Sons

Stevenson O. (2007) Neglected Children and their Families, 2nd edition. Oxford, Blackwell

Waterman C, Fowler J. (2004) Plain Guide to the Children Act 2004. Slough, National Foundation for Educational Research (NFER)

133

Chapter 8

Cytotoxic drugs

Chapter contents

Procedure guideline

The Great Ormond Street Hospital Manual of Children's Nursing Practices, First Edition. Edited by Susan Macqueen, Elizabeth Anne Bruce, Faith Gibson.
© 2012 Great Ormond Street Hospital for Children NHS Foundation Trust. Published 2012 by Blackwell Publishing Ltd.

Chemotherapy administration

Legislation

The *Manual of Cancer Services* (2008) (National Cancer Action Team 2009), an integral part of the NHS Cancer Plan (Department of Health (DoH) 2000), Cancer Reform Strategy (DoH 2007) and modernisation of cancer services aims to support quality assurance of cancer services and enable quality improvement. Within this strategy, a national programme of peer review for cancer services aims to improve care for people with cancer and their families by:

- Ensuring services are as safe as possible
- Improving the quality and effectiveness of care
- Improving the patient and carer experience
- Undertaking independent, fair reviews of services
- Providing development and learning for all involved
- Encouraging dissemination of good practice.

Peer review measures pertaining to safe practice with cytotoxic drugs include the *Chemotherapy Specific Measures* (National Cancer Action Team 2004) and more recently the *Children's Cancer Measures* (National Cancer Action Team 2009). Both of these documents clearly specify training requirements for pharmacists, doctors and nurses involved in the prescription, preparation and administration of chemotherapy within cancer services. Each hospital Trust must have its own policy and guidelines on the safe handling and administration of cytotoxic drugs. With the advent of Cancer Networks, these policies are becoming network wide and may also extend across a number of networks within a large geographical area (Houlston 2008).

Two authoritative reports published in 2008 (*The cancer reform strategy: maintaining momentum, building for the future – first annual report* (DoH 2008a) and *For Better or Worse – a report of the National Confidential Enquiry into Patient Outcome and Death* (2008) reviewing the care of patients who died within 30 days of receiving systemic anticancer therapy) highlighted concerns regarding the quality and safety of chemotherapy services. Cytotoxic medication, regardless of dosage or the condition for which it is being administered, is toxic to any rapidly dividing cells and therefore any errors in administration can be very significant. The National Chemotherapy Advisory Group's (2009) report on ensuring the quality and safety of chemotherapy services in England has issued a number of key recommendations aimed not only at reducing the risk of administration errors occurring but also ensuring that each service has robust policies and procedures in place in relation to the safety and quality of chemotherapy administration.

Consent

In accordance with the Department of Health Guidance on informed consent, written consent must be obtained from the child's parent or carer prior to commencing a course of chemotherapy or participating in any clinical trial (DoH 2001). In order to demonstrate adherence with the Children's Cancer Measures, any consent form, which patients or carers sign prior to starting a course of chemotherapy, should enable them to acknowledge that they have received generic written information covering the action they should take, whom they should contact for advice and the symptoms that should prompt this, with regards the following complications of chemotherapy:

- neutropoenic sepsis
- cytotoxic extravasation
- nausea and vomiting
- stomatitis, other mucositis and diarrhoea
- care of venous access device (National Cancer Action Team 2009).

If applicable, patients and their parents/carers should receive written information specific to the chemotherapy regimen they are to receive (this regimen should be specified on the consent form) (National Cancer Action Team 2009).

Safe handling

Safety of the child, staff and environment should be paramount when using cytotoxic therapy to minimise the risks of contamination. Research into the effects of cytotoxic drugs on animals has demonstrated that they are carcinogenic, mutogenic and teratogenic, and consequently this potential risk is transferred to those who prepare and administer cytotoxic drugs (Health and Safety Executive 2003). Cytotoxic drugs may contaminate the individual in various ways such as inhalation or absorption through the skin and/or mucous membranes. Contamination may also occur under differing circumstances such as during drug preparation and administration or when dealing with contaminated waste (RCN 1996a, 1996b, 1998). Employers and practitioners working in areas where cytotoxic drugs are prepared, administered, handled, transported and disposed of must ensure they are aware of and comply with all relevant legislation relating to safe handling of these substances. Employers must ensure standard operating procedures are in place for activities involving cytotoxic drugs and that these describe safe systems of work that meet all current applicable legislative requirements, including those of:

- The Medicines Act (1968)
- The Health and Safety at Work Act (1974)
- The Environmental Protection Act (1990)
- The Hazardous Waste Regulations (2005)
- The Control of Substances Hazardous to Health Regulations (COSHH 2002)
- Management of Health and Safety at Work Regulations (MHSW 1999)
- The Reporting of Injuries, Diseases and Dangerous Occurrences Regulations (RIDDOR 1995)
- The Personal Protective Equipment at Work Regulations (PPE 1992).

Employees have a responsibility to only carry out any potentially hazardous activity when suitably trained, confident and competent to do so (Management and Awareness of the Risks of Cytotoxic Handling [MARCH] 2009).

Reconstitution and preparation of chemotherapeutic agents

Knowledge of safety precautions and risks associated with administering chemotherapy begin at the point of reconstitution.

MARCH guidelines recommend that preparation of cytotoxics should be centralised in the pharmacy or in a pharmacy-controlled facility in a clinical area (MARCH 2009). Preparation is most appropriately undertaken by trained pharmacy staff using a negative-pressure pharmaceutical isolator designed for the purpose.

Personal protective equipment

An important aspect of safety when administering chemotherapy is the use of Personal Protective Equipment (PPE) for all staff. The employer should provide PPE to all staff who are involved in administering cytotoxic drugs (the Personal Protective Equipment at Work Regulations 1992). A local COSHH (2002) risk assessment should be carried out for each handling activity that might result in exposure (MARCH 2008). Gloves and a gown or apron should be worn on receipt of any raw materials, during setting up and checking of chemotherapy, during preparation and administration of chemotherapy and during waste disposal and managing a cytotoxic spillage (MARCH 2008). While the Health and Safety Executive (2003) advise that no one type of glove has been found to give unlimited protection against cytotoxic contamination, there is now some evidence to suggest that nitrile gloves offer good operator protection (Gross and Groce 1998, Singleton and Connor 1999). Eye protection should be worn during disposal of waste, when dealing with a cytotoxic spillage and during administration if there is a risk of spraying, splashing or aerosols (MARCH 2008). Eye protection should fully enclose the eyes, meet British Standard BS EN 166 and, where possible, should be disposable or capable of undergoing decontamination cleaning (British Standards 2002). Disposable gowns or aprons are preferable PPE when handling cytotoxic drugs and should have:

- Closed front
- Long sleeves
- Elastic or knit cuffs (MARCH 2008).

Work practices

Disposal of waste

All areas providing a chemotherapy service (both inpatient and outpatient) should have a policy detailing the disposal of cytotoxic waste products that complies with all relevant legislation (British Standards Institute 1990, Health and Safety Executive, DoH 2006). Cytotoxic waste includes:

- All equipment and materials used for cytotoxic spillage
- 'Frank' chemotherapy such as a syringe, infusion set and/or bags of cytotoxic chemotherapy not administered
- All equipment and materials used to prepare chemotherapy
- Empty syringes
- Disposable PPE
- Infusion sets once a non-cytotoxic flush has been administered (the entire set must be disposed of in a designated cytotoxic waste bag/bin)
- Nappies
- Any used ampoules, vials or needles used in the preparation of 'frank' chemotherapy should be disposed of in a designated cytotoxic sharps bin.

In the hospital setting, staff dealing with children's excreta (urine, vomit, faeces) should always wear gloves and should dispose of any nappies in a designated cytotoxic waste bin for 7 days after the administration of chemotherapy. Families/caregivers should be advised to wear gloves when handling their child's excreta for the same period of time (the use of washing up gloves or equivalent should be advised in the home).

Spillage and contamination

In order to ensure the safety of all staff working in clinical areas where cytotoxic medication is administered and to comply with relevant health and safety legislation, standard operating procedures detailing the appropriate actions staff should take in the event of a cytotoxic spillage. All staff should be familiar with local standard operating procedures and be regularly trained to deal with cytotoxic spillages. Cytotoxic spill kits should be available in all areas where cytotoxics are handled and should include:

- Absorbent granules/pads/sheets/paper towels
- Two pairs of powder-free gloves (gloves containing powder may enhance absorption of cytotoxic materials)
- Protective gown
- Disposable shoe coverings
- FFP2 or FFP3 filtered face piece respirator
- Safety glasses BS EN 166
- Cytotoxic waste disposal bag
- Plastic tweezers (to pick up any sharp materials or broken glass)
- Sign to identify the spill (MARCH 2007).

The spillage kit should also contain detailed instructions for dealing with both large and small spillages. The spillage should be recorded on an accident/incident reporting form as soon after the event as is practicable. New or expectant mothers should never be involved in the management of a cytotoxic spillage. If chemotherapy spills onto clothes, the individual should be advised to remove their clothes and thoroughly wash the affected area with soap and water. The contaminated clothing should then be washed at a high temperature and ideally should be washed separate to other non-contaminated clothes. Parents/carers who deliver home chemotherapy for their child should be provided with the information and equipment necessary for them to adequately deal with a spillage in the home.

Safe administration of chemotherapy

Training

The Manual for Cancer Services Children's Cancer Measures indicate that a nurse training programme in oncology skills and chemotherapy administration should be agreed by the Children's Cancer Network Chemotherapy Group (a sub group of the Children's Cancer Network the functional unit for children's cancer services within a specific geographical area) (NCAT 2009). Training requirements for nurses working in different settings (e.g. primary treatment centres, paediatric oncology shared care units) vary but should, as a minimum, meet the following requirements:

External: university-accredited to 20 credits at first degree level:

- type 1 – chemotherapy administration and oncology skills for paediatric oncology Internal: Children's Cancer Network (CCN) – agreed, RCN competency-based
- type 2 'full' – chemotherapy administration and oncology skills
- type 3 'foundation' – oncology skills for nurses not administering chemotherapy
- type 4 'low risk' – chemotherapy competencies focused only on administration of a CCN-agreed limited list of low-risk regimens.

Further detailed information on the competencies that should be included within each 'type' of training, along with specifications detailing minimum requirements for the types of training and numbers of trained nurses by location and setting are available within the Children's Cancer Measures (NCAT 2009).

Assessment

Prior to administering chemotherapy, a thorough nursing assessment must be undertaken and should consider:

- The child's diagnosis and disease presentation
- Pre-existing conditions
- Existing chemotherapy-induced toxicity
- The child's past experience with the prescribed drugs
- Anticipation of side-effects (probability, timing, prevention strategies, previous success (and failures) and assessment methods)
- Preparation of the child and family
- Identifying the family's desired level of involvement in care
- Record pre-assessment and level of family involvement.

Meeske and Ruccione (1987)

Preparation

Chemotherapy treatment protocols should specify investigations and tests that should be carried out before the administration of specific drugs to establish a results baseline. The investigations are then repeated after administration of the cytotoxic drugs. Treatment records should be maintained for each patient in which details of any investigations necessary prior to starting a whole course of chemotherapy and investigations that should be performed serially during the course (to detect/monitor any toxicity and response) and their intended frequency should be verified and recorded. Any short-term side effects as a result of the drug can be monitored, and, if necessary, modifications to the drug dosage or even the drugs being given can be made to the next block of treatment (Houlston 2008). Failure to verify that the results of recent tests are satisfactory prior to the commencement of further chemotherapy can lead to increased toxicity, which may, in some instances, result in permanent disability or even death. Nausea and vomiting, one of the most common side effects of chemotherapy is potentially avoidable. It is therefore imperative to give appropriate antiemetics before chemotherapy and to plan patient care accordingly (Houlston 2008). Drugs such as ifosfamide, cisplatin and methotrexate have toxic side effects that necessitate the administration of adequate pre- and post-hydration fluids. Written guidelines/protocols should be agreed by the head of the chemotherapy service for the treatment and/or prevention of regimen-specific complications such as the use of MESNA with ifosfamide and folinic acid rescue with high-dose methotrexate (NCAT 2009). Accurate recording of fluid balance is vital in order to prevent and/or detect toxic complications of chemotherapy treatment.

Principles table 8.1 Prescribing chemotherapy

Principle	Rationale
1. Medical staff must have received appropriate in-house education and training in order to be competent when prescribing chemotherapy.	1. To ensure those prescribing have knowledge of cytotoxic therapy.
2. As a result of a number of adverse incidents involving the maladministration of intrathecal chemotherapy, the Department of Health (DoH 2008b) has recommended that intrathecal chemotherapy should only be prescribed by appropriately trained Consultants or Specialist Registrars.	**2a)** To minimise the risk of a prescribing error. **b)** In accordance with Department of Health Guidelines (2008b). **c)** To minimise the risk of error.
3a and b) Chemotherapy dosages are calculated on the child's body surface area. This is usually calculated by a nomogram, which requires height and weight measurements. Many paediatric oncology centres also use the Children's Cancer and Leukaemia Group, Medical Research Council (CCLG) body surface area chart.	

(Continued)

Principles table 8.1 (*Continued*)

Principle	Rationale
3a and b) Certain protocols require doses to be prescribed in mg per kg this is usually for smaller children.	**3a)** To minimise the risk of cytotoxic drug toxicity. **b)** To ensure the dosages are accurate for the body surface area.
4. Chemotherapy should be prescribed according to a recognised (CCLG) standard protocol.	**4.** To ensure the most appropriate treatment is given.
5. If the patient is being treated 'off protocol' this should be documented on a designated 'off protocol' paperwork and/or documented clearly within the patient's medical records. N.B. 'Off protocol' refers to patients being treated with a chemotherapy regimen because it is not yet recognised as an established treatment plan.	**5.** To ensure appropriate documentation is used minimising the risk of error.
6. Intrathecal chemotherapy should always be prescribed on a separate drug chart to other intravenous chemotherapy.	**6.** To minimise the risk of inadvertent administration of intravenous drugs via the intrathecal route.
7a) All relevant demographic details should appear on the patient's chemotherapy prescription including; full name of patient, date of birth, unique patient hospital identification number and/or NHS number, any known allergies, height/weight/surface area, name of drug, dosage frequency, route of administration and sequence of drugs, length of treatment. **b)** Ensure all chemotherapy prescriptions are written clearly, in capital letters with all medication names written in full. Only black ink should be used when prescribing and the contact number of the prescriber should be recorded.	**7a and b)** To minimise the risk of error.
8a) Hydration fluids should be prescribed at the same time as the chemotherapy on an appropriate fluid prescription chart. **b)** This should include the type of fluid required, the amount needed (in millilitres) and the duration of hydration. Any additives required should also be clearly prescribed.	**8a)** To maintain an adequate fluid intake. **b)** To minimise the risk of error.
9. Bolus drugs, e.g. mesna, should be prescribed in the 'stat drugs' section of the drug chart including the date, times and dose to be administered.	**9.** To minimise the risk of error.
10. Antiemetic therapy should be prescribed according to local antiemetic policy and individual patient requirements. It is important to be aware of administering antiemetic therapy at an appropriate time for the patient.	**10.** To ensure emesis is adequately managed as early intervention is known to influence success (Selwood *et al* 1999). Emetic potential of individual agents are known, therefore appropriate anti-emetics can be prescribed (Selwood *et al* 1999).

Routes of administration

The oral route

Some cytotoxic agents used in the treatment of children's cancers such as methotrexate and mercaptopurine may be given via the oral route. Oral administration is generally economical, convenient and less invasive than other routes (Goodman and Riley 1997). However, it may also be unreliable and impractical in children for whom swallowing tablets is difficult and/or adherence an issue. Staff handling oral cytotoxic agents should ensure adequate safety precautions are taken. Appropriate gloves should always be worn when dispensing oral chemotherapy and hands must be washed after each dispensing. If dose administration aids are used they should be filled and labelled by a pharmacist trained in chemotherapy, and must contain only oral chemo-therapy. Crushing or cutting of oral chemotherapy should be avoided, if at all possible. If crushing or cutting of oral chemo-therapy is required, it should be carried out by trained staff in a class II drug safety cabinet (Society of Hospital Pharmacists of Australia 2007). If tablets need to be dissolved, the safest method is to place the tablet into a syringe with some sterile water and leave to disperse. A cap or bung should be placed onto the syringe tip to ensure that no spillage of cytotoxic medication can occur. If parents/carers are required to administer oral chemo-therapy at home, they should also be aware of the necessary safety precautions and may wear household rubber gloves or two

pairs of non-sterile gloves, which must only be used for this reason (HSE 2000, RCN 1998).

The intravenous route

It is generally accepted that children who are to receive long-term cytotoxic treatment should have a central venous access device (CVAD) inserted to facilitate treatment (Dougherty 2000). Hickman™ and Broviac™ catheters are commonly used in paediatric along with implantable ports and more recently PICCs (Peripherally Inserted Central Catheters) (Cowley 2004, McIntosh 2003).

Principles table 8.2 Techniques for administering intravenous cytotoxic medication (adapted from MARCH 2009)

Principle	Rationale
1. Prior to administering intravenous cytotoxics, the patency of the intravenous access device in use must be established by checking for blood return.	1. Ensuring patency by checking for blood return greatly reduces the risk of extravasation.
2. When administering bolus cytotoxics via a peripheral cannula, it is advisable to: • Administer vesicants first (after any required premedication), because the integrity of the vein is greatest at this time. • Wherever possible, use a newly inserted cannula.	2. As vesicants are routinely administered via a newly inserted peripheral cannula early administration of the vesicant ensures the integrity of the vein is at its greatest thereby minimising the risk of extravastion injury.
3. To reduce the risk of splash or spillage from cytotoxic infusions: • Administration sets should be inserted into infusion bags over a tray, and never into bags hanging from an infusion stand. • Administration sets should contain a burette so that cytotoxic infusions can be flushed with a compatible fluid prior to disconnection.	3. Reducing the risk of splashing or spillage during disconnection of the completed cytotoxic infusion from the administration set.

Extravasation

Extravasation is the inappropriate or accidental administration of vesicant chemotherapy into the subcutaneous or subdermal tissues, rather than into the intravenous compartment (MARCH 2009). Injuries can range from apparently insignificant erythematous reactions to severe necrosis (MARCH 2009). Extravasation injuries are well documented within the field of haematology/oncology as many of the cytotoxic drugs used are classified as vesicants (Hallquist *et al* 1999, Schulmeister and Camp-Sorrell 2000). Vesicants are drugs that have the potential to cause blistering and ulceration and which when left untreated, can lead to the more serious side effects of extravasation such as tissue destruction and necrosis (Ener *et al* 2004). Additional precautions should be taken when administering vesicant chemotherapy to ensure the procedure is completed safely. Trusts should have policies and guidelines in place for staff as to the best practice when administering vesicant chemotherapy and

these should be reviewed and updated regularly. The guidelines should detail the procedure to follow should an extravasation injury occur, and a policy for the treatment of extravasation injuries should also be available. Vesicant drugs can cause serious damage if inadvertently administered into the subcutaneous tissue, and for this reason are not often administered by nurses via the peripheral route (NIOSH 2004). Nursing staff who do deliver vesicant drugs peripherally should have received additional training and be competent in cannulation. They should also gain consent of the medical and management teams to undertake these extended practices to ensure they are adequately covered by the Trust where they work. Annual updates should be made available for nurses undertaking these procedures to ensure the most up-to-date evidence-based practice is delivered. Extravasation can be difficult to determine in some instances as signs and symptoms can be similar to phlebitis and/or infection. Patients may not always experience pain or discomfort if vesicant cytotoxic drugs extravasate (Pan

Birmingham Cancer Network Site Specific Group 2007). Consequently, all healthcare professionals involved in the administration of vesicant drugs should possess skills to assess possible incidents. While there is some controversy regarding the specific treatment of extravasation of some vesicants, extravasation guidelines recently published by the European Oncology Nursing Society (2007) recommend the same initial treatment regardless of the nature of the drug.

Procedure guideline 8.1 **Extravasation**

Statement	Rationale
1. Stop the infusion immediately. DO NOT remove the cannula at this point.	
2. Disconnect the infusion (not the cannula/needle).	
3. Leave the cannula/needle in place and try to aspirate as much of the drug as possible from the cannula with a 10 ml syringe. Avoid applying directed manual pressure to the suspected extravasation site to prevent any further extravasation of the vesicant.	**3.** By withdrawing as much of the vesicant from the site as possible the extent of the extravasation injury may be minimised. Avoiding direct manual pressure may also minimise injury by preventing spread of the vesicant within the tissues.
4. Mark the affected area and take digital images of the site.	**4.** To enable ongoing assessment of the injury.
5. Remove the cannula/needle.	
6. Collect the extravasation kit, notify the medical team and seek advice from local experts.	**6.** Expert advice is essential when treating extravasation injuries in order to prevent further damage to the site. In order to comply with The Children's Cancer Measures every clinical area involved in the administration of cytotoxic chemotherapy should hold a local policy regarding the recognition and treatment of cytotoxic extravasation (NCAT 2009).
7. Administer pain relief if required. Complete required documentation.	**7.** To manage local pain.

Intrathecal route

A number of chemotherapy protocols used in the treatment of childhood leukaemia and lymphoma involve the use of cytotoxic drugs injected intrathecally. These types of cancer often relapse within the central nervous system as the vast majority of cytotoxic drugs are unable to cross the blood brain barrier. Delivery of cytotoxic drugs directly into the intrathecal space can prevent against relapse within the central nervous system and has therefore been a vital factor in improving survival rates in childhood leukaemias and lymphomas. Only a small number of cytotoxic drugs can be safely administered into the intrathecal space (e.g. cytarabine). At least 55 incidents are known to have occurred around the world (a number in England) where the intravenous vinca alkaloid drug vincristine has been injected intrathecally during the chemotherapy treatment (DoH 2008). These incidents have resulted in the paralysis or death of the patients involved. The Government agreed a target to reduce the number of patients dying or being paralysed by intrathecal injections of vinca alkaloids to zero by the end of 2001 (DoH 2008). National guidance (HSC 2001/022) was issued in November 2001 to support this target. This was updated and reissued in October 2003 (HSC 2003/010). Further updated national guidance on the safe administration of intrathecal chemotherapy was issued in August 2008 (HSC 2001/001). The key requirements of this updated guidance are as follows:

- a written local policy covering all aspects of the national guidance
- a register of all trained and competent staff
- annual review of competence
- a designated area for the administration of intrathecal injections
- under normal circumstances intrathecal chemotherapy should only be administered within normal working hours
- intravenous chemotherapy drugs should be administered after intravenous chemotherapy drugs and should only be issued following written confirmation that any intravenous drugs have already been administered. The only exceptions are:
  ○ where intrathecal chemotherapy is being given to a child under general anaesthesia or
  ○ where the paediatric protocol/regimen requires that intrathecal chemotherapy is given first.
- If a regimen involves intrathecal chemotherapy combined with continuous intravenous chemotherapy, it is only acceptable to issue intrathecal chemotherapy once there is evidence that the infusional intravenous chemotherapy has started.

Any nurse involved in checking intrathecal chemotherapy prior to administration must have undergone a designated training programme and appear on a local register of designated as competent to check intrathecal chemotherapy.

References

British Standards (2002) Personal eye protection specification. BS EN 166

British Standards Institute (1990) Specific of sharps containers (BS7320). (Available at http://standards.mackido.com/bs/bs-standards24_view_6208.html (accessed February 2010)

Control of Substances Hazardous to Health Regulations (COSHH 2002) Available at http://www.opsi.gov.uk/si/si2002/20022677.htm (accessed February 2010)

Cowley K. (2004) Make the right choice of vascular access device. Professional Nurse, 19(10), 43–46

Department of Health (2000) The NHS Cancer Plan: a plan for investment, a plan for reform. London, DoH

Department of Health (2001) HSC/2001/023 Good Practice in Consent: Achieving the NHS Plan Commitment to Patient-centred Consent Practice. London, DoH

Department of Health and Human Sciences Centers for Disease Control and Prevention, National Institute for occupational safety and health (NIOSH) (2004) NIOSH Alert – Preventing Occupational Exposures to Antineoplastic and other hazardous drugs in the health care setting, Ohio. Available at www.cdc.gov/niosh

Department of Health (2006) Health Technical Memorandum 07-01: Safe Management of Healthcare Waste. Available at http://www.dh.gov.uk/en/PublicationsandStatistics/Publications/PublicationsPolicyAndGuidance/DH_063274 (accessed January 2010)

Department of Health (2007) Cancer Reform Strategy. London, Department of Health

Department of Health (2008a) The Cancer Reform Strategy: maintaining momentum, building for the future – first annual report. London, DoH

Department of Health (2008b) HSC 2001/001 Updated National Guidance on the Safe Administration of Intrathecal Chemotherapy. London, DoH

Dougherty L. (2000) Central venous access devices. Nursing Standard, 14(43), 45–50

Ener R A, Meglathery SB, Styler M. (2004) Extravasation of systemic hemato-oncological therapy. Annals of Oncology, 15, 858–862

European Oncology Nursing Society (2007) Extravasation Guidelines. Available at www.cancerworld.org (accessed February 2010)

Goodman M, Riley MB. (1997) Chemotherapy administration. In Groenwald SL, Frogge M, Henke Yarbro C. (eds) Cancer Nursing, 4th edition, pp. 317–404. Boston, Jones & Bartlett

Gross ER, Groce DF. (1998) An evaluation of nitrile gloves as an alternative to natural rubber latex for handling chemotherapeutic agents. Journal of Oncology Pharmaceutical Practice, 4, 165–168

Hallquist P, Yamamoto DS, Geyton JE. (1999) Extravasation of infusate via implanted ports: two case studies. Clinical Journal of Oncology Nursing, 3(4), 145–151

The Hazardous Waste Regulations (2005) Available at http://www.opsi.gov.uk/si/si2005/20050894.htm (accessed February 2010)

Health and Safety Executive (2000) Monitoring of Strategies for Toxic Substances, 2nd edition. London, HSE

Health and Safety Executive (2003) Safe Handling of Cytotoxic Drugs. London, DoH

Houlston A. (2008) Administration of chemotherapy. In Gibson F, Soanes L. (eds) Cancer in Children and Young People. Chichester, John Wiley & Sons

Management of Health and Safety at Work Regulations (MHSW 1999) Available at http://www.opsi.gov.uk/si/si1999/19993242.htm (accessed February 2010)

Management and Awareness of Risks of Cytotoxic Handling (MARCH) (2007) Spillages: management and containment available at: http://www.marchguidelines.com/members/guidelines/PNF1_Spillages.aspx (accessed Jan 2010)

Management and Awareness of Risks of Cytotoxic Handling (MARCH) (2008) Personal protective equipment (PPE): selection and use. Available at http://www.marchguidelines.com/members/guidelines/PNF1_PersonalProtectiveEquipment.aspx (accessed February 2010)

Management and Awareness of Risks of Cytotoxic Handling (MARCH) (2009) Extravasation. Available at http://www.marchguidelines.com/members/guidelines/Extravasation.aspx (accessed February 2010)

McIntosh N. (2003) Central venous catheters: reasons for insertion and removal. Paediatric Nursing, 15(1), pp. 14–18

Meeske K, Ruccione K. (1987) Cancer chemotherapy in children: nursing issues and approaches. Seminars in Oncology Nursing, 3(2), 118–127

National Cancer Action Team (2004) National Cancer Peer Review Programme Manual for Cancer Services 2004: Chemotherapy Specific Measures. London, DoH

National Cancer Action Team (NCAT) (2009) National Cancer Peer Review Programme Manual for Cancer Services 2008: Children's Cancer Services. London, DoH

National Cancer Advisory Group (2009) Chemotherapy Services in England: ensuring quality and safety. London, DoH

National Confidential Enquiry into Patient Outcome and Death (2008) For better, for worse? London, NCEPOD

Pan-Birmingham Cancer Network Site Specific Group (2007) Guidelines for the Management of Extravasation. Available at http://www.birminghamcancer.nhs.uk (accessed February 2010)

The Personal Protective Equipment at Work Regulations (PPE 1992) London, The Stationery Office. Available at http://www.opsi.gov.uk/SI/si1992/Uksi_19922966_en_1.htm (accessed February 2010)

The Reporting of Injuries, Diseases and Dangerous Occurrences Regulations (RIDDOR) (1995) Available at http://www.opsi.gov.uk/SI/si1995/Uksi_19953163_en_1.htm (accessed February 2010)

Royal College of Nursing Cancer Nursing Society (1996a) Guidelines for Good Practice in Cancer Nursing. London, RCN

Royal College of Nursing Cancer Nursing Society (1996b) A Structure for Cancer Nursing Services. London, RCN

Royal College of Nursing (1998) Clinical Practice Guidelines – The Administration of Cytotoxic Chemotherapy. London, RCN, p. 6

Schulmeister L, Camp-Sorrell D. (2000) Chemotherapy extravasation from implanted ports. Oncology Nursing Forum, 27(3), 531–538

Selwood K, Gibson F, Evans M. (1999) Side effects of chemotherapy. In Gibson F, Evans M. (eds). Paediatric Oncology Nursing: Acute Nursing Care. London, Whurr

Singleton LC, Connor TH. (1999) An evaluation of the permeability of chemotherapy gloves to three cancer chemotherapy drugs. Oncology Nursing Forum, 22(9), 1491–1496

Society of Hospital Pharmacists of Australia (2007) Standards of practice for the provision of oral chemotherapy for the treatment of cancer. Journal of Pharmacy Practice Research, 37, 149–152

Chapter 9

Fluid balance

Chapter contents

Procedure guidelines

The Great Ormond Street Hospital Manual of Children's Nursing Practices, First Edition. Edited by Susan Macqueen, Elizabeth Anne Bruce, Faith Gibson.
© 2012 Great Ormond Street Hospital for Children NHS Foundation Trust. Published 2012 by Blackwell Publishing Ltd.

Introduction

Fluid and electrolyte homeostasis is an essential requirement for optimal cellular and organ function; the kidneys play an essential role maintaining this balance. In health they regulate the volume and composition of body fluids by actively absorbing and excreting fluids, electrolytes and the unwanted end-products of metabolism. Correction and maintaining of fluid and electrolyte in children and infants presents unique challenges. New-born infants are at particular risk of fluid and electrolyte imbalance because of the immature mechanisms for thirst and urine concentration.

The content and distribution of total body water changes with age (Willock and Jewkes 2000). To assess these changes, it is important to note that body fluids are split into two main compartments, the intracellular (ICF) and the extracellular fluid (ECF) compartments. The ECF is then further divided into the intravascular (plasma), interstitial compartments (fluid surrounding tissues) and transcellular (cerebrospinal fluid, sinovial, pleural, peritoneal). It is important to remember that age-related changes affect both body water content and distribution (Table 9.1). Three-quarters of water distribution in the ECF is located in the interstitial space and one-quarter in the plasma (Willock and Jewkes 2000).

Maintenance of fluid requirements

Fluid loss consists mainly of urine, insensible losses (skin and respiratory tract), sweat, vomit and stool. Fluid balance is normally achieved in infants by maintaining adequate fluids, nutrition and warmth. The mechanisms to maintain homeostasis are highly sophisticated and finely balanced by many complex systems of movement of fluids and electrolytes between the vascular space and the body tissues. This involves osmosis and diffusion with a complex process of oncotic and hydrostatic forces moving fluid around the body compartments.

Infants and preterm babies are particularly vulnerable to any imbalance of fluids and electrolytes; this is partly due to their large percentage of ECF (Table 9.1), their immature compensatory mechanisms and high metabolic rate during the first few months of life. Any small insult during this time can upset this fine balance resulting in impaired renal function. Fluid and electrolyte maintenance or replacement will depend on the type and amount of fluid being lost. This must be calculated on an individual basis according to the child's fluid status and electrolytes (Table 9.2). Fluid requirements to maintain health are listed in Table 9.3.

In sick infants the recording of accurate fluid balance is particularly important, an imbalance can lead to mild, moderate or severe renal failure, requiring some form of intervention. The most common causes of acute kidney injury are trauma, septicaemia, fluid and electrolyte disturbances and obstructions. The treatment of which may include renal replacement therapy in the form of peritoneal dialysis, continuous veno-venous haemofiltration (HF) or haemodialysis (HD). The focus of this chapter will be fluid balance and the treatment of acute kidney injury.

Fluid balance in the ill child

A child's fluid balance (fluid input/output) must be measured and calculated according to their clinical condition. A child's weight and height are required to calculate the fluid requirements by surface area. This may need to be estimated if the child is critically ill. The first assessment should be the child's fluid status and base line observations (Table 9.4 and 9.5). Samples for blood and urine electrolytes may be required if the child is considered to have severe dehydration or bloody diarrhoea (Table 9.2).

Table 9.1 Approximate total body water (% of body weight)

Approximate total body water (% of body wt)	Pre-term	Term	1–2years	Adult male
Water content	90%	70–80%	64%	60%
ICF	48%	48%	34%	40%
ECF	27%	27%	30%	20%

Modified from Metheny and Snively 1983.

Table 9.2 Blood serum levels

Sodium	135–145 mmol/l
Chloride	100–108 mmol/l
Potassium	3.4–5.3 mmol/l
Total CO_2	20–30 mmol/l
Glucose	4–7 mmol/l
Albumen	34–52 g/l
Urea	2.5–6.0 mmol/l
Creatinine	20–50 umol/l
Calcium	2.22–2.51 mmol/l
Phosphate	1.2–1.8 mmol/l

This range results from consensus of opinion at GOSH.

Table 9.3 Average oral fluid requirements for a healthy infant

Age	New born	2 days	3 days	4 days	5 days	1 week–8 months	9–12 months
Average total fluid requirement in 24 hours (ml/kg)	30	60	90	120	150	150	150

Davenport 1996.

Table 9.4 Assessing hydration (modified from Advanced Life Support Group 1997 and Davenport 1996, cited in Willock 2000)

Assessment	Normal hydration	Mild dehydration <5%	Moderate dehydration 5–10%	Severe dehydration >10%	Hypervolaemia
General appearance	Alert, good muscle tone	Alert, good muscle tone. May be thirsty	May be irritable or lethargic, sunken eyes, sunken anterior fontanelle	Confused, floppy, sunken eyes, reduced eyeball turgor, sunken anterior fontanelle	Lethargic, puffy,
Colour	Consistent, pink lips, palms of hands, nail beds	Pink lips, palms of hands	Pale	Mottled/pale/grey	Normal
Temperature of extremities (in warm environment)	Warm	Normal or cool	Cool	Cold	Cool or warm depending on degree of overload
Peripheral pulses	Strong	Strong	May be weak	Weak	May be strong
Mucous membranes	Pink, moist	May be dry	Dry	Pale, dry	Pink, moist
Capillary refill time (in warm environment)	1–2 seconds	1–2 seconds	May be >2 seconds	>2 seconds	1–2 seconds
Respiration	Normal for age	Normal for age	Normal or elevated	Elevated	May be elevated
Skin turgor/observable oedema	Pinched skin immediately falls back to normal	Pinched skin immediately falls back to normal	Pinched skin slowly falls back to normal	Pinched skin remains tented	May have peri-orbital/abdominal/leg oedema
Heart rate	Normal for age	Normal for age	May be raised	Marked tachycardia	May be normal or tachycardia
Urine output	Infant 2 ml/kg/hr; Child 1 ml/kg/hr; Adolescent 0.5 ml/kg/hr	Reduced	Reduced	Reduced or anuric	Reduced or anuric
Urine S.G	1.005–1.020	May be >1.020	>1.020	>1.020	<1.005 before treatment of diuretics
Blood pressure	Normal for age	Normal	Normal	May be normal or low	Usually raised
Temperature gap	<2°C in warm environment	<2°C	May be wide	Wide	Usually >2
SPO$_2$	97–100%	97–100%	97–100% if recordable	May not be recordable	May be low
Chest X-ray	Clear	Clear	Clear	Clear	May show pulmonary oedema/enlarged heart
Abdominal X-ray	Normal	Normal	Normal	Normal	May show ascites/hepatomegaly
CVP (Rt. Atrium	0–5 mmHg	Normal	Normal	Normal or low	>5 mmHg
Body weight	Fairly stable (<1% body weight gain or loss per day)	Weight loss <50 g/kg	Weight loss 50–100 g/kg	Weight loss >100 g/kg	Weight gain >1%

Table 9.5 Degree of dehydration

Degree of dehydration	Estimated loss of body weight in a child/infant	Approximate loss of body weight (ml/kg) in infant	Estimated loss of body weight in older children and adolescents	Approximate loss of body weight (ml/kg) older children and adolescents
Mild	<5%	50 ml/kg	3%	30 ml/kg
Moderate	5–10%	100 ml/kg	6%	60 ml/kg
Severe	10–15%	150 ml/kg	9%	90 ml/kg

Willock and Jewkes 2000.

144

Principles table 9.1 Assessing fluid balance

Principle	Rationale
1. Once the fluid status has been ascertained a careful plan of fluid replacement may be calculated, the choice of solution replacing the salt and water is critical in dehydrated children (Tables 9.6 and 9.7).	**1.** To adequately hydrate the child preventing further damage to the vital organs (kidneys/heart/liver/brain).
2. General observations (Table 9.4): **a)** Assessment of a child includes general well-being. **b)** Dry mouth and skin. **c)** Sunken eyes and fontanelle, skin colour that appears mottled	**2.** **a)** Recognition of a child becoming seriously ill can sometimes be quite challenging. The parents/carers will often give the nurse valuable pointers to the child's unusual behaviour, e.g. 'they never usually remain still like this', 'they seem slightly confused' or are 'hallucinating'. These can be essential markers to assess a child's general condition and can initially be very subtle. **b)** Dry mucous membranes and skin are signs of dehydration. **c)** Indicate a moderate to severe level of dehydration (Tables 9.4 and 9.5).
3. Vital signs: the frequency of measurement will be dependent on a child's clinical condition: **a)** Capillary refill. **b)** Respiratory rate. **c)** Heart rate. **d)** Blood pressure. **e)** Measure peripheral and skin temperature gap. **f)** Oxygen saturations. **g)** CVP. **h)** Observe the child for oedema. This is often seen around the eyes, ankles, abdomen and scrotal area.	**3.** Measurement and interpretation of vital signs are tools to help assess a child's fluid status. **a)** 1–2 seconds would indicate that a child hydration status may be normal; >2 seconds may indicate a level of dehydration. **b)** Can be elevated with dehydration. **c)** Often elevated during dehydration as the body naturally shuts down to the peripheries directing blood to the vital organs. **d)** Blood pressure may be low in dehydration. As the child's condition deteriorates, a slight elevation may be seen as the body tries to compensate for the fluid loss (flight or fight response). Severe hypertension with a low urine output and warm peripheries are signs of fluid overload and acute kidney injury (AKI) (2006). **e)** A very simple way to monitor a child's fluid status is to measure the gap between the peripheral and core temperature. If this is >2°C in a child who has been well wrapped in a blanket, this may indicate dehydration (vasoconstriction). **f)** A low oxygen saturation may indicate dehydration/fluid overload. **g)** CVP is generally low in dehydration and high in fluid overload. **h)** If the child is oedematous, fluid is leaking from the ICF to the ECF. If the child has a low serum albumin, they can be intravascularly depleted. Care should be taken to distinguish the difference between the two (Table 9.4).

145

Principles table 9.1 (Continued)

Principle	Rationale
4. A child's weight should be recorded daily during the acute stage. Bed scales can be useful if the child is unstable. If the child is in renal failure a weight should be taken before and after any renal replacement intervention.	**4.** A child's weight gain/loss will be age and condition dependent and is an important requirement for assessing fluid replacement.
5. An early morning urine should be sent for urinary electrolytes and osmolarity.	**5.** The body desperately tries to reabsorb fluids by retaining sodium. This results in reduced sodium in the urine and can be a sign that the child is not adequately rehydrated. Measuring the specific gravity and osmolarity can assist in the assessment of fluid requirements.
6. Perform blood test (urea and electrolytes (U&Es)/FBC/ blood glucose/blood gases as required).	**6.** Blood results will help guide the experienced clinician to prescribe the appropriate fluid and electrolyte requirement. Haematocrit, serum osmolarity and plasma sodium and potassium are particularly useful when assessing levels of fluid and electrolyte imbalance (Table 9.2).

146

Table 9.6 Fluid replacement choice for hypovolaemia

Fluid choice	
Isotonic crystalloid fluid	**Colloid fluids**
Fluid replacement for hypovolaemia	
Saline 0.9%	4.5% albumin
Saline 0.45%	20% albumin
Saline 0.45% and dextrose 2.5%	Gelofusine
Saline 0.18% dextrose 4%	Haemaccel
Hartmann's solution	

Renal replacement therapy

Monitoring fluid balance in sick children is a basic requirement as they are often at high risk of developing a fluid imbalance secondary to their illness or treatment intervention. Early recognition and replacement of fluids during this time can reduce the risk of AKI and the need for renal replacement therapy (RRT). RRT may be a transient or permanent requirement depending on the severity or cause of kidney failure; recovery of renal function after a period of dialysis is never guaranteed. The choice of renal replacement therapy will depend on the expertise available in the area. The decision to embark on RRT is often dependent on the availability of resources in the local area. Children requiring dialysis are usually transferred to specialised renal units or to a paediatric intensive care unit. All forms of dialysis require nurses to have considerable expertise in this area and are not available in all paediatric units.

Peritoneal dialysis (PD) is performed via a catheter being inserted into the peritoneum, haemodialysis (HD) or haemofiltration (HF) requires vascular access. Dialysis is used as a supportive therapy until kidney function recovers; however, in end stage renal failure (ESRF) renal function is irreversible and

Table 9.7 IV fluid and electrolytes requirements in AKI

Initial management for rehydration in AKI

Dehydrated	0.9% NaCl	Fluid resuscitation 10–20 ml/kg over 30 minutes, assess urine output and repeat as necessary
Hypovolaemia	Hartmann's (APLS guidelines) or 4.5% albumin	10–20 ml/kg isotonic solution
Fluid overload AKI	Frusemide 2–4 mg/kg	IV dialysis if no response

Maintenance fluids

Daily IV requirement	Weight (kg)	IV fluid (ml)
	3–10 kg	100 ml/kg
	11–30 kg	100 ml/kg plus 50 ml/ kg for each additional kg >10 kg
	>30 kg	1500 ml plus 20 ml/ kg for each additional kg >30 kg

Sodium, potassium and chloride requirements

Weight	<10 kg	11–30 kg	>30 kg
Sodium, potassium and chloride daily requirement	2.5 mmols/kg	2 mmols/kg	1.5 mmols/kg

Rees *et al* 2006.

Procedure guideline 9.1 Fluid input/output

Statement	Rationale
1. Record an accurate fluid balance.	**1.** To assess fluid status, and enable an early detection of positive or negative balance.
2. There are a number of ways to calculate fluid requirements: **a)** Insensible losses ($400\,ml/m^2/24\,hrs$) plus previous day's urine output. **b)** A basic calculation of ml/kg (Table 9.3): • Babies prescribed phototherapy or overhead heating will require additional fluids.	**2.** To enable good renal perfusion and a well-hydrated child. **a)** This calculation is required if a child is on renal replacement therapy as they often do not have a urine output. **b)** To maintain homeostasis as babies receiving phototherapy have increased insensible losses.
3. Assess fluid status hourly during the acute stage.	**3.** Early recognition of oliguria/anuria indicates fluid depletion or acute kidney injury <1 ml/kg.
4. Administer IV fluids and assess type of fluid and volume requirements before administration (Table 9.6).	**4.** To rehydrate and expand the intravascular space. Prevention of potential fluid overload.
5. All fluid loss should be recorded as total output including vomit/nasogastric aspirate and stool/colostomy fluid and urine.	**5.** >1 ml/kg/hr of urine output should be expected if the child is adequately hydrated. A reduction of urine output could indicate dehydration or AKI.
6. Measurement of urine output is vital during the acute phase of illness. A urinary catheter may be required initially to accurately measure the output; however, weighing nappies is also a very adequate measurement and reduces the risk of infection.	**6.** Accurate fluid output is essential in assessing a child's fluid status. A urinary catheter can be considered to be a high-risk infection risk in children who are oliguric/anuric.
7. Calculate hourly urine output as ml/kg/hr based on a child's normal weight.	**7.** An urinary output of >2 ml/kg/hr in infants and 1 ml/kg/hr in children is within normal limits (Glasper *et al* 2006).

147

dialysis replaces renal function. The causes of paediatric AKI are birth trauma, sepsis, haemolytic uremic syndrome (HUS), glomerular diseases such as glomerulonephritis, obstructive uropathy within the urinary tract, major surgery and side effects of medicines such as chemotherapy and antibiotics (Table 9.8).

Dialysis is a 'method of separating particles of different dimensions in a liquid mixture using a thin semi-permeable membrane whose pores are too small to allow the passage of large particles, such as proteins, but large enough to permit the passage of dissolved crystalline material' (http://www.oup.com/uk/orc/bin/9780199551927/resources/glossary/glossary_medical). All renal replacement modalities use diffusion across a semi-permeable membrane to clear waste products from the blood, plus ultra-filtration to remove excess fluid from the body. This chapter will focus on dialysis in acute kidney injury only.

Haemofiltration (HF)

Haemofiltration (HF) is an extracorporeal treatment usually available in the critical care setting. Its use in paediatrics has increased significantly since the late 1990s. It is a highly effective

Table 9.8 Causes of AKI

Pre-renal	Renal	Post renal
Diarrhoea and vomiting	Bloody diarrhoea (HUS)	Urethral obstruction, e.g. PRV
Cardiac impairment	Hypovolaemia	Polydipsia and polyuria
Birth asphyxia	Hypovolaemia	Poor urinary output
Umbilical catheters	Infection	Poor urinary output
Bilateral renal arterial or venous thrombosis	Poor blood supply	Poor urinary output
Drugs	Drugs	

Rees *et al* 2006.

means of dialysis, but it is technically demanding and requires specialist training. Continuous veno-veno haemofiltration (CVVH) allows for continuous fluid and solute removal that is generally less aggressive than HD and would often be the treatment of choice in many paediatric intensive care units (Craig 1998, John and Eckardt 2007, Sefton *et al* 2001). Continuous arterio-venous haemofiltration (CAVH) can also be used for fluid removal. This is dependent on the difference between the child's arterial and venous pressure to drive blood through an extra-corporeal circuit. The process of filtration is dependent on good arterial pressures and would be extremely difficult if the child is on inotropic support (Flynn 2002, Lowrie 2000, Warady and Bunchman 2000).

Haemodialysis (HD)

HD is a procedure in which blood is pumped out of the body, from a specially created vascular access, and around an extracorporeal circuit where it passes through the haemodialyser before it is returned to the patient. The haemodialyser consists of a semi-permeable membrane across which bloods flows on one side and dialysis fluid on the other. The process of diffusion allows excess solutes to be removed from the blood; excess water is removed by the process of ultrafiltration. HD is a very effective method of RRT. It can be used either for children in AKI or ESRF.

Preparing the child for dialysis access

The child may have deranged electrolytes, which will have to be stabilised before the child goes to theatre for dialysis access. All forms of dialysis need access of one form or other and this usually requires an anaesthetic. Most children require stabilisation before going to theatre to reduce the high risk of complications. The side effect of correcting acidosis is low calcium. The ionised calcium levels must be known before giving IV sodium bicarbonate as this will result in lowered calcium levels, which affect muscle contraction, cardiac function and blood clotting.

The first-line treatments for hyperkalaemia and acidosis are:

- Calcium resoneum (oral/rectal)
- Nebulized ventolin
- IV bicarbonate
- Insulin and dextrose infusion.

These are effective methods of reducing the serum potassium and/or forcing extracellular potassium into the cells, thereby lowering the serum potassium temporally to enable the child to have a surgical procedure (line insertion).

For hypocalaemia, calcium gluconate 10% is administered. Care must be taken when giving calcium. Ideally this should be given as an infusion over 30 minutes by a central line (concentration 100 mg in 1 ml), and if the child only has peripheral access the calcium needs to be diluted to 20 mg in 1 ml to avoid extravasation, as calcium salts can cause serious tissue necrosis.

Starting extracorporeal treatments HD/HF

Calculation of extracorporeal volume (ECV)

The dialysis nurse must first estimate the child's total blood volume (Table 9.9), before the extracorporeal volume (ECV) can be calculated. The ECV is estimated as being 8–10% of the total blood volume (Mactier et al 2009). Once the ECV has been calculated, suitably sized dialysis lines and haemodialyser can be selected to ensure this volume is not exceeded. If the child is

Table 9.9 Estimated blood volumes

Estimated blood volumes

Age	Neonates	Infant	Child	Adult
Blood ml/kg	90	80	80	65

Davenport 1996.

grossly oedematous, allowances should be made to their weight to avoid over estimation of the ECV, which could result in too big a circuit being selected. A range of circuit sizes (neonatal, paediatric and adult) are available. In cases when the smallest circuit available is still greater than the child's ECV it is necessary to prime the circuit with bank blood. This avoids any adverse cardiovascular effects on the child and allows them to be safely dialysed. Usually the blood is not returned at the end of the session as it is extra to their circulating volume.

For example, a child of 10 kg will have a TBV of 800 ml (wt × 80) and an ECV of 64–80 ml (8–10% of TBV). Therefore, the volume of blood in the dialyser and circuit must not exceed 80 ml (Table 9.8).

The haemodialyser

The haemodialyser is selected according to the child's surface area. The surface area of the membrane in the dialyser should not exceed that of the child (Mactier et al 2009) and varying sized dialysers, ranging from $0.2 \, m^2$ to $1.7 \, m^2$ and greater are available to allow correct selection. A standard chart is available to calculate the child's surface area. The haemodialyser is composed of a modified cellulose membrane or synthetic material. Variations in dialyser membrane design, size and thickness result in different solute and fluid clearances allowing for a choice of product.

The ECV also indicates the blood pump speed for the dialysis session. Thus, the 10 kg child will have a maximum blood pump speed of 80 ml/min (Rees et al 2008).

Anticoagulation of the circuit

The dialysis circuit is routinely anticoagulated with unfractionated heparin to prevent clotting in the dialyser membrane or the circuit itself (European Best Practice Guidelines 2002). The dose of heparin is titrated to the child's weight and their individual requirements. Doses range from 0–25 units/kg/hour. It is given continuously during dialysis and a bolus dose may also be given at the start of the session. Heparin-free dialysis is possible for those children who have just had or who are about to have surgery. The circuit is flushed with saline regularly to help keep the fibres clear (European Best Practice Guidelines 2002).

Dialysis fluid for HD

Water is required to dilute the dialysis fluid and must meet national standards for microbiological and chemical purity. Water is softened and filtered and passed through a reverse osmosis membrane before it is used. The dialysis fluid, or dialysate, enables diffusion to take place across the dialyser. The HD machine dilutes concentrated bicarbonate and acidic component with the purified water and ensures the correct concentration is produced. It warms it to 37°C and pumps it around the dialyser allowing diffusion to occur. Sodium, bicarbonate, potassium, glucose and calcium levels can be adjusted to ensure an optimal mix for the child. The selection of dialysate values should be made in conjunction with the child's biochemical results. For example, a child with a serum potassium level of 3.0 mmol/L would lose more potassium through diffusion if the standard solution of 2 mmol/l was used, but this can be prevented or reversed if a higher potassium containing solution is selected.

Dialysis sessions

Children with AKI may require daily dialysis to cope with fluid gains and provide adequate solute clearance. Sessions vary in length and are dictated by the need for dialysis. For example, in children with a serum urea >40 umol/l it is necessary to limit dialysis length to less than 2 hours to avoid the risk of solute disequilibrium. Disequilibrium occurs if there is a discrepancy between the serum urea and the urea level in the brain, which can occur if the serum urea is reduced too quickly. To compensate, water moves across the blood-brain barrier to lower the brain urea causing swelling with potentially catastrophic neurological effects. Conversely, a child needing to be dialysed for the hyperkalaemia and hyperphosphataemia resulting from tumour lysis will be dialysed until the rate of lysing falls and their own renal function can cope.

Fluid loss

The amount of fluid to be removed during the dialysis session is calculated every session. The saline used to prime the lines at the start and at the end of the session is known as the wash-back. This should be added to total fluid removal as its volume can be as much as 400 ml.

Fluid input, output and balance of the previous day in addition to the previous day's weight and current blood pressure will help in the calculation of the amount of fluid that needs to be removed. The maximum amount of fluid removed should not exceed 5% of the child's body weight (Rees *et al* 2008). Excessive fluid loss will result in hypotension, nausea and cramps.

Vascular access

Central venous catheters can be single or dual lumen and should be of sufficient diameter size to allow for high blood flows. However, use of a single lumen catheter requires a larger blood circuit, which may be less optimal for young children.

An arterio-venous (AV) fistula is a permanent form of access used in children receiving chronic haemodialysis. This is created by the surgical anastemosis of an artery and a vein in the arm, most commonly the radial artery and cephalic vein. An AV fistula can be used as access acutely, however the focus of this chapter is dialysis in the acute setting only and most fistulas are formed for chronic usage.

149

Procedure guideline 9.2 Preparation of the child and family for HD/HF

Statement	Rationale
1. HD and HF must only be performed by staff who are: • Confident in caring for the acutely ill child • Able to develop expertise in HF and or HD and maintain competence • Familiar with the equipment • Able to manage the side-effects of HF/HD. (Clevenger 1998, Craig 1998, Sefton *et al* 2001).	1. To ensure that the treatment is performed safely and effectively, and to reduce the likelihood of side-effects and complications.
2. Ensure the child and family are prepared for the procedure using: • written information • verbal explanation • visual demonstration of the procedure where possible.	2. To minimise anxiety and to clarify their understanding of the procedure. To ensure effective communication between staff and parents/carers.
3. The child should be assessed and the therapy planned around their individual needs, taking into account underlying illness, severity of illness and the advantages and disadvantages of the therapies that are available (Flynn 2002, Schetz 2001). This should be clearly documented (Craig 1998).	3. To ensure that the treatment prescribed is appropriate for the child's needs (Bunchman 2002, Flynn 2002).
4. Ensure that the child and family understand the need for the choice of treatment and are aware of the risks and benefits of the procedure.	4. To minimise anxiety and ensure informed consent to treatment (Craig 1998).

Procedure guideline 9.3 Inserting a catheter (HD/HF)

Statement	Rationale
1. Appropriate vascular access should be inserted following local guidelines.	**1.** Good vascular access is essential for all extracorporeal treatments. Inadequate blood flows will result in sub-optimal dialysis. Adequate vascular access is one of the most important determinates in ensuring effective treatment (Bunchman 2002, Headrick 1998).
a) Central venous catheter (CVC) cuffed.	**a)** Cuffed lines last longer and the risk of displacement is reduced. However, they will need a GA to be removed once dialysis is no longer required.
b) Central venous catheter (CVC) uncuffed. Uncuffed central venous catheters are used for short-term use of 2 weeks or less. This is held in place by sutures.	**b)** Suitable for short-term use as the risk of infection is high and displacement is higher, however they do not require a general anaesthetic to be removed.
2. Cuffed CVC should be used if HF or HD treatment required for long periods, i.e. for more than 10 days.	**2.** Risk of displacement or accidental removal is reduced in cuffed catheters.
3. The catheter should be placed into the jugular vein with the tip cited in the right atrium.	**3.** Optimal placement is essential for adequate dialysis.
4. The catheter is tunnelled percutaneously under the skin.	**4.** The cuff acts as a physical barrier to external microbial entry and anchors the catheter in place.
5. Care should be taken when placing catheters in children who may require long-term dialysis.	**5.** The subclavian vein should never be used for catheter placement in children in end stage renal failure, as this causes a high incidence of vessel stenosis as well as compromising the formation and use of a fistula in that side (Mactier et al 2009).
6. Careful handling of the line is required and usage should be confined to dialysis only.	**6.** To minimise the risk of infection (Goldstein et al 1997, Sharma et al 1999).
7. The catheter usage should be restricted to dialysis only if possible.	**7.** Bacterial colonisation of the biofilm inside a catheter can occur and result in a shower of toxins into the child's bloodstream when the catheter is used. This results in a rigor, followed closely by a high temperature. Confirmation of the infection is by blood cultures. If the child is symptomatic of a line infection, broad spectrum intravenous antibiotics are given until specific sensitivities are obtained and treatment required as per hospital protocol.
8. If the child suffers a persistent pyrexia, the catheter may need to be removed, with replacement into a new access site.	
9. If there is a blockage or poor flow, it should be possible to withdraw blood freely out of either catheter lumen and re-infuse it back with minimal resistance.	**9.** A blockage can be due to thrombosis stenosis.
10. If a catheter has poor flow or has a high resistance to re-infusion, instillation of tissue plasminogen activator (TPA) can be used.	**10.** This helps to dissolve thrombus.
11. The child's pre-treatment status should be assessed and documented. This includes: • Vital sign recording, accurate blood pressure and core and peripheral temperature (Table 9.4) • Fluid balance • Weight • Biochemical, haematological and blood gas results • General overall condition.	**11.** To assess if the child is fit to undergo the treatment and provide a baseline to monitor the child during the procedure.

150

Haemofiltration

Haemofiltration (HF) has the advantage of continuous fluid and solute removal that is generally better tolerated and can be delivered by intensive care staff who have undergone specific training (Craig 1998, John and Eckardt 2007, Sefton *et al* 2001). There may also be a therapeutic value from CVVH during sepsis syndrome associated with the removal of harmful inflammatory mediators (Saudan *et al* 2006).

Continuous arterio-venous haemofiltration (CAVH) uses the difference between the patient's arterial and venous pressure to drive blood through an extra-corporeal circuit. As the clearance of waste is dependant on blood flow, it is of limited use with children because blood pressure is lower during childhood (Craig 1998, Reeves *et al* 1994). To overcome these issues, continuous veno-venous haemofiltration (CVVH) is increasingly considered as the RRT of choice in the Paediatric Intensive Care Unit (Flynn 2002, Lowrie 2000, Warady and Bunchman 2000).

During CVVH, a double lumen central venous line is inserted and blood is removed from one lumen (the arterial lumen), pumped around an extracorporeal circuit, passing through a haemofilter and returned to the second lumen (referred to as the venous lumen). The resulting pressure difference within the haemofilter leads to water and permeable solutes passing through the haemofilter membrane by convection and diffusion to form a filtrate, a process similar to glomerular filtration in the human body (Forni and Hilton 1997). As the haemofilter is only permeable to solutes with a molecular mass less than 50,000 daltons, solutes such as urea, creatinine, potassium, sodium, ionised calcium and almost all drugs not bound to proteins pass through the membrane, but larger substances, such as red blood cells and plasma proteins do not (Craig 1998, Headrick 1998, Ricci *et al* 2006).

The higher the rate of filtrate production, the greater the clearance of solutes and fluid. However, in order to produce sufficient filtrate to reduce urea and creatinine levels, the fluid and essential electrolyte loss would be too great. Therefore a physiologi-cally balanced solution is administered back to the patient, replacing these essential electrolytes and fluid, but not the waste produces such as urea, creatinine, ammonia and so on (Forni and Hilton 1997). If fluid is to be removed, the volume of replacement fluid is reduced, leading to a net loss of fluid from the child. This allows large volumes of parentral or enteral nutrition to be administered, as restriction of fluid intake is unnecessary (Flynn 2002, Headrick 1998).

The replacement fluid is infused into the CVVH circuit, but it can be given before (pre-dilution) or after (post-dilution) the haemofilter. Pre-dilution provides the added advantage of flushing the haemofilter by effectively diluting the blood before the filter, which may prolong circuit life by reducing the risk of clotting. This is at the expense of solute clearance which is reduced because of the haemodilution effect (Dirkes 2000, Headrick 1998). Alternatively, administering a dialysate fluid counter current through the filter will increase the movement of solutes across the membrane by diffusion and is referred to as continuous veno-venous haemodialysis (CVVHD). If both techniques are combined, this is known as haemodiafiltration (CVVHDF) and this may be more suitable for the highly catabolic patient (Saudan *et al* 2006). The site of fluid replacement and whether or not a dialysis fluid is employed remains the choice of individual clinicians and local guidelines.

The risks of CVVH are mainly around issues relating to the extracorporeal circuit. Constant vigilance is required to prevent severe haemorrhage due to circuit rupture or disconnection. Heat loss may also be significant, requiring the blood to be warmed before returning to the patient (John and Eckardt 2007). As anticoagulation may be required to prevent circuit clotting, the child may be at risk of systemic haemorrhage. Careful attention to the rates of filtrate production and fluid replacement will minimise the risk of severe fluid or electrolyte imbalance. Staff should be trained in the management of both circuit and patient related problems to reduce the risks to the patient and ensure the therapy is effective (Craig 1998, Sefton *et al* 2001).

Procedure guideline 9.4 **Preparing the equipment (HF)**

Statement	Rationale
1. An appropriate haemofiltration machine should be selected and checked according to local policy and manufacturers' recommendations.	**1.** To ensure effective treatment and prevent equipment malfunction and complications (Craig 1998).
2. Suitable haemofiltration lines and haemofilter should be selected based on the child's weight and clinical condition (Craig 1998). The haemofiltration circuit should be assembled according to the manufacturer's recommendations and local policy.	**2.** To minimise complications and ensure that the technique is delivered safely.
3. The circuit should be primed according to the manufacturer's recommendations and local policy.	**3.** To detect circuit leaks or malfunctions. To remove air and traces of sterilising agents reducing the risk of air emboli and anaphylaxis.

(Continued)

Procedure guideline 9.4 (*Continued*)

Statement	Rationale
4. The amount and type of anticoagulant should be assessed and prepared for use.	**4.** To reduce the risk of circuit clotting and anticoagulation of the child.
5. The amount and type of haemofiltration fluid should be assessed and prepared for use. Factors to take into account include the child's age, diagnosis, metabolic status and liver function.	**5.** Incorrect choice of haemofiltration fluid can lead to ineffective treatment and deterioration of the child. Complications include metabolic, electrolyte and acid-base imbalances (Ellis *et al* 1997, Soysal *et al* 2007). Infants and children with liver dysfunction cannot metabolise the lactate present in most replacement fluids and a bicarbonate base solution should be selected (Naka and Bellomo 2004). This should also be considered in children with severe metabolic derangement (particularly acidosis).
6. The need for further electrolyte supplements (such as potassium or phosphate) should be assessed and prepared for use.	**6.** To reduce complications and potential electrolyte imbalance as a result of haemofiltration.
7. Consider the rate of fluid exchange and the amount of fluid loss per hour.	**7.** To calculate the settings needed after treatment has commenced.
8. If the circuit volume exceeds more than 10% of the child's total circulating blood volume, the circuit should be primed with whole blood just before the start of treatment (Headrick 1998). The blood should be as 'fresh' as possible and local policy for administration of blood products must be followed (Parshuram and Cox 2002).	**8.** To prevent haemodilution and cardiovascular instability. Blood which has been stored for longer periods may have elevated potassium levels, especially if irradiated ,and the rapid administration of large volumes, which is required in haemofiltration, may cause hyperkalaemia. Hypocalcaemia may also be a complication due to the use of citrate in blood bank storage (Parshuram and Cox 2002).

Procedure guideline 9.5 **Preparation for HF**

Statement	Rationale
1. Ensure that all equipment is prepared and assembled for use and the haemofiltration machine is primed and ready.	**1.** To ensure the procedure goes smoothly and to minimise complications.
2. Using non-touch technique, clean the CVC and attach a syringe to each lumen.	**2.** To establish that the CVC is patent.
3. Remove the heparin from each lumen and discard.	**3.** To prevent heparin being administered and to check for clots in the CVC.
4. Attach a 10 ml syringe, release the CVC clamps and check each lumen for patency by withdrawing blood. Establish which lumen allows withdrawl of blood most easily and use this to attach to the 'arterial' side of the circuit.	**4.** Adequate fluid removal and dialysis are dependent on adequate flow rates.
5. Attach a 3-way tap (primed with saline) to each lumen and flush with 0.9% sodium chloride solution.	**5.** To establish if both lumens are patent and allow each lumen to be clamped independently.
6. If either lumen is blocked, follow local guidelines for checking and re-establishing patency (as above for HD).	**6.** Two patent IV access ports are required to perform haemofiltration.
7. Using the 3-way taps and lumen clamps, ensure both lumens are securely clamped.	**7.** To prevent blood loss from the CVC and prepare to start haemofiltration.

Procedure guideline 9.6 Starting CVVH

Statement	Rationale
1. Commencing haemofiltration is a two staff procedure. At least one member should be a competent haemofiltration practitioner.	1. To maintain patient safety.
2. Resuscitation equipment and appropriate intravenous fluid should be available.	2. Commencing haemofiltration can cause clinical instability which requires prompt intervention and resuscitation (Uchino *et al* 2007). The child may also react to the membrane of the haemofilter, leading to severe hypotension (Flynn 2002).
3. Administer oxygen for 2 minutes prior to starting haemofiltration. If the child is receiving artificial ventilation, increase the oxygen level as agreed with the medical team.	3. Starting haemofiltration can lead to hypoxia, especially in younger children.
4. If the child is receiving vasoactive or inotropic drugs, discuss with the medical team and experienced staff whether the doses need to be increased.	4. Due to the presence of the extra-corporeal circuit and large fluid/blood shifts, haemofiltration can lead to reduced plasma levels of drugs, which may need to be increased to maintain stability (Headrick 1998, Uchino *et al* 2007).
5. Stop the haemofiltration pump and clamp both the arterial and venous lines close to the tip.	5. To prevent leakage from the circuit and air entrapment.
6. Using non-touch technique, connect both lines to the relevant CVC lumen (selected as above), ensuring a bubble-free connection.	6. To prevent infection and air emboli.
7. Check the child for any signs of clinical instability before proceeding. The child's vital signs should be observed throughout the 'start-up' process (Uchino *et al* 2007).	7. To minimise complications as haemofiltration can exacerbate instability.
8. Release the clamps and 3-way taps from both the haemofiltration lines and the VAD.	8. To allow blood to flow in/out of the CVC.
9. Start the blood pump on the slowest possible speed. Observe the venous lumen closely for air and be prepared to clamp the lumen to prevent it entering the patient.	9. To detect air and minimise complications. Any air in the circuit will enter via the venous lumen.
10. If prescribed, administer a bolus of heparin into the haemofiltration circuit just after the blood pump is started.	10. To maintain/promote the integrity of the circuit and prevent clotting (Schetz 2001).
11. Reassess the child. If they are stable, slowly increase the blood pump speed to the desired level. Treat any signs of instability or complications as clinically appropriate.	11. To minimise complications.
12. Commence the anticoagulant infusion if prescribed.	12. To anticoagulant the extra-corporeal circuit to minimise circuit clotting which reduces the effectiveness of the therapy (Bunchman 2002, Ricci *et al* 2006, Uchino *et al* 2007).
13. Set the fluid exchange rate according to the calculated values based on the child's clinical condition, local policy and multi-disciplinary team guidance.	13. To commence the therapy. Exchange rate determines the efficiency of the treatment and should be individually assessed (Headrick 1998).
14. Set the amount of fluid loss to be achieved during the haemofiltration session.	14. To commence the therapy and reduce fluid overload.
15. Set appropriate machine alarm limits.	15. To minimise complications and maintain patient safety.

153

Procedure guideline 9.7 Monitoring and maintaining HF

Statement	Rationale
1. Throughout haemofiltration the nurse should be present at the bedside at all times.	**1.** The child is at risk of significant blood loss/air emboli if the circuit becomes accidentally disconnected or ruptures.
2. At least two sets of clamps should be available at the child's bedside.	**2.** To clamp the circuit in the event of leakage or rupture.
3. The child should be fully monitored before, during and after HF. Continuous ECG, invasive blood pressure, central venous pressure, respiratory rate, peripheral and core temperature and saturation monitoring are generally accepted as the minimum. The Glasgow coma score (GCS) should be recorded if the child is sedated and/or paralysed.	**3.** To ensure early detection of complications and side effects (Headrick 1998).
4. The childs observations should be recorded hourly or more frequently if clinically indicated.	**4.** To monitor the child for signs of clinical deterioration and/or complications including haemorrhage from either the circuit or from the child, anaphylaxis, hypoxia, hypothermia, fluid, electrolyte and acid-base imbalances, hypothermia and infection (Craig 1998, Headrick 1998, John and Eckardt 2007).
5. Arterial blood gas, full blood count, urea and electrolytes and clotting screen should be obtained 1 hour after haemofiltration has commenced and 6–8 hourly thereafter.	**5.** To detect for abnormalities due to haemofiltration (Headrick 1998, Parshuram and Cox 2002).

6. The circuit should be monitored continuously and the filter and bubble-trap inspected hourly. The ultrafiltrate fluid should also be monitored.	**6.** Changes in ultrafiltrate colour may indicate filter membrane rupture or haemolysis.
	  To detect potential circuit rupture early to minimise the risk of rapid severe blood loss.
	  To detect for early signs of circuit clotting (Ahsan Ejaz et al 2007).

7. The following should be documented hourly: • Blood pump speed • Arterial pressure • Venous pressure • Transmembrane pressure (TMP) • Fluid type.	**7.** To maintain patient safety, and to detect trends that may identify early signs of circuit clotting (Ahsan Ejaz et al 2007).
8. If heparin is being used, the circuit activated clotting time (ACT) should be assessed 1 hour after starting haemofiltration and 4 hourly thereafter.	**8.** To monitor anticoagulation of the circuit.
9. If the ACT is below the recommended level (generally 180–200 s) the dose of heparin should be increased in line with local guidelines (Bunchman 2002, Headrick 1998).	**9.** A low ACT indicates that the circuit is at risk of clotting.
10. If the ACT is above the recommended level, the dose of heparin should be decreased in line with local guidelines.	**10.** A high ACT indicates that the circuit is over-anticoagulated. This may lead to the child also being anticoagulated, increasing the risk of complications, such as bleeding (Monchi et al 2004, Schetz 2001).

Procedure guideline 9.8 Discontinuing HF

Statement	Rationale
1. At the end of the treatment session or if the circuit becomes clotted, haemofiltration will need to be discontinued.	1. To complete or re-start treatment.
2. Assess whether the child can be disconnected from the circuit immediately or needs to have the extra-corporeal blood 'washed-back'. Influencing factors include the child's weight, current haemoglobin level, overall clinical condition, current fluid balance, ongoing need for haemofiltration and whether the circuit was blood primed at the start.	2. 'Washing-back' the extra-corporeal blood may be beneficial in increasing the child's haemoglobin level without the need for another blood transfusion. This needs to be balanced against the additional fluid volume that the child will receive as a result.
3. To discontinue haemofiltration, stop the blood pump and clamp the arterial and venous lines and the CVC lumens.	3. To prevent blood loss and discontinue therapy.
4. If the circuit blood is to be washed-back, disconnect the arterial end from the CVC and attach a bag of 0.9% sodium chloride. Release all clamps and start the blood pump slowly.	4. To draw 0.9% sodium chloride solution into the circuit to flush out the blood and return to the child.
5. Continue the blood pump until the circuit is coloured 'salmon pink'.	5. This indicates that most of the red blood cells have been returned to the child.
6. Clamp both lines.	6. To prevent infection and blood leakage.
7. For both wash-back and discontinuation techniques, disconnect the lines from the CVC using aseptic non-touch technique. Attach a 10 ml syringe with 0.9% sodium chloride to each VAD lumen.	7. To disconnect the extra-corporeal circuit and maintain CVC patency.
8. After opening the CVC clamps, flush both lumens with the 0.9% sodium chloride and reclamp. Release the CVC clamps and inject 1000 units' heparin to fill the exact volume of each lumen and reclamp. Close off each lumen with an IV device cap.	8. To maintain CVC patency for future use.

155

Procedure guideline 9.9 Commencing HD

Statement	Rationale
1. Wash hands.	1. Following local hand hygiene policy.
2. Prepare the assembled equipment and dialysis machine when ready to perform the procedure: a) Ensure the dialysis machine is disinfected/clean and ready for patient use. b) Prime and prepare the circuit with 0.9% sodium chloride according to the manufacturer's instructions. c) Prepare the dialysate and connect it to the dialyser. d) Perform baseline vital observations: As above.	2. a) To avoid potential cross-contamination between children. b) To expel air and to rinse out any remaining sterilant. c) To prime the dialysate compartment and to prepare the semi-permeable membrane for dialysis. d) To assess the child's condition and allow for comparison during and following HD.
2. Using a non-touch technique, connect the vascular access to arterial and venous lines of the circuit.	2. To minimise the risk of infection.

(Continued)

Procedure guideline 9.9 (*Continued*)

Statement	Rationale
3. Start the cleaning cycle of the HD machine.	**3.** To ensure the machine is disinfected prior to use in accordance with manufacturer's instructions. This cycle can take 40 minutes.
4. Gather equipment together.	**4.** To be efficient undertaking the procedure.
5. When the cleaning cycle is completed, select the dialysis mode and connect the bicarbonate and acidic dialysis concentrates once the initial safety function check has been carried out.	**5.** To confirm the finish of the clean cycle and to signify the intention to start a new HD cycle. The machine performs safety checks and begins to prepare the dialysis concentrate for delivery.
6. Attach the saline.	**6.** These are used to prime air from the circuit and later allow infusion of saline to the circuit during recirculation and wash-back.
7. Place the dialyser in the holder. Connect the arterial line to the arterial (red) end of the dialyser. Clamp the patient end of the line and spike the 1L 0.9 NaCl. Connect the venous line to the venous (blue) end of the dialyser and hang the waste bag on the IV pole. Feed the pump segment into the pump; ensure the luer lock connections on the dialyser and the pressure transducers are securely attached.	**7.** To assemble the circuit and dialyser and place correctly on the machine. Always refer to manufacturer's instructions for further guidance. The saline will prime from the 1L bag, through the arterial line, through the dialyser, into the venous line and collect in the waste bag. During priming the blue end is uppermost to facilitate air removal.
8. Unclamp the arterial line and start the blood pump to commence priming the air from the circuit. Raise the level of saline in the venous drip chamber to three-quarter full and arm the air detector.	**8.** To expel air from the circuit and ready the fibres in the dialyser for blood.
9. Prepare the heparin/saline solution. The heparin is drawn up according to individual requirements, dose approx 10–25 units/kg/ml. Label and attach the syringe to the arterial circuit and place in the syringe driver.	**9.** To facilitate heparin delivery during the procedure to prevent clotting of the circuit.
10. Prime the infusion line and then attach to the arterial infusion port.	**10.** To allow infusion of saline if required during the procedure and to enable the wash-back later.
11. Gently clamp the venous line to expel air bubbles.	**11.** To de-airate the dialyser to enhance diffusional area.
12. Attach the dialysate ports to the dialyser when the function checks are complete and the dialysis fluid is ready.	**12.** To allow dialysis fluid to come into contact with the dialyser. This can only be done once the function checks are complete.
13. Start the dialysis fluid flow around the dialyser.	**13.** To start dialysing across the membrane to prepare the membrane for blood.
14. Pressure test the circuit by clamping the venous line to reach a pressure of 200 mmHg and then release the clamp.	**14.** To ensure the patency of the fibres in the dialyser so any blood leak will be detected.
15. When the circuit is primed with all the saline, stop the pump, clamp the A and V lines, disconnect the waste bag and the empty 1.0 litre bag of saline and connect them with the supplied female/female connection.	**15.** Now priming has finished, the circuit can be completed.
16. Unclamp, start the blood pump and recirculate the saline in the circuit, ensuring the 500 ml saline is unclamped.	**16.** As soon as fluid is on both sides of the membrane dialysis will occur and saline losses can be topped up from the 400 ml saline bag.

Procedure guideline 9.9 (*Continued*)

Statement	Rationale
17. Set the session length, required fluid loss, and heparin rate and infusion stop time (if required). Start HD.	**17.** Once these are entered, the machine is ready to start dialysis.
18. The following should be documented hourly: • Blood pump speed • Arterial pressure • Venous pressure • Transmembrane pressure (TMP) • Fluid type.	**18.** To maintain patient safety and to detect trends that may identify the early signs of circuit clotting (Ahsan Ejaz *et al* 2007).
19. The length of time a child is on HD is dependent on their general condition. Usually 2–4 hour sessions are sufficient for safe HD. At the end of HD the nurse needs to decide if the child requires the extra-corporeal blood 'washed-back'. Influencing factors include the child's weight, blood pressure, current haemoglobin level, overall clinical condition, fluid balance, ongoing need for HD and whether the circuit was blood primed at the start.	**19.** HD in acute children required continuous monitoring and evaluation of the session. The initial goals of fluid and waste product removal should be assessed before disconnection the circuit.

Procedure guideline 9.10 Discontinuing HD

Statement	Rationale
1. Towards the end of HD reduce blood pump speed to 100 ml/min.	**1.** This gives more time to return the blood to the child and clear the circuit of blood.
2. When the dialysis session has been completed the blood pump is stopped and the circuit clamped.	**2.** In preparation for the blood in the circuit to be returned to the child.
3. Using 0.9% sodium chloride 'wash-back' the blood in the circuit then stop the pump and clamp the access.	**3.** This ensures all the blood is returned to the child to prevent anaemia.
4. Disconnect the circuit from the vascular access using aseptic non-touch technique.	**4.** To minimise the risk of infection.
5. Instil appropriate anticoagulant agent, e.g. heparin into vascular access, then cap off.	**5.** To maintain patency of the access between sessions.
6. Dispose of circuit and equipment in accordance with local and national guidelines.	**6.** To reduce the risk of cross-infection.
7. Evaluate the procedure and record the information in the child's healthcare records.	**7.** To aid communication and ensure continuity of care.
8. Where possible weigh the child and complete the record of the dialysis session.	**8.** The post-HD weight is part of the information that will help the team assess the effectiveness of the HD session.
9. Remove the lines and empty the dialyser from the machine according to manufacturer's instructions before commencing the cleaning programme.	**9.** The machine should be disinfected between patients to minimise risks of cross-infection.
10. Discard equipment appropriately.	**10.** To observe local and national policies on correct disposal of clinical waste.

Patient complications

The commonest patient complication associated with haemodialysis is that of hypotension. This is caused if the quantity of fluid ultrafiltrated from the child during the HD session is too much or if fluid is removed too rapidly. For the fluid to be removed, it must be within the vascular space and if the rate of fluid removal is greater than the rate of vascular refill then hypotension results.

The ideal weight of a child is called the 'dry' weight. At this weight the blood pressure should be within normal limits for age and the fluid balance deemed isovolaemic. Clinical features of dehydration include hypotension, yawning, light-headedness, tachycardia, pallor, nausea and vomiting, cramp and cold and clammy peripheries. If left untreated the child can destabilise. A bolus infusion of 0.9% sodium chloride will instantly increase the circulating volume and correct the signs and symptoms. If a child is severely affected and collapses, administration of saline is the first priority.

Peritoneal dialysis

Peritoneal dialysis (PD) requires the insertion of a dialysis catheter into the peritoneum. This is then used to flush dialysate solution into and out of the peritoneum. The peritoneum is used as an autogenic semi-permeable membrane, filtering waste products and electrolytes from the blood via diffusion. As the dialysate used is glucose-based, it also allows fluid to be drawn from the blood into dialysate via osmosis and waste products, electrolytes and excess fluid are then removed via the catheter.

PD is the preferred treatment for children, this is primarily because of the difficulties accessing and maintaining vascular access for HD and HF, especially in small children (MacLeod 2002). There are instances where PD may not be viable and HD or HF may be required; for example if children have had extensive abdominal surgery, adhesions, peritonitis or significant gut involvement in haemolytic ureamic syndrome, pancreatitis and acites.

Types of PD

Manual dialysis is often used in children with AKI in non-dialysis units and in the neonatal period as initial fill volumes are too small for the automated machines. It is an extremely time-consuming treatment and has the potential for high infection rates because of the type of connections within the circuit. Once the infant can tolerate fill volumes of 60 ml per cycle they can be switched onto an automated dialysis machine. These are usually only available in hospitals who have dedicated paediatric renal units on site.

Peritoneal dialysis (PD) may be used in the management of both acute and chronic renal failure patients within the hospital or home environment. Peritoneal dialysis can be further divided into different modalities such as automated peritoneal dialysis (APD) used for overnight dialysis; continuous cycling PD (CCPD) used for acute kidney injury or chronic overload; tidal dialysis, which is cycling overnight with a constant volume of fluid left in the peritoneum; optichoice, which is APD with an additional exchange during the day for children who require additional dialysis; and CAPD, which is a manual method of dialysis for ESRF.

Continuous ambulatory PD (CAPD) is a system that is not dependent on a machine; requires minimal equipment; and is a very simple procedure to learn. The child usually requires four manual exchanges during the day. It can be used in the management of ESRF children at home. This type of dialysis is usually only suitable for adolescents who still have reasonable urine output.

Assessment of a child requiring PD

There are many factors that are taken into consideration when assessing a child's requirement for dialysis. Blood values (specifically creatinine, potassium, sodium and urea) (Table 9.2) fluid status, blood pressure and urine output are the main areas for consideration. Once all other medication interventions have failed to resolve the anuric phase, dialysis of some form will be indicated. The type of dialysis suitable will be dependent on the child's vital signs and the availability of PD. A full physical assessment and accurate patient history is essential at this stage.

All individuals performing PD should be appropriately trained and competent to ensure that the child receives the best form of treatment by nurses who have been trained in this area.

Procedure guideline 9.11 Preparation (PD)

Statement	Rationale
1. Assess the need for dialysis (Table 9.10).	1. To ensure that the infant/child is suitable for PD and that all other medical treatments for anuria/oliguria have been explored prior to insertion of the PD catheter.
2. Prepare the child and family for the procedure: using verbal, visual and written interpretation, dolls and toys if appropriate, offering time for questions and discussion.	2. To minimise anxiety and to clarify their understanding of and consent to the procedure.
3. Choose an appropriate sized Tenckhoff catheter (3 sizes available suitable for infants of 1 kg and above).	3. PD is dependent on a functioning Tenckhoff catheter.

Procedure guideline 9.11 (*Continued*)

Statement	Rationale
4. Make sure the child is not constipated.	**4.** To minimise complications of catheter displacement and mechanical problems with the catheter drainage.
5. Dietary assessment made and a nasogastric tube inserted at the same time as the Tenckhoff catheter if necessary.	**5.** Adequate nutrition and good albumen levels are vital to the efficiency of fluid removal on PD. Adequate nutrition will help reduce the urea level and lead to a faster recovery.
6. Monitor vital signs as often as condition requires. If vital signs or blood levels are outside the normal range they must be continually monitored.	**6.** Abnormal vital signs usually require the team to change the dialysis prescription.
7. Interpretation of vital signs pre peritoneal dialysis: **a)** A increasing peripheral/core temperature gap. **b)** A increasing pulse rate and respiratory rate. **c)** Hypertension. **d)** Weight gain/loss.	**7.** **a)** Temperature gap should be <2°C when the infant is adequately wrapped up, >2°C may be a sign of peripheral shutdown due to hypovolaemia or sepsis. **b)** Potential sepsis, pain or pulmonary oedema, anaemia. **c)** Fluid overload. **d)** Weight loss usually indicates good ultrafiltration/ improved urine output, weight gain can indicate inadequate dialysis.

159

Table 9.10 Indications for dialysis

Indications for dialysis	
Hyperkalaemia	K > 6.5 mmol/l
Severe fluid overload	Not responding to furosemide
Urea	Ur >40 mmol/l
Severe hyper/hyponatraemia	<118 mmol/l or
Acidosis	HCO_3 < 16 mmol/l
Multi-system failure	
Prolonged oliguria	<1 ml/kg/hr

Rees *et al* 2006.

Procedure guideline 9.12 Preparation for surgery (PD)

Statement	Rationale
1. Psychological preparation and support is extremely important to initiate in the early stages of this process.	**1.** Liaise with a play specialist.
2. Pre-insertion of PD catheter: **a)** Ensure that the child is safely prepared and transferred to theatre following local policies and protocols. **b)** Ensure antibiotic cover is prescribed. **c)** Supply theatres with necessary equipment needed for insertion of catheter and dressing of the new catheter.	**2.** To ensure that care is standardised and meets the child's needs. **b)** To reduce the risk of infection. **c)** To ensure the correct catheter is inserted and that the site is dressed appropriately to ensure that PD can be performed effectively and reduce the risk of infection at the exit site.

Procedure guideline 9.13 Starting PD for AKI

Statement	Rationale
Manual	
1. Setting up manual PD, collect following equipment: • Dialysis prescription and record chart • Drip stand • Heater for PD fluid • Manual PD giving set neonatal/paediatric • Dialysis fluid (Table 9.11) • Povidone–iodine or alternative disinfectant • Antimicrobial hand wash • Dressing pack • Sterile gloves • Trolley • Alcohol wipes • Apron.	1. To ensure the procedure goes smoothly and to minimise complications.
2. Explain procedure to child and family.	2. To minimise anxiety and to clarify their understanding of and consent to the procedure.
3. Wash hands for 1 minute.	3. To reduce the risk of infection.
4. Collect equipment.	4. To ensure the procedure goes smoothly and minimise complications.
5. Clean trolley with hard surface wipes, wash hands for 1 minute.	5. To reduce the risk of infection.
6. Open PD giving set, dressing pack, onto a sterile field and open the PD fluid bag into sterile field.	6. Maintaining a sterile field can reduce the risk of cross-contamination.
7. Open sterile gloves onto cleaned work surface.	7. Reduce the risk of contaminating the sterile field with your hands.
8. Wash hands for 1 minute and put on sterile gloves.	8. To reduce the risk of infection.
9. Clamp clamps of giving set, spike fluid bag with end of giving set and hang the bags of fluid onto stand.	9. If the fluid runs through the giving set before it is hanging on a stand the filters may become wet and this will affect the efficiency of the dialysis.
10. Prime set with dialysis fluid, keep the burette upright when full. Care must be taken not to wet the air filters of the burette as this will cause problems when filling and draining the burettes.	10. If the filter becomes wet, a vacuum is produced inside the burette and then will be unable to fill or drain the burette, in this situation the PD giving set may need to be changed. An air inlet placed into the filter may be helpful in this situation.
11. Place coil in warmer.	11. PD fluid should be warmed before it is run into the peritoneum for comfort and to prevent a drop in core temperature of the child.
12. Place sterile field under catheter, pour povidone–iodine solution into the pot, submerge catheter for 3 minutes.	12. Povidone–iodine solution is used to disinfectant the catheter and prevent infections by pathogens.
13. Connect set to PD catheter.	13. To start dialysis.
14. Hang drain bag below the level of the child.	14. Drainage from the peritoneum is dependent on gravitational force.
15. Re-check BP.	15. It is important to have a base line BP before starting dialysis, as blood pressure is one of the most important observations to accurately assess fluid balance.

160

Procedure guideline 9.13 (*Continued*)

Statement	Rationale
16. Open drain clamp and allow any fluid in situ to drain for 10 minutes and then clamp.	**16.** To ensure the peritoneum is empty.
17. Fill chamber with the prescribed amount of fluid to fill the child.	**17.** The fluid prescription should start at 10 ml/kg and be increased as tolerated.
18. If the drainage is blood stained the catheters should be flushed continuously, with 10 ml/kg of 1.36% dialysis fluid (with 200 units/l heparin added), until the dialysate clears becomes clear, cycling can then begin.	**18.** Placing of a PD catheter can cause a small amount of trauma to the tissues and bleeding occurs. Flushing will prevent the formation of a clot in the catheter.
19. Open clamp to allow the fluid to fill over approximately 10 minutes and re-clamp.	**19.** When starting PD it is important to administer fluid slowly at a reduced discomfort and minimise the risk of leakage. The dialysis settings are adjusted according to age, condition, biochemistry and vital signs. Young children are usually high transporters so fluid and electrolytes move across the peritoneum faster so their cycles are shorted. If a child presents with a very high urea slow dialysis is recommended as reducing the urea too quickly can cause disequilibrium (Rees *et al* 2006).
20. Leave fill in situ for prescribed length of time starting with dwells of 30 minutes. Care should be taken at this time to observe for leaking around the catheter; if this occurs the fill volume may need to be reduced.	**20.** A dwell time of 30 mins is usually sufficient for good clearance of electrolytes and fluid removal, however a fill of 30–50 ml/kg is usually required for adequate acute dialysis, the rate at which the fill can increase is dependent on the success of the catheter, if the catheter leaks the risk of infection increases and therefore the fill volume should be increased with caution.
21. Open drain clamp and allow to drain for 10 minutes; fluid from the peritoneum should drain by gravity.	**21.** Fluid should drain freely from the child when the clamps are open.
22. Start to record the dialysis in, out and ultrafiltration (UF).	**22.** Accurate recording of dialysis fluid in and out is essential to determine fluid balance.

Automated machine (home choice)

Statement	Rationale
1. Standard prescription: fill volumes for a newly inserted PD catheter should start on 10 ml per kg of 1.36% dialysis fluid, increasing to 40–50 ml/kg or 800 ml/m^2 in the under 2 years age group and 1.1–1.4 l/m^2 from 2 years upwards. The fluid volume is increased as tolerated over a 48 hour period in AKI.	**1.** Increasing the fill time gradually reduces the risk of complications of pain on filling and potential leakage.
2. Starting automated dialysis: Program: Total volume of fluid : 800 ml–1.4 l/m^2 Start with continuous cycles Length of cycles.	**2.** The dialysis program is adjusted according to age, condition, biochemistry and vital signs. As a rule young children are high transporters so fluid and electrolytes move across the peritoneum faster so their cycles are shorted. If a child presents with a very high urea, slow dialysis is recommended as reducing the urea too quickly can cause disequilibrium (Rees *et al* 2006).
3. Dwell time-30–40 minutes for babies 50–80 minutes depending on clinical condition.	**3.** The dwell time influences the process of osmosis and diffusion. This needs to be titrated according to the child's blood results and vital signs.

(*Continued*)

161

Procedure guideline 9.13 (*Continued*)

Statement	Rationale
4. Set up machines for peritoneal dialysis according to manufacturers' instructions and hospital policy for clean no-touch technique. Prime circuit with dialysis fluid according to manufacturers' instructions.	**4.** All equipment used in the delivery of therapies should comply with standards for medical equipment and hospital policy if good practice is to be maintained.
5. Connect PD: • Using clean non-touch technique, access PD catheter and connect circuit. • Open all clamps and initiate dialysis; always flushing post-drain prior to filling.	**5.** The non-touch technique has been adopted in the clinical area to reduce the risk of infection.
6. Ensure that the child is comfortable.	**6.** It is important to make sure the dialysis is running effectively and that the child is comfortable before leaving the bedside.

162

Table 9.11 Choice of PD fluids available

Type of dialysis fluid	Glucose dianeal	Bicarbonate/lactate physioneal	Starch derived glucose polymer icodextrin 7.5%	Amino acid neutrineal
	PD4-Ca 1.25 mmol/l	Physioneal 40 Ca-1.25 mmol/l		
	PD1-Ca 1.75 mmol/l	Physioneal 35 Ca-1.7 5 mmol/l	Extraneal Ca-1.75	
Concentration	1.36% 2.27% 3.86%	1.36% 2.27%	One concentration used only for last bag fill or long dwell periods	1.36% only
Bag size	0.25–5 l bags	2.5 l only		2 L only
Estimated blood volumes				
Age	Neonates	Infant	Child	Adult
Blood ml/kg (Davenport 1996)	90	80	80	65

PD prescription

Using collated information, plan the dialysis regimen. Collation of blood pressure, respiratory rate and pulse, U&Es, weight and clinical assessment dictates dialysis regimen and concentration and the type of fluids required. The dialysis fill volume in AKI starts at 10 ml/kg and can be increased up to 30–50 ml/kg over the next 48 hours if the catheter does not leak. The dwell time starts at 30 minutes for manual dialysis and is then changed according to the child's individual clinical needs. Ultra filtration in small babies is normally more rapid than in older children. This is due to the large surface area of the peritoneum; for this reason they require a shorter dwell time to ultra filtrate effectively. Ultra filtration (UF) in PD is the process whereby fluid (mostly water and electrolytes) moves across the peritoneal membrane as a result of a pressure gradient. The glucose concentrations come in 1.36%, 2.27% and 3.86% (Table 9.11). In general high glucose concentration removes greater amounts of fluids (Rees *et al* 2006).

Procedure guideline 9.14 Patient care on PD

Statement	Rationale
1. Accurate fluid balance is essential. Record the ultra filtration (UF), fluid input/output hourly during the acute phase.	**1.** UF is the fluid removed by dialysis. The amount of fluid removed will be dependent of the child's fluid balance.
2. Calculate the fluid restriction daily based on the urine output + UF + insensible loss of the previous day.	**2.** Fluid restrictions are essential to prevent the child becoming fluid overloaded (Rees *et al* 2006).

Procedure guideline 9.14 (*Continued*)

Statement	Rationale
3. Make the following observations hourly if unstable: • Core and peripheral temperature • CVP is sometimes required in ITU • Blood pressure • Neuro observations for HUS • Pulse • Respiratory rate • ECG monitoring • Bloods for U&E and FBC daily once stable • Blood sugars.	**3.** Helps assess fluid balance. Hyperglycemia can develop due to the high concentration of glucose in the dialysis fluid or as a secondary complication to HUS.
4. Provide adequate nutrition by TPN or NGF.	**4.** Adequate nutrition will help lower the urea and speed up recovery (Rees *et al* 2006).
5. Monitor the weight twice daily.	**5.** This is important to assess the effectiveness of the dialysis prescription.
6. Introduce play and stimulation.	**6.** If the child is well enough encourage play and distraction as the environment can be quite frightening for a child.

Interventions

Statement	Rationale
1. Connection and disconnection of all PD lines should be done with great care according to hospital policy. When a child requires continuous dialysis the lines should be changed every 24 hours for manual PD and 48 hours for home choice PD.	**1.** Risk of infection leading to peritonitis is high in this group due to having the perfect medium for growth of bacteria (warm with high glucose levels).
2. PD specimens should be taken if the child becomes pyrexial or the fluid in the drainage bag appears cloudy.	**2.** To avoid high risk of infection. If white cell count is $>100 \times 10^{6}/l$ possible peritonitis.
3. Wound site The wound dressings for acute sites should be kept clean and dry, only change if exudate is observed.	**3.** Exit site infections can lead to infections and peritonitis.

Procedure guideline 9.15 Special considerations (PD)

Statement	Rationale
1. Signs and symptoms of infection are: • Cloudy PD effluent • Abdominal pain • Pyrexia • Vomiting • Hypotensive.	**1.** Early detection of peritonitis. If the only symptom is cloudy fluid, the sample should be sent to haematology for analysis as cloudy fluid can result from an allergic response post insertion of the catheter or in response to the PD fluid. In this situation a raised esoinophil count is usually detected the PD specimen and full blood count of the child.

(*Continued*)

Procedure guideline 9.15 (*Continued*)

Statement	Rationale
2. Observe the exit site regularly for signs of inflamed or exudate, swabs should be taken if necessary. Should a tunnel infection be suspected, this should be confirmed on ultrasound scan and treated with appropriate antibiotic treatment.	2. To enable prompt treatment of exit site infections and prevent tunnel infection and peritonitis.
3. Signs and symptoms of disequilibrium are observed: confusion, convulsion, drowsy.	3. A rapid fall in the urea level can result in cerebral oedema due to failure to equalise the blood brain barrier. The dialysis should be reduced at this point by significantly increasing the dwell time (Rees *et al* 2006).
4. Constipation should be avoided and laxatives prescribed if necessary.	4. This causes problems with drainage, reducing efficiency of dialysis and leading to overload. Constipation also leads to discomfort and pain on dialysis.
5. If the waste fluid contains long white fibres (fibrin), monitor closely and treat with heparin if the quantity increases.	5. To prevent catheters becoming blocked, thus reducing efficiency of dialysis and leading to overload.
6. **Alarms:** Low UF can be caused by a number of factors: • Kinked lines • Failing peritoneum • Hypotension • Leakage • Need for a more concentrated dialysis • Fluid retention • Constipation • Low albumin.	6. It is necessary to identify the reason for a failing dialysis session and resolve the problem to prevent a life-threatening situation (Rees *et al* 2006).

164

Procedure guideline 9.16 Discontinuing PD

Statement	Rationale
1. Follow the procedure below: • Wash hands for 1 minute.	1. Reduce the risk of infection.
2. Collect equipment • Clean trolley with hard surface wipes • Wash hands for 1 minute • Open PD cap • Open sterile gloves onto cleaned work surface • Wash hands for 1 minute and put on sterile gloves • Close clamps of PD catheter and set • Place connection into povidone–iodine solution • Disconnect • Replace cap onto catheter • Disconnect set and dispose of used dialysis set.	2. On completion of dialysis equipment should be available close to the dialysis machine to ensure the child is disconnected for the dialysis machine safely and prevent the risk of infections. Disposable equipment should be disposed of according to your hospital policy.

References

Ahsan Ejaz A, Komorski RM, Ellius GH, Munjal S. (2007) Extracorporeal circuit pressure profiles during continuous venovenous haemofiltration. Nursing in Critical Care, 12(2), 81–85

Bunchman TE. (2002) Plasmapheresis and renal replacement therapy in children. Current Opinion in Pediatrics, 14(3), 310–314

Clevenger K. (1998) Setting up a continuous venovenous hemofiltration education program. Critical Care Nursing Clinics of North America, 10(2), 235–244

Craig M. (1998) Continuous venous to venous hemofiltration: Implementing and maintaining a program: Examples and alternatives. Critical Care Nursing Clinics of North America, 10(2), 219–233

Davenport M. (1996) Peadiatric fluid balance. Care of the Critically Ill, 12(1), 26–-31 Cited in Willock J, Jewkes F, (2000) Making sense of fluid balance in children. Paediatric Nursing, 12(7), 37–42

Dirkes SM. (2000) Continuous renal replacement therapy: Dialytic therapies for acute renal failure in intensive care. Nephrology Nursing Journal, 27(6), 581–589

Ellis EN, Pearson D, Belsha CW, Berry PL. (1997) Use of pump-assisted hemofiltration in children with acute renal failure. Pediatric Nephrology, 11, 196–200

European Best Practice Guidelines (2002) Haemodialysis Part 1. Nephrology Dialysis & Transplant, 17(Suppl 7), S1–S111

Flynn JT. (2002) Choice of dialysis modality for management of pediatric acute renal failure. Pediatric Nephrology, 17, 61–69

Forni LG, Hilton PJ. (1997) Continuous haemofiltration in the treatment of acute renal failure. The New England Journal of Medicine, 336(18), 1303–1310

Glasper EA, McEwing G, Richardson J. (2006) The Oxford Handbook of Children's and Young People's Nursing. Oxford, Oxford University Press, p 140

Goldstein SL, Macierowski CH, Jabs K. (1997) Hemodialysis catheter survival and complications in children and adolescents. Pediatric Nephrology, 11(1), 74–77

Headrick CL. (1998) Adult/Pediatric CVVH: The Pump, the patient, the circuit. Critical Care Nursing Clinics of North America, 10(2), 197–207

John S, Eckardt K-U. (2007) Renal replacement strategies in the ICU. Chest, 132(4), 1379–1388

Lowrie LH. (2000) Renal replacement therapies in pediatric multiorgan syndrome. Pediatric Nephrology, 14, 612

MacLeod L. [Chair] (2002) The Treatment of Adults and Children with renal Failure (3rd edition). Standards and measures. London, Royal College of Physicians and Renal Association

Mactier R, Hoenich N, Breen C. (2009) Clinical Practice Guidelines for Haemodialysis, 5th edition. Petersfield, UK Renal Association. Available at http://www.renal.org/Clinical/GuidelinesSection/Haemodialysis.aspx (last accessed 28th October 2011)

Metheny NM, Snively WD (1983) Nurses handbook of fluid balance. In Willock J, Jewkes F. (2000) Making sense of fluid balance in children. Paediatric Nursing, 12(7), 37–42

Monchi M, Berghmans D, Ledoux D, Canivet JL, Dubois B, Damas P. (2004). Citrate vs heparin for anticoagulation in continuous venovenous hemofiltration: a prospective randomized study. Intensive Care Medicine, 30, 260–265

Naka T, Bellomo R. (2004) Bench-to-bedside review: Treating acid-base abnormalities in the intensive care unit- the role of renal replacement therapy. Critical Care, 8, 108–114

Parshuram CS, Cox PN. (2002) Neonatal hyperkalaemic-hypocalcaemic cardiac arrest associated with initiation of blood-primed continuous venovenous hemofiltration. Pediatric Critical Care Medicine, 3(1), 67–69

Rees L, Webb N, Brogan P. (2006) Paediatric Nephrology (Oxford Specialist Handbook in Paediatrics). Oxford, Oxford University Press pp 359–369.

Rees L, Feather S, Shroff R. (2008) Haemodialysis Clinical Practice Guidelines for Children and Adolescents. Available at http://www.bapn.org/

assets/clinical_standards/BAPN%20HD%20Standards%20and%20Guidelines.pdf (last accessed 28th October 2011)

Reeves JH, Butt WB, Sathe AS. (1994) A review of venovenous haemofiltration in seriously ill infants. Journal of Paediatrics and Child Health, 30, 50–54

Ricci Z, Ronco C, Bachetoni A, D'amico G, Rossi S, Alessandri E, Rocco M, Pietropaoli P. (2006) Solute removal during continuous renal replacement therapy in critically ill patients: convection versus diffusion. Critical Care, 10, R67

Saudan P, Niederberger M, De Seigneux S, Romand J, Pugin J, Perneger T, Martin PY. (2006) Adding a dialysis dose to continuous hemofiltration increases survival in patients with acute renal failure. Kidney International, 70, 1312–1317

Schetz M. (2001) Anticoagulation for continuous renal replacement therapy. Current opinion in Anaesthesiology, 14, 143–149

Sefton G, Farrell M. Noyes J. (2001) The perceived learning needs of paediatric intensive care nurses caring for children requiring haemofiltration. Intensive and Critical Care Nursing, 17, 40–50

Sharma A, Zilleruelo G, Abitbol C, Montane B, Strauss J. (1999) Survival and complications of cuffed catheters in children on chronic hemodialysis. Pediatric Nephrology, 13(3), 245–248

Soysal DD, Karabocuoglu, Citak A, Ucsel R, Uzel N, Nayir A. (2007) Metabolic disturbances following the use of inadequate solutions for hemofiltration in acute renal failure. Pediatric Nephrology, 22, 715–719

Uchino S, Bellomo R, Morimatsu H, Morgera S, Schetz M, Tan I, Bouman C, Macedo E, Gibney N, Tolwani A, Oudemans-van Straaten H, Ronco C, Kellum JA. (2007) Continuous renal replacement therapy: A worldwide practice survey. Intensive Care Medicine, 22, 1563–1570

Warady BA, Bunchman TE. (2000) Dialyis therapy for children with acute renal failure: survey results. Pediatric Nephrology, 15, 11–13

Willock J, Jewkes F. (2000) Making sense of fluid balance in children. Paediatric Nursing, 12(7), 37–42

Further reading

British Association of Paediatric Nephrology Clinical standards in paediatric nephrology. Available at http://www.bapn.org/clinical_standards.html (last accessed 15th February 2012)

National Kidney Foundation (KDOQI) guidelines. Available at http://www.kidney.org/professionals/kdoqi/guidelines (last accessed 15th February 2012)

Nephrology Dialysis Transplantation European Best Practice Guidelines. Available at http://www.oxfordjournals.org/our_journals/ndt/era_edta.html (last accessed 15th February 2012)

NICE clinical guideline 84 Quick reference guide 2 Diarrhoea and vomiting in children. National Institute for Health and Clinical Excellence, MidCity Place, 71 High Holborn, London, WC1V 6NA. Available at http://www.nice.org.uk/nicemedia/live/11846/43843/43843.pdf (last accessed 15th February 2012)

Quinlan C, Cantwell M, Rees L. (2010) Eosinophilic peritonitis in children on chronic peritoneal dialysis. Pediatric Nephrology, 25(3), 517–522

UK Renal Association (2007) Clinical practice guidelines for haemodialysis. Available at http://www.renal.org/Clinical/GuidelinesSection/Haemodialysis.aspx (last accessed 15th February 2012)

Walters S, Porter C, Brophy PD. (2009) Dialysis and pediatric acute kidney injury (AKI): choice of renal support modality. Pediatric Nephrology, 24(1), 37–48

Chapter 10

Personal hygiene and pressure ulcer prevention

Chapter contents

Procedure guidelines

The Great Ormond Street Hospital Manual of Children's Nursing Practices, First Edition. Edited by Susan Macqueen, Elizabeth Anne Bruce, Faith Gibson.
© 2012 Great Ormond Street Hospital for Children NHS Foundation Trust. Published 2012 by Blackwell Publishing Ltd.

Introduction

Personal hygiene is an important consideration in the holistic care of both the healthy child and one who has specific needs and compromise due to illness, surgery and hospitalisation. A good standard of hygiene is an integral component of daily life and is necessary to maintain dignity and self-esteem as well as to prevent infection. It is essential that maintaining such a standard continues during a child's time in hospital. Maintaining hygiene can also assist to promote normality in a sick child, enhance comfort and aid psychological well-being.

For any child in hospital, the importance of involving the family in care is paramount in relation to all areas (Heimann 2000, Hockenberry and Wilson 2010, Hopper 2000, Swallow and Jacoby 2001), including the personal and hygiene needs of the child. Parents/carers should be encouraged to participate in the basic care of their children as much as the child's condition allows. The child's usual routine should be discussed and continued as much as possible to facilitate family interaction and participation (Davis *et al* 2003, Griffin 2001, Peate and Whiting 2006, POPPY Steering Group 2009, Savage 2000, Tran *et al* 2009) in line with a 'partnership' approach. The nurse has a role in facilitating the involvement of the child and family in undertaking as much care as they are able or indeed wish to do. This role also extends to the support of the child and family through teaching and advising on matters such as hygiene. Moreover, the nurse should be available and open to teach and guide support workers and students in best practice by example and providing theory to support practice. Integral to this, there is the need to ensure that practice remains evidence based, even for such basic aspects of care such as personal hygiene.

Ascertaining the child and family's normal routine and negotiating care should be an important component of the assessment process when first admitted to hospital. Assessment is essential for the appropriate planning of care for each individual. Moreover, it should continue on an ongoing basis throughout the child's stay in hospital.

An example of the importance of assessment can be shown by the frequency of hygiene practices a child undergoes. How often care-giving practices are carried out is influenced by many factors such as individual preference, normal routine, age, culture and, most importantly in the sick child, the physiological state relating to illness. Healthy children will continue their normal routine as much as possible in hospital. However, in those with an acute illness in high-dependency, intensive care or following surgery, preventing any further physiological stress or unnecessary handling should take precedence and personal hygiene occurs less frequently that normal. The sick child should be assessed for the ability to cope with care procedures on a regular basis and if they are not able to tolerate these, then they should be kept to an absolute minimum or left until a later time.

The low birth weight or premature baby provides a key example to illustrate this point. These babies, due to their size and/or gestation are generally not as able to tolerate prolonged and frequent episodes of handling exhibiting signs of stress and temperature instability (Ellis 2005, Knobel and Holditch-Davis 2007, Sherman *et al* 2006, Thomas 2003a, Waldron and MacKinnon 2007). Therefore, the concept of 'minimal handling'; i.e. long periods of rest with minimal stimulation (Bauer 2005,

Khurana *et al* 2005) is commonplace. The same principle can apply to any child who is acutely unwell. For these reasons above, there are no firm guidelines on how often care giving is performed as this should be individualised and based on ongoing assessment and evaluation.

Cultural considerations, including norms and variations, also need attention and are incorporated into both the assessment process and individual care regimes. Muslim girls, for example, may wish to request assistance from female carers only and it may not be appropriate to perform bathing and other routines on particular religious days such as the Sabbath within the Jewish population.

Attending to hygiene needs should be made as fun and enjoyable as possible with the use of appropriate toys as recommended. In the older child, independence should also be encouraged particularly in adolescence when self-consciousness and body image issues are more common. Maintaining privacy and dignity is paramount for the child at any age, particularly with regard to personal matters. An example is illustrated in relation to elimination where lack of privacy can lead to embarrassment, which, in turn, could result in retention of faeces and constipation.

This example highlights the important links between relevant issues. Hygiene practices also interlink; for example, toileting and bathing/washing can be addressed simultaneously such as in a baby where nappy care and bathing or 'topping and tailing' are often performed together. In any child, nail and eye care is incorporated into their overall daily hygiene routine along with washing and/or bathing.

Overall, it is imperative that individual, family, cultural and societal needs are considered and acknowledged for all the above mentioned areas of personal hygiene (Hewitt 2000, Murphy and Macloed Clark, 1993), as well as both physical and emotional needs.

Finally, although the focus is hygiene of the child, staff hygiene must also be acknowledged. Universal precautions should be remembered whenever one is in contact with body fluids to minimise cross-infection (Lawson 2001): for example, the use of gloves during nappy care, correct disposal of body fluids and handwashing or the use of alcohol hand-rub between patients (Moralejo and Jull 2003). See Chapter 12 on Infection Prevention and Control.

Bathing

Bathing and/or washing are essential elements of basic personal hygiene (Trigg and Mohammed 2006), not only to promote a child's comfort and well-being but also to minimise infection via the skin.

The skin forms a structural boundary and interface for any organism (Visscher *et al* 2002). It consists of three layers – epidermis, dermis and subcutaneous tissue (Tortora and Derrikson 2008, Tortora and Grabowski 2003). The subcutaneous layer is comprised of fatty tissue for insulation and serves as fuel for heat production. The middle layer – dermis – is composed of elastin fibres, collagen and fibrous protein. The top layer, the epidermis, is the most important for infection control as this is the protective layer caused by the impermeability to both water and bacteria of the outermost part, the stratum corneum (Jackson 2008,

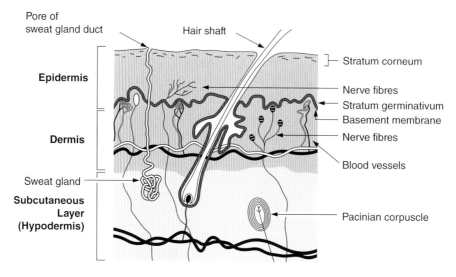

Pore of sweat gland duct

Hair shaft

Epidermis

Dermis

Sweat gland

Subcutaneous Layer (Hypodermis)

Stratum corneum

Nerve fibres
Stratum germinativum
Basement membrane
Nerve fibres

Blood vessels

Pacinian corpuscle

Figure 10.1   Diagram of the skin. http://www.nurse-prescriber.co.uk/visual_library.htm © 2005 Cambridge University Press, UK.

Tortora and Derrikson 2008, Tortora and Grabowski 2003) (Figure 10.1).

Resistance to substances and bacteria relies on the skin being both intact and sufficiently developed. From birth, the skin of a term neonate has a well-developed stratum corneum complete with keratin formation.

Following assessment of readiness and safety aspects, bathing commences and is carried out throughout development with the main change being that of dependency.

In some cases, bathing is not appropriate and so alternatives should be considered until such time that one can be performed in a timely and safe fashion appropriate to the neonate's condition (Behring *et al* 2003). For example, in a newborn baby, daily bathing is not necessary. At birth, the full-term neonate has a skin pH of 6.4, which falls to 4.9 (adult value) in the first four days (Irving 2001). This acidity creates an 'acid mantle' providing natural protection against infection (Blincoe 2006a, 2006b, Hale 2007). Bathing within the first 24 hours of life and daily bathing thereafter up to 10–14 days old can mean this process is delayed and can slow the separation of the umbilical cord due to the delay of normal skin flora colonisation (Franck *et al* 2000, Hopkins 2004, Mainstone 2005). In addition, it is widely recognised that the newborn baby can lose body heat rapidly in the first days of life and exposure for bathing can potentially cause the body temperature to drop (Bergstrom *et al* 2005, Medves and O'Brien 2004). 'Topping and tailing' (in other words, washing the face, body and nappy area separately) can be carried out on days that bathing is not performed.

In addition, the preterm neonate has physiological differences in their skin compared with the full term (Walker *et al* 2005a, 2005b). The neonate born less than 34 weeks gestation lacks sufficient keratin and so barrier function is limited in the first 10–14 days after birth (Chin 2000, Irving *et al* 2006, Jackson 2008, Walker *et al* 2005a). Moreover, skin acidity takes significantly longer to fall, often taking weeks rather than days, and delaying the acid mantle formation (Blincoe 2006a, 2006b, Mancini 2004, Quinn *et al* 2005). Skin frailty and susceptibility

to damage and infection along with greater physiological and temperature instability means that bathing is not appropriate for a significant length of time until weight and condition allow and the neonate can maintain their body temperature sufficiently outside an incubator. Close observation and careful washing of the skin if necessary is recommended here (Mainstone 2005, Hale 2007).

Bathing is also not recommended in healthy, very low birth weight babies (<1.5 kg) for at least 7 days after birth (Behring *et al* 2003, Medves and O'Brien 2004, Quinn *et al* 2005) for the same reasons. Again, 'topping and tailing' is recommended until condition, weight and temperature stability allow.

Similarly, in the older child, systemic illness and immobility may prevent bathing due to safety issues involved in transferring the child and excessive handling during illness. Bed bathing or washing the skin gently is recommended in line with physiological stability. In addition, showering can be a suitable or preferred alternative in the older child or adolescent.

Whatever method of cleansing is appropriate, it is important to assess the skin's integrity and cleanliness (McGurk *et al* 2004). Close observation of the skin is paramount, particularly in the sick child as skin breakdown can occur due to a variety of factors including oedema, pressure, friction, immobility, malnutrition and obesity. Washing or bathing a child provides a good opportunity to observe the skin and to attend to other aspects such as response to stimulation, movements, pressure areas and elimination function.

Washing and bathing are often appropriate times to communicate with a child. Baby bathing, for example, is a time for promoting parent–baby interaction by tactile communication and can be a positive experience for both. The baby's behaviour and the bath experience are used to engage parents/carers with their neonates (Hockenberry and Wilson 2010, Odio *et al* 2001). In the toddler or preschool child, the nurse and/or family can use this time to teach hygiene practices, reinforcing behaviours such as cleaning, hair washing, drying and dressing. In the older child, assistance with washing or bathing is a chance to give advice on and teach health promotion in relation to hygiene; for example, appropriate frequency, use of products like deodorant and shampoo. It is important to remember that there may be individual cultural norms to address with respect to frequency, which should assist with hygiene and the issue of privacy.

For any age, it is also an ideal opportunity to involve parents/carers in care giving and to facilitate parent–child interaction. For many children, normal bathing routines at home include elements of play, learning and close physical contact with their parents and carers.

Bathing: Assessment and preparation

Assessment applies to readiness of the child for bathing as well as assessing the environment and safety aspects.

Procedure guideline 10.1 Assessment for bathing

Statement	Rationale
The neonate and infant (up to age 1 year)	
1. In the term neonate less than 24 hours old, bathing is not absolutely necessary providing the baby is not covered in thick meconium or blood (Trigg and Mohammed 2006).	1. Due to the potential for temperature instability and to avoid the disruption of normal skin mantle/acidity (Johnson and Taylor 2010). This acidity along with vernix (Hale 2007, Hoath 1997, Tollin *et al* 2005) allows protection from pathogens.
2. If a bath is given to the newborn in the first 24 hours (e.g. if meconium/blood covered) the body temperature must be greater than 36.5°C, once stabilised after 2–4 hours of life.	2. Exposure to body fluids may predispose health professionals to contamination. A central (axilla) temperature of > 36.5°C is safe (Odio *et al* 2001).
3. In the neonate greater than 24 hours old, body temperature must be stable at the normal range of 36.6–37.2°C (Fellows 2010).	3. To avoid thermal instability from exposure and excess heat loss.
4. Assess the baby's readiness for a bath (physiological state and temperature stability) and consider environmental factors such as safety and room temperature (see below).	4. For maintenance of safety and to minimise risk (Behring et al 2003, Jackson 2008).
5. Room temperature must be at 20–25°C with no draughts (Odio *et al* 2001).	5. Allows a thermal balance to be achieved with minimal energy spent on heat production (Gardner et al 2010).
6. Note weight of the baby. If less than 1250–1500 g, bathing should not be done for the first week of life.	6. To avoid thermal instability.
7. Assess the behavioural state of the neonate who should be awake, alert and calm, and bathing should be before feeding (Trigg and Mohammed 2006).	7. For the neonate and infant to be safe and to facilitate appropriate stimulation and interaction.
Children	
1. Assess the child and family's ability for self-care in relation to age, illness and mobility.	1. To promote self-care and independence when appropriate for child's age.
2. Assess ease of movement and mobility.	2. Children unable to move easily get cold very quickly when undressed due to skin exposure and immobility.
3. Assess and ensure normal body temperature of 36. –37.2°C (Gardner et al 2010, Hockenberry and Wilson 2010) in a room temperature of at least 20°C.	3. To avoid thermal instability.
4. In cold rooms, apply additional safe heating.	4. For room temperature to be adequate as stated above.
5. Assess the need for support aids.	5. Children who require support to sit will require aids.
6. Assess the bath height and weight of the child and adjust as necessary.	6. To ascertain whether aids are required for lifting and to avoid back injuries.

(Continued)

169

Procedure guideline 10.1 (*Continued*)

Statement	Rationale
General	
1. At any age, assess the child and family's normal routine in order to incorporate this into care as much as is appropriate within the hospital setting. Discuss washing/bathing and care giving routines with the child and family and any specific requirements that are needed.	**1.** To continue hygiene routine as normal for the family. However, some practices are not appropriate in the hospital environment, for example some parents bathe with their children at home.
2. Document the child's normal routine and specific needs in the nursing notes.	**2.** To encourage a partnership approach to care between nurse and family. For all carers to be aware of the child's needs.
3. Assess and observe for any culture-specific variations in practices.	**3.** It is imperative that cultural and societal norms are incorporated into care regimes within the hospital setting.

The baby bath

Procedure guideline 10.2 Baby bathing

Statement	Rationale
1. Assemble equipment together as required – baby bath, soft cloth, towel(s), and nappy (also soap, shampoo, creams and baby wipes if desired by the parents/carers following discussion with nursing staff).	**1.** For adequate preparation, readiness and ease of procedure.
2. Use water to clean the skin. Soap, shampoo or baby bath is not necessary in the first 1–2 months unless parents/carers specifically request.	**2.** Although there are some differing opinions in the literature (Blincoe 2005, 2006a, 2006b, Walker *et al* 2005b) as to whether products or water alone should be used, it is generally accepted that cleaning skin with water is as effective as other skin cleansing solutions (Beal 2005, Fernandez *et al* 2003, Johnson and Taylor 2010, Stokowski 2006, Trigg and Mohammed 2006, Trotter 2004, 2006, 2007a, 2007b, 2008) in babies within the first month of life.
3. If parents/carers choose to use one of the wide range of skin care products available, this should be discussed with the relevant health professional. The latter should check all products are suitable for use in neonates.	**3.** Parents/carers may have preferences for the use of specific preparations, which should be recommended for use in the neonate (Walker *et al* 2005b).
4. If soap or emollients are used, they should have a neutral pH, used 2–3 times per week (Camm 2006, Hale 2007, Mainstone 2005, Walker *et al* 2005a, 2005b).	**4.** To prevent the loss of acid mantle of the skin and minimise infection (Hale 2007).
5. Baby wipes can be used if preferred but they must be neutral and unperfumed (Atherton 2009, Odio *et al* 2001). Again, the nurse should check the neutrality.	**5.** These have been shown to be effective for skin cleaning in neonates (Atherton 2009, Odio *et al* 2001).

Procedure guideline 10.2 (*Continued*)

Statement	Rationale
6. In addition, avoid the use of talcum powder unless medically indicated. Advise parents/carers, should they bring powder into hospital, that adequate drying suffices to keep a baby's skin dry and that prevention of infection is paramount.	6. Talcum powder can be an infection risk and so parents/carers should be advised of this.
7. Fill baby bath one-quarter to one-half full with water that feels comfortable warm (29–32°C) to the skin (using elbow). Fill with cold water first, and then apply hot water.	7. To avoid extremes of temperature that could harm the baby.
8. Place bath at a comfortable height on a safe, secure stand or place on the floor.	8. To avoid back injury and strain and to avoid the bath becoming unstable or falling.
9. Undress the baby to the nappy and wrap in towel.	9. To keep the baby warm.
10. Firstly, clean face starting with the area around the eyes with clean or sterile water and dry (Figure 10.2a).	10. As stated above, water is an effective cleaning agent and soap is not recommended for the delicate skin of the face (Johnson and Taylor 2010).
11. Only perform eye care if there is discharge. This need not be done routinely (see section below on eye care). However, if there is encrustation, discharge or a known eye problem, perform eye care at this stage.	11. Routine eye care can be traumatic and is unnecessary unless there is evidence of a known condition that requires attention. However, parents/carers may choose to incorporate eye care into the normal hygiene routine.
12. Do not use cotton wool for the face.	12. Cotton wool may leave strands on the face and eyes.
13. Clean the face including the nose, the skin creases around the neck and under the chin, and the contours of the ears. In neonates, there is no need to attempt to clean deep inside the ear canal and poking a cloth or cotton bud into the actual ear drum should be avoided (www.babyworld.co.uk). Remove ear wax only once it is easily accessible.	13. Debris such as milk and saliva can collect in certain areas such as skin creases and may cause soreness or harbour infection if not cleaned away. The ear will naturally rid itself of any wax over time.
14. Wash hair if necessary holding baby over the bath and use corner of towel to dry (Figure 10.2b).	
15. Unwrap the towel, remove nappy and holding securely, place baby gently into the bath. This is done by using one of your arms to place underneath to support the baby's neck/shoulders and by holding the upper arm of the baby on opposite side. Your other arm should grasp the baby's feet or placed underneath the buttocks (Figure 10.2c). This hand becomes free when the baby is in the bath (Figure 10.2d).	15. For adequate support for the baby's head and neck and for maintenance of safety.
16. Do not leave the baby unsupported until they are able to sit without support. Never leave a neonate/infant unsupervised in a bath. They must be observed at all times. The use of non-slip mats is recommended.	16. To maintain the safety and well-being of the neonate/infant at all times. From age 8–10 months, although this should be assessed for each individual baby due to variations, a baby will be able to sit unsupported in the bath.
17. Use soft cloth or wash wipe to wash baby with free hand, attending to skin creases.	17. Skin creases are more likely to harbour micro-organisms.

171

(*Continued*)

Procedure guideline 10.2 (*Continued*)

Statement	Rationale
18. Watch for signs of stress in the baby such as increased agitation, colour changes, muscle tone changes, increased respiratory rate, excessive crying and jitteriness (Boxwell 2010, Gardner *et al* 2010, Thomas 2003a). Also watch for heat loss by observing colour and temperature of the skin (Thomas 2003b). Stop the bath if signs of stress or cooling are evident.	**18.** To maintain safety for the baby.
19. Wrap in towel and dry body thoroughly.	
20. During the whole procedure, observe for rashes, marks or other abnormalities that may require attention. If dry skin and/ or a 'cradle cap' are observed, apply baby oil or olive oil gently to affected parts.	**20.** To identify any skin condition that may require attention. Baby oil or olive oil can help maintain soft, moist skin and prevent flakiness and excessive dryness (Trotter 2004).
21. Apply clean nappy fastening underneath umbilical cord if this is still not separated.	**21.** To facilitate drying of the cord (see section below on nappy care and Chapter 17).

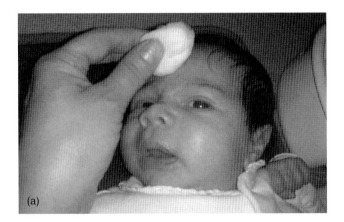
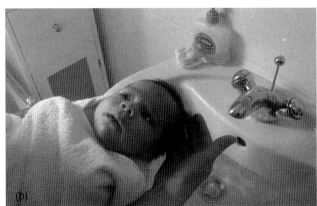
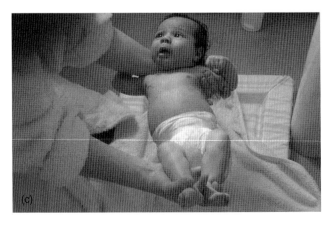
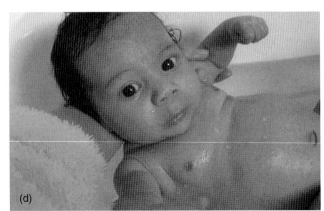

Figure 10.2 (a–d) Baby bathing.
Please note that these figures are of a parent/carer providing care hence why no gloves are being worn. In a hospital environment, in view of infection control, staff must wear gloves. Also, a soft gauze swab should preferably be used as cotton wool may leave strands of cotton on the skin or eyelids. Photograph courtesy of Julia Petty.

Topping and tailing

Procedure guideline 10.3 **Topping and tailing**

Statement	Rationale
1. Assemble all equipment – bowl of warm water, soft flannel or cloth, towel, clean nappy (nappy creams and other products if used – see Statements 2–5 in Nappy care section above) and if necessary clean clothes.	1. For adequate preparation.
2. Fill bowl with water at 29–32°C (see Baby bathing section previously).	2. For safe temperature and to avoid thermal stress.
3. Place baby on towel and keep wrapped or keep the baby dressed.	3. To maintain body temperature.
4. Repeat Statements 10–13 in Baby bathing for washing the face, neck, eyes and ears using warm water. Dry face.	4. As for baby bathing.
5. Clean hands and nails, under arms and around the umbilical cord stump, again using water only.	5. See chapter on umbilical cord care (Chapter 17). Water alone is recommended for cleaning the cord stump (Dunn 2009, Trotter 2008, Trotter 2008, Zupan and Gardner 2004).
6. Unwrap or undress the baby and remove nappy.	6. To prevent heat loss from exposing the body for too long.
7. Clean baby's body with warm water and a soft cloth observing for rashes, marks, etc. (for use of soap and shampoo, see above in Baby bathing).	
8. Clean nappy area last, cleaning from the front to the back in females (away from the genitalia towards the anus); see section on nappy care for greater detail.	8. To prevent cross-infection from stool or bowel bacteria to the urinary tract.
9. Dry the body thoroughly.	
10. Place clean nappy on, securing under the umbilical cord stump and dress the baby.	10. See section on nappy care and Chapter 17.

173

Washing and bathing the child

The toddler, preschool child and older child or adolescent will require a daily bath or shower and hair washing once every 2–3 days. Teeth and nail care are also pertinent areas of hygiene. As the child gets older, the potential for self-consciousness and embarrassment may arise and this should be minimised by ensuring privacy and dignity is maintained at all times, taking cultural factors into account.

Children are developing independence and so they need to be taught care procedures appropriately according to age and development. However, in hospital, busy schedules and time constraints may make encouraging independence difficult. Therefore, parents/carers have a central role to play in a busy ward environment (www.disabledliving.org.uk). This is an ideal chance to reinforce partnership and negotiation between child and family. Unless there are good clinical reasons for changes to the child's normal daily routine, every effort should be made to keep practices as normal as possible when in hospital.

Full independence with self-care develops over time in most children, providing the child is able-bodied and well. The individuality in children's development also needs to be recognised in relation to growing independence with bathing or dressing ability. Choice should also be allowed, for example in the older child or adolescent who may prefer showering or washing to bathing.

Bath time is usually a time of fun and an opportunity to play. This should not be any different for a sick, immobile or disabled

Procedure guideline 10.4 Washing and bathing the child

Statement	Rationale
Toddler and preschool child	
1. Accompany the child at all times during bathing.	1. To ensure safety of the child at all times.
2. The face and body can be cleaned with gentle soap and flannels/cloths and a shampoo recommended for use in children for the hair. Ears should be gently cleaned when necessary using a soft cotton bud to gently remove any earwax that is accessible.	2. Milder products that are recommended for use in children are less likely to cause skin reactions. Do not push the cotton bud inside the canal as this may cause damage or push ear wax further into the canal causing blockage and loss of hearing.
3. Nails should also be cleaned (see section on nail care).	3. Nails are a particular source of colonisation for bacteria.
4. Clean teeth twice a day – morning and evening with recommended child soft toothbrush.	4. See section on Oral hygiene.
5. Use play, toys and involve siblings as appropriate.	
6. Use non-slip mats in the bath.	
School age	
1. Older children (generally over the age of 7 years but variations do exist and must be recognised) will be taught and will become able in time to perform washing and bathing. This should include such activities as cleaning teeth, drying and dressing independently with supervision (Hockenberry and Wilson 2010).	1. To encourage health promotion and independence.
The older child/adolescent	
1. There will be independence with self-care if fully mobile and well, with all aspects of hygiene. This may include independent showering and hair washing practices.	1. As above.
2. Maintain privacy at all times and continue individual hygiene routines as well as cultural considerations.	2. To respect the child's dignity and avoid embarrassment.

child although the physiological condition of the child will influence when and how this is carried out.

The bed bath

If the child/adolescent is not fully able-bodied or sick, then a bed bath may be necessary. Parents/carers can be taught the procedure.

The child with a disability or special need

Personal cleaning and bathing should continue in the child with special needs and equipment or adaptations may be necessary, such as bath lifts, hoists or supports.

Toileting

Attaining continence is a developmental milestone, which generally takes place over the first few years of life. For some, reaching this milestone comes later than expected or for others, continence may never be achieved for a specific reason, e.g. cognitive impairment, severe learning difficulties, neurogenic bladder, trauma, congenital malformation or surgical intervention. There may also be a loss of continence at some later point in development, be it transient or permanent (Sanders 2002).In order to attain continence, children must learn to attend to their own elimination needs. This ability develops over time as independence and cognitive maturity increases (Schum et al 2002). Continence, both urinary and bowel, is learnt and develops over time as a complex sequence of events. Generally, achievement of 'normal' milestones

Procedure guideline 10.5 **Bed bathing**

Statement	Rationale
1. Discuss the bed bath with the child.	1. For full consent, understanding and cooperation.
2. Ensure a warm, private environment prior to the procedure and that the bed is a comfortable height.	2. To ensure the environment is conducive to protecting privacy and dignity and safety considerations.
3. Ensure a surface is cleared for equipment.	
4. Assist child/adolescent to undress and cover with towels.	4. To ensure privacy and dignity and prevention of exposure before necessary.
5. Clean eyes (see eye care section), face and teeth.	
6. Expose and wash/dry upper body while legs and feet are covered.	6. As above.
7. Then vice versa, cover upper body and clean and dry legs and feet.	7. As above.
8. Observe particular parts of the body that may warrant greater attention such as ears, axilla, groin, skin creases and genitalia (see below).	8. Certain body areas harbour more dirt, debris and pathogens.
9. Check the pressure areas and general skin condition.	9. This is most appropriate and convenient time.
10. Change washcloth and water if it is very dirty. Then clean genitalia prior to the anal area.	10. Cleaning genitalia prior to the anal area prevents cross-infection from stool and bowel bacteria.
11. For boys (only from age 1 upwards), ensure the foreskin is clean and retract very gently if necessary to clean.	11. Care must be taken with retracting the foreskin during infancy but can be done in the older boy to ensure cleanliness in this area.
12. For girls, wipe from front to back on females, followed by anal area.	12. Again, to prevent cross-infection from stool and bowel bacteria to the genitalia.
13. Assistance may be needed in large children/adolescents with rolling over to gain access to the back of the body.	13. To prevent injury to oneself.
14. Dry thoroughly and cover.	14. To maintain dignity at all times
15. Assist to dress as necessary.	
16. Change sheet if necessary with assistance to roll child from side to side.	16. As above, to prevent injury to oneself and the child.
17. Hair can be washed over the end of the bed if needed.	
18. Perform passive limb exercises if appropriate or recommended according to guidelines.	18. In the immobile child, this may be an ideal time to perform such manoeuvres in order to exercise the limbs, encourage circulation and prevent complications with immobility.
19. Talk/interact and/or play with the child as appropriate.	19. To put the child at ease and encourage interaction.
20. Throughout the procedure, observe the child's vital signs.	20. To ensure the child is not compromised physiologically from the interventions performed.

175

Procedure guideline 10.6 Bathing the child with special needs

Statement	Rationale
1. Assess the need for equipment in children with special needs (see previous section: Assessment for bathing) and check the bath is the correct size to take supportive bathing equipment.	1. To ensure readiness and ensure safety.
2. If the child is not able to mobilise, it may be preferable to bath/wash as quickly as possible and play after the bath.	2. If the child requires assistance with bathing, drying and dressing, heat loss may be increased by any unnecessary delay.
3. Consider safety for children with poor head control or epilepsy.	
4. Consider equipment for protection of parent's/carer's back by reducing the need to lift the child in and out of the bath, e.g. bath stands, bath overlays, bath lifts and hoists, adjustable height baths, bath boards and seats.	4. To minimise risk and injury to child and parent/carer. See Chapter 16 on Moving and Handling.
5. Use appropriate bathing equipment for the child who needs support in a semi-reclined position, e.g. foam supports, hammock supports, bath cushions and inserts, mouldable supports.	5. As above.
6. For the child who needs support in a sitting position (i.e. cannot sit unaided), e.g. sitting supports, suction backrests and grab bars (www.disabledliving.org.uk).	6. As above.
7. Liaise and gain advice from other members of the multidisciplinary team, e.g. occupational therapists, physiotherapists, play specialists.	7. Such health professionals can give specific expert advice to assist in the care of special needs from different disciplines within a holistic team approach.
8. Bed bathing is a safe alternative for immobile, heavier children (see previous section) or a shower may be easier.	8. To maintain the child's safety by selecting an appropriate method of bathing.
9. Ensure manual handling techniques are maintained.	9. To minimise risk and injury.

176

for complete toilet training occurs from 18 months up to 3–4 years but it must be emphasised that significant variations exist between individual children. It is more important to observe for stages rather than ages (www.babycentre.co.uk/toilettraining). However, the following serves as a guide.

Firstly, bladder control: in infancy, the bladder is controlled by a spinal reflex arc as part of the autonomic nervous system. The bladder fills up and the detrusor muscle sends sensory messages to the sacral bladder zone within the spinal cord. Impulses return to the muscle of the bladder to cause relaxation while the sphincter is closed. When the bladder is full, motor impulses lead to the opposite situation; the detrusor muscle contracts, the sphincter relaxes and urine can be passed (Choby and George 2008, Dewar 2010, Heron *et al* 2008, Joinson *et al* 2008, 2009, Mota and Barros 2008, Rogers 2002a, Tennant 2010, Vermandel *et al* 2008, Wu 2010). Over time, a child comes to learn to interpret the feelings of having a full bladder and so can then inhibit urination until an appropriate time (Rogers 2000). Development of this pathway occurs over the first 18–20 months of life.

From 2 years of age, a child's cognitive maturity grows so that the interpretation of signals and the self-control of voiding are linked together and co-ordinated. From 2 years, a child should have commenced cooperation in toilet training and by 3 years should have daytime bladder control. Night bladder control should also start to mature from 3 years of age.

Secondly, bowel control is based on relaxation of the internal anal sphincter and simultaneous increased activity of the external sphincter in response to faeces within the rectum, again under reflexive control. During toilet training, the child will come to voluntarily contract the external sphincter until an appropriate time for elimination.

In the healthy child, the aim is to achieve self-toileting at an expected stage of development in line with the physical development of urinary and bowel function. The child is then deemed 'toilet trained' (Rogers 2002a). Even a child who is not continent for physical reasons can still be taught to be independent, e.g. to attend to a stoma or in-dwelling catheter. Most children, even those with learning difficulties can, with patience, be toilet trained (Disabled Living Foundation 2003, Rogers 2002b). The concept of early and thorough child and family education is of utmost importance here (Boucke 2003).

In some cases, however, the child is unable to attend to their own toileting needs, e.g. disabled children who are not fully able bodied, the child with severe learning disabilities (Rogers 2002b), or the child who is immobilised. The nurse must assist with toileting in the appropriate way while maintaining privacy and dignity at all times. In addition, differences in cultural and societal norms must always be considered and integrated into care regimen for the individual child and family.

Assessment of toileting needs

Assessment of toileting needs should be carried out in children of all ages in order to identify any potential problems. In addition, it is done so that care can be given according to normal routine and stage of development. In order to assess the normal toileting pattern of a child, it is important to understand how continence and toilet training develops as described above.

It may be useful to utilise an appropriate tool or framework to assess the child's continence level as recommended by the *National Service Framework for children, young people and maternity services* (DoH 2004a) proposing that an accessible, high-quality assessment strategy is provided for children and their parents/carers in any setting. A framework for assessment is also included as part of the good practice in paediatric continence services – benchmarking in action that sets out an *Essence*

of Care best practice tool (DoH 2000). The continence foundation emphasises the importance of individual assessment to specify the type of incontinence if applicable, in order to provide an appropriate management strategy for toileting (www. continence-foundation.org.uk). Specific writers propose checklists for continence assessment (Boucke 2003, Brazleton and Sparrow 2004, Canadian Pediatric Society 2000, Rigby 2001, Rogers 2002a,2002b). Rogers (2000, 2002a, 2002b), for example, suggests an assessment checklist for the child specifically, which comprises evaluation of motor, cognitive and language development as well as toileting ability.

It should be remembered that the complex pattern of continence does not always occur as expected. Children with special needs or disabilities may differ widely in terms of their developmental level. Assessment of toileting patterns unique to their specific needs is the key to deciding what management strategy to implement for these children (AAP 2009, Bakker *et al* 2002, Barone *et al* 2009, Blum *et al* 2003, Dewar 2010, Horn *et al* 2006, Rogers 2002a , 2002b, Schmidt 2004).

Assessment must also include the child's normal privacy requirements along with any issues of embarrassment experienced by the child particularly during adolescence, for example, in girls that are menstruating. The wide variation in norms must be acknowledged; for example toileting frequency. There should also be a link made between nutrition and hydration in relation to elimination. Certain situations may alter normal elimination; for example, illness, infection, medication, immobility, fear and anxiety, lack of privacy and loss of consciousness.

Procedure guideline 10.7 Assessment of toileting needs

Statement	Rationale
1. Ascertain the child's developmental level in relation to toileting ability and the stage of toilet training attained.	**1.** To facilitate and continue the child's normal pattern as much as possible.
2. Assessment should be thorough and systematic and should include the following: medical history of elimination problems (e.g. urinary tract infections, constipation, presence of pre-existing stomas, catheters); factors that alter normal elimination (illness and hospitalisation, infection, medication, immobility, fear and anxiety, lack of privacy and loss of consciousness); details of age-appropriate milestones; language development and delay; mobility level; presence of any existing problems such as bedwetting; daytime enuresis (Rogers 2000).	**2.** For complete and holistic care of the child's condition.
3. It may be valuable to assess the child's level of continence using a specific tool/checklist if necessary such as that proposed by Rogers (2002a, 2002b). Consider:	**3.** To account for the many factors that may influence toileting ability while the child is hospitalised. In addition, a tool/ checklist may assist the nurse to assess level of continence more thoroughly and ensure that no important elements are forgotten.

(Continued)

Procedure guideline 10.7 (*Continued*)

Statement	Rationale

• **Motor development**
  ◦ Non-mobile child: can they sit with or without support?
  ◦ Mobile child: does the child attempt to squat without losing balance? Is independent walking developing?
• **Cognitive development**
  ◦ Does the child search actively and appropriately for toys by means such as eye Do they initiate an action?
  ◦ Do they engage in make-believe play, for example – sitting a doll on a potty
• **Language development**
  ◦ Does the child understand a simple request such as 'Where's Mummy/Daddy?'
  ◦ Are they able to communicate needs with words, signs and/or gestures
• **Toileting ability**
  ◦ Does the child stay dry for at least an hour?
  ◦ Is he/she aware of what a potty or toilet is for?
  ◦ Does he/she show awareness of when they are wet or soiled?
	It is vital that toileting procedures and expectations on behaviour are applicable to the current level of child's development in relation to motor, cognitive and language domains.
	
	If toilet training has commenced at home, it is important to continue as much as possible. Assistance with toileting can then be tailored to the individual child and their developmental level.

4. If the child is known to be incontinent or has a specific toileting problem, the nurse needs to find out as much as possible about the condition as part of the assessment process. Again, a tool or checklist can be used for this considering, for example: • Onset of incontinence • Frequency of micturition and opening bowels, fluid intake and necessity for particular medication; for example, laxatives for constipation • Symptoms such as urgency, nocturia, poor urinary stream, pain, warning of the need to void • Method of continence management; for example, frequent toileting, use of pads, urine collection devices • Environmental factors; for example, accessibility of toilet and availability of assistance • Impact on the individual and family including effect on mood, self-esteem, social activity • Identification of conditions that might exacerbate incontinence (Rigby 2001).	4. Again, as above, a tool/checklist may assist the nurse to assess the level of incontinence and what the specific problems are.
5. Assess the child's ability for self-care as well as the ability to verbalise the need for voiding.	5. To determine the level of dependency on parents/carers.
6. Assess the child's needs for privacy in line with specific cultural and societal requirements.	6. To minimise embarrassment and loss of dignity/self-consciousness.
7. Following initial assessment of needs, regular and ongoing assessment is required particularly if the child is dependent on parents/carers, non-verbal or immobilised.	7. The more dependent and vulnerable children will require parents/carers to assess when to assist with toileting.
8. During assisting with toileting, the urine and stool can be observed for normality and any potential problems. Specimens can be taken as required during toileting sessions (see Chapter 14 Investigations).	8. To assess for normality along with any potential problems related to alteration to normal elimination as brought about by illness, hospitalisation, medication, and infection to give some examples.

Procedure guideline 10.7 (*Continued*)

Statement	Rationale
9. At any age, assess the child and family's normal routine and incorporate this as much as is appropriate within the hospital setting. Discuss toileting routine with the child and family and any specific requirements that are needed.	**9.** To continue hygiene routine as normal for the family.
10. Document the child's normal routine and specific needs in the nursing notes.	**10.** To encourage a partnership approach to care between nurse and family and for all parents/carers to be aware of the child's needs.
11. Assess and observe for any culture-specific requirements or variations in practices.	**11.** It is imperative that cultural and societal norms are incorporated into care regimes within the hospital setting.

Toileting the child

For the continent child, individual toileting routine should be maintained as much as possible during hospital stay. For the child with special needs, incontinence may be an issue and this should be dealt with sensitively and within a multidisciplinary framework. Incontinence results from many different 'special needs' and may relate to a physical problem such as neuropathic bladder or congenital malformation, or may relate to a learning difficulty leading to developmental delay. Children who are anxious or fearful may regress and day and/or night wetting may occur. Nurses and the family must be aware of these changes and act accordingly. Other toileting issues that may be present are constipation, the presence of a stoma (see chapter on bowel care (Chapter 5)) and enuresis, either nocturnal or daytime wetting (Rhodes 2000).

Procedure guideline 10.8 **Toileting the child**

Statement	Rationale
Toileting the continent child	
1. Assess the child's age and developmental level in relation to toilet training – see section on assessment of toileting needs.	**1.** To ensure that toilet training and normality is continued as much as possible within the hospital setting.
2. Acknowledge the possibility of developmental regression in children who are hospitalised – for example, temporary loss of continence particularly in children with recently acquired skills in this area.	**2.** To ensure the effects of hospitalisation are recognised and minimised.
3. Continue with toilet training programme as much as possible within the constraints of hospital routine and current treatment, e.g. sitting on potty as certain times, use of a reward system when a potty is used successfully (AAP 2009, Bakker *et al* 2002, Barone *et al* 2009, Blum *et al* 2003, Dewar 2010, Horn *et al* 2006, Schmidt 2004).	**3.** As for rationale 1 above.
4. If the child is continent but immobilised following trauma, anaesthesia/surgery, or intensive care for example, then support the parents/carers to assist with the use of a bedpan, helping the child to roll onto the bedpan or to sit up onto it.	**4.** The child will not be able to mobilise and use the toilet due to illness and treatment.
5. Follow manual handling guidelines at all times (e.g. do not bend over or stretch beyond normal capability, ensure the bed is the correct height). See Chapter 16 on Moving and Handling.	**5.** To prevent injury to staff.

(Continued)

Procedure guideline 10.8 (*Continued*)

Statement	Rationale
6. Ensure a private environment by the use of screens if the child is not in a cubicle or curtains when applicable.	**6.** To maintain the child's privacy and dignity throughout the hospital stay.
7. Encourage the child and/or family to verbalise the need for assistance if appropriate.	**7.** The child will not be able to get to the toilet for the above reasons and so rely on the nurse to assist with this.
8. Wear non-sterile gloves and aprons when handling and disposing of body fluids.	**8.** To adhere to universal precautions policy. See Chapter 12 on Infection Prevention and Control.

Toileting the child with a disability or specific need

1. Following assessment, ascertain individual toileting problem and formulate a plan after discussion with parents/carers.	**1.** To continue the child's normal pattern in line with a partnership approach.
2. Follow local or national guidelines, if applicable, for the management of specific problems, e.g. catheter care (Simpson 2001), constipation (NHS 2003, NICE 2010) and stoma care.	**2.** For safe, evidence based practice. See separate chapters on catheter care (Chapter 29) and bowel care (Chapter 5).
3. Liaise with the multidisciplinary team, e.g. occupational therapist, physiotherapist, stoma nurse, and incontinence advisor, in relation to the management of specific problems.	**3.** For holistic and thorough assessment of the child's special needs and to utilise expert assistance for best practice.
4. Administer relevant prescribed medication as necessary, e.g. laxatives, antibiotics, drugs to increase motility.	**4.** Certain drugs may be part of the child's care and may also have side effects that may affect toileting, e.g. loose stools.
5. Gain advice on products and special equipment from the multidisciplinary team and/or appropriate charities and organisations such as the Disabled Living centre (Sanders 2002, www.Disabledliving.org.uk).	**5.** Again for expert advice on best practice.

Nappy care

A newborn baby will pass urine between 5 and 20 times each day and can have a bowel movement following each feed. During illness and in certain medical and surgical conditions children may experience increased frequency (Philipp *et al* 1997, Price 2000, Turner 2000). Skin integrity in the neonate and young infant may make it physically more susceptible to irritation, breakdown and attack from infective agents (Adam 2008, Adam *et al* 2009, Bayliss 1998, Borkowski 2004, Prasad *et al* 2003, Scheinfeld 2005) particularly when that child is sick. Therefore, any infant or child who is incontinent, requiring the use of nappies, is at risk of developing nappy rash (Atherton 2004, 2005, Atherton and Mill 2004).

When skin is exposed to urine and faeces for prolonged periods an excess of moisture builds up and skin becomes waterlogged.

This then becomes soft and fragile with an increased friction coefficient making it vulnerable to frictional damage (Irving *et al* 2006). In addition, the combination of ammonia in urine and bacteria in faeces creates a chemical cocktail that increases skin pH and releases proteolytic enzymes causing irritation. This results in the painful redness and rawness (inflammation) known as nappy rash (Adam 2008, Adam *et al* 2009, Atherton 2004, 2005, Atherton and Mill 2004, Bayliss 1998, Borkowski 2004, Prasad *et al* 2003, Scheinfeld 2005).

Skin damage and increased skin pH affect the body's natural defence mechanisms against harmful micro-organisms. In extreme cases, a secondary infection can occur, complicating the condition and its treatment and resulting in further skin breakdown. In the hospital environment any skin breakdown increases the risk of hospital acquired infection.

In general the incidence of nappy rash relates to the length of time skin is in contact with dampness, urine, faeces and the susceptibility of an individual's skin to these factors (Allison 2000). When dealing with a complex system such as skin, which is affected by both internal and external stressors as well as emotional and systemic factors, identification of cause can sometimes be extremely difficult. There will always be situations where a causative agent cannot be found, and despite the best of care, nappy rash can still occur (Berg 1998). The aim of nursing care is to prevent nappy rash through regular and thorough cleaning, drying and airing and should the condition arise, the application of protective, medicated or soothing creams (Blincoe 2005, 2006a, 2006b, Camm 2006, Jackson 2008, Trotter 2006).

Treating nappy rash

During outbreaks of nappy rash, the frequency of nappy changes should be increased to reduce contact with irritant substances (Berg 1998). A dabbing motion should be used to clean and dry the skin to prevent frictional damage caused by overzealous scrubbing and wiping. In severe cases, a spray applicator should be used or the skin should be bathed (Allison 2000).

Periods of skin airing should be introduced during nappy changes and for more prolonged periods in severe cases as this promotes dryness so allowing skin repair to occur. Airing can be successfully accomplished with minimal mess by laying sleeping children on an open nappy with protective sheeting beneath (Bayliss 1998). During the day the infant can be placed without a nappy in a towel/protective lined bath or play pen for periods of directly supervised play. In hospital the use of wall air/oxygen at nappy changes to gently and effectively dry the nappy area can also be beneficial. The use of hairdryers even on a cool setting should not be used as they can lead to second degree burns. The application of barrier creams may be beneficial when nappy rash is present (Walker *et al* 2005a, 2005b). Encouraging a good nutritional intake will provide essential vitamins to aid cell repair. Homeopathic tablets and creams, as well as complementary therapies, acupuncture and acupressure, are being increasingly used successfully. Referral to a specialist may be worth considering in persistent or severe cases (Herreboudt and Sigalov 1997).

In all cases of nappy rash an appropriate pain assessment should be carried out and adequate analgesia prescribed and administered. The involvement of a pain nurse specialist may be invaluable in severe cases (Scardillo and Aronovitch 1999).

Nappies

The choice of nappy system, whether disposable or reusable, makes little difference to the incidence of nappy rash if used correctly. Individual limitations should be considered when planning frequency of nappy changes and assessing the causes of nappy rash outbreaks (Blincoe 2005, 2006a, 2006b).

Disposable nappies are effective in drawing fluid away from the skin and can be changed less frequently in the absence of stools, making regular application of barrier creams unnecessary in most children. If used, creams should be applied sparingly with the skin remaining visible through the cream.

This will reduce the risk of skin nappy transfer, which can block the nappy lining so compromising nappy absorbency and function (Price 2000). There is now a new generation of disposable nappies on the market whose inner layer is impregnated with a built-in barrier cream of zinc oxide and petrolatum, which is thought to transfer to infant skin through body warmth and movement thus providing a water resistant protective layer on the skin, but not compromising nappy absorbency (Turner 2000).

Cloth nappies are less efficient at keeping moisture away from skin and therefore may require more frequent changing and the regular use of a barrier cream. Careful laundering is required to kill bacteria and ensure removal of possible irritant washing agents. Fabric conditioner should not be used, as this will reduce nappy absorbency as well as being a potential irritant to infant skin (Allison 2000).

All nappies can be pre-weighed to enable monitoring of urine/fluid output using the conversion of 1 gram weight = 1 ml urine/stool output (Gardner *et al* 2010).

Skin cleansers

As stated in the section on bathing, water alone applied with cotton wool or a soft cloth is adequate for cleaning the skin of the nappy area (Trotter 2008), as it is least likely to cause irritation, sensitivity or disrupt the pH of the skin, thus avoiding soap. If alternatives to water for cleansing are sought, the use of aqueous cream, liquid paraffin or oil (e.g. olive oil) as cleaning agents are less abrasive than soap and will not affect skin pH. However, nurses should be aware that they may affect the adherence of certain barrier creams. Use of nut based oils (e.g. arachis or peanut oil) is not generally recommended as its use has been shown to be a possible causative factor in the development of peanut allergy (Lack *et al* 2003). Some brands of baby wipes have been shown to cleanse as gently as water and may contain additives that may help to maintain the barrier properties of the skin (Atherton 2009, Jones 2000, Turner 2000). Alcohol based wipes should be avoided as they will cause obvious distress if used on broken/irritated skin.

Creams, lotions, topical medications/applications

There is recent agreement in the current literature that water alone is sufficient for skin cleansing and products are generally avoided (Beal 2005 Fernandez *et al* 2003, Johnson and Taylor 2010, Stokowski 2006, Trotter 2004, 2006, 2007a, 2007b, 2008, Trigg and Mohammed 2006). However, there are some conditions that require topical application, either as a treatment or to provide a skin barrier so preventing further excoriation.

The majority of barrier creams are either preparations containing water repellent silicones such as dimethicone, or waterproof ingredients such as petroleum, which creates a protective layer between skin and nappy contents. Barrier creams are less effective when applied to broken skin and should be ideally used as a preventative measure (Atherton and Mill 2004) or in the early stages of irritation. They require frequent application to be effective, some adhering more effectively than others and trials to find one that suits the needs of an individual child may be required. Creams may also include ingredients with known soothing, antiseptic or astringent properties (Allison 2000, Price 2000, Williams 2001). If using creams whose effectiveness lies in the application of a thick layer then they should be applied during periods of airing rather than applying before using a disposable nappy due to the risk of nappy lining blockage interfering with the absorbency of the nappy (Willis 1997).

Children with bowel disruptions related to medical treatment, or who are undergoing surgery resulting in a period of altered bowel activity, may benefit from a regimen of preventative application of barrier products and periods of airing as a routine precaution to prevent outbreaks. The use of the antacid, aluminium hydroxide, dried onto the skin with air or oxygen in the presence of acidic stool (easily tested with pH paper) may also

181

be helpful until the bowel function stabilises. In situations where faecal or urine skin erosions have occurred, the application of sucralfate (mixed as an emollient or dried onto the skin with air or oxygen) is beneficial.

Sucralfate binds to basic fibroblast growth factor, which occurs during skin repair and has been shown to promote healing in these cases, and it is also thought to help combat bacterial infection (Lyon *et al* 2000, Markham *et al* 2000).

Creams and sprays designed to protect skin against watery irritant stoma output may be beneficial for use in children whose causative irritant is watery diarrhoea, or for use in patients who require minimal handling or are too unwell to tolerate repeated frequent changes. These preparations are designed to adhere to the skin for long periods to enable fixture of stoma bags. They are non-greasy and less likely to rub off the skin during nappy changes or cause nappy lining blockage. They have the advantage of creating a tough barrier requiring less frequent application, but in turn are more expensive than more traditional barrier creams and are currently only available on prescription, or from stoma care nurses (Scardillo and Aronovitch 1999, Williams 2001).

Hydrocolloid dressings and pastes, which due to their impermeable nature facilitate rehydration and promote granulation, if skilfully applied can be used to protect raw areas of skin from irritant output (Scardillo and Aronovitch 1999). Another useful dressing, Mepiform, is a thin flexible dressing, which adheres gently to fragile tissue and is vapour-permeable and waterproof (Scardillo and Aronovitch 1999). Corticosteroids are powerful anti-inflammatory agents, which can accelerate healing and consequently may be of benefit for treating severe nappy rash (Borkowski 2004). They are more readily absorbed in infants, especially when applied in the occluded environment of the nappy, and therefore a low potency formula should be applied very sparingly. Professionals remain divided on their use because of their associated immunosuppressive properties, which decrease the skin's ability to fight infection and increase the risk of developing Candida dermatitis. There is also the potential risk of causing pituitary-adrenal suppression, which is particularly dangerous in infants. It is generally agreed that if necessary their use should be kept to a minimum and restricted to serious cases that do not respond to other treatments.

Antifungal creams, used most commonly for Candida rashes (thrush), should be considered in cases that are not responsive to standard nappy rash treatment (Borkowski 2004).

During bouts of nappy rash there is a disruption of the normal skin barrier and irritant or allergic contact dermatitis may occur more readily. It is important to remember that any topical application contains preservatives and ingredients, which may be potential sensitisers and in turn can result in skin irritation (Allison 2000, Scardillo and Aronovitch 1999). The possibility of peanut oil allergy arises again, as some common topical nappy creams may contain as much as 30% arachis oil as a base (Lack *et al* 2003). Parents/carers should be aware of these issues and check ingredients in a pharmaceutical formulary and in 'product supplied' information when selecting a cream for patient use. Evaluation of any products used is essential and should be carried out following 3–4 days of continuous use, unless obvious reaction or deterioration occurs beforehand.

Assessment for nappy rash

The cornerstone of successful treatment of any outbreak of nappy rash is the accurate assessment of various possible etiological factors and the treatment of precipitating or perpetuating causes (Atherton 2004, 2005, Atherton and Mill, 2004). The nurse should be aware of predisposing factors (Box 10.1). During the initial nursing history assessment, potential 'at risk' patients can be identified before rashes occur and appropriate preventative measures can be implemented (Adam 2008, Adam *et al* 2009).

Outbreaks can vary considerably between individuals (Allison 2000) so careful assessment and evaluation of rash and subsequent treatment using an assessment tool is vital. One example is the validity scale in Table 10.1 (Jordan *et al* 1986).

As well as assessing rash severity and response to treatment the nurse should be able to distinguish between nappy rash and other common skin conditions (Adam 2008, Atherton 2004, Cooper 2000, Jordan *et al* 1986) (see Table 10.2).

Nappy care

Nappy care applies to the neonate, infant and toddler up to the point of completed toilet training. In addition, some children who have developmental delay and have not yet reached this stage, or those with incontinence during the day and/or at night may require nappies. Nappies should be changed regularly depending on age, frequency of stools and individual routine. This principle also applies to the use of incontinence pads in the older child. See the following section on Nappy care for further detail.

Box 10.1 Predisposing factors to development of nappy rash

Contact with ammonia in urine or bacteria in faeces
Abrasion (chafing on clothes or nappy)
Infrequent nappy changes
Fungal infections (e.g. thrush or Candida)
Plastic pants
Sensitivity to:

- Household chemicals e.g. fabric conditioner/washing powders
- Creams, lotions and bath additives
- Materials (e.g. elastic/latex)
- New foods/dietary changes (e.g. when weaning)
- Prescribed medication.

Immunisation
Teething
Cold or infection
Incorrectly washed reusable nappies
Over application of creams blocking pores in nappy linings
High body temperature increasing humidity in wet nappy
Riboflavin deficiency (causing scrotal or vulval dermatitis, inflammation in genital region)
Surgical gut resection or nutritional deficiency resulting in watery stool (Zsolway *et al* 2002).
Zinc deficiency (Zsolway *et al* 2002)
Immunological deficiency conditions and immune suppressed patients

Table 10.1 Diaper rash severity scale

	Skin integrity	Skin eruptions	Skin redness			
Grade	Ulceration	Scaling	Lesions (papules, vesicles)	Oedema	Spotty	Continuous
0	–	–	–	–	–	–
0.5	–	Vsl	–	–	Vsl	Vsl
1.0	–	Sl	–	–	Sl	Sl
1.5	–	Mod	Vsl	Vsl	Mod	Mod
2.0	–	Sev	Sl	Sl	Mod sev	Mod sev
2.5	Sl	–	Mod	Mod	Sev	Sev
3.0	Mod	–	Mod sev	Mod sev	–	–
3.5	Mod sev	–	Sev	Sev	–	–
4.0	Sev	–	–	–	–	–

Vsl = very slight; Sl = slight; Mod = moderate; Mod sev = moderate to severe; Sev = severe.
Slight nappy rash = grade less than 1.0; moderate = grade 1.0 to <2.0; severe = grade above 2.0.
Severity of rash is graded according to type and severity of individual symptoms The score is then adjusted one half grade upward or downward depending on size of area affected to obtain overall score (Jordan *et al* 1986).

Procedure guideline 10.9 **Assessing nappy rashes**

Statement	Rationale
1. Assess temperature.	1. To identify bacterial infection and or temperature as cause.
2. Establish how long the patient has been suffering with nappy rash.	2. To identify acute nature and severity of rash, and possible presence of secondary bacterial and fungal infections.
3. Check for links with any predisposing factors (Box 10.1).	3. Identification of predisposing factors can aid treatment and be used to prevent further outbreaks.
4. Check current frequency of nappy changes.	4. To assess skin sensitivity to rash outbreaks and to determine frequency of nappy changes during treatment.
5. Ascertain if discomfort is limited to nappy changes/passing of urine/stool or is the child generally irritable?	5. To differentiate between infected and irritant nappy rash and systemic infection. 　To enable assessment of type and regularity of pain relief required.
6. What does the rash look like? 　Is the skin intact? 　Note any spots: size and colour, whether they are raised or flat, have a head, are weeping or crusting (Figure 10.3).	6. To enable identification and differentiation of nappy rash from other skin conditions/skin infections. 　To determine treatment/need for medical input.
7. Treatment already implemented and success/improvement achieved.	7. To evaluate treatment success. 　Identify product sensitivity and/or possibility of secondary fungal/bacterial infection.
8. Document severity of rash using an appropriate tool.	8. To enable assessment and evaluation of subsequent care/treatment.
9. Obtain history of pre-existing skin conditions. Examine other skin areas for rashes including trunk, head, knee, elbow and neck crevices.	9. To identify general skin condition such as eczema or psoriasis as opposed to nappy rash; will determine treatment regime/need for medical input.
10. Does the baby look generally well? For what condition/treatment is the child in hospital?	10. Nappy rash, which fails to respond to conventional treatment in the presence of other conditions, may have a more complex diagnosis attributable to gut function, or nutritional deficiencies.
11. Swab unresolving/severe rashes for bacterial and fungal organisms.	11. To aid diagnosis.

Table 10.2 Types of nappy rash, their aetiology, appearance and treatment

Type of nappy rash	Aetiology	Appearance	Therapy
Contact (irritant) early stage	Moisture, friction, prolonged contact with urine and stool	Generalised superficial red rash (erythematous), commonly sparing skin folds	General nappy care. Iincreased frequency of changes, meticulous cleaning and drying and airing of nappy area with use of barrier creams
Jaques napkin rash/eruption	Acidic urine/stool output, chronic diarrhoea, or urinary dribbling with associated genitourinary abnormality or malformation (Allison 2000). Sometimes complicated with secondary infection	Acute irritant nappy rash with open raw sore areas punctuate sores eruption or rashes	General nappy care. Use of antacids (Markham et al 2000), and stoma barrier products. Periods of nappy airing. Bathing or gentle dabbing as opposed to wiping during changes using oil or aqueous cream and water as cleaning agents. Treatment of any secondary infection
Bacterial	Staphylococcus, Streptococcus	Warm, broken, scratched skin weeping shallow ulcers with collaret of scale. With oedema/swelling/pyrexia and infant irritability (Allison 2000, Zsolway et al 2002)	General nappy care. Swabbing for lab assessment. Prescribed topical/oral antibacterial for local infection, intravenous antibiotics in severe cases
Intertrigo	Moisture trapped in skin folds. Commonly seen in children with watery/loose diarrhoea or inadequate cleaning/drying (Allison 2000)	Redness, soreness or rash limited to areas where two surfaces of the skin are in close contact, e.g. inner walls of buttocks, by anal opening	Meticulous drying of skin folds during changes. Frequent changes and periods of airing.
Fungal	Candida albicans	Bright/beefy red/angry looking sometimes scaly and sharply demarcated rash; satellite lesions spreading into skin creases or beyond the margins of the nappy area. Can also present as contact irritant rash, which is unresponsive to treatment or becomes suddenly worse. Classical white patches surrounded by red skin are less common but possible	General nappy care. Antifungal creams.
Refractory nappy rash	Nutritional deficiencies of essential fatty acids, biotin, riboflavin, pyridoxine, copper or zinc (possibly presenting with a low alkaline phosphatase, which is a zinc dependant enzyme) (Zsolway et al 2002).	Unresolving nappy rash, unresponsive to antifungal treatments, in hospitalised or generally unwell patient (Zsolway et al 2002).	Assessment and rectification of any nutritional deficiencies. General nappy care. Use of barrier products
Atopic dermatitis	Unknown aetiology (Zsolway et al 2002).	Scaly rash, which may also appear on other areas of body including face and flexures of arms and legs with evidence of rubbing/scratching in older infants (Zsolway et al 2002).	General nappy care using prescribed creams used for treatment of eczema on rest of body. Referral to paediatrician/dermatologist
Allergic dermatitis	Babies' skins can develop a sensitivity reaction to any products used for nappy care	Starts with a red area, which can become raised and itchy (can be confused with eczema). Long-term eruptions have whitened central areas surrounded by reddened skin	Discontinued use of offending product and antihistamine to relieve symptoms
Seborrhoea eczema	Inflammatory condition, unknown aetiology	Erythematous, greasy, salmon coloured, well-demarcated, scaly plaques	General nappy care. Referral to dermatologist
Psoriasis		Rarely affecting children under 4 years. Irritant rash, salmon pink lesions with clearly defined edges and covered in silvery scale possibly with symptoms of psoriasis on other skin areas	Referral to dermatologist

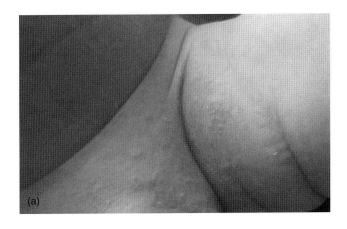

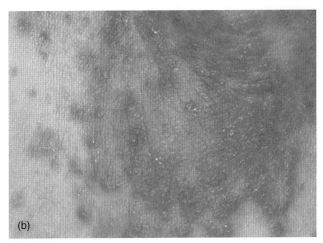

Figure 10.3 (a, b) Typical clinical diaper dermatitis. Photograph courtesty of Julie Petty.

Procedure guideline 10.10 **Routine nappy care**

Statement	Rationale
1. Nappy care to be carried out as soon as possible after soiling: • After feeds • Before long periods of sleep • In the hospital setting check patient's nappy area 3–4 hourly unless otherwise indicated • 6–8 hourly in the case of premature infants • At first sign of nappy rash increase frequency of changing.	1. To prevent prolonged periods of skin contact with irritants known to cause nappy rash. To ensure nappy area is checked regularly in the absence of family carer. Nappies should be changed at least six times over 24 hours (Price 2000). Sick premature neonates require minimal handling. To combat further breakdown/damage. Increased frequency has been shown to decrease outbreaks and speed up recovery and resolution of condition.
2. Ensure you have everything ready before starting: • Nappy • Gloves, apron • A toy/mobile • A warm, dry and clean environment • A changing mat, or towel to lay the baby on • Any creams which you wish to use • Bag/bin for disposal of the old nappy • Wash and dry your hands.	2. To prevent having to leave baby unattended during procedure, maintaining universal precautions and not to distract the baby.
3. Lay the baby on a towel or changing mat. Undo the bottom half of the baby's clothes and lift them out of the way.	3. To prevent soiling.
4. Unfasten nappy tabs and fasten them back onto the nappy, fold nappy over and underneath bottom.	4. To prevent tabs sticking to the baby's skin.
5. As for Bathing guidelines, using water and cotton wool clean the front of the nappy area first (the genital area before the anal area)	5. To reduce the possibility of bacteria from the bowel/anal area being transferred to and entering the urethra causing urinary tract infection.

(Continued)

Procedure guideline 10.10 (*Continued*)

Statement	Rationale
6. For girls always wipe from front to back – away from the vagina towards the perineal area (anus). For boys clean the penis but do not retract the foreskin: this applies to the infant in the first year. From age 1 upwards, gentle retraction can be done to check for cleanliness	**6.** As above
7. Clean between the folds of the groin and thighs thoroughly.	**7.** Common areas where nappy rash occurs.
8. Lift both of the legs by the ankles and clean the bottom.	
9. Dry the bottom thoroughly from front to back.	
10. Apply a clean nappy.	
11. As stated in the Bathing section, water alone can be used to clean the nappy area without the necessity for skin products. This also applies to the routine use of barrier creams on the skin. The skin can be left without a barrier cream unless parents/carers request a particular product, which should be checked for suitability in neonates (Walker *et al* 2005a, 2005b). In the case of a rash developing however, it may be necessary to use a specific product.	**11.** Water alone has been shown to be sufficient for cleansing the skin certainly in the first 1–2 months and the benefits of routine barrier creams have not been agreed.
12. If applying creams in the case of nappy rash or other skin conditions requiring topical treatment, loosely tape up the nappy and wash your hands before applying; alternatively measure out cream prior to nappy change.	**12.** To prevent introduction of micro-organisms into cream pot/tube.
13. Carefully apply cream taking special care around the vagina and applying again from front to back.	**13.** To prevent transfer of bowel bacteria to urethra.
14. In newborns, the umbilical cord stump should be observed at each nappy change and cleaned if necessary with water.	**14.** Water has been shown to be effective for cleaning the cord stump (Zupan and Gardner 2004).
15. As stated in the Bathing section, avoid, if possible, covering the umbilical cord with the nappy until the stump has separated and has been removed (a notch can be cut at the front top edge of the nappy if necessary or the nappy can be folded at the top).	**15.** To prevent the cord becoming moist, aiding drying of the stump and reducing risk of infection (Dunn 2009). (See Chapter 17.)
16. In boys tuck the penis facing downwards.	**16.** To prevent upward leaks.
17. Fasten the nappy at both sides with the tapes, making sure it is snug, but not so tight that it pinches the skin.	**17.** A nappy that is too tight can cause chaffing abrasive friction and discomfort.

18. Re-tape the soiled nappy around the contents and put in plastic bag or bin. Remove faecal matter from reusable nappies and place in sanitising bin.
   Wash hands thoroughly and re-dress baby.
   In all cases of nappy rash ensure appropriate pain relief is prescribed and given.
	18. To maintain universal precautions.

186

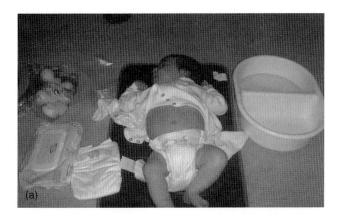
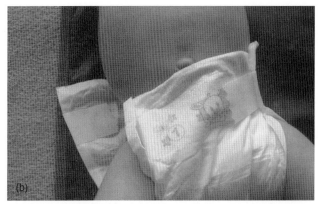
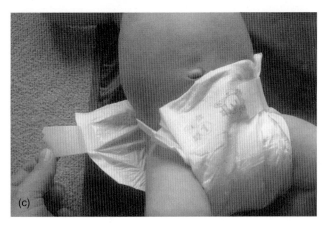
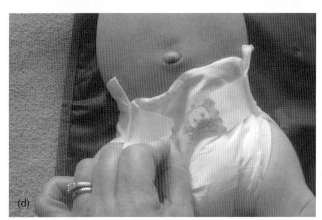

Figure 10.4 (a–d) Application of nappy.
Note that these figures are of a parent/carer providing care, hence why no gloves are being worn. In a hospital environment, in view of infection control, staff must wear gloves. Photograph courtesty of Julie Petty.

Nail care

The nails are horny plates of modified epithelium that serve to protect the tips of fingers and toes (Watson 2005). The nail apparatus is composed of several parts (www.physsportsmed.com) including the nail matrix, the plate or the actual nail itself and the surrounding proximal and lateral nail folds. The areas underneath the nail comprise the nail bed, the hyponychium where the nail plate separates from the nail matrix and the sub-ungual space underneath the whole nail (Figure 10.5).

Finger and toenails can be a potential source of infection and personal hygiene principles must apply to these body parts in the child who is either healthy or sick. Transient flora is acquired from the environment which is carried on the hands, feet and nails and then transferred to other parts of the body by cross transmission (Lawson 2001). The sub-ungual space under the nail is particularly prone to harbouring micro-organisms and there may be a higher concentration at this site than elsewhere.

Therefore, nail care should be considered when attending to the holistic personal hygiene needs of any child. In addition, there are specific times when nail cleanliness is paramount, for example when attending to other procedures such as wound care, during mealtimes, after outside play in mud or sand and as

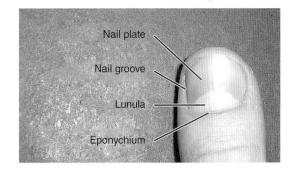

Figure 10.5 A sagittal view of the nail demonstrating the structure of the nail unit and the underlying tissues and bone.

part of pre-operative preparation for the child when infection risk must be minimised as much as possible.

Although the main focus here is on the child, nail cleanliness in relation to the hands is also an essential component of general hygiene for staff (Arrowsmith *et al* 2001, Rothrock 2006, WHO 2005) (see Chapter 12 Infection Prevention and Control).

Micro-organisms carried on hands and nails can be transferred between patients by cross-transmission if adequate hand-washing policies are not adhered to (Lawson 2001). Normal hand washing, the aim of which is to remove dirt, organic debris and microorganisms as quickly as possible (Boyd 2003) may be ineffective to remove the pathogens from nails and sub-ungual space.

Long and/or artificial nails further increase the risk of infection via this source, the presence of nail varnish (Boyd 2003) and breaks in continuity between the skin and nail bed (Watson 2005). Several studies have demonstrated how nails are a rich source of infection in the clinical area (Foca *et al* 2000, Hedderwick *et al* 2000, Jeannes and Green 2001).

Nail assessment

As part of the general assessment of hygiene status of the child, the nails should be observed carefully so that appropriate care can be given. Nail assessment needs to include the changing presentation of finger and toenails as a child grows. Baby nails are much softer and thinner than the older child growing from a more fragile nail bed. This needs to be taken into account when caring for the delicate nails of the newborn and infant. In the older child, nails are thicker, more robust and there may be cultural and age specific decorations such as varnish, false nails and jewellery.

Procedure guideline 10.11 **Nail assessment**

Statement	Rationale
1. Assess nails as part of the child's overall hygiene routine along with the parents/carers.	1. To incorporate nail care into daily routine of the child and family.
2. Observe all aspects of the nails and nail bed, including the sub-ungual area of both fingers and toes.	2. For holistic and thorough assessment of hygiene status of the nails.
3. Observe for dirt and debris on and under the nail.	3. Presence of dirt serves as an infection source.
4. Observe nail for length and for the presence of jagged or broken edges.	4. Long, jagged/broken nails can further increase infection risk and cause trauma (Boyd 2003).
5. Observe and note the presence of nail varnish, false nails and jewellery.	5. Nail decoration such as these increases the risk of infection (Boyd 2003).
6. Observe whether there is any evidence of nail-biting or damage to the skin around the nail area	6. Loss of continuity between skin and nail can harbour micro-organisms (Watson 2000). In addition, this point plus the above two points may be areas to advise the child and family in relation to health promotion.
7. Observe the colour of the sub-ungual area checking it is pink, with adequate capillary refill without presence of cyanosis.	7. Colour of the nail beds provides useful information on oxygenation and perfusion.
8. Assessment must be carried out pre-operatively.	8. To minimise infection within the sterile surgical area.
9. Assess for presence of disease such as fungal infection, redness, swelling, abnormal growth, trauma, hardened nails that may indicate skin conditions as well as any gross abnormalities that may affect appearance and growth of the nails.	9. Nail problems can stem from many sources on fingers and/or toes.

10. At any age, assess the child and family's normal routine in order to incorporate this into care as much as is appropriate within the hospital setting. Discuss and document care-giving routine in relation to nail care with the child and family and any specific requirements that are needed.	10. To continue hygiene routine as normal for the family. However, some practices may not be appropriate in the hospital environment; for example, some parents/carers bite their infants/child's nails for them at home. Therefore alternative advice should be offered.
	    To encourage a partnership approach to care between nurse and family.
	    For all parents/carers to be aware of the child's needs.

11. Assess and observe for any culture-specific variations in practices; for example, the colour of the sub-ungual and surrounding area, presence of rings.	11. In some cultures, discolouration may be due to different foodstuffs or substances; for example, henna. It is imperative that cultural and societal norms are incorporated into care regimes within the hospital setting.

Prevention of nail problems is based on thorough assessment and good nail hygiene. Both the finger and toenails must be included.

Nail hygiene

For children of all ages, nail hygiene is an important hygiene consideration. For fingernails, these can be cleaned during hand washing or bathing. In addition, the toe nails need attention and cleaning. This is best carried out during bathing or wash times.

Oral hygiene

The mouth is important for eating, drinking, speech, communication, taste, breathing and defence against infection. Oral

Procedure guideline 10.12 Nail care

Statement	Rationale
1. For all ages, assess nails at bath or hand wash times according to assessment criteria in the previous section.	1. Assessment is the first stage in order to plan subsequent care.
2. For any aged baby or child it may be necessary to teach the parents/carers nail care by performing the practice followed by supervising them.	2. Some parents/carers (for example, those with a first baby) may be unsure and may require teaching and support for even the most basic of care tasks.
3. For any aged baby or child, if nails require cutting, discuss with the parents/carers and gain consent or support them to carry out the procedure.	3. This aids the negotiation of care in the context of a partnership between nurse and family.
4. In the neonate/baby, check and clean nails during bathing or topping and tailing using water and a soft flannel/cloth.	4. For the integration of care practices.
5. Check the neonate's finger nails and cut to the level of the top of the finger using small baby nail scissors or clippers. Alternatively, nails can be gently filed using a soft, small emery board.	5. Cutting too close to the skin may cause trauma and damage to the nail bed. Equipment specially designed for babies should be used to minimise such damage.
6. For the preschool child, wash the child's hands and nails or assist them to do so, during hand washing and/or bathing, using a soft brush if necessary (AORN 2009).	6. As above, for the integration of care practices.
7. In the child of any age, cut nails using nail scissors to length indicated above, paying particular attention to jagged edges. Cut/trim or file nails straight across. Provide reassurance at all times.	7. The child may be fearful of the procedure and so continual reassurance may be required.
8. Teach the child hand and nail care during the procedure.	8. To encourage independence and health promotion.
9. For the older child and adolescent, observe hand and nail washing technique, teaching and giving guidance as necessary.	9. Generally speaking, children after the age of 5 will be able to perform their own hygiene if able and healthy.
10. If the older child is unable to perform nail care due to special needs, illness, immobility, lack of dexterity, perform the procedure during bed bathing/washing.	
11. Prior to surgery remove any nail varnish with recommended solution, any jewellery and false nail or cut the nails as stated before (Rothrock 2006, AORN 2009).	11. To minimise infection in the operating theatre and to be able to observe perfusion of finger tips.
12. Emphasise the importance of cleaning under the nail with the use of a brush (AORN 2009).	12. The area underneath the nail is a potential source for pathogens to harbour.
13. Attend to, and clean, both finger and toe nails.	13. Toe nails particularly are a source of infection and certain conditions so should not be missed.

hygiene is an integral part of total care in which nurses play a pivotal role. Systematic assessment forms the basis of all care undertaken and is essential so that any changes are monitored and appropriate treatment implemented. Planned interventions help to minimise or reverse changes in the oral cavity. The frequency of oral care and the tools used to perform safe and effective care are often debated in the literature. Nonetheless there is evidence that states that oral care and dental hygiene should begin as the primary teeth erupt. National guidelines verify the importance of good oral hygiene from as early as possible (DoH 2007), which is further supported by emerging guidance through online resources (Growing Kids.co.uk, AboutDentistry.com, HygieneExpert.co.uk). Even babies with no teeth require consideration, as erupting primary teeth can decay like permanent teeth if not looked after properly.

The principle objective of oral hygiene is to maintain the mouth in a good condition. It specifically aims to:

- Achieve and maintain a clean, healthy oral cavity
- Prevent the build up of plaque on oral surfaces, thus helping prevent dental caries
- Keep oral mucosa moist
- Maintain mucosal integrity and promote healing
- Prevent infection
- Prevent broken or chapped lips
- Promote patient comfort and well-being
- Maintain normal oral function.

For the nurse to provide a good standard of oral hygiene, knowledge and understanding of the normal anatomy and physiology of the mouth, teeth, gums, tongue and lips is required (Figure 10.6).

The anatomy and physiology of the mouth is complex. There are two major functions of the mouth: digestion and defence. The oral cavity is the first part of the gastrointestinal tract. The structures visible on examination are: the mucosal lining, the lips, the tongue and the teeth.

The **mucosal lining** is continuous with the gastrointestinal tract and protects the underlying tissues. The mucous membranes, via the salivary glands, secrete mucus and saliva. Saliva

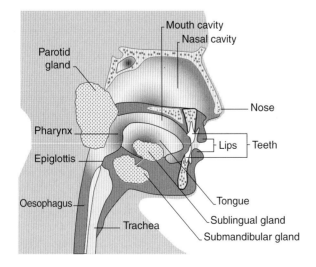

Figure 10.6 The mouth.

is formed mainly of water (99% of total) and normally has a pH of 6.8–7.0. It does, however, become more alkaline as the secretory rate increases during chewing. Saliva contains lysozyme, which has an antiseptic action; immunoglobulin (IgA), which has a defensive function; and , salivary amylase, which is a digestive enzyme. These properties result in keeping the oral mucosa moist, smooth, clean and shiny with the buffering capacity to minimise change in overall pH maintaining the balance of the microbial flora.

The **lips** form a muscular entrance to the mouth; they are covered by squamous, keratinized epithelial tissue, which is vascular and very sensitive. They are necessary for ingestion of food, enunciation of words and convey the mood of a person, e.g. smiling and grimacing.

The **tongue** is covered with mucous membrane from which project numerous papillae and taste buds on the upper surface. The muscles of the tongue afford it great mobility, which is essential for speech and swallowing; its other main function is interpreting taste sensations.

The **teeth** consist of enamel, dentine, cementum and pulp. The first tooth normally erupts around 6 months of age with full complement of 20 deciduous primary teeth being acquired by the age of 2 and a half years.

Permanent dentition begins at 5 and 6 years and the full number of 28 teeth have normally appeared by 13–15 years. The four wisdom teeth erupt later, usually by the age of 25, making the full complement of 32 teeth.

In addition to this knowledge, nurses must also understand the importance of adequate hydration and nutrition, microbiology and oral infections, the effects of various drugs on the oral mucosa, treatments and diseases (Thurgood 1994). For example, antibiotics alter the flora in the mouth and increase the risk of opportunistic infections, antihistamines reduce salivary production, any fever may result in halitosis and thumb sucking may alter the position of the teeth.

Children with a number of conditions may have compromised oral well-being, for example children with cerebral palsy or disability and epidermolysis bullosa (a genetically based disease characterised by chronic, painful blistering: the skin and mucous membranes are so fragile that the slightest touch can cause severe blistering – inside and outside the body); special consideration will need to be give to identify the optimum method for oral hygiene to be performed (see later section on compromised oral health). Assessment and identifying the child's 'usual' oral care is crucial in children with special needs or other long-term conditions that may compromise oral health. The child's role and the assistance they might require to maintain normal oral hygiene must be made explicit in a plan of care. As far as possible, the child should be assisted to maintain their normal pattern of care.

Consideration will need to be given to identify the optimum method for oral hygiene to be performed (see later section on compromised oral health). Assessment and identifying the child's 'usual' oral care is crucial in children with special needs or other long-term conditions that may compromise oral health. The child's role and the assistance they might require to maintain normal oral hygiene must be made explicit in a plan of care. As far as possible, the child should be assisted to maintain their normal pattern of care.

Oral assessment

Oral assessment is considered to be central to planning effective care and begins with a history of previous dental care, which includes the child's usual brushing and cleaning regimen, as well as recording any previous oral problems. Based on this assessment an individualised care plan can then be developed which identifies either prophylactic or treatment specific measures. The use of an oral assessment tool can facilitate the development of a care plan. Assessment has the potential to provide baseline data; predict, prevent or minimise oral complications; and evaluate nursing interventions (Coyne *et al* 2010, Hockenberry and Wilson 2010).

Oral hygiene tools for children with primary/secondary teeth

Regular brushing is imperative in plaque removal and although some studies have shown that nurses prefer using foam sponges (Pearson 1996), there is a general agreement that a small headed, soft, multi-tufted, nylon bristled toothbrush is the best tool for cleaning the teeth (Pearson and Hutton 2002) and massaging gingiva. Teeth should be cleaned effectively twice a day, as soon as possible after a meal if eating, and before bedtime, with a soft toothbrush and toothpaste. The more frequently and the longer teeth are cleaned the greater the probability of effective plaque removal. Even when the child is not eating, regular and thorough

Procedure guideline 10.13 **Oral assessment**

Statement	Rationale

1. An oral assessment, e.g. the Nebraska tool adapted for use in children (Table 10.3) is useful if recording the status of the oral cavity and can be applied or adapted to suit all ages.
   An effective oral assessment should involve the examination of the eight aspects of the mouth:
• Each category is given a score of 1 (being normal)
• A change being indicated as a rise in a score above 1
• The highest score being 3
• A normal mouth scores 8 and the highest score obtainable is 24.
	1. To identify specific problems.
	   To enable appropriate advice to be given.
	   To facilitate effective management.
	   To promote oral health.

2. Assessment of the oral cavity must be performed thoroughly & systematically.	2. To monitor changes and prescribe appropriate interventions.
3. The assessment procedure should be explained to the child and family, including why the assessment is necessary and what it entails.	3. To obtain informed consent. Communication helps to ensure success.

4. Whenever possible the child should be involved in the assessment.
   When assessing the mouth of a young child it is advisable to have a second adult present to support the child's head.
	4. To help ensure success.
	   To teach the child about good mouth care.
	   For comfort and reassurance.

5. A good source of light is required to examine the oral cavity, e.g. pen torch.	5. To enable good visualisation of the mouth.
6. Standard (universal) precautions should be adopted and non-sterile gloves worn.	6. To minimise the risk of cross-infection.
7. The teeth should, if possible, be cleaned prior to examining the oral cavity.	7. To remove plaque and debris. To aid observation and assessment.

8. It is important to accurately record the assessment in the child's healthcare record and on the oral assessment score sheet.	8. To monitor any changes.
	   To implement appropriate treatment.
	   To ensure continuity.
	   To evaluate care.

9. Special skills of observing 'in an instant' maybe required when undertaking oral assessment in children with special needs.	9. To undertake assessment quickly To explain and gain collaboration to undertake the assessment.

Table 10.3 Oral assessment guide in children

Category	Method of assessment	1	2	3
Swallow	Ask the child to swallow or observe the swallowing process. Ask the parent/carer if there are any notable changes	Normal Without difficulty	Difficulty in swallowing	Unable to swallow at all. Pooling, dribbling of secretions
Lips and corner of mouth	Observe appearance of tissue	Normal Smooth, pink and moist	Dry, cracked or swollen	Ulcerated or bleeding
Tongue	Observe the appearance of the tongue using a pen-torch to illuminate the oral cavity	Normal Firm without fissures (cracking or splitting) or prominent papilla. Pink and moist	Coated or loss of papillae with a shiny appearance with or without redness and/or oral *Candida*	Ulcerated, sloughing or cracked
Saliva	Observe consistency and quality of saliva	Normal Thin and watery	Excess amount of saliva, drooling	Thick, ropy or absent
Mucous membrane	Observe the appearance of tissue using a pen-torch to illuminate the oral cavity	Normal Pink and moist	Reddened or coated without ulceration and/or oral *Candida*	Ulceration and sloughing, with or without bleeding
Gingivae	Observe the appearance of tissue using a pen-torch to illuminate the oral cavity	Normal Pink or coral with a stippled (dotted) surface. Gum margins tight and well defined, no swelling	Oedematous with or without redness, smooth	Spontaneous bleeding
Teeth (If no teeth score 1)	Observe the appearance of teeth using a pen-torch to illuminate the oral cavity	Normal Clean and no debris	Plaque or debris in localised areas	Plaque or debris generalised along gum line
Voice	Talk and listen to the child. Ask the parent/carer if there are any notable changes	Normal tone and quality when talking or crying	Deeper or raspy	Difficult to talk, cry or not talking at all

Oral assessment guide – Adapted from Eilers, J. Berger, A. and Peterson, M. (1988). © Great Ormond Street Hospital 2004. NB if score >8 introduce pain assessment instrument.

mouth care is vital. However, there may be times when an optimal oral hygiene regimen is sacrificed for patient comfort.

Rinsing the oral cavity after brushing is also important. This activity removes loose debris and further irrigates the tissues (Madeya 1996). It also reduces the likelihood of ingestion of toothpaste, which can lead to fluorosis. Tap water, or for some children sterile water, is the most common mouth rinse. Only those patients at high risk of mucosal deterioration (e.g. following chemotherapy) are advised to use an antibacterial mouth rinse such as chlorhexidine 0.2%. It should be rinsed and remain in contact with the mucosal membrane for at least 30–90 seconds to be effective (BMA/RPSGB 2010). It should not be rinsed with water after its use. The rationale for using an antibacterial mouth rinse in this small group of children is that many of the micro-

organisms responsible for causing systemic infections can be isolated from the oral cavity. In addition to tooth brushing and rinsing with water/chlorhexidine, children who are profoundly neutropenic and at risk of developing fungal infections should use a prophylactic anti-fungal agent. Children wearing orthodontic braces should be encouraged to rinse with a fluoride mouthwash at night in addition to cleaning their teeth normally twice a day.

The general guidelines of oral hygiene outlined in this section and throughout this chapter are examples of best practice that would benefit from being shared with all children receiving care from healthcare professionals. Underpinning this practice is the need to explore and document the child's 'usual' oral hygiene routine (Beal 2005, DoH 2007).

Principles table 10.1 Oral hygiene tools

Principle	Rationale
Tooth brushes	
1. A small headed, soft, multituft nylon bristled toothbrush should be used to brush/clean teeth and oral tissues.	1. They provide the most effective method for removing plaque.

Principles table 10.1 (*Continued*)

Principle	Rationale
2. They can potentially cause gum haemorrhages.	**2.** Children at risk of low platelet count should use a soft toothbrush.
3. They are for single patient use and should be kept clean.	**3.** They should therefore be rinsed and stored once dry. Toothbrushes should be changed every 12 weeks (when bristles become frayed or bent) or daily whilst undergoing bone marrow transplantation.

Powered toothbrushes

Principle	Rationale
1. These have a rotating, oscillating and vibratory action.	**1.** Considered to achieve a modest reduction in plaque and gingivitis compared to manual toothbrushing (Heanue *et al* 2003).
2. The bristles are hard and are not advisable for children with a fragile mucosa.	**2.** Their efficacy is not yet proven in cancer care.
3. Useful for physically impaired children.	**3.** However, to be effective advice and instruction on use is essential (Renton-Harper *et al* 2001).

Fluoride toothpaste

Principle	Rationale
1. It strengthens tooth enamel and decreases risk of dental caries.	**1.** Clear evidence exists that it is efficacious in preventing caries (Marinho *et al* 2003, 2004).
2. It can have a drying effect if left in contact with oral mucosa.	
3. Check fluoride content of water supply prior to introducing supplements.	**3.** Excessive fluoride may result in very tough teeth and produce unsightly spotting, i.e. fluorosis.

Foam cleaning sponges

Principle	Rationale
1. These may be used as a temporary measure, or combined with a toothbrush to remove debris and cleanse the mouth when a child: • Has no teeth; For example in the neonate / infant prior to appearance of teeth, foam sponges soaked first in clean water (use sterile water in the neonate) can be used to clean and moisten the lips, tongue and inside the mouth. For the very small neonate, cotton wool buds can provide an alternative. Liquid paraffin or Vaseline can also be applied in this way to moisten dry lips when the neonate/infant is unable to lubricate their own lips; for example when intubated or sedated in intensive care • Has severe mucositis preventing them from brushing their teeth • A platelet count below 20 × 109/l with associated bleeding • Is in the terminal stages of illness when comfort is the only intended outcome • Has a reduced level of consciousness.	**1.** They are: • Ineffective at removing plaque (Pearson and Hutton 2002) • Soft, unthreatening and easy to use • Able to be squeezed into difficult places • Able to deliver fluids to specific places.
2. Mouth care packs should be disposed of once opened.	**2.** To avoid the risk of infection.

Dental floss

Principle	Rationale
1. Combined with a toothbrush, it is the most effective method of removing plaque. It reaches parts that toothbrush bristles are unable to reach. It must be used with care. It is not advised in children less than 10 years (Lloyd 1992).	**1.** Dexterity is needed to manipulate floss. It is difficult to floss someone else's teeth. There are some conditions, which may cause bleeding and increased risk of infection.

193

(Continued)

Principles table 10.1 (*Continued*)

Principle	Rationale
Vaseline	
1. It can be applied to the lips to soothe dryness. It is the most acceptable method to prevent dry, cracked lips (Campbell *et al* 1995).	**1.** It provides an occlusive barrier, which retains moisture.
2. It is easy to apply and will remain in place for many hours if not licked off!	
3. It should not be used in the following circumstances: • Oxygen therapy • Smoking • Babies under phototherapy.	**3.** It is highly flammable and traps bacteria.
Chlorhexidine based mouthwash (0.2% solution)	
1. It is absorbed into the cell wall of micro-organisms and is active against yeast, fungi and gram-negative and gram-positive organisms.	**1.** It can be used prophylactically and therapeutically for identified high-risk patients. It should remain in contact with the mucous membranes for 30–90 seconds and then spat out.
2. If the mucosal membrane is inflamed or broken rinse with chlorhexidine based mouthwash after cleaning teeth.	
3. Dilution of the mouthwash should be avoided but during episodes of severe mucositis, the solution may be mixed with 50/50 water and chlorhexidine, continuing until after the mouth is healed. Dilution should be stopped as soon as possible.	**3.** Dilution reduces its efficacy.
Anti-fungal agents	
Nystatin	
1. Action of nystatin is purely topical and needs frequent administration.	**1.** It requires a long contact time with the oral mucosa.
2. Nystatin has not shown to be prophylactic against the incidence of localised or systemic candidiasis (Clarkson *et al* 2009).	**2.** There is no overall evidence to support the use of drugs not absorbed from the GI tract for the prevention of oral candidiasis in either adults or children (Clarkson *et al* 2009, Worthington *et al* 2008).
3. The treatment dose is 1 ml orally four times a day.	
4. Nystatin pastilles are preferable because they remain in contact with the oral mucosa for longer.	
5. It should be given an hour after the use of chlorhexidine.	
6. Children need to abstain from eating and drinking for 20–30 minutes after using nystatin.	**6.** To allow the nystatin to be absorbed.
Fluconazole	
1. Used as a therapeutic agent and prophylaxis for children at risk of developing a yeast or fungal infection. It should only be used for patients who are profoundly neutropenic (Chandrasekar and Gatny 1994). Easily tolerated as a once a day dose.	**1.** Indiscriminate use can cause a growth of micro-organisms such as *Candida glabrata*, *Klebsiella*.
2. It can cause a feeling of nausea.	

194

Preparation and performing oral care

One of the most effective means of preventing dental caries is a regimen of proper oral health tailored to the individual child by the dentist (Hockenberry and Wilson 2010). Children should be taught to carry out their own oral care under the supervision and guidance of parents/carers. In some situations parents/carers may need to be taught proper brushing techniques along with their children. Young children will need to have their teeth brushed for them, up to an age when the parent or carer feels they have the dexterity to do it properly for themselves. The easiest and most effective way is for the adult to sit down and have the child stand in front with the child's head against the adult's chest and brush the teeth (Lloyd 1994). For neonates and very young children they may lie in the adult's lap. In the case of an ill child who is confined to their bed or sofa, it is more appropriate to find a position that is most comfortable for them.

In the situation of a very young child, in children who have not been used to regular dental care or children with learning disabilities, play therapy can be a useful medium through which to introduce a regular regimen. Allowing the child to handle the mouth-care products in a non-threatening environment that includes performing mouth care on a favourite toy, their parent/carer or a nurse, are useful techniques to reduce anxiety. Play specialists can help provide a supportive role in this aspect of care. Aids such as specially designed brushes or electric toothbrushes may be required in order for the child with special needs to be enabled to undertake effective cleaning of their teeth. See Chapter 24 Play as a Therapeutic Tool.

In the case of older children and teenagers they may need to be reminded that mouth care should remain part of their daily hygiene routine. This group of patients have increased concern regarding body image and sexuality. They may be anxious or embarrassed by changes in their oral cavity such as: gingival enlargement; increased salivation; inability to swallow or speak effectively; halitosis. They may be angry about these changes and direct their anger towards staff or even reject treatment measures. The following issues should always be considered:

- Where possible allow them control, for example, let them choose the timing of mouth care.
- Respect their need for privacy when undertaking any aspect of oral care.
- Involve them in planning their oral care so that they will understand its importance and thus be more receptive to health teaching; ideally, they should be accepted as a vital member of the healthcare team.

Ensure explanations are age appropriate and reinforced with written information.

Procedure guideline 10.14 Performing oral care

Statement	Rationale
1. The nurse's role is to facilitate family-centred care, therefore, whenever possible oral care should be performed by the child and/or family member/carer.	1. To reduce anxiety. To allow time for questions.
2. Whenever possible encourage the child to take control of their mouth care, e.g. choosing the time to do it.	2. To increase adherence.
3. In the case of a well neonate, oral care will simply involve observation of the mouth, tongue and lips. If clean and moist, no further intervention is required. As stated earlier, liquid paraffin or Vaseline can be applied to the neonate's dry lips if necessary.	3. A neonate prior to the appearance of teeth does not need routine mouth care unless there is an indication to do so (e.g. dryness or presence of any Candida or other conditions). A well neonate will be able to lubricate their own mouth and lips.
4. Once teeth start to appear within the first year, gentle cleaning with a soft toothbrush and low-fluoride toothpaste, both suitable for use in babies, should be carried out on a daily basis.	4. To prevent any potential for tooth decay at the earliest possible age.
5. If the neonate is unwell, it may be necessary to perform more regular mouth care to lubricate the mouth and lips (see Compromised health).	
6. Play specialists can help prepare older children for mouth care procedures.	6. To ensure age appropriate preparation.

(Continued)

Procedure guideline 10.14 (*Continued*)

Statement	Rationale
7. The child should be encouraged to handle the mouth care products in a non-threatening environment and perform mouth care on a favourite toy, parent/carer or nurse.	**7.** To reduce anxiety.
8. Ensure explanations are age appropriate and reinforced with written information.	**8.** To ensure that the child understands why mouth care is important and what it will mean if they do not adhere to guidance.
9. Their need for privacy must be respected when undertaking any aspect of oral care.	**9.** To decrease anxiety or embarrassment from changes in their oral cavity, e.g. gingival enlargement, increased salivation, inability to swallow or speak effectively, halitosis.
10. Older children and/or teenagers have increased concern regarding body image and sexuality.	**10.** To increase receptiveness to health teaching.
11. Involve them in planning their oral care so that they will understand its importance.	**11.** Empowering teenagers to manage their own care.
12. Dental check-ups should begin as soon as primary teeth erupt.	**12.** Primary teeth can decay the same as permanent teeth.
13. The child's mouth should be assessed and appropriate mouth care given.	
14. Normal practice from home may be continued if appropriate.	
15. Teeth should be cleaned once they erupt with a special soft baby toothbrush.	**15.** Good teeth cleaning habits benefit the child for life (Lloyd 1994).
16. Teeth should be cleaned effectively twice a day.	**16.** Bedtime brushing is especially important, as there is more time for interaction between oral bacteria and unremoved substrate on the tooth substance.
17. The child's mouth should be assessed daily using an oral assessment guide.	**17.** To accurately and regularly monitor the child's mouth, used specifically in compromised health.
18. Prior to performing oral hygiene the nurse should: • Put on an apron • Perform a clinical handwash • Put on a pair of non-sterile gloves.	**18.** To meet standard precautions. To minimise the risk of cross-infection. Oral fungal infections are often asymptomatic. *Candida albicans* can be transmitted between patients on the hands of staff.
19. The gloves should be powder and latex free.	**19.** To prevent allergic reaction.
20. Children under 7 years should position their heads so that parents/carers can access their mouth whilst stabilising their head. This is achieved by the child having their back to the adult, whilst the adult cups their chin with one hand and brushes the child's teeth with the other. This is known as the 'Starkey' position.	**20.** The teeth of children under 7 years are most effectively cleaned if it is done by their parents/carers (Lloyd 1994). To facilitate access ensuring effectiveness of cleaning.

Procedure guideline 10.14 (*Continued*)

Statement	Rationale
21. Fluoride toothpaste should be used as follows: • Use a small pea sized amount on a toothbrush. • Supervise use of toothpaste to prevent swallowing of excessive amounts. • It should be spat out and rinsed thoroughly with water.	21. Fluoride can build into the enamel to increase resistance to decay.
22. The toothbrush should be used by: • Placing the tips of bristles at 45° against teeth and gums. • Moving the brush backwards and forwards in a gentle but vibratory motion. • To clean the inner (lingual) surfaces place toothbrush vertical to teeth and move up and down against the gums. • Always start and finish in the same spot. • It is important that the gums as well as the teeth are cleaned. • Teeth should be cleaned for 2–3 minutes	22. To ensure adequate cleaning action. To ensure a thorough and complete cleaning.
23. Using an electric toothbrush requires less dexterity.	23. The bristles do the action and therefore the brush needs to be moved around all areas of the mouth
24. Using a toothbrush with timer is more effective.	24. Ensures teeth are cleaned for a recommended effective period.
25. Dental floss is used by pulling gently downwards and upwards against each tooth to clean both above and below the gum.	25. Flossing removes bacteria that escape normal tooth brushing. Daily use recommended.
26. If the child has been assessed as having dry, cracked or ulcerated lips apply Vaseline. Vaseline if required should be used sparingly and applied with a gloved finger.	26. To maintain integrity and comfort.
27. Each container of Vaseline is for single patient use.	27. To prevent cross-contamination.
28. All used equipment should be cleaned, disinfected and stored safely.	28. As per local policy.

197

Health promotion and oral care

For the nurse there is an important role in informing, advising, helping with the acquisition of skills, assisting with the process of clarifying beliefs, enabling the adaptation of life-style, promoting change in the structures and organisations that influence health status (Coutts and Hardy 1995). Dental decay is one of the most common childhood diseases. From newborn, to toddler, to the young and older child, any childcare health professional has an important role in encouraging and shaping good oral health care practices (Daly *et al* 2002, DoH 2004b, 2004c, NICE 2004). The main cause of dental decay is sugars in the diet. While any simple sugars, in theory, can be metabolised by plaque bacteria to generate acid, the ones most implicated are the non-milk extrinsic sugars, for example sugars added during processing or preparation, or prior to consumption of food and beverages. Honey is also in this category. Non-milk extrinsic sugars do not include lactose in milk, dairy products or fructose found naturally within fruit and vegetables (intrinsic sugars). Starch products such as bread are only slowly degraded in the mouth to sugars, and together with fruit, vegetables and dairy products are not strongly linked to caries (Health Education Authority 1996). It is both the presence of non-extrinsic sugars in the diet and the frequency of their consumption that are the basic cause of dental caries (Moynihan 2002, Watt and McGlone 2003). The factors associated with caries incidence are (SIGN Publication 47 2000, Levine and Stillman-Lowe 2009):

- Amount of fermentable carbohydrate consumed
- Sugar concentration of food
- Physical form of carbohydrate
- Length of time teeth are exposed to decreased plaque pH
- Frequency of eating meals and snacks
- Length of interval between eating
- Sequence of food consumption.

To produce tooth decay three factors are required: a susceptible tooth, bacteria and sugar. Establishing good oral care and dental practices early in life encourages children to believe in the importance of healthy teeth. Healthcare professionals and schoolteachers have an important role to play in the ongoing education of children and the whole family (see www.3dmouth.org for education resources for schools produced by the British Dental Association).

Compromised health and oral care

This group includes those with a condition that makes dental and oral care more hazardous or difficult and includes infants, children and teenagers with:

- Cardiac disease
- Immunosuppression, as a result of cancer therapies and HIV
- Haemophilia and other bleeding disorders
- Reduced level of consciousness
- Developmental delay/learning disability
- Impaired dexterity
- Health disorders requiring medium to long-term use of medication
- Conditions necessitating intensive care/artificial ventilation by oral intubation.

Children in these groups may be more susceptible to poor oral health and subsequent caries development (see Table 10.4, taken from Gibson and Nelson 2000). [.] Minimising trauma, reducing risk of infection, ensuring oral comfort and maximising oral health will be the focus of an individualised mouth care regimen.

Principles table 10.2 Oral health promotion

Principle	Rationale
1. For snacks between meals encourage non-sugary foods, e.g. cheese, fresh vegetables or water.	**1.** Sugar promotes dental caries. Frequent exposure to sugar increases the incidence of caries.
2. If sugary foods are consumed, ensure they are part of main meals and completed before teeth are brushed.	**2.** Sugar can contribute to dental caries, especially when given at night. Saliva flow is greatly reduced at night so the sugar remains in contact with the teeth for longer periods.
3. Involve the dietician in the child's care. Many children with chronic illness require a diet high in refined carbohydrates to ensure adequate energy intake.	**3.** Liaise with the dietician before advising any reduction in sugar content.
4. Avoid sugary medicines.	**4.** Paracetamol syrups and cough mixtures are commonly used paediatric medicines and are available sugar free.
6. Encourage regular dental checkups at least annually.	**6.** Should begin around 1 year of age. Children, particularly those at risk of oral problems, should have check-ups more frequently. Dentists can assess manipulative skills and special needs of children to prescribe the best brushing technique and regimen. Good dental habits are important to family health.
7. Trauma to the teeth is not uncommon in childhood.	
8. Do not leave a child unattended while brushing their teeth.	**8.** To prevent injury as an inpatient.

Table 10.4 General conditions that may compromise oral well-being

General conditions that may compromise oral well-being	Specific examples	Oral complications that may be experienced
Impaired/altered physical dexterity	Cerebral palsy Accidents or other illness causing: • neurological damage • unconsciousness • loss of limb maxillofacial injury.	Difficulty or inability to perform oral hygiene resulting in: • build-up of plaque • dental caries • halitosis. Ataxia or spasticity may increase risk of damage to mucosa and soft tissue structures
Physical complications	Restricted oral access due to: • orthodontic or maxillofacial surgery • enlarged, protruding tongue • respiratory problems • epidermolysis bullosa • restricted movement of tongue due to surgery or pain • chronic constipation • cleft palate (may have prosthesis). Intubated and nursed in the intensive care environment particularly for neonates or infants that are orally intubated	May cause difficulty in performing oral hygiene (as above) Mouthbreathing causing dry mucosa Increased risk of mucosal deterioration Ineffective removal of debris Foul mouth and odour Lips, gums, palate prone to pressure sores; retention of food debris under prosthesis
Fragile mucosa	Effects of chemo/radiotherapy Epidermolysis bullosa Preterm neonate	Mucositis, ulceration, causing: • pain • infection • -bleeding
Children with special needs	Down's syndrome and other disabling conditions	Tendency towards thick, ropy, sticky saliva which adheres to the surface of teeth and forms plaque Deformed teeth may retain plaque
	Habitual licking or biting of lips	Dry, cracked or inflamed lips Discomfort
	Teeth alignment abnormalities	Require effective cleaning to avoid build-up of debris
Children with reduced level of consciousness	Child who is dying Following epileptic seizure Head injury Post-surgical procedure Physical injury Infection Toxic injury Sedation during intensive care and intubation for mechanical ventilation	Oral care should be performed twice daily by healthcare professional/parent/carer, since the mouth can become dry or coated with mucus
Immunodeficiencies	HIV Post cytotoxic therapy Combined immune deficiency	Reduced production of protective immunoglobulins in saliva resulting in increased risk of infection Persistent *Candida* infections
Common childhood illnesses and dental habits	Measles Fever Grinding of teeth Thumb sucking	Koplik, white spots Dryness, coated tongue, halitosis Mild/severe loss of tooth surface Alteration to position of teeth (upper, anterior)
Poor nutritional intake	Anorexia Dehydration Chronic disorders requiring high intake of refined oral carbohydrates, e.g. glycogen storage disease	Vitamin deficiency, tissue vulnerability Dryness, halitosis Increase in dental caries Oral ulceration
Foreign body in nose	Commonly inserted are peas, peanuts and small toys	Sudden foul odour in the mouth

(Continued)

199

Table 10.4 (*Continued*)

General conditions that may compromise oral well-being	Specific examples	Oral complications that may be experienced
Drugs	Antibiotics	Altered oral flora, increased risk of opportunistic infections
	Antihistamine	Reduced salivary production
	Atropine	Reduced salivary production
	Chlorhexidine based mouthwash	Temporary brown staining of teeth
		Stinging/burning sensation
		Bitter taste, altered after taste
		Delayed healing of tissue
	Corticosteroids	Gum hyperplasia
	Cyclosporin	Altered taste perception (often metallic)
	Cytotoxic agents	Saliva absent or ropy
	Diuretics	Altered salivary function
	Insulin	Altered salivary function
	Iron supplements	Temporary green/black staining of teeth
	Long-term, high sugar content medication, e.g. lactulose	Increased incidence of dental caries
	Morphine	Dry mucosa
	Nifedipine	Gingival enlargement
	Oxygen therapy	Dry mucosa
	Phenytoin	Gingival hypertrophy

Principles table 10.3 Oral care during compromised health

Principle	Rationale
1. If the child has been assessed as having swallowing difficulties: • Commence a fluid balance chart • Consider monitoring their weight • Contact the child's dietician • Use a local anaesthetic spray if prescribed. Discuss pain management with appropriate personnel.	1. To maintain adequate hydration. To ensure nutritional adequacy.
2. If the child has been assessed as having plaque or debris on their teeth: • Consider referral to the dentist • Consider a dietary referral • Commence health education as and when appropriate.	2. Risk factors are available against which to assess children and teenagers (SIGN 2000).

Immuno-compromised children

1. All children, regardless of diagnosis, should use a soft toothbrush and toothpaste twice a day.	1. To ensure that all children undergoing chemotherapy receive appropriate mouth care.
2. An oral care protocol should be in place.	2. Ensures standardised and appropriate care is given (Gibson *et al* 1997, Nelson *et al* 2001).
3. When the oral cavity lies within the treatment field, radiotherapy will exert a direct effect, decreasing cell renewal with the resulting complications.	3. Decreased cell renewal results in: • Epithelial thinning • Inflammation • Ulceration • An increased risk of secondary infection.
4. A number of the chemotherapy agents used are known to cause oral stomatitis.	4. Reduced bone marrow activity results in an increased risk of: • Bleeding due to thrombocytopenia • Infection due to neutropenia.

Principles table 10.3 (*Continued*)

Principle	Rationale
Oral phobia	
1. Children who have been, or who are intubated are known to experience problems having oral hygiene carried out, leading to oral phobia.	
2. Oral care should be assessed on an individual basis but intubated children should: • Have their teeth cleaned as normal • Have Vaseline applied to their lips.	
3. The endotracheal tube will need to be repositioned to the opposite side of their mouth if they are intubated orally. Liaise with appropriate nurse specialist.	
Children with epidermolysis bullosa	
1. Only the use of a mouthwash may be possible.	1. To ensure the mucosal integrity is maintained.
2. Some mouth washes contain alcohol and therefore sting.	
3. Strong flavours should be avoided.	
4. A small toothbrush or foam cleaning sponges may be used.	4. To prevent infection.
5. An electric toothbrush (small round oscillating head) may be used for front teeth and wherever access permits.	5. To maintain comfort and dignity of the patient.
Stomatitis due to *Candida albicans*	
1. This is quite common in childhood and is treated with oral nystatin. *Candida albicans* appears as slightly raised white patches, generally starting on the tongue, spreading to the mucous membranes of the gums cheeks and palate.	1. It may be associated with: • Gastrointestinal disturbances when children are cutting teeth • Antibiotic therapy • Immunosuppresion • A lack of cleanliness.
The neonate/infant in high dependency or intensive care	
1. Neonates and infants within the intensive care environment may be intubated orally or may be receiving oxygen therapy. Regular cleaning and moistening of the lips and all parts of the mouth should be done using foam sponges or cotton wool buds soaked in sterile water followed by liquid paraffin (see section on performing oral care).	1. Oral intubation and the presence of an artificial tube renders lubrication of the mouth and lips difficult and debris may build up. Oxygen is also likely to cause further dryness of the lips, tongue and mucous membranes.
2. This should be done at regular intervals depending on age and gestation and how the sick neonate tolerates interventions; ideally 4–6 hourly if condition allows. This will be less frequent in the preterm/low birthweight neonate (8 hourly).	2. The sick preterm neonate is more prone to physiological stress during interventions and the concept of 'minimal handling' should be considered (Bauer 2005, Khurana *et al* 2005)
3. The neonate/infant who is compromised in this way should have close observation of their lips and mouth for excoriation from the presence of tubes as well as for the presence of *Candida* inside the mouth.	3. Artificial tubes (endotracheal or feeding) can cause friction particularly during movement or if they are in place for significant time periods. In addition, any such tube in place is a potential infection risk.

201

Eye care

Eyes should be clean and free of any discharge or debris. If this is the case, cleaning the eyes should not be routine and restricted to the presence of certain conditions such suspected or actual infection, encrustation, excessive stickiness or any other known specific disease. In addition, eye care may be necessary when the baby/child is unable to naturally lubricate the eyes themselves due to surgery or when receiving muscle relaxants, leading to potential dryness and damage.

However, it must be acknowledged that parents/carers may incorporate eye care into their baby or child's hygiene routine at home. If appropriate, gentle cleansing can be performed unless there is any reason for the eyes not to be touched, such as existing damage or avoidance of unnecessary handling in an unstable patient. This should be discussed with the parents/carers and reasons explained.

If eye care is performed, aseptic technique principles should always be adhered to in the hospital environment. In healthy or the older child where cleaning the eyes is part of the overall washing routine, it need not be aseptic. The use of clean, tap water suffices in this case.

Procedure guideline 10.15 Eye care

Statement	Rationale
General eye cleansing (aseptic)	
1. Prepare all equipment – sterile water or boiled, cool tap water, sterile gauze swabs and galipot or an eye care pack, sterile gloves.	1. For adequate preparation.
2. Ensure the baby or child is in an appropriate position and is stable enough to undergo the procedure – e.g. is not stressed from too much handling and is exhibiting vital signs within normal limits. In addition, explain and reassure the procedure to the parents/carers or child if they are old enough to understand.	2. For ease of procedure and accessibility of the baby or child. To prevent causing any undue or further stress. The child/parent may be fearful of the procedure so reassurance is essential to minimise anxiety.
3. Pour sterile water or cooled, boiled water into a sterile galipot.	3. To prevent infection from bacteria present in non-sterile water.
4. Wet sterile gauze swabs, one by one, and gently wipe across bottom lid of eye from inner to outer corner. Use one swab for each swipe and discard. Clean until discharge has been removed.	4. To avoid cross-infection between each eye.
5. Clean both eyes in this way ensuring that separate swabs are used for each eye.	5. As above.
6. Repeat as necessary. Eye cleansing is usually carried out during hygiene/care sessions (Johnson and Taylor 2010) – this will be determined by the condition of the eyes and the baby/child's normal routine as discussed.	6. Frequency should be individualised to each baby/child.
7. During any eye care at any age, assess and observe eyes for stickiness, discharge, encrustation, dryness, trauma and redness.	7. To identify potential infection, damage or other condition that warrants specific eye care/treatment.
Specific eye care	
1. If the above occurs, specific eye treatment is necessary. Firstly, if there is discharge or excess stickiness present, take a swab for culture and sensitivity and send to the microbiology laboratory. Consider if it may be a viral infection and take appropriate sample (see Chapter 14 Investigations).	1. For appropriate antibiotics to be commenced following culture.
2. For any age, in the presence of infection or other known disease, apply prescribed eye cream to bottom of each eyelid using a separate pack for each eye. Similarly, eyes drops may be prescribed – one vial for each eye. Apply by gently retracting the upper and lower eye lid and dropping one drop to each eye.	2. Eye creams may have antibiotic properties and should form part of the total eye care regimen. Having separate vials/packs avoids cross-infection between each eye. Gentle application is necessary to avoid damage to the delicate area around the eyes.

Procedure guideline 10.15 (*Continued*)

Statement	Rationale
3. Eye ointment or drops should be applied in the same way to the baby or child who is receiving muscle relaxants or requires care for excessive dryness. In a baby/child who is totally immobilised, moist, lubricating gel pads can be used and replaced regularly according to recommended guidelines for use.	**3.** Some eye preparations are designed for lubrication of the eye to prevent dryness and corneal damage.
4. If there is discharge with persistent tearing but no infection is diagnosed, there may be a blocked tear duct (dacryostenosis). Discharge should be wiped away (as above for general cleansing) when this builds up and the side of the nose can be gently massaged.	**4.** This condition is common in newborns and infants and should diminish within the first year of life.
5. If cleaning is required more than 4–6 times a day, antibiotics may be required (www.keepkidshealthy.com).	**5.** Infection may be a secondary occurrence.
6. In any child, specific eye diseases will warrant individual care regimes as prescribed by the medical staff; some examples are: • Contagious conjunctivitis (bacterial or viral); antibiotics/antiviral agents will be required • Allergic reaction resulting in redness, swelling, itching and tearing; antihistamines or drops will be required and possibly steroids • Stye (infection at the base of the eyelash); warm compress and antibiotics • Corneal abrasions will require lubricating and antibiotic ointment • Trauma, chemical burns, lacerations and cuts will require immediate medical attention (www.mcg.edu/pediatrics).	**6.** For specific treatment to be tailored to the individual eye condition that the baby or child presents with.
7. For eye care in relation to any of the above-mentioned conditions, repeat as necessary with subsequent care sessions (Johnson and Taylor 2010) or as conditions warrants. If prescribed drops or ointments are administered, continue according to pharmacists' recommendations.	
8. When no further discharge, infection or immobility is present, review and assess the eyes for continuing problems, discontinuing treatment on consultation with the medical team.	

Administration of eye drops

Topical drug delivery for the treatment of eye disease remains the preferred route, as many regions of the eye are relatively inaccessible to systemically administered drugs. Drugs are delivered to treat infections, to provide intraocular treatment for diseases such as glaucoma, and pre and post surgical procedures.

Topical drug delivery is itself complicated by effective removal mechanisms that include the blinking reflex, tear turnover and low corneal permeability. Further complications include patient anxiety and the difficulty found in administering them.

Drugs administered as eye drops penetrate directly into the cornea. The cornea is considered to be the main pathway for the permeation of drugs into the eye. The cornea is an optically transparent tissue that conveys images to the back of the eye and covers about one-sixth of the total surface area of the eyeball (Agarwal *et al* 2002, Bartlett and Jaanes 2008, Wilson *et al* 2005). The concentration of drug in the precorneal area provides the driving force for its transport across the cornea via passive diffusion. Thus, efficient ocular drug absorption requires good corneal penetration as well as prolonged contact with the corneal tissue.

As previously mentioned, eye drops are used to treat conditions such as glaucoma and conjunctivitis, and are used pre and post surgical procedures, for conditions such as cataracts, glaucoma and squints.

Glaucoma refers to increased pressure on the inside of the eyeball. The increased pressure is usually caused by an obstruction to or the absence of the aqueous drainage system. Conservative treatment usually consists of anti-inflammatory eye drops such as Betoptic, which works by decreasing the production of aqueous humour. Surgical management aims to create a drainage system through performing a goniotomy or a

203

trabeculectomy, following which steroid and antibiotic eye drops would be administered (Agarwal *et al* 2002, Bartlett and Jaanes 2008, Wilson *et al* 2005).

Squint repair involves surgery that moves the muscles back to their correct alignment through resecting the muscles of the eyeball. Maxitrol drops are given post operatively to reduce the swelling and assist prevention of infection in the newly repaired squint.

Types of drops used for eye treatment include:

- Mydriatic-cycloplegic
- Coricosteroids

- Antibiotics.

A mydriatic drug dilates the pupil and is used for pre surgical procedures that require visualisation of structures behind the iris such as cataract extraction and vitrectomy. Drugs used would be atropine or cyclopentolate.

Combinations of corticosteroids and antibiotics are used to suppress inflammation following ophthalmic surgery. Examples include betamethasone (Betnesol) and dexamethasone (Maxitrol) (Agarwal *et al* 2002, Bartlett and Jaanes 2008, MA/RPSGB 2010, Wilson *et al* 2005).

Procedure guideline 10.16 Administration of eye drops

Statement	Rationale
1. Ensure the drops have been prescribed correctly on the child's prescription chart.	1. To adhere to hospital drug policy.
2. Prepare the patient and family explaining the procedure, including information about the drops.	2. To relieve anxiety and determine the level of cooperation.
3. Liaise with the family as to how the child will be positioned, i.e. is someone needed to help hold the child in a safe position or do they needed to be wrapped in a blanket.	3. To ensure the safety of the child and accurate instillation.
4. Ensure a separate bottle for each eye is available if both eyes require treatment.	4. To prevent cross-infection.
5. Ensure the drops used are for the named patient only and have not been used for other patients.	5. To prevent cross-infection.
6. Advise parents/carers of the importance of correct instillation.	6. To enhance their understanding of effective technique.
7. Wash your hands thoroughly.	7. To adhere to hospital infection control policy and to prevent infection.
8. Tilt the child's head back or lie them flat.	8. To ensure accurate instillation.
9. With your forefinger gently pull down the lower eyelid to form a pocket.	9. To ensure accurate instillation.
10. Place the dropper close to the child's eye (avoid touching the eye, eye lashes or any other surface) and administer the correct amount of drops into the lower eyelid.	10. To ensure accurate instillation.
11. Release the lower eyelid and allow the child to blink.	11. To ensure the whole eye is covered by the drug.
12. Wipe away any excess fluid.	12. To prevent irritation to the surrounding area.
13. If another drop or another type of drug is required repeat the same process waiting for a few minutes before proceeding.	13. The fornix can only accommodate one drop. Extra will overspill possibly leading to systemic absorption.
14. If an ointment is required prepare the child as above and apply by squeezing a thin line of the ointment starting at the inside corner of the eye and allow the child to blink.	14. To ensure accurate administration.
15. If using drops and ointments, use the drop first then wait 5 minutes before applying the ointment.	15. To prevent overspill and ensure accurate administration.

Contact lenses

Children of all ages may wear contact lenses instead of spectacles although those in the younger age group (less than 8 years old) are likely to have had their lenses fitted in a hospital eye department.

Contact lenses are small, thin optical lenses worn on the front surface of the eye to correct refractive eye problems, such as myopia, hyperopia and astigmatism. There are two types of contact lenses: soft lenses and rigid gas permeable (RGP) lenses. Soft lenses are larger than the diameter of the cornea, whereas RGPs have a diameter smaller than that of the cornea. Contact lenses are not to be worn while asleep, as this can cause irreversible changes to the cornea.

Children may have to wear contact lenses as a consequence of surgical removal of congenital cataracts, high refractive error, or congenital anterior segment abnormalities. They may have very high prescription soft lenses or they may have a cosmetic lens with a painted iris to camouflage an abnormal iris.

As well as fitting lenses to help improve the eyesight, contact lenses are occasionally used to act as a bandage on the eye for example after surgery or injury. These lenses may be thinner and larger than standard contact lenses. They are inserted and removed in the same way as other soft lenses but this may be more difficult as the eye can be particularly uncomfortable.

Inserting and removing the lenses is usually done by the patient or parent/carer but at times the lens may need to be dealt with by the nursing staff, for example if a child is going to theatre. In a young child who is upset, it is easier to insert and remove the lenses when they are asleep.

Some patients may wear daily disposable lenses which are thrown away after every use and require no solutions, just instructions to always wash the hands before touching either the eyes or the lenses and never to reuse the lens on a second day. If the lenses are not daily disposable, there are likely to be between one and three special solutions that are used to clean and disinfect contact lenses. Tap water should never be used on the lenses as it may contain various organisms that can cause eye infections.

Maintaining contact lens hygiene is paramount. The parents/carers and patient should have been made aware of the importance of keeping the contact lenses clean since eye infections associated with contact lenses can result in the vision being affected and in rare instances can lead to blindness (BCLA 2011, Ventocilia and Wicker 2010).

In an emergency, soft lenses can be removed using a pair of round ended forceps and rigid lenses can be removed using a rubber sucker (if available). This should be performed by a skilled practitioner.

Procedure guideline 10.17 Insertion of contact lenses

Statement	Rationale
1. Wash hands thoroughly.	1. To reduce risk of lens contamination
2. Remove the lens from the case and make sure it is clean.	
3. Position the lens on the tip of the index finger of your right hand (left hand if left-handed). Make sure the lens is right side out.	3. To ensure accurate insertion.
4. Hold upper eyelid with your left hand. Pull lower lid downward with the middle finger of right hand.	4. To ensure accurate insertion.
5. Place the lens gently on the eye. If inserting a lens in a child's eye, you may need to push the lens under the upper lid first. The lens will naturally centre on the eye once the lids are closed.	5. To ensure accurate insertion.
6. Release lower eyelid first and then gradually release the upper eyelid.	6. To ensure lens is not blinked out.

Procedure guideline 10.18 Removal of soft contact lenses

Statement	Rationale
1. Wash your hands thoroughly.	1. To reduce risk of lens contamination.
2. Hold the upper eyelid with your left hand. Pull your lower lid downward with the middle finger of your right hand.	2. To ensure accurate removal.
3. Use the index finger and thumb of your right hand to pinch the lens gently out of the eye. To remove soft contact lenses from a young child, see directions in next section.	3. To ensure accurate removal.

Procedure guideline 10.19 **Removal of gas permeable contact lenses and all contact lenses from children**

Statement	Rationale
1. Wash your hands thoroughly.	**1.** To reduce risk of lens contamination.
2. Hold upper eyelid with your left hand. Pull lower lid downward with a finger or thumb of your right hand.	**2.** To ensure accurate removal.
3. Push both lids against globe and towards each other. The lens will be pushed out by the pressure from the lids.	**3.** To ensure accurate removal.

206

Procedure guideline 10.20 **Care of contact lenses**

Statement	Rationale
1. Cleaning: immediately after removing the lens from the eye, rub in the palm of the hand with cleaning solution.	**1.** To remove build up of daily debris.
2. Rinsing: after cleaning the lens, rinse the lens with saline.	**2.** To ensure cleaning solution has been removed.
3. Disinfecting: place the clean lens in a clean lens container filled with fresh disinfecting solution to store the lens.	**3.** To prevent infection. The case should be cleaned, rinsed and air dried before new disinfecting solution is used. Contact lens cases are a common source of infection and need to be cleaned inside and outside after each use.
4. Ensure that the right and left contact lenses are placed in appropriate sections of case.	**4.** To ensure correct lens is used.

Ear care

Children who have an obstruction in the ear such as wax or dried blood (post surgery) or have an infection may need to have ear drops to remove the obstruction. These may be simple softening drops or drops that contain antibiotics with or without anti-inflammatory properties.

Ear drops can be used if there is an infection of the outer ear canal (otitis externa) or the middle ear (otitis media) if the ear drum is perforated.

Otitis externa

This is an inflammation of the ear canal between the ear drum and the outside of the ear. Because of its warm dark environment, the ear canal is a perfect medium for bacteria and fungus to grow. With otitis externa children will complain of an 'itchy ear' and the ear feeling full or plugged up. Following this the ear will become red, swollen and extremely painful. It can be treated by cleaning out the ear and administering ear drops.

Otitis media

Normally the middle ear is filled with air and relies on three tiny bones to transmit the sound signals to the inner ear. In the case of infection, pus, fluid and inflammation are produced in the middle ear, the area behind the eardrum. With otitis media, older children will complain of ear pain, ear fullness, dizziness or hearing loss. Younger children may demonstrate irritability, fussiness, tugging of the ear, or have difficulty in sleeping, feeding or hearing. Children of any age may have a high temperature.

Antibiotics are an effective treatment for otitis media if it is caused by bacterial infection and Augmentin would be the drug of choice. In association with these oral medications, ear drops can be employed, after medical assessment. If there is a perforation of the ear drum, Ciprofloxacin hydrochloride is used, primarily because of its anti-inflammatory properties. If the ear drum is unperforated, Sofradex can be useful.

In situations where the otitis media is not caused by a bacterial infection symptomatic treatment is undertaken, namely analgesia and ear drops.

Ear drops that may be prescribed are:

- Chloramphenicol 5% – 2–3 drops, 3 times daily
- Gentisone HC – 2–4 drops, 3–4 times daily and once at night

- Betnesol N – 2–3 drops, 3–4 times daily; reduce when getting better
- Sofradex – 2–3 drops, 2–4 times daily
- Genticin – 2–3 drops, 3–4 times daily and once at night
- Ciprofloxacin hydrochloride- 3 drops, 2 times daily, for 7 days.

Procedure guideline 10.21 **Administration of ear drops**

Statement	Rationale
1. Inform the child if they are old enough to understand, and their family, that you are going to administer the ear drops.	**1.** To obtain verbal consent for the procedure. To obtain their cooperation if they are old enough.
2. Answer any questions they may have about their ear drops.	**2.** To allay any worries that they may have. To address their information needs.
3. Check prescription.	**3.** To minimise risk of drug error.
4. Check that the eardrops are prescribed according to the policies used by the hospital.	
5. Ensure that: • The correct ear drops are written on the drug chart • The correct route and instruction, i.e. one or both ears, is written on the drug chart • The correct strength is stated • The number of drops is stated • The frequency is stated.	**5.** To minimise risk of drug error.
6. Prepare the drug.	
7. Prepare the equipment to administer the drops: the correct ear drops, some cotton wool or gauze swabs on a tray.	
8. Prior to the procedure wash your hands.	**8.** To minimise the risk of cross-infection.
9. The procedure: **a)** Check that the name of the patient and hospital number on their identity bracelet matches that on the prescription chart and that their name is also on the bottles of drops **b)** Tilt the head to one side making sure the child is comfortable and ensuring their head is supported. **c)** Gently pull the ear lobe out and upwards to straighten the ear canal. **d)** Place the ear drops in the ear canal – if necessary squeeze the bottle gently to allow the drops to fall. **e)** Keep the head tilted for at least 2 minutes to allow the drops to reach the area required. **f)** If required, repeat for the other ear. **g)** If there is any oozing from the ear, dab it dry with the cotton wool or gauze. **h)** Re-wash hands after the ear drops have been administered.	**9.** **a)** To ensure the drops are given to the correct patient. Single patient use bottles must be used to prevent cross-contamination.
10. Sign the child's drug prescription chart.	**10.** To determine responsibility for administration.
11. Record the administration of the drug in the child's daily healthcare records	**11.** To maintain an accurate record.

Pressure ulcer prevention

Pressure ulcers are areas of localised damage to the skin, which can extend to underlying structures such as muscle and bone (Allman *et al* 1995, 1997). Damage is believed to be caused by a combination of factors including pressure, shear, friction and moisture (Allman *et al* 1995). Pressure ulcers can develop in any area of the body (Rycroft-Malone and McInnes 2000) but generally occur over bony prominences (Jones *et al* 2001, Murdoch 2002, Willock *et al* 1999).

In young children the head (occiput, ears) is particularly at risk due to its disproportionate size in infancy. Pressure ulcers may also arise due to the incorrect use, fixation or application of equipment or medical devices, e.g. splints, chest braces, probes, catheters, etc (*Willock et al* 1999).

Individuals at particular risk of pressure ulcer development include those undergoing surgery, in critical care, with orthopaedic conditions or with spinal injury (NICE 2005).

Potential risk factors associated with pressure ulcer development included (adapted from NICE 2005):

- Pressure
- Shearing
- Friction
- Impaired or restricted mobility/immobility
- Sensory impairment
- Reduced level of consciousness
- Reduced skin /tissue perfusion secondary to disease process or medication, e.g. inotropes
- Incontinence, urinary or faecal (inappropriate to age and/or developmental stage) and other sources of moisture, e.g. oedema, sweat, wound exudate
- Acute, chronic and terminal illness
- Posture
- Cognition, psychosocial status
- Previous history of pressure ulceration
- Malnutrition/dehydration
- Co-morbidity (for example, assess systemic signs of infection, blood supply, pain, medication).

The development of pressure ulcers can be exacerbated by:

1. Disease processes (including depression and mental illness). Many disease processes predispose children to pressure ulcer formation by precipitating the risk factors described above. Emotional disturbance and psychiatric conditions can affect motivation, the ability to self-care or the ability to cooperate with care being provided.
2. Infection. Infection can lead to the deterioration of otherwise minor lesions particularly if the immune system is compromised.
3. Changes in environment, carer or equipment. Skin breakdown associated with changing circumstances is primarily influenced by failures in communication. On discharge or transfer of the 'at risk' child, the following should be communicated: level of risk; equipment/prevention strategies required; size, grade, position and treatment regimen of any existing pressure ulcers (Figure 10.7). This information should be provided in writing and verbally at the time of discharge/transfer (RCN 2005).

Pressure ulcers are, in most cases, avoidable provided adequate early assessment takes place and preventative measures are implemented. Pressure damage is dependent on the application of a force, i.e. pressure, shear, friction or a combination of these (Bridel 1993). Early assessment should identify the potential exposure of each child to these forces and allow for intervention before damage occurs in vulnerable children (Quigley and Curley 1996).

Assessment: risk

Risk assessment should be used as an adjunct to clinical judgment and not as a tool in isolation from other clinical features. A guide to completing a risk assessment should be at the bedside of all patients (see Figure 10.8). The assessment should take place within 6 hours of admission using the agreed tool (see Figure 10.9).

Pre-admitted patients and patients admitted on the day of surgery should be reassessed on return from recovery. ICU patients need to be assessed daily, but daycase patients do not need to be assessed.

The risk assessment must be documented, signed and dated by the assessor. The use of an assessment tool has been proven to identify patients that are at risk of developing a pressure ulcer. Early research has shown that there are paediatric based assessment tools that have proven to be sensitive and specific in certain paediatric populations (Gray 2004).

The child's parent/carer should be involved in the assessment process and advised regarding their role in identifying the early stages of skin breakdown. The child's parent/carer will often be the first to notice any skin changes given their level of interaction with the child and familiarity with skin through dressing, changing nappies, bathing, etc. Education regarding the early signs of pressure damage will assist the parent/carer in protecting their child long term from such complications. Information provided should be targeted at parents/carers where the child is identified as at risk in order to avoid creating unnecessary concerns in unaffected families. All parents/carers should, however, have access to relevant educational materials on request.

Assessment: skin

All children should have their skin assessed for pre-existing damage on admission and the findings documented. It is important to obtain a baseline skin assessment when a child arrives in a clinical area so that any damage if present can be identified and promptly treated. (RCN 2005). Early skin assessment will also avoid confusion regarding when and how the damage occurred if it is later the subject of a complaint or clinical incident.

In certain instances this may not be possible due to:

- The nature of the presenting illness
- Objection of child/carer
- Religious/cultural reasons
- Issues related to the maintenance of the privacy and dignity of the child.

Reasons for the assessment not taking place should also be documented.

Intact skin

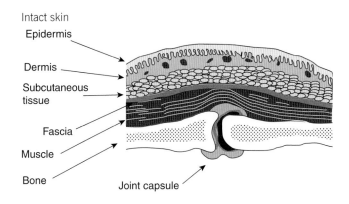

Grade 1 Non-blanchable erythema of intact skin. Discolouration of the skin, warmth, oedema, induration or hardness may also be used as indicators particularly on darker skin

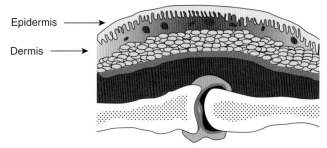

Grade 2 Partial thickness skin loss involving epidermis or dermis or both. The ulcer is superficial and presents clinically as an abrasion or blister

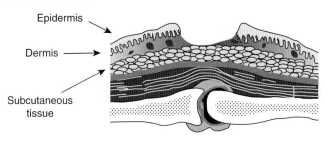

Grade 3 Full thickness skin loss involving damage to or necrosis of subcutaneous tissue that may extend down to, but not through, underlying fascia

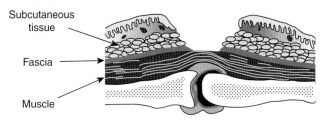

209

Grade 4 Extensive destruction, tissue necrosis, or damage to muscle, bone or supporting structures with or without full thickness skin loss

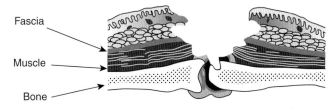

Figure 10.7 Images based on material from the European Pressure Ulcer Advisory Panel (1999) Pressure Ulcer Prevention Guidelines.

Pressure ulceration generally occurs over bony prominences. Children under 2 years have proportionally larger heads, less hair and less occipital subcutaneous tissue, when compared to older children and adults. This leads to an increased risk of skin breakdown over the occipital region when lying supine (Solis 1988, Neidig 1989).

The assessor should pay particular attention to the:

- Occiput (back of head)
- Ears
- Heels
- Sacrum.

Identifying the early signs of pressure ulcer formation allows healthcare professionals to intervene quickly, preventing significant loss of tissue and associated complications.

The assessor should be aware of:

- Persistent erythema (redness of the skin)
- Non-blanching erythema (red skin that does not go white and return to red following the application of light finger pressure)

- Blisters
- Discolouration
- Localised heat, oedema or induration (hardness of skin).

Very careful assessment is required for children with darkly pigmented skin

The following signs may indicate pressure damage in darkly pigmented skin:

- Early stages:
  - purplish/bluish localised areas of skin
  - localised heat.
- More advanced:
  - localised coolness
  - localised oedema and induration.

Note: Skin temperature is assessed as relative to surrounding skin.

The child's general skin condition should also be noted (e.g. dryness, cracking, erythema, maceration, excoriation, fragility, temperature, swelling, fluid leakage). Any impairment of skin

**Paediatric Pressure Ulcer
Risk Assessment Tool**

Great Ormond Street **NHS**
Hospital for Children
NHS Trust

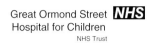

Notes for use:
- Look at the categories. Look across and read the acuity of illness statements in each box. Match the score to the statement that reflect your patient's current condition. Total the scores for the five categories and your patient with then have a 'at risk' score.
- Scores of 10 or less indicate your patient is <u>at risk</u> of developing a pressure ulcer. You will need to <u>implement</u> the <u>nursing interventions</u> that can be found <u>below</u> and also on the front page of the Risk Assessment documentation record.
- A copy of this tool should be kept at the beside of each patient within their nursing notes

Risk factor	Score 1	Score 2	Score 3	Score 4
Mobility	**Completely immobile** – does not make changes in body or extremity position without assistance. Patient cannot physiologically tolerate position changes.	**Very limited** – Makes occasional slight changes in body or extremity position but unable to turn self independently.	**Slightly limited** – Makes frequent changes in body or extremity position independently.	**No limitations** – Makes major changes in position without assistance.
Activity	**Bed bound** – Confined to bed.	**Chair bound** – Ability to walk is severely limited or non-existent. Cannot bear own weight. Needs help to get into chair or wheelchair.	**Walks occasionally** – Walks occasionally for short distances with or without help. Spends majority of shift in bed or chair.	**All patients too young to walk or patient walks frequently** – Walks frequently.
Sensory perception	**Completely limited** – Unresponsive to painful stimuli due to altered GCS or sedation. Inability to feel pain over most of body surface.	**Very limited** – Responds to painful stimuli. Cannot communicate discomfort verbally or has sensory impairment, limiting ability to feel pain over half of body.	**Slightly limited** – Responds to verbal commands but cannot always communicate discomfort. Has sensory impairment, limiting ability to feel pain or discomfort in 1 or 2 extremities.	**No impairment** – Responds to verbal commands. Has no sensory deficit that limits ability to feel or communicate pain or discomfort.
Moisture	**Constantly moist** – Skin is kept moist almost constantly, by perspiration, urine, drainage etc. Dampness is detected every time patient is moved. Linen, nappy/pad or dressing changes are constant.	**Very moist** – Skin is often but not always moist. Linen, nappy/pad or dressing changes every 2 to 4 hours.	**Occasionally moist** – Skin is occasionally moist. Nappy/pad changes as routine. Dressing/linen change every shift.	**Rarely moist** – Continent. Dressing changes as routine. Linen changed every 24 hours.
Tissue perfusion	**Extremely compromised** – Hypotensive or patient is requiring inotrope support. Patient requires mechanical ventilation. Patient cannot physiologically tolerate position changes.	**Compromised** – Normotensive. Oxygen saturation of <95%. Haemoglobin may be <10mg/dl. Capillary refill may be >2 seconds. Serum pH is <7.35.	**Adequate** – Normotensive. Oxygen saturation of <95%. Haemoglobin may be <10mg/dl. Capillary refill may be <2 seconds. Serum pH is normal.	**Ideal** – Normotensive. Oxygen saturation normal. Normal haemoglobin level. Capillary refill <2 seconds. Normal serum pH.

Version No: 1.0	Version date: 18/12/07	Document development lead: Mathew Garner

**Paediatric Pressure Ulcer
Care Plan for 'at risk' patients**

Great Ormond Street **NHS**
Hospital for Children
NHS Trust

Tool adapted from: Quigley SM and Curley MA (1996) Skin integrity in the pediatric population:
preventing and managing pressure ulcers. Journal of the Society of Pediatric Nurses 1(1) pp7–18

Nursing interventions required for a child scoring 10 or lower must include:

- Daily inspection of skin and bony prominences. The prophylactic use of a barrier film (e.g. Cavilon®) for children in nappies or pads

- A plan for re-positioning, ideally every 2 hours, except when the patient cannot physiologically tolerate position changes. The patient's skin should also be checked at these times. If the patient cannot be repositioned then the clinician who made this decision needs to document the reasons why in the medical notes.

- Use of repositioning record chart. ITU areas to use electronic documentation systems i.e. CareVue.

- Use of Repose® mattress. If the child has blanching/non-blanching erythema on this mattress, then an alternated air *mattress is indicated*

- Give family/carer a copy of the GOSH 'Looking after your child's skin advice leaflet'.

- Completed moving and handling assessment to reduce friction and shear

- Completed nutritional assessment to identify adequate dietary intake

- Reassessment must be recorded daily for all patients scored 'at risk'

Please refer to the Pressure Ulcer Clinical Guideline for further information; this is available through the Clinical Guidelines website. In addition you may wish to contact your Tissue Viability link nurse or the Clinical Nurse Specialist for Tissue Viability on ext 5929, or bleep 0982 if you have any further enquiries.

Figure 10.8 Paediatric pressure ulcer risk assessment tool. Kindly reproduced with permission from Great Ormond Street Hospital for Children NHS Foundation Trust.

Name:

Hosp #:

DOB:

Ward:

(Affix patient label)

Paediatric Pressure Ulcer Risk Assessment

Great Ormond Street **NHS**
Hospital for Children
NHS Trust

Date of assessment:	
Time of assessment (24 hour clock):	
Assessed by:	
Score on Admission:	
A score of 10 or lower indicates that the child is at risk of developing a pressure ulcer. Nursing interventions need to be implemented	
Documentation of reassessment – SEE REVERSE	

Notes for use

- Inspect skin and complete assessment tool within 6 hours of admission and then weekly or when significant change occurs.
- Pre-admitted patients and patients admitted through Dinosaur ward should be reassessed on return from Recovery.
- ICU patients should be assessed daily or when significant change occurs e.g. change in GCS or on extubation.
- Observe for signs of:
  - Blanching or non-blanching erythema
  - Blisters, oedema and existing pressure ulcers
  - Pay attention to occiput, ears, heels and sacrum
- Children with skin breakdown on admission should be treated as 'at risk' patients
- Also detail child's general skin condition, e.g. dry, eczematous, macerated, excoriated, healthy

Date Reassessed	Score	Initials	Date Reassessed	Score	Initials	Date Reassessed	Score	Initials	Date Reassessed	Score	Initials

Nursing interventions required for a child scoring 10 or lower must include:

- Daily inspection of skin and bony prominences. The prophylactic use of a barrier film (e.g. Cavilon®) for children in nappies or pads
- A plan for re-positioning, ideally every 2 hours, except when the patient cannot physiologically tolerate position changes. The patient's skin should also be checked at these times. If the patient cannot be repositioned then the clinician who made this decision needs to document the reasons why in the medical notes.
- Use of repositioning record chart. ITU areas to use electronic documentation systems, i.e. CareVue.
- Use of Repose® mattress. If the child has blanching/non-blanching erythema on this mattress, then an *alternating airmattress is indicated*
- Give family/carer a copy of the GOSH 'Looking after your child's skin advice leaflet'.
- Completed moving and handling assessment to reduce friction and shear
- Completed nutritional assessment to identify adequate dietary intake
- Reassessment must be recorded daily for all patients scored 'at risk'

A LAMINATED ASSESSMENT TOOL SHOULD BE KEPT AT THE BEDSIDE OF EACH PATIENT WITHIN THEIR NURSING NOTES

Figure 10.9 Paediatric pressure ulcer risk assessment chart. Kindly reproduced with permission from Great Ormond Street Hospital for Children NHS Foundation Trust.

integrity exposes the child to an increased risk of infection and may contribute to the risk of pressure damage by reducing the skin's capacity to resist the effects of pressure, shear and friction.

Re-assessment should take place weekly or following significant changes in the child's health status or environment (e.g. moves ward). Regular reassessment will take into account changes in the child's condition and the influences of changing physical circumstances. If a child is at risk their skin needs to be assessed every time they are repositioned.

Planning

A score of 10 or below on the Braden Q assessment tool constitutes a child being at risk.

If the child is identified as being at risk of developing a pressure ulcer a plan of care must be provided.

Care for a child scoring 10 or lower, must include:

- Daily inspection of skin and bony prominences
- The prophylactic use of a barrier film (e.g. Cavilon®) for children in nappies or pads. Barrier films protect the skin from moisture, shear, and friction, which can contribute to pressure ulcer development
- A plan for re-positioning at least every 2 hours, except when the patient cannot physiologically tolerate position changes (NICE 2005). If the child cannot be turned the child's consultant should explain the reason for this to the family and document this is the child's medical record
- Use of repositioning record chart. Early assessment should identify the potential exposure of each child to these forces and allow for intervention before damage occurs in vulnerable children (Quigley and Curley 1996)
- Use of specialist mattresses, e.g. Repose® mattress. Pressure-reducing base mattresses have been demonstrated to significantly reduce the incidence of pressure ulceration (Collins and Shipperley 1995). The mattress should be impervious to body fluids, cleaned regularly and checked annually for cover damage in order to avoid cross-contamination between patients (Cullum et al 2000). The mattress should not impact on any child's ability to rest or sleep
- Completed moving and handling assessment to reduce friction and shear
- Completed nutritional assessment to identify adequate dietary intake
- Give family/carer a copy of the local information leaflet on Looking after your child's skin advice leaflet (GOSH 2011).
- Children at significant risk of pressure ulcer development should be identified at shift changes and if the child is transferred to another ward area, unit or healthcare provider. This ensures prevention strategies are maintained.

Management: repositioning

Consider mobilising, positioning and repositioning interventions for all patients (including those in beds, chairs and wheelchair users). Acceptability to the patient and needs of the parent/carer should be considered (NICE 2005). Pressure ulcers occur primarily due to a sustained application of pressure, which reduces oxygenation and causes tissue distortion, leading to cell death (Bridel 1993).

All patients with pressure ulcers should actively mobilise or change their position or be repositioned frequently (NICE 2005). Frequent repositioning relieves pressure over vulnerable sites.

Minimise pressure on bony prominences and avoid positioning on pressure ulcer if present (NICE 2005). Any individual who is assessed to be at risk of developing pressure ulcers should be repositioned if it is medically safe to do so (European Pressure Ulcer Advisory Panel 1999).

Frequency of repositioning may be restricted by the child's medical condition, level of comfort and attached medical devices, e.g. IV cannulae and external fixators. In cases where patients cannot be adequately repositioned a suitable support surface should be used.

The minimum suggested time interval between repositioning is 2 hours. However, this should be adjusted according to the response of the child's skin to pressure, i.e. if the skin reddens after 2 hours reduce the time interval and reassess (European Pressure Ulcer Advisory Panel 1999). Capillary pressure varies between individuals (NICE 2005). Dermal capillary pressure may be compromised by impaired cardiac function, peripheral shutdown, ambient temperature and drug therapies, etc. An ill child may have significantly reduced dermal capillary pressure when compared to a healthy child (Landis 1930).

If there is no evidence of erythema, then turning may not be necessary, but a child still ought to be assessed every 2 hours.

Three of the possible positions and tilts used with patients are shown in Figure 10.10(a–c). The term '30° tilt' describes the use of pillows to position a patient off their bony prominences (hips and sacrum) so that weight is redistributed over the larger surface area of the buttocks. The tilt positions should not be used exclusively but to offer alternative positions to the traditional side-to-side turns. By having five alternative positions, the time period any part of the body is exposed to pressure is reduced (Figure 10.10(d–e)). It may be possible to extend the time period between 30° tilt positions as the pressure is spread over a greater surface area. Also because the patient does not need to be physically rolled it is often possible to reposition the patient without assistance.

Having placed the patient in the 30° tilt position it should be possible to place a hand beneath the patient and touch the sacrum ensuring that it is free of pressure (Figure 10.10f). Limb elevation is integral to 30° tilt. One or two pillows should be used (depending on limb size) to elevate the lower limbs leaving the heels extended over the end completely free of pressure (Figure 10.10g). This position should be adopted routinely for all at risk patients even if they are on a pressure-relieving mattress. (Most pressure relieving mattresses provide inadequate pressure relief at the heel.)

Tilting the foot end of the bed by 10–15° will prevent the patient slipping down the bed (Figure 10.10h). This has the dual effect of reducing exposure of the skin to shear and friction, thereby limiting the need for moving and handling by nursing staff. Nursing staff should be aware that this may increase pressure over the sacrum/buttocks, which may initially require more frequent observation. However, with a Repose® mattress (or similar) in situ increased risk of breakdown is negligible.

It is important to recognise the effects on the skin caused by manual handling and to minimise friction and shear by limiting the potential for rubbing or dragging the child's skin during

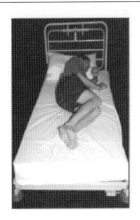
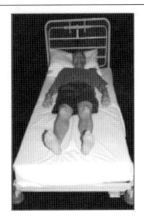
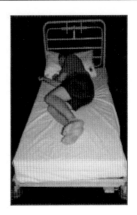

There are more than the three positions (above) into which patients can be repositioned.

30° tilt describes the use of pillows to position a patient off their bony prominences (hips & sacrum) so that weight is redistributed over the larger surface area of the buttocks

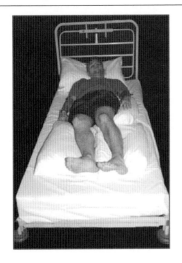

The "tilt" positions should not be used exclusively but offer alternative positions to traditional side-to-side turns. By having 5 alternative positions the time period any part of the body is exposed to pressure is reduced.

It may be possible to extend the time period between 30° tilt positions as the pressure is spread over a greater surface area.

Also because the patient does not need to be physically rolled it is often possible to reposition the patient without assistance.

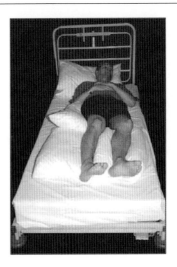

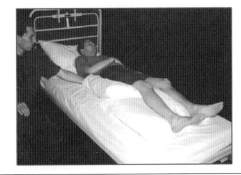

Having placed the patient in the 30° tilt position you should be able to place a hand beneath the patient and touch the sacrum ensuring that it is free of pressure.

Figure 10.10 Various positions and tilts.

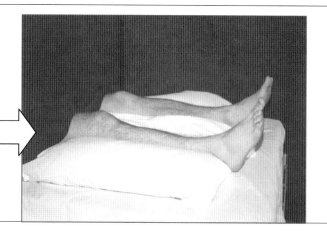

Limb elevation is integral to 30° tilt.
1 or 2 pillows should be used (depending on limb size) to elevate the lower limbs leaving the heels extended over the end completely free of pressure.

This position should be adopted routinely for all at risk patients even if they are on a pressure-relieving mattress. (Most pressure relieving mattresses provide inadequate pressure relief at the heel.)

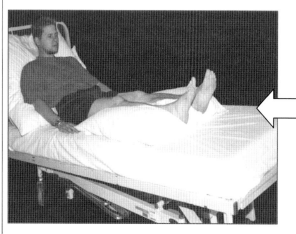

Tilting the foot end of the bed by 10-15° will prevent the patient slipping down the bed.

This has the dual effect of reducing exposure of the skin to shear and friction and limiting the need for moving and handling by nursing staff.

Nursing staff should be aware that this may increase pressure over the sacrum /buttocks which may initially require more frequent observation. However with a Repose® mattress (or similar) in situ increased risk of breakdown is negligible.

Figure 10.10 (*Continued*)

repositioning. Devices to assist manual handling, e.g. sliding sheets, hoists, should be used where possible to reduce the potential of skin damage to the child and injury to parents/carers.

Young children are encouraged to sit out of bed on their parent/carer's laps. This should not be discouraged in those at risk of pressure damage. Sitting out on the parent/carer's lap provides a positional change and is important for the child as it provides comfort and reassurance.

Older children at risk of pressure ulcer development should avoid sitting in chairs for prolonged periods. The agreed period of time should be recorded in the care plan and will generally be no longer than 2 hours (NICE 2002). The sitting position places susceptible children at particular risk due to the concentration of body weight upon the relatively small surface area of the buttocks (Bennett 1985).

Management: support surfaces – mattresses, cushions and other equipment

There are two main forms of pressure relieving support surface:

1. Continuous low pressure (CLP): The surface contours to the shape of the user thus spreading pressure over a larger surface area and reducing pressure at bony prominences. The surface may be air, gel, foam or fluid filled (or a combination of these).

2. Alternating pressure (AP): Alternate air cells inflate and deflate over a 7–10 minute cycle. The inflated cells support the user's weight while the deflated cells provide pressure relief.

All children irrespective of risk or medical status are entitled to a base mattress (for cot or bed) that is pressure reducing, comfortable, waterproof, clean and intact. Pressure-reducing base mattresses have been demonstrated to significantly reduce the incidence of pressure ulceration (Collins and Shipperley 1995). The mattress should be impervious to body fluids, cleaned regularly and checked annually for cover damage in order to avoid cross-contamination between patients (Cullum et al 2000).

Children identified as being at risk of developing pressure ulcers but who cannot be repositioned should be supplied with an appropriate pressure relieving support surface (see Figure 10.11 for an example of this type of mattress). Consult your local policy for alternative mattresses and for the hire of specialist beds/mattresses.

A manually inflated pressure relieving overlay mattress available in bed, cot and thermacot sizes. It is currently the first line mattress for the prevention & treatment of pressure ulcers at Great Ormond St Hospital but may also be used to promote comfort.

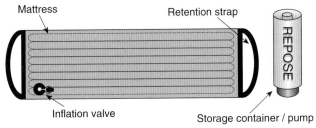

Method of use:
• Open canister & remove rolled up mattress.
• Unroll mattress onto a flat surface with the valve facing up.
• Put the canister back together to form the pump
• Attach the pump nozzle to the mattress valve securely and pump air into the mattress
• Full inflation is indicated by a backflow of air escaping from the valve.
• Once inflated the mattress should be laid on top of the base mattress with the valve at the foot end facing downwards. (To avoid disturbing patient if further inflation required)
• The retention straps should be fitted around the base mattress to secure it in place.
• The mattress can be used with or without a sheet. If a sheet is used it should be loosely tucked in. Despite being 'plastic' the mattress cover is breathable and sweat should not build up next to the skin. The mattress is particularly effective without a sheet when used for the prevention and management of occipital / ear pressure ulcers.
• If the mattress is punctured it cannot be repaired and should be thrown away.
• Check mattress is fully inflated at least once a week by adding 2–3 pumps of air and ensuring backflow occurs.
• The mattresses are for use on multiple patients provided usual infection control procedures are followed (see Chapter 12 Infection Prevention and Control).

Cleaning:
• After routine patient (i.e., no identified or suspected infection risk): Clean with neutral detergent and water and rinse thoroughly.
• After patient with identified infection risk (e.g. MRSA): Clean with hypochlorite solution & rinse thoroughly.
• N.B: Some topical agents may stain the mattress cover this does not mean that the mattress is dirty or unsuitable for use as long as routine cleansing has been performed.

To deflate in event of cardiac arrest pierce mattress with a sharp object

Figure 10.11 The Repose® mattress.

Comfort and the promotion of rest is a primary objective in respect to most disease processes, provision of equipment to support this goal is therefore justified.

Pillows, foam wedges, gamgee, etc, can be used to help maintain position but care should be taken that these do not interfere with the action of any other support surface in use. Many children by virtue of their disease process or developmental stage may have difficulty maintaining position (Ndawula and Brown 1990).

Pressure relieving mattresses should be covered by no more than a single, unfolded sheet that is not tucked in, in order to ensure effectiveness. Layers of bed linen between the child and a CLP support surface will prevent the surface contouring to the child's body shape leading to increased interface pressures. In the case of AP, excess bed linen can fill the space vacated by the deflated cells limiting the delivery of pressure relief. Tucking sheets in can, in both cases, cause problems. The taut bed sheet either limits contouring (CLP) or forms a bridge between inflated cells limiting the pressure relief provided by the deflated cells (AP).

There is no evidence that any of the following items listed are able to relieve pressure effectively and they may in some circumstances increase interface pressures (NICE 2002):

• Water filled gloves (Nichols 1996)
• Synthetic/genuine sheepskins (Lockyer-Stevens 1993)
• Doughnut-type devices
• Fibre-filled overlay mattresses, e.g. 'Spenco' (Lockyer-Stevens 1993).

In rare circumstances it is acceptable to use genuine/synthetic sheepskin or fibre-filled overlays but only to promote comfort not as, or in place of, a pressure-relieving device (Medical Devices Agency 1994).

Cleaning of mattresses

Always consult manufacturer's instructions before cleaning any equipment. If damage occurs manufacturers are reluctant to replace any faulty item if these instructions are not followed. Some central decontamination units will take on this role as quality control of the cleaning process is standardised and recorded centrally.

1. For routine use: clean cover with neutral detergent and water and dry well. Ensure there are no tears or leakage in the mattress. If this occurs the mattress should be replaced.
2. If contaminated with body fluids or following use by a patient with highly transmissible micro-organisms: after cleaning, as above, disinfect with 1000 ppm sodium hypochlorite solution.

Use of certain cleaning agents can damage the waterproofing of cover material. This applies especially to alcohol-based products, which should not be used under any circumstances.

Management: skin care

Soaps should be avoided when cleansing the skin of all children at risk of pressure ulceration. The recommended cleansing agent is aqueous cream. Soaps have a drying effect on the skin caused by the removal of natural oils. Normal skin is naturally acidic (pH 4.9). This environment provides a degree of antibacterial protection. Soap products can alter the pH of the skin. Many products contain preservatives and perfumes that can cause irritation/sensitisation (Irving 2001).

In neonates even aqueous cream should be avoided unless skin cracking is imminent. The temperature and humidity controls of modern incubators preclude the use of additional moisturisers in most circumstances (Irving 2001).

Nappy rash is a significant cause of skin breakdown in children (see Nappy rash section).

Education

Educational programmes for the prevention of pressure damage should be structured, organised and comprehensive, and made available at all levels of healthcare providers, patients and family or caregivers. This will raise awareness and facilitate prevention of nappy rash (Allman 1997, Bridel 1993, Rycroft-Malone and McInnes 2000).

The educational programme should include information on the following items:

- The skin (including differences between prenatal, post natal and older child)
- Pathophysiology and risk factors for pressure damage
- Risk assessment tools and their application
- Principles of positioning to decrease risk of pressure damage
- Documentation of assessment (the child, risk status and condition of skin), planning, implementation and evaluation of subsequent care
- Selection and instruction in the use of pressure relieving and other devices
- Clarification of responsibilities for all concerned with this problem
- Development and implementation of guidelines.

Family and carers need to be made aware of the Trust's commitment to reducing the occurence of pressure ulcers and the severity of those which do occur. Families and carers of those who are identified as a risk should be given appropriate information on pressure ulcers.

Management: pressure ulcers

In the event that a pressure area of Grade 1–4 is identified by hospital staff, the following actions should be taken.

Grade 1

Non-blanching erythema of intact skin. Discolouration of the skin, warmth, oedema, induration or hardness can also be used as indicators, particularly on individuals with darker skin.

1. Record in the nursing notes and inform nurse in charge.
2. Review pressure risk assessment, and positioning/turning frequency.
3. Involve parents/carers in care if possible, ensuring that they have the local information leaflet.
4. Review the need for placing child on a Repose® or other pressure-relieving mattress.
5. Continue to observe, being aware that the extent of the pressure damage may not be clear for up to 72 hours.
6. Complete clinical incident form – include grade, site of injury, specialty and all requested information.

Grade 2

Partial thickness skin loss involving epidermis, dermis, or both. The ulcer is superficial and presents clinically as an abrasion or blister.

Carry out numbers 1–6 as above, plus:

7. Complete tissue viability referral if not already done so.
8. Review nutritional status – refer to dietician if necessary.
9. Take photograph of the pressure ulcer for the case notes (consent required).

Grade 3/4

Grade 3: full thickness skin loss involving damage to or necrosis of subcutaneous tissue that may extend down to, but not through, underlying fascia.

Grade 4: extensive destruction, tissue necrosis, or damage to muscle, bone or supporting structures with/without full thickness skin loss.

Carry out numbers 1–9 as above, plus:

10. Follow the local guidance for reporting for Grade 3 and 4 pressure ulcers.
11. The patient's consultant may wish to refer the patient to the Plastic Surgery team.

Pressure ulcer identified on or within 72 hours of admission to hospital

In the event that a pressure area of Grade 1–4 is identified by hospital staff on or within 72 hours of admission, follow steps 1–9 above.

Pressure ulcers must be reported as Clinical Incidents (see Figure 10.12).

Management after discharge

When the patient is ready for discharge from hospital and the pressure ulcer has not completely healed, a referral to the GP or community team should be made, giving background and details of care required.

Conclusion

This chapter has provided general information and guidance on a range of personal hygiene issues and pressure ulcer prevention

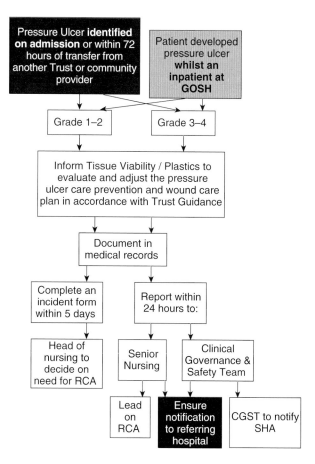

Figure 10.12 Pressure ulcer reporting flow chart. RCA, root cause analysis.

to ensure the care of both the well and sick child in hospital. Health professionals and parents/carers alike must strive to give the best possible care in these basic but essential areas, recognising the individuality of each child in relation to the sex, age, culture, religion and clinical condition. Care planning should be adjusted accordingly to such specific needs with parents/carers being mindful of privacy and dignity at all times. Finally, both child care professionals and parents/carers should work together to facilitate best practice for child in these fundamental aspects of nursing care.

References

Adam R. (2008) Skin care of the diaper area. Pediatric Dermatology, 25(4), 427–433

Adam R, Schnetz B, Mathey P, Pericoi M, de Prost Y. (2009) Clinical demonstration of skin mildness and suitability for sensitive infant skin of a new baby wipe. Pediatric Dermatology, 26(5), 506–513

Agarwal S, Agarwal A, Apple DJ, Buratto L. (2002) Textbook of Ophthalmology, Volume 1. Philadelphia, Lippincott Williams and Wilkins

Allison F. (2000) Nappy Rash an overview. Practice Nursing, 11(17), 17–19

Allman RM. (1997) Pressure ulcer prevalence, incidence, risk factors, and impact. Clinical Geriatric Medicine, 13(3), 421–36

Allman RM, Goode PS, Patrick MM, Burst N, Bartolucci AA. (1995) Pressure ulcer risk factors among hospitalized patients with activity limitation. Journal of the American Medical Association, 273(11), 865–870

American Academy of Pediatrics (AAP) (2009) Parenting Corner Q and A: Toilet Training When is the right time to start toilet training? Available at http://www.aap.org/publiced/BR_ToiletTrain.htm (last accessed 9th September 2010)

Association of periOperative Nurses (AORN) (2007) Standards, Recommended Practices and Guidelines. Denver, USA, AORN.

Arrowsmith.VA, Maunder JA, Sargent RJ, Taylor R. (2001) Removal of nail polish and finger rings to prevent surgical infection. Cochrane Library, 3, update software

Atherton DJ. (2004) A review of the pathophysiology, prevention and treatment of irritant diaper dermatitis. Current Medical Research Opinion, 20(5) 645–649

Atherton D. (2005) Maintaining healthy skin in infancy using prevention of irritant napkin dermatitis as a model. Community Practitioner, 78(7), 255–257

Atherton DJ. (2009) Managing healthy skin for babies. Infant, 5(4), 130–132

Atherton D, Mill K. (2004) What can be done to keep babies' skin healthy? RCM Midwives, 7(7), 288–290

Bakker E, van Gool JD, van Sprundel M, van der Auwera JC, Wyndaele JJ. (2002) Results of a questionnaire evaluating the effects of different methods of toilet training on achieving bladder control. British Journal of Urology, 90, 456–461

Barone JG, Jasutkar N, Schneider D. (2009) Later toilet training is associated with urge incontinence in children. Journal of Pediatric Urology, 5(6), 458–461

Bartlett JD, Jaanes SD. (2008) Clinical Ocular Pharmacology, 5th edition. Oxford, Butterworth Heineman

Bauer K. (2005) Effects of positioning and handling on preterm infants in the neonatal intensive care unit. In Sizun J, Browne JV. (eds) Research on Early Developmental care for preterm neonates. Paris, John Libbey Eurotext

Bayliss J. (1998) Nappy rash an age old problem. Practice Nursing, 9(19), 33–36

Beal JA. (2005) Evidence for best practices in the neonatal period. American Journal of Maternal Child Nursing, 30(6), 397–403

Behring A, Vezeau TM, Fink R. (2003) Timing of the newborn first bath: A replication. Neonatal Network. The Journal of Neonatal Nursing, 22(1), 39–46

Bennet L, Lee B. (1985) Pressure versus shear in pressure sore causation. In Lee BY. (ed.) Chronic Ulcers of the Skin. New York, McGraw Hill

Bentley E. (1994) Views about preventive dental care for infants. Health Visitor, 67(3), 88–89

Berg R. (1998) Etiology and pathophysiology of diaper dermatitis. Advances in Dermatology, 3, 95–98

Bergstrom A, Byaruhanga R, Okong P. (2005) The impact of newborn bathing on the prevalence of neonatal hypothermia in Uganda: a randomized, controlled trial. Acta Paediatric, 94(10), 1462–1467

Blincoe AJ. (2005) Cleansing and caring for the skin of neonates. British Journal of Midwifery, 13(4), 244–247

Blincoe AJ. (2006a) Protecting neonatal skin: cream or water. British Journal of Midwifery, 14(12), 731–732, 734

Blincoe AJ. (2006b) Caring for neonatal skin and common infant skin problems. British Journal of Midwifery, 14(4), 213–216

Blum NJ, Taubman B, Nemeth N. (2003) Relationship between age at initiation of toilet training and duration of training: A prospective study. Pediatrics, 111, 810–814

Borkowski S. (2004) Diaper rash care and management. Pediatric Nursing, 30(6), 467–470

Boucke L. (2003) Infant Potty Basics. Lafayette, CO, White-Boucke Publishing

Boxwell G. (ed) (2010) Neonatal Intensive Care Nursing, 2nd edition. London, Routledge

Boyd S. (2003) Hands that rock the cradle: Nail hygiene in the NICU. Journal of Neonatal Nursing, 9(2), 41–44

Brazelton TB, Sparrow JD. (2004) Toilet training the Brazelton way. Cambridge, MA, deCapo Press

Bridel J. (1993) The aetiology of pressure sores. Journal of Wound Care, 2(4), 230–238

British Dental Association www.3dmouth.org (last accessed 9th September 2010)

British Contact Lens Association (2011) Buying cosmetic contact lens. General Optical Council see www.bcla.org.uk

British Medical Association and Royal Pharmaceutical Society of Great Britain (2010) British National Formulary for Children. London BMA/RPSGB. Available at http:bnfc.org/bnfc/bnfc/current

Camm J. (2006) Skincare for newborns: guidelines and advice. RCM Midwives, 9, 126

Campbell ST, Evans MA, Mactavish F. (1995) Paediatric Oncology Nursing Forum Guidelines For Mouthcare. London: Royal College of Nursing

Canadian Pediatric Society (2000) Toilet learning: Anticipatory guidances with a child-oriented approach. Paediatrics and Child Heath, 5, 333–335

Chandrasekar PH, Gatny CM. (1994) Effect of fluconozole prophylaxis on fever and use of amphotericin in neutropenic patients. Chemotherapy, 40(2), 136–143

Chin GY. (2000) Neonatal physiology and skincare. Journal of Paediatrics and Obstetric Gynaecology, March/April, 23–27

Choby BA, George S. (2008) Toilet training. American Family Physician, 78(9), 1059–1064

Clarkson JE, Worthington HV, Eden OB. (2009) Interventions for preventing oral mucositis or oral candidiasis for patients with cancer receiving chemotherapy (excluding head and neck cancer) (Cochrane Review). Cochrane Library, 3, Oxford, update software

Collins F, Shipperley T. (1995) Assessing the seated patient for the risk of pressure damage. Journal of Wound Care, 8(3), 123–126

Cooper P. (2000) The use of Clinisan in the skin care of the incontinent patient. British Journal of Nursing, 9(7), 445–448

Coutts L, Hardy L. (1995) Teaching for Health, 2nd edition. Edinburgh, Churchill Livingstone

Coyne I, Neill F, Timmins F. (2010) Clinical Skills In Childrens Nursing. Oxford, OUP

Cullum N, Deeks J, Sheldon T, *et al* (2000) Beds, mattresses and cushions for preventing and treating pressure sores (Cochrane review). Oxford, Cochrane Library Issue 1

Daly B, Watt R, Batchelor P, Treasure E. (2002) Essential Dental Public Health. Oxford, Oxford University Press

Davis L, Mohay H, Edwards H. (2003) Mothers involvement in caring for their premature infants: an historical overview. Journal of Advanced Nursing, 42(6), 578–586

Department of Health (2000) Essence of Care, NHS Modernisation Agency. London, Department of Health

Department of Health (2004a) National Service Framework for children, young people and maternity services. London, Department of Health

Department of Health (2004b) Choosing Health: Making Healthy Choices Easier – Executive Summary. London, Department of Health

Department of Health (2004c) NHS Dentistry: Delivering Change –Report by the Chief Dental Officer (England) July. London, Department of Health

Department of Health (2007) Improving Oral Hygiene. Available at http://www.dh.gov.uk/en/Publicationsandstatistics/Publications/Publications PolicyAndGuidance/Browsable/DH_5536407 (last accessed 4th January 2012)

Dewar G. (2010) The right potty training age; whats best for your child. Available at http://parentingscience.com/potty-training-age.html – (last accessed 15th November 2011)

Disabled Living Foundation (2003) Available at www.disabledliving.org.uk (last accessed 15th November 2011)

Dunn PM. (2009) Managing the umbilical cord at birth. Infant 5(3), 73

Ellis J. (2005) Neonatal hypothermia. Journal of Neonatal Nursing, 11, 76–82

European Pressure Ulcer Advisory Panel (1999) Pressure Ulcer Prevention Guidelines. Oxford, EPUAP

Fellows P. (2010) Management of thermal stability. In: Boxwell G. (ed.) Neonatal Intensive Care Nursing, 2nd edition. London, Routledge

Fernandez R, Griffiths R, Ussia C. (2003) Water for wound cleansing, (Cochrane review). Cochrane Library, 3, Oxford, update software

Foca M, Jakob K, Whittier S. (2000) Endemic pseudomonas aeruginola infection in a NICU. New England Journal of Medicine, 343, 495–700

Franck L, Quinn D, Zahr L. (2000) Effect of less frequent bathing of preterm infants on skin flora and pathogen colorization. Journal of Obstetric. Gynecologic and Neonatal Nursing, 29(6), 584–589

Gardner SL, Carter BS, Enzman-Hines MI, Hernandez JA. (2010) Merenstein and Gardners Handbook of Neonatal Intensive Care, 7th edition. St Louis, Mosby

Gibson F, Nelson W. (2000) Mouth care for children with cancer. Paediatric Nurse, 12(1), 18–22

Gibson F, Horsford J, Nelson W. (1997) Oral care: practice reconsidered within a framework of action research. Journal of Cancer Nursing, 1(4), 183–190

Gray M. (2004) Which pressure ulcer risk scales are valid and reliable in a paediatric population? Journal of Wound, Ostomy and Continence Nursing, 31(4), 157–163

Great Ormond Street Children's Hospital (GOSH) (2004) Mouth Care. Clinical Practice Guideline. Available at http://www.childrenfirst.nhs.uk/health-professionals/clinical-guidelines/mouth-care (last accessed 18th November 2011)

Great Ormond Street Children's Hospital GOSH (2011) Available at http://www.gosh.nhs.uk/medical-conditions/procedures-and-treatments/looking-after-your-childs-skin-during-a-hospital-stay/ (last accessed 15th November 2011)

Griffin T. (2001) Nurses and Families in the NICU – Parental visits and infant care: Understanding parents' needs. Neonatal Network, 20, 1

Hale R. (2007) Protecting neonates' delicate skin. British Journal of Midwifery, 15(4), 231–232, 234–235

Health Education Authority (1996) A Handbook of Dental Health for Health Visitors, Midwives and Nurses. London, Health Education Authority

Heanue M, Deacon SA, Deery C, Robinson PG, Walmsley AD, Worthington HV, Shaw WC. (2003) Manual versus powered toothbrushing for oral health (Cochrane Review). Cochrane Library, 1, Oxford, update software

Hedderwick SA, McNeil SA, Lyons MJ, Kauffman CA. (2000) Pathogenic organisms associated with artificial fingernails worn by healthcare workers. Infection Control and Hospital Epidemiology, 21(8), 505–509

Heimann K. (2000) Family Needs ; How do we know what they want? Paediatric Nursing, 12(7), 31–35

Heron J, Joinson C, Croudace T,von Gontard A. (2008) Trajectories of daytime wetting and soiling in a United Kingdom 4–9 year old population birth cohort study. Journal of Urology, 179(5), 1970–1975

Herreboudt A, Sigalov J. (1997) Nappy rash at a glance: From top to bottom. British Journal of Midwifery, 5(7), 42–46

Hewitt D. (2000) Child-centred care; Ethno friendly or ethnocentric? Paediatric Nursing, 12(6), 6–8

Hoath SB. (1997) The stickiness of newborn skin: bioadhesion and the epidermal barrier. Journal of Pediatrics, 131, 338–346

Hockenberry MJ, Wilson D. (2010) Wong's Nursing Care of Infants and Children, 9th edition. St Louis, Mosby

Hopkins J. (2004) Essentials of newborn skin care. British Journal of Midwifery, 12(5), 314–317

Hopper A. (2000) Sources of Stress for parents of a sick neonate: A literature review. Paediatric Nursing, 12(4), 29–32

Horn IB, Brenner R, Rao M, Cheng TL. (2006) Beliefs about the appropriate age for initiating toilet training: Are their racial and socioeconomic differences? Journal of Pediatrics, 149, 165–168

Irving V. (2001) Caring for and protecting the skin of preterm neonates. Journal of Wound Care, 10, 253–256

Irving V, Bethell E, Burton F. (2006) Neonatal Wound Care – Minimising Trauma and Pain. Wounds UK, 2(1), 33–41

Jackson A. (2008) Time to review neonatal skin care. Infant, 4(5), 166–168

Jeannes A, Green J. (2001) Nail art: A review of current infection control issues. Journal of Hospital Infection, 49, 139–142

Jethwa K. (1994) Nappy Rash: A pharmaceutical approach Professional Care of Mother and Child Oct 219–220

Johnson R, Taylor W. (2010) Skills in Midwifery Practice, 3rd edition. Edinburgh, Churchill Livingstone

Joinson C, Heron J, Von Gontard A, Butler U, Emond A, Golding J. (2008) Early childhood risk factors associated with daytime wetting and soiling in school age children. Journal of Pediatric Psychology, 33(7), 739–750

Joinson C, Heron J, Von Gontard A, Butler U, Emond A, Golding J. (2009) A prospective study of age initiation of toilet training and subsequent bladder control in school age children. Journal of Developmental and Behavioral Pediatrics, 30(5) 385–393

Jones K. (2000) Baby skincare wipes pass no more tears mildness test. British Journal of Midwifery, 8(9), 577–580

Jones I, Tweed C, Marron M. (2001) Pressure area care in infants and children: Nimbus Paediatric System. British Journal of Nursing, 10(12), 789–795

Jordan WE, Lawson KD, Berg RW, Franxman JJ, Marrer BS. (1986) Diaper dermatitis: Frequency and severity among a general infant population. Pediatric Dermatology, 3(3), 198–207

Khurana S, Whit Hall R, Anand KJS. (2005) Treatment of pain and stress in the neonate NeoReviews, 6(2), e76. Available at http://neoreviews.aappublications.org/ (last accessed 15th November 2011)

Knobel R, Holditch-Davis D. (2007) Thermoregulation and heat loss prevention after birth and during neonatal intensive-care unit stabilization of extremely low-birthweight infants. JOGNN, 36, 280–287

Lack G, Fox D, Northstone K, Golding J. (2003) Factors associated with the development of peanut allergy in childhood. New England Journal of Medicine, 348(11), 977–985

Landis EM. (1930) Micro injection studies of capillary blood pressure. Heart, 15, 209–278

218

Lawson LG. (2001) Handwashing: a neonatal perspective. Journal of Neonatal Nursing, 7(2), 42–46

Levine R, Stillman-Lowe C. (2009) The Scientific Basis of Oral Health Education, 6th edition. London, British Dental Journal/British Dental Association

Lloyd S. (1992) Brushing up on children's mouth care. Professional Care of Mother and Child, 2(1), 16–17

Lloyd S. (1994) Teaching parents to look after children's teeth. Professional Care of Mother and Child, 4(2), 34–36

Lockyer-Stevens N. (1993) The use of water filled gloves to prevent decubitus ulcers on heels. Journal of Wound Care, 2(5), 282–287

Lyon C, Stapleton M, Smith A, Griffiths C, Beck M. (2000) Topical sucralfate in the management of peristomal skin disease; an open study. Clinical and Experimental Dermatology, 25(8), 584–588

Madeya ML. (1996) Oral complications from cancer therapy: part 2-nursing implications for assessment and treatment. Oncology Nurses Forum, 23(5), 808–820

Mainstone A. (2005) Maintaining infant skin health and hygiene. British Journal of Midwifery, 13(1), 44–47

Mancini AJ. (2004) Skin. Pediatrics, 113(4) (supplement) 1114–9

Marinho VCC, Higgins JPT, Sheiham A, Logan S. (2003) Fluoride toothpastes for preventing dental caries in children and adolescents (Systematic Review). Cochrane Library, 3, 2007, Oxford, update software

Marinho VCC, Higgins JPT, Sheiham A, Logan S. (2004) One topical fluoride (toothpastes, or mouthrinses, or gels, or varnishes) versus another for preventing dental caries in children and adolescents. [Systematic Review] In the Cochrane Library Issue 3, 2007 Oxford

Markham T, Kennedy F, Collins P. (2000) Topical sucralfate for erosive irritant diaper dermatitis. Archives of Dermatology, 136(10), 1199–1200

McGurk V. Holloway B, Crutchley A. (2004) Skin integrity assessment in neonates and children. Paediatric Nursing 16 3, 15–18

Medical Devices Agency (1994) Number PS2: Stati Mattress overlays. London, Department of Heath

Medves JM, O'Brien B. (2004) The effect of bather and location of first bath on maintaining thermal stability in newborns. Journal of Obstetric, Gynecologic, and Neonatal Nursing, 33(2), 175–182

Moralejo D, Jull A. (2003) Hand rubbing with an alcohol based solution reduced healthcare workers' hand contamination more than hand washing with antiseptic soap. Evidence-Based Nursing, 6(2), 54

Mota DM, Barros AJ. (2008) Toilet training; methods, parental expectations and associated dysfunctions. Journal of Pediatrics, 64(1) 9–17

Moynihan PJ. (2002) Dietary advice in dental practice. British Dental Journal, 193, 563–568

Murdoch V. (2002) Pressure care in the paediatric intensive care unit. Nursing Standard, 17(6), 71–6

Murphy K, Macleod Clark J. (1993) Nurses experiences of caring for ethnic minority clients. Journal of Advanced Nursing, 18, 442–450

National Institute for Clinical Excellence (2002) NICE guideline on pressure ulcer risk management and prevention(Guideline B). www.guidance.nice.org.uk/pdf/clinicalguidelinepressuresoreguidancenice.pdf. Viewed on: 9/5/11

National Institute of Clinical Excellence (2004) Dental Recall: Recall Interval between Routine Dental Examinations, Clinical guideline 19. London, National Institute of Clinical Excellence

National Institute for Clinical Excellence (2005) The prevention and management of pressure ulcers – clinical guideline. Available at www.guidance.nice.org.uk/CG29/quickrefguide/pdf/English (accessed 9th May 2011)

National Institute of Clinical Excellence (2010) Constipation in Children and Young people. Clinical guideline 99. London, National Institute of Clinical Excellence

Ndawula E, Brown L. (1990) Matresses as reservoirs of epidemic methicillin-resistant staphylococcus aureus. Lancet, 337, 448

Neidig J, Kleiber C, Oppliger R. (1989) Risk factors in the paediatric patient following open heart surgery. Progress in Cardiovascular Nursing, 4, 99–106

Nelson W, Gibson F, Hayden S, Morgan N. (2001) Using action research in paediatric oncology to develop an oral care algorithm. European journal of Oncology Nursing, 5(3), 180–189

Quinn D, Newton N, Piecuch R. (2005) Effect of less frequent bathing on premature infant skin. Journal of Obsteterics, Gynecology Neonatal Nursing, 34(6), 741–746

Nichols DS. (1996) The development of postural control. In Case-Smith J, Allen AS, Nuse-Pratt P. (eds) Occupational Therapy for Children, 3rd edition. St Louis, Mosby-Yearbook

Odio M, Streicher-Scott J, Hansen RC. (2001) The interactive newborn bath: using infant neurobehaviour to correct parents and newborns. The American Journal of Maternal & Child Nursing, 24(6), 280–286

Pearson LS. (1996) A comparison of the ability of foam swabs and toothbrushes to remove dental plaque. Implications for nursing practice. Journal of Advanced Nursing, 23(1), 62–69

Pearson LS, Hutton JL. (2002) A controlled trial to compare the ability of foam swabs and toothbrushes to remove dental plaque. Journal of Advanced Nursing, 39(5), 480–489

Peate F, Whiting P. (2006) Caring for Children and Families. Chichester, John Wiley & Sons

Philipp R, Hughs P, Golding J. (1997) Getting to the bottom of nappy rash. British Journal General Practice, 47, 421, 493–497

POPPY Steering Group (2009) Family-centred care in neonatal units. A summary of research results and recommendations from the POPPY project. London, NCT

Prasad HR, Srivastava P, Verma KK. (2003) Diaper dermatitis – an overview. Indian Journal of Pediatrics, 70(8), 635–637

Price S. (2000) A practical guide to preventing and treating nappy rash. British Journal of Midwifery, 8(11), 702–704

Quigley S, Curley M. (1996) Skin integrity in the peadiatric population: preventing and managing pressure ulcers. Journal of the Society Paediatric Nurses, 1(1), 7–17

Renton-Harper P, Addy M, Newcombe RG. (2001) Plaque removal with the un-instructed use of electric toothbrushes; comparison with a manual brush and toothpaste slurry. Journal of Clinical Periodontology, 28(40), 325–330

Rhodes C. (2000) Effective management of daytime wetting. Paediatric Nursing, 12(2), 14–17

Rigby D. (2001) Integrated continence services. Nursing Standard, 16(8), 46–55

Rogers JM. (2000) Promoting continence; the child with special needs. Paediatric Nursing, 12(4), 37–42

Rogers JM. (2002a) Toilet training: lessons to be learnt from the past. Nursing Times, 98(43), 56–57

Rogers JM. (2002b) Learning Disability Nursing; continence care award; solving the enigma: toilet training children with learning disabilities. British Journal of Nursing, 11(14), 958–962

Rothrock JC. (2006) What Are the Current Guidelines About Wearing Artificial Nails and Nail Polish in the Healthcare Setting? Available at http://www.medscape.com/viewarticle/547793 (last accessed 9th September 2010)

Royal College of Nursing (2005) Pressure Ulcer Risk Assessment and Prevention: Clinical Practise Guidelines. Available at www.rcn.org.uk/development/practice/clinicalguidelines/pressure_ulcers (last accessed 9th May 2011)

Rycroft-Malone J, McInnes E. (2000) Pressure Ulcer Risk Assessment and Prevention – technical report. London, Royal College of Nursing

Sanders C. (2002) Choosing continence products for children. Nursing Standard, 16(32), 39–43

Savage E. (2000) Family nursing; minimising discontinuity for hospitalised children and their families. Paediatric Nursing, 12(2), 33–37

Scardillo J, Aronovitch SA. (1999) Successfully managing incontinence-related irritant dermatitis across the lifespan. Ostomy/Wound Management, 45(4), 36–44

Scheinfeld N. (2005) Diaper dermatitis; a review and brief survey of eruptions of the diaper area. American Journal of Dermatology, 6(5), 273–281

Schmidt BA. (2004) Toilet training: Getting it right the first time. Contemporary Pediatrics, 21, 105–119

Scottish Intercollegiate Guidelines Network (SIGN) (2000) Preventing dental caries in children at high caries risk. Edinburgh, SIGN. Available at http://www.sign.ac.uk/pdf/sign47.pdf (last accessed 15th November 2011)

Schum TR, Kolb TM, McAuliffe TL, Simms MD, Underhill RL, Lewis M. (2002) Sequential acquisition of toilet-training skills: a descriptive study of gender and age differences in normal children. Pediatrics, 109(3), 48–54

Sherman TI, Greenspan JS, St Clair N, Touch SM, Shaffer TH. (2006) Optimising the neonatal thermal environment. Neonatal Network, 25(4), 251–260

Simpson L. (2001) Indwelling urethral catheters. Nursing Standard, 15, 46, 47–54

Solis I, Krouskop T, Trainer N, Marburger R. (1988) Supine interface pressure in children. Archives of Physical and Medical Rehabilitation, 69(7), 524–526

Stokowski LA. (2006) Neonatal skin: back to nature? Midwifery Today, 78, 34–35

Swallow VM, Jacoby A. (2001) Mother's evolving relationships with doctors and nurses during the chronic illness trajectory. Journal of Advanced Nursing, 36(6), 755–764

Tennant S. (2010) Toilet training more beneficial when started early. Urology Times, April, 22–25

Thomas KA. (2003a) Preterm infant thermal responses to care giving differ by incubator control mode. Journal of Perinatology, 23(8), 640–645

Thomas KA. (2003b) Infant weight and gestational age effects on thermoneutrality in the home environment. Journal of Obsterics, Gynecology and Neonatal Nursing, 32(6), 745–752

Thurgood G. (1994) Nurse maintenance of oral hygiene. British Journal of Nursing, 3(7), 332–353

Tollin M, Bergsson G, Kai-Larsen Y, et al (2005) Vernix caseosa as a multi-component defence system based on polypeptides, lipids and their interactions. Cell Molecular Life Sciences, 62(19–20), 2390–2399

Tran C, Medhurst A, OConnell B. (2009) Support needs of parents of sick and/or preterm infants admitted to a neonatal unit. Neonatal, Paediatric and Child Health Nursing, 12(2), 12–17

Trigg E, Mohammed TA. (2006) Practices in children's nursing – guidelines for hospital and community, 2nd edition. Edinburgh, Churchill Livingstone

Tortora GJ, Grabowski S. (2003) Principles of Anatomy and Physiology, 10th edition. Chichester, John Wiley and Sons

Tortora GJ, Derrikson BH. (2008) Principles of Anatomy and Physiology, 12th edition. Chichester, John Wiley and Sons

Trotter S. (2004) Care of the newborn : proposed new guidelines. British Journal of Midwifery, 12(3), 152–157

Trotter S. (2006) Neonatal skincare: why change is vital. RCM Midwives, 9(4), 134–138

Trotter S. (2007a) Baby products – it's all in the labelling. MIDIRS Midwifery Digest, 17(2), 263–266

Trotter S. (2007b) Baby care – back to basics&trade, TIPS Limited Scotland

Trotter S. (2008) Neonatal skin and cordcare – the way forward. Nursing in Practice, 40, 40–45. Available http://www.sharontrotter.org.uk/NIP 2008new.htm (last accessed 9th September 2010)

Turner A. (2000) Healthy infant skin: Focus on nappy rash and sensitive skin. British Journal of Midwifery, 8(5), 306–310

Ventocilia M, Wicker D. (2010) Contact Lens Complications. Available at http://emedicine.medscape.com/article/1196459-overview (last accessed 15th November 2011)

Vermandel A, Van Kanpen M, Van Gorp C, Wyndaele JJ. (2008) How to toilet train healthy children? A review of the literature. Neurourology and Urodynamics 27(3), 162–166

Visscher MO, Chatterjee R, Ebel JP, LaRuffa A, Hoath SB. (2002) Biomedical assessment and instrumental evaluation of healthy infant skin. Pediatric Dermatology, 19(6), 473–481

Waldron S, MacKinnon R. (2007) Neonatal thermoregulation. Infant, 3(3), 101–104

Walker L, Downe S, Gomez L. (2005a) Skin care in the well-term newborn: two systematic reviews. Birth, 32(3), 224–228

Walker L, Downe S, Gomez L. (2005b) A survey of soap and skin care product provision for well term neonates. British Journal of Midwifery, 13(12), 768–772

Watson R. (2000) Anatomy and Physiology for Nurses, 11th edition. London, Baillière Tindall

Watson R. (2005) Anatomy and Physiology for Nurses, 12th edition. London, Baillière Tindall

Watt RG, McGlone P. (2003) Prevention. Part 2. Dietary advice in the dental surgery. British Dental Journal, 195, 27–31

Williams C. (2001) 3M Cavilon durable barrier cream in skin problem management. British Journal of Nursing, 10(7), 469–472

Willis J. (1997) Avoiding and treating the skin irritations of babies and children. Nursing Times, 93(51), 55–56

Willock J, Hughes J, Tickle S. (1999) Pressure sores in children – the acute hospital setting. Journal of Tissue Viability, 10(2), 59–65

Wilson E, Trivedi R, Pandey SK. (2005) Pediatric Cataract Surgery; Techniques, Complications and Management. Philadelphia, Lippincott Williams and Wilkins

World Health Organization (WHO) (2005) Guidelines on Hand Hygiene in Health Care. Geneva, World Health Organization. Available at http://www.who.int/patientsafety/events/05/HH_en.pdf (last accessed 9th September 2010)

Worthington HV, Clarkson JE, Eden OB. (2008) Interventions for preventing oral candidiasis for patients with cancer receiving treatment (Cochrane Review). Cochrane Library, 1, 2008, Oxford, update software

Wu HY. (2010) Achieving urinary continence in children. Nature Reviews Urology, 7(7), 371–377

Zsolway K, Harrison A, Honig P. (2002) Diaper rash in a young infant. Pediatric Case Reviews, 2(4), 220–225

Zupan J, Gardner P. (2004) Topical Umbilical cord care at birth. Cochrane Review, Issue 3, Oxford, update software

Useful websites

www.nurse-prescriber.co.uk/education/visual_lib/pp42.

http://www.sharontrotter.org.uk/index.htm (Midwife, Breastfeeding Consultant and Neonatal Skincare Advisor)

http://www.tipslimited.co.uk/ (Trotters Independent Publishing Services Ltd: expert parenting advice and independent reviews of mother and baby products)

www.babyworld.co.uk

www.babyworld.co.uk/information/baby/bathing/bathing_new_baby

www.babyworld.co.uk/information/baby/bathing/top_and_tail.asp

www.babyworld.co.uk/information/baby/changing/Image/changing1

http://www.babyworld.co.uk/information/baby/bathing/top_and_tail.asp

www.babycentre.co,uk

www.babycentre.co.uk/toilettraining

http://factsheets.disabledliving.org.uk

www.keepkidshealthy.com

www.mcg/edu/pediatrics/CCNotebook/chapter2/eye.htm

www.continence-foundation,org,uk/campaigns/goodpracticecontinence.pdf

http://www.thailabonline.com/blood/nail

http://www.physsportsmed.com/issues/1999/09/tanzi.htm

http://dentistry.about.com/od/childrensdentistry/a/kidsdental.htm

http://www.growingkids.co.uk/DevelopingGoodOralHygiene.html
www.keepkidshealthy.com/symptoms/eyeproblems.html
http://bnfc.org/bnfc/bnfc/current (British National Formulary for Children 2010–2011)
http://bcla.org.uk/en/consumers/consumer-guide-to-contact-lenses/cosmetic-contact-lenses-coloured-and-special-effects.cfm British Contact Lense Association

Eyes

British Journal of Opthalmology p. 480, Eyedrop Instillation for Reluctant Children
BNF, administration of drugs to the eye, 2010

Burrows *et al*, Drug Delivery to the Eye
Robinson 1993 Ocular anatomy and physiology relevant to ocular drug delivery, Opthalmic Drug Delivery Systems

Ears

Medicines Information, Pharmacy Department, Great Ormond Street Hospital, London
Medicines for Children (2003) Royal College of Paediatrics and Child Health, London
Betnesol leaflet, Celltech Pharmaceuticals Ltd, Slough, 2001
British National Formulary (2010) British Medical Association and Royal Pharmaceutical Society of Great Britain

Chapter 11

Immunisations

Chapter contents

Procedure guideline

The Great Ormond Street Hospital Manual of Children's Nursing Practices, First Edition. Edited by Susan Macqueen, Elizabeth Anne Bruce, Faith Gibson.
© 2012 Great Ormond Street Hospital for Children NHS Foundation Trust. Published 2012 by Blackwell Publishing Ltd.

Introduction

Immunisation has proved to be one of the most successful public health interventions. In countries with effective immunisation programmes there has been a significant decline in the incidence of vaccine-preventable infectious diseases. Globally, smallpox was declared eradicated in 1980. Poliomyelitis has been eliminated from the Americas and the Western Pacific and, in June 2002, the European Region was certified polio-free (unfortunately in 2010, polio was reintroduced when wild poliovirus was confirmed in seven samples from children with acute flaccid paralysis in Tajikistan (WHO 2010)). In 2009, polio was endemic in only four countries in the world (Global Polio Eradication Initiative 2010). In Finland, where a two dose policy of MMR vaccine has been in place since 1982, indigenous measles, mumps and rubella were eliminated in 1996 (Heinonen *et al* 1998, Peltola *et al* 2000). In the UK, high uptake of childhood vaccines has resulted in an all time low incidence of most vaccine preventable diseases. Within a few years of introducing the new conjugate vaccines, *Haemophilus influenzae* type b (Hib) in 1991 and meningococcal C in 1999, there was a dramatic decline in invasive disease caused by these organisms (Heath and McVernon 2002; Ruggeberg and Heath 2003). In 2008/9 there only 13 cases of meningococcal C disease compared with 955 in 1998/99, a 99% reduction (HPA 2009).

Perhaps ironically, this reduction in childhood infectious disease has created new challenges and has led some parents/carers and professionals to focus more on the risks attached to vaccines rather than on the complications of disease. This has resulted in some parents/carers rejecting specific vaccines (Smailbegovic *et al* 2003). This is a cause for concern. In the mid-1970s fears over a possible link with brain damage led to a large reduction in acceptance of pertussis vaccine. This was followed by three large epidemics, providing a sharp reminder of the importance of immunisation and of the effectiveness of the vaccine. It took nearly 15 years before the previous high levels of vaccine uptake were once more achieved, and in that period hundreds of children suffered unnecessarily and many died because of the scare (Baker 2003). More recently, concerns that MMR vaccine may be linked with the development of autism and bowel disorders took hold in 1998, resulting in rejection of the vaccine by many parents/carers. The research that triggered these concerns is now discredited, and a significant body of research shows evidence for no such link, but in the intervening years, the fall in vaccine uptake rates resulted in dramatic increases in numbers of cases of measles disease and two deaths.

All professionals involved in giving immunisations should be fully informed of the benefits and, where they exist, the side effects of all vaccines so that they can advise parents/carers appropriately. The actual administration of the vaccine is only a minor part of the process. The overwhelming majority of vaccines are given in the community setting and it is a practice which is largely undertaken by practice nurses and health visitors. However, hospital staff need to be familiar with the routine schedule, indications and contraindications and current issues as they will often be asked for advice by parents/carers. It should also be standard practice for hospital staff seeing children in Accident & Emergency and outpatients' departments, as well as those admitted as in-patients, to consider children's immunisation status. For some children, often the most vulnerable, this will provide an important opportunity to catch up on incomplete immunisations or to remind their parents/carers that further immunisations are due (Walton *et al* 2007).

Routine childhood immunisation schedule in UK – 2010

The routine schedule (Table 11.1) in the UK is based on advice from the Joint Committee on Vaccination and Immunisation (JCVI) and published in *Immunisation Against Infectious Diseases* ('The Green Book') (Department of Health (DoH) 2006) and letters from the Chief Medical Officer (CMO) and Chief Nursing Officer (CNO). As guidance changes the web

Table 11.1 Routine childhood immunisation schedule in United Kingdom (2010)

Age	Vaccine	
8 weeks	Diphtheria/tetanus/acellular pertussis/inactivated polio vaccine/*Haemophilus influenzae* type b (DTaP/IPV/Hib)	One injection
	and	
	pneumococcal conjugate vaccine (PCV)	One injection
12 weeks	DTaP/Hib/IPV	One injection
	and	
	meningococcal C (Men C)	One injection
16 weeks	DTaP/Hib/IPV	One injection
	and men C	One injection
	and PCV	One injection
12 months	Hib/men C booster	One injection
13 months	Measles/mumps and rubella (MMR)	One injection
	PCV booster	One injectiion
3 years 4 months	d(D)TaP/IPV (pre-school booster)	One injection
	MMR (second dose) (can be given earlier)	One injection
12–13 years (girls only)	Human papillomavirus vaccine (HPV) (3 doses)	One injection per dose
13–18 years	Tetanus/low dose diphtheria/IPV (Td/IPV) (school leaver's booster)	One injection

based version of the Green Book is updated (http://www.publications.doh.gov.uk/greenbook/).

There have been significant changes to the routine schedule in recent years.

Since 2004 the primary schedule has included acellular pertussis vaccine rather than whole cell pertussis vaccine and inactivated polio vaccine (IPV) rather than oral polio vaccine at all ages (DoH 2004). IPV is a killed vaccine, administered by injection and is given combined with other injectable vaccines. In 2005 the universal BCG programme for school children was discontinued and BCG is now indicated for all neonates living in areas with a high incidence of TB and for other individuals in high-risk groups (DoH 2005).

In 2006 further changes were made to the routine primary vaccine schedule with the introduction of pneumococcal conjugate vaccine (PCV), a reduction of the number of doses of meningococcal C vaccine (men C) from three to two, and the introduction of boosters of Hib andMen C at 12 months and PCV at 13 months (DoH 2006). Most recent guidance is that these boosters can be administered all at the same time with MMR vaccine. In 2008, human papillomavirus vaccine (HPV) was added to the schedule, to be offered to girls aged 12–13 years, with a catch-up programme for older girls (DoH 2008).

Special risk groups

Some children are at increased risk of complications from infectious diseases. These children fall into two main groups:

1. Children with conditions where they are at increased risk from the complications of diseases and therefore in whom it is particularly important to ensure a full course of the **routine vaccines** is administered at the recommended times. This includes premature and small-for-dates babies, children with asthma, chronic lung or congenital heart disease, children with Down syndrome and those with impaired immune systems. Children with congenital or acquired immunodeficiency, such as due to agammaglobulinaemia, HIV infection, some forms of chemotherapy, etc, fall into this latter group.
2. Children who have specific conditions or are in particular circumstances that place them at increased risk of developing other vaccine-preventable diseases. Examples include:
   • All infants born in areas where the incidence of TB is 40 per 100,000 or greater. Children whose parents/carers or grandparents were born in a country with a high incidence of TB and previously unvaccinated new immigrants from a high prevalence country. BCG is recommended for all these groups.
   • Children born to women who are carriers of Hepatitis B virus or who had acute hepatitis B infection during pregnancy require hepatitis B vaccine.
   • Children with absent or severely dysfunctioning spleens, chronic renal, liver or heart disease, immunosuppression, individuals with cochlear implant or who have had a cerebrospinal fluid leak, chronic respiratory disease including asthma requiring repeated use of inhaled or systemic steroids should have pneumococcal vaccine indicated. This will include both the pneumococcal conjugate vaccine for children under the age of 5 years and the pneumococcal polysaccharide vaccine for those over the age of 2 years.

Children over the age of 6 months with chronic lung disease, including asthma, chronic heart or renal disease, diabetes or immunosuppression due to disease or treatment are recommended to have influenza vaccine

More detail of all these indications is available in the relevant chapter of the Green Book (DoH 2006).

Immunity

For almost as long as diseases have been studied, it has been noted that there are some diseases that very rarely recur in the same person. After the first attack, the body seems to become immune. This is due to the presence of primed memory cells which are able to respond rapidly to a second attack so that the causative organism cannot multiply and produce the disease. Immunity from infection can be induced by either active or passive means.

Passive immunity

Passive immunity follows when an injection of pre-formed antibodies is administered or a baby acquires antibodies transplacentally. Injected antibodies are in the form of an immunoglobulin preparation derived from the plasma of individuals who have either encountered a particular infection or who have been vaccinated. The immunity acquired is immediate but short lasting, usually 3–6 months. A number of forms of immunoglobulin are available:

• Human normal immunoglubulin given to immunosuppressed individuals in contact with measles
• Specific immunoglobulins against:
  ○ herpes zoster – given to pregnant women, some neonates and immunosuppressed individuals after exposure to chickenpox
  ○ hepatitis B, rabies and tetanus – given to normal individuals after exposure to these infections.

Further details can be obtained from the Health Protection Agency (HPA) http://www.hpa.org.uk/infections/topics_az/immunoglobulin/menu.htm

Active immunity

Active immunity results when the body is stimulated by an antigen to produce antibodies and/or memory cells specific to a particular infection. This may be achieved either by natural infection or by immunisation. Although the protection against future disease acquired from natural infection may in a few cases be greater than that from a vaccine, the disadvantage is that it puts an individual at risk from the complications of disease and it may even result in death. When a vaccine is administered it stimulates the production of memory cells and usually antibodies. If the organism is encountered, immunological memory enables the body to produce antibodies or cells specific to that infection which then neutralise the infecting organisms or their toxin. Active immunity is usually long lasting, although for some infections e.g. diphtheria, tetanus and polio it may need to be boosted at intervals.

Table 11.2 Types of vaccines

	Live (Attenuated)	Inactivated or component	Toxoid
V	Measles/mumps/rubella (MMR)	Hepatitis A	
I	Polio (oral – OPV)	Hepatitis B	
R	Varicella	Influenza	
A	Yellow fever	Human papillomavirus vaccine (HPV)	
L		Japanese encephalitis	
		Polio (inactivated – IPV)	
		Tick-borne encephalitis	
B	BCG	Anthrax	Diphtheria
A	Typhoid (oral)	*Haemophilus influenzae* type b (Hib)	Tetanus
C		Meningococcal C (conjugate)	
T		Meningococcal A&C (plain)	
E		Meningococcal A, C, W135 & Y (plain and conjugate)	
R		Pertussis (acellular)	
I		Plague	
A		Pneumococcal (plain and conjugate)	
L		Typhoid (inactivated)	

Types of vaccine

Vaccines can be categorised as to whether they are live or 'killed'; viral or bacterial; killed whole organism, toxoids or components (Table 11.2). On the basis of knowing the type of vaccine, one can predict both the likely contraindications and adverse effects.

Live vaccines

These contain live but attenuated (weakened) organisms. To produce an immune response, the organism replicates (grows) over a period of a few days or weeks after being administered. Except for live polio vaccine, which is now rarely used outside resource-poor countries, the viruses are not transmissable. Immunity is usually (possibly even for life) long lasting and a mild form of the disease can occur as a result of vaccination. For example, fever, rash and being off food have been reported in about 5% of recipients of MMR 7–10 days after its administration, with about 1% having parotitis 21 days following the vaccine. After BCG, a live bacterial vaccine, disseminated BCG may occur in immunosuppressed individuals with serious disorders such as Severe Combined Immunodeficiency Syndrome (SCIDS).

Toxoids

These are vaccines prepared from the toxin produced by the organism. It has been chemically inactivated so that, although it still produces an immune response, it is not capable of causing disease.

Whole cell vaccines

These vaccines are prepared from the complete organism, which has been killed and rendered non-pathogenic. They are uncommonly used now.

Conjugate vaccines

These are prepared by taking the polysaccharide (sugar) capsule of the organism and attaching a protein. The polysaccharide by itself is poorly immunogenic in young children, but the addition of the protein renders it highly immunogenic. Examples of conjugate vaccines, in routine use, are Hib, meningococcal C and pneumococcal vaccines.

Component vaccines

These are prepared from components of the organisms. Examples are acellular pertussis and some influenza vaccines.

Genetically engineered vaccines

Hepatitis B and Human Papillomavirus vaccines are manufactured using recombinant technology. A strain of yeast or similar organism is used to produce the antigen. It is likely that in future more vaccines will be produced in this way.

General considerations

Contraindications to childhood immunisation

Contraindications to all vaccines are detailed in the guidance produced by the Department of Health (DoH 2006). There are very few genuine contraindications to vaccines and most children who have permanent true contraindications will be under the care of a paediatrician. There are general contraindications that apply to all vaccines and those which apply only to specific vaccines or to children with specific conditions.

General contraindicationsare:

- Immunisation should not be carried out in an individual who has a history of an anaphylactic reaction to a preceding dose.
- Immunisation should be postponed in an individual who is suffering from an acute illness. Minor illness such as coughs

and colds, without fever or systemic upset, are not sufficient reason to postpone immunisation.

- Some vaccines should be postponed in the presence of an evolving neurological disorder.

The latter two are to avoid wrongly attributing the progression of the disorder to the vaccine and arrangements should be in place to ensure immunisation takes place once they have recovered, or the disorder has stabilised.

In addition to these general contraindications some live vaccines may pose a risk to individuals with altered immunity. In addition to guidance from the Department of Health, a best practice statement on immunisation of the immunocompromised child has been developed by the Royal College of Paediatrics and Child Health (RCPCH) (http://www.rcpch.ac.uk/publications/recent_publications.html). This provides detailed guidance on children with primary immunodeficiency, those being treated with standard and intensive chemotherapy, solid organ recipients, children being treated with immunosuppressive drugs for inflammatory disease and children with HIV infection.

Live vaccines should either be given at the same time or with a minimum interval of 4 weeks. Immunoglobulin may reduce the response to a live vaccine. As a generalisation:

- If a live vaccine is given before immunoglobulin, an interval of 4 weeks should be left.
- If immunoglobulin precedes a live vaccine, an interval of 3 months should be allowed.

Adverse reactions and safety of vaccines

All vaccines can give rise to side effects. These are usually mild and self-limiting, for example, swelling and redness at the injection site are common. By remembering whether a vaccine is live or 'dead', it is possible to predict, in general terms, the likely adverse effects and contraindications. In addition to mild local reactions, most vaccines can cause systemic upset of varying degrees. Live vaccines may also produce the disease, but almost always in a mild form.

It may be difficult to distinguish a coincidental illness from an adverse reaction and often the tendency is to assume the latter. Only good studies can estimate the true incidence of adverse reactions. Following the first dose of MMR vaccine a proportion of children develop mild measles, mumps or rubella. In a study involving 581 pairs of twins, one twin received MMR vaccine and the other a placebo. Three weeks later the roles were reversed. Low rates of systemic effects thought due to the vaccine were reported (Peltola and Heinonen 1986). Fever greater than $38.5°C$ occurred at a maximum rate 9–10 days after the vaccine among 4.9% of vaccinees compared with 1.0% after placebo. After the same interval, 4.3% of vaccinees developed a rash, compared with 3.0% given placebo. Children who received the vaccine were more likely to be irritable and drowsy although cough and/or cold were more common following the placebo.

Other studies have confirmed these findings. For MMR and other combined vaccines there is evidence that there is little, if any increase in the rate of reactions in comparison with giving the antigens separately. However, combining some antigens may change the immune response for better or worse, depending on the combination.

Serious adverse reactions following vaccination are rare. Studies involving large numbers of children are necessary to determine the frequency of such reactions. These are usually performed after the vaccine has been in use for some time and are part of postmarketing surveillance. Studies linking hospital records with immunisation records have reported that 1 in 3,000 children have a febrile convulsion due to MMR vaccine (Farrington et al 1995) and 1 in 32,000 develop idiopathic thrombocytopenic purpura due to it (Miller et al 2001). These are a tenth of the rates after the diseases.

All significant adverse events following immunisation (AEFIs) should be reported to the local immunisation lead and to the Medicines and Healthcare products Regulatory Agency (MHRA) using the 'Yellow Card' system.

Efficacy of vaccines

No vaccine is 100% effective. Before any vaccine is introduced, trials are conducted to ensure it is of high efficacy. After a first injection of combined MMR vaccine about 10% of children are not protected against measles (Ramsay et al 1994), a higher proportion, perhaps as high as 30%, are not protected against mumps (Harling et al 2005) and a smaller proportion, 1–2%, not protected against rubella. This means that there will always be some cases of disease if only one dose is given. In an outbreak of measles in Quebec City in 1989, of 62 siblings of cases of measles who developed measles themselves, 41 (66%) were immunised. At first sight this might suggest that the vaccine was poorly effective, however closer examination shows this not to be the case. Of 17 unvaccinated siblings all (100%) developed measles, compared with only 41 of 441 (9%) vaccinated siblings. This gives a vaccine efficacy of 91%. If none of the children had been vaccinated, there would have been a further 400 cases (De Serres et al 1995).

It is important to remember that not all preparations of a vaccine are the same. Although there is little variation in the measles vaccines used in the developed world, the efficacy of different pertussis vaccines varies enormously. Trials in the 1990s showed that one variety of whole cell pertussis vaccine had an efficacy of 35–40%, whereas the whole cell vaccine that was used in the UK had an efficacy of 90% (Miller 1999). The Jeryl Lynn mumps vaccine used in the UK has an efficacy of 70–90%, whereas studies have shown that the Rubini strain offered no protection (e.g. Schlegel et al 1999). The efficacy of BCG vaccine has also been found to vary widely from nil to 80% (Fine and Rodrigues 1990).

To monitor the effectiveness of vaccines, all cases of the routine vaccine-preventable diseases should be notified to the local Consultant in Communicable Disease Control. Some, for example, tuberculosis, Hib, pneumococcal and meningococcal infections, are also the subject of enhanced surveillance schemes. These are more accurate and allow detailed study of the characteristics of cases of the diseases.

Herd immunity

If a high enough rate of protection can be achieved, by high vaccine uptake with an effective vaccine, a disease becomes so uncommon that even those still susceptible are at little risk. This is known as 'herd immunity' and it provides protection not only to immunised individuals but also to those who have not been immunised. This is an important way of protecting children who cannot be immunised because they are too young, those in whom vaccines are contraindicated, and some who have been immunised but who still remain unprotected due to 'vaccine failure'. The uptake needed to attain herd immunity will depend on the disease, the vaccine and the population. The more infectious the disease and the more mixing within the population, the greater the level of immunisation that will be required to achieve herd immunity. The exception to this is tetanus, as the disease is not transmitted from person to person, each individual needs their own immunity to be protected and there is no herd immunity.

The aim of any vaccination programme is to reduce the incidence of disease. However, characteristics of the disease, the population and the vaccine will determine to what extent this is possible and how it might be achieved.

The options for vaccination programmes are:

- Eradication – a situation where the disease and its causal agent are completely and permanently removed worldwide. The only example of a disease that has been eradicated is naturally occurring smallpox.
- Elimination – may refer to the regional eradication of an infection, e.g. polio in the western hemisphere, or to the disappearance of human disease but persistence of the organism in the environment.
- Containment – reduction of morbidity and mortality to levels which are no longer considered to be a public health problem, e.g. diphtheria in the UK.

The aim of the MMR vaccination programme is to eliminate the infections. To achieve this very high levels of immunity are needed. For example, in the case of measles, which is highly infectious, 95% of the population need to be immune to prevent circulation of the disease. Since the vaccine is about 90% effective against measles, if 88% of children are given MMR vaccine, only 79% of each birth cohort would be protected against measles. It is therefore recommended that children receive two doses of MMR vaccine. The second dose is needed to protect those who did not respond to the first dose. High rates of protection against measles (99%) are seen with a two-dose schedule (Hennessey et al 1999).

Specific diseases and the vaccines

Diphtheria

Organism

Corynebacterium diphtheriae and, less commonly, *Corynebacterium ulcerans*. Most isolates do not produce toxin, i.e. are non-toxigenic.

Disease

Clinical: significant disease only results from infection with a strain producing the toxin, i.e. a 'toxigenic' strain. After an incubation period of 2–4 days, one of three clinical pictures may occur – nasal, tonsillar or laryngeal. In each case an exudate appears at the relevant site. There may or may not be constitutional upset. The main complications are respiratory obstruction, myocarditis and muscle paralysis. Treatment is with antitoxin, antibiotics and supportive therapy.

Morbidity: between 1986 and 2005 there were 211 notifications of the organism, but only 24 were toxigenic.

Mortality: this is approximately 5%, the last death due to *C. diphtheriae* in the UK was in 2008 in an unimmunised child (Health Protection Agency 2008).

Vaccination

Nature of vaccine: the toxin is chemically detoxified to produce a toxoid. When used as a vaccine it prevents the complications of the disease, but doesn't prevent infection. The vaccine is not available separately.

Efficacy: 87–96%

Contraindications: as for any killed vaccine.

Adverse effects: local reactions and mild systemic upset are fairly common. More severe effects are rare. The low dose vaccine must be used in individuals who are 10 years of age or older.

Haemophilus influenzae type b (Hib)

Organism

Haemophilus influenzae type b (Hib). Other serotypes rarely cause invasive disease.

Disease

Clinical: following a short incubation period, meningitis, epiglottitis, septic arthritis, pneumonia, pericarditis, bacteraemia or cellulitis may occur. The disease is less common after the 4th birthday but still sufficiently common for the vaccine to be recommended for all children up to their 10th birthday. Treatment with antibiotics and supportive therapy is usually effective. Between 10% and 30% of children with meningitis are left with a significant neurological or auditory disability.

Morbidity: prior to the introduction of immunisation, there was a 1 in 600 chance of contracting the disease before the age of 5. In 1998, 6 years after vaccination started, there were 29 cases of Hib meningitis as opposed to over 400 per year in the pre-vaccine era. There was a small increase in cases in the late 1990s for a number of reasons. A cohort of children under 4 years were offered a booster dose of vaccine in 2003 and since 2006, all children are offered a booster dose at 12 months of age. Hib infection is now uncommon.

Mortality: approximately 5% for meningitis and higher for epiglottitis. There used to be 65 deaths per year, but now there are very few.

Vaccination

Nature of vaccine: the polysaccharide (sugar) capsule is attached ('conjugated') to a protein (tetanus toxoid or diphtheria toxoid derivative). The vaccine is not available separately.

Efficacy: over 95%. In areas where it has been used, the disease is very uncommon.

Contraindications: as for any killed vaccine.

Adverse effects: other than mild local reactions, these are very uncommon.

Hepatitis B

Organism

A virus of the genus *Hepadnavirus*.

227

Disease

Clinical: the infection may be passed from mother to infant around the time of delivery ('vertical' spread), by blood products or from person to person during sexual intercourse ('horizontal spread'). There is also some spread within families, the mode of transmission not always being clear. When acquired vertically the infant is usually asymptomatic but may become a carrier and develop liver disease later in life. Adults acquiring the disease may develop an acute hepatitis and not become carriers.

Morbidity: depends on the population. The carrier state is noted in 1 in 1500 blood donors, but 1 in 100 mothers in some inner city areas. There were almost 700 reports of acute Hepatitis B in 2003.

Mortality: accurate figures are not available.

Vaccination

Nature of vaccine: recombinant DNA product prepared from yeast.

Efficacy: depends on the age and general health of the recipient. It is very effective in infants, but less so in adults or those with chronic illnesses, e.g. renal failure. It is available as a separate vaccine.

Contraindications: as for any killed vaccine.

Adverse effects: uncommon.

Human papillomavirus

Organism

A double stranded DNA virus with about 100 strains. HPV viruses are classified as either 'high-risk' or 'low-risk' depending on whether or not they are oncogenic (cancer causing) strains.

Disease

Clinical: HPV is extremely prevalent and most people are infected in their life-time. The virus infects squamous epithelia, including the skin and mucosae of the upper respiratory and anogenital tracts. Most infections are self-limiting and asymptomatic. Persistent genital infection with a high-risk strain can result in cancer of the cervix. About 40 strains infect the genital tract, with 70% of cervical cancers being caused by two strains: HPV16 and HPV18. Of genital warts over 90% are caused by two types, HPV6 and HPV11. The viruses causing problems in the genital area are usually spread by sexual intercourse. HPV can also cause laryngeal papillomatosis (polyps in the voice box), but this is rare. Each year, in spite of the screening programme, there are about 1100 deaths due to cervical cancer. In 2006, there were over 83,700 new cases of genital warts.

Vaccination

Two vaccines are available; one with two strains of the virus (16 and 18 – Cervarix) and the other with four (6, 11,16 and 18 – Gardasil). Both are produced using recombinant technology. The vaccine in routine use in the UK is Cervarix. Three doses of vaccine are needed over 6 months. For maximum benefit, the vaccine needs to be given before infection has occurred, i.e. before sexual debut.

Efficacy: The vaccine is highly effective (over 99%) at preventing infection in susceptible young women. Current studies suggest protection is maintained for at least 6 years.

Adverse effects: Most common side effects are pain and swelling at the injection site.

Influenza

Organism

There are three types of influenza virus: A, B and C. Influenza A and influenza B are responsible for most clinical illness. Changes in the principal surface antigens of influenza A, make these viruses antigenically labile. Minor changes (antigenic drift) occur progressively from season to season. Major changes (antigenic shift) occur periodically, resulting in the emergence of a new subtype. In 2009, a new influenza virus H1N1 was detected, this was referred to as 'swine flu' as the virus showed some similarities to the virus that infects pigs. This virus spread quickly from person to person worldwide and H1N1 vaccines were developed rapidly. Fortunately the disease was mild in most people.

Disease

The organism is highly infectious and transmitted by aerosol, droplets or direct contact with respiratory secretions of someone with the infection. The incubation period is 1–3 days. The infection spreads rapidly, especially in closed communities. Most cases in the UK tend to occur during a 6–8 week period during the winter. The timing, extent and severity of this 'seasonal' influenza can all vary. Symptoms include sudden onset of fever, chills, headache, myalgia and extreme fatigue. Other common symptoms include a dry cough, sore throat and stuffy nose. In healthy individuals, influenza is an unpleasant but usually self-limiting disease with recovery in 2–7 days. Serious illness and mortality from influenza are highest among neonates, older people and those with underlying disease, particularly chronic respiratory and cardiac disease, or those who are immunosuppressed.

Morbidity: Even in a low incidence year, 3000–4000 deaths have been attributed to influenza.

Vaccination

The World Health Organization (WHO) monitors influenza viruses throughout the world. Each year the WHO makes recommendations about the strains to be included in seasonal flu vaccines for the forthcoming winter. To provide continuing protection, annual immunisation with vaccine against the currently prevalent strains is necessary.

Influenza vaccines are prepared using virus strains in line with the WHO recommendations. Current vaccines are trivalent, containing two subtypes of influenza A and one type B virus.

The viruses are usually grown in embryonated hens' eggs, chemically inactivated and then further treated and purified.

Efficacy: 70–80% protection.

Contraindications: as for any killed vaccine. As the vaccine is usually manufactured in hens' eggs, if possible, an egg-free preparation should be used for people who have had a previous anaphylactic reaction to egg products. If this is not available, expert advice should be sought.

Adverse reactions: pain, swelling or redness at the injection site, low grade fever, malaise, shivering, fatigue, headache, myalgia and arthralgia are among the commonly reported symptoms of vaccination. These symptoms are also similar to those of influenza infection and some individuals claim that the vaccine has given them "flu' but as the vaccine is killed this is not plausible.

Measles

Organism
A virus of genus *Morbillivirus* of the Paramyxoviridae family.

Disease
Clinical: after an incubation period of about a week, sore eyes, a dry cough and rash develop. Complications occur in 1 in 15 cases, with convulsions in 1% and encephalitis in 1 in 1000. A fatal progressive neurological disorder (subacute sclerosing panencephalitis-SSPE) may develop many years later. Prior to the introduction of immunisation measles epidemics occurred every 2 years.

Morbidity: there were almost 80,000 notified cases a year in the 1980s. Since many cases of notified measles are not later confirmed to be the disease, oral fluid testing on all notified cases of measles, mumps and rubella has been in place since 1995. This allows laboratory confirmation of the initial clinical diagnosis. In 2005 there were 2114 notified cases of measles but fewer than 5% were confirmed. As a result of a decline in uptake of MMR vaccine, confirmed cases of measles increased from 56 in 1998 to a peak of 1370 in 2008.

Mortality: 120 people died from measles in the 1980s, but only 18 in 1990-9 and most of these were due to the late effects. Until 2006 the last confirmed deaths due to acute measles was in 1992. However, a child died in 2006 and another in 2008 from acute measles. These were both teenagers who, due to treatment that rendered them immunosuppressed, could not be given MMR vaccine. This is a potent example of the importance of herd immunity to protect individuals who cannot be immunised.

Vaccination
Nature of vaccine: live attenuated vaccine given as MMR.

Efficacy: 90-95% for the measles component. For this reason, and because measles is highly infectious, from October 1996 the standard immunisation schedule has included two doses of MMR with a minimum separation of 1 month except when a child is under 18 months old, when the interval should be 3 months.

For mumps, the efficacy is usually quoted as 85–90%. However, recent work suggests it may be as low as 64%. There is also evidence to suggest that the immunity from mumps vaccine may wane over time. In contrast, the efficacy of the rubella component is greater than 95%.

Contraindications: as for any live vaccine. It can be given to anyone who is HIV positive, but if they have AIDS, advice should be sought from their consultant. MMR vaccines in use in most countries contain small quantities of egg and so there has been concern about giving the vaccine to children who are allergic to egg for fear that they might have a serious reaction to it. However, there is a lot of experience of using the vaccine in such children without any untoward effects. Therefore, the most recent advice from the Department of Health (2006) suggests that where there is a history of confirmed anaphylactic reaction to food containing egg paediatric advice should be sought with a view to immunisation under controlled conditions such as in an hospital setting. This is rather to reassure the parents/carers than of

medical necessity. There is no good evidence that skin testing helps in the management of these children. The vaccine should not be given to anyone who has had an anaphylactic reaction to neomycin or gelatin.

Adverse effects: mild measles occurs in about 5%, at 5–11 days after immunisation. Mild mumps or rubella occurs somewhat later. None is infectious. Vaccination is complicated by convulsions after 1 in every 3000 doses and idiopathic thrombocytopenic purpura (ITP) after 1 in every 32,000. Adverse reactions are much less frequent after revaccination than after the first dose (Virtanen *et al* 2000).

Two brands of vaccine were withdrawn in 1992 because the mumps strain used ('Urabe') gave rise to a mild meningoencephalitis, but with no long-term sequelae.

Meningococcal C

Organism
Neisseria meningitidis serogroup C.

Disease
Clinical: meningitis and/or septicaemia are the most serious manifestations of the infection. Multi-organ failure with gangrene of extremities, which may require amputation, can occur. Treatment is with antibiotics and general organ support. Even with intensive treatment there is a high mortality. When the vaccine was introduced in 1999 there were 724 cases in under 19 year olds, of whom about 10% died. Since 1999 there has been a 99% decrease in the number of laboratory-confirmed cases in people under 20.

Vaccination
Nature of vaccine: polysaccharide conjugate, along the same lines as Hib. The UK was the first country to introduce the conjugate vaccine in November 1999.

Efficacy: 95%+ in the first year of life, but wanes rapidly, so a booster is given at 12 months old. It is only available as a separate vaccine.

Contraindications: as for any killed vaccine.

Adverse effects: local, fever general malaise, etc. Significant adverse effects are rare.

Mumps

Organism
A virus of the paramyxovirus group

Disease
Clinical: the most common presentations are parotitis and pancreatitis. It used to be the commonest form of viral meningoencephalitis in children and young people and was a significant cause of sensorineural deafness.

Morbidity: it only became officially notifiable with the introduction of the MMR vaccine. There were 20,713 cases notified in 1989 but only 500 in 2002. Cases started to increase in 2004, this peaked in 2005 when there were 43,378 confirmed cases. These occurred mainly among older adolescents and young adults who had either never received MMR vaccine or only one dose. The epidemic highlighted the need for two doses of MMR vaccine.

Mortality: before the vaccine came into use there were 2–5 deaths each year.

Vaccination
See measles.

Pertussis

Organism
Bordetella pertussis.

Disease
Clinical: varies from a cold to frequent bouts of coughing terminated by vomiting and the characteristic whoop. Convulsions and permanent neurological sequelae occur. It may be an unrecognised cause of cot death.

Morbidity: 7158 notifications between 2000–2008 but probably under notified.

Mortality: there were 34 official notifications between 2000 and 2008, but there is reason to think that this was an underestimate and that about nine children a year die from pertussis. Most deaths from pertussis are in babies under the age of 6 months.

Vaccination
Nature of vaccine: the main vaccine used in infants in the UK was changed in 2004 from the killed whole bacterial preparation ('whole cell' vaccine) to an acellular vaccine. The acellular vaccines contain a limited number of components as opposed to the whole cell vaccines, which, as the name suggests, contain the whole, but inactivated bacterium, with approximately 3000 components. In comparison with the previously used whole cell vaccine, acellular or 'component' vaccines have been shown to have about the same incidence of side effects when given at 2, 3 and 4 months, but, except for the five component vaccine, a lower efficacy. In older children these vaccines have fewer side effects than the conventional vaccine. A five component vaccine is given as the primary course and a three component vaccine as the pre-school booster.

Efficacy: over 90% for the traditional whole cell vaccines used in UK and the five component acellular vaccine. However, there is evidence to suggest possible waning of immunity after vaccination, hence the need for one or more boosters in childhood.

Contraindications: as for any inactivated vaccine. If prone to convulsions, special care should be taken to advise about the management of pyrexia and convulsions. The vaccine, as with other childhood vaccines, should be withheld in those children with an evolving neurological disorder.

Adverse effects: local reactions and pyrexia are common within 48 hours after vaccination. Convulsions occur in approximately 1 in every 60,000 doses after whole cell vaccine, when given at 8, 12 and 16 weeks. These are far less common after acellular vaccine (Le Saux *et al* 2003). Long-term damage occurs rarely if ever.

Pneumococcal disease

Organism
Streptococcus pneumoniae has over 90 serotypes. About 20–30 account for the majority of disease, with seven serotypes responsible for 82% of invasive disease in UK children under 4 years old.

Disease
Clinical: pneumonia, bacteraemia and meningitis are the most important forms of invasive disease. The contribution to acute otitis media is also significant.

Morbidity: in 2004/5, 252 cases of meninigitis, of which 104 were in children less than 5 years old; 6287 cases of bacteraemia of which 731 were in children under 5 years old; and about 70–80,000 cases of pneumonia. Approximately one in three infants has otitis media each year, of which 25–30% are due to the pneumococcus. Approximately 25% of those surviving meningitis have a significant disability. In the first 30 months following the introduction of PCV it has been estimated that up to 959 cases of serious illness and up to 53 deaths caused by invasive disease were prevented.

Mortality: 15–20% for those with meningitis and about 7% for those with other invasive disease.

Vaccination
Nature of vaccine: a plain polysaccharide vaccine is prepared from 23 serotypes and a conjugate vaccine (PCV) from 13 serotypes (when PCV was introduced in 2006, it was a 7 serotype vaccine). These are available only as separate vaccines. In the first 30 months following the introduction of PCV(7) it was estimated that up to 959 cases of serious illness and up to 53 deaths caused by invasive disease were prevented.

Contraindications; as for any killed vaccine.

Efficacy: the plain polysaccharide vaccine, as with any such vaccine, is ineffective in young children, whereas the conjugate vaccine is highly effective, but, if given to infants, needs a booster to maintain immunity.

Adverse effects: as for any killed vaccine.

Poliomyelitis

Organism
An enterovirus with three antigenically distinct types.

Disease
Clinical: most polio infections are asymptomatic, but it may cause meningitis or paralysis.

Morbidity: 10 cases 1994–2003, all vaccine-associated. The disease has nearly been eradicated worldwide.

Mortality: rare in UK.

Vaccination
Nature of vaccine: injected killed (IPV) replaced oral live attenuated (OPV) vaccine in the UK in 2004, the latter is reserved for use in outbreaks.

Contraindications to IPV: as for any killed vaccine.

Efficacy: very high.

Adverse effects: killed vaccine - local reactions and fever occasionally. Oral vaccine - paralytic polio in 1 in 2-3 million recipients or unimmunised contacts.

Rubella

Organism
The rubivirus is a togavirus of the Togaviridae family.

Disease

Clinical: in most people, the illness is mild but if acquired in the first trimester of pregnancy, it gives rise to numerous malformations in the majority of fetuses.

Morbidity: only became notifiable with the introduction of the MMR vaccine. There were 133 confirmed cases in the 5 year period 2005–2009, and only three cases of congenital rubella syndrome reported 2005–2007.

Mortality: uncommon.

Vaccination

See measles.

Tetanus

Organism

Clostridium tetani.

Disease

Clinical: also known as 'lockjaw', the disease is usually acquired from dirt in a skin wound. It is not spread from person to person and so herd immunity is not relevant. It causes painful spasms, which may affect the respiratory muscles and be fatal.

Morbidity: 45 cases notified between 2000 and 2008. During 2003 a cluster of tetanus cases occurred in injecting drug users. Two of these patients died.

Mortality: four deaths reported 2000–2008.

Vaccination

Nature of vaccine: purified toxoid prepared using the same principles as diphtheria toxoid. Not available separately.

Efficacy: highly effective.

Adverse effects: local reactions, fever and general malaise occur in a small proportion of recipients. Significant adverse effects are rare.

Tuberculosis

Organism

Mycobacterium tuberculosis, a slow growing bacterium.

Disease

Clinical: spread is from person to person and can affect almost any organ in the body. The prevalence of disease is higher in association with HIV infection and deprivation. Treatment is with antitubercular drugs.

Morbidity: between 1991 and 2000 there were 53,236 cases notified and over the last 5 years there has been a steady increase to 8047 cases in 2005. This rise was seen mainly in London.

Mortality: 4080 deaths between 1991 and 2000. In spite of the rise in cases the number of deaths fell to 300 in 2007.

Vaccination

Nature of vaccine: the vaccine used is not prepared from the TB organism (*Mycobacterium tuberculosis*), but a related bovine organism (*Mycobacterium bovis*). Bacillus Calmette-Guérin (BCG) is a live attenuated vaccine.

Efficacy: studies have had very variable outcomes, but in UK school children it was about 80%. The dominant effect is to prevent dissemination of the disease and severe forms of disease such as meningitis, rather than infection per se.

Contraindications: as for any live vaccine. In addition, it should not be given to anyone with a positive tuberculin test, a history of previous BCG and a scar, or a history of TB, itself.

Adverse effects: an ulcer at the site of immunisation occurs frequently and occasionally the organism may become disseminated, especially in the immunosuppressed.

Vaccines not in general use in UK

- Varicella zoster virus (VZV) – a live attenuated vaccine is in use in the USA; although it is licensed in the UK, it is not in routine use and remains under consideration.
- Rotavirus – a live attenuated oral vaccine was introduced in the USA in 1999, but withdrawn after a few months because of a causal association with intussusception. A new type of rotavirus vaccine was introduced into the universal vaccine schedule in the USA in 2006.
- Meningococcal B – a vaccine to protect against meningococcal B infection is highly desirable but is proving much more difficult to develop than meningococcal C vaccine. Recent clinical trials in UK have produced encouraging early results but it is difficult to predict when a meningococcal B vaccine may be available (Sadarangani and Pollard 2010).
- Respiratory syncitial virus – passive immunisation (monoclonal antibodies) is available and used in high-risk infants, however there is still controversy as to its value.

Storage and administration of vaccines

Storage

All vaccines are temperature and light sensitive to varying degrees. If stored outwith the optimum temperature range, usually 2–8°C, the efficacy of the vaccine may decline and, less commonly, may give rise to more adverse reactions. If a glass vial of vaccine is frozen, it may develop hairline cracks allowing pathogens to enter and result in injection site infections. All vaccines must be kept in special refrigerators, whose temperature should be recorded at least once each working day and ideally twice. This should be done with a maximum and minimum thermometer so the extremes of temperature can be noted. From the time that a vaccine leaves the manufacturer to the time it enters the patient (the 'cold chain'), the temperature at which it is stored should be checked and recorded. Vaccines should spend the least possible time out of the refrigerator.

Ensuring good uptake

It is important that high uptake of vaccines is achieved and maintained to ensure the protection of individual children as well as to achieve herd immunity. In the UK over 90% of 1-year-old children have received the full primary course of vaccines. However, there is a considerable range in uptake between Primary Care Organisations (PCOs) and even in PCOs with high uptake, there are pockets with lower coverage. Children who are less likely to be fully immunised include low birthweight children, those born prematurely (Jessop *et al* 2010), with disabilities and chronic conditions and children who are hospitalised (Samad *et al* 2006). These are also the groups of children who are more likely to be more seriously affected by an infectious

231

Procedure guideline 11.1 Administration of vaccines

Statement	Rationale
1. Before embarking on the vaccination process, informed consent should be sought from someone with parental responsibility, or from the young person, if 'Fraser/Gillick' competent. Whether or not the latter applies, the procedure should be explained in an age-appropriate manner. Written consent is not required, but it must be fully informed. Full details may be obtained from Chapter 2. Immunisation Against Infectious Diseases (Department of the Health 2006a).	
2. After consent has been obtained, the presence of any contraindications should be excluded and then the vaccine prepared. The individual vaccine container and where appropriate, diluent should be checked to ensure it is the right vaccine, of the right strength and that it is within its expiry date.	
3. It is not necessary or practical to attempt to sterilise the skin, however, it should be visibly clean. If alcohol is used to clean the skin, it should be allowed to dry before the injection is given, otherwise it may be more painful and it could inactivate a live vaccine. With the exception of BCG vaccine, injections should normally be given by deep subcutaneous or intramuscular (IM) injection, using a 23G needle, 25 mm in length. A 16 mm long needle should be reserved for premature or very small babies only.	
4. Children with bleeding disorders should not be given IM injections. Intramuscular and subcutaneous injections should be given in the deltoid or anterolateral thigh. Vaccines should not be given in the buttock, unless a large volume injection of immunoglobulin is needed, in which case the buttock may be used. BCG vaccine is given intradermally at the insertion of the left deltoid, using a 26G needle 10 mm long	
5. Once the vaccine has been given, the name of the vaccine, its batch number, the dose and the site of immunisation should all be recorded. Ideally this information should be given to the carer in the child's personal child health record, the GP and whatever local agency is responsible for providing immunisation statistics.	**5.** This information is necessary to ensure that: • The individual child receives the correct number of all the necessary immunisations, in a timely fashion • Any local reaction after one of two injections can be attributed to the correct vaccine • If there is a problem with one or more batches of vaccine, the recipients can be traced • Coverage of vaccination can be monitored and appropriate action taken if it is inadequate.

disease. Poor immunisation uptake among these children is likely to be due to a combination of frequent hospitalisations leading to routine care being overlooked, or the belief by health professionals or parents/carers that vaccines are contraindicated because of their condition. This is rarely the case.

One of the most important factors affecting uptake is parental attitudes and beliefs about vaccine safety and efficacy and about the seriousness of diseases (Bennett and Smith 1992, Peckham *et al* 1989, Sutton and Gill 1998). These are shaped by a range of influences including previous experience, the advice of family and friends, attitudes to health more generally, the media and advice from health professionals. Surveys have shown that although the majority of parents/carers are satisfied with their

experience of the immunisation 'process', a proportion feel they are not given sufficient information (Bedford and Lansley 2006, Evans *et al* 2001, Harrington *et al* 2000). To make an informed decision about immunisation, parents/carers need to have information in a language they can understand and an opportunity to have their questions answered. This can be time-consuming for health professionals, but it is time very well spent. Many good written resources exist. These can be used by health professionals to keep themselves informed as well as being useful for parents/carers.

One important strategy for ensuring that children are protected is to check immunisation status when they attend for other reasons, for example children attending accident and emergency departments, outpatients' departments or on admission to hospital. Although it may not always be feasible to offer opportunistic immunisation, it is good practice to remind parents/carers and to follow this up with a letter to the GP and/or health visitor. Children with complex health needs in particular, often have their immunisation status overlooked and nurses have a particularly important role in ensuring that these children, as well as all others, have the opportunity to be fully immunised (Walton *et al* 2007).

The Personal Child Health Record (PCHR), which is issued to parents/carers for all children at or soon after birth, should contain a record of all immunisations the child has received and all serious conditions from which the child suffers. This is a valuable tool for parents/carers as well as for health professionals allowing them to review children's immunisation status.

In September 2009, NICE issued guidance on improving the uptake of vaccines. The guidance focused on increasing immunisation uptake among children and young people aged under 19 years in groups and settings where immunisation coverage is low and on improving uptake of the hepatitis B vaccination programme for babies born to mothers infected with hepatitis B

The guidance ephasised the importance of the following areas:

- Good immunisation programmes (provision, access and support)
- Accurate information systems
- Training for professionals
- The contribution of nurseries, schools, colleges of further education
- Targeting groups at risk of not being fully immunised
- The organisation of programmes for hepatitis B immunisation of high risk infants.

The importance of opportunistic immunisation in hospital settings was endorsed in these guidelines (NICE 2009)

Vaccine safety scares

It is often difficult to distinguish a coincidental event following a vaccine from an adverse reaction due to a vaccine (temporal vs causal connection). This has led to major scares in relation to pertussis and MMR vaccines. In a paper published in 1974 (Kulenkampff *et al* 1974), it was suggested that in some children brain damage could result from the administration of whole cell pertussis vaccine. Following adverse media coverage the uptake of the vaccine plummeted to 30% and lower in some areas. As a result, there was a resurgence of the disease with thousands of extra cases and many tragically avoidable deaths (Baker 2003). It took at least 15 years for uptake rates to return to their previous level.

More recently, a paper linking autism and bowel problems was widely interpreted as suggesting a possible link with MMR. However the authors were very clear in stating: 'We did not prove an association between MMR vaccine and the syndrome described' (Wakefield *et al* 1998 (retracted)). One of the authors voiced his concern that there might be a link and advised the use of separate antigens rather than the combined MMR vaccine. This view received disproportionate publicity and understandably many parents/carers and health professionals became confused and concerned. Since publication of this paper a significant

body of research has found evidence for no link between MMR vaccine and autism or bowel disease (Elliman and Bedford 2007). However, the uptake of MMR vaccine declined overall and there were outbreaks of measles among unimmunised children (Asaria and MacMahon 2006). Although the original research is now discredited, and MMR uptake rates are improving, work must continue to fully restore parents'/carers' confidence in the safety of MMR vaccine.

These examples show how easy it is, on the basis of poor research and media attention, to destroy confidence in the vaccine programme. It is therefore essential that health professionals are properly informed before advising parents/carers. Once the seeds of doubt have been sown, it is very difficult to reverse the effects.

Immunisation of healthcare professionals

Healthcare professionals (HCPs), by the nature of their jobs, are exposed to many infections, but they may also act as a source of infection for patients and well children. For both reasons it is important that all possible measures are taken to prevent infection. Immunisation plays an important part in this. The guidance on this occupies chapter 12 of the Green Book.

All healthcare workers should be up to date with the routine immunisations. This includes tetanus, diphtheria, polio and MMR. The MMR vaccine is of particular importance as staff may transmit measles or rubella infections to vulnerable groups. It is also important for their own protection. An example of this was the case of a doctor working on an oncology unit in 2008 who was confirmed as having measles (Health Protection Agency 2008). Satisfactory evidence of protection would include documentation of having received two doses of MMR or having had positive antibody tests for measles and rubella. However, following suspected mumps cases in an acute hospital setting, only 7% of 42 healthcare worker contacts had a documented history of two doses of MMR vaccine (Williams *et al* 2010).

BCG, if not previously given, is indicated for healthcare workers who have close contact with infectious patients. This is particularly important for staff working in maternity and paediatric departments and departments in which the children are likely to be immunocompromised In the absence of a BCG scar and a history of receiving the vaccine, the HCP or student should have a tuberculin skin test and if negative (and no reason to assume impaired immunity), they should be given BCG.

All HCPs and students who will be exposed to blood, blood-stained body fluids or patients' tissues should be offered hepatitis B vaccine if not known to be already immune. Most occupational health departments offer boosters of vaccine, either at set intervals or if the antibody levels fall below a certain titre. There is convincing evidence that once immune, boosters are not needed.

Chickenpox is more serious in adults and immunosuppressed individuals than in children. All HCPs without a clinical history of chickenpox or herpes zoster should have serology performed. If not immune, and in the absence of contraindications, they should receive a course of vaccine (two doses as opposed to the one required for children).

Regarding influenza, annual vaccination is recommended for HCPs directly involved in patient care as it not only helps to prevent influenza among staff but may also reduce transmission of the infection to vulnerable children. Unfortunately uptake of influenza vaccine among healthcare workers is also reported to be poor, possibly because of a lack of understanding on the part of many staff (Canning *et al* 2005).

Conclusion

Immunisation is a highly effective intervention, which has protected literally millions of children worldwide from disability and death. Although immunisation is largely carried out in the community, hospital staff have an important role to play in ensuring that their patients are fully protected as appropriate. In some cases this will involve offering vaccines in a hospital setting. For others, their parents/carers may need reminding of the importance of vaccines. In the case of children with complex conditions, primary care staff may value advice on the child's suitability for immunisation. In an era when vaccine preventable diseases are uncommon, and the public has forgotten how serious they can be, hospital staff may be the only group with experience of the diseases. This can be a valuable asset in discussing the importance of immunisation. It is also imperative that healthcare workers ensure that they too are fully immunised. This is for their own protection as well as that of their patients.

References

Asaria P, MacMahon E. (2006) Measles in the United Kingdom: can we eradicate it by 2010? British Medical Journal, 333(7574), 890–895

Baker JP. (2003) The pertussis vaccine controversy in Great Britain, 1974–1986. Vaccine, 21, 4003–4010

Bedford H, Lansley M. (2006) Information on childhood immunisation: Parents' views. Community Practitioner, 79(8), 252–255

Bennett P, Smith C. (1992) Parents attitudinal and social influences on childhood vaccination. Health Education Research Theory and Practice, 7(3), 341–348

Canning HS, Phillips J, Allsup S. (2005) Health care worker beliefs about influenza vaccine and reasons for non-vaccination – a cross-sectional survey. Journal of Clinical Nursing, 14(8), 922–925

Department of Health (2004) New vaccinations for the childhood immunisation programme. Available at http://www.dh.gov.uk/AboutUs/Heads OfProfession/ChiefMedicalOfficer/CMOLetters/fs/en (last accessed 26 August 2004)

Department of Health (2005) Changes to the BCG programme. Available at http://www.dh.gov.uk/assetRoot/04/11/49/96/04114996.pdf (last accessed 3rd January 2012)

Department of Health (2006a) Salisbury D, Ramsay M, Noakes K. (eds) Immunisation against infectious disease. London, The Stationery Office. Available at http://www.doh.gov.uk/greenbook/index.htm (last accessed 15th June 2010)

Department of Health (2008) Introduction of Human Papillomavirus vaccine into the national immunisation programme. Available at http://www.immunisation.nhs.uk/publications/CMO020508.pdf (last accessed 15th June 2010)

De Serres G, Boulianne N, Meyer F, Ward BJ. (1995) Measles vaccine efficacy during an outbreak in a highly vaccinated population: Incremental increase in protection with age at vaccination up to 18 months. Epidemiology of Infection, 115, 315–323

Elliman D, Bedford H. (2007) MMR: where are we now? Archives of Diseases of Childhood, 92(12), 1055–1057

Evans M, Stoddart H, Condon L, Freeman E, Grizzell M, Mullen R. (2001) Parents' perspectives on the MMR immunisation: a focus group study. British Journal of General Practice, 51(472), 904–910

Farrington P, Pugh S, Colville A, Flower A, Nash J, Morgan-Capner P, Rush M, Miller E. (1995) A new method for active surveillance of adverse events from diphtheria/tetanus/pertussis and measles/mumps/rubella vaccines. Lancet, 345, 567–569

Fine PEM, Rodrigues LC. (1990) Mycobacterial diseases. In Richard Moxon E. (ed.) A Lancet Review. Modern Vaccines. London, Edward Arnold

Global Polio Eradication Initiative (2010) Wild poliovirus weekly update. Available at http://www.polioeradication.org/casecount.asp (last accessed 15th June 2010)

Harling R, White JM, Ramsay ME, et al (2005) The effectiveness of the mumps component of the MMR vaccine: a case control study. Vaccine, 23, 4070–4074

Harrington PM, Woodman C, Shannon WF. (2000) Low immunisation uptake: Is the process the problem? Journal of Epidemiology and Community Health, 54, 394

Health Protection Agency (2008) Death in a child infected with toxigenic Corynebacterium diphtheriae in London. Health Protection Report, 2(19)

Health Protection Agency (2009) 10 years of meningitis C vaccine: outstanding health protection measure of the past decade. Available at http://www.hpa.org.uk/NewsCentre/NationalPressReleases/2009PressReleases/09112310yearsofmeningitisCvaccine/

Heath PT, McVernon J. (2002) The UK Hib vaccine experience. Archives of Diseases of Childhood, 86(6), 396–399

Heinonen OP, Paunio M, Peltola H. (1998) Total elimination of measles in Finland. Annals of Medicine, 30(2), 131–133

Hennessey KA, Ion-Nedelcu N, Craciun D, Toma F, Wattigney W, Strebel PM. (1999) Measles epidemic in Romania, 1996–1998: assessment of vaccine effectiveness by case-control and cohort studies. American Journal of Epidemiology 150(11), 1250–1257

Jessop LJ, Kelleher CC, Murrin C, Lotya J, Clarke AT, O'Mahony D, et al (2010) Determinants of partial or no primary immunisations. Archives of Diseases of Childhood, 95(8), 603–605

Kulenkampff MM, Schwartzman JS, Wilson J. (1974) Neurological complications of pertussis inoculation. Archives of Diseases of Childhood, 49, 46–49

Le Saux N, Barrowman NJ, Moore DL, Whiting S, Scheifele D, Halperin S. (2003) Canadian Paediatric Society/ Health Canada Immunization Monitoring Program-Active (IMPACT). Decrease in hospital admissions for febrile seizures and reports of hypotonic-hyporesponsive episodes presenting to hospital emergency departments since switching to acellular pertussis vaccine in Canada: a report from IMPACT. Pediatrics, 112(5), e348

Miller E. (1999) Overview of recent clinical trials of acellular pertussis vaccines. Biologicals, 27, 79–86

Miller E, Waight P, Farrington CP, Andrews N, Stowe J, Taylor B. (2001) Idiopathic thrombocytopenic purpura and MMR vaccine. Archives of Diseases of Childhood, 84, 227–229

National Institute for Health and Clinical Excellence (2009) PH 21 Reducing the differences in the uptake of immunisations: quick reference guide. Available at http://www.nice.org.uk/nicemedia/pdf/PH21QuickRefGuide.pdf (last accessed October 2011)

Peckham C, Bedford H, Senturia Y, Ades A. (1989) The Peckham Report. National Immunisation Study: Factors affecting immunisation in childhood. Horsham, Action Research

Peltola H, Heinonen OP. (1986) Frequency of true adverse reactions to measles-mumps-rubella vaccine. A double-blind placebo-controlled trial in twins. Lancet, 1, 939–942

Peltola H, Davidkin I, Paunio M, Valle M, Leinikki P, Heinonen OP. (2000) Mumps and rubella eliminated from Finland. Journal of the American Medical Association, 284(20), 2643–2647

Ramsay ME, Moffatt D, O'Connor M. (1994) Measles vaccine: a 27-year follow-up. Epidemiology of Infection, 112(2), 409–412

Royal College of Paediatrics and Child Health (RCPCH) (2002) Immunisation of the Immunocompromised Child: Best Practice Statement.

London, RCPCH. Available at http://www.rcpch.ac.uk/publications/recent_publications.html

Ruggeberg J, Heath PT. (2003) Safety and efficacy of meningococcal group C conjugate vaccines. Expert Opinion on Drug Safety, 2(1), 7–19

Sadarangani M, Pollard AJ. (2010) Serogroup B meningococcal vaccines-an unfinished story. Lancet Infectious Disease 10(2), 112–124

Samad L, Tate AR, Dezateux C, Peckham C, Butler N, Bedford H. (2006) Differences in risk factors for partial and no immunisation in the first year of life: prospective cohort study. British Medical Journal, 332, 1312–1313

Schlegel M, Osterwalder JJ, Galeazzi RL, Vernazza PL. (1999) Comparative efficacy of three mumps vaccines during disease outbreak in Eastern Switzerland: cohort study. British Medical Journal 7, 319(7206), 352

Smailbegovic MS, Laing GJ, Bedford H. (2003) Why do parents decide against immunisation? The effect of health beliefs and health professionals. Child Care Health Development, 29(4), 303–311

Sutton S, Gill E. (1998) Immunisation uptake: the role of parental attitudes. In: Hey V (ed.). Immunisation Research: a summary volume. London, Health Education Authority

Virtanen M, Peltola H, Paunio M, Heinonen OP. (2000) Day-to-day reactogenicity and the healthy vaccine effect of measles-mumps-rubella vaccination. Pediatrics, 106(5), E62

Wakefield AJ, Murch SH, Anthony A, Linnell J, Casson DM, Malik M, Berelowitz M, Dhillon AP, Thomson MA, Harvey P, Valentine A, Davies SE, Walker-Smith JA. (1998) Ileal-lymphoid-nodular hyperplasia, non-specific colitis, and pervasive developmental disorder in children. Lancet, 351(9103), 637–641 (RETRACTED)

Walton S, Elliman D, Bedford H. (2007) Missed opportunities to vaccinate children admitted to a paediatric tertiary hospital. Archives of Diseases of Childhood, 92(7), 620–622

Williams CJ, Liebowitz LD, Levene J, Nair P. (2010) Low measles, mumps and rubella (MMR) vaccine uptake in hospital healthcare worker contacts following suspected mumps infection. Journal of Hospital Infections, 76(1), 91–92

World Health Organization (2010) Outbreak of poliomyelitis in Tajikistan in 2010: risk for importation and impact on polio surveillance in Europe? European Surveillance, 15(17). Available at http://www.eurosurveillance.org/ViewArticle.aspx?ArticleId=19558 (last accessed 16th June 2010)

Further resources

Anon. Travel Health Sites. http://www.healthcentre.org.uk/hc/pages/travel.htm

Centers for Disease Control, USA http://www.cdc.gov/node.do/id/0900f3ec8000e2f3. *This is a very good USA website*

Department of Health website on immunisation. http://www.immunisation.net/ *Contains information on all the vaccines, The Green Book (Immunisation against Infectious Disease), factsheets and other infor-mation can be downloaded.* www.mmrthefacts.nhs.uk. *The MMR website has a question and answer section*

Department of Health (2001) Health Information for Overseas Travellers (the Yellow Book). London, The Stationary Office http://www.archive.official-documents.co.uk/document/doh/hinfo/travel02.htm Advice about overseas travel. Is somewhat out of date now

Great Ormond Street Hospital/Institute of Child Health http://www.ich.ucl.ac.uk/immunisation/ An independent website for parents and professionals

Health Protection Agency. Immunisation website. http://www.hpa.org.uk/infections/topics_az/vaccination/vacc_menu.htm

Health Protection Agency. Vaccination of individuals with uncertain or incomplete immunisation status http://www.hpa.org.uk/infections/topics_az/vaccination/algorithm_2006_Septl.pdf.

Kassianos GC. (2001) Immunization. Childhood and Travel Health. Oxford, Blackwell. Covers all aspects of immunization in primary care

Medical Research Council (2001) Review of autism research. Epidemiology and Causes. 2001. MRC. http://www.mrc.ac.uk/Utilities/Documentrecord/index.htm?d=MRC002394

Miller E, Andrews N, Waight P, Taylor B. (2003) Bacterial infections, immune overload, and MMR vaccine. Measles, mumps, and rubella. Archives of Diseases of Childhood, 88(3), 222–223. http://adc.bmj.com/cgi/reprint/88/3/222. *This research study looked to see if children were more likely to get serious infections after having MMR vaccination*

National Travel Health Network and Centre. http://www.nathnac.org/pro/index.htm

The National Travel Health Network and Centre (NaTHNaC) promotes standards in travel medicine, providing travel health information for health professionals and the public

Offit PA, Quarles J, Gerber MA, Hackett CJ, Marcuse EK, Kollman TR, *et al* (2002) Addressing parents' concerns: do multiple vaccines overwhelm or weaken the infant's immune system? Pediatrics, 109, 124–129. http://pediatrics.aappublications.org/cgi/reprint/109/1/124. *A review*

Offit P A, Hackett C J. (2003) Addressing parents' concerns: do vaccines cause allergic or autoimmune diseases? Pediatrics, 111(3), 653–659. http://pediatrics.aappublications.org/cgi/reprint/111/3/653. *A review*

Offit PA, Jew RK. (2003) Addressing parents' concerns: do vaccines contain harmful preservatives, adjuvants, additives, or residuals? Pediatrics, 112(6 Pt 1), 1394–1397. http://pediatrics.aappublications.org/cgi/reprint/112/6/1394. *A review*

Offit PA, Coffin SE. (2003) Communicating science to the public: MMR vaccine and autism. Vaccine, 22(1), 1–6. *Review*

Ramsay ME, Rao M, Begg NT. (1992) Symptoms after accelerated immunisation. British Medical Journal, 304(6841), 1534–1536

World Health Organization. Immunisation website http://www.who.int/topics/immunization/en/

World Health Organization (2005) International Travel and Health. Geneva, World Health Organization, http://www.who.int/ith/en/

Chapter 12

Infection prevention and control

Chapter contents

Procedure guidelines

The Great Ormond Street Hospital Manual of Children's Nursing Practices, First Edition. Edited by Susan Macqueen, Elizabeth Anne Bruce, Faith Gibson.
© 2012 Great Ormond Street Hospital for Children NHS Foundation Trust. Published 2012 by Blackwell Publishing Ltd.

Introduction

In May 2004, the 57th World Health Assembly approved the creation of an international approach to patient safety (the World Alliance to Patient Safety). The topic chosen for the first Global Patient Safety Challenge was healthcare associated infections. The World Health Organization (WHO) chose Hand Hygiene in Health Care as the first guideline (World Health Organization 2009).

In 2005, the World Health Organization launched the Clean Care is Safer Care initiative and invited all Member States to participate. Many countries have pledged their support to address healthcare associated infection including antibiotic resistance. Through this process a strong message is being delivered on the global commitment to address this problem.

The potential threat to health from infectious diseases is diverse and includes: the threat of new or previously unrecognised diseases such as Sudden Acute Respiratory Syndrome (SARS); the threat of animal diseases that can transmit to humans such as Creutzfeld Jacob Disease (CJD); the threat from poor hygiene, inept disease control measures or disreputable standards of nursing and medical care. Assessing and managing the risk of healthcare associated infection (HCAI) is fundamental in any healthcare setting. NHS bodies must comply with all relevant legislation such as the Health and Safety at Work Act 1974 (HSE 2003a) and the Control of Substances Hazardous to Health Regulations (COSHH) 2002 (HSE 2009).

The Medicines and Healthcare product Regulatory Agency (MHRA) are responsible for enhancing and safeguarding the health of the public by ensuring medicines and medical devices work and are acceptably safe. No product is risk free. Any adverse event involving a medicine, medical device or blood must be reported to the MHRA. See reporting adverse incidents and disseminating medical devices alerts DB 2011(01) www.mhra.gov.uk. Local policies must be followed.

Recent legislation, the Health and Social Care Act (2008), which came into force in April 2009, brings a modern approach to governance in the UK. The new system will enable a joined up regulation for health and social care along with mental health, helping to ensure better outcomes for the people who use these services. Registration under the H&SCA 2008 will be extended to include all provider healthcare services such as prison healthcare services, NHS Blood Transfusion and Transplant, independent healthcare and adult social care providers, primary dental care, private ambulance providers and by April 2012 primary medical care providers.

The Care Quality Commission (see www.cqc.org.uk) is responsible for regulation of three previous bodies (the Commission for Health Care, Audit and Inspection – known as the Healthcare Commission; The Commission for Social Care Inspection; and The Mental Health Act Commission) to ensure safety, quality and performance assessment of commissioners and providers. They ensure that regulation and inspection activity across health and social care and mental health is co-ordinated and managed under a single, integrated regulator. This includes a need to register all health and social care providers, including NHS providers, with the Care Quality Commission in order to provide services. For staff working in provider organisations, the new regulatory system provides a much clearer composition of exactly which requirements they must meet in order to provide services. The risk-based approach means that regulation activity will be targeted where action is required. If providers do not comply with the standard required, such as cleanliness and infection prevention and control, then the CQC can impose specific conditions responding to specific risks. This may include issuing a warning notice, imposing conditions on registration such as closing a ward or service until safety requirements are met to total suspension of services where absolutely necessary. This could lead to prosecution with heavy financial penalties.

Various documents outline ways of working to aim for 'no avoidable infections'. A one-stop shop for NHS staff to access the latest tools, resources, news and ideas can be found at www.clean-safe-care.nhs.uk. An example is using The Saving Lives Tools, which gives an overview, a self-assessment tool, a balanced score care, how to use high impact interventions (care bundles) and resources with further information. Information on clinical and non-clinical infection control guidelines, including for the community and the home, can also be found at the National Resources for Infection Control at www.nric.org.uk.

Healthcare providers have a duty of care to ensure that appropriate engineering governance is in place and are managed effectively. All Healthcare Technical Memorandum (HTM) are supported by the initial document HTM 00, which embraces the management and operational policies from previous documents and explores risk management issues (see www.csc.org.uk/index_files/pages683.htm). They take into account International and European Standards along with standards in industry.

Financial burden of hospital acquired infection

It is estimated that around 9% of hospital in-patients acquire an infection while in hospital, culminating in approximately 100,000 hospital infections per year. As many as 5000 patients in England alone die due to a hospital acquired infection, with a further 15,000 where infection might be attributable (CMO 2002). This is probably an underestimation due to lack of comprehensive data. Hospital acquired infections (HAI) cost the NHS £1billion per year in England culminating, on average, in 11 extra days in hospital per case. HAI cost 2.9 times more than an uninfected patient and is estimated at £4,000–10,000 per case. Urinary tract infections, the most common HAI, are estimated at £1327 per case whereas blood stream infections, which have a more serious morbidity, are estimated to cost £5397 per case. This rises to £9152 per case when the patient has more than one HAI (Plowman *et al* 1999). Surgical site infections (SSI) comprise up to 20% of HCAI and at least 5% of patients undergoing surgery develop a surgical site infection (NICE 2008). Approximately 15–30% of hospital acquired infection could be prevented by improved application of knowledge and adherence to infection prevention and control procedures (CMO 2002).

A prospective surveillance study of nosocomial infections (NI) in a neonatal unit (Urrea *et al* 2003) indicated the incident rate was 1.6 per 100 patient days (accumulative rate was 32.7 per 100 admissions). Bacteraemia (28.4%), conjunctivitis (19.5%). respiratory infection (10.2%) and urinary tract infection (7.9%) were the most common episodes observed. The main pathogens were Gram-positive bacteria (76.4%) with coagulase negative

237

Staphylococcus (72.5%) being the main pathogen. Intrinsic risk factors related to NI were low birth weight (<1000g), urinary and peripheral venous catheters.

In healthcare the normal body defences are often invaded with sophisticated technology or lowered by the use of drugs, such as chemotherapy, thus increasing the risk of infection. The risk may be from foetal monitoring equipment (low risk) to the high risk of implanted materials in cardiac surgery or transplantation. However this should not be an excuse for poor practice or for neglecting to monitor outcomes of care.

All clinicians (nurses, doctors and professions allied to medicine) should partake in working together to build on improving the outcome of care. This then informs the child and family of the potential risks of infection in a given pathway of care.

Freedom of information

The Freedom of Information Act (2000) allows all members of the public the right to obtain information held by public authorities, this includes healthcare acquired infections, unless there are good reasons to keep it confidential. Therefore, when receiving or giving health care:

The child and family should:

- Expect the risk of infection to be explained to them and for that risk to be minimised
- Plan their living around their hospital stay. If HCAI occurs this may cause increase cost and disruption to family life
- Expect the hospital to be a clean and safe environment
- Wish to be empowered, through adequate written information and discussion. They would like to be able to discuss with healthcare workers, when infection control standards fall below the standard they expect, action is taken and the situation is rectified. An example is healthcare staff not washing their hands between patients
- Expect to know that when a member of staff sustains an inoculation injury the parents and/or child will be asked for consent to test the child's blood for blood-borne viruses – hepatitis B and C and HIV (Department of Health 2008b)
- Expect staff to have taken all precautions to avoid preventable infections in themselves, e.g. immunisations.

The staff should:

- Be offered and encouraged to take up immunisations against preventable infectious diseases
- Maintain competencies in infection prevention and control standards through learning programmes and from information easily available to them
- Know common bacteria, viruses and fungi that cause most HCAI along with those affecting the immune-compromised host
- Know about the prevalence of antibiotic resistant micro-organisms, such as meticillin resistant Staphylococcus aureus (MRSA) both in the community and hospital setting (Khairulddin et al 2004) and how they are acquired and cross-transmitted
- Ensure all children have a risk assessment for infection and it is documented. It should include a birth history with gestational age and complications, an immunisation history, exposure to any infectious disease including seasonal diseases such

as chickenpox or respiratory syncitial virus (RSV), travel abroad and any infectious diseases in the family or close friends, such as tuberculosis or diarrhoea and vomiting
- Ensure personal protective equipment is available for all staff to minimise the risk of infection to themselves and others through contamination with blood and body fluids (UK Health Departments 1990)
- Ensure the environment is clean and well maintained to aid all healthcare workers to practice adequate infection prevention and control (NPSA 2009b)
- Ensure all clinical equipment purchased is either single-use, single patient use or easily cleanable and adequate for its use to minimise infection risks (MDA DB2000 (04) (MDA 2000))
- Ensure equipment posing any risk of infection is cleaned and decontaminated between each patient use. Documentation of this process must be available for audit trails. There must be adequate equipment available to comply with this standard. Manufacturer's instructions must be followed
- Ensure the child and family are informed, if appropriate, when they have been exposed to an incident involving an infection risk
- Know when to contact the Infection Control Team for advice, which must be available 24 hours a day
- Ensure clinical staff receive microbiological surveillance data feedback to aid interpretation and encourage intervention when necessary
- Have access to a Director of Infection Prevention and Control (DIPC), if providing NHS services, who communicates closely with the Consultant in Communicable Disease Control (CCDC) covering local primary care facilities and other appropriate public health officials. The DIPC is responsible for producing an annual infection control report and making it available to the public.

Bioterrorism

The risk of bioterrorism is a modern day problem. The Centers for Disease Control and Prevention (CDC) has designated the agents that cause anthrax, smallpox, plague, tularemia, viral hemorrhagic fevers, and botulism as Category A (high priority). These agents can be easily disseminated environmentally and/or transmitted from person to person; can cause high mortality and have the potential for major public health impact; might cause public panic and social disruption; and require special action for public health preparedness. For updated information see www.cdc.gov or www.hpa.org.uk.

The chain of infection

The transmission of infection requires three main elements:

1. A source of an infecting micro-organism.
2. A susceptible host.
3. A means of transmission for that micro-organism.

Developments in molecular techniques, along with typing of the micro-organism and additional deoxyribonucleic (DNA) sequencing, has improved epidemiological investigation and understanding of the transmissibility and invasiveness of specific micro-organisms.

Source

Micro-organisms are present in natural ecosystems such as air, soil and water. Those which cause infections in the host with depressed resistance are known as opportunistic pathogens.

Micro-organisms are mainly divided into bacteria, viruses, fungi and parasites. The six main characteristics of these micro-organisms are:

1. Pathogenicity – the ability to cause disease.
2. Infectivity.
3. Invasiveness.
4. Virulence.
5. Properties of adherence to invasive devices such as *Staphylococcus epidermidis* on synthetic materials.
6. Susceptibility or resistance to antimicrobial agents.

Antimicrobial chemotherapy and bacterial resistance

Antibiotics can be either bacteriostatic, where they do not kill the bacteria but prevent them from reproducing and allowing the host defences to kill the bacteria, or bactericidal where the bacteria are destroyed. Spencer (2007) describes how groups of antibiotics act in different ways and through overuse have developed resistance to treatment. Antibiotics act by:

- Prevention of cell wall formation – penicillins, cephalosporins and glycopeptides (e.g. vancomycin and teicoplanin)
- Alteration of cell membrane permeability – cyclic peptides (e.g. polymixin)
- Interference with protein synthesis – tetracyclines, aminoglycosides, macrolides. fucidic acid and mupiricin
- Interference with nucleic acid synthesis – rifampicin and nitrofurans
- Interference with folic acid synthesis – sulphonamide, trimethroprim.

There are fewer agents for treating viral infections but they act by blocking the synthesis of ribonucleic acid (RNA) or deoxyribonucleic acid (DNA) or by prevent viral uncoating. Examples are acyclovir, given in varicella zoster (shingles), which blocks the DNA synthesis, and amantadine, used in influenza or human immuno-deficiency disease, which acts by preventing uncoating.

The choice of antimicrobial treatment is guided by the probable site of infection and the likely causative micro-organism. Where an infective micro-organism is suspected but not known then broad spectrum antibiotics are often given. Due to the risk of bacterial resistance developing as soon as the likely micro-organism is identified in the laboratory, narrow spectrum antibiotics should be given (DoH 1998).

The antigenic make up of micro-organisms may be altered through the use of antibiotics. Spencer (2007) describes how bacteria resist the action of antibiotics by:

- Altering the permeability of the cell membrane to prevent the drug from entering the cell
- Preventing the drug from reaching its target site once inside the cell by either pumping out the drug or by trapping the drug inside the bacterial cell
- Inactivating or modifying the drug by use of an enzyme
- Altering the target site for the action of the drug.

Bacteria are resistant to antibiotics in a number of ways:

- Inherent resistance – this is due to the specific bacterial composition in relation to antibiotic action, e.g the make-up of the cell wall. It can also be due to the possession of a resistant gene that is only activated when there is exposure to a specific antibiotic
- Genetic mutation – this is spontaneous mutation during the process of multiplication and does not require exposure to antibiotics
- Transfer of genetic material. This can happen in three ways:
  1. Conjugation – a resistant bacterium transfers the resistant gene(s), which maybe on a plasmid (a strand of DNA), to a non-resistant bacterium through a pilus. This is not species specific and the resistance can be passed between different species of micro-organisms.
  2. Transformation – a resistant bacterium is killed or dies and its genetic material is released into the environment. A non-resistant bacterium picks up that genetic material and becomes resistant.
  3. Transduction – a resistant bacteria is infected by a virus (bacteriophage). This bacteriophage acquires the resistant gene from the bacteria during replication. The bacteriophage, carrying the resistant genetic material, is mixed with the bacterial cell's non-resistant DNA during replication. If the cell does not die it passes the resistant DNA to non-resistant cells by binary fission.

Although inevitable, the emergence of antibiotic resistance is a serious problem. It is important to slow the process down by adherence to antibiotic policies, to use narrow spectrum antibiotics where possible and to administer them in accordance with appropriate prescribing with regard to the correct length of time and dose. The reason for giving antibiotics should be recorded in the child's clinical notes and this must be reviewed daily.

Exogenous infection

Exogenous sources of infection (originating from outside the body), especially in the hospital setting, are mainly from:

1. **People** (staff, other children, parents and visitors)
   - Those incubating infectious diseases such as chickenpox
   - Those with infected lesions such as herpes simplex or *Staphylococcus aureus*
   - Those colonised with pathogenic micro-organisms, e.g meticillin resistant *Staphylococcus aureus* (MRSA), but not displaying disease (asymptomatic carriers). Some people carrying *Staphylococcus aureus* are known as 'super shedders' and disperse large amounts of skin scales, which carry these organisms into the environment causing gross contamination
   - Those who are chronic carriers of infectious agents such as Salmonella
   - Those who act as vectors and transmit micro-organisms from one patient to another through lack of handwashing.
2. Environment
   - Inadequate decontamination of equipment such as endoscopes, beds, thermometers, IV pumps, blood pressure cuffs or inadequate sterilisation of surgical instruments
   - Poor building design such as inadequate numbers of sinks or too little storage space for sterile goods
   - Building work with inadequate dust control
   - Poor maintenance of the environment such as descaling of taps or shower heads, cracked sinks/baths which harbour micro-organisms

239

- Poor pest control such as infestation of cockroaches, flies, pigeons or mice
- Inadequate monitoring of standard control measures for water including hydrotherapy pools, piped gases, steam, sterilisation and decontamination processes, catering, laundry and domestic services.

A susceptible host and risk factors

An individual risk assessment for the prevention of infection should be performed on each child.

If the child or family are the source of infection then this assessment must include the risk to other children, staff and visitors.

$$\text{The risk of infection} = \frac{\text{micro-organism} + \text{virulence} + \text{invasiveness}}{\text{host susceptibility}} \times \text{environment}$$

The host risk factors (Macqueen 2006) include: gestational age, low birth weight, method of nutrition, umbilical stump, congenital abnormalities and congenital infections, and state of immunisation.

Gestational age

At less than 32 weeks gestation the stratum corneum is permeable to bacteria (at 37 weeks the skin is a good barrier to infection). The skin of babies born full term has a pH of 6.4 which reduces to 4.6 over a few days as the body develops its protective mantle, a natural antibacterial protection. This can take up to 3 weeks in the pre-term infant.

The humoral defence mechanism, complement, is only 20–40% of adult values (for a full term infant it is 50–80% of adult values). Maternal immunoglobulin G (IgG) begins passing transplacentally at approximately 15 weeks gestation but does not reach its optimum until about 33 weeks. The foetus begins to synthesis immunoglobulin M (IgM) at about 30 weeks gestation.

Low birth weight

The risk of infection is less in babies weighing more than 2500g as opposed to those weighing less than 1000g.

Method of nutrition

Infection occurs less in breast-fed babies because of protection from maternal antibody transference. Infection occurs more in bottle-fed babies because of the lack of hygiene in equipment, preparation and storage of feeds.

Umbilical stump

The risk of infection is increased by delay in cord separation, inadequate sterilised equipment used for cutting and clamping the cord or the placement of umbilical catheters.

Congenital abnormalities and congenital infections

The risk of infection increases with syndromes with abnormal immune function such as Di George, Downs and severe combined immune deficiency; abnormalities such as cardiac and renal disease; and congenital infection such as rubella, cytomegalovirus, hepatitis or human immunodeficiency virus.

Immunisation

Immunisation programmes can prevent many infectious diseases. See Chapter 11.

Mode of transmission

The Centres for Disease Control and Prevention (CDC) Guidelines for isolation precautions in hospital (Siegal *et al* 2007) cites the main routes of transmission for micro-organisms as: contact, droplet, airborne and environment.

Contact

Direct contact transmission is body surface to another body surface. This may happen when lifting a child or changing a nappy. Scabies can be transmitted via this route. Indirect contact transmission involves the contact of a susceptible host with a contaminated article such as a dirty instrument, dirty environment or equipment. Antibiotic resistant micro-organisms or norovirus can be transmitted by this route.

Droplet

Droplets are generated through sneezing, coughing or talking or through procedures which generate aerosols such as suction or bronchoscopy. Transmission occurs when micro-organisms from an infected person are propelled a short distance through the air (between 3–6 feet) onto the mucosal surfaces (conjunctiva, nasal surface or mouth) of the host. The droplets do not remain suspended in the air. An example is influenza or pertussis (whooping cough).

Airborne

Transmission occurs by dissemination of either airborne droplet nuclei (5 nanometres or less) or dust particles that contain micro-organisms from an infected person, which are then inhaled by a susceptible host. These may remain suspended in the air and transmitted over longer distances by air currents or through air handling units. *Mycobacterium tuberculosis* or *Varicella* viruses can be transmitted by this route.

Environment

Micro-organisms such as *Aspergillus* sp. are found ubiquitously in the environment but may cause disease in immune-compromised children.

Standard precautions

Standard precautions (previously known as universal precautions) are meant to reduce the risk of transmission of blood-borne viruses and a wide variety of other pathogens from both recognized and unrecognized sources. They are the basic level of infection prevention and control precautions that are to be used, as a minimum, in the care of all patients. They include:

- Hand hygiene and skin protection
- Personal protective equipment
- Isolation nursing
- Aseptic non-touch technique
- Management of exposure to blood and body fluid spillages including inoculation injury
- Decontamination of equipment and the environment
- Laundry arrangements

- Waste disposal
- Pest control.

Hand hygiene and skin protection

Hand washing is one of the most important procedures for preventing the spread of disease. The Healthcare Infection Control Practice Advisory Committee and the HICPAC/SHEA/APIC/IDSA Hand Hygiene Task Force have published a review of practice (Boyce and Pittet 2002). The current spread of antibiotic-resistant organisms along with the increasing recognition of HCAI can be partly attributed to a failure by healthcare professionals to wash their hands either as often or as efficiently as the situation requires. An example is the role of understaffing, lack of attention to hand hygiene and associated central venous catheter-associated infections (Fridkin *et al* 1996).

Kampf (2004) wrote about the six golden rules to improve adherence in hand hygiene:

1. Select an alcohol-based hand rub that has good skin tolerance.
2. The hand rub should be easily available.
3. Implement teaching and promotion of hand hygiene.
4. Create a hospital budget that covers all costs involved with preventable nosocomial infection. Combine this with the budget for hand hygiene products.
5. Get the senior staff to set a good example in order to motivate junior staff because negligence seems to correlate with the number of professional years (Maury *et al* 2000).
6. Have the patient–staff ratios well balanced. It has been shown that staff shortages decrease hand hygiene compliance (Harbouth *et al* 1999, Vicca 1999).

Well-defined hand hygiene programmes have demonstrated a change of behaviour and sustained adherence in long-term follow up (Boyce and Pittet 2002).

Some detergents may occasionally cause dermatitis (HSC 2007). Any forms of contact dermatitis should be reported to the Occupational Health Department in order to provide the individual with alternative agents and to monitor possible side effects of hospital antiseptics/detergents.

Principles table 12.1 Equipment required for hand washing

Principle	Rationale
1. It is essential hand washing facilities are easily available in all patient areas, treatment rooms, sluices and kitchens.	1. To encourage personnel to wash their hands.
2. Basins should have elbow-operated mixer taps or automated controls such as an electronic eye.	2. This minimises recontamination of hands when turning off the tap.
3. Liquid soap or antiseptic soap dispensers should hold disposable cartridges to avoid 'topping up' and should be elbow, foot or electronically operated.	3. Dispensers have been associated with contamination of contents and containers causing cross infection (Archibald *et al* 1997).
4. Paper hand towels should be available in the clinical setting, not cloth towels or hot air hand dryers.	4. Cloth hand towels are a source of contamination. Disposable paper towels are quicker and less noisy than hot air hand dryers (Redway *et al* 1994). Soft paper towels are preferred by nurses (Gould 1995).
5. Waste bins should be foot operated with a lid.	5. To avoid recontamination of the hands when lifting the lid.

Principles table 12.2 General hand care

Principle	Rationale
1. Healthcare workers are prone to sore hands due to the number of times they are required to wash their hands.	1. Bacterial counts increase when the skin is damaged.
2. Always wet hands before applying soap or antiseptic solutions, rinse and dry well.	2. This minimises any contact dermatitis or allergic reaction that may occur.
3. Apply a good hand cream regularly – non-ionic base (Walsh *et al* 1987).	3. Hand creams should be applied regularly to protect the skin from drying (Pratt *et al* 2007).
4. Open cuts or abrasions should be covered with a waterproof plaster.	4. To prevent micro-organisms from entering or leaving the wound.

(Continued)

Principles table 12.2 (*Continued*)

Principle	Rationale
5. Keep nails short and clean. Do not wear false nails or nail polish. If nails can be seen above the finger tips when looking at the palm of the hand then they are too long.	**5.** To avoid scratching the child. Microbes found beneath the fingernails have caused cross-infection (Jeanes and Green 2001).
6. Avoid wearing rings with ridges or stones, watches or bracelets, and roll up your sleeves.	**6.** Skin scales with micro-organisms become lodged on rough surfaces. The wrists should also be included in hand washing. It may be necessary to wash the forearms as they may have become contaminated. 'Bare below the elbows' is a practice adopted by professional bodies (DoH 2007a).
7. Healthcare workers who suffer from chronic skin diseases, such as eczema, should consult with Occupational Health for advice when working in the clinical situation.	**7.** Healthcare workers with chronic skin disease should avoid those invasive procedures which involve sharp instruments or needles when their skin lesions are active, or if there are extensive breaks in the skin surface. A non-intact skin surface provides a potential route for blood-borne virus transmission, and blood–skin contact is common through glove puncture that may go unnoticed (DoH 2007b).

242

Principles table 12.3 **When to wash your hands**

Principle	Rationale
1. Routine hand washing removes transient micro-organisms from soiled hands.	**1.** Transient micro-organisms are located under the surface of the skin and beneath the superficial cells of the stratum corneum. They are termed 'transient' because direct contact with other people, equipment or body sites all result in the transfer of micro-organisms to and from the hands (Mackintosh and Hoffman 1984).
2. It is essential to decontaminate the hands after they become contaminated with micro-organisms or before clean activities such as an aseptic technique (Infection Control Nurses Association 2002a). This may include: • Before and after commencing work • Whenever hands are visibly dirty • Any situation that involves direct patient contact, e.g. bathing, toileting • Before entering and leaving an isolation cubicle • Before and after handling wounds, indwelling devices, such as urethral catheters or intravenous lines • Before preparing, handling or eating food • After visiting the toilet • After bed-making • After removing gloves • Before any sterile procedure • Before and after administration of medication • After any possible heavy microbial contamination such as nappy changing • Before and after emptying urinary drainage bags • Before caring for susceptible children (immune-compromised) • After handling contaminated laundry and waste.	**2.** To remove transient micro-organisms which are likely to contaminate hands from touching children or the environment in which they are nursed. To avoid contaminating clean areas such as the sites of indwelling devices, surgical wounds, equipment or the environment. The times that hand hygiene should be performed have been summarised into the '**Your 5 Moments for Hand Hygiene**' as these are considered the most fundamental times for the levels of hand hygiene to be undertaken during care delivery and daily routines (NPSA 2009a, Sax *et al* 2007).

Principles table 12.3 (*Continued*)

Principle	Rationale
3. Hands should always be washed after removing gloves and before sterile gloves are worn (Pratt *et al* 2007).	**3.** Hands may become contaminated on removal and gloves may be accidentally perforated during use (Pratt *et al* 2007).
4. Gloved hands should not be washed or cleaned with alcohol hand rubs, gels or wipes.	**4.** This may spoil the integrity of the glove material (Doebbeling *et al* 1988) and organisms may adhere to the material.

Principles table 12.4 **Choice of cleansing agent**

Principle	Rationale
1. Liquid soap containing an emollient and water should be available in all clinical and non-clinical areas for routine social hand washing.	**1.** Staff are more likely to wash their hands with a product that does less harm to the skin. Liquid soap removes most transient micro-organisms. It should always be used when nursing children with *Clostridium difficile* or norovirus as alcohol gel is ineffective against these micro-organisms (Chadwick *et al* 2000, HPA 2007, Saving Lives 2007).
2. Bar soap should not be used in clinical areas.	**2.** Bar soap stored in wet areas contains more micro-organisms (Kabara and Brady 1984).
3. Alcohol gel containing an emollient is useful on visibly clean hands. It is not a cleansing agent but can be used when rapid hand disinfection is required, such as on a ward round.	**3.** It can be used after a routine hand wash as an adequate method of decontaminating the hands prior to aseptic procedures such as IV drug administration, dressings or minor surgery.
4. There are a number of antiseptic solutions but the most commonly used in the UK (ICNA 2002) are: **a)** Chlorhexidine gluconate. **b)** Iodophors.	**4.** These will further reduce bacterial counts on the skin and destroy transient micro-organisms. They can be used when a higher level of disinfection is required such as in surgery. **a)** This has an intermediate range of activity, is initially slow-acting, has persistent chemical activity (up to 6 hours), is minimally affected by organic matter and is less irritating than iodophors. **b)** These have a wide range of microbial activity, have persistent chemical activity, are neutralised in the presence of organic material, can cause skin irritation and are frequently used for surgical scrubbing.

Procedure guideline 12.1 **Hand decontamination technique**

Statement	Rationale

1. Social hand wash:
    Wash hands using soap and running water for 10–15 seconds (ICNA 2000). The same time applies for washing with aqueous antiseptics solutions or alcohol hand rubs, gels or wipes.
	1. The social or routine hand wash is the most commonly used technique and removes most transient micro-organisms. It is used in all non-clinical areas and in most clinical areas.
	    Use before and after performing any procedure and especially if hands are visibly dirty or after performing a dirty task such as changing nappies.

(*Continued*)

243

Procedure guideline 12.1 (*Continued*)

Statement

2. Use a six-step hand wash (Ayliffe *et al* 1978):

  a) Wet hands under running water.
  b) Dispense one dose of soap into cupped hands and apply the soap covering all surfaces. Vigorously rub all surfaces of lathered hands for 10–15 seconds (see Figure 12.1).
  - Rub palm to palm
  - Right palm over left dorsum and left palm over right dorsum
  - Palm to palm fingers interlaced
  - Back of fingers to opposing palms with fingers interlaced
  - Rotational rubbing of right thumb clasped in left palm and vice versa
  - Rotational rubbing back and forwards with clasped fingers of right hand in left palm and vice versa.
  c) Rinse hands under running water to remove residual soap.
  d) Dry hands thoroughly.

3. Alcohol hand rub or gel:
  Rub hands systematically, as above, covering all areas with alcohol solution for approximately 10–15 seconds and allow to dry.

4. Surgical scrub or hand wash:
  This is essential before all surgical operations and invasive procedures.

  a) Use elbow or sensor operated taps.
  b) Rinse with water, apply antiseptic detergent to the hands and wrists and wash for at least 1 minute up to the elbow.

  c) A sterile brush maybe used for the first application of the day but continual use is inadvisable. Using a pre-packed sterile brush, clean under the nails (only) of both hands.
  d) Rinse thoroughly.
  e) Apply a second application of antiseptic solution and wash hands and two-thirds of the forearms with either:
    i) Povidone–iodine for at least 1 minute
    ii) Chlorhexidine gluconate for at least 2 minutes.
  f) Rinse thoroughly.
  g) One sterile towel should be used to blot dry your first hand and arm and another sterile towel for the second hand and arm.

5. After the initial surgical scrub an alternative method is the application of an alcoholic solution, with or without an antiseptic solution. Two 5 ml are amounts applied to the hands and wrists using standardised technique and rubbed completely dry (National Association of Theatre Nurses 2004).

Rationale

2. During hand washing particular attention should be given to areas of the hands most commonly missed (Taylor 1978).

  c) This helps prevent dermatitis or allergic reactions.

4. It is intended to remove or destroy transient micro-organisms and substantially reduce detachable resident micro-organisms. It is intended to decrease the risk of wound infections should surgical gloves become damaged.
  a) To avoid re-contaminating hands after washing.
  b) The level of your hands should always remain above your elbow when performing a surgical scrub (National Association of Theatre Nurses 2004) to prevent contaminated water from the arms running onto the hands.
  c) Damage to the skin may occur if scrubbing too often thus increasing the microbial colonisation of the skin.

  e) According to manufacturer's guidelines.

  g) Skin scales could be disturbed if a rubbing action is used (National Association of Theatre Nurses 2004).

244

Procedure guideline 12.2 Hand drying techniques

Statement	Rationale
1. Always dry hands thoroughly using disposable paper towels in the clinical area.	1. Wet hands transfer micro-organisms more effectively than dry ones. Paper towels are quicker at 7–9 seconds compared with 25.4 seconds with dryers (Redway *et al* 1994). Newer dryers are more efficient but remain noisy. Paper towels rub away transient micro-organisms and old, dead skin cells loosely attached to the surface of the hands.
2. Foot-operated waste disposal pedal bins with lids should be used.	2. To prevent re-contamination of hands if the lid is touched.
3. Warm air hand dryers can be used in non-clinical areas.	3. The noise that the machines make is less invasive to children outside clinical areas and requires less input for domestic services.
4. Communal cloth roller towels must not be used.	4. These increase the risk of cross-contamination of hands due to the moisture retained in the material.
5. When applying alcohol gel allow to dry naturally on the skin.	5. This maximises the decontamination of the antiseptic solution on the skin.

245

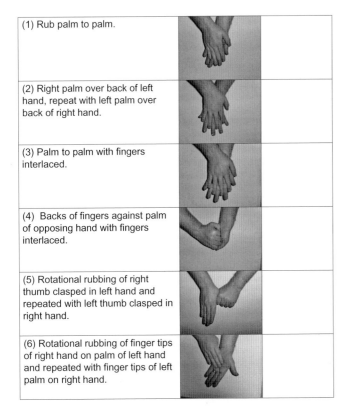

(1) Rub palm to palm.	
(2) Right palm over back of left hand, repeat with left palm over back of right hand.	
(3) Palm to palm with fingers interlaced.	
(4) Backs of fingers against palm of opposing hand with fingers interlaced.	
(5) Rotational rubbing of right thumb clasped in left hand and repeated with left thumb clasped in right hand.	
(6) Rotational rubbing of finger tips of right hand on palm of left hand and repeated with finger tips of left palm on right hand.	

Figure 12.1 Flow chart for hand hygiene (after Ayliffe *et al* 1978)

Personal protective equipment

Personal protective equipment (PPE) is defined in the Personal Protective Equipment at Work Regulations 1992 (HSE 2005) as all equipment (including clothing affording protection against the weather) that is intended to be worn or held by a person at work and that protects them against one or more risks to health or safety.

This protects the wearer's body from:

- Contamination such as chemicals
- Infection such as blood borne viruses, bacteria and fungi
- Injury such as inoculation injury through splashing of body fluids into the mucosal surfaces or by needle-stick injury
- Fine particles such as from powdered drugs or from dust during building work.

Employers are required to provide PPE free of charge where there are risks to health and safety that cannot be adequately controlled by other means.

Employers are required to assess the risks presented by these substances and put into place appropriate measures to prevent or control exposure. This may require modification of work practices, staff training, use of suitable PPE or replacement with safer alternatives. All chemicals used in the workplace are required to have an accompanying COSHH data sheet that provides technical, composition and first aid information which can be used in the event of exposure (HSE 2009). This includes chemicals such as chlorhexidine, alcohol (as in alcohol hand gel) and mercury as found in sphygmomanometers.

Employers need to consider what PPE is available in order to select the most suitable for controlling the risks. PPE must also be suitable for the user and the conditions in which it is to be used (e.g. fits correctly and is compatible with other items of PPE). The Personal Protective Equipment at Work Regulations 1992 requires this to protect employees from occupationally acquired hazards, which could lead to prosecution of the employer. Reporting of Injuries, Diseases and Dangerous Occurrences Regulations (RIDDOR) (1995) require any major injuries, illnesses or accidents occurring in the workplace to be reported (RIDDOR – Report an Incident). This includes diseases such as hepatitis or human immune-deficiency virus (HIV) through inoculation injury, latex sensitivity or tuberculosis.

Employers must ensure that PPE is properly maintained and that there are proper facilities for its storage. This ensures all equipment is fit for purpose and does not become damaged. Out of date, excess heat, humidity, dampness or ozone generating equipment (in use electrical generators or X-ray equipment), can alter the integrity of some materials.

Employees must be adequately instructed and trained in the safe and proper use of any PPE required for their work. This ensures all staff are aware of their personal health and safety and the legal reasons as to why PPE must be worn.

Employees must report any defect in any PPE to their employer and to return PPE to the correct storage place after use. This enables the employer to take immediate action and ensure safety equipment is easily obtainable.

PPE should be selected on the basis of an assessment of the risk of transmission of micro-organisms to the patient, and the risk of contamination of healthcare worker's clothing and skin by patients' blood, body fluids, secretions and excretions. This applies to all staff who must follow local guidelines.

PPE should be removed carefully to avoid contamination of the healthcare worker or the environment. Casanova *et al* (2008) looked at transfer of either bacteriophage or fluorescent marker as a method of tracking contamination from PPE to skin. The results demonstrated that there was frequent transfer of the tracer to clothes and skin on removal of PPE when using the algorithm designed by the CDC. Healthcare institutions should implement the use of PPE removal protocols. This should be considered for surgery and emphasis should be placed on the need for hand washing after removal. This is recommended by Casanova *et al* (2008) and the Department of Health guidance on pandemic influenza (NHS 2007, NHS 2008).

All PPE must conform to European Community (CE) standards to ensure it is of an acceptable standard and safety quality.

Principles table 12.5 Disposable gloves

Principle	Rationale
1. Disposable gloves for clinical use are available in latex (non-powdered low protein latex) and synthetic materials (nitrile, vinyl, Elastryn, neoprene, polyisoprene, Tactylon), in sterile and non-sterile form and with or without powder.	1. Changes in health and safety legislation, the recognition of increased risks to healthcare workers from blood-borne viruses (BBVs) and the introduction of Standard Precautions has resulted in significant increase in use of gloves and other types of equipment containing natural rubber latex (NRL).
2. Latex is classed as a hazardous substance. Under the COSHH regulations (HSE 2009) organisations have a duty to eliminate, substitute, and limit and control exposure to latex, unless there is a need to use it (NPSA 2005).	2. Due to the increase in latex allergy in healthcare workers and children.
3. Healthcare workers (up to 17%) or patients (up to 65% in children with spina bifida) exposed to latex or other synthetic materials found in gloves may display signs of skin rashes; hives; flushing; itching; nasal, eye or sinus symptoms; asthma; and, rarely, anaphylactic shock (HSE 2008a).	3. Some children are more likely to become latex sensitive such as those who have frequent exposure to latex from medical/surgical procedures. These include children born with spina bifida, anomalies of the urinary tract and those who have multiple surgery. Children with certain food allergies may be prone to latex allergy (HSE 2008a).
4. Alternatives to NRL gloves must be available for use by practitioners and patients with NRL sensitivity.	4. To avoid sensitisation. While there is little difference in the barrier properties of unused intact gloves, studies have shown repeatedly that vinyl gloves have higher failure rates than latex or nitrile gloves when tested under simulated and actual clinical conditions (Siegal *et al* 2007).
5. Powdered gloves and polythene gloves should not be used in healthcare activities.	5. Latex allergens released from gloves and bound to airborne cornstarch powder have been shown to cause respiratory allergy in healthcare workers. Polythene gloves often split and do not stay on the hand.
6. Hands must be washed after removing gloves.	6. Wearing gloves does not replace the need for hand washing. Gloves may have small unapparent defects or become torn during use and hands can become contaminated during removal of gloves.

Principles table 12.5 (*Continued*)

Principle	Rationale
7. Gloves must be worn for invasive procedures, contact with sterile sites, and non-intact skin, mucous membranes, and all activities that have been assessed as carrying a risk of exposure to blood, body fluids, secretions and excretions; and when handling sharp or contaminated instruments (Pratt *et al* 2007).	**7.** Sterile gloves must be worn for all sterile procedures, such as insertion of intravascular lines or during surgery. Boxed, clean, non-sterile, non-latex gloves can be used for routine use (Rossoff *et al* 1993).
8. Gloves should be worn as single use items. Put gloves on immediately before an episode of patient contact or treatment and remove them as soon as the activity is completed.	**8.** It is important to change gloves between different care/treatments on the same patient to avoid contamination. For example after suctioning a patient and before doing a dressing. Work with the principle of 'clean' to 'dirty'. Failure to change gloves between patients is an infection control hazard.
9. When gloves are worn in combination with other PPE, such as a gown, they are put on last.	**9.** Gloves that fit snugly around the wrist are preferred for use with a gown because they will cover the gown cuff and provide a more reliable continuous barrier for the arms, wrists, and hands.
10. Gloves must not be washed for subsequent reuse nor should alcohol hand rubs be used on the gloves.	**10.** Microorganisms cannot be removed reliably from glove surfaces and continued glove integrity cannot be ensured (Doebbeling *et al* 1988).
11. Gloves must be disposed of as clinical waste in the hospital setting.	**11.** Follow the local policy.

Disposable aprons and gowns

The Centers for Disease Control and Prevention (CDC) Guidelines for Isolation Precautions Preventing Transmission of Infectious Agents in Healthcare Settings (Siegal *et al* 2007) advocates the use of gowns. However, there is not sufficient evidence to support the total use of gowns instead of aprons (Health Protection Scotland 2008). The use of gowns versus aprons is dependent on the nature of the situation and therefore good practice should dictate whether exposure to a high degree of environmental and surface contamination is expected. If gross contamination is likely then waterproof gowns or those with waterproof panels should be worn.

Principles table 12.6 Disposable aprons and gowns

Principle	Rationale
1. It is good practice to wear disposable aprons for all care episodes where the risk of contamination exists both in the hospital and community setting.	**1.** Contamination of the healthcare workers' clothing may occur with blood and body fluids, skin scales, colonisation with antibiotic resistant micro-organisms or other infectious agents.
2. Colour-coded aprons maybe used for different tasks.	**2.** Colour-coded aprons may be used for specific tasks such as when serving food or for children in isolation. This reminds people to complete the task before going onto another.
3. Non-permeable long-sleeved gowns should be worn where the risk of transmission of micro-organisms is increased such as in desquamating skin diseases and MRSA or excessive blood loss and blood borne viruses.	**3.** To avoid contamination of the healthcare worker.
4. The routine donning of aprons or gowns on entry into an intensive care unit or other high-risk area is not necessary.	**4.** Evidence suggests this does not prevent or influence potential colonisation or infection of patients in these areas (Siegel *et al* 2007).

Facial protection – masks, visors, goggles

Patients, staff and visitors should be encouraged to adopt hygienic practices during coughing and sneezing to reduce transmission of common infectious agents such as colds and influenza.

Good hygiene measures are:

a) Cover nose and mouth with disposable single-use tissues when sneezing, coughing or wiping and blowing noses.
b) Dispose of used tissues promptly in the nearest waste bin.
c) Wash hands after coughing, sneezing, using tissues or contact with respiratory secretions and contaminated objects.
d) Keep hands away from the eyes, mouth and nose.
e) Some patients (e.g. older people and children) may need assistance with containment of respiratory secretions; those who are immobile will need a receptacle (such as a paper bag) readily at hand for immediate disposal of tissues and a supply of hand wipes and tissues.

Full facial protection should be worn when:

- There is a risk of splashing/spraying of blood or body fluids into mucosal surfaces (nose, mouth, eyes) or broken skin areas on the face. There is a risk of infectious agents, including blood-borne viruses, being absorbed through mucosal surfaces and broken skin. Accidents with splashing/spraying may occur when attending to children involved in trauma, children receiving dialysis (highest risk when putting them on the machine and when taking them off), during intensive care, if bleeding occurs, or when taking a blood sample from a child.
- If a child has a respiratory infection and aerosolised procedures are being performed. Procedures that stimulate coughing and promote the generation of aerosols include aerosolised or nebulised medication administration, diagnostic sputum induction, bronchoscopy, airway suctioning, endotracheal intubation, positive pressure ventilation via face mask (e.g. Continuous Positive Airway Pressure – CPAP, Bi-level Positive Airway Pressure – BiPAP or Variable Positive Airway Pressure – VPAP), and high-frequency oscillatory ventilation. Droplet nuclei may land on mucosal surfaces of the HCW increasing the risk of infection.
- During surgery when drilling bone or using diathermy. Surgical smoke is produced by thermal destruction of tissue. The smoke produced has been shown to be mutagenic and can contain bacteria and viruses (papilloma virus, hepatitis and HIV). Furthermore, these particles are small enough to penetrate deep within the respiratory tract (Spearman *et al* 2007).

The choice of facial protection depends on the risk factors. Healthcare workers must be aware of the risks of infection to themselves as well as, if infected, the risk to others including patients. Personal eyeglasses and contact lenses are not considered adequate eye protection. Eyeglasses do not shield the eye completely and contact lenses do not cover the entire mucosal surface.

Principles table 12.7 Choice of facial protection

Principle	Rationale
1. Eye protection, such as goggles, which are appropriately fitted, indirectly-vented with anti-fog coating and good peripheral vision should be available.	1. They should be available in different sizes to aid a snug fit for all shapes/sizes of face for best protection. These provide the most reliable practical protection from splashes, sprays and respiratory droplets. Some goggles fit over prescription glasses with minimal gaps. Goggles do not protect other mucosal surfaces of the face.
2. Face shields are commonly used as an infection control alternative to goggles and protect the eyes, nose and mouth.	2. To provide better face and eye protection from splashes and sprays, a face shield should have crown and chin protection and wrap around the face to the point of the ear, which reduces the likelihood that a splash could go around the edge of the shield and reach the eyes. Disposable face shields for clinical personnel made of light-weight films that are attached to a surgical mask or fit loosely around the face should not be relied on as optimal protection.
3. Safety glasses provide impact protection but do not provide the same level of splash or droplet protection as goggles and generally should not be used for infection control purposes.	
4. Full-face piece elastomeric respirators and powered air-purifying respirators (some with high efficiency particulate air filters – HEPA filters) are designed and used for respiratory protection, but because of their design incidentally provide highly effective eye protection as well.	4. Selection of this type of PPE should be based on an assessment of the respiratory hazard in an infection control situation, but will also provide, as an additional benefit, optimal eye protection. They may be used when performing aerosolised procedures for children with pandemic influenza.

Principles table 12.7 (*Continued*)

Principle	Rationale
5. The European Standard EN149:2001 defines the following classes of filtering in half masks: • P1 filters at least 80% of airborne particles with <22% inward leakage • P2 filters at least 94% of airborne particles with <8% of inward leakage • P3 filters a least 99.95% of airborne particles with <2% inward leakage.	**5.** Generally P2 masks should be worn when attending a child with an airborne or droplet infections and P3 should be worn if performing aerosolised procedures. Healthcare workers who wear a P3 mask must undergo fit testing prior to use (HSE 2003b).
6. Surgical masks are plain masks that cover the nose and mouth and are held in place by straps around the head. In healthcare settings, they are normally worn during medical procedures to protect not only the child but also the healthcare worker from the transfer of microorganisms, body fluids and particulate matter generated from any splash and splatter. While they will provide a physical barrier to large projected droplets, they do not provide full respiratory protection against smaller suspended droplets and aerosols.	**6.** They are not regarded as personal protective equipment (PPE) under the European Directive 89/686/EEC (PPE Regulation 2002 SI 2002 No. 1144).
7. Wear a mask when entering a child's room and performing direct patient care. A mask should be worn once and then discarded. **a)** Change masks when they become moist. **b)** Do not leave masks dangling around the neck. **c)** On touching or discarding a used mask, perform hand hygiene.	**7.** If patients are cohorted in a common area or in several rooms on a nursing unit, such as in RSV or pandemic influenza cases, and multiple patients must be visited over a short time, it may be practical to wear one mask for the duration of the activity; however, other PPE (e.g. gloves, gown, aprons) must be removed between patients, and hand hygiene must be performed between each patient episode of care.

249

Isolation nursing

CDC Guideline for Isolation Precautions: Preventing Transmission of Infectious Agents in Healthcare Settings (2007) cites numerous studies of the epidemiology of HAIs in children and has identified unique infection control issues in this population. Additionally, there is a high prevalence of community-acquired infections among hospitalised infants and young children who have not yet become immune either by vaccination or by natural infection. The result is more patients and their sibling visitors with transmissible infections present in paediatric healthcare settings. Seasonal infections, such as respiratory syncitial virus (RSV), influenza, varicella (chickenpox) and viral gastro-enteritus such as norivirus, cause regular outbreaks.

Close physical contact between healthcare personnel and infants and young children (e.g. cuddling, feeding, playing, changing soiled nappies, and cleaning copious amounts of uncontrolled respiratory secretions) provides abundant opportunities for transmission of infectious material. Practices and behaviours, such as congregation of children in play areas where toys and bodily secretions are easily shared and family members living-in with infants and young children, can further increase the risk of transmission. Children in chronic care settings or in nurseries may have increased rates of colonisation with resistant micro-organisms and may be sources of introduction of resistant organisms to acute care settings.

Infection control management and the need for isolation is dependent on local decisions, which are informed by the risk to the population at the time, data regarding institutional experience/epidemiology, trends in community and institutional HAIs, local, regional, and national epidemiology, and emerging infectious disease threats. (See Table 12.1.)

Trusts need to have a bed management system that not only helps to find the most appropriate bed for a child but also helps to prevent cross-infection by tracking the use of single rooms for potentially infected children. Insufficient single rooms will lead to children with infections being 'housed' in open ward areas. If insufficient single rooms are available, cohort nursing, i.e. placing children with the same infection but no other infection, in a discrete clinical area where they are cared for by staff who are restricted to those children, helps to prevent the spread of infection to other clinical areas. This is more easily achieved where wards are divided into small bays of 2-4 beds which can be isolated further by the closure of doors at the entrance/exit and which have en suite sanitary facilities. Areas must be kept uncluttered, free from unnecessary equipment and have a high standard of cleanliness maintained.

Health Building Note 4 (HBN 4): Supplement Isolation Facilities in Acute Settings (HBN 2005) outlines the requirements for isolation facilities with separate air management systems, an ante-room and en-suite facilities.

Table 12.1 Isolation Precautions required for specific infections or clinical conditions [adapted with kind permission from Barbara Brekle, Clincal Nurse Specialist in Infection Control, Infection Control Department, GOSH]

Infection/Condition	Isolation Precaution	Incubation and Duration	Infective Material	Comments
Adenovirus – Conjunctivitis – Gastroenteritis – Respiratory tract disease	Contact Contact Contact Droplet	Incubation: 2–14 days Contagious: duration of virus shedding	Eye secretions Faeces Respiratory secretions	Isolation precautions indicated for the duration of the hospitalisation
Aspergillosis	Standard	Incubation: unknown	Building work, dust	**Contact** precautions and **Airborne** precautions if massive soft tissue infection with copious drainage and repeated irrigations required. Prevention of aspergillosis in immunocompromised child is paramount
Bronchiolitis	(See specific viral agents)		Respiratory secretions	(See specific viral agents)
Brucellosis	Standard Contact precautions for children with draining wounds	Varies from less than 1 week to several months. Most patients become ill within 3–4 weeks of exposure	Infected animals. Unpasteurised milk or milk products from infected animals	UK statutory notifiable disease. Not transmitted from person to person except rarely via banked spermatozoa and sexual contact. Provision antimicrobial prophylaxis following laboratory exposure
Campylobacter	Contact	Incubation: 1–11 days	Infected domestic animals. Unpasteurised milk. Raw or undercooked meat	UK statutory notifiable disease
Chickenpox (varicella)	(See Varicella)			(See Varicella)
Clostridium difficile	Contact	Incubation: unknown Contagious: duration of illness	Faeces	Soap and water must be used for hand washing as alcohol gel is ineffective for removing spores.
Conjunctivitis	Standard		Eye secretions	
Creutzfeldt-Jakob disease	Standard	1.5 years to more than 30 years	Brain, CSF, eyes, spinal cord, tonsils	No person-to-person transmission reported. Use disposable instruments for contact with tissues associated with high levels of infectivity. For current information see: http://www.cjd.ed.ac.uk
Croup (acute laryngotracheobronchitis)	(See specific viral agents)		Respiratory secretions	(See specific viral agents)
Cryptosporidium	Contact	Incubation: 2–14 days Contagious: until 7 days after symptoms resolve	Faeces Faeces of infected animals	Oocysts resist standard chlorination. People with a diagnosis of cryptosporidiosis should not use swimming pools for 2 weeks after symptoms resolve
Cytomegalovirus (CMV) infection	Standard	Incubation for horizontally transmitted infections is unknown	Blood, breast milk, cervical secretions, saliva, semen, tears, urine	No additional precautions for pregnant healthcare workers
Epstein–Barr virus infection (including infectious mononucleosis)	Standard	Incubation: 30–50 days Intermittent excretion is life long Period of communicability indeterminate	Saliva, blood, respiratory secretions	

Disease/Organism	Precautions	Incubation/Contagious	Source	Comments
E. coli (enterovirulent, including E. coli O157) (including haemolytic-uraemic syndrome)	Contact	Incubation: 10 hrs to 6 days; Contagious: duration of illness	Animals faeces. Contaminated food	UK statutory notifiable disease for haemolytic-uraemic syndrome
Giardia lamblia	Contact	Incubation: 5–25 days; Contagious: duration of illness	Faeces	Oocysts
German measles	(See Rubella)			(See Rubella)
Haemophilus influenzae	(See Meningitis; Pneumonia)			(See Meningitis; Pneumonia)
Hand, foot and mouth disease	Contact; Droplet	Incubation: 3–6 days; Contagious: duration of illness	Nasopharyngeal secretions, faeces	
Hepatitis:				
– Type A	Contact	Incubation: 15–50 days	Blood, faeces	
– Type B	Standard	Incubation: 45–160 days	Blood, body fluids	
– Type C	Standard	Incubation: 2 weeks to 6 months	Blood, body fluids contaminated with blood	
– Type D	Standard	Incubation: 2–8 weeks	Blood	Seen only with hepatitis B
– Type E	Contact	Incubation: unknown	Faeces	
– Type G	Standard	Incubation: unknown	Blood	
Herpes simplex:				
– Encephalitis	Standard			
– Mucocutaneous, disseminated or primary, severe	Contact	Contagious: until lesions dry and crusted	Skin lesions	
– Neonatal	Contact	Contagious: until lesions dry and crusted	Skin lesions	Also, for asymptomatic, exposed infants delivered vaginally or by C-section and if mother has active infection and membranes have been ruptured for more than 4–6 hrs until infant surface cultures obtained at 24–36 hrs of age after 48 hrs incubation
Herpes zoster (shingles)	(See Varicella zoster)		Skin lesions	(See Varicella zoster)
Human immunodeficiency virus (HIV)	Standard	Development of serum antibody to HIV: 6–12 weeks	Blood, breast milk, cervical secretions, semen	See www.dh.gov.uk for HIV post exposure prophylaxis guidance from UK Chief Medical Officers' Expert Advisory Group on AIDS
Impetigo	Contact	Contagious: when lesions appear and until crusted and healed or 48 hours after commencing antibiotic treatment.	Skin lesions	Infection is usually caused by Staphylococcus or Streptococcus bacteria. Avoid communal use of towels, flannels, sheets or clothes as highly infectious.
Infectious mononucleosis	(See Epstein–Barr virus)			(See Epstein–Barr virus)
Influenza:				
– Human (seasonal influenza including H1N1 strain)	Droplet; Contact	Incubation: 1–3 days; Contagious: duration of illness	Nasopharyngeal secretions	P2 masks to be worn; plus face shields when performing aerosol generating procedures
– Avian (e.g. H5N1 strain)		Incubation: 3–7 days	Faeces and secretions of infected birds	Limited evidence that suggests person-to-person transmission. See www.hpa.org.uk for current avian influenza guidance

(Continued)

Table 12.1 (Continued)

Infection/Condition	Isolation Precaution	Incubation and Duration	Infective Material	Comments
– Pandemic influenza	Droplet Contact	Incubation: 1–3 days Contagious: duration of illness	Nasopharyngeal secretions	P3 masks (fit-tested) to be worn. See www.hpa.org.uk for current pandemic influenza guidance
Lice	(See Pediculosis)			(See Pediculosis)
Malaria	Standard		Blood	Not transmitted from person to person except rarely through transfusions
Measles (rubeola)	Airborne	Incubation: 8–12 days Contagious: during prodromal signs (coryza, cough, conjunctivitis, pyrexia) – usually 2–4 days until 3–4 days after onset of maculopapular rash	Respiratory droplets	UK statutory notifiable disease. Non-immune healthcare workers should not enter room
Meningitis:				
– Aseptic (nonbacterial or viral)	Contact			
– Bacterial	Standard			
– Fungal	Standard			
– *Haemophilus influenzae,* type B	Droplet	Incubation: unknown Contagious: 24 hrs after initiation of effective treatment	Respiratory droplets	See www.hpa.org.uk for recommendations for prevention of secondary cases of *Haemophilus influenzae* (Hib) disease
– *Neisseria meningitidis*	Droplet	Contagious: 24 hrs after initiation of effective treatment	Respiratory droplets	See www.hpa.org.uk for provision of post-exposure prophylaxis for contacts
– *Streptococcus pneumoniae*	Standard			
– Meningitis tuberculosis	Standard (Airborne – see comment)			UK Statutory notifiable disease. Airborne precautions if concurrent active pulmonary disease and until active tuberculosis ruled out in family members See www.hpa.uk for current information and follow up of contacts
Meningococcal disease (sepsis, pneumonia, meningitis)	Droplet	Incubation: 1–10 days Contagious: 24 hrs after initiation of effective treatment		UK statutory notifiable disease for meningococcal septicaemia See www.hpa.org.uk for provision of post-exposure prophylaxis for contacts
MRSA (meticillin-resistant *Staphylococcus aureus*)	Contact		From the environment or people who are carriers	See www.dh.gov.uk for MRSA screening of patients. All children and young people coming into hospital should be screened
Multidrug-resistant Gram negative organisms (e.g. vancomycin resistant enterococci (VRE), extended spectrum beta-lactamases (ESBLs))	Contact			All patients should be isolated in an acute setting

Condition	Precautions	Incubation/Contagious	Route of transmission	Comments
Mumps (infectious parotitis)	Droplet	Incubation: usually 16–18 days, cases may occur from 12 to 25 days. Contagious: from 2 days before until 9 days after onset of parotid swelling	Respiratory secretions	UK statutory notifiable disease. Non-immune healthcare workers should not enter the room
Mycobacteria, non-tuberculosis	Standard			Not transmitted person to person
Norovirus	Contact	Incubation: 12–48 hours	Faeces, vomit	Known as 'winter vomiting disease' and is highly infectious with person to person transmission or through contaminated environment. Hands must be washed with soap and water as alcohol hand gel is ineffective
Necrotising enterocolitis	Standard		Faecal	Isolate in acute illness
Parainfluenza virus infection	Contact Droplet	Incubation: 2–6 days. Contagious: duration of illness	Respiratory droplets	
Parvovius B19 (erythema infectiosum)	Contact Droplet	Incubation: 4–21 days. Contagious: duration of illness	Respiratory droplets	Pregnant healthcare workers should not provide care
Pediculosis (lice)	Contact	Incubation: 6–10 days. Contagious: until treated effectively	Hair	See www.hpa.org.uk for current information
Pertussis (whooping cough)	Droplet	Incubation: 6–21 days, usually 7–10 days. Contagious: until 5 days after initiation of effective treatment	Respiratory droplets	UK statutory notifiable disease. Wear P2 respirators. See www.hpa.org.uk for post-exposure prophylaxis for contacts. Cough may persist for several weeks
Pinworm infection (enterobiasis)	Standard			
Pneumonia:				
– Adenovirus	Contact; Droplet Standard	Contagious: duration of virus shedding		
– Bacterial (not listed elsewhere)				
– B. cepacia (in CF patients, including respiratory tract colonisation)	Contact	Unknown		Avoid exposure to other patients with CF
– B. cepacia (in patients without CF)				(See Multidrug-resistant organisms)
– Fungal	Standard			
– Haemophilus influenzae, Type B	Droplet	Incubation: unknown. Contagious: until 24 hrs after initiation of effective treatment	Respiratory droplets	See www.hpa.org.uk for recommendations for prevention of secondary cases of Haemophilus influenzae (Hib) disease.
– Meningococcal	Droplet		Respiratory droplets	(See Meningococcal disease)
– Mycoplasma (primary atypical pneumonia)	Droplet	Incubation: 2–3 weeks. Contagious: duration of illness	Respiratory droplets	
– Pneumococcal pneumonia	Standard		Respiratory droplets	Use droplet precautions if evidence of transmission within patient care facility

(Continued)

254

Table 12.1 (Continued)

Infection/Condition	Isolation Precaution	Incubation and Duration	Infective Material	Comments
– Pneumocystis jiroveci (Pneumocystis carinii)	Standard			Avoid placement in same room with an immunocompromised child
– Staphylococcus aureus	Standard			See www.hpa.org.uk for Panton–Valentine leukocidin (PVL) staphylococci contacts
– Streptococcus Group A	Droplet	Contagious: until 24 hrs after initiation of effective treatment	Respiratory droplets	Also contact precautions if skin lesions present
– Viral				(See specific viral agent)
Poliomyelitis	Contact	Incubation: 7–21 days Contagious: duration of illness	Faeces	UK statutory notifiable disease for acute polio
Prion disease				(See Creutzfeld–Jakob disease)
Respiratory syncytial virus (RSV)	Contact Droplet	Incubation: 2–8 days Contagious: duration of illness	Respiratory secretions	Common in UK during October–March
Rhinovirus	Contact	Incubation: 2–3 days, occasionally up to 7 days Contagious: duration of illness	Nasal secretions	Transmission occurs predominantly by person-to-person contact with self-inoculation by contaminated secretions on hands
Ringworm	(see Tinea)			(See Tinea)
Rotavirus	Contact	Incubation: 2–4 days Contagious: duration of illness	Faeces	
Rubella (German measles)	Droplet	Incubation: 14–23 days Contagious: 7 days before until 7 days after the onset of the rash	Nasopharyngeal secretions	UK statutory notifiable disease. Non-immune healthcare workers should not enter the room. Non-immune pregnant women should not enter the room. Administer vaccine within 3 days of exposure to non-pregnant susceptible individuals
Salmonella	Contact	Incubation: for GE: 6–48hrs; for enteric fever: 3–60 days Contagious: duration of illness	Faeces Contaminated food	UK statutory notifiable disease if associated with food poisoning In children with typhoid fever precautions should be continues until 3 negative stool cultures obtained at least 48hrs after cessation of antimicrobial therapy
Scabies	Contact	Incubation: 4–6 weeks Contagious: until 24hrs after initiation of effective treatment	Skin	Rash may persist for several weeks even after treatment
Scarlet fever	(See Streptococcal disease)			(See Streptococcal disease)
Severe acute respiratory syndrome (SARS)	Airborne Droplet contact	Incubation: Generally 4–5 days but can be up to 10 days	Respiratory secretions. Faeces	UK statutory notifiable disease FFP3 masks (fit-tested) and face shields to be worn in suspected cases See: www.hpa.org.uk/ for current SARS guidance
Shigella	Contact	Incubation: 1–7 days Contagious: duration of illness	Faeces	UK statutory notifiable disease if associated with food poisoning
Shingles	(See Herpes zoster)			(See Herpes zoster)

Disease	Precautions	Incubation / Contagious period	Source / Route	Comments
Staphylococcal disease:				
– Food poisoning	Contact	Incubation: 30 min to 8hrs. Contagious: duration of illness	Contaminated food	UK Statutory notifiable disease
– Pneumonia	Droplet	Contagious: until 24hrs after initiation of effective treatment	Respiratory secretions	
– Scalded skin syndrome	Contact	Contagious: duration of illness	Wound secretions	
– Skin, wound, burn	Contact	Contagious: duration of illness	Wound secretions	
Streptococcal disease (Group A):				
– Skin, wound or burn	Contact	Contagious: until 24hrs after initiation of effective treatment		UK Statutory notifiable disease if associated with invasive disease
– Pharyngitis	Droplet	Contagious: until 24hrs after initiation of effective treatment	Respiratory secretions	
– Pneumonia	Droplet	Contagious: until 24hrs after initiation of effective treatment	Respiratory secretions	
– Scarlet fever	Droplet	Incubation: 1–7 days. Contagious: until 24hrs after initiation of effective treatment	Respiratory secretions	UK Statutory notifiable disease
Streptococcal disease (Group B):				
– Neonatal	Standard			All pregnant women should be screened for vaginal/rectal colonisation. Intrapartum chemoprophylaxis as indicated
Tapeworm disease	Standard	Incubation: 2 days to months, most cases within 14 days		Not transmitted from person-to-person
Tetanus	Standard	Incubation: unknown		UK Statutory notifiable disease. Not transmitted from person-to-person
Tinea (ringworm)	Standard			
Toxoplasmosis	Standard	Incubation: 4–21 days		Transmission from person to person is rare
Toxic shock syndrome	*Strep. pyogenes:* Contact droplet. *Staph. aureus:* Standard	Contagious: until 24hrs after initiation of effective treatment		
Tuberculosis:				
– Extrapulmonary, draining lesion	Airborne; Contact	Incubation: from infection to a positive TST result: 2–12 weeks; Risk of developing TB highest during 6 months after infection and remains high for 2 years	Lesion	UK statutory notifiable disease. See www.hpa.org.uk for current information. Isolate patient in negative pressure room; wear P2 masks (P3 for MDR TB)
– Cavitary pulmonary, laryngeal disease; positive sputum AAFB smears	Airborne	Contagious: until 3 sputum smears for AAFB negative	Sputum; respiratory secretions	Isolate patient in negative pressure room; wear P2 masks (P3 for MDR TB)
– Extrapulmonary, no draining lesion	Standard			

(Continued)

255

Table 12.1 (Continued)

Infection/Condition	Isolation Precaution	Incubation and Duration	Infective Material	Comments
– Skin-test positive with no evidence of current active disease	Standard			
Typhoid fever				Is a statutory notifiable disease (See Salmonella)
Varicella (chicken pox)	Airborne Contact	Incubation: 8–21 days (after use of varicella zoster immunoglobulin – VZIG–extend up to 28 days) Contagious: 48 hrs before appearance of the first lesions until lesions are crusted	Skin lesions	Non-immune healthcare workers should not enter room See www.hpa.org.uk for varicella zoster immunoglobulin (VZIG) for exposed immunocompromised persons
Varicella zoster (shingles) – Disseminated disease in any patient – Localised disease in immunocompromised patient	Airborne Contact	Contagious: when rash appears until lesions are crusted	Skin lesions Respiratory	Non-immune healthcare workers should not enter the room. See www.hpa.org.uk for varicella zoster Immunoglobulin (VZIG) for exposed immunocompromised persons
– Localised in patient with intact immune system with lesions that can be contained/covered	Contact	Incubation: when rash appears until lesions crusted over	Skin lesions	Non-immune healthcare workers should not provide care
Whooping cough (pertussis)	(See Pertussis)			(See Pertussis)

There are three main reasons for isolation rooms:

1. Source isolation to separate an infected child from other children and visitors in a single room to help prevent the spread of infection.
2. Protective isolation to separate an immunosuppressed child to minimise the acquisition of an exogenous infection.
3. Cohort source isolation to segregate a number of children with the same infection together in one area or ward when there are inadequate number of single rooms, to help prevent the spread of infection.

Single rooms are often used as an alternative for isolating children with an infection depending on the risk assessment. The air flow should be neutral or slightly negative to the corridor to minimise cross-transmission.

If en-suite facilities are not available then, where necessary, a designated toilet facility should be made accessible. This will depend on the type of infection and mode of spread. The use of fans should be carefully reviewed as this may increase the risk of cross-transmission with micro-organisms such as varicella, MRSA or TB.

The Communicable Disease Centre sets out guidelines for Environmental Infection Control in Healthcare Facilities (MMWR 2003). For severely immune-suppressed children such as those undergoing bone marrow transplant, the risk of environmental micro-organisms such as *Aspergillus* sp. must be considered. These children must be nursed in mechanically ventilated single rooms or areas with a high-efficiency particulate air (HEPA) filter. This is an air filter that removes >99.97% of particles >0.3µm (the most penetrating particle size) at a specified flow rate of air. HEPA filters may be integrated into the central air handling systems, installed at the point of use above the ceiling of a room, or used as portable units (MMWR 2003).

The following check list should be considered before isolating children:

- Does the child and parent/carer know why they are being isolated and have they been given the opportunity to ask questions?
- Do all staff understand about the infection and the mode of transmission?
- Do all staff know what personal protective equipment to wear, when to wear it, how to wear it and how to dispose of it safely?
- Do visitors have to wear aprons and gloves or any other PPE?
- Does the isolation room door need to be closed all the time or can it be left open?
- Can all staff explain the need for isolation clearly and consistently so confusing messages are not given?
- Does the child have their own examination equipment, weighing scales and any other relevant equipment and, if not, do the staff know how to decontaminate the equipment?
- Do staff know to keep charts/notes outside the cubicle?
- Can the child leave their room for short walks?
- Are staff encouraged to enter the child's room other than to provide physical care?
- Is the family and the child, as appropriate, asked each day how they feel?
- Is the care plan up to date and relevant play therapy or school work built into the day plan?

- Is anyone reviewing on a daily basis whether the child still needs to be isolated?

Aseptic non-touch technique

Aseptic practices minimise the potential introduction of micro-organisms during any clinical procedure which has a risk of introducing infection. Definitions of aseptic technique are often ambiguous with confused terminology. This has led to variable clinical practice (Aziz 2009).

The ANTT Practice Framework for ANTT provides ten foundation principles for healthcare organisations and health professionals to apply safe aseptic technique, whether in the operating theatre for complex surgery or in the community for simple clinical procedures. The traditional paradigm of sterile, aseptic, non-touch or clean techniques is discounted. This is because 'sterile' (free from all microorganisms) techniques are not possible in typical health care settings, and the term 'clean' is not a satisfactory quality standard for invasive clinical procedures. In ANTT, the aim is always to prevent the introduction of pathogenic organisms into the patient (asepsis).

ANTT is based upon the principle of key-part and key-site protection. Practice is based upon the technical demands of individual clinical procedures, namely, how difficult it is to protect key-parts. This is risk-assessed according to defined criteria, rather than the subjective assessment of individual health professionals (Rowley et al 2010). This risk assessment is easily reproducible between health care workers and subsequently promotes standardised practice. Determined by this risk-assessment, practice is defined as being Standard-ANTT or Surgical-ANTT.

- Standard-ANTT:
  ◦ Key-parts/key-sites are protected with Micro Critical Aseptic Fields and a non-touch technique
  ◦ A suitably decontaminated 'general aseptic field' is used to further promote asepsis
  ◦ Employment of standard precautions (hand washing, gloves and other appropriate personal protective equipment)
- Surgical-ANTT:
  ◦ Due to the number or size of key-parts, a critical aseptic field is employed. This will require the use of sterilised gloves to maintain asepsis.
  ◦ Whilst standard precautions are still utilised, additional precautions are required such as surgical hand scrub, sterilised gowns, full barrier precautions.

Rowley and Clare (2009) describe how 150–250 NHS hospitals have adopted ANTT. Evidence consistently demonstrates that the risk of infection declines following the standardisation of aseptic care and increases when the maintenance of intravascular catheters is undertaken by inexperienced healthcare workers (Pratt et al 2007).

Resources for ANTT can be found on www.antt.org.uk.

Many organisations translate ANTT principles into practice by utilising ANTT Clinical Guidelines for common clinical procedures. For example, intravenous therapy is generally performed using a Standard-ANTT approach. It is invariably technically uncomplicated with few key-parts that are easily protected using non-touch technique and Critical Micro Aseptic Fields (e.g. caps and covers). The ANTT Clinical Guideline for IV therapy is outlined below.

257

Procedure guideline 12.3 **ANTT for intravenous therapy**

Statement	Rationale
1. Ensure the area where the procedure is to be performed is uncluttered and clean. At least 30 minutes should elapse after completion of bed making and domestic cleaning.	1. To minimise the risk of contamination with dust (Dougherty and Lister 2008).
2. Risk assess the procedure to determine the level of infective precautions and which ANTT approach is appropriate.	2. If touching key-parts/key-sites cannot be avoided use a critical aseptic field and manage the procedure 'critically' using sterilised gloves and suitable infective precautions, otherwise Standard-ANTT is both safe and efficient.
3. Clean the preparation area, allow to dry, creating a 'general aseptic field' promoting asepsis.	3. Effective decontamination will help to remove microorganisms and organic material, creating an area free from pathogenic microorganisms.
4. Collect appropriate equipment ensuring all items are in date and packaging is intact.	4. To ensure the integrity and sterility of the products.
5. Clean hands with alcohol hand rub or soap and water.	5. To reduce the risk of key-part contamination following the gathering and before the assembly of equipment.
6. Apply non-sterile gloves and a disposable apron. Use sterile gloves if you must touch key-parts.	6. An apron helps to protect from splashes. Hands are a major source of contamination; gloves protect the health professional during the preparation of medications.
7. Open sterilised equipment and ensure that any aseptic 'key parts' only come into contact with other aseptic key-parts.	7. To ensure asepsis of key-parts is maintained.
8. Clean the neck of the glass ampoules or vial with a rubber bung with 2% chlorhexidine in 70% alcohol for 30 seconds and allow to dry. Break glass ampoules with the wipe to protect from sharps injuries.	8. To promote asepsis and reduce potential contamination or injury.
9. Draw up the prescribed medicine using ANTT. Protect key-parts with Micro Critical Aseptic fields (e.g. an aseptic hub/cap or a sheathed non-sharp needle) and place into the general aseptic field.	9. Where 'key parts' are left exposed contamination can occur by airborne microorganisms or through touching non-aseptic parts.
10. If taking blood or giving IV medication ensure that the injection ports are cleaned using a friction technique with 2% chlorhexidine in 70% alcohol for 30 seconds and allowed to dry (Soothill et al 2009). Access an intravenous line using a non-touch technique, flushing and appropriately 'locking' the device according to local policies.	10. To disinfect the injection port and minimise the potential introduction of microorganisms. A non-touch technique ensures the asepsis of the key-parts of the procedure.
11. If at any time you think you may have contaminated a key-part, dispose of it immediately and use a new piece.	11. The risk of introducing infection is too high.
12. Collect equipment used and dispose of all sharp/glass equipment in a sharps bin. Used equipment should be disposed of according to local waste disposal policies.	12. To ensure compliance with waste regulations (DoH 2006).
13. Clean hands with either soap and water or alcohol hand rub immediately after discarding gloves.	13. This hand clean is placed here because gloved hands will have sweated deep and low-lying organisms to the surface of the skin. This will help in breaking any chain of infection.

Management of exposure to blood and body fluids

This section deals with the management of exposure to blood and body fluid spillages, including inoculation injury. Injuries due to needles and other sharps have been associated with transmission of hepatitis B virus (HBV), hepatitis C virus (HCV) and human immune deficiency virus (HIV) to healthcare personnel (UK Health Departments 1998). The prevention of sharps injuries has always been an essential element of Standard Precautions (Universal Precautions). These include measures to handle needles and other sharp devices in a manner that will prevent injury to the user and to others who may encounter the device during or after a procedure. Avoid sharps usage wherever possible and consider the use of alternative methods.

The following principles should be applied when handling and disposing of sharp instruments or equipment (a sharp):

- Whoever uses a sharp is responsible for its safe disposal
- Never bend, break or re-sheath a used needle
- Ensure that the sharps containers comply with British Standard 7320:1990 Specification for Sharps Containers and/or are type-approved in accordance with the Carriage of Dangerous Goods (Classification, Packaging and Labelling) and Use of Transportable Pressure Receptacles Regulations 1996 (Statutory Instrument 1996 No. 2092)
- Sharps bins should be assembled safely according to manufacturer's instructions and the appropriate written information filled in on the bin label. This prevents spillage if the sharps bin accidentally dismantles and ensures a record of the audit trail
- Sharps bins must never be filled above the 'full line' on the bin. Users are responsible for locking the bin when full and for ensuring the correct identification of the source area is on the bin (ward/unit area, hospital/PCT/source building, date of disposal and the signature of the person disposing the sharps bin). Staff must not push down sharps in the bin or attempt to retrieve an article from the bin as this increases the risk of injury. The temporary closure of the bin after each use should prevent accidental access
- Sharps bins should be located at an appropriate height, never on the floor or above shoulder height. Brackets can be used, as appropriate, to secure sharps bins. They should be out of access to the general public and kept in a safe place out of reach of children when in use
- Filled sharps bins waiting for disposal should be kept in a locked, safe place
- Staff transporting filled sharps bins must wear suitable protective clothing, carry the container by the handle and avoid carrying the bin close to their body.

The Eye of the Needle (2005), a Health Protection Agency report on surveillance of significant occupational exposure to blood borne viruses in healthcare workers, indicated percutaneous injury (78%) was the most common reported type of exposure, with nursing related professions representing 45% of the initial reports and medical and dentistry professionals accounting for 37%. Injuries occurring after a procedure and during disposal of equipment were predominately related to failure to comply with procedures for the safe handling and disposal of sharps and clinical waste and were mostly preventable.

Ongoing surveillance of inoculation injuries in healthcare workers and the risk of blood borne virus transmission can be obtained from www.hpa.org.uk .The approximate transmission rates are:

1. For HBV, approximately 300 per 1000 (30%) after percutaneous exposure from a donor who is HBeAg +ve, for a non-immune healthcare workers.
2. For HCV, approximately 30 per 1000 (3%) after percutaneous exposure from a HCV +ve donor.
3. For HIV, approximately 3 per 1000 (0.32%) after percutaneous exposure & less than 1 per 1000 (0.1%) after mucocutaneous exposure result in transmission from an HIV +ve donor.

See Box 12.1 for list of body fluids which pose a risk for HIV transmission.

It has been considered that there is no risk of HIV transmission where intact skin is exposed to HIV-infected blood (DoH 2008). Testing and follow-up for other infections (hepatitis B and C) as appropriate should be undertaken, and the need for post-exposure prophylaxis for hepatitis B should be considered.

For non-blood contamination, for example medications, information can be obtained from the UK National Poisons Centre, open 24 hours tel 0844 892 0111. This service is for professional use only and employees must not contact this number about themselves. However, the Occupational Health Nurse Advisor, an attending doctor, the nurse in charge or a clinical department manager may contact this number for information on behalf of the exposed employee.

If a child has been exposed, specialist advice from a paediatrician experienced in the field of HIV should be sought. PEP guidelines for children exposed to blood-borne viruses can be found on the website of the Children's HIV Association of UK and Ireland (www.chiva.org.uk/protocols/pep.htlm).

Decisions about testing the infection status of children and young people or incapacitated patients, after a needle-stick or other injury to a healthcare worker, must take account of the current legal framework governing capacity issues and the use

---

Box 12.1

Below is a list of body fluids and materials which may pose a risk of HIV transmission if significant occupational exposure occurs (Guidance from the UK Chief Medical Officers' Expert Advisory Group on AIDS (2008) HIV Post-Exposure Prophylaxis)

Amniotic fluid
Blood
Cerebrospinal fluid
Exudative or other tissue fluid from burns or skin lesions
Human breast milk
Pericardial fluid
Peritoneal fluid
Pleural fluid
Saliva in association with dentistry (likely to be contaminated with blood, even when not obviously so)
Semen
Synovial fluid
Unfixed human tissues and organs
Vaginal secretions
Any other body fluid if visibly bloodstained

of human tissue. In England, Wales and Northern Ireland this area is covered by the Human Tissue Act 2004 and the Mental Capacity Act 2005 (E&W only). In Scotland this area is covered by the Adults with Incapacity (Scotland) Act 2000 and the Human Tissue (Scotland) Act 2006. Updated advice should be followed according to Guidance from the UK Chief Medical Officers' Expert Advisory Group on AIDS (DoH 2008b) No blood from a baby or young person should be tested for blood borne viruses when investigating an inoculation injury without consent.

Reporting of injuries, diseases and dangerous occurences regulations

The Reporting of Injuries, Diseases and Dangerous Occurrences Regulations (RIDDOR) 1995 (HSE 2008b) place a legal duty on an employer, self-employed people and people in control of premises, to report certain work-related injuries, such as acute illness requiring medical treatment, where there is reason to believe that this resulted from exposure to a biological agent or its toxins or infected material. This can include inoculation injury. The information enables the Health and Safety Executive (HSE) and local authorities to identify where and how risks rise and to investigate ways to reduce injury and ill health acquired at work. The reporting system is online (see www.hse.gov.uk/riddor) and requires certain information to be reported on F2508 – Report of an Injury an F2508A – Report of a Case of Disease. Staff must follow their local policy as the necessary information must be collated. Failure to protect staff from work related injury can result in a financial penalty or prosecution (HSE 2002).

Blood spillage

National guidance recommends the use of a chlorine based disinfectant (UK Health Departments 1998). Contamination should be wiped up with paper towels soaked in freshly prepared hypochlorite solution, chlorine releasing tablets or granules containing 10,000 ppm (1%) available chlorine.

Blood spillage and other body fluids should be cleared up promptly taking care to avoid splashing:

- Make the area safe while getting the appropriate kit to clear the spillage. Use a 'wet floor' sign until the area is safe
- Ensure the area is well-ventilated when using a disinfectant
- Always wear appropriate personal protective equipment; gloves and disposable apron as a minimum. Mouth and eye protection should be worn if there is any risk of splashing
- Cover the spillage with disposable paper roll or cloths in order to soak up and contain the spillage
- Once contained, the spill and disposable paper roll should be carefully placed into a clinical waste bag
- If the spillage contains glass or other sharp objects the disposable roll should be collected using a scoop or other object that avoids handling the contaminated sharps'. If shards of glass cannot be safely wrapped they should be disposed of into a sharps bin instead of the clinical waste bag
- Use a chlorine releasing agent to soak up the spillage and follow manufacturer's instructions along with local policies. Clean the area with a detergent afterwards. There are combined chlorine agents and detergents on the market which make it a one step process
- Do not use a chlorine releasing agent on urine as this may causes toxic fumes.

Procedure guideline 12.4 Blood or body fluid spillage

Statement	Rationale
1. In case of any incident involving inoculation with blood or body fluids, splashes to broken skin, eyes, mouth or nose, or a bite, perform first aid immediately: • Encourage free bleeding of any wound but DO NOT suck the wound • Wash skin wounds with soap and copious running water. DO NOT scrub • Flush mucosal contamination such as eyes, nose and mouth with copious amounts of running water. If contact lens are used flush before and after removal.	**1.** This reduces the risk of infection to the recipient.
2. The manager should ensure a risk assessment occurs immediately and by following local policy such as: **a)** Sending staff to Occupational Health Department (OHD) during normal hours or **b)** Discussion with on-call Microbiologist/Infectious Disease Doctor (outside of OHD hours) or **c)** Sending staff to their local A&E department **d)** Completing an incident form and the RIDDOR form *(form F2508)* according to local policy.	**2.** All healthcare workers should have immediate 24 hour access to advice on post-exposure prophylaxis (PEP), to appropriate drugs and support. **d)** The RIDDOR reporting is a legal requirement to monitor accidents at work.

Procedure guideline 12.4 *(Continued)*

Statement	Rationale
3. Healthcare workers must not attempt to do a risk assessment on themselves or obtain consent for testing blood samples.	**3.** They may not have up-to-date knowledge of current advice and obtaining consent could be seen as coercion.
4. If the source patient is known, they or their parents/carers will be counselled and if in agreement their blood will be tested for hepatitis B, hepatitis C and HIV.	**4.** To ascertain their infectivity status and to plan the treatment, if necessary, for the injured healthcare worker.
5. The injured healthcare worker's blood will be taken and stored.	**5.** This provides a baseline for future testing if any related illness occurs in the future.
6. If post exposure prophylaxis for HIV is required then this must be started as soon as possible (preferably within 1 hour of the injury) but can be given up to 72 hours after the exposure (DoH 2008).	**6.** This is the optimal time to prevent sero-conversion.
7. If the healthcare worker is not immune to hepatitis B, passive immunity in the form of specific immunoglobulin or active immunity in the form of an accelerated course of hepatitis B vaccination can be considered. Healthcare workers previously vaccinated but at risk from hepatitis B following an inoculation accident may require a booster dose of hepatitis B vaccine. They should report to the OHD.	**7.** Although all healthcare workers should be vaccinated against hepatitis B, there is a small failure rate. The risk of transmission to an unvaccinated individual from a hepatitis B e antigen positive source is 1:3. Healthcare workers must be aware of their immunity status.
8. Hepatitis C remains the most commonly transmitted virus through inoculation injury as there is no vaccination.	**8.** Follow-up of healthcare workers may be needed when the donor's results are known.
9. Occupational Health Departments should counsel the healthcare worker in terms of work activities, safe sex and blood donations during the follow-up period.	**9.** During the incubation period of any likely disease the healthcare worker may be infectious but asymptomatic, and may inadvertently pass the infection to others.
10. All managers must ensure their staff are aware of local policies and comply with the advice	**10.** Various legislation indicates managers must ensure all staff are aware of health and safety regulations.

Decontamination of equipment and the environment

Under the Health and Social Care Act 2008 all institutions providing health care must give assurance that all decontamination of re-usable devices in those institutions is carried out to an acceptable standard. This includes equipment sent for inspection, service or repair (Device Bulletin 2006(05)). Areas that perform these duties are inspected regularly and undergo an accreditation scheme that ensures they are safe to practice. This includes endoscopy suites. There must be a designated named lead in decontamination. The Decontamination Lead is responsible for ensuring that policies exist, there is a quality assurance programme and that they take account of best practice and national guidance. The remit of decontamination includes:

• The environment, including cleaning and disinfection of fabric, fixtures and fittings of a building along with walls, floors, ceiling and bathroom facilities
• Equipment, including cleaning and disinfection of items that come into contact with the child or service user but are not invasive devices, e.g. beds, mattresses, incubators, commodes, hoists and slings
• Reusable medical devices including cleaning, disinfection and sterilisation of invasive medical devices such as surgical instruments and endoscopy equipment.

All equipment must be cleaned prior to disinfection or sterilisation. There are three levels of decontamination:

1. Sterile (at point of use) – where there is a high risk of infection such as in surgical operations or when entering a sterile body area.
2. Sterilised or high level disinfection (having been through a sterilising or high level disinfection process but does not have to be sterile at point of use) – where equipment is used on a non-sterile body area or cavity such as in colonoscopy or intubation.
3. Clean (free of visible contamination) such as in incubators, beds and other such equipment.

Sterile goods should always be checked to ensure they are in date and the wrapping is intact before use.

If equipment is decontaminated at ward or unit level there must be a documented audit trail of the process. Outbreaks of infection have cited equipment being involved in transmission (Coovadia *et al* 1992), such as basinettes, thermometers, suction apparatus, specimen form box, sinks and pedal bins. Other commonly used equipment, such as blood pressure cuffs, have been associated with outbreaks of *Clostridium difficile* (Manian *et al* 1996). Equipment used which is not fit for purpose, such as wooden tongue depressors used as IV splints in young babies, has caused serious fungal infection (Holzel *et al* 1998). The environment within the incubators was moist and warm enhancing the growth of environmental fungal spores on the wood of the tongue depressor, which had been harvested in untreated forests (normally the wood used is heated in kilns prior to use in factories).

Children's toys easily become contaminated and can be a cause of cross-contamination (McKay and Gillespie 2000). Toys that are to be shared in the healthcare setting should be cleanable (hard surface rather than cloth or fluffy toys). Cleaning of toys should be performed after a known case of infection and also on a regular basis. Any broken or difficult to clean toys should not be used. Computer games should have a key board that can be easily cleaned.

In healthcare the designated leads for cleaning involves the Director of Nursing and Modern Matrons. These designated leads work closely with the Director of Infection Prevention and Control, Infection Control Team, Facility Managers and Estate Management to ensure a clean and safe environment are maintained. The nurse or other persons in charge of any children or residential area has direct responsibility for ensuring cleanliness standards are maintained throughout the shift. All areas should have a service level agreement (SLA).

Although the environment has been cited in incidents of cross-infection the proof that it is a direct cause is limited. However, it is important to note that hands can be contaminated by the environment and act as a vehicle for micro-organisms to the child. The hospital environment is different from the home and the literature indicates a clean environment is a safer environment (Dancer 1999).

Laundry management

All healthcare providers must ensure that there is adequate segregation, transportation, decontamination and delivery of clean laundry and linen (HSG 1995). A fact sheet for clothing, laundry and home hygiene is provided for families by Health Protection Scotland (2008). Clean and dirty linen should be transported separately. Linen should be stored in clean cupboards. Follow local policies for the management of laundry arrangements.

Linen is normally segregated into the following categories:

1. Used linen – linen that has been used but is not contaminated with blood, body fluids or from infectious children.
2. Soiled or foul linen – linen that has been contaminated with blood or body fluids.
3. Infected linen – linen that has been used on a known or possible infected child or which has been heavily soiled with blood or body fluids known to contain highly transmissible micro-organisms.
4. Other types of laundry – theatre scrubs or theatre linen not under the above categories. Baby clothes and other delicate material may be separated and a service level agreement made with the laundry service.

Principles table 12.8 Principles of safe handling of laundry

Principle	Rationale
1. Clean linen must be stored in a clean, dry area and protected from dust. It should not be stored in the dirty utility room.	1. Baby clothes and nappies are often stored in these areas and there is a risk of contamination.
2. Clean linen should not be dropped on the floor or be placed on waste bins or linen skips.	2. Linen can become contaminated by the high micro-biological load in these areas.
3. Never shake linen when making beds.	3. This action disperses skin scales and micro-organisms into the air which will contaminate surfaces or children at risk.
4. Always put dirty laundry in the linen skip or directly into an appropriate coloured polythene bag.	4. Never hug dirty linen to the body when carrying it as this will contaminate uniforms/clothing.
5. Protective clothing such as aprons and gloves should be used when handling used or contaminated laundry.	5. This helps prevent contamination of uniforms/clothing and hands.
6. Always wash hands after handling used or contaminated laundry.	6. Hands may become heavily contaminated from skin scales or soiled linen.

Nappies

Although the cost of using nappy laundering services is about the same as using disposables, it is felt to be more environmentally friendly, although this is debatable. Some local councils in the UK subsidise a nappy laundering service, which makes it cheaper for home use. However, in a healthcare institution it is probably more efficient to use disposable nappies. Outbreaks of *Bacillus cereus* have been associated with the soaking of nappies in a maternity unit (Birch *et al* 1981).

Uniforms

Guidance on uniforms has been published by the Royal College of Nursing (RCN 2009). Although there is no conclusive evidence that uniforms and work wear play a direct role in spreading infection, the Department of Health's uniform and work wear guidance (DoH 2010) set out good practice.

Effective hygiene and preventing infection are absolutes in all healthcare settings. Despite lack of conclusive evidence of the risk of uniforms spreading infection, they may become contaminated when performing care (Callaghan 1998). Patients and the wider public expect a uniform to be clean and professional in appearance. Uniforms should be changed daily. Public attitudes to wearing uniform outside the workplace indicate that it is good practice for healthcare workers to either change at work or to cover their uniform as they travel to and from work.

All elements of the washing process contribute to the removal of micro-organisms on fabric. Detergents (either powder or liquid) and agitation of water release any soiling from the clothes, which is then removed by the volumes of water during rinsing. Temperatures also play a part both during washing and ironing. The DoH guidelines (DoH 2010) indicate that scientific observations and tests, literature reviews and expert opinion suggest that:

- There is little effective difference between domestic and commercial laundering in terms of removing micro-organisms from uniforms and work wear (Wilson *et al* 2007)
- Washing with detergent at 30°C will remove most gram positive micro-organisms including MRSA

- A 10 minute wash at 60°C is sufficient to remove almost all micro-organisms. In tests only 0.1% of any *Clostridium difficile* spores remain. Microbiologists carrying out the research advise that this level of contamination on uniform and work wear is not a cause of concern.

Washing machines and tumble dryers should be maintained and cleaned regularly in accordance with manufacturer's instructions. This maintains the efficient working of the machines and reduces the risk of rubber seals or the outside of the machines becoming soiled and risking contamination of clean laundry.

Waste disposal

Healthcare waste refers to any waste produced by, and as a consequence of, healthcare activities. The document HTM 07-01: Safe Management of Healthcare Waste (2006) outlines as best practice guide to the management of healthcare waste. The document also applies to offensive/hygiene and infectious waste produced in the community from non-NHS healthcare sources. It includes colour-coded segregation so it is important to refer to local policies.

Healthcare waste (the term 'Special Waste' is used in Scotland) is waste from natal care, diagnosis, treatment or prevention of disease in humans/animals. Examples are infectious waste, laboratory cultures, anatomical waste, sharps waste, medicines waste and laboratory chemicals.

Offensive/hygiene waste is waste that:

- May cause offence due to the presence of recognisable healthcare waste items or body fluids
- Does not meet the definition of infectious waste
- Is not identified by the producer or holder as needing disinfection or any other treatment to reduce the number of micro-organisms present.

Examples of offensive/hygiene waste are incontinence and other waste produced from human hygiene, sanitary waste, nappies, medical items and equipment which do not pose a risk of infection including gowns, plaster castes.

263

Principles table 12.9 Principles of waste disposal

Principle	Rationale
1. Waste must be disposed of immediately into the correct receptacle. This includes tissues that have been used for nasal discharge and may contain infectious agents.	1. The environment will become contaminated if waste is left lying around on surfaces or the floor.
2. Clinical waste must be segregated from other waste at point of source and at all stages of the waste disposal process.	2. This reduces accidental incidents of waste being disposed of inappropriately.
3. Healthcare workers or others handling waste must wear protective clothing according to a local risk assessment of likely contamination on the type of waste handled, e.g. clinical waste, sharps bins.	3. This avoids contamination or injury.
4. Clinical waste bins should have foot operated or electronic operated lids. These bins must be decontaminated on a regular basis.	4. This reduces the risk of contamination of hands when disposing of paper hand towels after washing.

(Continued)

Principles table 12.9 (*Continued*)

Principle	Rationale
5. Waste bags must not be over-full and must be secured adequately to avoid spillage.	**5.** Over-filling increase the risk of contamination of the outside of the bag.
6. Clinical waste bags and sharps bins must be labelled.	**6.** This is to ensure an adequate audit trail should an incident occur.
7. Receptacles containing liquid clinical waste such as disposable chest drains, should have rigid, leak-proof clinical waste bins.	**7.** To avoid spillage.
8. Clinical waste awaiting collection must be stored securely away from members of the public.	**8.** To avoid inadvertent contamination/injury or the public searching for needles/syringes/drugs.

Sharps disposal

Sharps are items that could cause cuts or puncture wounds. They include needles, hypodermic needles, scalpels and other blades, knives, infusion sets, saws, broken glass and nails. To ensure safety is maintained an approved sharps bin should be used and correctly assembled. They must be locked when ready for disposal. All the documentation on the bin should be filled in to maintain an audit trail. Further identification is often used by applying an additional tag.

Sharps bins must be kept out of reach of children. They should be stored in a safe, locked area to avoid abuse. They should be changed when about two-thirds full or between each patient's use.

In 2002, a London Hospital was successfully prosecuted by the Health and Safety Executive for contravening section 3(1) of the Health and Safety at Work Act 1974, in that it failed to ensure, so far as was reasonably practicable, the health and safety of persons not in their employment including a child aged 21 months, due to a failure to control the risk of injury or infection by leaving a sharps bin in a place accessible to members of the public. The Trust was given a heavy fine (HSE Press release E111:02).

Pest control

Pests such as flies, cockroaches, rats and mice can cause transmission of infection. Healthcare providers should ensure they have in place a system for monitoring and treating pests on a regular basis. There should be continuous improvement indicators to ensure adherence with the NHS Service Level Specification on Pest Control (NHS 2009).

Ward/unit staff must report any sighting of pests to the pest control officer according to their local policy.

Pests, such as cockroaches and flies, are known to inhabit dirty areas and therefore may become contaminated with organisms commonly found in faeces or rotting material. Flies are known to carry organisms such as *Salmonella* and *Shigella* species (Ugbogu *et al* 2006) causing concern in places such as food premises. Cockroaches have been cited in the possible transmission of multiple antibiotic resistant micro-organisms in a neonatal unit (Cotton *et al* 2000).

References

Archibald LK, Corl A, Shah B, Schultze M, Arduino MJ, Aguero S, Fisher DJ, Stechenberg BW, Banerjee SN, Jarvis WR (1997) Serratia marcescens outbreak associated with extrinsic contamination of 1% chlorxylenol soap. Infection Control Hospital Epidemiology 18(10), 704–709

Aziz AM. (2009) Variations in aseptic technique and implications for infection control. British Journal of Nursing, 18(1), 26–31

Ayliffe GAJ, Babb JR, Quoraishi AH. (1978) A test for hygienic hand disinfection. Journal of Clinical Pathology, 31, 923

Birch BR, Perera BS, Hyde WA, Ruehorn V, Ganguli LA, Kramer JM, Turnbull PCB (1981) Bacillus cereus cross-infection in a maternity unit. Journal of Hospital Infection vol 2; 349–354

Boyce JM, Pittet D. (2002) Recommendations of the Healthcare Infection Control Practice Advisory Committee and the HICPAC/SHEA/APIC/IDSA Hand Hygiene Task Force: Guidelines for Hand Hygiene in Health-Care Settings. Infection Control and Hospital Epidemiology 23(12), S3–S40

British Standards Institute (1990) BS7320; 'Specification for Sharps Containers'. London, BSI

Callaghan I. (1998) Bacterial contamination of nurses' uniforms: a study. Nursing Standard, 13(1), 37–42

Casanova L, Alfano-Sobsey E, Rutala WA, Weber D J, Sobsey M. (2008) Virus transfer from personal protective equipment to healthcare employees' skin and clothing. Emerging Infectious Diseases, 14, 1291–1293

Chadwick PR, Beards G, Brown D, Caul EO, Cheesbrough J, Clarke A, Currey I, Currey A, O'Brien SO, Quigley K, Sellwood J, Westmoreland D. (2000) Report of the Public Health Laboratory Service Viral Gastro-enteritis Working Party. Management of hospital outbreaks gastro-enteritis due to small round structured viruses. Journal of Hospital Infection, 45, 1–10

Chief Medical Officer (CMO) (2002) Getting Ahead of the Curve: A Strategy for Infectious Diseases (including other aspects of health protection). London, Department of Health

Coovadia YM, Johnson AP, Bhana RH, Hutchinson GR, George RC, Hafferjee IE. (1992) Multiresistant *Klebsiella pneumonia* in a neonatal nursery: the importance of maintenance of infection control policies and procedures in the prevention of outbreaks. Journal of Hospital Infection, 22, 197–205

Cotton MF, Wasserman E, Pieper CH, Theron DC, Van Tubbergh, Campbells G, Fang FC, Barnes J. (2000) Invasive disease due to extended spectrum beta-lactamase-producing *Klebsiella pneumoniae* in a neonatal unit: the possible role of cockroaches. Journal of Hospital Infection, 44, 13–17

Dancer SJ. (1999) Mopping up hospital infection. Journal of Hospital Infection, 43, 85–100

Department of Health, Standing Medical Advisory Committee Sub-group on Antimicrobial Resistance (1998) The Path of Least Resistance. London, DoH

Department of Health (2006) Environmental and Sustainability: Health Technical Memorandum 07-01: Safe Management of Healthcare Waste. London, DoH

Department of Health (2007a) Uniform and Workwear. An evidence base for developing local policy. London, DoH

Department of Health (2007b) HIV Infected Health Care Workers: guidance on management and patient notification. Available at http://www. dh.gov.uk/Publicationsandstatistics/PublicationsPolicyAndGuidance/ Browsable/DH_4118230 (last accessed 6th June 2011)

Department of Health (2008a) The Health and Social Care Act 2008: Code of Practice for health and adult social care on the prevention and control of infections and related guidance. London, DoH

Department of Health (2008b) HIV post-exposure prophylaxis guidance from the UK Chief Medical Officer's Expert Advisory Group on AIDS. London, Department of Health

Department of Health (2010) Uniforms and workwear: Guidance on uniforms and workwear policies for NHS employers. London, DoH

Doebbeling BN, Pfaller MA, Houston AK, Wenzel RP. (1988) Removal of nosocomial pathogens from the contaminated glove. Implications for glove reuse and handwashing. Annals of Internal Medicine, 109(5), 394398

Dougherty L, Lister S. (eds) (2008) The Royal Marsden Hospital Manual of Clinical Procedures. 7th edition. Oxford, Wiley-Blackwell

European Directive (2002) 89/686/EEC. PPE Regulations 2002 SI2002 No. 1144. Available at http://www.county-safety-services.com/_docs/89-686-EEC.pdf (last accessed 6th June 2011)

Fridkin SK, Pear SM, Williamson TH, Galgiani JN, Jarvis WR (1996) The role of understaffing in central venous catheter-associated bloodstream infections. Infection Control Hospital Epidemiology 17(3),150–158

Gould D. (1995) Hand decontamination nurses' opinions and practices. Nursing Times, 91(17), 42–45

Harbouth S, Sudre P, Dharan S, Cadenas M, Pittet D. (1999) Outbreak of *Enterobacter cloacae* related to understaffing, over crowding and poor hygiene practices. Infection Control Hospital Epidemiology, 20, 598–603

HBN (2005) Health Build Note 4, Supplement 1: Isolation Facilities in Acute Settings. Available at http://microtrainees.bham.ac.uk/lib/exe/fetch.php?media=hbn4.pdf (last accessed 6th June 2011)

Healthcare Infection Control Practice Advisory Committee – HICPAC (2007) Guideline for Isolation Precautions: Preventing Transmission of Infectious Agents in Healthcare Settings. Centers for Disease Control and Prevention, Atlanta

Health Protection Agency (2005) The Eye of the Needle: Surveillance of Significant Occupational Exposure to Blood-borne Viruses in Healthcare Workers. Centre of Infection; England, Wales and Northern Ireland Seven-year Report. London, HPA

HPA Regional Microbiology Network (2007) A good practice guide to control *Clostridium difficile*. Available at www.hpa.org.uk (last accessed 6th June 2011)

Health Protection Scotland (2008) Transmission Based Precautions – Literature Reviews – Gowns versus Aprons. Available at www.documents. hps.scot.nhs.uk/hai/infection-control/transmission-based-precautions/ literature-reviews/mic-lr-gowns-2008-04.pdf (last accessed 25th August 2010)

HSE (2002) Press Release E111:02 12th June 2002. Available at http://www. hse.gov.uk/press/2002/e02111.htm (last accessed 6th June 2011)

HSE (2003a) Health and Safety Regulation: a short guide. London, Health and Safety Executive

HSE (2003b) Fit testing of respiratory protective equipment facepieces. OC282/28. Health and Safety Executive. Available at http://www.hse.gov.uk/ foi/internalops/fod/oc/200-299/282_28.pdf (last accessed 6th June 2011)

HSE (2005) A short guide to the Personal Protective Equipment Regulations 1992. Health and Safety Executive. Available at http://www.hse.gov.uk/ pubns/indg174.pdf (last accessed 6th June 2011)

Health and Safety Executive (2007) Preventing Contact Dermatitis at Work. HSC, UK

HSE (2008a) Royal College of Physicians and NHS Plus. Latex Allergy Occupational aspects of management – a national guideline see http://www. hse.gov.uk/healthservices/latex/allergyguide.pdf (last accessed 6th June 2011)

HSE (2008b) A guide to the Reporting of Injuries, Diseases and Dangerous Occurrences Regulations 1995, 3rd edition. London, Health and Safety Executive

HSE (2009) Control of Substances Hazardous to Health Regulations 2002: What you need to know about COSHH. London, Health and Safety Executive

HSG (1995) (18) Hospital laundry arrangements for used and infected linen. London, National Health Service Executive, Department of Health

Health Protection Scotland (2008) Washing .clothes at home. Information for people in hospitals or care homes and their relatives. Available at http:// www.silverguard.co.uk/static/contentfiles/pdf/hsg9518.pdf (last accessed 6th June 2011)

Holzel H, Macqueen S, MacDonald A, Alexander S, Campbell CK, Johnson EM, Warnock DW. (1998) Rhizopus microspores in wooden tongue depressors: a major threat or minor inconvenience? Journal of Hospital Infection, 38, 113–118

Infection Control Nurses Association (2002) Guidelines for Hand Hygiene. Bathgate, Infection Control Nurses Association. Available at www.ips.uk.net

Ingram P, Murdoch MF. (2009) Aseptic non-touch technique in intravenous therapy. Nursing Standard, 24(8), 49–57

Jeanes A, Green J. (2001) Nail art: a review of current infection control issues. Journal of Hospital Infection, 49, 139–142

Kabara JJ, Brady MB. (1984) Contamination of bar soaps under 'in use' conditions. Journal of Environmental Pathology Toxicology and Oncology, 5(4–5), 1–14

Kampf G. (2004) The six golden rules to improve hand hygiene. Journal of Hospital Infection, 56, S3–S5

Khairulddin N, Bishop L, Lamagni TL, Sharland M, Duckworth G. (2004) Emergence of methicillin resistant Staphylococcus aureus (MRSA) bacteraemia among children in England and Wales, 1990–2001. Archives of Diseases in Childhood, 89, 378–379

Mackintosh CA, Hoffman PN. (1984) An extended model for the transfer of micro-organisms and the effect of alcohol disinfection. Journal of Hygiene, 92, 345–355

Macqueen S. (2006) Control of infection. In Trigg E, Mohammed TA. (eds), Practices in Children's Nursing: Guidelines for Hospital and Community, 2nd edition. London, Elsevier Churchill Livingstone

Manian FA, Meyer L, Jenne J. (1996) *Clostridium difficile* contamination of blood pressure cuffs: a call for a closer look at gloving practices in the era of universal precautions. Infection Control and Hospital Epidemiology, 17, 180–182

Maury E, Alzieu M, Baudet JL, Haram N, Barbut F, Guidet B, Offenstadt G. (2000) Availability of an alcohol solution can improve hand disinfection compliance in an intensive care unit. American Journal of Respiratory Critical Care Medicine, 162(1), 324–327

McKay J, Gillespie LA. (2000) Bacterial contamination of children's toys used in a general practitioner's surgery. Scottish Medical Journal, 45, 012–013

Medical Devices Agency (MDA) (2000) Single-use Medical Devices: Implications and Consequences of reuse. MDA DB2000(4). London, MDA

Medicines and Healthcare products Regulatory Agency (MHRA) (2011) Reporting Adverse Incidents and Disseminating Medical Device Alerts. DB 2011(01). London, Department of Health

MMWR (2003) Guidelines for Environmental Infection Control in Healthcare. Available at http://www.cdc.gov/mmwr/preview/mmwrhtml/ rr5210a1.htm (last accessed 6th June 2011)

National Association of Theatre Nurses (2004) Standards and recommendations for safe peri-operative practice. Harrogate, National Association of Theatre Nurses

NHS (2009) Service Level Specification. Standard Output Specification on Pest Control. London, Department of Health

265

NHS (2007) Pandemic Influenza: Guidance for Infection Control in Hospital and Primary Care settings. London, Department of Health

NHS (2008) Pandemic Influenza: Guidance for Infection Control in Critical Care Settings. London, Department of Health

NHS (2009) Service Level Specification. Standard Output Specification on Pest Control. London, Department of Health

NPSA (2005) Protecting people with allergy associated with latex. National Patient Safety Agency Information, reference NPSA/2005/8. London, NPSA. Available at http://www.nrls.npsa.nhs.uk/resources/?EntryId45=59791 (last accessed 23rd October 2011)

NPSA (2009a) Your 5 Moments for Hand Hygiene. Available at www.npsa.nhs.uk/cleanyourhand (last accessed 23rd October 2011)

National Patient Safety Agency (NPSA) (2009b) The NHS Cleaning Manual. London, National Patient Safety Agency

NICE (2008) Surgical Site Infection: prevention and treatment of surgical site infection. London, National Institute for Clinical Excellence

Plowman R, Graves N, Griffin M, Roberts JA, Swan AV, Cookson B, Taylor L. (1999) The Socio-economic Burden of Hospital Acquired Infection. London, Public Health Laboratory Service

Pratt RJ, Pellowe CM, Wilson JA, Loveday HP, Jones SRLJ, McDougall C, Wilcox MH. (2007) The epic2 Project: National evidence-based guidelines for preventing healthcare associated infections in NHS hospitals in England. Journal of Hospital Infection, 65(suppl.1, Feb), S1–64

RCN (2009) Guidance on uniforms and workwear. London, Royal College of Nursing

Redway K, Knights B, Bozoky Z. (1994) Hand Drying: A study of bacterial types associated with different hand drying methods and with hot-air hand dryers. London, University of Westminster

Reporting of Injuries, Diseases and Dangerous Occurrences Regulations (RIDDOR) (1995) Report and Incident. Available at http://www.hse.gov.uk/riddor/ (last accessed 23rd October 2011)

Rossoff LJ, Lams S, Hilton E, Borenstein M, Isenberg HD. (1993) Is the in use of boxed gloves in an intensive care unit safe? American Journal of Medicine, 94, 602–607

Rowley S. (2001) Theory to practice. Aseptic non-touch technique. Nursing Times, 97(7), VI–VIII

Rowley S, Clare S. (2009) Improving standards of aseptic practice through an ANTT trust-wide implementation process: a matter of prioritisation and care. Journal of Infection Prevention, 10(Suppl 1), s18–s23

Rowley S, Sinclair S. (2004) Working towards an NHS standard for aseptic non-touch technique. Nursing Times, 100(8), 50–52

Rowley S, Clare S, Macqueen S, Molyneux R. (2010) ANTT v2: An updated practice framework for aseptic technique. British Journal of Nursing, 19(5, suppl) S5–S11

Saving Lives: Reducing infection, delivering clean and safe care(2007) High Impact Intervention no. 7 Care bundle to reduce the risk from *Clostridium difficile*. Available at www.dh.gov.uk (last accessed 6th June 2011)

Sax H, Allegranzi B, Uckay I, Larson E, Boyce J, Pittet D. (2007) 'My five moments for hand hygiene': a user-centred design approach to understand, train, monitor and report hand hygiene. Journal of Hospital Infection, 67, 9–21

Siegel JD, Rhinehart E, Jackson M, Chiarello L, and the Healthcare Infection Control Practices Advisory Committee (2007) Guideline for Isolation Precautions: Preventing Transmission of Infectious Agents in Healthcare Settings. Available at http://www.cdc.gov/ncidod/dhqp/pdf/isolation2007.pdf (last accessed 6th June 2011)

Spearman J, Tsavellas G, Nichols P. (2007) Current attitudes and practices towards diathermy smoke. Annals of the Royal College of Surgeons of England, 89,162–165

Spencer RC. (2007) Microbes, infection and immunity. In Perry C. (ed.) Infection Prevention and Control. Oxford, Blackwell

Soothill JS, Bravery K, Ho A, Macqueen S, Collins J, Lock P. (2009) A fall in bloodstream infections followed a change to 2% chlorhexidine in 70% isopropanol for catheter connection antisepsis: A pediatric single centre before/after study on a hemopoietic stem cell transplant ward. American Journal of Infection Control, 37, 626–630

Statutory Instrument (1996) No. 2092 The Carriage of Dangerous Goods (Classification, Packaging and Labelling) and use of Transportable Pressure Receptacles Regulations. See www.legislation.gov.uk/id/uksi/1996/2092 (last accessed 6th June 2011)

Taylor L. (1978) An evaluation of handwashing techniques. Nursing Times, January 12th, 54–55Ugbogu OC, Nwachukwi NC, Ogbuagu UN. (2006) Isolation of Salmonella and Shigella species from house flies (Musca domestica l) in Utura, Nigeria. African Journal of Biotechnology, 5(11), 1090–1091

UK Health Departments (1990) Guidance for Clinical Health Care Workers: Protection Against Infection with HIV and Hepatitis Viruses. London, HMSO

U K Health Departments (1998) Guidance for Clinical Healthcare Workers: Protection Against Infection with Blood Borne Viruses. London, The Stationery Office

Urrea M, Iriondo M, Thio M, Krauel X, Serra M, LaTorre C, Jimenez R. (2003) A prospective incidence study of nosocomial infections in a neonatal unit. American Journal of Infection Control, 31, 505–507

Vicca AF. (1999) Nursing staff workload as a determinant of meticillin-resistant Staphylococcus aureus spread in an adult intensive therapy unit. Journal of Hospital Infection, 43, 109–113

Walsh B, Blackmore PH, Drabu YJ. (1987) The effect of hand cream on the antibacterial activity of Chlorhexidine Gluconate. Journal of Hospital Infection, 9, 30–33

Wilson JA, Loveday HP, Hoffman PN, Pratt RJ. (2007) Uniform: an evidence review of the microbiological significance of uniforms and uniform policy in the prevention and control of healthcare-associated infections. Report to the Department of Health (England). Journal of Hospital Infection, 66(4), 301–306

World Health Organization (2009) Guidelines on Hand Hygiene in Healthcare. First Global Patient Safety Challenge: Clean Care is Safer Care. Available at http://whqlibdoc.who.int/publications/2009/9789241597906_eng.pdf (last accessed 6th June 2011)

Further reading

American Academy of Pediatrics (2006) Report of the Committee on Infectious Diseases. In Pickering LK, et al. (eds) Red Book, 27th edition. AAP, Elk Grove Village, USA

Anderson RE, Young V, Stewart M, Robertson C, Dancer SJ. (2011) Cleanliness audit of clinical surfaces and equipment: who cleans what? Journal of Hospital Infection, 78(3), 178–181

Centers for Disease Control and Prevention (CDC) (2007) Guideline for Isolation Precautions: Preventing Transmission of Infectious Agents in Healthcare Settings. Available at http://www.cdc.gov/ncidod/dhqp/pdf/Isolation2007.pdf (last accessed 2nd January 2012)

Center for Disease Control and Prevention (CDC) (2011) Guide to infection prevention for outpatient settings: Minimum expectations for safe care. Atlanta, CDC

Department of Health (2009) Health Technical Memorandum 01-05: Decontamination in primary care dental practices. London, Department of Health

Health Protection Agency (HPA) Infectious Diseases. Available at http://www.hpa.org.uk/Topics/InfectiousDiseases/ (last accessed 2nd January 2012)

National Patient Safety Agency (2009) WHO Surgical Safety Checklist. London, Nationl Reporting and Learning Service

Royal College of Nursing (2011) Wipe it out. One chance to get it right. Infection Prevention and Control: Information and Learning Resources for health care staff. London, Royal College of Nursing

Chapter 13

Intravenous and intra-arterial access

Chapter contents

Procedure guidelines

The Great Ormond Street Hospital Manual of Children's Nursing Practices, First Edition. Edited by Susan Macqueen, Elizabeth Anne Bruce, Faith Gibson.
© 2012 Great Ormond Street Hospital for Children NHS Foundation Trust. Published 2012 by Blackwell Publishing Ltd.

Intravenous access

Intravenous access is frequently required in children with significant health problems for a wide range of reasons that include blood sampling, drug and fluid administration and parenteral nutrition. It may be part of a planned sequence of events and investigations or it may have to be carried out speedily, in an emergency situation. The implications of cannulation should not be underestimated. The introduction of a foreign body into the vein is an extraordinary intervention, with potentially serious infection risks. It is traumatic, painful and stressful for both the child and their family. Whilst the insertion of a cannula is a routine event for health professionals, many children and families associate it with dramatic events and serious illness (Bruce 2009). Children and parents/carers will require support and encouragement to deal with the procedure. Children often state that the 'needle' is one of the most feared items of equipment that they are likely to encounter in hospital (Bruce 2009). It is recommended that for the insertion of peripheral devices and when accessing all devices an aseptic non-touch technique (ANTT) is used to minimise infection risks. Insertion of central venous access devices requires the use of a sterile technique (Rowley 2001). Many factors need to be considered, some of which are summarised here.

This chapter looks at a range of vascular access devices (VADs) commonly used in children, the criteria for selecting alternative devices and the nursing care required to maximise child safety while the device remains in place (Table 13.1). The choice of device will depend on several factors and these are also explored in this chapter. Cannulation techniques and care of peripheral lines are presented in detail. Four types of central catheters, percutaneous (non-tunnelled) catheters, tunnelled catheters (Broviac and Hickman lines), and implantable ports are explained. Any specific considerations that differ from peripheral line management for the care and management of these lines are highlighted. Non-surgical insertion of central lines is an advanced nursing skill requiring specialist training, the techniques for which are outlined for both non tunnelled short-tem catheters in intensive care patients and peripherally inserted central venous catheters (PICC lines) inserted using interventional radiology (see Chapter 14).

Midline catheters in the veins of the upper arm are generally not used in children as they offer little advantage over peripheral lines due to the small size of the arm veins (Kaye *et al* 2000). Catheters designed for haemodialysis or those inserted into the pulmonary artery, the left atrium, the umbilical vein or artery are not discussed in this general text either. What follows is a comprehensive description that will inform decision making, clinical care and support of children and families in relation to three approaches to IV access:

1. Peripheral venous catheters.
2. Central venous access catheters.
3. Arterial lines.

First this section begins with information regarding IV access and training.

Peripheral venous catheters

Peripheral catheters are the most commonly used VAD. They are principally used for short term infusions of fluids, blood products and drugs, as well as blood sampling. An intravenous cannula consists of a plastic catheter, which is inserted with the aid of a stylet or needle placed in the lumen of the catheter with the sharp point protruding from the end, known as 'over the needle' cannula; they are available in a range of sizes, lengths and materials. Size of cannula chosen will depend on the size of the vein and the volume of fluid likely to be infused. For example, size 24 G is suitable for small volumes for neonatal veins, while size 22 G is commonly used in young children. Peripheral venous catheters should be left in place until IV therapy is completed unless there are signs of phlebitis or extravasation (Centre for Disease Control and Prevention [CDCP] 2002).

Table 13.1 Catheters commonly used for venous access in children

Catheter type	Entry site	Length	Usual lifespan of device	Comments (CDCP 2002)
Peripheral venous catheter	Usually veins of hand, forearm, feet or ankle	<8 cm	1–8 days (CDCP 2002)	Phlebitis with prolonged use, rarely associated with blood stream infection
Non-tunnelled central venous catheters	Percutaneous insertion into a central vein (femoral, subclavian internal jugular)	≥8 cm	≤2 weeks (Kaye *et al* 2000)	Increased risk of blood stream infections. Heparin bonded recommended
Peripherally inserted central venous catheters (PICC)	Inserted into basilic, cephalic or brachial veins and enter the superior vena cava	≤20 cm	1–6 weeks	Lower rates of infection than non-tunnelled CVCs
Tunnelled central venous catheters	Implanted into subclavian, internal jugular or femoral vein	≥8 cm	Long term	Lower risks of infection than non-tunnelled catheter – cuff inhibits migration of organisms. Surgery required for removal
Implanted ports	Tunnelled beneath the skin to subclavian or internal jugular with a subcutaneous port accessed via a needle	≥8 cm	Long term	Lowest risk for infection. Improved body image, no site care needed when line not in use, not recommended for children who are needle phobic

Principles table 13.1 Selection of an appropriate device

Principle	Rationale
The choice of device will depend on the following questions.	
1. What is the child's clinical condition?	1. In emergency settings rapid access is required for life support procedures and wide bore peripheral venous or intraosseous cannula are recommended (Advanced Life Support Group 2001). Treatment protocols will frequently determine the type of access required.
2. Which sites are available?	2. Peripheral veins on the dorsum of the hand, the forearm, the dorsum of the feet and the saphenous vein on the ankle are all suitable, but children with long-term conditions may have poor peripheral access (Advanced Life Support Group 2001).
3. What drugs will be administered through the intravenous line?	3. Some drugs must be delivered centrally, e.g. chemotherapy, inotropes.
4. How many drugs and fluids may require concurrent administration?	4. Treatment may require central devices with multiple lumens to meet drug and fluid requirements.
5. What is the local trust policy?	5. Standard local policy and practices may stipulate the use of certain devices.
6. What is the anticipated time period for treatment?	6. Different devices are available: • Short-term devices: peripheral and non-tunnelled central lines • Medium-term: PICC lines • Long-term devices: tunnelled or implanted ports.
7. What choice can be offered to the child and family?	7. Advantages such as a PICC line in preference to multiple re-sitings of peripheral lines or tunnelled versus implanted ports should be discussed with the child and family to ensure the most appropriate device is chosen.
8. Will the age of the child influence choice of device?	8. Specific considerations apply to premature and neonatal infants where additional hazards relate to vessel size and increased infection risks (CDCP 2002). Accessing and maintaining VADs in preschool children can be challenging, requiring age specific skills in psychological care, site selection and vigilance in safely securing any VADs.

Principles table 13.2 Planning and preparation: staff training issues

Principle	Rationale
1. Only a practitioner who has been trained in the skill should undertake the cannulation of a child. This training may be ward-based and provided by an experienced practitioner or it may be a more structured, classroom-based training with practical and theoretical elements (UKCC 1996).	1. Cannulation is a complex skill that cannot be learned from a book or a guideline, therefore appropriate education is required.
2. The trainee should read appropriate literature and research around the subject of cannulation. Nurses who take on new or expanded roles should be responsible for ensuring that they work within guidelines of the Code of Professional Conduct (NMC 2009) and that they identify their own moral and legal accountability.	2. To develop a sound theoretical base and to assist professionals with problem solving in practice.
3. Training in peripheral cannulation should include the opportunity to practice the skill on a manikin and/or willing colleagues, before the trainee attempts the cannulation of a child.	3. The trainee should feel confident before cannulating to maximise the potential for success.

269

(Continued)

Principles table 13.2 (*Continued*)

Principle	Rationale
4. Any training should acknowledge that the physical act of inserting a catheter into the child's vein is only a part of this procedure. Training should incorporate the sequence of events and psychological considerations (Claar *et al* 2002).	**4.** Cannulation and the sequence of events is a complex procedure requiring numerous skills. The potential for distress to the child, family and practitioners involved should not be underestimated.
5. Once the essential skills have been taught the trainee must have opportunities to practice as soon and as frequently as possible.	**5.** This will develop their skills while their knowledge is fresh and allow them to gain confidence in their abilities (Frey 1998).
6. The newly trained practitioner should continue to make themselves aware of developments in practice, research and available products.	**6.** To ensure that knowledge remains valid, up to date and practice remains safe and effective. (NMC 2010b).

Procedure guideline 13.1 **Planning and preparation: child and family (cannulation)**

Statement	Rationale
1. Explain the entire procedure to the child and family including the reason for the cannulation, avoiding medical jargon and complex language. Information must be given according to the child's age and developmental understanding. There is evidence that tolerance to pain increases with age and maturity when the child no longer perceives medical interventions as punitive (Haslam 1969).	**1.** To ensure that the child and family understand the reason for the procedure and are psychologically prepared. Well-informed parents/carers are more likely to stay calm and will be in a position to support their child (Frederick 1991). The better informed the child, the better able they will be to develop coping strategies (Sclare and Waring 1995).
2. For communication to be effective, the non-verbal aspects of the practitioner–parent/carer–child relationship must be understood.	**2.** Active listening appears to be demonstrated mainly through non-verbal communication (Magnusson 1996).
3. Obtain verbal consent from the child and family for the procedure (DoH 2009, Orr 1999, UN General Assembly 1989).	**3.** To ensure that they agree in principle to the proposed cannulation (Power 1997).
4. Written consent must be obtained for surgical insertion of central catheters requiring general anaesthetic.	**4.** To ensure a written record of informed consent and to comply with local policy.
5. Provide play preparation if appropriate, involving a play specialist where possible. Consider involvement of a clinical psychologist if appropriate, particularly if previous procedures have been very stressful for the child (Claar *et al* 2002).	**5.** To enable explanation in a non-threatening manner and give the child the opportunity to express fears in a familiar environment (Action for Sick Children 2003, Broome 1990, Landsdown 1993).
6. Prepare appropriate methods of distraction for the child to use during the procedure itself. Attempt to discover from the child and family what techniques are most likely to consume their attention, e.g. pop-up books, musical books, blowing bubbles and guided imagery where the child is encouraged to imagine something pleasant, e.g. a favourite holiday.	**6.** To prevent the child's whole attention being centred on the invasive procedure. These techniques can help to distract and relax the child (Heiney 1991, Langley 1999).
7a) Consult the child and family on previous successes and failures and the best veins to use. Consider which hand the child favours and avoid using if possible. **b)** Establish whether the child sucks his thumb and to which he shows a preference (Van Cleve *et al* 1996).	**7a)** Many families will have had previous experiences of cannulation and/or will understand how their child copes with a stressful situation. **b)** Thumb-sucking will be an important coping strategy during the stressful experience of hospitalisation (Dougherty 1996).

Procedure guideline 13.1 (*Continued*)

Statement	Rationale
8. Do not make promises to use sites that you know you will not be able to access.	**8.** This would represent a betrayal of the child's trust (Frederick 1991).
9. Avoid selecting veins adjacent to joints if possible.	**9.** Increased risk of extravasation and phlebitis may occur at these sites (Davies 1998).
10. Consult the child and family on the use of local anaesthetic cream or spray for **peripheral access,** and check for previous allergic reactions. If used ensure that it remains in place for the appropriate length of time.	**10.** Application of local anaesthetic will reduce the pain of the procedure (Association of Paediatric Anaesthetists of Great Britain and Ireland 2008).
11. Apply anaesthetic cream or spray and leave for a minimum of 45 minutes.	**11.** Follow the manufacturer's guidelines, for example 45 minutes may achieve analgesia to pinprick but not loss of sensation or touch and pressure (anaesthesia). The optimal application time for EMLA® to achieve 95% anaesthesia to the area is 90 minutes. This is due to the nerve fibre size and is particularly relevant in the age group 1–5 years (Arrowsmith and Campbell 2000, Biccard 2001).
12. A suitable peripheral vein will be palpable or visible, of good width and length with a brisk refill capacity. Straight, non-tortuous veins, without valves, are preferable. Cover cream with a clear dressing or cling film if preferred. It may be useful to also cover the dressing with a bandage if the child is likely to fiddle with the cream and dressing.	**12.** Using clingfilm avoids the discomfort of removing the dressing later.
13. The child should not be permitted to lick the cream.	**13.** Absorption by mucous membranes is rapid and is against manufacturer's recommendations. Additionally, inadvertent biting of the tongue and lips may occur. It may also induce a local allergic reaction.
14. If an allergic reaction is noted, ensure that a detailed account of the event and materials used is entered in the child's health record. Consider copying this account for the family's health records.	**14.** To minimise the risk of exposure to allergens in the future and to ensure that the child's health record is comprehensive.

271

Procedure guideline 13.2 Preparation of equipment and environment (cannulation)

Statement	Rationale
1a) Avoid using the child's own bed-space or room.	**1a)** All equipment is close at hand and better task lighting is available in a clinical area. Risk of unsafe disposal of sharps will be reduced.
b) Use a procedure room where possible.	**b)** To ensure the child's own bed remains a safe haven (Frederick 1991). Greater privacy for the child and family is also assured.
2. If it is impossible to use a clinical room, arrange equipment, etc. as far as possible as they would be found in the treatment room.	**2.** To ensure equipment is close at hand and the child and nurse are comfortably positioned. To reduce risk of introducing infection.

(*Continued*)

Procedure guideline 13.2 (*Continued*)

Statement	Rationale
3. Prepare the following equipment on a clean tray but do not open the packaging until a few minutes before needed. Check the expiry dates and sterility of all products and equipment selected. 1× alcohol impregnated swab 1× appropriate cannula 2× cotton wool balls 1× T connector primed with 0.9% sodium chloride 1× 10 ml syringe containing 0.9% sodium chloride for flushing 1× needle-less port 1× packet of Steri-strips (optional) 1× IV3000® or similar 1× cotton bandage 1× appropriate splint 1× Smith & Nephew insertion record (if available).	**3.** To ensure that the most appropriate size and type of cannula is used (Murdoch and Bingham 1990). Select the correct size and type of cannula for the child. Selection should be based on the needs of the patient and the intended use and position of the cannula (Dougherty 1996).
4. Prepare personal protective clothing, i.e. clean gloves and apron.	**4.** To prevent cross-infection and possible contamination of clothing.
5. Gloves should be of a comfortable fit but tight to the skin, particularly at the fingertips.	**5.** To allow easier palpation of the vein.

Principles table 13.3 **Staff provision and roles**

Principle	Rationale
1. Seek the assistance of a colleague to hold the child's limb, assist with securing the device and to provide distraction if appropriate.	**1.** The assistance of a colleague will help to maximise the chance of a successful insertion procedure (Fulton 1996, Robinson and Collier 1997, Turner 1989).
2. Allow the child's parents/carers to be as involved as they wish but also give them the option of being absent if they prefer (Dearmun 1992, Kumar and Russell 1995, Shaw and Routh 1982).	**2.** The parents/carers will be able to assist with holding their child, assist with distraction and will provide emotional support for the child throughout the procedure.
3. If the parents/carers choose not to be present or are unavailable it is advisable to recruit another colleague to assist with the procedure. However, older children, particularly those familiar and relatively comfortable with cannulation may be so cooperative that the practitioner performing the procedure will not require assistance: an expert nurse will be able to assess this easily.	**3.** To provide comfort for the child.
4. All practitioners involved should be aware of the level of holding and restraint that will be required for the individual child. However, they should also have a good knowledge of ethics and policy on the issue of restraint (Brenner 2007, Pearch 2005, RCN 2003).	**4.** A degree of restraint will be necessary and appropriate for most children, for the purpose of maintaining the safety of the child and all others present and to prevent the need for repeated attempts at cannulation (RCN 2003, Robinson and Collier 1997). The age of the child and their possible competence to assent or consent to the procedure must also be considered (Gillick *vs* West Norfolk and Wisbech area HA 1985 http://www.bailii.org/uk/cases/UKHL/1985/7.html).

Procedure guideline 13.3 Cannulation: the procedure

Statement	Rationale
1a) Position the child on a chair, on a treatment couch or on their parent's/carer's lap as appropriate.	**1a)** To reduce the trauma of the procedure.
b) Whenever possible allow the child the freedom to select their chosen position. Ensure that the chosen position will be comfortable for the child, parents/carers and staff for the duration of the procedure.	**b)** To maximise the chance of a successful insertion procedure and aid adherence by the child.
2. Perform a surgical hand wash.	**2.** To prevent cross-infection.
3. Put on personal protective clothing and ensure that any staff assisting are similarly attired.	**3.** To prevent cross-infection and contamination of clothing.
4. Place yourself in a comfortable position, sitting facing the child and family.	**4.** So that good eye contact can be maintained and to aid adherence with the procedure.
5. Remove the local anaesthetic cream if used and wipe dry with a tissue or gauze.	
6. If an Opsite IV3000 dressing was used, remove by stretching parallel with the skin.	**6.** This breaks the glue, causing less irritation and pain.
7. Confirm with the child if appropriate that the cream has caused numbness of the skin effectively.	**7.** To re-assure the child that the pain of the procedure will be reduced.
8. Apply an appropriate size of tourniquet 5–8 cm above the chosen vein but not so tight to occlude arterial supply. Indications of occluded arterial supply include: loss of colour, compromised pulse and pain. Lightly tapping the vein or instructing the child to clench or pump the fist can encourage further venous filling.	**8.** To facilitate filling of the vein, enhance visualisation and allow the assisting nurse to have hands free for other tasks (Millam 1992).
9. Palpate the chosen vein.	**9.** To ensure that it can still be found and is still considered suitable. To ascertain the calibre and direction of the vein.
10. Cleanse the skin at the site where it is intended to insert the needle, working outwards, with an alcohol-impregnated swab for at least 30 seconds.	**10.** To clean the skin and prevent introduction of infection.
11. Do not fan or blow-dry or otherwise attempt to accelerate the drying process.	**11.** To prevent re-contaminating the skin (Franklin 1998).
12. Do not re-palpate the vein once the skin has been sterilised.	**12.** To prevent re-contaminating the skin.
13. Un-sheath the cannula and hold it firmly so that the two component parts cannot become separated. Examine the cannula for faults. If any are found reject but retain for inspection by clinical supplies advisor and complete incident report.	**13.** To reduce the risk of foreign particles or material entering the blood stream and potentially causing particle embolism.
14. Gently stretch the skin over the vein.	**14.** To ensure easy penetration of the skin and to immobilise and anchor the vein, making it easier to insert the cannula.

(Continued)

273

Procedure guideline 13.3 (*Continued*)

Statement	Rationale
15. Insert the cannula through the skin at an angle of 10–45° depending on the depth of the vein to be entered. On entering the vein, a first flashback of blood into the chamber of the stylet will be observed (called primary flashback).	**15.** The cannula can be inserted in various ways and the choice depends on the cannula length, vein location and skill of the practitioner (four possible methods are described in Box 13.1). Whatever method is used the cannula should enter the skin at such an angle that the needle punctures the vein wall and enters the lumen without piercing the opposite wall (Millam 1992). Catheters have the ability to soften once in the vein, allowing it to be firm when inserted but soft and therefore less traumatic once inserted.
16. GO SLOWLY. It is imperative that this stage of the procedure is not rushed.	**16.** To ensure adequate filling of the hub and to prevent a failed procedure.
17. Decrease the angle of the cannula so that it is resting on the skin and withdraw the stylet slightly: a second flashback of blood will be observed up the shaft of the cannula (called secondary flashback). Slowly advance the cannula without advancing the stylet until it is fully inserted.	**17.** There are various documented techniques for this (floating, two-handed, one-step and pushing off the stylet). These are described in full in Box 13.2. Individual practitioners will discover their favourite technique through experience (Millam 1992).
18. Release the tourniquet.	**18.** To restore usual venous blood flow.
19. Taking care to hold the cannula in position to avoid extravasation, position a piece of clean cotton wool or gauze beneath the end of the cannula to absorb any blood that may escape. Remove the stylet while applying digital pressure over the cannula with one finger.	**19.** To prevent blood return and contamination of the surrounding area, avoid creating an environment in which bacteria could thrive.
20. Place the stylet safely in a tray.	**20.** To avoid accidental needle-stick injury.
21. Continuing to protect the cannula, connect a 'T' extension and flush with 2–5 ml of 0.9% normal saline, using a 10 ml syringe.	**21.** To ensure cannula is correctly inserted, ensure patency and prevent clotting. A 10 ml syringe prevents excessive pressure being exerted on the vein (Todd 1998).
22. Clamp the extension set, remove the syringe and apply a smartsite or alternative needleless port to the end of the 'T' extension.	

274

Box 13.1 Approaching the vein

1. **Approaching the vein from the top:**
   Insert the cannula at a 15–25°angle depending on the vein depth. Take care not to insert it too far into the lumen or it may penetrate the back wall.
2. **Approaching the vein from the side:**
   Position the cannula tip adjacent to the vein aimed towards it. This method, which is preferred if you have injected a local anaesthetic, prevents piercing the vein's back wall.
3. **Approaching below a bifurcation:**
   A bifurcated vein looks like an inverted 'V' It may be easier to cannulate than a single vein because it is more stable and less likely to roll. Insert the cannula about 1 cm below the bifurcation, then tunnel it into the vein at the inverted 'V'. This approach prevents you from entering the vein at too steep an angle, reducing trauma to the vein wall on insertion. You are also less likely to pierce the vein's opposite wall.
4. **Approaching a vein that is palpable but only visible for a short segment:**
   This technique may help you to cannulate a vein that extends into the deep tissues where you cannot see or feel it. Insert the cannula about 1 cm in front of the vein's visible segment, then tunnel the cannula through the tissue to enter the vein. Tunnelling may reduce trauma to the vein wall on insertion.

Box 13.2 Advancing the cannula; four options (Millam 1992)

The four options for advancing the cannular (Millam 1992) are given below.
1. **Floating the cannula into the vein**
   With this method you will remove the stylet before fully advancing the cannula. It is a good technique to use if you are inexperienced – you will be less likely to puncture the vein's opposite wall because you will advance the catheter only after you see adequate blood return (secondary flashback). Also the fluid flow helps to float the catheter into place.
   - Perform venepuncture and advance the cannula about one-third to a half of its length into the vein or when you observe primary flashback in the hub
   - Place a piece of gauze or cotton wool under the catheter hub to catch any blood that escapes when you remove the stylet
   - Release the tourniquet and remove the stylet
   - Attach the tube and start the IV infusion at a slow rate
   Use one hand to maintain vein stretch while advancing the cannula with the other hand.
2. **The two-handed technique**
   Many practitioners use this technique because the stylet partially obstructs the cannula as you advance the cannula. This method reduces blood spillage.
   - Insert the cannula into the vein approximately half the length of the cannula or until primary flashback is visible in the hub
   - With one hand hold the hub of the cannula while retracting the stylet about halfway with the other hand
   - While maintaining vein stretch advance the cannula until it is inserted fully
   - Remove the tourniquet. If the vein is small leave the tourniquet tied to increase vein size during cannula advancement.
   Remove the stylet and attach the IV tubing or flush with 1–2 ml of 0.9% sodium chloride and attach the T connector.
3. **One-step technique**
   You might choose this method if you are experienced in venepuncture and the vein you are accessing is straight, even and superficial. An experienced, skilful practitioner can place the cannula in the vein lumen with one deft motion without injuring the vein.
   - In one step enter the skin and advance the cannula into the vein completely up to the hub
   Remove the stylet and attach the IV tubing or T connector.
4. **Pushing the cannula off the stylet**
   This technique is recommended when using a cannula with a raised lip on the hub, e.g. quik-cath.
   - Advance the cannula halfway into the vein
   - Pressing your forefinger or thumb against the hub's lip slide the cannula forward, so it moves off the stylet and into the vein
   Discard the stylet, remove the tourniquet, and attach the IV tubing or T connector.

Procedure guideline 13.4 **Dressing of the cannula**

Statement	**Rationale**
1. Taking care at all times to protect the cannula, apply a sterile clear dressing, preferably Opsite IV3000 1 hand ported®. Do not use opaque tapes or elastoplast.	1. To facilitate easy observation and prevent contamination of the cannula insertion site (Millam 1992, Oldham 1991).
2. For extra security, particularly if the child is likely to sweat excessively or in the case of babies, Steri-strips can be applied prior to the clear dressing.	2. This will help to prevent mechanical phlebitis and extravasation and avoid the distress of re-cannulation (McCann 2003).
3. Apply an appropriate size splint to the adjacent joint if necessary and bandage the entire area.	3. To immobilise the limb, preventing movement that may cause occlusion, extravasation and phlebitis (Livesley 1993).
4. The child's fingers and toes should remain visible.	4. To facilitate checks of the child's circulation.
5. Dispose of all sharps and other waste appropriately and perform a clinical hand wash.	5. To comply with hospital policies.

Procedure guideline 13.5 **Summary points (cannulation)**

Statement	Rationale
1. Take time to plan the procedure. Be aware of the reasons why cannulation can be less than successful on some occasions (Table 13.2).	**1.** Time spent planning the procedure will pay off. To maximise the chance of a successful insertion procedure and aid adherence by the child.
2. The practitioner should evaluate and record the procedure in the child's health record including a note of the techniques used, their relative success and failure and the level of tolerance to the stress, exhibited by the child and family. Additionally, type and size of cannula, lot number, expiry date of equipment, number of attempts and site should be recorded.	**2.** To ensure that the child's health record is comprehensive and to provide information to other practitioners who may need to cannulate the child either later in this admission or at a later time.
3. Ensure that the cannula is securely bandaged and protected at all times and that the family are briefed on action required in the event of possible complications, e.g. the cannula becoming dislodged or falling out.	**3.** To give the child and family confidence, to assist them in following as normal a routine as possible and to improve the child's experience of hospitalisation.
4. In the event that the first attempt at cannulation was unsuccessful the same practitioner should have no more than **one further attempt.** If this attempt is unsuccessful an experienced colleague should be asked to perform the procedure.	**4.** Repeated attempts by the same practitioner will damage the self-confidence of the practitioner and reduce the confidence the child and family might have in them.
5. In the event that repeated attempts by various practitioners are unsuccessful the team should consider and discuss with the child and family: • The relative importance and urgency of the procedure • The reasons why a cannula is required • Other staff who may be able to help, e.g. senior colleagues, anaesthetists • Equipment and products that may make the procedure easier, e.g. different types of cannula, a light source • The need to preserve veins for future use • Alternative methods of venous access, e.g. long and PICC lines • The ability of the child to tolerate further attempts and interventions • Alternative therapies not requiring venous access • The possibility of rebooking the procedure for a future date.	**5.** Repeated attempts at cannulation are stressful for all involved, family, child and staff and the team must attempt to maintain a realistic perspective.
6. If after consideration and discussion it is concluded that further attempts will be made, the child should be allowed a break if possible.	**6.** This will allow the child to regain their composure and the staff to reflect and re-evaluate the procedure.
7. Dispose of sharps in the appropriate receptacle immediately.	**7.** To prevent accidental needle-stick injury.
8. Always ensure that all practitioners perform a surgical hand wash prior to the procedure and a clinical hand wash following the procedure.	**8.** To prevent infection.

Table 13.2 Cannulation trouble-shooting guide (RCN 2010)

Problem	Cause	Suggested action
1. Missed vein	1. Inadequate anchoring Wrong positioning Poor lighting Less than 100% concentration	1. Withdraw the needle almost to the bevel and manoeuvre gently to realign needle and vein Try again but if it becomes painful, remove Make certain you are better prepared next time
2. Spurt of blood on entry	2. Bevel tip of needle entering vein before entire bevel is under skin, due to vein being superficial	2. Ignore Reassure the patient if a small blood blister develops
3a) Blood flow stops	3a) Over shooting vein or advancing needle while withdrawing blood	3a) Gently ease the needle back and continue. Manoeuvre gently
3b) Blood flow stops	3b) Vein collapses due to contact between the needle and the valve or vein wall Poor blood flow	3b) Release and re-tighten tourniquet and continue As above and massage above the needle tip to pull blood into vein
4a) Haematoma	4a) Perforation of posterior wall of vein	4a) Insert the needle at the correct angle and stop when flashback is seen in the syringe or tubing of winged infusion device. Do not advance the needle during the taking of a sample
4b) Haematoma	4b) Forgetting to remove tourniquet before removing needle	4b) Remember to remove the tourniquet next time
4c) Haematoma	4c) Inadequate pressure on puncture site	4c) Apply pressure. Supervise the patient doing the same
5. Hardening of veins due to scarring and thrombosis	5. Prolonged use of one site	5. Assess patency Alternate venepuncture sites to prevent this Do not use hard veins, as this is often not successful and will cause the patient pain
6. Mechanical problems	6. Faulty equipment, for instance, bent needle tips, cracked syringes	6. Check carefully before use and discard (adverse incident reporting)
7. Transmittable diseases	7. Viruses pose the major risk – hepatitis B, cytomegalovirus, HIV	7. All blood should be handled with care and caution, especially when handling specimens of infected blood Gloves may be worn when taking blood and handling samples Local hospital policy should be strictly followed. Universal precautions
8. Needle inoculation	8. Lack of caution. Overfilling of 'sharps' containers.	8. Dispose of equipment safely to prevent inoculation Keep up-to-date with relevant vaccinations If this does occur, follow accident procedure and report the incident immediately. An injection of hepatitis B immunoglobulin may be required or triple therapy

Procedure guideline 13.6 Positive reinforcement and reward (cannulation)

Statement	Rationale
1. Time should be taken to give positive feedback to the child for tolerating the invasive procedure (Action for Sick Children 2003).	1. To hand control back to the child.
2. The parents/carers should also be given positive feedback for their valuable contribution.	2. To acknowledge the value of their involvement and teach parents/carers mastery of the event, equipping them with coping strategies for future occasions.
3. If a story or game has been used for distraction purposes, allow the child to complete the activity.	3. To conclude the procedure with a positive outcome.
4. Any reward, however small, will help the child to feel a sense of achievement and control, such as certificates and sticker charts. For a list of suppliers of certificates and stickers please see Appendix 13.1.	4. Children respond well to a reward system.

Care of the cannula: Visual infusion phlebitis

It is recognised that intravenous therapy involves significant risks of damaging side effects. However, infection of IV sites and phlebitis in children are an infrequent occurrence (Hecker 1988, Jackson 1998, Nelson and Garland 1987). Infusion phlebitis is defined as the acute inflammation of the vein directly linked to the presence of an intravenous access device. Phlebitis affects the inner endothelial layer (intima) of the vein, and results from chemical, physical or mechanical irritation (Lamb 1995, Richardson and Brusco 1993). It is characterised by pain and tenderness along the course of the vein, erythema and inflammatory swelling with a feeling of warmth at the site (Perdue 1995, Perucca and Micek 1993). The incidence of phlebitis is 20–80%, 60% occurring within 8–16 hours of insertion (Perucca and Mieck 1993). The standard recommendation is 5%.

Complications increase hospital stays, duration of therapy and can put patients at risk of further medical problems. This has an impact on resources if a patient acquires septicaemia. Additionally, the patient experiences pain and could become needle phobic (Kolk *et al* 1999). Pain has been reported up to 6 months post cannula removal and everyday activities, e.g. wearing a wristwatch or leaning on forearms, may be affected for some time afterwards. Future access points may be reduced. Fibrotic veins and scarring results in an altered body image for the child, with possible limb immobility (CPC extravasation guideline) (Berry and Bravery 2005).

The three most common causes of irritation are:

1. **Chemical:** Properties of fluids or drugs. Children may be at increased risk of chemical phlebitis. Children's veins are smaller and subject to reduced blood flow around the device (Goodwin and Carlson 1993, Weinstein 1993).
2. **Physical:**
   - Irritant cannula material, length or gauge of the cannula
   - An inexperienced practitioner lacking the skill of cannula insertion
   - Poor site placement of the cannula, e.g. use of the antecubital fossa
   - The use of too large a cannula, occluding the vein and limiting blood flow around the cannula
   - Prolonged duration of the cannula.
3. **Mechanical:**
   - Associated with poor fixation of the cannula allowing movement such as rubbing against the vessel wall
   - Activity of the child or manipulation by the child may contribute to the development of phlebitis, e.g. cannula in the foot of a walking child
   - Experimental studies have ruled out infection as being the major cause of phlebitis (Maki 1976)
   - Contamination by microscopic particles may be transferred to the child by infusion fluids and drugs. After insertion of a plastic cannula into a vein a loosely formed fibrin sheath collects around the device within 24–48 hours forming a nidus (Weinstein 1993) This helps the bacteria to adhere to the cannula and microbial agents in the blood, which means it is difficult to treat cannula related infections without removing the device.

Procedure guideline 13.7 Prevention of infection (cannulation)

Statement	Rationale
1. Prevention should have no single focus. Be aware of possible causes, use appropriate monitoring tools and audit practice.	**1.** Being aware of the common reasons for irritation that will facilitate early intervention.
2. Refrain from using veins in areas over joints and splint if unavoidable.	**2.** Movement of the cannula in the vein is a significant cause of infusion phlebitis.
3. Select veins with ample blood volume when infusing irritant substances.	**3.** The larger the blood volume and flow, the lower the risk of infusion phlebitis.
4. Securely anchor the cannula and replace loose or contaminated dressings.	**4.** To prevent movement.
5. Frequently inspect and monitor the IV site, at least daily.	**5.** To achieve early detection of infusion phlebitis.
6. Remove the cannula at the first sign of discomfort and inflammation (score of 2 or above on VIP scale, see below).	**6.** To prevent further deterioration, extravasation and infection of the IV site.
7. Whenever the bandage and/or splint are removed the opportunity should be taken to assist the child to wash the previously covered area of their hand. The nurse should also inspect the skin for sore areas and skin integrity.	**7.** To maintain personal hygiene and reduce the risk of infection and damage to the skin.

Procedure guideline 13.7 *(Continued)*

Statement	Rationale
8. **Standard:** All children with an IV access device in situ should have the site inspected **at least daily** for signs of infusion phlebitis. The subsequent score and action taken if any should be documented in the child's health record. Additionally the cannula site should be observed when: • Bolus injections are administered • IV flow rates are checked and altered • Solution containers are changed.	8. Good clinical practice.
9. **Visual infusion phlebitis (VIP) score. (Dinley grading scale)** The VIP score is based on a traffic light design:	9. The VIP score improves the process of checking the cannula site. It provides a mechanism for recording objectively, rather than the term 'satisfactory'. The practitioner should know what to look for, be aware of the risks of IV cannulation and therapy and available treatments. This will help to reduce IV related complications.
0 = IV site appears healthy. **OBSERVE CANNULA SITE**	In adults it has been recommended that routine replacement of the cannula should be undertaken every 72 hours. To reduce the risk of bacterial sepsis (Maki and Ringer 1991). However, various studies have challenged this assertion and shown that prolonged cannulation did not increase the complications of phlebitis, infection and obstruction (Jackson 1998, Lai 1998, Phelps and Helms 1987). It is common practice in child health nursing to leave the cannula in situ until treatment is discontinued or infiltration occurs (Phelps and Helms 1987).
1 = *One* of the following is evident: Slight pain near IV site *or* slight redness near IV site.	
CAUTION 2 = *Two* of the following are evident: Pain at IV site, with erythema, swelling or both.	
RESITE CANNULA. 3 = *All* of the following signs are evident: Pain along the path of the cannula, erythema, induration or a palpable venous cord less than 5 cm above the IV site.	
RESITE CANNULA 4 = *All* of the following signs are evident and extensive: Pain along the path of the cannula, erythema, induration or a palpable venous cord more than 5 cm above the IV site.	
RESITE CANNULA – CONSIDER TREATMENT 5 = *All* of the following signs are evident and extensive: Pain along the path of the cannula, erythema, induration, a palpable venous cord and pyrexia.	

Procedure guideline 13.8 Cannula dressing change

Statement	Rationale
1. Change the clear dressing on a peripheral cannula only if it becomes potentially or actually ineffective in securing the cannula and keeping the site of entry clean.	1. To delay or possibly prevent the trauma of insertion of a new cannula.
2. Opsite IV3000 1 hand ported® or a similar proprietary product, such as or Tegaderm IV® should always be used.	2. To reduce the risk of dislodgement, mechanical phlebitis and cross-infection and to allow for easy observation of the entry site (Needham and Strehle 2008).
3. Explain the procedure to the child and family and prepare to use distraction techniques that may be helpful in gaining the child's cooperation and trust. Involve the play specialist where possible. Collect all the necessary equipment on a clean tray: • 1× packet of sterile gauze • 1× sachet of sodium chloride for irrigation • 2× sterile cotton wool balls (in case of inadvertent removal of cannula) • 1× packet of Steri-strips (optional) • 1× IV3000® or similar.	3. To prepare the child for what is about to happen, support them during the procedure, and ensure preparation allows timely procedure.
4. Ask a colleague to assist in the changing of the dressing.	4. The assistance of a colleague with the technique will reduce the risk of the cannula becoming dislodged during the procedure.
5. If possible, use a procedure room for this intervention.	5. To ensure that the child's bed area remains a 'safe haven.'
6. Carefully remove the old dressing, holding the cannula in place at all times. Take the opportunity to thoroughly inspect the site of entry of the cannula for any sign of infection.	6. To prevent accidental dislodgement or removal of the cannula.
7. If necessary, clean the area using sterile gauze soaked in 0.9% sodium chloride and then dry with sterile gauze.	7. To ensure effective adhesion of the replacement dressing.
8. Apply the new clear dressing remembering to protect the cannula at all times. Steri-strips may be used for extra security but do not use opaque tapes or Elastoplast®. Re-apply the splint and bandage ensuring that all is secure.	8. A clear dressing allows the site to be easily observed for signs of phlebitis or extravasation (McCann 2003, Oldham 1991).
9. Record the procedure in the child's health record and document any other important information.	9. To ensure that the child's health record is comprehensive so as to provide information to other practitioners that may be required to change the dressing at a later time.
10. Give the child positive reinforcement for tolerating this procedure.	10. Children respond well to positive encouragement.

Administration of a drug by bolus injection and flushing the cannula

This section outlines the procedure for administering an intravenous (IV) bolus drug via a peripheral line. It includes the administration of IV 0.9% sodium chloride flush to maintain cannula patency where no regular infusions of fluid or bolus drugs are prescribed. The practitioner's aim should be to maintain the patency of the cannula for as long as possible.

Re-cannulation should be avoided where possible, as this will cause the child and family further distress. There is no limit to the length of time that a cannula may remain in situ and with appropriate care, several days may be possible (Bregenzer 1998, Lai 1998). Studies recommend 8–12 hourly flushing (Dunn and Lennihan 1987, Goode et al 1991, Gyr et al 1995, Kleiber et al 1993).

Procedure guideline 13.9 Administration of an IV drug by bolus injection

Statement	Rationale
1. Collect the required equipment: • 1× 0.9% sodium chloride for injection • 1× 10 ml syringe for 0.9% sodium chloride flush • 1× 21 G (green) needle for drawing up 0.9% sodium chloride • 1× alcohol impregnated swab • Additional syringe(s) and needle(s) to prepare prescribed drug(s) as required • Drug(s) to be administered • Clean plastic tray for preparation • Medication chart of the child.	1. To ensure the procedure is undertaken safely and efficiently.
2. Clean all surfaces of plastic tray with an alcohol wipe. Allow to dry naturally.	2. To prevent cross-infection.
3. Explain to the child and family the reason for the procedure and what it will entail. Ensure the patient is ready in a suitable environment (according to local policy).	3. To gain their confidence and trust and empower the child (UN General Assembly 1989, Charles-Edwards 2003).
4. Put on a plastic apron and perform a surgical hand wash.	4. To prevent cross-infection and contamination of clothing.
5. Put on non sterile gloves.	5. To comply with protective precautions.
6. Open the syringes and needles ensuring key sterile parts are not contaminated. Connect needles to syringes and place in plastic tray with the syringe tips uppermost.	6. To prevent contamination of key sterile equipment.
7. Check the drug(s) to be given against the prescription including: • Correct name in full • Correct date of birth • Correct ID number • Correct drug and dosage for age/weight • Route of administration • No known relevant drug allergies • Prescription is signed and dated by prescriber • Prescription is clear and legible • Time drug is due to be given • Time previous dose administered • Correct drug • Drug expiry date.	7. To ensure correct administration of drug(s). Local policy determines the need for a second nurse to check these details.
8. Calculate correct volume of drug to be prepared.	8. To ensure correct dose administered.
9. Using a non-touch technique prepare drug(s) according to the manufacturer's instructions.	9. To maintain sterility of the drugs.
10. Prepare a minimum of 1–2 ml 0.9% sodium chloride to flush the cannula.	10. To clear any drugs through the cannula and maintain cannula patency.
11. Take the tray and prescription chart to the patient in the location where the drug is to be administered.	11. To adhere to local policy and practice.

281

(Continued)

Procedure guideline 13.9 (*Continued*)

Statement	Rationale
12. Prior to administration check the patient's ID band to confirm patient's full name, date of birth and hospital ID against the prescription chart.	**12.** To adhere to local drug administration policy.
13. Remove the bandage from over the cannula.	**13.** So that the site of entry of the cannula may be observed throughout the procedure.
14. Take the opportunity to thoroughly inspect the site of entry of the cannula for any sign of phlebitis, infiltration or infection. Assess the entry site using the visual infusion phlebitis (VIP) score, described in section 13.7.	**14.** To ensure drug(s) can be administered via the site.
15. Clean the injection hub with an alcohol impregnated wipe.	**15.** To prevent introduction of infection.
16. Allow the hub to dry naturally. Do not fan or blow dry.	**16.** To prevent re-contamination of the port (Franklin 1998).
17. Attach the syringe containing 0.9% sodium chloride to the port, open the clamp and slowly flush the cannula with 1–2 ml of 0.9% sodium chloride.	**17.** To check patency of the cannula. Studies suggest that 1–2 ml is sufficient (Gyr *et al* 1995, Goode *et al* 1991, Dunn and Lennihan 1987).
18. Ask or observe the child for any signs of pain or discomfort experienced and, while flushing, observe the cannula entry site and surrounding area for any sign of swelling, phlebitis or extravasation.	**18.** To check patency of the cannula.
19. Clamp the 'T' extension, while still flushing, to create positive pressure.	**19.** To prevent occlusion and blood backflow into the 'T' extension (Kleiber *et al* 1993).
20. If a drug is to be administered attach the syringe to the hub and administer the drug following the manufacturer's instructions.	**20.** To give the drug safely and minimise risk of adverse reactions.
21. If more than one drug is due ensure adequate flushing with recommended solution between each drug.	**21.** To ensure drug is flushed from the catheter to avoid any drug precipitation.
22. When the final drug has been administered, attach a syringe containing 0.9% sodium chloride and flush the cannula, clamping the 'T' extension while still flushing.	**22.** To ensure all medication has been flushed from the cannula and into the bloodstream of the child.
23. In the event that resistance is felt while flushing, attempt turbulent flushing technique, delivered in a pause-push action.	**23.** This is used as a method of preventing catheter occlusion (Goodwin and Carlson 1993).
24. If resistance is so strong that it is not possible to flush the cannula, replace the 'T' extension, having first primed with 0.9% sodium chloride and repeat the process above.	**24.** Blockages may occur in the T extension due to backflow or inadequate flushing. Cannulae smaller than 22 gauge do not include a valve, making backflow and blockage more likely (Danek and Norris 1992).
25. If it is impossible to flush the cannula using the techniques described, remove it according to the guidelines below. Ascertain the continued need for the cannula, reviewing treatment, management and investigations with the multi-disciplinary team.	**25.** The cannula should be removed if it is no longer required (Phelps and Helms 1987).
26. Ensure the splint is still in the correct position and re-bandage the area over the cannula.	**26.** To ensure the patency for collection of the next blood sample or administration of the next drug.

Procedure guideline 13.9 (*Continued*)

Statement	Rationale
27. Give the child positive reinforcement for tolerating this procedure.	27. Children respond well to encouragement.
28. Take a plastic tray containing all equipment used to an area where it can be disposed of safely.	28. To ensure correct disposal of clinical waste according to local policy.
29. Place all syringes and needles into a sharps bin.	29. To minimise the risk of needle-stick injury and contamination.
30. Clean plastic tray with alcohol impregnated wipe and return to storage.	30. To adhere to local guidelines.
31. Record the VIP score as described previously, in the child's health record and document any important information, e.g. relative ease of flushing, any pain experienced.	31. To ensure that the child's health record is comprehensive and to provide information to other practitioners that may flush the cannula at a later time.
32. If the cannula is being accessed regularly for the administration of medication or blood sampling (at least 8 hourly) no further flushing will be required. However, in the event of infrequent access, the cannula should be flushed on an 8 hourly basis using the technique described above.	32. Studies recommend 8–12 hourly flushing with 0.9% sodium chloride (Dunn and Lennihan 1987, Goode *et al* 1991, Gyr *et al* 1995, Kleiber *et al* 1993).

Administration of an intravenous fluid or drug infusion

This section describes the procedure for giving a prescribed fluid or drug infusion via a peripheral cannula to a child. Drugs administered to children as an intravenous infusion may be inserted into a bag of intravenous fluid, the burette of an infusion set for administration via a volumetric infusion pump or in a syringe for use in a syringe driver. The most appropriate method should be selected depending on volume of diluent required and available infusion device.

Procedure guideline 13.10 **Administration of an intravenous fluid or drug infusion**

Statement	Rationale
1. Collect the required equipment: • Clean plastic tray for preparation • 1 ampoule of 0.9% sodium chloride for injection • 1× 10 ml syringe for 0.9% sodium chloride flush • 1× 21 G (green) needle for drawing up 0.9% sodium chloride • 1× alcohol impregnated swab • Additional syringe(s) and needle(s) to prepare prescribed drug as required • Drug to be administered • Prescribed intravenous fluid or diluent • Appropriate infusion set or syringe and extension tubing • Intravenous fluid prescription and/or prescription chart of the child • Infusion device and drip stand.	1. To ensure the procedure is undertaken safely and efficiently. A flush solution of 0.9% sodium chloride will be required to check for line patency and to clear the cannula before and after any drug infusion to avoid drug precipitation. When an intravenous infusion is being routinely changed it is not necessary to routinely flush the cannula at that time.
2. Clean all surfaces of the plastic tray with an alcohol wipe. Allow to dry naturally.	2. To prevent cross-infection.

(*Continued*)

Procedure guideline 13.10 (*Continued*)

Statement	Rationale
3. Explain to the child and family the reason for the procedure and what it will entail. Ensure the patient is ready and in a suitable environment (according to local policy).	**3.** To gain their confidence and trust and empower the child (Charles-Edwards 2003, UN General Assembly 1989).
4. Put on a plastic apron and perform a surgical hand wash.	**4.** To prevent cross-infection and contamination of clothing.
5. Put on non-sterile gloves.	**5.** Protective precautions.
6. Open the sterile equipment ensuring key sterile parts are not contaminated (e.g. syringe hubs, needles and additive ports). Connect needles to syringes and place in plastic tray with the syringe tips uppermost. Ensure the clamps on the giving set are closed.	**6.** To prevent cross-infection.
7. Check the drug(s) and fluid to be given against the prescription including: • Correct patient name in full • Correct date of birth • Correct ID number • Correct drug and dosage for age/weight • Route of administration • No known relevant drug allergies • Prescription is signed and dated by prescriber • Prescription is clear and legible • Time period over which the drug or fluid is due to be given • Time previous dose administered • Correct drug • Drug expiry date • Adhesive drug administration label.	**7.** To ensure the correct dose is administered to the correct child. Local policy determines the need for a second nurse to check these details.
8. Calculate correct volume of drug and fluid to be prepared.	**8.** To administer as prescribed.
9. Prepare drug and fluids according to the manufacturer's instructions using a non-touch technique throughout.	**9.** To clear any drugs through the cannula and maintain cannula patency. To maintain sterility of the drugs.
10. Prepare a minimum of 1–2 ml 0.9% sodium chloride to flush the cannula.	**10.** To clear any drugs through the cannula and maintain cannula patency.

11. Either (a) inject prepared drug into infusion fluid bag via the additive port and mix well by shaking the bag.
   Without contaminating the key parts insert the spike on the administration set into the septum of the infusion bag and proceed to point 14 below.
	11. To ensure even distribution of drug in the bag of fluid.
	   To prepare infusion correctly.

12. Or (b) To dilute the drug in a smaller volume via a buretted giving system. Hang the bag of infusion fluid and gradually open the roller clamp to allow 20 ml of fluid into the burette. Inject the prescribed drug into the burette via the additive port. If further dilution is required, reopen the roller clamp between infusion bag and burette and fill to required amount. Close roller clamp. Ensure the drug is well mixed in burette by shaking the burette. Proceed to point 14 below.	**12.** To prepare infusion correctly.
13. Or (c) To administer the drug via a syringe driver draw up required volume of diluent in appropriate size syringe and then pull back the syringe plunger to enable you to inject the drug into the syringe using a non-touch technique. Ensure the drug is well mixed in the syringe by gentle shaking.	**13.** To prepare infusion correctly.

Procedure guideline 13.10 *(Continued)*

Statement	Rationale
14. Prime the giving set or syringe extension set according to manufacturer's instructions without any loss of drug mixture.	**14.** To ensure correct volume of drug given to the patient and to avoid any external hazards associated with the drug.
15. Attach a completed drug label detailing the drug, dose, diluent, volume of diluent, date, time and your signature(s).	**15.** To adhere to local policy.
16. Prepare a syringe of 1–2 ml 0.9% sodium chloride to flush the cannula as required.	**16.** To check line patency or to flush line to prevent drug precipitation.
17. Take the tray of prepared infusion and prescription chart to the patient in the location where the drug is to be administered.	**17.** To adhere to local policy and practice.
18. Prior to administration check the patient's ID band to confirm the patient's full name, date of birth and hospital ID against the prescription chart.	**18.** To adhere to local drug administration policy.
19. Remove the bandage from over the cannula.	**19.** So that the site of entry of the cannula may be observed.
20. Take the opportunity to thoroughly inspect the site of entry of the cannula for any sign of phlebitis, infiltration or infection. Assess the entry site using the visual infusion phlebitis (VIP) score, described in section 13.7.	**20.** To ensure drug/fluid can be administered via this site.
21. Clean the injection hub with an alcohol impregnated wipe.	**21.** To prevent introduction of infection.
22. Allow the hub to dry naturally; do not fan or blow dry.	**22.** To prevent re-contamination of the port (Franklin 1998).
23. Attach the syringe containing 0.9% sodium chloride to the port, open clamp and slowly flush the cannula with 1–2 ml of 0.9% sodium chloride.	**23.** To check the patency of the cannula. Studies suggest that 1–2 ml is sufficient (Dunn and Lennihan 1987, Goode *et al* 1991, Gyr *et al* 1995).
24. Ask or observe the child for any signs of pain or discomfort experienced and while flushing, observe the cannula entry site and surrounding area for any sign of swelling, phlebitis or extravasation.	**24.** Observing the child throughout the procedure will allow problems to be picked up earlier.
25. Clamp the line, while still flushing, to create positive pressure.	**25.** To prevent occlusion and blood backflow into the 'T' extension (Kleiber *et al* 1993).
26. Gently remove the sterile cap protecting the end of the infusion tubing without contaminating key parts. Attach to 'T' extension and screw together securely.	**26.** To maintain sterility of key parts.
27. Position infusion into infusion device following manufacturer's instructions.	**27.** To prepare the infusion correctly.
28. Set infusion device with required infusion rate, volume limit, pressure alarm limits.	**28.** To minimise drug infusion errors.
29. Open the clamps on infusion line and set the pump to run.	**29.** To prepare infusion correctly.
30. Ensure the splint is still in the correct position and re-bandage the area over the cannula.	**30.** To check on-going safety.
31. In the event that the infusion device alarms high pressure check the cannula for signs of redness or swelling.	**31.** Drug may have infiltrated surrounding soft tissue.

(Continued)

285

Procedure guideline 13.10 (*Continued*)

Statement	Rationale
32. If there are signs of infiltration stop the drug infusion and follow local policy.	**32.** To minimise tissue damage.
33. Check the line and cannula are not clamped or kinked. Ensure flow is not inhibited by any positioning or movement of the child.	**33.** To pick up early on any potential blockage.
34. Check the pressure alarm is set according to the manufacturer's guidelines.	**34.** For safety.
35. If the cannula has become blocked attempt to clear the blockage with a flush of 0.9% sodium chloride as described above.	**35.** To clear the cannula.
36. When a drug infusion is complete, stop infusion device and close line clamps.	
37. Ensure the drug is adequately flushed through the administration system at the prescribed rate using the administration techniques described above as follows:	**37.** To ensure the correct dose is administered.
38. Either (a) replace the infusion bag with prescribed, compatible infusion fluid to flush drug through the giving set.	**38.** To ensure the drug is flushed safely.
39. Or (b) If using a burette system add 18–20 ml of 0.9% sodium chloride to the burette and infuse this flush solution.	**39.** To ensure the drug is flushed safely.
40. Or (c) If using a syringe driver, replace drug syringe with syringe containing 5–10 ml 0.9% sodium chloride flush and infuse this solution.	**40.** To ensure the drug is flushed safely.
41. When flush infusion is complete close all clamps. Disconnect the infusion administration set and leave 'T' extension secure under the bandage.	**41.** To ensure the cannula and 'T' extension is well protected.
42. Take the plastic tray containing all equipment used to an area where it can disposed of safely.	**42.** To minimise the risk of needle-stick injury and contamination.
43. Place all syringes and needles into a sharps bin.	**43.** To adhere to local guidelines
44. Clean the plastic tray with an alcohol impregnated wipe and return to storage.	**44.** To prevent cross-infection.
45. Record the administration of the drug or infusion fluid on prescription chart. Record fluid administered on the fluid balance chart. Record VIP scores as described below in section 13.7, in the child's health record and document any important information, e.g. any change in patient status associated with the drug administration.	**45.** To ensure the child's healthcare record is comprehensive so as to provide information to other practitioners who may subsequently be caring for the child.

Principles table 13.4 **Principles of blood sampling**

Principle	Rationale
1. Taking blood samples from an existing peripheral cannula reduces the trauma of blood tests for the child and family. The technique is particularly useful when it is necessary to take blood regularly over a period of time, for example, when performing diagnostic tests. It may be appropriate to insert a cannula specifically for the purposes of blood sampling if this is likely to be more convenient.	1. Minimal literature can be found on this subject so these guidelines are largely based on experience and current practice on a Programmed Investigation Unit where the technique is employed on a daily basis (Kleiber *et al* 1993).
2. Only nurses who have been formally assessed as competent IV givers should attempt this technique, following demonstration and training by an experienced practitioner.	2. To follow good clinical practice.

Principles table 13.4 (*Continued*)

Principle	Rationale
3. It should be noted, however, that some tests cannot be performed on blood sampled from a peripheral cannula. Examples are: • Blood glucose cannot be monitored when the cannula has been used for the administration of any glucose solution • Lines used for giving antibiotics cannot be used for measurement of levels of that drug • Blood results taken for clotting levels may be affected when the line has been flushed with 0.9% sodium chloride with 10 units heparin. Consult local pathology department for advice.	3. To ensure the correct sample is taken. • Dextrose adheres to the lining of the cannula resulting in inaccurate results • The antibiotic adheres to the lining of the cannula resulting in inaccurate results • The heparin present can lead to the result suggesting prolonged clotting times.
4. It remains worthwhile flushing a peripheral cannula with 0.9% sodium chloride if it is to be used for blood sampling.	4. Assists in maintaining patency of the line and allows sampling from the cannula for longer than would be possible (Gyr et al 1995, Kleiber et al 1993).
5. Keep the cannula splinted if it is positioned adjacent to a joint.	5. To prevent the cannula from bending causing occlusion, phlebitis or extravasation.
6. Always wear personal protective clothing when blood sampling from a peripheral cannula and employ an aseptic, non-touch technique.	6. To prevent cross-infection and contamination of clothing.
7. Always insert as large a cannula as possible when it is to be used for blood sampling. Generally, cannulae smaller than 22G (blue) are unsuitable.	7. Small cannulae (24G) do not allow easy sampling of blood and can become occluded during the procedure (Danek and Norris 1992).
8. If any samples are collected for the purposes of research studies, the child and family must have consented to this using the appropriate process and documentation.	8. To ensure that no samples are taken without the full approval of the child and family.

287

Procedure guideline 13.11 Blood sampling technique

Statement	Rationale
1. Collect all necessary equipment on a clean tray: • 1× alcohol impregnated swab • 1× 2ml syringe for extraction of 'dead space' • 2ml syringes adequate to extract required quantity of blood if required • The appropriate blood containers and connectors • 1× 0.9% sodium chloride for injection • 1× 10ml syringe • 1× 21G (green) needle for drawing up 0.9% sodium chloride • Request forms • Polythene specimen bags as required.	1. To be well prepared for the procedure.
2. Ensure laboratory guidelines for taking and sending samples are adhered to.	2. Some tests must be undertaken by the laboratory within a specified time or delivered to them under certain conditions.
3. Explain to the child and family the reason for the procedure and what it will entail.	3. To gain their confidence and trust and empower the child (United Nations General Assembly 1998, Charles-Edwards 2003).

(Continued)

Procedure guideline 13.11 (*Continued*)

Statement	Rationale
4. Remove the bandage from over the cannula.	**4.** So that the site of entry of the cannula may be observed throughout the procedure.
5. Perform a surgical hand wash and put on personal protective clothing.	**5.** To prevent cross-infection and contamination of clothing.
6. Apply an appropriate size of tourniquet 5–8cm above the cannula but not so tight to occlude arterial supply. Indications of occluded arterial supply include: loss of colour, compromised pulse and pain.	**6.** To assist filling of the vein, improving blood flow from the cannula.
7a) Clean the port and needle-less system (if in use) with an alcohol impregnated wipe. **b)** Allow the port to dry naturally; do not fan or blow dry.	**7a)** To prevent introduction of infection. **b)** To prevent re-contamination of the port (Franklin 1998).
8. Using a 2ml syringe withdraw 1ml of blood and discard.	**8.** To withdraw saline or heparinised saline used previously.
9. Either: Using 2ml syringes, slowly withdraw the required quantity of blood. Transfer the required quantities of blood from the syringe to the appropriate blood containers.	**9.** 2ml syringes cause less vacuum and are less likely to collapse the vein.
10. Or: Attach an appropriate needle-less system and collect the required samples directly into the appropriate bottles, either using the vacuum method or using the containers as syringes.	**10.** This method, being a closed system, should be favoured as it reduces the risk of contamination and splash injuries.
11. Release the tourniquet.	**11.** To restore usual venous blood flow.
12. Flush the cannula with 1–2ml of heparinised saline immediately and clamp the 'T' extension while still flushing to create positive pressure.	**12.** To prevent occlusion and blood backflow into the 'T' extension (Kleiber *et al* 1993).
13. Ensure the splint is still in the correct position and re-bandage the area over the cannula.	**13.** To ensure patency for collection of next sample or administration of the next drug.
14. Check that the correct quantities of blood have been collected into the correct containers, label the containers, ensuring the name and hospital number correspond on both form and bottle(s) and place both the form and the bottle(s) into a specimen bag.	**14.** To prevent errors and to ensure that the appropriate care and treatment are given to the child.
15. Check the name and hospital number on the sample and request form against the name and hospital number on the child's ID bracelet.	**15.** To ensure that the sample has been collected from the correct child and to prevent critical incidents.
16. Send the samples with the completed request forms to the correct laboratory.	**16.** To ensure the correct test is undertaken.
17. Explain to the child and family the implications of any results, when they are likely to be available and who will communicate the results to them.	**17.** To keep them fully informed of their care, management and the possibility of any change in treatment.

288

Procedure guideline 13.11 (*Continued*)

Statement	Rationale
18. Record the blood collected and tests performed, in the child's health record.	**18.** To ensure that the child's health record is comprehensive and to provide information to other practitioners who may collect samples from the cannula at a later time.
19. Give the child positive reinforcement for tolerating this procedure.	**19.** We know that children respond well to positive feedback.

Procedure guideline 13.12 **Removal of the cannula**

Statement	Rationale
1. There are four possible reasons for removal of the cannula: • Extravasation • It may no longer be required • It may no longer be functioning effectively or it may be causing the child excessive discomfort • A VIP score of 2 or above.	**1.** For further information about and advice on management of extravasation see also Berry and Bravery (2005) and Chapter 8.
2. Collect all the required equipment on a clean tray. • 1× packet of sterile gauze • 1× sachet of 0.9% sodium chloride for irrigation • 4× sterile cotton wool balls • 1× appropriate plaster • Micropore® (2.5 cm).	
3. Always employ an aseptic, non-touch technique.	**3.** To prevent cross-infection.
4. If possible, use a procedure room for this intervention.	**4.** To ensure that the child's bed area remains a 'safe haven.'
5. Explain the procedure to the child and family.	**5.** To gain their confidence and trust.
6. Remove the bandage and splint.	
7. Perform a surgical hand wash and put on personal protective clothing.	**7.** To prevent cross-infection and contamination of clothing.
8. Inspect the exit site and assess for infiltration, phlebitis or infection utilising the VIP scoring system. If there is cause for concern alert senior colleagues and medical staff.	**8.** Further treatment may be required.
9. Carefully remove the old dressing, holding the cannula in place at all times.	
10. Hold a piece of sterile gauze or cotton wool over the exit site but do not apply pressure.	**10.** Pressure should not be applied until the needle has been fully removed or it will cause the needle to be dragged out of the vein causing pain and venous damage.
11. Slowly withdraw the cannula, maintaining a neutral angle with the child's skin.	

289

(Continued)

Procedure guideline 13.12 (*Continued*)

Statement	Rationale
12. Immediately apply gentle digital pressure to the exit site for 3–4 minutes.	**12.** To absorb any blood that escapes and to prevent the formation of a haematoma.
13. Examine the cannula and place it carefully into a tray.	**13.** To ensure that no particles or cannula parts remain in the vein and to prevent possible inoculation injury.
14. Lift the soiled gauze/cotton wool and inspect the exit site to check that bleeding has ceased.	
15. Do not wipe the exit site with the gauze/cotton wool.	**15.** This could re-activate bleeding by dislodging the thrombus.
16. If necessary, clean the area using sterile gauze soaked in 0.9% sodium chloride but avoid the exit site.	**16.** The exit puncture site is a potential entry point for infection.
17. Assist the child to wash the previously splinted and bandaged area thoroughly, using soap and water.	**17.** To cleanse and provide comfort.
18. Apply a sterile plaster, child friendly if available, directly over the exit site and a sterile cotton wool ball secured with micropore® tape over the plaster.	**18.** To create a pressure dressing.
19. If the child prefers, they may choose only sterile cotton wool and tape without a plaster.	**19.** To reduce trauma to the child when the plaster is removed and to empower the child (Charles-Edwards 2003, Van Cleve *et al* 1996).
20. Advise the child and family that the plaster/cotton wool and tape should remain in situ for 24 hours. The pressure dressing of cotton wool/micropore® may be removed after 4 hours.	
21. Dispose of the cannula in a sharps container or a yellow clinical waste bag.	**21.** The used cannula is not technically a sharp but does require disposal by incineration due to the inoculation risk that exists.
22. Perform a clinical hand wash.	**22.** To prevent cross-infection.
23. Document the procedure, date of removal, duration of cannula, VIP score and action taken in the child's health record.	**23.** To ensure that the child's health record is comprehensive.
24. Give the child positive reinforcement for tolerating this procedure (Box 13.3).	

Peripherally inserted central catheters

There are a number of different central catheters used to gain IV access, these are described below.

The peripherally inserted central venous catheter (PICC) is a catheter designed for mid-term access requirements, from 3 days to 6 weeks. The PICC provide a less invasive, minimal risk alternative to other forms of central venous access devices. It is suitable for children with poor peripheral access, when children have had other long-term access devices temporarily removed due to infection, or when a child's condition prohibits the insertion of a tunnelled catheter via a chest site.

It is inserted at or above the antecubital vein, usually into the cephalic or basilic vein, with the tip residing in the superior vena cava (SVC) (Camara 2001, Flynn 1999, Gabriel 1996a, 1996b, Goodwin and Carlson 1993, Ryder 1993, Todd 1998, Weinstein 1993). Insertion is normally via a peripheral vein, most commonly the basilic, cephalic, or median cubital veins and threaded up through the axillary vein, into the lower third of the superior vena cava. Insertion can also be via the internal jugular vein when peripheral venous access is poor (similar to Hickman tunnelled catheters). The PICC is tunnelled under the skin on the chest and usually enters the internal jugular vein with the tip threaded down to the superior vena cava. Two incisions are made:

1. The **insertion site** where the catheter enters the central venous system.

> **Box 13.3** Best practice standard for cannulation and venepuncture in children
>
> - The practitioner must be competent and confident that in performing these skills, must satisfy the NMC guidelines for practice as this is in the best interest of the child (UKCC 1996)
> - The practitioner must be skilled and trained in the technique (Heiney 1991, Millam 1992)
> - The opinion of the child must be considered and respected (Alderson and Montgomery 1996, Charles-Edwards 2003, DoH 2001, 2003, Fulton 1996, UN General Assembly 1989)
> - Time must be taken to assess the child's veins to ensure that the appropriate site is used prior to applying local anaesthetic (Sclare and Waring 1995)
> - The preparation must be structured and tailored to the individual child and family (Action for Sick Children 2003, Heiney 1991)
> - Children should be allowed to choose their pain site and choice of equipment, for example a butterfly or a cannula, whenever possible (Van Cleve *et al* 1996)
> - Paediatric nurses must be trained in when and how to hold a child still and they should have an understanding of their legal responsibilities (RCN 2003, Robinson and Collier 1997)
> - Children's nurses must prepare the parent/carer so that they can make an informed decision about whether to accompany their child during the cannulation/venepuncture (Bradford and Singer 1991)
> - Children's nurses must utilise the parent/carer–child bond during the procedure to help stress and build mastery over the event (Dearmun 1992, Shaw and Routh 1982)

2. The **exit site** on the chest wall where the catheter exits the skin tunnel. The skin tunnel provides a barrier against infection.

PICCs are true central lines, so they can be used for all types of IV drugs and fluids including vesicant therapy, as the SVC has a large blood flow to dilute these medications. PICCs should not be confused with the term PIC sometimes used to describe a peripherally inserted catheter, i.e. a peripheral cannula; or Midline catheters (long lines) which are also placed peripherally, but are not suitable for vesicant therapy as the catheter tip resides in a much smaller vein (Todd 1999).

Several different companies manufacture PICCs, each with varying guidance for usage. The type of PICC discussed in this chapter is a Bard Groshong® closed ended valve PICC. It is made of soft medical grade silicone rubber tubing and has a closed rounded tip. Unlike open ended PICCs, the closed end has a three position, pressure sensitive Groshong® valve. The valve is located near the rounded closed radiopaque catheter tip. Positive pressure into the catheter will open the valve outwards, allowing fluid infusion. Negative pressure will cause the valve to open inwards, to allow blood aspiration, but remains closed when not in use at normal intrathoracic pressures, this maintains patency by reducing the risk of blood backflow, clotting and air embolism. It is therefore not necessary to clamp or heparinise the line (Bard Access systems 2003). This increases patient safety and reduces the cost of ongoing maintenance. The translucent nature of the Groshong® PICC allows visualisation of any blood residue in the catheter, allowing adequate flushing to reduce the risk of occlusion. Open ended PICCs need flushing with heparinised 0.9% sodium chloride, every 4–24 hours, depending on the catheter size (see individual manufacturer's guidelines). PICCs have one or two lumens. Bard Groshong® PICC's range from 3 to 5 French gauge (Fr). Size 4 is recommended especially if blood sampling is required. The 5 Fr catheter is a dual lumen device for multiple infusions. The valves are staggered and rotated, allowing the concurrent infusion of incompatible drugs. Each lumen must be treated separately (i.e. separate flushes for each lumen, etc).

The Groshong® valve is designed to remain closed between −7 and 80 mmHg. Normal central venous pressure in the SVC is 0–5 mmHg. If the pressure were greater than 80 mmHg it would cause the valve to open, allowing backflow of blood into the catheter. This is confirmed using image intensification or a chest X-ray.

The advantages of the catheter are:

1. It does not require needles to initiate access.
2. It reduces the need for repeated venepuncture and cannulation, which can cause the child and family psychological distress.
3. There is less risk of extravasation compared to an implantable port.
4. It can be used for the administration of IV fluids, drugs including cytotoxic and vesicant drugs, parenteral nutrition and blood products.
5. The preferred method of placement involves minimal risk, (Dougherty 2000, Gabriel 1996a, 1996b) less than placement of an implant able port or tunnelled central catheter. (Todd 1998).
6. The PICC preserves the patient's peripheral veins for essential venepuncture (Todd 1998).
7. Elimination of the need for heparin flushing or clamping, to maintain patency (Bard Access Systems 1994).
8. There are fewer colony-forming units of skin flora on the arm than the chest (Maki and Ringer 1991).
9. The catheter can be repaired easily if breakage occurs, provided enough external catheter remains undamaged.
10. The device can be easily removed on the ward by a trained healthcare professional (see section on removal of catheter).

The disadvantages of the catheter are:

1. It can occasionally be difficult to obtain blood from the catheter.
2. The usual site for placement is the ante cubital fossa at the elbow joint, which is often flexed and can cause kinking of the catheter.

3. The catheter can break easily if excessive force is applied or if the dressing is inadequately positioned.
4. The catheter is not designed for long-term use.

In children, PICCs are often inserted under a general anaesthetic by an interventional radiologist or surgeon, more recently specialist nurses are being trained to place PICCs, reflecting an example of Advanced Level Nursing (DoH 2010). Nurses are now able to technologically advance their practice, allowing them to augment their individual professional practice in the best interests of their patients (Gabriel 1996b). This development in practice increases professional responsibility and accountability, but also liability, as it is essential that nurses can produce evidence to justify their practice (Todd 1998).

All personnel who use PICC's must be trained and competent in the techniques involved. to minimise potential complications associated with these devices (Todd, 1998).

Non-tunnelled short-term percutaneous central venous catheters

Non-tunnelled short-term, central venous lines are used for the care of acutely ill children usually in intensive care or high-dependency settings (Kaye et al 2000). They are used to give drugs that need to be administered rapidly and reliably into large veins with a high blood flow rate. Rapid administration of intravenous fluids or blood products can be provided for children with severe shock and to monitor the central venous pressure. A central catheter may also be inserted for temporary cardiac pacing, the administration of total parenteral nutrition and when there is a lack of peripheral venous access (Henderson 1997, Woodrow 2002). As these patients often require multiple infusions these lines have at least two or three access ports. They are technically easier to insert than PICCs. However, there is a higher risk of severe infection than with peripheral lines and nursing staff must be trained and competent in managing these lines (Capka et al 1993). These lines are designed to last for approximately 2–3 weeks and patients requiring long-term central access may require a tunnelled or subcutaneous port (Kaye et al 2000).

The insertion of a short-term central catheter is carried out at the child's bedside or following induction of anaesthesia in theatre frequently using the Seldinger technique (Hijazi et al 1997). Single, double, triple and quadruple lumen lines may be used, depending on the child's condition. Each lumen will open at a different point along the catheter to allow for multiple drug and fluid administration. Catheters are most commonly inserted into the superior or inferior vena cava or right atrium via the internal jugular, subclavian or femoral vein.

The femoral vein has easily identifiable anatomical landmarks, direct pressure can be applied easily in the event of bleeding and it is easily accessible during resuscitation (Advanced Life Support Group 2001, Chiang and Baskin 2000). Several studies in children have found a low incidence of mechanical complications and despite the risk of infection from soiled nappies (Kaye et al 2000), infection rates are no higher than for non-femoral catheters (CDCP 2002). Although avoidance of this site after major abdominal trauma has been recommended (Fuhrman and Zimmerman 1998). The subclavian vein is avoided in children with high intrathoracic pressure and in small infants to avoid inad-

vertent puncture of the pleural space and life-threatening pneumothorax or haemothorax (Hijazi et al 1997). The right internal jugular is the largest and safest neck vein to use in children (Kaye et al 2000). Although it should be avoided in patients with raised intracranial pressure (ICP) as the catheter may impede venous return and further increase the ICP (Hijazi et al 1997).

Early complications of short-term central venous catheters include, catheter malposition, cardiac perforation, arrhythmias, pneumothorax, haemothorax, brachial plexus injury, thoracic duct injury when subclavian or jugular veins are used; subcutaneous emphysema, haematoma at the puncture site, arterial damage and inadvertent arterial cannulation. Extravasation injuries, although less common, can occur at any stage. Other complications seen are infection, haemorrhage, air embolism, nerve damage, occlusion, venous thrombosis, catheter fragmentation and catheter migration (Henderson 1997, Kaye et al 2000).

Tunnelled central venous catheters: Hickman and Broviac lines

Hickman® catheters were first introduced into healthcare in the 1960s. They are widely used in children requiring long-term intravenous therapy. A Hickman® catheter is a tunnelled single, dual or triple lumen catheter made of radiopaque silicone. A Broviac® catheter is single lumen and is smaller in French size than Hickman® catheters and therefore used for infants and children (Bard Access Systems 1994). Some centres especially in bone marrow transplant units, use triple lumen catheters in children. The size of catheter required for the child will depend upon age, weight and venous anatomy.

Until a few years ago the insertion of central venous catheters was a surgical procedure; now, interventional radiologists and nurses are placing Hickman® catheters, using ultrasound and percutaneous insertion techniques (see Chapter 14). CVADs are inserted under sedation or anaesthetic and often only minimal analgesia is required post insertion. Surgical placement of the device requires the surgeon to make an incision in the chest wall and tunnel the catheter under the skin. The catheter tip is then placed via a large central vein usually the external/internal jugular, subclavian, axillary, long saphenous or femoral vein, into the superior vena cava, or right atrium (Dougherty 2000, Dougherty and Lamb 1999). Percutaneous insertion involves the location of the chosen access vein (external/internal jugular or subclavian vein) by the use of ultrasound. Once the vein is located, a small puncture is made and the catheter tip is inserted directly into the vessel. It is then threaded via the access vein into its correct position with the tip sitting within the right atrium or superior vena cava. Both insertion techniques verify catheter tip placement via image intensification after insertion. Sutures may be used both internally and/or externally to help secure the catheter. Hickman® catheters have a SureCuff® cuff attached which helps to prevent dislodgement of the device (Bard Access Systems 1994). The cuff enables fibrous tissue in-growth, which secures the device and also acts as a barrier to bacteria. Tissue in-growth into the cuff takes up to 3 weeks, but this may be delayed or impaired in the immunocompromised patient. The care and maintenance of the Broviac® and Hickman® catheter is often dependent on local hospital policy and manufacturer's guidelines. Policies should include research-based practice supporting clinical procedures relating to central venous access devices, and the care and maintenance required. Nursing and medical staff who use CVADs should also ensure they are adequately trained and educated in relation to the use of these devices. Asepsis should be adhered to at all times when accessing CVADs and an aseptic non-touch technique (ANTT) should be used wearing sterile or non-sterile gloves (Weinstein 1993).

Implantable ports

An implantable port is a totally implanted central venous access device used for long-term intravenous therapy. The port consists of two parts, a silicone catheter, which is attached to a dome shaped chamber with a silicone septum. Implanted ports have been single ported, however, in the last decade dual ports have been introduced into the CVAD market although their use in children within the UK is limited (Bard Access Systems 1994).

Implantable ports are available in two catheter French gauge sizes, 6.6F or 9.6F. The size of the actual port (domed shaped device) is also available in two different sizes, low profile port or adult port. All children who have an implantable port inserted must be assessed for the amount of subcutaneous tissue, which will cover the port once inserted to determine the correct size.

Ports maybe sited in the chest or just under the arm. Chest placement can provide greater security as the port is sutured to the muscles between the ribs and this prevents it from becoming mobile. A mobile implanted port has an increased risk of needle displacement, extravasation/infiltration and possible damage to the silicone septum (Dougherty and Lamb 1999, Weinstein 1993).

As these ports are totally implanted, a specially designed needle is required to access the device to avoid damage the silicone septum of the port. They are often referred to as 'huber' or 'non-coring' needles and under no circumstances should any other type of needle be used when accessing the device (Bard Access Systems 1994). Winged infusion sets and gripper needles are two types of Huber needle used, and the choice is often down to patient preference. Access needles may remain in situ for between 7–14 days depending on the child's clinical condition and their level of immunosuppression (Dougherty 2000). In haematology and oncology units port needles should be changed every 7 days as the immunosuppressive effects of the disease and its treatment places the patient at an increased risk of infection. However, in children suffering from cystic fibrosis implantable port needles are often changed only every 14 days, as these patients are not at high risk of infection.

293

Procedure guideline 13.13 Central catheters: perioperative care

Statement	Rationale
1. Inform the family of the following: • That a catheter is necessary • The reason for the catheter • What it entails • The potential risks associated with the catheter • The length of time it is likely to be in situ.	1. To ensure the child and family are kept fully informed.
2. If necessary, contact an appropriate Play Specialist or nurse to work with the child.	2. To help to prepare the child for the procedure.
3. Supply the patient and their parents/carers with the appropriate information leaflets.	3. To address any information requirements.
4. Children usually require a general anaesthetic for the insertion of a central venous catheter.	4. To prevent the child becoming distressed during the procedure.
5. Follow local policies for routine perioperative care.	5. To maintain patient safety.
6. The child may be sore for a few days in the area surrounding any skin tunnel, exit and insertion sites. Analgesia may be required.	6. To maintain patient comfort (Marcoux *et al* 1990).
7. Where lines are inserted straight into a vein it is unlikely that the child will experience pain.	7. Clinical experience suggests this is an accurate assessment.
8. For those lines inserted via a skin tunnel in the chest, specific points about the insertion site should be noted: • Dissolvable sutures may be used at the insertion site • Steristrips, if used, should normally be removed after a week.	8. Lines inserted via this route require special considerations. • After 5–7 days sufficient wound healing should have occurred.

(Continued)

Procedure guideline 13.13 (Continued)

Statement	Rationale
9. Specific points about the catheter exit site to note include: **a)** The suture wings are used to secure the PICC by suturing the wings to the patient's skin. **b)** An occlusive dressing will be applied following insertion. **c)** The dressing should cover the whole of the external catheter and hub of the catheter. **d)** The site should be cleaned and re-dressed at least weekly using an aseptic non-touch technique or and when the dressing is loose, damp or soiled.	9. **a, b)** To reduce the risk of accidental dislodgement. There is an increased risk of catheter migration, phlebitis, granuloma and infection if the catheter is not adequately secured (Gabriel 2001). **c)** To prevent kinking or tugging of the catheter (Todd, 1998) and minimise the risk of accidental fracture of the catheter. **d)** To minimise the risk of infection and to enable care to be planned.
10. If the child bleeds around the site: **a)** Apply a pressure dressing over the theatre dressing. **b)** Repeat the pressure dressing as required. **c)** Remove and change all dressings 24 hours later taking care not to dislodge the catheter.	10. **a)** To stop bleeding. **b)** To stop bleeding. **c)** Blood left underneath the dressing increases the risk of infection (Hindley 1997, Marcoux *et al* 1990).
11. The size of the catheter should be recorded in the child's notes.	11. • To be aware of catheter volumes for drug administration, blood sampling, alteplase or urokinase administration and to facilitate catheter repair.
12. The position of the catheter tip must be checked by X-ray or image intensification before the catheter is used. This is usually performed at the time of insertion. The operative record should state whether this has occurred or if a chest X-ray is required on return to the ward.	12. To check catheter and tip position (Royal College of Nursing 1995).
13. For patients with long-term devices, safety issues must be discussed with the family. These include: • General advice regarding how to look after the catheter • What to do if the catheter is accidentally removed or dislodged • What to do if the catheter breaks • What to do if the cap falls off.	13. To ensure the family are prepared for any eventuality thereby ensuring the child's safety.
14. For patients with long-term devices a safety pack should be given to the family. This should contain: • 2 pairs of blue clamps • Spare occlusive dressing • Small occlusive dressing • Sterile gauze • Spare Steri-strips • Spare caps • Alcohol wipes.	14. To ensure that the family can safely deal with any situation that arises.

Procedure guideline 13.14 **Femoral vein cannulation**

Statement	Rationale
1. Preparation of the child and family. Children are fully sedated and ventilated patients may require muscle relaxants (for further details of preparation of child and family see Arterial lines).	1. To facilitate venous access (Kaye *et al* 2000).

Procedure guideline 13.14 (*Continued*)

Statement	Rationale
2. Only a suitable trained and competent medical practitioner or specialist nurse should undertake the central venous cannulation.	**2.** To ensure patient safety. Experienced operators have a higher success rate and lower infection rates and associated complications (CDCP 2002, NICE 2002). In elective situations NICE (2002) recommend the use of ultrasound guidance by trained operators.
3. Sterile, barrier precautions, based on local policy, should be used for the procedure.	**3.** Standardised sterile techniques reduce infection risks (Centers for Disease Control and Prevention, 2002).
4. Standard (universal) precautions should be used and a visor is recommended.	**4.** To minimise cross-infection risks (DoH 2001).
5. Prepare the following equipment: • Sterile CVC insertion pack • Appropriate sized heparin bonded central venous catheter (check that the correct size and length catheter pack has been selected) • Sterile gown and gloves • 0.9% sodium chloride for injection • Sterile syringes and needles • Sterile lancet • Chlorhexidine solution • Lidocaine 1% • Percutaneous entry needle, e.g. 20 or 22 Abbocath™ • Three way taps • 3/0 Skin sutures • Occlusive dressing.	**5.** To ensure equipment is available. Heparin bonded catheters have a reduced incidence of thrombotic and infective complications (Pierce et al 2000).
5. Select the most appropriate vein to cannulate (see introduction).	
6. Ensure child is adequately sedated with appropriate continuous monitoring of airway, breathing and circulation.	**6.** Child's condition may be critical and at risk of cardiopulmonary arrest.
7. Children should be positioned supine with the groin exposed and leg slightly abducted at the hip; a small roll (such as a towel) under the hips may help.	**7.** To facilitate access and achieve a more palpable pulse (Advanced Life Support Group 2001, Fuhrman and Zimmerman 1998).
8. Perform surgical hand wash and put on sterile clothing.	**8.** Standardised sterile techniques reduce infection risks (CDCP 2002).
9. Clean skin with chlorhexidine solution.	**9.** To reduce infection risks.
10. Establish sterile field.	**10.** To reduce infection risks.
11. Identify the puncture site. The femoral vein is found by palpating the femoral artery.	**11.** The vein lies medial to the artery (Advanced Life Support Group 2001, Fuhrman and Zimmerman 1998).
12. Infiltrate skin with 1% lidocaine (maximum dose 4 mg/kg i.e. 0.4 ml/kg).	**12.** To provide local anaesthetic.
13. Attach a syringe to the entry needle and attempt to cannulate the vein (use a 22 G Abbocath™ for size 4 Fr or a 20 G Abbocath™ for size 5 Fr). In infants a 22 G Abbocath™ can be used and a 0.18″ Kimal™ guide wire can be passed through it and the 5 Fr line can then be sited by passing it over the guide wire.	**13.** To access the vein.

(*Continued*)

Procedure guideline 13.14 (*Continued*)

Statement	Rationale
14. With one finger on the artery to mark its position, insert the needle at a 45° angle towards the patient's head, with the syringe in line with the femoral vein.	**14.** To access the vein.
15. Advance the needle, and at the same time pull back on the syringe plunger.	**15.** To identify successful cannulation.
16. When blood flows back into the syringe ask assistant to open the catheter pack.	**16.** To avoid wastage of catheter. To maintain sterile procedure.
17. Apply pressure to occlude blood flow through the needle and remove the syringe.	**17.** To avoid blood loss.
18. Advance the Seldinger wire into the vein through the needle to one-fourth to one-third of its length.	**18.** To ensure adequate positioning (Hijazi *et al* 1997).
19. Withdraw needle taking care not to dislodge the wire.	
20. Insert the full length of the catheter over the wire into the vein.	**20.** To minimise accidental displacement.
21. Withdraw wire and aspirate and flush all lumens with 0.9% sodium chloride.	**21.** To prime all the catheter lumens and check line patency.
22. Suture the catheter in place.	**22.** To secure catheter.
23. Apply a sterile clear occlusive dressing.	**23.** To facilitate observation and reduce risk of infection.

Procedure guideline 13.15 Care of central venous lines: maintaining a closed system

Statement	Rationale
1. Ensure all intravenous connections are secure and tight.	**1.** To prevent air embolism or haemorrhage Luer-lock fittings are recommended (Dougherty 2000).
2. Ensure lines and infusions are carefully positioned to avoid tangling or traction on the site.	**2.** To ensure patient safety and to avoid accidental disconnection.
3. Ensure all infusions and lines are clearly labelled.	**3.** To ensure patient safety.
4. Ensure any lines not in use are securely clamped and capped off.	**4.** To prevent backflow of blood.

Procedure guideline 13.16 Care of central venous lines: observations

Statement	Rationale
1. The catheter site should be monitored for any of the following: • Redness • Swelling • Pus formation • Pain or discomfort • Bleeding.	**1.** To recognise signs of infection, dislodgement or haemorrhage.

Procedure guideline 13.16 (*Continued*)

Statement	Rationale
2. Lines that have been inserted via a skin tunnel, the skin over the catheter (i.e. the skin tunnel) should be monitored for any of the following: • Redness • Inflammation • Red tracking following the path of the catheter • Pain or discomfort.	2. To recognise signs of a skin tunnel infection.
3. The general condition of the child should be monitored.	3. To detect signs of catheter related infection.
4. If the child has a pyrexia, the medical staff should be informed.	4. Blood cultures should be ordered and antibiotics may be required.
5. Any rigor following use of the catheter should be reported. Microorganisms in the catheter, or retained in a thrombus or fibrin sheath, may have been flushed into the body.	5. To effectively monitor the child and recognise signs of infection.
6. Observe the child for any of the following: • Oedema of the face, neck, hands, arms or shoulders • Venous distension • Pain, aching or tenderness proximal to the catheter • Numbness or tingling of the fingers, hands or arms • Skin discolouration, particularly of the arms and hands.	6. These are signs of a thrombosis (Brown-Smith *et al* 1990).

Procedure guideline 13.17 **Central venous lines: infection control**

Statement	Rationale
1. Principles of asepsis should be adhered to whenever a catheter is accessed. Accessing the catheter should be kept to a minimum.	1. To minimise the risk of infection an aseptic non-touch technique should be used (Rowley 1997, 2001).
2. If an infection is suspected antibiotic administration should where possible be administered via the catheter.	2. To treat the infection effectively (Wiener 1998).
3. If the catheter is a dual lumen device, alternate lumens must be used for antibiotic administration, even if only one lumen shows positive cultures.	3. To ensure each lumen is treated for infection, and to prevent cross contamination.
4. Central venous catheters should be removed when a catheter related blood stream infection is suspected and the patient is haemodynamically unstable.	4. To remove the source of the infection (CDCP 2002).

Procedure guideline 13.18 **Central venous lines: dressings**

Statement	Rationale
1. The catheter is normally covered with a transparent semipermeable polyurethane film.	1. This dressing allows secure fixation of the device and easy visual inspection of the exit site. It provides a sterile barrier yet is permeable to water vapour in order to prevent the growth of local microflora.

(*Continued*)

Procedure guideline 13.18 (*Continued*)

Statement	Rationale
2. A gauze dressing such as Mepore® can be used if the child cannot tolerate an occlusive dressing or if the exit site is infected or has significant exudate.	**2.** Mepore® is an absorbent dressing, which will absorb any exudates. No difference in catheter related infections have been found between transparent and gauze dressings (CDCP 2002).
3. If Mepore® is used because the site is infected, it should be changed daily.	**3.** To monitor the site.
4. Criteria for dressing selection include: skin allergies, the condition of exit site and patient preference.	**4.** Alternative dressings can be used if the child has a severe skin complaint.
5. The site should be cleaned and re-dressed at least weekly using an aseptic non-touch technique and/or when the dressing is loose, damp or soiled.	**5.** To allow the site to be observed and to minimise colonisation rates (CDCP 2002).
6. Criteria for cleaning solution selection include: known skin allergies, condition of exit site, e.g. discharge, patient preference/ activities.	
7. The exit site may be cleaned with 0.9% sodium chloride or an alcohol based cleaning solution, e.g. 0.5% chlorhexidine.	**7.** Chlorhexidine 0.5% has good activity against bacteria viruses and most fungi (Bravery and Hannan 1997, Maki *et al* 1991, Royal College of Nursing 1995:).
8. Chlorhexidine should not be used more frequently than twice weekly on long-term sites. 0.9% Sodium chloride can be used in the interim periods.	**8.** It can excoriate the skin.
9. Extra security can be achieved by: **a)** Ensuring the dressing covers the entire catheter up to the hub. **b)** A vest or armband made out of surgifix or a similar product may be used for additional protection in active children. **c)** Looping the catheter and securing the loop to the skin with Steri-strips or a dressing.	**9.** To give extra protection and **a)** To minimise the risk of catheter fracture. **b)** To minimise the risk of accidental removal. **c)** To minimise the risk of accidental removal.

Procedure guideline 13.19 **Accessing the catheter: general information**

Statement	Rationale
1. Inform the family of the following: • That the catheter needs to be accessed • The reason for the access • What it entails • The likely duration of the procedure.	**1.** To obtain 'consent' and aid adherence.
2. The child may require play and distraction techniques to be utilised while accessing the catheter.	**2.** To minimise anxiety.
3. Prepare a working surface and wash hands according to local infection control policy.	**3.** To remove surface debris and clean the surface.
4. Prepare all the equipment required to complete the procedure using an aseptic non-touch technique. This could include: • Preparation of 0.9% sodium chloride and drugs for administration • Priming administration sets.	**4.** To ensure adequate preparation. To clear the dead space and reduce the risk of air embolism.

Procedure guideline 13.20 **Accessing central venous catheters: maintaining patency**

Statement	Rationale
1. Line patency is maintained by continuous intravenous infusions.	1. Keeping the line open for any further emergency use.
2. Alternatively intermittent flushing with 2 ml 0.9% sodium chloride after blood sampling or drug administration should be performed for PICC and for non-tunnelled percutaneous central catheters according to local policy.	2. To ensure the line is cleared of blood. Catheter obstruction is usually due to thrombus formation on the vessel wall or a fibrin sleeve around the catheter (Polderman and Girbes 2002); 2 ml will accommodate the catheter priming volume (Intravenous Nurses Society 1990).
3. When not in use Groshong PICC lines will require 0.9% sodium chloride to be injected once a week.	3. The use of prophylactic sodium chloride with heparin 10 units per ml is recommended for tunnelled catheters and implantable ports.
4. The Groshong catheter has a 3-way valve incorporated into the tip that prevents blood entering the catheter (Bard Access Systems 1994).	4. Heparin reduces the incidence of thrombus formation and infectious complications and is also used in non-heparin bonded non-tunnelled percutaneous catheters (CDCP 2002).
5. 0.9% sodium chloride with heparin 10 units per ml is used in devices that are regularly accessed.	5. To maintain patency.
6. 0.9% sodium chloride with heparin 100 units per ml is used in ports that will not be accessed for 4 weeks.	6. To maintain patency over 4 weeks.
7. Flushing volumes for catheters used in children vary, adhere to manufacturer's guidelines and local policy.	7. Hickman® and Broviac® catheters are supplied at a standard adult length but are often cut down to fit children.
8. Flushing volumes for implantable ports are: • 4.2 ml for low profile ports • 5.4 ml for large ports.	8. To accommodate the catheter priming volume. See the manufacturer's guidelines.
9. A pulsated, stop-start, positive pressure technique is recommended when flushing central catheters.	9. To maintain catheter patency. This method of flushing creates turbulence within the catheter lumen, clearing debris from the catheter wall (Dougherty 2000, Todd 1998). The maintenance of positive pressure helps to prevent a vacuum forming after completion of the flush, preventing blood being sucked back into the catheter, thereby helping to prevent catheter occlusion (Goodwin and Carlson 1993).

Procedure guideline 13.21 **Cap change**

Statement	Rationale
1. There are different sorts of caps that can be used, e.g. injectable, non-injectable or needleless, e.g. Bionectors™ and Smartsite™.	1. Selection criteria include: reason for access, frequency of access, to reduce the risk of needle-stick injury, local policy.
2. A needle-less access cap is preferred as it allows access via Luer slip and Luer lock syringes: a) It is a closed system. b) It is a needle free system. c) It is a latex free system.	2. Allows secure fittings of syringes, which reduces the risk of drug spillage of hazardous substances, e.g. cytotoxic, tetragenic and mutogenic drugs. a) Reduced risk of infection and air embolism. b) Reduced risk of needle-stick injuries. c) Protection of children from latex exposure.

(Continued)

Procedure guideline 13.21 (*Continued*)

Statement	Rationale
3. Luer lock syringes are recommended.	**3.** To minimise the risk of accidental removal resulting in haemorrhage and air embolism.
4. Caps should not be accessed/punctured in excess of manufacturer's recommendations.	**4.** To meet manufacturer's recommendations and specifications for use to avoid cap damage (Royal College of Nursing 1995).
5. The cap must also be changed at least weekly or if blood is retained within the cap.	**5.** To minimise the risk of infection.
6. The cap is normally changed immediately after the catheter has been accessed.	**6.** To reduce the risk of infection by limiting access to the catheter.
7. To change a cap use an aseptic non-touch technique: • Remove used cap • Clean exposed hub with an alcohol impregnated swab • Allow to dry • Attach new cap.	**7.** To minimise risk of infection: • To minimise risk of infection • To ensure effectiveness of cleaning agent (Dougherty 2000, Rowley 2001).

300

Procedure guideline 13.22 Assessing catheter patency

Statement	Rationale

1. Equipment required:
  a) 10 ml syringes.
	1.
	  a) To facilitate access without rupturing the catheter. Syringes smaller than 10 ml should **not** be used. Smaller syringes generate very high internal pressures with very little force. The back pressure from an occlusion may not be felt when using a small syringe until damage to the catheter has occurred. Syringes less than 10 ml exert pressures in excess of 25 psi. Pressures of between 25–40 psi may rupture the catheter, especially if it is occluded.

b) Needles.
  c) 0.9% Sodium chloride for injection – 10 ml.
	b) To prepare solutions.
	  c) To ascertain patency.

2. Assess the function and position of the catheter using an aseptic non-touch technique:
  a) *For non-injectable caps:* remove the cap, clean the catheter hub using an alcohol based cleaning solution and allow to dry.
  b) *For a needle-less system:* clean the cap using an alcohol based cleaning solution and allow to dry.
  c) Attach the syringe of 0.9% sodium chloride to the catheter.
  d) Flush with at least 2 ml of 0.9% sodium chloride.
	2. To minimise the risk of infection.
	
	  a, b) To enable the catheter to be accessed. To minimise damage to the catheter/cap and to ensure effectiveness of the cleaning agent (Dougherty 2000, Rowley 2001).
	
	  c) To prepare to inject fluid to check catheter function and integrity. To enable the system to be accessed.
	  d) To check catheter function/position.

3. Assistance should be sought from an experienced nurse or doctor if any of the following occur: • Resistance is felt • The child reports pain • You are unable to inject sodium chloride • Swelling is observed along the skin tunnel or in the neck area • Leakage of fluid from the catheter or exit site.	**3.** These signs could indicate: • Catheter rupture/damage • A blockage/fibrin sheath • Catheter malposition • Thrombosis • An infiltration/extravasation (Gabriel 1997, Holcombe *et al* 1992, Mayo and Pearson 1995, Reed and Philips 1996, Rumsey and Richardson 1995).

Procedure guideline 13.23 **Flushing off medium- and long-term devices**

Statement	Rationale
1. Equipment required: as for assessing catheter patency (see above).	1. To be adequately prepared.
2. To flush off the catheter access the catheter, assess catheter function and then: • Attach empty 10 ml syringe • If catheter has not been accessed for a week, withdraw 2 ml of fluid • Disconnect syringe and discard withdrawn waste • Attach a syringe of sodium chloride 0.9% to the catheter • Inject the sodium chloride 0.9% in a stop-start pulsating method while maintaining positive pressure • **For tunnelled catheters and ports only:** Attach syringe containing 0.9% sodium chloride with 10 units heparin per ml, and inject in a stop-start pulsating method while maintaining positive pressure • While the last 0.5 ml is injected disconnect the syringe • Attach a new cap if required.	2. • To prepare to remove old saline • To reduce the risk of introducing microorganisms into the patient's bloodstream, as microorganisms and fibrin may be present • To reduce the risk of infection. • To prevent infusion of blood clots • To prepare to flush off the catheter • To clear the catheter of debris and minimise the risk of blood back tracking into the catheter tip, which could cause a blood clot and a blockage in the catheter (Dougherty 2000) • To prevent blood within the catheter from clotting. This is not required for Groshung® PICC catheters • To ensure positive pressure is maintained (Dougherty 2000).
3. All lumens should be flushed weekly using this procedure.	3. To maintain patency.
4. Assistance should be sought from an experienced nurse or doctor if any abnormal signs listed in assessing catheter patency noted in 13.22 (3) are observed.	4. To maintain patient safety.

301

Procedure guideline 13.24 **Blood sampling**

Statement	Rationale
1. Extra equipment required: • Blood bottles • Three 10 ml syringes • 0.9% Sodium chloride for injection – 10 ml • Green needles (21 G).	
2. To obtain a blood sample from a catheter through a needle-less system or exposed hub: • Clean the catheter using an aseptic non-touch technique • Connect the empty 10 ml syringe • Withdraw 2–4 ml of fluid • Disconnect syringe and discard withdrawn waste (Bravery and Hannan 1997) • In some instances neonatal and intensive care patients will have the waste blood returned, if so this should be done through a three-way tap • Connect a new 10 ml syringe • Withdraw required amount of blood • Disconnect syringe • Connect syringe of saline • Inject the saline in a stop-start pulsating method whilst maintaining positive pressure (Dougherty, 2000) • While the last 0.5 ml is injected disconnect the syringe.	2. • To prepare to withdraw fluid • To remove saline that may dilute sample • To ensure the sample is uncontaminated • To reduce the risk of infection • To prevent infusion of blood clots • To minimise the risk of contamination (MacGeorge et al 1988) • If blood loss exceeds 5–10% of the circulating blood volume, blood replacement may be necessary (Hazinski 1992a,b) • To obtain sample • To obtain sample • To prepare to flush catheter • To flush catheter • To clear the catheter of debris and minimise the risk of blood back tracking into the catheter tip, which could cause a blood clot and a blockage in the catheter (Dougherty 2000) • To ensure positive pressure is maintained (Dougherty 2000).

(Continued)

Procedure guideline 13.24 (*Continued*)

Statement	Rationale
3. Blood must be put into the appropriate bottles.	**3.** To facilitate testing.
4. The blood sample may need to be shaken.	**4.** To prevent clotting.
5. When taking blood cultures the first blood withdrawn (waste blood) must be used for the blood cultures.	**5.** To ensure that the internal contents of the catheter can be tested for infection.
6. Where possible three-way taps should be avoided in any intravenous system, however if it is likely that the further access will be needed a three-way tap should be used to avoid disconnecting the system.	**6.** There is an increased risk of infection.
7. Assistance should be sought from an experienced nurse or doctor if any abnormal signs listed in Assessing Catheter Patency noted in 13.22 (3) are observed.	

Procedure guideline 13.25 Administration of a bolus drug via a central venous catheter

Statement	Rationale
1. Put on a plastic apron and wash hands thoroughly using an antibacterial hand wash. Dry hands thoroughly using paper towels.	**1.** To minimise the risk of possible contamination to patient. To adhere to Infection Control Hospital Policy.
2. Collect a plastic tray and clean all surfaces inside and out with an alcohol wipe. Allow alcohol to dry naturally.	**2.** To ensure the tray is cleaned of possible bacteria. Alcohol is an effective cleaning agent only if left to dry before use.
3. Collect equipment required for the procedure and undertake any calculations necessary. The equipment you will need is: • 2× 10 ml syringes • 2× needles • 1× 5–10 ml of 0.9% sodium chloride • 1× vial of heparinised 0.9% sodium chloride 10 units per ml • 1× alcohol wipe • Drug(s) to be administered and any diluent(s) required • Medication chart of patient requiring the drug.	**3.** To adhere to the guidelines for ANTT. To ensure the procedure is undertaken safely and efficiently.
4. NB Flushing volumes for catheters used in children vary; adhere to local policy for flushing volumes.	**4.** Bard® catheters are a standard length in order to fit the adult sized patient. Subsequently, Hickman® and Broviac® catheters are often cut down in length to fit the child.
5a) Wash hands thoroughly using an antibacterial hand wash for at least 1 minute. **b)** Ensure all surfaces of the hands and digits are cleaned. **c)** Rinse and dry hands thoroughly using paper towels.	**5a)** To reduce possible bacteria present on hands after cleaning plastic tray and collecting equipment. **b)** To adhere to ANTT guidelines. **c)** To adhere to Infection Control Hospital Policy.
6. Put on non-sterile gloves.	**6.** To adhere to ANTT guidelines and to adhere to Infection Control Hospital Policy.
7. Open the syringes and needles ensuring that the key parts of the equipment are not contaminated. Connect needles to syringes and place into plastic tray with the syringe tips uppermost.	**7.** To adhere to ANTT guidelines.

Procedure guideline 13.25 (*Continued*)

Statement	Rationale
8a) Open ampoules of 0.9% sodium chloride and 0.9% sodium chloride with 10 units per ml heparin. **b)** Check the ampoule for the solution type, strength and expiry date. **c)** Draw up the required amount of solutions ensuring not to contaminate any of the key parts.	**8a)** To ensure all solutions used are appropriate for the CVAD. **b)** To minimise the risk of possible error. **c)** To adhere to Hospital Policy for Drug Administration and to adhere to ANTT guidelines.
9. Check the drug(s) to be given against the child's prescription chart including: • Correct patient name in full • Correct date of birth • Correct patient ID number • Correct drug and dosage for age/weight • Expiry date and time of drug • Route of administration • Any allergies known • Prescription is signed and dated by prescriber • Prescription is written in a clear, legible manner.	**9.** To adhere to Hospital Policy for Drug Administration. To minimise the risk of possible drug error.
10. Calculate the amount required in ml for the dose of drug prescribed using the standard drug formula.	**10.** To adhere to Hospital Policy for Drug Administration and to minimise the risk of possible drug error.
11. Prepare the drug(s) as required and draw up the required amount(s) in ml. Use a 10 ml syringe if possible, but a smaller syringe may be used for accuracy. If a drug is pre-made ensure the syringe contains the correct amount of the drug in ml for the dose prescribed.	**11.** To adhere to Hospital Policy for Drug Administration and to minimise the risk of possible drug error.
12. Take the tray containing drug(s) and medication chart to the patient's cubicle, or area where drug(s) are to be administered.	**12.** To adhere to Hospital Policy for Drug Administration.
13. Prior to administration, double-check the patient's ID band to confirm patient's full name, date of birth and hospital ID number against the prescription chart.	**13.** To adhere to Hospital Policy for Drug Administration.
14. Locate the catheter and required lumen. Clean the hub/needle-less system with an alcohol wipe, leave to dry naturally for 20–30 seconds.	**14.** To adhere to ANTT guidelines and to prevent possible contamination.
15. Attach the syringe containing 0.9% sodium chloride to the catheter, open clamp and flush the catheter with 2–5 ml. Observe for any signs of pain, redness, swelling or leakage.	**15.** To check patency of device.
16a) Attach syringe(s) to the hub/needle-less system of the catheter and administer drug(s) over the necessary period of time. **b)** If more than one drug is due at the same time, ensure adequate flushing with an appropriate diluent between each drug.	**16a)** To administer medication safely and prevent possible drug reactions and/or adverse effects **b)** To ensure drug is flushed from catheter and to prevent drug(s) mixing within the catheter leading to possible drug precipitation.
17. When the final drug has been administered, attach syringe containing 0.9% sodium chloride and flush catheter with 2–5 ml.	**17.** To ensure all medication has been flushed from the catheter and into the patient. To adhere to ANTT guidelines.
18a) Attach syringe containing heparin solution and administer into the catheter using a pulsed method of flushing. **b)** Instil 2–4 ml, closing the clamp of the catheter while flushing in the last 0.5 ml as this creates positive pressure within the device.	**18a)** To minimize the risk of blockage. **b)** To clear the internal lumen of catheter from any residue and to minimise blood entering the catheter.

(*Continued*)

Procedure guideline 13.25 (*Continued*)

Statement	Rationale
19. Take plastic tray containing all equipment used to an area where it can be safely disposed of.	**19.** To ensure correct disposal of equipment according to hospital policy.
20. Place all syringes and needles into a sharps bin and dispose of all waste appropriately.	**20.** To minimise the risk of needle-stick injury. To minimise the risk of contamination.
21. Clean plastic tray with alcohol impregnated wipes and return to storage.	**21.** To adhere to ANTT guidelines.

Procedure guideline 13.26 Administration of a drug infusion via a central venous catheter

Statement	Rationale
1a) Put on a plastic apron and wash hands thoroughly using an antibacterial hand wash. **b)** Dry hands thoroughly using paper towels.	**1a)** To minimise the risk of possible contamination to patient. **b)** To adhere to Infection Control Hospital Policy.
2a) Collect a plastic tray and clean all surfaces inside and out with an alcohol wipe. **b)** Allow alcohol to dry naturally.	**2a)** To ensure the tray is cleaned of possible bacteria. **b)** Alcohol is an effective cleaning agent only if left to dry before use.
3. Collect equipment required for the procedure and undertake any calculations necessary. The equipment you will need is: • 1× 10 ml syringes • 1× needles • 1× 5–10 ml of 0.9% sodium chloride • 1× Alcohol wipe • 1× infusion set with burette • Drug(s) to be administered and any diluent(s) required • Medication chart of patient requiring the drug.	**3.** To adhere to the guidelines for ANTT. To ensure the procedure is undertaken safely and efficiently.
4. NB Flushing volumes for catheters used in children vary, adhere to local policy for flushing volumes.	**4.** Bard® catheters are a standard length in order to fit the adult sized patient. Hickman® and Broviac® catheters are often cut down in length to fit the child.
5a) Wash hands thoroughly using an antibacterial hand wash for at least 1 minute. **b)** Ensure all surfaces of the hands and digits are cleaned. **c)** Rinse and dry hands thoroughly using paper towels.	**5a)** To reduce possible bacteria present on hands after cleaning plastic tray and collecting equipment. **b)** To adhere to ANTT guidelines. **c)** To adhere to Infection Control Hospital Policy.
6. Put on non-sterile gloves.	**6.** To adhere to ANTT guidelines. To adhere to Infection Control Hospital Policy.
7. Open the syringe(s) and needle(s) ensuring that the key parts of the equipment are not contaminated. Connect needle(s) to syringe(s) and place into plastic tray with the syringe tips uppermost. Open infusion set with burette and a bag of compatible diluent. Ensure all clamps on set are clamped closed. Without contaminating the key parts, insert the spike on set into the septum of the infusion fluid bag.	**7.** To adhere to ANTT guidelines.

Procedure guideline 13.26 (*Continued*)

Statement	Rationale
8a) Hang the bag of infusion fluid up and gently open the roller clamp between the fluid bag and burette. Allow 20 ml of fluid into the burette and then close the roller clamp.	**8a)** The infusion tubing requires 18 ml in order to prime it thoroughly.
b) Squeeze the drip chamber below the burette until fluid reaches the half-way line. NB In some situations it may be necessary to add the drug to the burette with the correct volume of diluent *before* priming the line. Follow local policy for this procedure.	**b)** To prevent air entering the infusion tubing. To avoid excess fluid infusion and to ensure the patient receives the drug immediately the infusion is commenced. Alternatively administration via a syringe driver is advised for intensive care patients especially for vasoactive drugs.
9a) Gently open the roller clamp below the burette and allow the fluid to prime the infusion tubing.	**9a)** To ensure all of infusion tubing is adequately primed.
b) Continually rub the air sensor panel on the infusion tubing whilst priming.	**b)** Gentle rubbing of the air sensor panel ensures air is dispelled from the infusion tubing.
10. Check the drug(s) to be given against the child's prescription chart including: • Correct patient name in full • Correct date of birth • Correct patient ID number • Correct drug and dosage for age/weight • Expiry date and time of drug • Route of administration • Any allergies known • Prescription is signed and dated by prescriber • Prescription is written in a clear, legible manner.	**10.** To adhere to Hospital Policy for Drug Administration. To minimise the risk of possible drug error.
11. Calculate the amount required in ml for the dose of drug prescribed using the standard drug formula.	**11.** To adhere to Hospital Policy for Drug Administration. To minimise the risk of possible drug error.
12. Clean the access site on top of the burette with an alcohol wipe and allow drying naturally for 20–30 seconds.	**12.** To minimise the potential for contamination. To adhere to ANTT guidelines.
13. Insert the syringe containing the drug into the additive port and inject drug into the burette.	**13.** To insert drug into infusion administration set.
14. If drug requires further dilution, open the roller clamp between infusion fluid bag and burette and fill to required amount.	**14.** To ensure drug is prepared according to manufacturer's instructions.
15a) Close the clamp on top of the burette and gently shake the burette.	**15a)** To ensure drug and diluent are adequately mixed.
b) Ensure line clamp is opened once drug and diluent are mixed.	**b)** To prevent air entry.
16. Attach a label to the burette detailing the drug, dose, date, time commenced and name of the individual who administered the drug.	**16.** To prevent possible drug errors.
17. Take the tray containing drug(s) and medication chart to the patient's cubicle, or area where drug(s) is to be administered.	**17.** To adhere to Hospital Policy for Drug Administration.
18. Prior to administration, double-check the patient's ID band to confirm patient's full name, date of birth and hospital ID number against the prescription chart.	**18.** To adhere to Hospital Policy for Drug Administration.

305

(*Continued*)

Procedure guideline 13.26 (*Continued*)

Statement	Rationale
19. Locate the catheter and required lumen. Clean the hub/needleless system with an alcohol wipe, leave to dry naturally for 20–30 seconds.	**19.** To adhere to ANTT guidelines. To prevent possible contamination.
20. Attach syringe containing 0.9% sodium chloride to the catheter, open clamp and flush the catheter with 2–5 ml. Observe for any signs of pain, redness, swelling or leakage.	**20.** To check patency of device.
21. Gently remove the sterile cap protecting the end of the infusion tubing without contaminating key parts. Attach to smartsite on the end of the child's catheter and screw together securely.	**21.** To adhere to ANTT guidelines. To prevent accidental disconnection of infusion to the child.
22. Hang the infusion fluid bag onto a drip stand containing infusion device to be used. Insert infusion administration set into the pump and set the necessary rates, pressure readings and volume limits.	**22.** To ensure the drug is delivered safely and efficiently to the child. To minimise the risk of possible drug infusion errors. To adhere to infusion device manufacturer's recommendations.
23. Open clamp on the child's catheter and set the pump to run. If required, the first 18 ml of fluid can be administered quickly to the child, as no drug is present. If this is done, ensure volume limits are set and the infusion is not left unattended.	**23.** If the drug is to be given at a low infusion rate, or is required immediately, this will reduce delay in the drug entering the child's system. To prevent inadvertent administration of drug too rapidly.
24a) It is essential that if this method is used, infusion rates should be re-checked after the 18–20 ml flush has been given and set at a rate appropriate to the infusion of the drug(s). **b)** Consideration should be given to neonates or children on strict fluid restrictions as too much fluid infused too rapidly could have implications.	**24a)** To minimise the chance of administering the drug(s) at the faster rate initially set for priming volume. This method should only be used if agreed at a local level. **b)** To reduce the risk of fluid overload.
25. When the drug has been infused add 18–20 ml 0.9% sodium chloride flush to the burette ensuring ANTT is adhered to. Ensure burette access site is cleaned with an alcohol wipe and allowed to dry naturally before accessing.	
26. When the flush has infused, disconnect the infusion tubing from the catheter and flush the device with 2–5 ml of 0.9% sodium chloride.	**26.** To ensure adequate flushing of the device.
27. Attach the syringe containing 0.9% sodium chloride with 10 units per ml heparin, and inject into catheter using a pulsed method of flushing.	**27.** To prevent blood within the catheter from clotting. Pulsed flushing creates more turbulence within the catheter and removes debris reducing risk of catheter blockage.
28. When down to the last 0.5 ml continue to inject, while closing the clamp on the catheter at the same time.	**28.** To create positive pressure within the catheter reducing backflow of blood into the catheter.
29. Take the plastic tray containing all equipment used to an area where it can be safely disposed of.	**29.** To ensure correct disposal of equipment according to hospital policy.
30. Place all syringes and needles into a sharps bin and dispose of all waste appropriately.	**30.** To minimise the risk of needle-stick injury. To minimise the risk of contamination.
31. Clean the plastic tray with alcohol impregnated wipes and return to storage.	**31.** To adhere to ANTT guidelines.

Procedure guideline 13.27 Troubleshooting (PICC)

Statement	Rationale
1. **Withdrawal occlusion** (able to flush in but not withdraw blood). If it is difficult to obtain blood but the catheter can be irrigated do the following while trying to aspirate: • Depending on catheter site: reposition child, i.e. from side to side or lying to sitting, or reposition limb • Raise the child's arms • Turn the child's head to each side • Ask the child to cough • Seek assistance if the problem persists.	1. Withdrawal occlusion can be caused by the catheter tip lying against the vein wall, catheter kinking, thrombus formation or fibrin sleeve formation (Gabriel 1997, Hadway 1998, Holcombe *et al* 1992, Mayo and Pearson 1995, Reed and Philips 1996, Rumsey and Richardson 1995).
2. **Total occlusion** (not able to flush anything in or aspirate blood) • Position of catheter tip can be confirmed by X-ray • Alteplase or urokinase can be instilled into the catheter by someone who has been trained to do so • Leave alteplase/urokinase in the catheter for the required length of time before attempting removal • Seek assistance if the problem persists.	2. • Due to the fragile nature of the catheter, it could burst if excessive force is used.
3. **PICCs catheter fracture (breakage)** PICCs can be repaired quite easily provided there is enough remaining external catheter. A minimum of 5 cm undamaged catheter below the suture wing is essential when repairing any PICC line.	

4. **Repairing a PICC**
a) Gather equipment:
  • Repair kit of appropriate size
  • Antiseptic: 70% chlorhexidine
  • Blue clamps
  • Gauze swabs
  • Sterile scissors
  • Dressing pack
  • Sterile gloves
  • 10 ml syringe x 2
  • Green needle (21 G) x 2
  • 10 ml ampoule 0.9% sodium chloride
  • Blood culture bottles
  • Steristrips
  • Large occlusive dressing
  • Cap.
	4.

b) Using sterile equipment and aseptic non-touch technique.	b) To minimise the risk of infection.
c) Clean the external segment of the catheter with antiseptic solution, allow to dry.	c) To minimise the risk of infection. To ensure effectiveness of the cleaning agent (Dougherty 2000, Rowley 2001).
d) Place cleaned segment on a sterile drape.	d) To maintain asepsis.
e) Using sterile scissors cut the PICC line cleanly above the damaged portion.	e) To ensure that all the damaged catheter is discarded.
f) Identify the two-tone coloured over-sleeve portion of the repair kit and advance it over the cut end of the remaining line. This should slide easily over the catheter and 2–3 cm of the line needs to exit the over-sleeve.	f) To facilitate catheter repair.
g) Gently insert the metal stent of the repair kit into the PICC line.	g) To facilitate catheter repair.

307

(Continued)

Procedure guideline 13.27 (*Continued*)

Statement	Rationale
h) Slide the over-sleeve portion up to the winged portion and align the 'grooves' between the 'wings'. Push together until a locking sensation is felt. This will ensure that the two pieces are fully engaged.	**h)** To ensure the repaired catheter is sturdy and ready to use.
i) Attach a 10 ml syringe and if possible aspirate blood for culture.	**i)** There is an increased risk of infection due to catheter breakage. Blood aspiration confirms line patency.
j) Flush gently with 10 ml 0.9% sodium chloride.	**j)** To ensure the repaired catheter is working and does not have any leaks.
k) Attach a cap.	**k)** To complete the procedure.
l) Dress with steristrips and an occlusive dressing (e.g. IV 3000) as appropriate to fully secure the line.	**l)** Ensuring the hub of the PICC is supported reduces the risk of further damage to catheter.
m) If there is any concern regarding the position of the line and/or aspiration is not possible, confirm placement with an X-ray.	**m)** To confirm catheter tip placement.

Procedure guideline 13.28 Removing PICC catheters

Statement	Rationale
1. Before removal of a central catheter is attempted, inform the family of what is going to happen. Explain that the child does not need a general anaesthetic for the removal of the catheter.	**1.** To ensure the child is adequately prepared.
2. Tunnelled catheters and ports are removed surgically.	**2.** For ease, comfort and safety.
3. Short-term non-tunnelled catheters can be removed using the procedure described below (in patients with normal clotting values) but should be withdrawn quickly before applying very firm pressure to the site.	**3.** To minimise risk of haemorrhage
4. A competent trained nurse or doctor can remove the catheter on the ward.	**4.** The practitioner must be aware of possible complications and their management (see complications below).
5. Ensure the child is in a relaxed position with the arm extended.	**5.** To enable ease of removal.
6. Gather the necessary equipment. This could include: • Stitch cutters • Sterile gauze • Occlusive dressing.	**6.** To ensure being adequately prepared.
7. Using an aseptic non-touch technique: • Remove the dressing. • Remove the sutures using a sterile stitch cutter.	**7.** • To enable removal of catheter.
8. Slowly start to ease out the PICC, pull out a small amount then release and do the same again.	**8.** This manoeuvre allows greater control because minimal pressure is exerted, removing the catheter without stretching it.
9. Continue to slowly remove the catheter in this way.	
10. When it is completely removed, sterile gauze should be placed over the site with pressure for 5–10 minutes.	**10.** To achieve homeostasis.

Procedure guideline 13.28 (*Continued*)

Statement	Rationale
11. NB If the catheter has been tunnelled under the skin, pressure should be applied to the insertion site, e.g. jugular vein, as well as the exit site.	**11.** To reduce the risk of bleeding into the neck.
12. Inspect the end of the catheter to ensure it has come out as one complete piece.	**12.** To ensure that the entire catheter was removed.
13. Apply a small occlusive dressing.	**13.** To ensure the wound is kept clean and dry.
14. Document procedure in the child's medical records.	**14.** To ensure that an accurate record is maintained.
15. Observe the wound for redness, pus and swelling.	**15.** These indicate a possible wound infection.
16. Observe the wound for bleeding.	**16.** This could indicate a haemorrhage.
17. If the catheter is removed because it is infected intravenous antibiotics may be required.	**17.** To clear infection.
18. Antibiotics should be administered via a peripheral catheter.	**18.** To enable infection to clear.
19. Ideally a new catheter should not be sited until the infection has cleared.	**19.** To prevent the new catheter becoming infected.
20. The wound should be cared for as advised by the surgeons and/or specialist nurse.	**20.** To promote wound healing.

309

Removal of central venous catheters: possible complications

Although removal of a PICC or non-tunnelled catheter is usually a straightforward procedure, difficulties can arise (Bard Access Systems 1996, Camara 2001). It is essential that the person removing the catheter is aware of all the possible complications (Macklin 2000) in order to recognise the signs of any complication at the earliest opportunity and act accordingly.

These signs include the following:

Bleeding

If a PICC was inserted via a skin tunnel, there is potential to bleed into the neck, from the jugular vein (vein used for insertion of PICC). Ensure that the child does not have abnormal clotting and that their platelet count is above 60.

Venous spasm in PICC line removal

This is the most common problem. If resistance is felt during removal, it is essential to stop, and allow the venous spasm to resolve. A warm compress can help to relax the muscle. If the problem persists, a more experienced practitioner should be called.

During removal, the catheter moves through various valve curves and the internal lumen of the vein which gradually narrows. Movement across the smooth muscle can stimulate the muscle, causing the vein to contract vigorously (Marx 1995). This can also be exacerbated by patient anxiety (Miall et al 2001).

Vagal reaction

The vagus nerve can be stimulated by emotional stress. Early sighs are: pallor, cold, sweating and nausea. It can lead to hypotension and sinus bradycardia, resulting in dizziness and fainting. If any of these symptoms occur, the child should have a cold compress applied to the forehead or back of the neck and a more experienced practitioner should be called. If the child has had a previous unpleasant experience this may cause them unnecessary fear of the procedure. If it is anticipated that the child may become anxious, it may help to involve a play specialist or specialist nurse.

Phlebitis (inflammation)

Phlebitis can be caused by different factors: insertion technique, vein size and condition, type of infusate administered (chemical phlebitis is rarely seen with PICCs due to the tip placement in the SVC; (Richardson and Bruso 1993), filtration of solutions, size and the material the PICC is made from (Frey 1995, James et al 1993). It is characterised by pain along the track of the PICC (Frey 1999). Phlebitis results from irritation of the vein (Gabriel 2001). Because PICCs are usually inserted peripherally through a narrow vein, it can restrict the blood from flowing freely around the catheter (Gabriel 2001). This can lead to irritation of the vein wall, i.e. mechanical phlebitis. This can also occur if each time the child extends the arm, the PICC is allowed to move in and out of the vein (Gabriel 2001). Redness and warmth along the vein can lead to the vein becoming hard and cord like (Frey 1999, Goodwin and Carlson 1993) Initial treatment is to apply a warm compress to the site, elevate the arm, and limit mobility of the joint (Frey 1999).

Thrombosis

Thrombosis is the development of blood clots at the end of the catheter, on the tip or outside the catheter on the vein wall. It can be characterised by a decreased flow rate, resistance when flushing, swelling in areas distal to the clot, e.g. hand, forearm, neck. If a thrombus is suspected the child's physician should be called. Removal should not be attempted until the size and location of the thrombus have been confirmed, usually by venogram.

PICC Catheter fracture/damage

Catheter fracture can occur as a result of the above complications, if the person removing the PICC continues to do so despite resistance being felt. This is extremely dangerous. If any resistance is felt on removal, it should be stopped, as the catheter is fragile and can easily break.

If the catheter breaks externally while the PICC is being removed, it may be possible to continue with careful removal. If the catheter breaks internally, it is possible for the remaining segment of catheter to migrate to the heart or even the pulmonary arterial system. This is a serious complication and can be characterised by anxiety, light-headedness, shortness of breath, confusion, pallor, tachycardia and hypotension. If this occurs place the child on their left side and call for the surgeon.

Arterial lines

Arterial lines are used to provide continuous accurate monitoring of blood pressure, access for frequent arterial blood gas analysis and other blood samples in theatres, intensive and high-dependency settings, and during the inter-hospital transfer of acutely sick children. They are normally sited in the radial, femoral or axillary arteries using percutaneous puncture. The umbilical artery may be used in newborns but are not included in these guidelines.

Patency of the cannula is maintained with an infusion of 0.9% sodium chloride, and 1 unit of heparin per ml be added to maintain patency and longevity of the line (Wynsma 1998). Drugs and hypertonic solutions must never be given via an arterial line, as these can cause severe tissue necrosis when the drug is delivered in a high concentration to the affected limb (Cardinal et al 2000, Lua et al 1997). Arterial lines must therefore be clearly labelled and the cannula site needs to be exposed and continually monitored. The child should not be left unattended at any time. Any bleeding at either the puncture site or from disconnected equipment can then be quickly identified.

The arterial line is connected to a transducer and haemodynamic monitor, which consists of an amplifier that enhances the signal and this is converted into a digital display and an oscilloscope trace. Arterial waveform analysis can provide valuable information as well as the absolute systolic and diastolic pressure (Hazinski 1992a,b). The blood pressure recordings may be compared to non-invasive blood pressure recording as required or according to local policy. However, invasive monitoring is normally more accurate, especially in the critically ill (Bur et al 2000) and will be 5–10 mmHg higher than non-invasive measurements.

All those involved in the siting and management of arterial cannula must be trained and competent in the techniques involved.

Procedure guideline 13.29 Preparation: system set up (intra-arterial infusion)

Statement	Rationale
1. There are two delivery methods of intra-arterial infusion available (Hazinski 1992a,b), which provide different levels of accuracy of fluid administration.	1. The correct system must be followed.
a) An optimal system that uses a syringe pump with a variable pressure alarm.	a) This is used when warranted by the patient's age and condition, e.g. neonates and intensive care patients when a very accurate record of fluid administration is required.
b) A non-optimal system that uses a high-pressure bag with manual pressure gauge, this provides a less accurate record of volume of fluid administered.	b) This system is used in other patients, e.g. peri-operative procedures where a moderately accurate record of fluid administration is sufficient.
2. The following equipment should be gathered to set up the system • Haemodynamic monitoring system (monitor) • Arterial line set • Heparinised 0.9% sodium chloride • Transducer • Pressure bag or syringe pump, dispensing pin, and 50 ml syringe.	2. An alarm monitor for prompt detection of occlusion and for blood pressure monitoring is required.

Procedure guideline 13.29 (*Continued*)

Statement	Rationale
3. Check the arterial pressure monitoring system for any faults or loose connections.	3. To avoid accidental disconnection.
4. Prime the system thoroughly with heparinised 0.9% sodium chloride. Ensure that: • Air is thoroughly removed • All connections are well secured • All ports are primed • The system is clearly labelled.	4. To prevent air embolism.

Procedure guideline 13.30 **Preparation: child and family (intra-arterial infusion)**

Statement	Rationale

1a) Explanation and preparation of children preoperatively should be included as part of the whole preoperative preparation.
 b) Where children have presented in emergency settings detailed explanations may have to be given or repeated for families after the initial resuscitation process. Normally the child will be anaesthetised or heavily sedated during this time.
    Occasionally the child may be conscious and some restraint may be necessary (please refer to your local hospital restraint guidelines), e.g. resiting of a line in the intensive care unit.
	1a) To ensure they understand the reason for the procedure and can give informed consent.
	 b) To ensure they are psychologically prepared, also well-informed children are able to develop coping strategies (Broome 1990).
	    Well-informed parents/carers are more likely to stay calm and be able to support their child (Landsdown 1993).

2. Explain the procedure to the child and family, avoiding medical jargon, including the following: • That a cannula is necessary • The reason for the cannula • What it entails • The potential risk of the cannula • The length of time it is likely to be in situ.	2. To comfort and distract a conscious child. To provide a safe environment for the child.
3. The child's parents/carers may be present but they should be given the option of leaving if they prefer. The practitioner inserting the cannula must be comfortable and willing to perform the procedure in the parents'/carers' presence.	3. Being present with their child through a difficult procedure should be negotiated.
4. Appropriate methods of distraction may be required for the semi-conscious child.	4. To prevent the child's whole attention being centred on the invasive procedure (Langley 1999).

Procedure guideline 13.31 **Cannulation (arterial)**

Statement	Rationale
1. Only a suitably trained and competent practitioner should undertake arterial cannulation.	1. To ensure the procedure is carried out safely and correctly.

(*Continued*)

Procedure guideline 13.31 (*Continued*)

Statement	Rationale
2. An aseptic non touch technique should be employed throughout the procedure. Standard (universal) precautions must be adhered to. An apron, gloves and a visor should be worn.	**2.** To minimise the risk of infection (DoH 2001, Pearson 1996, Wynsma 1998).
3. Prepare the following equipment on a clean surface or tray • Dressing pack • 0.9% sodium chloride for injection • 2 × 2 ml syringes • 1 × 5 ml syringe • 3 × 21 G needles • 2 × cannula, e.g. Abbocath™ size 22 G • Sterile lancet • 1 × short 15 cm low compliance extension tubing, e.g. Lectrocath™ • Three-way tap • Alcohol based povidone–iodine solution • Lidocaine 1% • Skin closures (e.g. Steri-strips™) • Transparent dressing (e.g. Opsite 3000™) • Splint.	**3.** To ensure equipment is readily available (Lua 1997).
4. Select the most appropriate artery to cannulate, in children the radial artery is preferred, but femoral or axillary arteries may be used.	**4.** Collateral blood supply is good. It s easily palpable. There is a reduced risk of infection compared with femoral access (Cronin *et al* 1990, Kirby *et al* 1997, Lua 1997).
5. The brachial artery is not recommended if other sites are available and the ulnar or posterior tibial vessels are not used.	**5.** The brachial is an end artery (Lua 1997). Cannulation of the ipsilateral radial or dorsalis pedis may result in the development of digital ischaemia (Lua 1997).
6. Intravenous analgesia and sedation may be required.	**6.** To reduce pain and fear and to ensure the patient remains still. Topical anaesthesia may be ineffective for arterial puncture (Lawson *et al* 1995).
7. Perform an Allen's test before using the radial artery to check that an ulnar artery is present and patent: • Occlude both arteries at the wrist • Release the pressure on the ulnar artery • Observe the circulation returning to the hand, i.e. that it will flush pink. If this does not happen, do not proceed with a radial puncture on that side.	**7.** To ensure an adequate circulation is maintained (Kirby *et al* 1997).
8. Seek the assistance of a colleague with the securing of the line and to position the child as follows: • Radial artery Hyperextend and restrain the wrist over a small roll. • Femoral artery Elevate buttocks with a small roll. • Axillary artery Rotate the arm to the 'how' position (i.e. hand to ear). Place rolled up towel under the chest to rotate the axilla upwards.	**8.** To maximise the success of the procedure. To provide better access.

Procedure guideline 13.31 (*Continued*)

Statement	Rationale
9. Perform a surgical hand wash.	**9.** To minimise the risk of infection.
10. Put on protective clothing.	**10.** To minimise the risk of infection.
11. Identify the vessel by palpation.	**11.** To ensure that it can be found and is suitable.
12. Establish a sterile field.	**12.** To minimise the risk of infection
13. Cleanse the skin at intended cannulation site with alcohol based povidone–iodine for at least 30 seconds and leave to dry.	**13.** To clean the skin and prevent the introduction of infection.
14. Unless the patient is a neonate infiltrate the skin with a very small volume of 1% lidocaine.	**14.** To avoid cardiac arrhythmias.
15. Examine the cannula for faults and attach a 2 ml syringe.	**15.** To ensure it will meet its purpose.
16. Gently stretch the skin over the artery.	**16.** To immobilise the vein.
17. Break the skin with a sterile lancet or 21 G needle.	**17.** An inadequate skin nick may cause significant resistance to cannula insertion.
18. Insert the cannula through the skin parallel to the vessel at an approach angle of 45° and advance it slowly.	
19. If the vessel is not entered, pull back slowly as an artery may be transfixed. If so advance after flashback of blood. If not pull back the skin and redirect, so that the needle does not become blocked thus preventing adequate flashback.	
20. When the artery is punctured blood will be seen to pulsate in the syringe.	
21. Collect the required amount of blood in the syringe for any urgent analysis.	
22. Decrease the angle of the cannula so that it is resting on the skin and withdraw the stylet slightly.	
23. A second flashback of blood will be observed up the shaft of the cannula, blood may rush back or be easily aspirated.	
24. Slowly advance the cannula over the needle with a twisting motion to achieve successful cannulation.	**24.** To ensure the cannula is correctly inserted. There is a risk of puncturing the cannula and embolising the tip.
25. If the artery is entered but the catheter cannot be fully advanced, a guide wire, e.g. Cook™ positive placement wire or a kumal™ guide wire (size 0.18 for a 22 G cannula) may help.	
26. Never re-advance the needle into the cannula.	**26.** The needle may puncture the cannula.
27. During attempted arterial cannulation sluggish back flow indicates either inadvertent venous cannulation or para-arterial placement, i.e. a haematoma.	
28. Press firmly on the artery to occlude the blood flow, keep the cannula in position and withdraw the stylet.	

313

(*Continued*)

Procedure guideline 13.31 (*Continued*)

Statement	Rationale
29. Continuing to protect the cannula, connect a 5 ml syringe and flush with 0.9% sodium chloride.	**29.** To prevent clotting and to check the patency of the line.
30. Check the site for swelling and skin blanching.	**30.** Prompt detection of extravasation.
31. Occlude the artery, remove the syringe and attach low compliance tubing primed with 0.9% sodium chloride.	**31.** To avoid blood loss from the cannula.
32. Taking care at all times to protect the cannula, apply 2 × 1 cm skin closures, e.g. Steri-strips, a sterile clear dressing. Some additional secure strapping of the tubing may be required to ensure adequate fixation while maintaining good site visualisation.	**32.** To facilitate observation of the cannula site and reduce the risk of infection (Millam 1992).
33. Apply an appropriate sized splint, according to local policy, ensuring the cannula remains visible for regular inspection. Radial lines should be splinted with the wrist extended.	**33.** To prevent movement, which may cause extravasation, phlebitis or cannula damage (Hazinski 1992a,b).
34. Attach the arterial line set to the transducer and monitor.	
35. Calibrate the transducer following the manufacturer's instructions (see also maintenance calibration).	**35.** To ensure accurate monitoring of blood pressure.
36. Observe arterial trace on the monitor for appropriate waveform.	**36.** Attempted femoral artery cannulation may result in inadvertent femoral venous line cannulation (Lua 1997).
37. Set appropriate alarm limits on the monitor.	**37.** To maintain patient safety.
38. Dispose of all used equipment according to local waste policy.	**38.** To minimise risk of infection or sharps injury.
39. Perform a surgical hand wash.	**39.** To minimise risk of cross-infection.
40. Document cannulation in the child's healthcare records.	**40.** To maintain an accurate record.
41. Following this procedure, time should be taken to give comfort and positive feedback to the aware child and the parents/carers.	**41.** To reassure them and acknowledge the parents/carers contribution.

Procedure guideline 13.32 **Maintenance: calibration**

Statement	Rationale
1. The transducer must be calibrated following the insertion of an arterial line, at the beginning of a nursing shift, when the child's position is changed or when an intra-arterial line has been accessed.	**1.** To ensure the haemodynamic measurements are accurate. A change in position can affect this accuracy Any intervention in the monitoring system may affect the accuracy of measurements (Hazinski 1992a,b).
2. For calibration the transducer must be level with the right atrium.	**2.** To ensure accurate measurement of intra-arterial pressures (Hazinski 1992a,b, Lua 1997).
3. Using the mid-clavicle as a guide, locate the 4th intercostal space and follow this space across the chest wall to the mid-axillary line. This is called the phlebostatic axis (Hazinski 1992a,b).	

Procedure guideline 13.32 (*Continued*)

Statement	Rationale
4. The position of the child can be either lying flat or their body not elevated by more than 45°.	**4.** The child's right atrium and the phlebostatic axis remain constant up to a 45° (Hazinski 1992a,b).
5. To calibrate the transducer, using a spirit level if necessary, follow the manufacturer's instructions:	
6. Silence alarms.	**6.** To prevent occlusion or pressure alarms.
7. Turn the three-way tap off to the child.	**7.** To isolate the transducer for calibration.
8. Turn the three-way tap on to the atmosphere (air).	**8.** To calibrate to atmospheric pressure.
9. Press the zero key on the monitor. When the monitor indicates that the process is complete close the three-way tap to the atmosphere and open the three-way tap to the child.	**9.** To calibrate to atmospheric pressure.
10. Select a suitable waveform scale on the monitor.	**10.** To provide a clear arterial pressure trace.
11. Select correct monitor label, e.g. arterial blood pressure = p1 (pressure line no.1).	**11.** To identify which pressure is being monitored.
12. Adjust monitor upper and lower limit alarms to an appropriate level for the child's age and condition.	**12.** To alert the practitioner to any significant changes.

315

Procedure guideline 13.33 **Maintenance: maintaining patency**

Statement	Rationale
1. A continuous pressurised infusion should be maintained through the cannula.	**1.** To keep the cannula patent. To reduce risk of back flow into the monitoring system (Hazinski 1992a,b).
2. Intermittent irrigation is not recommended.	**2.** The cannula would become obstructed.
3. Heparinised 0.9% sodium chloride or an approved fluid should be prescribed.	**3.** Heparin may prolong cannula life and maintain patency (Wynsma 1998).
4. Heparin may be omitted especially in patients with severe bleeding disorders.	**4.** To reduce risk of haemorrhage and contamination of blood samples (Blackmore *et al* 1998, Cardinal *et al* 2000, Gamby and Bennett 1995, Heap *et al* 1997, Lua 1997).

Procedure guideline 13.34 **Maintenance: observations**

Statement	Rationale
1. Check the monitor is set to display the arterial pressure trace and numerical values.	**1.** To ensure accurate and continuous monitoring of the arterial blood pressure.
2. Check for a normal waveform, which should have a sharp peak systole upstroke, a clear dicrotic notch and a definite end diastole (Hazinski 1992a,b).	**2.** To ensure accurate and continuous monitoring of the arterial blood pressure.

Procedure guideline 13.34 (*Continued*)

Statement	Rationale
3. Record volume of fluid administered via the line each hour on the child's fluid balance chart.	**3.** To maintain accurate records.
4. The cannula site must be exposed and observed by a trained competent practitioner. The patient must not be left unattended.	**4.** To check for adequate blood supply. To reduce the risk of cannula dislodgement or loss of patency and to reduce risk of blood loss due to disconnection.
5. Any abnormalities must be reported to medical staff immediately.	**5.** The cannula may need to be replaced.
6. The circulation of the cannulated limb should be continuously monitored for signs of the following: Cyanosis, decreased pulse, blanching, cool extremities, sluggish capillary refill or bleeding.	**6.** To detect deceased circulation distal to the cannula site, arterial spasm or clot formation (Hazinski 1992a,b, Lua 1997, Wynsma 1998).
7. The cannula must be removed if there is sustained blanching to the limb distal to the cannula site.	**7.** To maintain circulation to the limb (Wynsma 1998).
8. Observe for signs of cannula displacement into the tissues including swelling, bleeding, lack of a normal arterial waveform, fluid leakage, blanching or pain.	**8.** To maintain patient safety and comfort (Hazinski 1992a,b, Lua 1997).
9. Observe the tissues around the cannula for signs of infection (Hazinski 1992a,b) including pain, redness, pus, temperature change and swelling.	**9.** For prompt recognition of signs of infection.
10. Observe for bleeding around cannula due to cannula movement within the vessel (there will still be a normal arterial waveform displayed on the monitor).	**10.** For prompt recognition of complications.
11. Ensure cannula is secure and immobilised.	**11.** To prevent further movement and maintain cannula.
12. If necessary clean site and re-secure dressing when bleeding has stopped.	**12.** To minimise risk of infection.
13. Accidental removal of the arterial cannula will require the immediate application of pressure to the site for 5–15 minutes or until bleeding has stopped (Hazinski 1992a,b). The site should be covered with a sterile dressing until it has healed.	**13.** To prevent blood loss.
14. The administration set and other tubing must be checked for unsecure connections and kinks in the tubing.	**14.** To ensure there are no loose connections. To avoid line occlusion.
15. Perform hourly assessment of the continuous infusion and for normal pressures within the infusion device.	**15.** The pressure bag may deflate.
16. Monitor the general condition of the child, any pyrexia should be investigated and acted on according to local policy.	**16.** To detect signs of cannula related infection (Pearson 1996). Antibiotics may be required.
17. The cannula should be re-sited when clinically indicated e.g. signs of inflammation, pyrexia, or positive blood cultures.	**17.** Micro-organisms in the cannula may have been flushed into the circulation (Pearson, 1996).
18. All observations must be recorded in the child's healthcare records.	**18.** To maintain an accurate record.

Procedure guideline 13.35 Blood sampling (arterial)

Statement	Rationale
1. Prepare the child and family by explaining: • That a blood sample is required • What the procedure will entail • The implications of any results • When the results will be available.	1. To obtain consent and adherence (Broome 1990, Landsdown 1993).
2. The child may require play or distraction during the procedure.	2. To minimise anxiety (Heiney 1991, Langley 1999).
3. Depending on the blood tests required gather suitable equipment, for example: • Injection tray, blood bottles, 5 ml syringe 10 ml syringe alcohol impregnated wipe, sterile hub cap, syringe cap, protective paper sheet or towel and non-sterile gloves.	3. To minimise infection risk.
4. Prepare working surface, wash hands according to local infection policy.	4. To minimise infection risk
5. Standard universal precautions must be adopted when blood sampling and gloves, visors and an apron should be worn (DoH 2001).	5. To minimise infection risk.
6. An aseptic non-touch technique should be used.	6. To minimise infection risk.
7. If it is difficult to obtain blood, seek assistance from a doctor or an experienced practitioner.	7. To avoid artery damage or artery occlusion.
8. Stop infusion line and silence alarms.	8. To prevent occlusion or pressure alarms.
9. Remove cap from sampling port and clean hub with alcohol impregnated wipe.	
10. Connect a 5 ml syringe.	
11. Open the three-way tap to patient and syringe and withdraw a minimum of 3 ml dead space.	11. To clear the system of heparin, old blood and small emboli (Hazinski 1992a,b, Lua 1997, Magnay et al 2000, Weiss et al 2000).
12. Turn the three-way tap off to hub/patient/infusion.	
13. Remove the syringe and place on a clean tray.	
14. Re-access the device using syringe or blood sample container.	
15. Open three-way tap to patient and syringe.	
16. Withdraw required quantity of blood.	
17. Turn the three-way tap off to the hub and remove syringe or blood sample container and cap sample.	17. To prevent backflow of blood and movement of infusion fluid (Hazinski 1992a,b).
18. Replace dead space fluid slowly if required.	18. To prevent arterial spasm and retrograde aortic flow (Hazinski 1992a,b).
19. Dead space fluid may be replaced if free of blood clots or debris.	19. To minimise unnecessary blood loss and iatrogenic anaemia (Andrews et al 1999).

317

(Continued)

Procedure guideline 13.35 (*Continued*)

Statement	Rationale
20. Turn the three-way tap off to patient and flush port from infusion device (Weiss *et al* 2000).	**20.** To prevent blood collection in hub.
21. Turn three-way tap off to hub and open to infusion and patient.	
22. Close hub and cover with a sterile hub.	
23. Flush the line from the infusion device to clear any blood.	**23.** Blood left in a line could cause a dampened trace with lower blood pressure readings (Hazinski 1992a,b).
24. Observe site for any blanching.	
25. Ensure infusion is turned on and unclamped.	
26. Switch all alarms back on.	
27. Observe monitor for normal trace.	
28. Ensure arterial line is secure.	
29. Dispose of all used equipment according to local waste policy.	**29.** To meet health and safety standards
30. Wash hands.	**30.** To reduce infection risks.
31. Perform bedside tests and/or send samples for laboratory analysis.	
32. Record blood samples taken in the child's healthcare records.	**32.** To maintain an accurate record.

Procedure guideline 13.36 Troubleshooting: dampened trace

Statement	Rationale
1. Assess and report changes in the patient's cardiovascular status, including pulse check, ECG waveform, pulse oximetry, and non-invasive blood pressure.	**1.** Patient may have inadequate or no cardiac output (pulseless electrical activity).
2. Check arterial line site, connections and infusion flow rate.	**2.** To prevent back flow of blood into line.
3. Check arterial line set for clots, air and black flow of blood and change system if necessary.	
4. Check that blood can easily be aspirated at access port.	**4.** Occlusion may be due to blood clot (Wynsma 1998).
5. Attempt to aspirate any clot, using 2 ml of 0.9% sodium chloride lightly bounce plunger of syringe to loosen blood clot.	**5.** To clear line occlusion.
6. Do not forcefully flush the catheter if resistance is high.	**6.** May traumatise vessel, release clot and damage local blood circulation.
7. Redress cannula site, check for kinks or poor positioning of the cannula.	**7.** To clear line occlusion.
8. Reposition patient or limb.	**8.** To clear line occlusion.

Procedure guideline 13.37 Troubleshooting: abnormal readings

Statement	Rationale
1. Abnormally high or low readings must be investigated promptly and any change in the patient's condition reported immediately to the medical staff.	1. Patient safety is paramount.
2. Assess the patient's cardiovascular status, including pulse check, ECG waveform, pulse oxymetry and non invasive blood pressure to determine whether it's a monitoring problem or a real change in the patient's condition.	2. Changes in arterial waveform frequently reflect pathological changes in the patient's condition, requiring urgent medical treatment, for example, hypovolaemia, cardiac compromise, hypertension (Andrews *et al* 1999, Campbell 1997).
3. Observe trace for catheter 'fling' (Hazinski 1992a,b).	3. Artificial elevation in peak systolic pressure trace may be noted.
4. Position transducer level with the mid-axilla.	4. To minimise distortion.
5. Ensure low compliance tubing of minimal length is used.	5. To ensure accurate measurements.
6. Recalibrate transducer.	6. Ensure accurate calibration.

Procedure guideline 13.38 Troubleshooting: puncture site bleeding

Statement	Rationale
1. If bleeding occurs at the puncture site apply firm pressure for 5–15 minutes (Hazinski 1992a,b).	1. To stop bleeding
2. Ensure catheter is securely strapped and the limb is immobilised.	2. To minimise catheter and limb movement.

Procedure guideline 13.39 Troubleshooting: circulation compromise

Statement	Rationale
1. If circulation is compromised distal to the puncture site decreased pulse, blanching cyanosis or cool skin may be seen.	1. This may be due to artery spasm.
2. Using a gentle irrigation technique maintain a continuous flush and ensure extremity is kept warm distal to the cannula site.	2. To promote vasodilation (Andrews *et al* 1999).
3. Check extremity for signs of adequate circulation. The cannula must be removed if there is sustained blanching to the limb.	3. To maintain circulation to the limb.

Procedure guideline 13.40 Troubleshooting: no waveform

Statement	Rationale
1. If there is no waveform visible on the monitor, assess and report changes in the patient's cardiovascular status, including pulse check, pulse oxymetry and ECG waveform.	1. To ensure patient safety.

(Continued)

Procedure guideline 13.40 (*Continued*)

Statement	Rationale
2. Check the system is correctly set up and attached according to manufacturer's guidelines (Hazinski 1992a,b).	
3. Check appropriate arterial scale is in use on the monitor.	
4. Check monitors display settings are correctly set.	
5. Try an alternative transducer and module.	**5.** To determine if equipment is faulty.
6. Consult a biomedical engineer.	**6.** To determine if equipment is faulty.

Procedure guideline 13.41 **Removal of arterial cannula**

Statement	Rationale
1. The arterial line should be removed when: • Limb circulation is compromised • The cannula is misplaced • It is no longer required for monitoring or frequent blood sampling • There are signs of infection (Cardinal *et al* 2000, Pearson 1996).	**1.** Minimise risks associated with arterial cannula.
2. Check for normal blood coagulation levels.	**2.** To avoid prolonged bleeding from site following cannula removal.
3. Patients with severe clotting disorders may require an infusion of depleted clotting factors (e.g. fresh frozen plasma) immediately prior to arterial cannula removal.	**3.** To avoid prolonged bleeding from site following cannula removal.
4. Inform the child and family of the following: • Why the arterial line needs to be removed • What this entails • Prepare the child using distraction techniques.	**4.** To obtain consent and adherence and to help the child cope with the procedure (Landsdown 1993, Langley 1999).
5. Standard (universal) precautions must be adopted including non-sterile gloves, visor and an apron.	**5.** To minimise infection risks (DoH 2001).
6. Use an aseptic non-touch technique throughout.	**6.** To minimise infection risks.
7. Gather the following equipment: • Clean tray • Non-sterile gloves • Sterile gauze • Surgical tape • Small sterile plaster (if required).	
8. Put on clean apron and visor.	**8.** To minimise infection risk (DoH 2001).
9. Perform hand wash.	**9.** To minimise infection risks.
10. Clean tray with an alcohol impregnated wipe.	**10.** To minimise infection risks.
11. Wash hands.	**11.** To minimise infection risks.
12. Put on gloves.	**12.** To minimise infection risks.

Procedure guideline 13.41 (*Continued*)

Statement	Rationale
13. Open packaging.	
14. Place equipment on tray.	
15. Loosen all dressings.	
16. Withdraw line from artery.	
17. Using sterile gauze immediately apply firm pressure for up to 5 minutes or until bleeding has stopped.	**17.** To stop the bleeding and reduce risk of haematoma formation.
18. Apply a sterile plaster or dressing over the site.	**18.** To protect site.
19. Dispose of all used equipment according to the waste policy.	**19.** To meet health and safety standards.
20. Wash hands.	**20.** To minimise infection risks.
21. Observe site for bleeding.	**21.** To detect further bleeding.
22. Record the procedure in the child's healthcare records.	**22.** To maintain accurate records.

321

References

Advanced Life Support Group (2001) Advanced Paediatric Life Support, 3rd edition. London, BMJ Books

Alderson P, Montgomery J. (1996) Health care choices: Making decisions with children. London, Institute of Public Policy Research

Andrews T, Waterman H, Hillier V. (1999) Blood gas analysis: a study of blood loss in intensive care. Anaesthesia, 30(4), 851–857

Arrowsmith J, Campbell C. (2000) A comparison of local anaesthetics for venepuncture. Archives of Disease in Childhood, 82(4), 309–310

Association of Paediatric Anaesthetists of Great Britain and Ireland (2008) Good practice in ostoperative and procedural pain management. Pediatric Anesthesia, 18(1), 1–81

Bard Access Systems (1994) Hickman, Leonard & Broviac catheters. Nursing Procedure Manual. Utah, Bard

Bard Access Systems (1996) Groshong® PICC and MID LINE Catheters. Instructions for use. Utah, Bard

Bard Access Systems (2003) Groshong® Peripherally Inserted Central Venous Catheter (P.I.C.C.) Nursing Procedure manual. Available at http://www.bardaccess.com/assets/pdfs/nursing/ng-grosh-nxt.pdf

Berry K, Bravery K. (2005) Extravasation and infiltration. GOSH Clinical Practice Guideline (updated 2010). Available at http://www.childrenfirst.nhs.uk/health-professionals/clinical-guidelines/extravasation-and-infiltration (last accessed 7th November 2011)

Biccard B. (2001) EMLA-1hr is not enough for venous cannulation. Anaesthesia, 56(10), 1027–1028

Blackmore M, Maundrill R, Lavies NG. (1998) Use of heparin in arterial lines. Anaesthesia, 53(1), 100

Bradford R, Singer H. (1991) Support and information for parents. Paediatric Nursing, 3(4) 18–20

Bravery K, Hannan J. (1997) The use of long-term central venous access devices in children. Paediatric Nursing, 9(10), 29–37

Bregenzer T. (1998) Is routine replacement of peripheral intravenous catheters necessary? Archives of Internal Medicine, 158, 151–156

Brenner M. (2007) Child restraint in the acute setting of pediatric nursing: an extraordinary stressful event. Issues in Comprehensive Pediatric Nursing, 31(1–2), 29–37

Broome ME. (1990) Preparation of children for painful procedures. Paediatric Nursing, 16(6), 537–541

Brown-Smith JK, Stoner MH, Barley ZA. (1990) Tunneled catheter thrombosis: factors related to incidence. Oncology Nurses Forum, 17(4), 543–549

Bruce E. (2009) Management of painful procedures. In Twycross A, Dowden S, Bruce E. (eds) Managing pain in children: a clinical guide. Oxford, Wiley-Blackwell

Bur A, Hirschl MM, Herkner H, Oschaatz E, Kofler J, Woisetschlager C, Laggner AN. (2000) Accuracy of oscillometric blood pressure measurement according to the relation between cuff size and upper arm circumference in critically ill patients. Critical Care Medicine, 28(2), 371–376

Camara D. (2001) Minimising risks associated with peripherally inserted central catheters in the NICU. MCN. The American Journal of Maternal/Child Nursing, 26(1), 17–22

Campbell B. (1997) Arterial waveforms: monitoring changes in configuration. Heart & Lung, 26(3), 204–214

Capka MB, Carey S, Marks D, Wison M, Bernard J. (1993) Nursing observations of central venous catheters: the effect on patient outcome. In Guzetta CE, Ahrens T, Fontaine D. (eds) The Best of Critical Care Nursing. St Louis, Mosby

Cardinal P, Allan J, Pham B, Hindmarsh T, Jones G, Delisle S. (2000) The effects of sodium citrate in arterial catheters on acid base and electrolyte measurements. Critical Care Medicine, 28(5), 1388–1392

Centres for Disease Control and Prevention (2002) Guidelines for the prevention of intravascular catheter related infections. Morbidity and Mortality Weekly Report, 51(RR-10), 1–29

Charles-Edwards I. (2003) Power and control over children and young people. Paediatric Nursing, 15(6), 37–43

Chiang VW, Baskin MN. (2000) Uses and complications of central venous catheters inserted in a pediatric emergency department. Pediatric Emergency Care, 16(4), 230–232

Claar R, Walker L, Smith C. (2002) The influence of appraisals in understanding children's experiences with medical procedures. Journal of Paediatric Psychology, 27(7), 553–563

Clarke S, Radford M. (1986) Topical anaesthesia for venepuncture. Archives of Disease in Childhood, 61, 1132–1134

Cronin WA, Germanson TP, Donowitz LG. (1990) Intravascular catheter colonization and related blood stream infection in critically ill neonates. Infection Control Hospital Epidemiology, 11, 301–308

Danek G, Norris E. (1992) Pediatric IV catheters; efficacy of saline flush. Pediatric Nursing, 18(2), 111–113

Davies S. (1998) The role of nurses in intravenous cannulation. Nursing Standard, 12(17), 43–46

Dearmun A. (1992) Perceptions of parental participation. Paediatric Nursing, 4(7), 6–9

Department of Health (2001) The epic project: developing national evidenced-based guidelines for preventing healthcare association infections phase 1: guidelines for preventing hospital-acquired infections. London, Department of Health

Department of Health (2003) Getting the Right Start; NSF for children. Emerging Findings. London, Department of Health

Department of Health (2009) Reference Guide to Consent for Examination or Treatment. London, Department of Health

Department of Health (2010) Advanced level nursing: a position statement. London, Department of Health

Dougherty L. (1996) Intravenous cannulation. Nursing Standard, 11(2), 47–51

Dougherty L. (2000) Central venous access devices. Nursing Standard, 14(43), 45–50

Dougherty L, Lamb J. (eds) (1999) Intravenous therapy in nursing practice. London, Churchill Livingstone

Dunn D, Lennihan S. (1987) The case for saline flush. American Journal of Nursing, 6, 689–699

Flynn S. (1999) Administering Intravenous Antibiotics at Home. Professional Nurse, 14(6), 399–402

Franklin L. (1998) Skin cleansing and infection control in peripheral venepuncture and cannulation. Paediatric Nursing, 10(9), 33–34

Frederick V. (1991) Pediatric IV therapy: Soothing the patient. RN, December, 43–47

Frey AM. (1995) Pediatric peripherally inserted central catheter program report: A summary of 4,496 catheter days. Journal of Intravenous Nursing, 18(6), 280–291

Frey A. (1998) Success rate for peripheral IV insertion in a children's hospital. Journal of Intravenous Nursing, 21(3), 160–165

Frey AM. (1999) PICC complications in neonates and children. Journal of Vascular Access Devices, Spring, 17–26

Fuhrman BP, Zimmerman JJ. (1998) Paediatric Critical Care, 2nd edition. St Louis, Mosby

Fulton Y. (1996) Children's rights and the role of the nurse. Paediatric Nursing, 8(10), 29–31

Gabriel J. (1996a) Care and Management of Peripherally Inserted Central Catheters. British Journal of Nursing, 5(10), 594–599

Gabriel J. (1996b) Peripherally Inserted Central Catheters: Expanding UK Nurses' Practice. British Journal of Nursing, 5(2), 71–74

Gabriel J. (1997) Fibrin sheaths in vascular access devices. Nursing Times, 93(10), 56–57

Gabriel J. (2001) PICC securement: Minimising potential complications. Nursing Standard, 15(43), 42–44

Gamby A, Bennett J. (1995) A feasibility study of the use of non-heparinised 0.9% sodium chloride for transduced arterial and venous lines. Intensive & Critical Care Nursing, 11, 148–150

Gillick vs West Norfolk and Wisbech area HA (1985) Available at http://www.bailii.org/uk/cases/UKHL/1985/7.html.

Goode C, Titler M, Rakel B, et al. (1991) A meta-analysis of effects of heparin flush and saline: quality and cost implications. Nursing Research, 40(6), 324–330

Goodwin M, Carlson I. (1993) The peripherally inserted central venous catheter. British Journal of Intensive Care, 12(4), 96–97

Gyr P, Smith K, Pontinous S, Burroughs T, Mahla C, Swerczek L. (1995) Double blind comparison of heparin and saline flush solutions in maintenance of peripheral infusion devices. Pediatric Nursing, 21(4), 383–389

Hadway LC. (1998) Major thrombotic and non-thrombotic complications. Loss of patency. Journal of Intravenous Nursing, 21(5S), 143–160

Haslam D. (1969) Age and perception of pain. Psychological Science, 15, 86–87

Hazinski MF. (1992a) Children are different. In: Ladig D, Van Schaik T. (eds) Nursing Care of the Critically Ill Child, 2nd edition. St Louis, Mosby

Hazinski MF. (1992b) Nursing care of the critically ill child 2nd edition. St Louis, Mosby

Heap MJ, Ridley SA, Hodson K, Martos FJ. (1997) Are coagulation studies on blood sampled from arterial lines valid? Anaesthesia, 52(7), 640–645

Hecker J. (1988) Improved technique in IV therapy. Nursing Times, 84(34), 28–33

Heiney P. (1991) Helping children through painful procedures American Journal of Nursing, November, 20–24

Henderson N. (1997) Central venous lines. Nursing Standard, 11, 49–56

Hijazi OM, Cheyney JJ, Guzzetta PC Jr, Toro-Figueroa LO. (1997) Venous access and catheters. In Levin DL, Morriss FC. (eds) Essentials of Pediatric Intensive Care (Vol 2), 2nd edition. New York, Churchill Livingstone

Hindley M. (1997) Reducing exit site infections and the risk of accidental removal of Hickman lines in children within the first month post insertion. Journal of Cancer Nursing, 1(1), 54–55

Holcombe BJ, Forloines-Lynn S, Garmhausen LW. (1992) Restoring patency of long term central venous access devices. Journal of Intravenous Nursing, 15(1), 36–41

Intravenous Nurses Society. (1990) Intravenous nursing standards of practice. Journal of Intravenous Nursing, 13, S1–S98

Jackson A. (1998) A battle in vein: Infusion phlebitis. Nursing Times, 94(4), 68–71

James L, Bledsdoe L, Hadaway LC. (1993) A retrospective look at tip location and complications of peripherally inserted central catheter lines. Journal of Intravenous Nursing, 16(12), 104–109

Kaye R, Sane SS, Towbin RB. (2000) Pediatric Intervention: an update-part 2. Journal of Vascular and Interventional Radiology, 11, 807–822

Kirby RR, Taylor RW, Civeta JM. (1997) Handbook of Critical Care, 2nd edition. Philadelphia, Lippincott-Raven

Kleiber C, Hanrahan K, Loebig Fagan C, Zittergruen M. (1993) Heparin vs. saline for peripheral IV locks in children. Pediatric Nursing, 19(4), 405–409

Kolk A, Hoof R, Fiedeldij Dop M. (1999) Preparing children for venepuncture. Child Care Health and Development, 26(3), 251–260

Kumar R, Russell H. (1995) Parental presence during procedures: A survey of attitudes amongst paediatricians. Journal of the Royal Society of Medicine, 88, 508–510

Lai K. (1998) Safety of prolonged peripheral cannula and IV tubing use from 72 hours to 96 hours. American Journal of Infection Control, 26(1), 56–70

Lamb J. (1995) Peripheral IV therapy. Nursing Standard, 9(30), 32–35

Langley P. (1999) Guided imagery: a review of the effectiveness in the care of children. Paediatric Nursing, 11(3), 18–21

Landsdown R. (1993) Playing monsters and dragons. Nursing Standard, 7(25), 11

Lawson R, Smart N, Gudgeon A, Morton N. (1995) Evaluation of an amethocaine gel preparation for percutaneous analgesia before venous cannulation in children. British Journal of Anaesthesia, 75(3), 282–285

Livesley J. (1993) Reducing the risks: management of paediatric intravenous therapy. Child Health, 1(2), 68–71

Lua L, Gonzales M, Guzzeta PC, Toro-Figueroa LO. (1997) Arterial access and catheters. In: Levin DL, Morris FC. (eds) Essentials of Paediatric Intensive Care, 2nd edition. New York, Churchill Livingston

MacGeorge L, Steeves L, Steeves RH. (1988) Comparison of the mixing and Reinfusion methods of drawing blood from a Hickman Catheter. Oncology Nursing Forum, 15(3), 335–338

Macklin D. (2000) Removing a PICC. American Journal of Nursing, 100(1), 52–54

Magnay JL, Tak A, Magnay AR. (2000) Supplementing near patient quality control schemes with clinical audit of specimen quality: a model form ensuring reliable results. Paper presented at the Paediatric Intensive Care Society Conference, Stoke on Trent, October

Magnusson S. (1996) Oh, for a little humanity. British Medical Journal, 313, 1601–1603

Maki D. (1976) Preventing infection in intravenous therapy. Hospital Practice, April, 104

Maki D, Ringer M. (1991) Risk factors for infusion-related phlebitis with small peripheral venous catheters. Annals of Medicine, 114, 845–854

Maki D, Ringer M, Alvarado CJ. (1991) Prospective randomised trial of povidone iodine, alcohol and chlorhexidine for prevention of infection associated with central venous and arterial lines. Lancet, 338, 339–343

Marcoux C, Fisher S, Wong D. (1990) Central venous access devices in children. Pediatric Nursing, 16(2), 123–133

Marx M. (1995) The management of the difficult peripherally inserted central venous catheter line removal. Journal of Intravenous Nursing, 18(5), 243–249

Mayo DJ, Pearson DC. (1995) Chemotherapy extravasation: a consequence of fibrin sheath formation around venous access devices. Oncology Nursing Forum, 22(4), 675–680

McCann B. (2003) Securing peripheral cannulae: evaluation of a new dressing. Paediatric Nursing, 15(5), 23–26

Miall LS, Das A, Brownlee K, Conway SP. (2001) Peripherally inserted central catheters in children with cystic fibrosis. Eight cases of difficult removal. Journal of Infusion Nursing, 24(5), 297–300

Millam DA. (1992) Starting IVs how to develop your venepuncture expertise. Nursing, September, 33–46

Murdoch L, Bingham R. (1990) Venous cannulation in infants and small children. British Journal of Hospital Medicine, 44(6), 405–407

National Institute for Clinical Excellence (2002) Guidance on the use of ultrasound locating devices for placing central venous catheters. Technology appraisal guidance No.49. London, NICE

Needham R, Strehle EM. (2008) Evaluation of dressings used with local anesthetic cream and for peripheral venous cannulation. Paediatric Nursing, 20(8), 34–36

Nelson D, Garland J. (1987) The natural history of Teflon catheter associated phlebitis in children. American Journal of Diseases in Children, 141, 1090–1092

Nursing and Midwifery Council (2009) Code of Professional conduct. London, Nursing and Midwifery Council

Nursing and Midwifery Council (2010a) Guidelines for records and record keeping. Nursing and Midwifery Council, London

Nursing and Midwifery Council (2010b) The PREP Handbook. London, Nursing and Midwifery Council

Oldham P. (1991) A sticky situation: Microbiological study of adhesive tape used to secure IV cannulae. Professional Nurse, 6(5), 268–269

Orr F. (1999) The role of the paediatric nurse in promoting paediatric right to consent. Journal of Clinical Nursing, 8(1), 291–298

Pearch J. (2005) Restraining children for clinical procedures. Paediatric Nursing, 17(7), 36–38

Pearson ML. (1996) Guidelines for the prevention of intravascular device-related infections. Hospital Infection Control Practices Advisory Committee. Infection Control Hospital Epidemiology, 17, 438–473

Perdue M. (1995) Intravenous complications. In Terry J, Bararanowski L, Lonsway R, Hedrick C (eds) Intravenous Therapy Clinical Principles and Practice. Philadelphia, W.B. Saunders

Perucca R, Micek J. (1993) Treatment of infusion related phlebitis: review and nursing protocol. Journal of Intravenous Nursing, 16(5), 282–286

Phelps S, Helms R. (1987) Risk factors affecting infiltration of peripheral venous lines in infants. The Journal of Pediatrics, 111, 384–389

Pierce C, Wade A, Mok Q (2000) Heparin bonded central venous lines reduce thrombotic and infective complications in critically ill children. Intensive Care Medicine, 26, 967–972

Polderman KH, Girbes ARJ (2002) Central venous catheter use Part 1. Mechanical complications. Intensive Care Medicine, 28, 1–17

Power K. (1997) Legal and ethical implications of consent to nursing procedures. British Journal of Nursing, 6(15), 885–888

Reed T, Philips S. (1996) Management of central venous catheter occlusions and repairs. Journal of Intravenous Nursing, 19(6), 289–294

Richardson D, Brusco P. (1993) Vascular access devices: Management of common complications. Journal of Intravenous Nursing, 16(5), 44–49

Robinson S, Collier J. (1997) Holding children still for procedures. Paediatric Nursing, 9(4), 12–14

Rowley S. (1997) A Safe and efficient Handling technique for Intravenous Therapy: Aseptic Non-Touch Technique. London, Great Ormond Street for Children NHS Trust

Rowley S. (2001) Aseptic non-touch technique. Nursing Times, 97(7), 6–8

Royal College of Nursing (1995) Leukaemia and Bone Marrow Transplant Forum. Skin tunnelled catheters guidelines for care. London, Royal College of Nursing

Royal College of Nursing (2003) Restraining, holding still and containing children and young people; Guidance for nursing staff. London, RCN

Rumsey KA, Richardson DK. (1995) Management of infection and occlusion associated with vascular devices. Seminars in Oncology Nursing, 11(3), 174–183

Ryder MA. (1993) Peripherally Inserted Central Venous Catheters. Nursing Clinics of North America, 28(4), P937–P971

Sclare I, Waring M. (1995) Routine venepuncture: Improving services. Paediatric Nursing, 7(4), 23–27

Shaw E, Routh D. (1982) Effect of mother's presence on children's reaction to aversive procedures. Journal of Pediatric Psychology, 7, 33–42

Smith & Nephew Ltd. (2003) Ametop® product information. http://wound.smith-nephew.com/uk/Standard.asp?NodeId=2742 (last accessed 7th November 2011)

Smith & Nephew Ltd. (2003) Opsite® product information. http://wound.smith-nephew.com/uk/node.asp?NodeId=3467 (last accessed 7th November 2011)

Todd J. (1998) Peripherally inserted central catheters (PICC). Professional Nurse, 13(5), 297–302

Todd J. (1999) Peripherally inserted central catheters and their use in IV therapy. British Journal of Nursing, 8(3), 141–148

Turner T. (1989) Catalogue of disaster. Nursing Times, 89(49), 19

United Kingdom Central Council for Nursing, Midwifery and Health Visiting (1996) Guidelines for Professional Practice. London, UKCC

United Nations General Assembly (1989) Convention on the Rights of the Child. Available at http://www.hrweb.org/legal/child.html (last accessed 9th November 2011)

Van Cleve L, Johnson L, Pothier P. (1996) Pain responses of hospitalised infants and children to venepuncture and intravenous cannulation. Journal of Pediatric Nursing, 11(3), 161–168

Weinstein S. (1993) Plumer's Principles and Practice of Intravenous Therapy, 6th edition. Philadelphia, Lippincott

Weiss M, Fischer JE, Neff T, Hug ML, Baenziger O. (2000) Always flush the sampling port before sampling the arterial line. Acta Anaesthesiology Scandinavica, 45(6), 729–733

Wiener E. (1998) Venous Access in Pediatric Patients. Journal of Intravenous Nursing, 21(5s), 122–133

Woodrow P. (2002) Central venous catheters and central venous pressure. Nursing Standard, 16, 45–52, 54

Wynsma L. (1998) Negative outcomes of intravascular therapy in infants and children. AACN Clinical Issues, 9(1), 49–63

Appendix 13.1 Suppliers of stickers and certificates

End to End Labels Ltd
Vale Road Industrial Estate
Vale Road
Spilsby
Lincolnshire
PE23 5HE
Tel: 01790 753473
Fax: 01790 752979
http://www.endtoendlabels.co.uk/
A range of stickers that can also be customised with individual
printing requests.

The Sticker Factory
The Granary
Walnut Tree Lane
Sudbury
Suffolk CO10 1BD
Tel: 01787 370950
Fax: 01787 371890
http://home.btconnect.com/sticker_factory/system/index.html
A range of stickers that can also be customised with individual
printing requests.

Chapter 14

Investigations

Chapter contents

Procedure guidelines

General introduction

This chapter aims to introduce the nurse to the range of investigations and associated nursing practice and clinical care associated with child health care.

Introduction to radiology

The aim of this section is to help nurses understand their role in preparing children for radiological investigation and assisting the radiologist to perform radiological investigations in children. Some radiology departments may have a designated radiology nurse who is experienced in all aspects of the department's work and the procedures that occur. When this facility is not available, the role will often fall on the ward nurse who accompanies the child to the radiology department. It is often the case that the most optimal imaging is achieved when the nurse caring for the child remains with them to support them, facilitate holding, provide advice on the child's condition, and build on previously established nurse-patient or parent/carer rapport. The role of the accompanying nurse therefore will be to support the child and the family, act as the patient's advocate and assist with the preparation of the child and carer based on a thorough assessment of the child and knowledge of the examination required. The nurse may also be involved in the preparation of equipment prior to the examination and assist the radiographer in ensuring that the child remains in the correct position. Any test can make a child or parent/carer apprehensive so reassurance that most tests are not painful, or uncomfortable is critical to avoid difficult or lengthy procedures due to an uncooperative or frightened child. It is important to avoid negative suggestions to the child such as 'barium doesn't taste nice' but rather 'you will need to drink a plain drink that we can add your favourite flavour to if you like'. Parents/carers may also inadvertently give their child negative messages without realising they are making it harder for their child. It is therefore important that the ward nurse has the knowledge to support the family through these commonly performed procedures.

If the child is an inpatient the preparation using toys to demonstrate the test can help, or parents/carers can be encouraged to do this at home prior to admission. The radiology department should have a room that is decorated in a suitable way for children, with toys to distract the child before and during the test. The X-ray room is a controlled environment where children can feel they have no say or choice about whether the procedure is performed (Fegley 1988). It may be helpful for the child to take a favourite toy or storybook with them to the X-ray department and to have small rewards available, such as stickers or certificates, to help to make it a positive experience and make it easier for any subsequent visits.

The X-ray room should be warm to avoid cooling of the child. Some clothing can be left in place, depending on the type of X-ray examination, and the nurse should check with the radiographer what is allowed. It is more common to remove any clothes with metal poppers or zippers beforehand.

The stability of the child's condition must be assessed before considering a move to the radiography department. The use of portable X-ray machines within intensive care units is well established. Children whose access to the department is difficult or

Table 14.1 Summary of radiology department tests

Radiology tests	Imaging material	Example
Plain X-rays	X-ray	Chest, knee, etc.
Fluoroscopy	X-ray	Barium, upper gastro-intestinal (GI) series, intravenous urography (IVU)
Ultrasound	Sound waves	Chest, abdomen
Computerised tomography	X-rays and computer	Brain
Nuclear medicine	Radionucleides (injection of radioisotope)	Renal studies
Magnetic resonance imaging	Magnetic field and computer	Chest, abdomen, brain
Interventional radiology	Ultrasound and fluoroscopy	Angiography Renal biopsy Also used for central venous line insertion

whose condition might be compromised, such as children in balanced traction or immune suppressed children being reverse barrier nursed, should also be considered for a portable X-ray machine.

Wall mounted oxygen and suction should be available in every radiology room as well as monitoring equipment. Full resuscitation equipment for all ages of children must be present within the department and trained personnel available.

Many tests in the radiology department use X-rays. X-rays use ionising radiation and in the setting of diagnostic radiology are generally very low or low dose. We are all exposed to background radiation all our lives and a child's chest X-ray is typically the equivalent of one day of background radiation, i.e. the child is one day 'older' in radiation terms which is negligible. Other tests such as computed tomography (CT) use a higher dose and are only performed after careful clinical consideration by the referring doctor and the radiologist, nevertheless the diagnostic benefit for the child usually far outweighs any potential risk from the radiation. A summary of radiology tests can be found in Table 14.1.

Factors to note:

1. The need for radiological information that can aid in clinical diagnosis or treatment must be balanced against the potential hazards of the exposure to radiation.
2. It is a legal requirement that tests involving ionising radiation can only be requested by a doctor or other specially trained person, such as a nurse practitioner (Department of Health 2000).
3. The X-ray examination is clinically directed by the radiologist or trained physicist.
4. The radiographer normally directs and is responsible for the examination.
5. All X-rays hold a potential risk.
6. It is important to remember that although the risk to the individual child is insignificant, it is a general philosophy

that the dose to the general public from medical use of ionising radiation should be reduced.

7. The net gain outweighs the risk, i.e. children undergoing frequent X-ray examinations.

8. Before any investigations are performed on any child the principles laid down in the Ionising Radiation (Medical Exposure) Regulations must be adhered to (Department of Health 2000).

9. The radiographer will ask all female patients over the age of 12 requiring X-rays of the abdomen, pelvis or spine whether they have started their periods and the date of their last

period in order to meet legal requirements (Department of Health 2000).

10. Nurses should take responsibility and act as an advocate for the child; e.g. ensure there is no possibility of pregnancy in girls of appropriate age.

11. Nurses or mothers who are pregnant should not assist with X-ray examinations in order to protect the unborn child.

12. Extensive information is available for parents/carers of children about to undergo radiological investigations on the GOSH web site (http://www.gosh.nhs.uk/gosh/clinical services/Radiology/InformationforFamilies/#H4_5662).

Principles table 14.1 Preparation of child and family

Principle	Rationale
1. The child and parents/carers should have a full explanation of why the imaging is being undertaken prior to arriving in X-ray and have been given details of the procedure, equipment and processes involved. This must include any activity expected of the child, e.g. drinking the medications, holding their breath and procedures such as cannulation or catheterisation.	1. Better understanding means it will be easier to be assured of adherence during imaging.
2. An assessment and care plan is recommended prior to complex procedures.	2. To ensure correct management of the child and minimise the effects of any pain or discomfort (Heiney 1991).
3. Books and leaflets written for children can help in explaining the type of equipment that will be used and the procedures involved. There are some very good inexpensive publications available that can be easily adapted by nursing and radiographic staff to the needs of their individual department. A photograph album with photographs of the various members of staff that the child and parents/carers will meet and the various pieces of equipment they may encounter can also be used by play specialists or nurses to prepare the family.	3. These will give a simple explanation of the process during the procedures and explain that the X-ray machines are large, can be mobile, i.e. move around the child during the procedure and may be frightening.
4. Check the name, date of birth and hospital number of the child is correct. In-patients must have a completed name band.	4. To help ensure the correct procedure is performed on the correct patient.
5. Girls who have passed the menarche should be asked in private if they might be pregnant.	5. X-rays can cause harm to an unborn foetus (Brent 1989).
6. The child should be weighed prior to the test.	6. To enable the correct doses of drugs and radiopaque dye to be given.
7. The accompanying adult should be aware that they may be required to immobilise their child by gently holding – therefore they should be both comfortable with this and not pregnant which would prevent their involvement.	7. It is very difficult to calm a child when the accompanying adult has obvious issues with holding. X-rays can cause harm to an unborn foetus.

Principles table 14.2 Care of the child undergoing a radiological investigation

Principle	Rationale
1. Privacy This is an important aspect of any procedure. All children should have their investigation in private and only people who are necessary for the investigation should remain in the X-ray room.	1. To maintain the privacy and dignity of the child and parent/carer (Casey 1995) and reduce the general exposure of individuals to radiation.
2. Protection The nurse and/or parent/carer must wear the lead covering apron and thyroid collar if assisting with an X-ray examination. Local protection for the child may be required, for example ovary pads/gonad pads. 　When X-rays are being taken on the ward using portable equipment, a safe zone should be established, ensuring that no unnecessary personnel are present in the area and that those who are required are wearing protective clothing.	2. To minimise radiation dose (Royal College of Radiologists 2008).
3. Positioning The radiographer will assist the nurse and/or parent/carer in achieving the position that is required. The radiographer may provide various adapted boxes or stools for the child to sit or lie on, to get the best exposure the first time. 　If only the mother is present, the nurse may be asked to get more involved if the mother is unwilling or pregnant and therefore unable to hold the child herself.	3. The correct positioning of the child and the maintenance of the position during the X-ray examination is one of the most important aspects of the care (http://www.enotes.com/nursing-encyclopedia/body-positioning-x-ray-studies). The difficulty in positioning is greater with a child under the age of 5 years (Gyll 1982) but it does become easier as the child gets older.
4. Restraint It is the nurse's role to ensure that the child is not restrained unecessarily or for any great length of time and that appropriate explanation and reassurance is given.	4. To comply with national restraint guidelines (Royal College of Nursing 2008).
5. Special Needs In the case of a child who is wheelchair-bound or physically disabled it is advisable to ask the child's usual carer how to move the child. It may not be possible to obtain particular X-rays on some physically handicapped children, because of their inability to move or maintain a particular position. The nurse should remember that they are the child's advocate on these occasions.	5. To avoid harm to the child, parent/carer or nurse. To comply with local lifting and handling policies.
6. Praise and reward At the end of any X-ray examination the child must be praised for their cooperation and, if appropriate, a bravery certificate or sticker awarded.	6. To provide positive feedback and reassurance to the child and parent/carer.

Principles table 14.3 Sedation and general anaesthetics

Principle	Rationale
1. It may be necessary to administer sedation or general anaesthetic (GA) to complete the required examination (NICE 2010).	**1.** The need for the child being examined to remain still and cooperate is paramount to obtaining accurate diagnostic images. As technology improves and advances, the need to keep children absolutely still during some X-ray procedures, remains the same, however the time necessary for them to remain still decreases as newer equipment completes the examination in a much shorter time.
2. Local sedation and GA policies regarding fasting, preparation and monitoring must be adhered to.	**2.** To maintain patient safety.
3. Invasive procedures require an appropriately trained nurse to remain with the child.	**3.** Any deterioration or distress may require prompt intervention.
4. In very young babies, i.e. those less than 6 weeks old, it is often worth feeding before any sedation is considered.	**4.** By feeding the baby their normal feed, wrapping them well and allowing them to fall asleep, the need for sedation may be avoided.
5. The doctor or nurse prescriber must prescribe the sedation. The type and method of administration should be adjusted according to the estimated length of the procedure.	**5.** To comply with local policy.
6. If children are attending as outpatients, sedation must be administered before they enter the examination room. If the radiology department does not have day stay facilities a day bed must be pre-arranged within the hospital.	**6.** To enable the child to fall asleep in a suitable and comfortable environment. To allow for full recovery in a safe environment.
7. Children who have been given sedation should arrive in the department already asleep or drowsy. Monitoring of these children is the responsibility of the nurse present. A set of observations should be taken, including colour, pulse, respiration and pre-sedation oxygen saturation. During the investigation the child must be constantly monitored for colour, O_2 saturation, pulse and respiration.	**7.** To maintain patient safety.
8. Appropriate resuscitation personnel and equipment must be available.	**8.** To maintain patient safety.
9. The child should be returned to the ward/day care area after the investigation with a full set of observations, and a complete handover should be given to the ward staff.	**9.** To maintain continuity of care.
10. Some units have developed nurse-led sedation programmes which are finely tuned to meet the sedation requirements of their particular unit. Great care must be exercised in adhering to the sedation policy of these units.	**10.** To ensure patient safety and to enable procedures to be carried out in an effective and timely manner.
11. A child who has an airway problem, raised intracranial pressure, is critically sick or has difficult behavioural problems must receive a general anaesthetic. General anaesthesia will be administered by an anaesthetist who will be responsible for all patient monitoring during and immediately after the procedure. Appropriate resuscitation personnel and equipment must be available.	**11.** To ensure patient safety.

329

(Continued)

Principles table 14.3 (Continued)

Principle	Rationale
12. Preparation of the child for anaesthetic should follow recommended guidelines, including fasting (see Chapter 23).	**12.** To maintain patient safety.
13. The ward nurse should accompany the child with the parents/carers into the anaesthetic area and check the child's name, hospital number and date of birth with the anaesthetic nurse. A consent form should also have been signed by the parents or carers prior to the investigation.	**13.** To ensure safe practice and to comply with local policies.
14. In most anaesthetic areas one parent/carer is usually allowed to stay with the child until they are asleep. Once the child is asleep the parent/carer and ward nurse should leave the anaesthetic area unless the ward nurse is required to assist with the investigation.	**14.** To enable the parent/carer to remain with their child to support and comfort them.
15. Following the procedure and extubation, the nurse must stay with the child until they are able to maintain their own airway and are rousable by speech.	**15.** To maintain patient safety.
16. New approaches to sedation and in fact approaches to minimising sedation are constantly been tried and evaluated, it will be important to keep up to date with new approaches (Parker *et al* 1997, Scott *et al* 2002).	**16.** To ensure the latest and safest approaches are in use.

General radiology

General radiography (X-rays) is the most commonly used of all the imaging modalities in any hospital. This is due to the fact that a patient (child or adult) will very often have a plain X-ray before moving on if necessary to other specialist modality. General X-rays can be used to look at anatomy, either bone or soft tissue in any part of the body. It uses ionising radiation generated by an X-ray tube to gain the most appropriate view of the affected area (e.g. knee, ankle, abdomen, chest). They are non-invasive and should not give any discomfort to the child. There is no preparation for a plain X-ray except sufficient explanation. Most plain X-ray examinations are for one or two images only, however lengthy examinations such as skeletal surveys (up to 15 images of different bones in the body) are also undertaken. These are done for a variety of bony abnormalities, but also for suspected non-accidental injury (NAI). The nurse looking after the child must always ensure that the child and the family have a full explanation of the process of what is going to be done before they arrive in the X-ray room. It is the responsibility of the radiographer to always get the best image possible, using the lowest dose of radiation.

Fluoroscopy

Modern fluoroscopy (also termed screening) uses pulsed X-rays to create a real time moving X-ray image, which can be viewed on a monitor beside the operator (usually a radiologist but sometimes a radiographer). It differs from a standard X-ray in that it gives dynamic information and if contrast is given, such as barium or a water-soluble contrast medium, this can be viewed within the patient such as in a barium swallow. The patient lies on the X-ray couch in the beam of the X-ray tube and images are acquired on an image intensifier on the other side of the patient.

As with other sources of ionising radiation the child, operators and carers need to be protected from X-rays during the procedure by wearing lead coats. The most common tests are described below.

Principles table 14.4 Fluoroscopy care

Principle	Rationale
1. The patient must not be pregnant (unless there are very extenuating circumstances and the radiologist is aware of these in advance).	1. X-rays may cause harm to an unborn foetus (DoH 2000).
2. Accompanying carers must not be pregnant if they are to be present in the room during the examination.	2. X-rays may cause harm to an unborn foetus (DoH 2000).
3. Only qualified operators may use the fluoroscopy machine at any time, under any circumstances.	3. This is a legal requirement (DoH 2000).
4. Only essential people should be present in the fluoroscopy room during the examination.	4. To reduce the general exposure of individuals to radiation (DoH 2000).
5. The radiologist or the radiographer will give instructions regarding radiation safety as appropriate.	5. These are trained personnel and there is a legal obligation to follow their instructions (DoH 2000).
6. Female patients over 12 years will be asked if they have started menstruating and if so if there is any chance they could be pregnant. A department policy and notices explaining that everyone will be asked helps make this less personal.	6. This is a legal requirement (DoH 2000) and while a potentially embarrassing and/or offensive question it needs to be asked, done in privacy with sensitivity this should reduce any problems.
7. High dose procedures (such as pelvic angiography) are only performed in the first 10 days after a period in female patients who have reached the menarche.	7. This is the '10 day rule' based on the assumption that ovulation and conception are unlikely to have occurred by Day 10 of a menstrual cycle and therefore there is no chance of the patient being unknowingly pregnant (Bury et al 1995).
8. Medium and low dose procedures are only performed in the first 28 days after a period in female patients who have reached the menarche unless pregnancy can be absolutely excluded in which case the procedure may take place at any time. If the patient knows she is pregnant the examination is usually deferred unless there is a pressing medical indication.	8. This is the '28 day rule' based on the assumption that pregnancy is unlikely and even if conception has occurred there is little if any risk to the foetus (Bury et al 1995).

Intravenous urography

An intravenous urography (IVU) is a test to examine the urinary tract (kidneys, ureters and bladder). The most common indication in children is to delineate pelvicalyceal anatomy, particularly in the context of renal calculi. On arriving in the department some local anaesthetic cream is applied at various sites suitable for a cannula. When this has had time to take effect the carer and the child will enter the examination room and the child will need to lie on the X-ray couch. An X-ray of the abdomen will be taken and an injection of contrast medium (a clear iodine based solution that is filtered and excreted by the kidneys and is radio-opaque) is given intravenously and a series of X-rays of the abdomen are taken at intervals. On most modern systems the child and carer will be able to see the images on the TV monitor. Most patients get a warm sensation with the injection and sometimes feel that they need to void.

The test usually takes about 20–30 minutes, but sometimes delayed pictures may be necessary, up to several hours later in certain circumstances.

Principles table 14.5 Intravenous urography care

Principle	Rationale
1. A history of allergies must be sought and the radiology staff be made aware of any allergies.	**1.** Allergic reaction to contrast medium is rare (1%) but may very rarely progress to anaphylactic shock (<0.05%) and may be fatal.
2. A previous anaphylactic reaction to contrast media is a contraindication.	**2. Risk of fatal anaphylaxis.**
3. The weight of the child must be known and recorded.	**3.** The volume of contrast medium given is dependent on the weight of the child.
4. The child must be well hydrated.	**4.** Dehydration increases the risk of nephrotoxicity from the contrast medium.
5. Local anaesthetic cream should be applied to at least four likely cannulation sites at least 30 minutes before the procedure (dorsum of hands and feet in children under 2 and additionally to the antecubital fossae in children over 2).	**5.** To reduce the pain of cannula placement. Hands and feet are most easily cannulated in younger children.
6. The child should have a cannula placed in advance, in the ward or day care setting.	**6.** Placing a cannula in advance reduces the stress for the child at the time of the examination. If children cry during cannula placement the swallowed air in the stomach and small bowel degrades the image.
7. Resuscitation equipment and anaphylaxis management guidelines must be available.	**7.** To treat an anaphylactic reaction to contrast medium (Tramer *et al* 2006).
8. The older child should be fasted for 3 hours. Children who are still breast/bottle fed should be fasted for an hour.	**8.** To reduce gas and stomach contents degrading the image (Royal College of Radiologists 2003).
9. The child should be changed into a hospital gown.	**9.** To avoid radio-opaque artefacts (buttons, zips, glittery motifs, etc) degrading the image.
10. The child should empty their bladder before the test.	**10.** To reduce the need for the child to get up from the table during the study.
11. The child should be reassured during the test.	**11.** To keep the child calm and thereby optimise the images.
12. There is no special aftercare.	**12.** The contrast medium is excreted in the urine and is usually completely cleared by 6 hours. The child can eat and drink directly after the test.

332

Micturating cystourethrogram

A micturating cystourethrogram (MCU) examines the bladder and urethra and may give information about the ureters and upper urinary tract if there is reflux of contrast. A catheter is passed into the bladder (usually via the urethra, although a suprapubic catheter can be used if it is already in place) and radio-opaque water soluble contrast is instilled. Images of the bladder are taken and images of the urethra are acquired when the child micturates. The most common indications for an MCU include looking for anatomical abnormalities of the lower urinary tract (such as posterior urethral valves in boys) and to look for ureteric reflux if other abnormalities have already been demonstrated on ultrasound. Current thinking is that it is not routinely indicated in the investigation of urinary tract infection or antenatal hydronephrosis. In female infants where detail of urethral anatomy is not required the direct isotope cystogram (DIC) provides information on reflux with a much lower radiation exposure. Once children are potty trained an alternative test, the indirect radionucleotide cystogram (IRC), may be used to assess reflux without the need for catheterisation and is therefore the preferred test in children over 3 years.

Principles table 14.6 Micturating cystourethrogram care

Principle	Rationale
1. If the child is already on antibiotics these should be continued and the dose doubled for five days starting from the day of the test. If the child is not on antibiotics these should be prescribed at the time of the study according to local protocol.	1. Despite using a sterile technique there is a possibility of introducing bacteria into the urinary tract during catheterisation. Antibiotics are increased/prescribed for prophylaxis (Coptcoat et al 1988).
2. The infant will need to change/be changed into a hospital gown and will need to have the nappy removed. Older children may prefer to keep their own T-shirts on. Parents/carers may like to bring a spare. Babygrows with poppers will need to be removed.	2. To allow access for catheterisation using a sterile technique. To avoid radio-opaque artefacts.
3. A sterile technique will be used by the radiologist, nurse or radiographer.	3. To reduce the risk of infection.
4. The infants and parents/carers arms and hands must be kept out of the sterile field.	4. To reduce the risk of infection.
5. The child will need to be turned on each side in turn with the help of the carers.	5. To obtain oblique images to assess the lower ureters and urethra which would otherwise be obscured by the contrast filled bladder.

333

Dysphagia swallow using videofluoroscopy

Dysphagia swallow with videofluoroscopy is used to assess swallowing safety and coordination and is usually performed by the radiologist or radiographer in conjunction with the speech therapist. The child is usually seated (or placed in a specially formed seat like a car seat) and a variety of consistencies from fluids through to solids mixed with barium are offered to the child. Swallowing is then observed with fluoroscopy and simultaneously recorded on videotape or DVD. The test usually takes 15 minutes.

Principles table 14.7 Dysphagia swallow using videofluoroscopy care

Principle	Rationale
1. The child must be fasted for at least 2 hours.	1. The children need to be hungry/thirsty so they will accept the range of consistencies offered.
2. Suction equipment must be available.	2. There is a risk of aspiration during the procedure.
3. The parents/carers should bring some food that they would normally feed the child and that the child likes.	3. Barium can be mixed with any liquid or foodstuff to make it radio-opaque. There is more chance of the child accepting what is offered if it is familiar.

Upper gastrointestinal series

An upper gastointestinal series (UGI) (which covers the older terms of barium/contrast swallow, barium/contrast meal) examines from the pharynx to the first loop of jejunum. Barium (or water soluble contrast medium) is given orally and observed as it transits the upper gastrointestinal (GI) tract. Several images will be acquired by the radiologist with the child in various positions on the table. It is usually performed supine in children (but erect in adults). The most common indications in children include looking for structural anatomical abnormalities such as malrotation and to observre gastro-oesophageal reflux. The examination takes approximately 15 minutes.

Principles table 14.8 Upper gastrointestinal series care

Principle	Rationale
1. The child must be fasted for 3 hours before the examination, babies who are still breast/bottle fed should be fasted for 1 hour.	1. To avoid stomach contents and bowel gas degrading the images and to ensure the child is hungry and thirsty so they will take the barium.
2. A history regarding allergies is not required.	2. Barium sulphate is an inert compound.
3. The child will need to change/be changed into a hospital gown but may keep their underwear on. Older children may prefer to keep their own T-shirts on. Parents/carers may like to bring a spare. Babygrows with poppers will need to be removed.	3. To protect the child's own clothing against spillage of barium and to reduce radio-opaque artefacts which degrade the image.
4. Ask the child if they have a favourite flavour of milkshake.	4. The barium solution can be flavoured with milk shake powders to make the taste more familiar.
5. Use a drinking vessel that is age appropriate and the child is used to, e.g. feeding bottle, beaker or cup and straw	5. Familiarity will help encourage the child to drink the barium.
5. The child should be reassured during the test.	5. To keep the child calm and thereby optimise the images.
6. The child should receive good hydration after the test.	6. Barium sulphate may be constipating in some children.
7. Inform the parents/carer that barium may be visible in the stools for up to 3 days.	7. Barium is inert and is excreted unchanged.

Tube oesophagram

A tube oesophogram examines the oesophagus in cases of possible tracheo-oesophageal fistula (for all other oesophageal studies an upper GI series is performed). The child is placed prone and water soluble contrast is injected into the oesophagus via a nasogastric tube placed with its tip in the mid oesophagus. Lateral images are acquired. If a fistula is present contrast will be seen to leak through from the oesophagus into the trachea. The test takes approximately 20 minutes, or 30 mintues if a nasogastric tube is not already in place.

Principles table 14.8 Tube oesophagram care

Principle	Rationale
1. The child should be starved for at least 2 hours before the procedure.	1. To reduce the risk of the child vomiting or refluxing.
2. A nasogastric tube can be passed in advance on the ward if the child is an inpatient.	2. A tube must be passed for the test. It is often less stressful for the child if this is positioned before arriving in the X-ray department and will reduce the time the child has to be on the X-ray table.
3. Suction equipment must be available.	3. If a fistula is present the child will aspirate and may need urgent airway suction.
4. The child must be positioned prone.	4. The contrast can then flow with gravity through the fistula from the posterior oesophagus to the more anterior trachea.
5. The X-ray tube must be positioned laterally.	5. To show the fistula in profile.

Barium follow through

A barium follow through examines the gut from the pharynx to the caecum. Its main purpose is to examine the small intestine as this cannot be reached by endoscopy. Like an upper GI series barium, it is usually given orally but may be given by nasogastric, nasojejunal or gastrostomy tube. A series of images will be acquired at intervals during the study. The child does not have to stay in the X-ray room all the time but will be brought in intermittently to monitor the progress of the barium. The most common indication is to look for mucosal abnormalities or strictures. The test usually takes between 45 minutes and 3 hours depending on how long the barium takes to transit the small bowel.

See the principles table for upper gastrointestinal series care for barium follow through care.

Barium enema

A barium enema is used to examine the large bowel from the rectum to the caecum. The most common indication in children is in unexplained chronic constipation or following surgery. The child will need to lie on the couch and will then be asked to turn on their side while the radiologist passes a thin soft plastic catheter a few centimetres into the rectum (older children may prefer their parents/carer to wait outside while this is done). The catheter is taped in place and barium solution is run through the catheter and around the large bowel. Barium is a thick, white liquid that is radio-opaque and gives images of the structure and mucosal surface of the large bowel. The radiologist follows its progress under screening until it reaches the appendix. This may involve turning the child onto their side, back and so on. The radiologist will take a limited series of X-ray images. The child and carer will usually be able to see the images on the TV monitor. The test normally takes about 30 minutes. After the test older children will want to go to the toilet straightaway. Babies and infants will pass the barium on the couch or into their nappies in the next few hours. In all children barium may be visible in the bowel motions for up to three days (see http://www.patient.co.uk/showdoc/40000225/ for example).

Principles table 14.9 Barium enema care

Principle	Rationale
1. The child must avoid foods with a high fibre content the day before the examination.	1. Optimal images are acquired with an empty bowel.
2. The child must be fasted for 3 hours before the examination, but they may still take clear fluids up to 1 hour before the test.	2. To avoid stomach contents and bowel gas degrading the images.
3. A history regarding allergies is not required.	3. Barium sulphate is an inert compound.
4. The child should be reassured during the test.	4. To keep the child calm and thereby optimise the images.
5. The child should receive good hydration after the test.	5. Barium sulphate may be constipating in some children.
6. Inform parents/carer that barium may be visible in the stools for up to 3 days.	6. Barium is inert and is excreted unchanged.

Contrast enema (and Gastrografin enema)

A contrast enema is used to examine the lower GI tract from the anus to the terminal ileum in cases where barium is inappropriate. It is most commonly used in neonates, pre-term infants, if there is a possibility of perforation or obstruction, or if the child is expected to undergo an operation in the 48 hours following the procedure. A contrast enema does not give mucosal information but gives information about the patency of the large bowel. A Gastrografin (a hyperosmolar contrast agent) enema is used in the treatment of meconium ileus. This procedure usually takes approximately 15 minutes. There is no specific preparation required.

In some sick children, the risks involved in contrast enemas are high and include perforation of the gut and respiratory distress in a child who is obstructed. The procedures should therefore not be undertaken lightly and must be under the direct supervision of a radiologist following a request from a surgical colleague. Oxygen, suction and full resuscitation equipment must be available and should include replacement fluids to counteract hypovolaemia should perforation of the gut occur.

Principles table 14.10 **Contrast enema care**

Principle	Rationale
1. No bowel preparation is needed.	1. This procedure is only performed in children who are very young and would not tolerate bowel preparation or in children whose condition implies the distal gut is likely to be collapsed and in whom no fine detail is required.
2. As child is undressed and often very small, the use of a warm air blanket and bubble wrap to cover the child should be considered.	2. Very small babies lose body heat very quickly and need to be kept warm during the procedure.
3. Water soluble contrast is used (not barium).	3. Water soluble contrast is less irritating if spilt into the peritoneum (in perforation or at surgery) and in cases of sub-total obstruction will not cause complete obstruction (http://www.patient.co.uk/doctor/Barium-Enema-Examination.htm).
4. If meconium ileus is diagnosed diluted Gastrografin (50:50) is used.	4. Gastrografin is hyperosmolar and therefore draws fluid into the lumen of the gut helping to loosen the sticky meconium and allowing it to be passed per rectum, thereby relieving the obstruction.
5. The child must be well hydrated. Some departments require venous access to be established if Gastrografin is to be given.	5. Non-isotonic contrast agents, especially Gastrografin, draw fluid into the gut and in pre-terms and neonates these fluid shifts can result in marked hypovolaemia.
6. Care should be taken when changing the infant's nappy after the procedure.	6. Most water soluble contrast agents are sticky and any passed per rectum after the procedure may cause the nappy to stick to the skin. Warm water should be used for cleaning.

Air enema

An air enema is performed to reduce an ileo-caecal intussusception. The diagnosis of intussusception is usually made by ultrasound and an air enema is only performed once the diagnosis has been made. A catheter is placed in the rectum and air is introduced at a continuous pressure under fluoroscopic guidance to push back (reduce) the intussuscepted bowel. Several attempts may be made at varying pressures until the intussusception is reduced or the procedure is abandoned. This procedure may take up to 30 minutes. The main complication is perforation of the bowel. Absolute contraindications are if a perforation is already present or if the child is not adequately fluid resuscitated before the procedure. Relative contraindications are a history of more than 48 hours, children less than 6 months or more than 3years, and an absence of blood flow on Doppler imaging on ultrasound: in which cases the clinical decision to proceed is made jointly by the surgeon and radiologist.

Principles table 14.11 **Air enema care**

Principle	Rationale
1. The child must have intravenous access.	1. To allow rapid resuscitation if there is a complication or if the child proceeds directly to the operating theatre.
2. The child must be adequately fluid resuscitated with intravenous fluid before the procedure.	2. To reduce the risk of complication from hypovolaemia.
3. The child must have been assessed by the surgeon.	3. The decision to perform an air enema is taken jointly by the radiologist and surgeon.

Principles table 14.11 (*Continued*)

Principle	Rationale
4. The parents/carers must be made aware of the risk of perforation of the bowel.	**4.** The risk of perforation is approximately 1:50 to 1:100. The bowel is oedematous and may be ischaemic or gangrenous and is at increased risk of perforation. The air enema may demonstrate a perforation that has already occurred or cause a perforation, which would then require surgery.
5. The use of sedation and/or analgesia is according to local practice.	**5.** Some centres use sedation but this may make it difficult to assess the clinical state of the child.

Tracheobronchography

Tracheobronchography, often called bronchography, is a technique used for imaging the airway. It is a simple and safe procedure, which is quick to perform. This examination is performed in the X-ray department because high-quality imaging is required for accurate diagnosis of airway abnormalities. The patient is either ventilated or given a general anaesthetic for the procedure. A contrast medium is introduced into the airway via a feeding tube or catheter and X-ray pictures are taken to demonstrate the trachea and main bronchi. The main abnormalities that can be identified with bronchography are a narrowing, or stenosis, of the airway and tracheobronchomalacia. Children who have tracheobronchomalacia have a softening of the cartilaginous rings and plates of the trachea and bronchi. This causes the airway to collapse leading to near death episodes or result in the child being unable to be weaned from the ventilator.

Stenosis of the airway can be caused by intralumenal abnormalities such as complete tracheal rings or by extralumenal (extrinsic compression) caused by congenital heart disease. Bronchography is an essential tool for assessing patients post surgical repair of their airway and is used for guidance for balloon dilatation and stent insertion.

Principles table 14.12 **Tracheobronchography care**

Principle	Rationale
1. A radiology request form must be completed.	**1.** Legal document required for any radiographic procedure.
2. Consent must be gained before the procedure.	**2.** Ensure the child and parents/carers receive appropriate information and are aware of the risks and benefits of the procedure.
3. Children who require a general anaesthetic must be fasted correctly according to hospital policy.	**3.** To minimise the risk of aspiration during general anaesthetic.
4. Continuous infusions of long acting muscle relaxants in ventilated patients should be discontinued.	**4.** Spontaneous breathing will need to be observed during the procedure.
5. There is no other specific preparation for children who are already ventilated.	**5.** This is not a painful or difficult procedure, or one that is likely to cause bleeding.
6. Ventilated patients are accompanied to the radiology department by an intensivist or anaesthetist.	**6.** To maintain the airway in transit to and from radiology and during the procedure.
7. Patients are either ventilated from intensive care units or given a general anaesthetic in the interventional radiology suite.	**7.** Patients are required to keep still for the procedure.

(Continued)

337

Principles table 14.12 (*Continued*)

Principle	Rationale
8. Patients will have either an endotracheal tube or a tracheostomy tube in place.	8. The endotracheal tube or tracheostomy tube allows easy access for the catheter or feeding tube used for the procedure as well as providing artificial ventilation if required.
9. Although intubated the child is required to be breathing spontaneously.	9. When assessing a child for tracheobronchomalacia the child must be breathing spontaneously to be able to visualise the collapse of the airway and assess its severity.
10. The child is placed supine on the X-ray table with their arms supported above their head.	10. Bi-plane imaging is used. The arms are positioned above their head to prevent the humerus over lying the trachea in the lateral projection.
11. A small feeding tube or catheter is passed into the trachea through a small valve in the ventilatory circuit. A radiopaque, isotonic contrast medium is injected in aliquots of 0.2 ml under fluoroscopic (X-ray) guidance.	11. The small feeding tubes or catheter provides a mean for injecting the contrast media into the airway. These are very small and therefore do not cause airway obstruction during the procedure. They are soft and do not damage the wall of the airway.
12. For tracheobronchomalacia, rapid sequences of images are taken at various levels of positive end expiratory pressure (PEEP) with the child breathing spontaneously.	12. The severity of the airway malacia is assessed by changing the level of PEEP within the ventilatory circuit. The higher the PEEP required to hold open the airway the more severe the malacia. This can provide essential information for the intensivists so that they can maintain a patent airway while the child is on a ventilator.
13. During the procedure oxygen saturations, respiratory rate, heart rate and blood pressure are monitored.	13. These children are often unstable so require close monitoring. The contrast medium injected into the airway and the changing levels of PEEP can cause oxygen desaturation.

Linogram

A linogram involves injecting intravenous contrast through a venous access line under fluoroscopy to check its position and integrity. Most commonly this is performed if there have been problems with injecting through the line or on drawing back. The test takes 15 minutes.

Principles table 14.13 Linogram care

Principle	Rationale
1. There is no preparation for this test.	1. Only images of the opacified line are required.
2. The test is performed under sterile conditions.	2. To reduce the risk of infection of the line.
3. The test is contraindicated if there has been a previous anaphylactic reaction to intravenous contrast media.	3. To avoid a further anaphylactic reaction.

Ultrasound

Ultrasound is an excellent imaging modality to examine parts of the body comprising soft tissue (e.g. liver, kidney, thyroid, testes, breast or musculoskeltal structures) or fluid containing structures such as the bladder, gall bladder or vessels. It is less useful in examining structures that contain gas such as the bowel. Ultrasound uses sound waves that are of too high a frequency to be heard by the human ear. A tranducer (probe) is used to both send and receive the returning ultrasound signal and this is then converted to an image on the screen. The child cannot feel the ultrasound waves and therefore this examination causes no discomfort to the child. Ultrasound jelly is used to ensure good contact between the probe and the child's skin, which may tickle the child a little. For many ultrasound examinations no preparation is necessary. The mother is often able to give the child a good explanation, as the procedure is similar to a pregnancy scan. However, examination of the bladder and/or pelvis requires that the bladder is full and examination of the biliary tree (as part of an abdominal scan) requires that the child is fasted. After the scan the gel is wiped off and the child is free to go.

Principles table 14.14 Ultrasound care

Principle	Rationale
1. For examination of the brain (in neonates), testes, thyroid, thymus, musculoskeletal soft tissues, breast, vascular system and heart (echocardiography) no preparation is needed.	1. These structures are easily examined and are unaffected by external factors.
2. For examination of the pelvis the child must have a full bladder and should therefore drink water before the scan.	2. A full bladder pushes loops of small bowel out of the pelvis and allows a 'transonic window' through the bladder for the examination.
3. For examination of the bladder the bladder must be full and the child should therefore drink water before the scan.	3. The bladder cannot be examined if it is not distended.
4. For examination of the biliary tree (as part of an abdominal scan) the child must be fasted.	4. The gall bladder needs to be distended to be examined. If the child is not fasted the gall bladder will be contracted in response to any fatty food or drink, including milk.

Computed tomography

The computed tomography scan, commonly known by its abbreviated name CT scan, has become a very important tool in diagnostic medicine. It is an X-ray procedure that combines many X-ray images with the aid of a computer to generate cross-sectional images and if needed, three-dimensional images of the internal structures of the body. CT scan is used to define normal and abnormal structures in the body and/or to assist in procedures by helping to guide the placement of instruments, as in biopsies. Compared with conventional radiography the images produced show superior tissue contrast definition and superimposed structures on the image are eliminated.

The scanner consists of a large doughnut shaped gantry within which lies an X-ray tube and special detectors that measure the non-absorbed X-rays passing through a given part of the anatomy. These detectors gather the information for reconstruction of the image by basically converting the X-rays into electrical pulses. The pulses are fed into a computer for processing and then a cross-sectional image or 'slice' is displayed on a television monitor.

Depending on the clinical indications for doing a scan and which body part is being examined a contrast material (an X-ray dye) may be used either orally or intravenously for highlighting certain structures. CT is a low-risk procedure, the most common problem being an adverse reaction to intravenous contrast media, which is iodine based. Care should be taken with children who have a positive history of allergy, asthma or untoward reactions to iodinated contrast media. Premedication with corticosteroids or histamine H1 and H2 antagonists might be considered in these cases (Singh and Daftary, 2008).

The analogy often used for understanding CT is that you imagine the body as a loaf of bread and each image or slice is like removing a slice and looking at it from underneath. While the scan is in progress the child needs to be very still as the scanner takes very fine slices through the body. Young or uncooperative children may need to be sedated or have a general anaesthetic if it is available. Alternatively if the patient is under 3 months of age a feed is usually adequate to settle them. Metal objects although not harmful to the child do cause artefacts on the images, therefore any jewellery, or clothes with metal fastenings need to be removed prior to the scan.

Principles table 14.15 Computed tomography care

Principle	Rationale
1. Assess whether the child will need sedation or anesthetic for the scan.	**1.** To ensure the child keeps still for the scan.
2. If sedation is to be used ensure there are no contra-indications to sedation.	**2.** Children should not be sedated if they have a condition that is contra-indicated in local policy.
3. In females of reproductive age check date of last menstrual period.	**3.** To ensure there is no risk of pregnancy (Department of Health 2000).
4. Remove any metal objects, jewellery or metal fastenings on clothes.	**4.** To ensure no artefacts on images.
5. Children requiring sedation or general anaesthetic should be fasted according to local policy.	**5.** To reduce risk of aspiration (RCN 2005).
6. For children needing oral contrast ensure that it is given to the child when advised to do so by the CT scan staff.	**6.** To ensure adequate opacification of the bowel.
7. If the child has a history of previous allergic reaction to iodinated contrast they may require steroid cover.	**7.** To prevent anaphylaxis.

Nuclear Medicine

Nuclear Medicine is part of the Radiology Department, so when reporting for an examination all patients should report to the main X-ray reception. Virtually every Nuclear Medicine examination involves the child having a radioisotope injection through either a butterfly needle or a requested cannula, which has been inserted on the ward. Central intravenous lines cannot be used as the injection (isotope) can become stuck to the inside of the lines.

Every radioisotope injection is patient specific, and is bought on the day of the examination (e.g. MIBG is imported from Belgium). Each isotope is calculated for a child's weight, examination and, most importantly, appointment time. As such each dose is ordered the day before and any cancellation after doses have been ordered incurs penalty charges for the referring clinician.

Nuclear Medicine is based on the principle that a radioisotope is an unstable substance that gives off energy (gamma radiation) as it decays into a stable compound. We are able to 'label' certain isotopes, e.g. technetium, allowing it to be specifically directed at one type of organ or cell type. After the injection the gamma camera detects the gamma rays being emitted from the isotope within the child. The amount of radiation used for these diagnostic tests are very small and there are no side effects. The 'decaying' process means that the energy of the isotope is constantly decreasing. If a child is late for their appointment their isotope may have decayed beyond the level required and their appointment will have to be cancelled: timing is crucial.

Procedure guideline 14.1 Nuclear Medicine care

Statement	Rationale
1. A radiology request form must be completed.	**1.** As required by law all examinations require an authorised member of medical staff to request any examination detailing the relevant clinical information (Department of Health 2000).
2. Weight and height of the child should be measured prior to the procedure.	**2.** All doses are calculated by weight.
3. Apply anaesthetic cream, to venous sites 30 mins prior to canulation.	**3.** This may reduce any pain felt from the cannula insertion.

Procedure guideline 14.1 (*Continued*)

Statement	Rationale
4. Children for renal studies need to be well hydrated before the scan. For MIBG, White Cell, milk, Gallium and Somatostatin studies, please contact the department for the appropriate preparation.	**4.** To ensure children receive the correct preparation.
5. Some examinations require specific preparation such as fasting. Appointment letters should explain this to parents/carers. Wards should be informed by a member of Nuclear Medicine staff the day before any appointment to confirm requirements for the study to go ahead. Children who require sedation or a general anaesthetic must be fasted correctly according to hospital policy.	**5.** Without the required fasting period no sedation or general anaesthetic can be administered.
6. For all studies it is imperative that children are kept as still as possible for imaging to occur.	**6.** Any movement of the child 'blurs' the image being taken at that time. Some images may take up to 10 minutes to complete for one picture.
7. Books, toys, tapes and videos should be available to distract and entertain the child. They should be encouraged to bring any favourite book or toy with them.	**7.** To help the child to remain still.
8. Some children do require additional help to obtain diagnostic images, e.g. sedation. Extra time is allowed for these examinations as sedation does require patience on all sides to be a complete success. If prior warning is not given to Nuclear Medicine staff then the appointment may have to be cancelled.	**8.** Children may not be able to lie still for long enough.
9. Sedation or a general anaesthetic can be considered for children undergoing these investigations but this must be communicated with the Nuclear Medicine staff in advance according to local policy.	**9.** To maintain child safety.
10. There are no side effects from these scans and the child can eat normally afterwards, unless otherwise directed by staff.	**10.** Be aware of any particular directions for individual children.
11. In most instances the isotope is excreted out of the body in the urinary system over the following 24 hours, so the following precautions must be followed: a) The child should drink more unless being fasted for sedation in which case IV fluid should be administered. b) The child should empty their bladder/have nappies changed, more frequently. c) Staff should wash hands thoroughly after changing nappies/going to the toilet. d) Give the toilet a double flush. e) Dispose of nappies according to local policy. f) Avoid contact with pregnant women.	**11.** The isotope is excreted by normal biological means. a) To ensure safe disposal of radioactive isotopes.
12. The above are routine precautions, which should be followed with all children having undergone a Nuclear Medicine examination. Any specific instructions should by given by Nuclear Medicine staff at the time of the appointment.	**12.** Be aware of any particular directions for individual children.
13. If the child becomes ill following any Nuclear Medicine injection this should be treated as any other normal illness would be treated and doctors informed.	**13.** Isotopes are not likely to be the cause of any illness.

Magnetic resonance imaging

Magnetic resonance imaging (MRI) is a way of looking inside the body without using X-rays. MRI can produce two- or three-dimensional images using a very large magnet, radio waves and a computer. The magnet is large enough to surround a child, which is why it is sometimes referred to as a tunnel. The magnetic fields used are not known to be harmful, which means that children can have someone with them, as long as they keep very still so that they do not disturb the magnet and radio waves.

There is no preparation required for an MRI scan, but everyone entering the magnetic area will be checked for metallic objects, which may not be taken into the room as they can damage the magnet or the child if they become projectile. No patients with a pacemaker or aneurysm clip may enter the scan room (http://www.bupa.co.uk/individuals/health-information/directory/m/mri-scan).

Children do not have to undress as long as they are not wearing clothes with zips or other metal parts. They can come in pyjamas or ziperless jogging suits. The child has to keep very still during the scan, as one movement can spoil all the images, unlike X-rays. This is because the images are built up from information collected during the whole of the scanning time. A child who is not able to keep still for about 30 minutes may have to be sedated. The child will be asked to lie on the table, will be made as comfortable as possible and will then be moved into the scanner. It can be frightening for a young child and they may need sedation. Children over the age of 5 years may find it quite interesting. They can take a favourite toy in with them, as long as there is no metal in it. There is a significant amount of information available for parents/carers to prepare their child (see http://www.youtube.com/watch?v=p9T6m21AZ80, http://www.gosh.nhs.uk/gosh_families/information_sheets/mri_scan/mri_scan_families.html).

Once the child is in the magnet, the machine starts to make a whirring and thumping noise, which can get very loud and this continues for the whole of the scan. The child can talk to the radiographer while in the magnet and they also have a bell to press should they wish to stop. In practice, many children go to sleep and have to be woken up when the scan is finished.

Occasionally it is necessary to inject a small amount of contrast, which does not contain iodine, into the arm. Allergic reactions are therefore rare.

No special care is required following a scan, provided the child has not received sedation. For those children requiring sedation, local sedation policies should be followed. (See also computed tomography section above and NICE guidelines (2010).

Interventional radiology

Interventional radiology is a medical specialty that uses image-guided, minimally invasive diagnostic and treatment techniques that are often an alternative to surgery. Interventional radiology will assist in the diagnosis and treatment of diseases using small catheters or other devices guided by radiological imaging. Procedures performed by interventional radiologists are generally less costly and are less traumatic to the child involving smaller incisions, less pain, and shorter hospital stays. Some procedures commonly performed in the interventional radiology department are as follows.

Central venous access

At many institutions a large proportion of the work carried out within Interventional Radiology is related to central venous access as the demand for long-term central venous access has risen. These devices are increasingly used for the administration of antibiotics and chemotherapeutic drugs, for total parenteral nutrition, and for providing high-flow access for hemodialysis and plasmapheresis. Indwelling catheters also offer the ability to obtain frequent blood samples, which may be needed in some children. As some children are reliant on permanent central venous access, repeated placement of these devices in children can prove to be a challenge when traditional venous access sites are used repeatedly, because of the resultant stenosis or occlusion of the central vessels. Placing these lines in the interventional radiology department equipped with dedicated ultrasound and fluoroscopic machines allows the planned vascular access site to be evaluated prior to catheter placement. Ultrasonograpic investigation of the neck may demonstrate multiple small collateral vessels instead of a single large jugular vein, which usually indicates a stenosis or occlusion of the main vein. In many instances, one of the collateral veins can be accessed under direct ultrasonographic visualisation. Therefore using fluoroscopic guidance, contrast material, guidewires and catheters an interventional radiologist can usually bypass these thrombosed or stenosed vessels and access the central circulation, thereby allowing placement of a catheter via vessels that could not be used otherwise.

Venous access under ultrasonographic and fluoroscopic guidance has the added advantage of significantly decreasing the rate of immediate complications such as inadvertent arterial puncture, pneumothorax, and catheter tip malpositioning.

Central venous line (CVL) insertion

This is a procedure that involves placement of a soft infusion catheter into a centrally located vein using vascular interventional techniques. The most commonly placed lines include, PICC (peripherally inserted central catheter), Hickman lines (single and double lumens), Port-a-caths, Vas caths and Perm cath.

Depending on the type of central venous access required it can either be carried out under local or general anaesthetic. For a PICC line or femoral vas cath local anaesthetic, with or without sedation, is sufficient in the older child. However, for tunnelled catheter insertion such as a Hickman catheter®, which requires a large amount of cooperation, a general anaesthetic is strongly recommended.

Renal biopsy

Renal biopsy is undertaken to identify a specific disease process, determine the extent of kidney damage, enable early detection of transplant rejection and assess transplant failure. The kidney to be biopsied is visualised using ultrasound guidance. The intended biopsy tract is infiltrated with local anaesthetic and a thin needle is passed through the skin into the area of the kidney. Inside the needle is a sharp cutting edge that slices and removes small pieces of the kidney. In older children this procedure is successfully performed with sedation or demand-valve equimolar nitrous oxide. If the child is young or not suitable for either sedation or Entonox a general anaesthetic is recommended. As there is a small risk of post-operative bleeding it is imperative that clotting results are obtained prior to the procedure and the operator is informed if the child is currently on aspirin. Post-operative observations should also include early detection of complications such as bleeding.

Angiography

Angiography is an X-ray examination of the arteries and veins to diagnose blockages and other blood vessel problems. The most common method for carrying out this procedure is to make a small nick in the groin, the femoral artery is punctured to allow insertion of a catheter which can be guided to the blood vessels of interest and an injection of contrast or dye gives the radiologist a clear picture of any abnormal vessels. One of the most common reasons for angiograms is to see if there is a blockage or narrowing in a blood vessel that may interfere with the normal flow of blood through the body. In many cases, the interventional radiologist can treat a blocked blood vessel without surgery at the same time the angiogram is performed. Interventional radiologists treat blockages with techniques such as angioplasty (a balloon is guided to the site of narrowing and expanded to overcome narrowing, sometimes a small metal stent is inserted to aid in keeping the vessel open). Other conditions that may indicate an angiogram are arteriovenous malformations, trauma, vasculitis, renovascular hypertension and cerebral aneurysms.

The age and cooperation of the child undergoing this procedure, in conjunction with reference to local policy should be made as to whether this procedure requires a general anaesthetic or sedation. Post-operatively, bed rest is encouraged for at least 6 hours or according to local policy to minimise risk of bleeding from puncture site. The circulation should also be assessed during routine post-operative observations.

Procedure guideline 14.2 Interventional radiology care

Statement	Rationale
1. Prior to requesting central venous access for a child in your care a decision should be made by the medical team caring for the child in conjunction with the child and main care givers as to the type of central venous access device required. (See Table 14.2 to guide you in making this choice.)	1. Ensure the appropriate device is inserted to fulfil the treatment requirements.
2. If children are having their PICC line, Hickman or Port-a-cath inserted under general anaesthetic they will need to be fasted according hospital policy.	2. Ensure safety during general anaesthetic and minimise risk of aspiration.
3. Consent must be obtained for all central venous access procedures.	3. Ensure the child and parents/carers receive appropriate information and are aware of benefits and potential problems.
4. If children are having their PICC line inserted under local anaesthetic a pre-procedural visit should be arranged with the nursing staff in interventional radiology. The use of Entonox (see Chapter 21) is also optional and depending on the child's medical condition may be a useful anxiolytic.	4. Ensure the child and parents/carers are aware of the procedure to be performed and aware of what to expect.
5. All children require recent full blood count with results within normal limits. If there is any deviation of blood results this should be discussed with the Interventional Radiology team and bloods corrected prior to the procedure.	5. To ensure safe procedure.
6. If the child is under 12 months, and a tunnelled PICC line is required or if they are having a Hickman or Port-a-cath inserted, they will also require a clotting screen and group and save. If the clotting screen is abnormal, this should be corrected prior to the procedure or discussed with the Interventional Radiology team and haematology registrar. If the group and save results show the child to be antibody positive they will require a cross match prior to the procedure.	6. Ensure safe procedure and the availability of blood should it be required.

Table 14.2 Catheters commonly used for venous access in children

Catheter type	Entry site	Length	Usual lifespan of device	Comments (Centers for Disease Control and Prevention, 2002)
Peripheral venous catheter	Usually veins of hand, forearm, feet or ankle	<3 inches	1–8 days (Centre for Disease Control & Prevention, 2002)	Phlebitis with prolonged use, rarely associated with blood stream infection
Non-tunnelled central venous catheters	Percutaneous insertion into a central vein (femoral, subclavian internal jugular)	≥8 cm	≤2 weeks	Increased risk of bloodstream infections. Heparin bonded recommended
Peripherally inserted central venous catheters (PICC)	Inserted into basilic, cephalic or brachial veins and enter the superior vena cava	≤20 cm	1–6 weeks	Lower rates of infection than non-tunnelled CVCs
Tunnelled central venous catheters	Implanted into subclavian, internal jugular or femoral vein	≥8 cm	Long term	Lower risks of infection than non-tunnelled catheter – cuff inhibits migration of organisms. Surgery required for removal
Implanted ports	Tunnelled beneath the skin to subclavian or internal jugular with a subcutaneous port accessed via a needle	≥8 cm	Long term	Lowest risk for infection. Improved body image, no site care needed when line not in use, not recommended for needle phobic children

344

Procedure guideline 14.3 Interventional radiology aftercare

Statement	Rationale
1. If the child has had a general anaesthetic, routine vital sign observations should be performed as per hospital policy.	1. To ensure safe recovery.
2. Observe the insertion and exit site for bleeding. If the child bleeds post-operatively apply a pressure dressing over the existing theatre dressing. If a child bleeds post-operatively after a tunnelled PICC insertion, pressure should be applied over the insertion site as this is the most likely cause of bleeding, as well as the exit site. This should be changed within 24 hours and subsequent dressing changes should be performed as per hospital policy.	2. To aid early detection. Blood left underneath the dressing increases risk of infection (Hindley 1997, Marcoux et al 1990).
3. The insertion site should be observed for redness, swelling, exudate, pain or discomfort or red tracking up the arm.	3. Early detection of possible line infection.
4. All central venous access lines are usually screened into position during insertion in the interventional radiology department; therefore the line may be used immediately unless otherwise stated.	4. Ensure line tip is in safe position for use immediately (RCN 2010).
5. Observe for pain and administer pain relief as required.	5. If a central venous catheter is tunnelled the child may be sore for a few days. Therefore maintain comfort of the child (Marcoux et al 1990).

Collection of microbiological specimens

Microbiological and virological laboratory testing has a key role in the management of children with infection. Accurate and rapid identification of significant micro-organisms is vital for guiding optimal anti-microbial therapy, and improving outcome from infectious disease. Laboratory diagnosis is also essential for effective infection control in both the hospital and community settings, as well as providing invaluable epidemiological data.

Clinicians have responsibility for the collection and safe transportation of samples to the laboratory. The validity of test results largely depends on good practice in the 'pre-test' stage and it is essential that documentation is accurate and comprehensive (Higgins 1994). Microbiological tests are not as standardised as some other lab tests; the way in which a sample is processed and the results are interpreted depend heavily on the information provided with the specimen. Contamination of samples, especially those from normally sterile sites such as blood or cerebro-spinal fluid, leads to misleading results, inappropriate antibiotic usage and unnecessary laboratory work. Prolonged periods of storage at ambient temperature and delay in transport of specimens to the laboratory may increase the number of contaminants present. It is therefore essential that every effort should be made to avoid these problems.

Rationale for specimen collection

Specimen collection is undertaken when laboratory investigation is required for the examination of material, e.g. tissue, body fluid or faeces to aid diagnosis.

Preparation

- Laboratory request forms are either:
  - Printed from the Patient Information Management System (PIMS) if at GOSH or a similar system in other trusts. Use the labels on the form to label the specimen accompanying the form. These are usually bar coded to aid the audit trail
  - Handwritten clearly on the relevant laboratory request form.
- All specimens must be clearly labeled to identify their source. **DO NOT pre-label specimen containers as this increases the risk of errors. The specimen must be labelled next to the child/patient when the sample is taken**. A laboratory request form with the following information must accompany the specimen. This aids interpretation of results and reduces the risk of errors.
  - Patient's name, age, ward/department/GP and hospital number
  - Type of specimen and the site from which it was obtained (where necessary)
  - Date and time collected
  - Diagnosis with history and reasons for request, such as returning from abroad (specify country) with diarrhoea and vomiting, rash, pyrexia, catheters in situ or invasive devices used, or surgical details regarding post operative wound infection
  - The question you wish to answer by having the sample tested
  - Any antimicrobial drug/s given
  - Consultant's name and cost code
  - Name/bleep number of the nurse/doctor who ordered the investigation, as it may be necessary to telephone preliminary results and discuss treatment before the final result is authorised.
- Always explain the procedure to the child and parent/carer and the reasons for taking the specimen. Separate permission must be obtained from the child and parent/carer if specimens are sought for research purposes. They have a right to refuse without any obligation (Royal College of Paediatrics and Child Health Ethics Advisory Committee 2000).
- Hands should be washed before and after specimen collection. Gloves should be worn when collecting or handling specimens to avoid skin contamination.

- When collecting certain specimens, e.g. catheter urines and cerebro-spinal fluid, every effort should be made to avoid infecting the child. An appropriate aseptic non-touch technique should be used.
- All pathological specimens must be treated as potentially infectious and local written laboratory protocols should be followed for the safe handling and transportation of specimens (Health and Safety Executive 2003). Specimens should be collected in sterile containers with close fitting lids to avoid contamination and spillage. All specimen containers must be transported in a double sided, self-sealing polythene bag with one compartment containing the laboratory request form and the other the specimen.
- Ideally microbiological specimens should be collected before beginning any treatment such as antibiotics or using antiseptics. However, treatment must not be delayed in serious sepsis.
- When collecting pus specimens obtain as much material as possible as this increases the chance of isolating micro-organisms that may be difficult to grow or are minimal in number, e.g. tuberculosis.
- Transport medium is used to preserve micro-organisms during transportation. Charcoal medium improves the isolation of bacteria by neutralising toxic substances such as naturally occurring fatty acids found on the skin. As many viruses do not survive well outside the body special viral transport medium is used.
- Specimens are generally delivered to the laboratories by relevant hospital personnel, via a pneumatic tube delivery system, by patients/relatives if from the community or by post.
- Specimens sent by post must be packed and sent according to World Health Organization regulations (2007). The laboratory will have the relevant equipment for packaging. It is imperative that the regulations are followed as the sender maybe liable (with a financial penalty) for any spillage that may occur.
- In children suspected of suffering from Category A pathogens such as viral haemorrhagic fevers (HPA online information) or Human Transmissable Spongiform Encephalopathies (ACDP 2003), the Infection Control Team or Consultant in Communicable Diseases Control (CCDC) must be consulted before any specimens are taken (Health and Safety Executive 2004).
- Chlorine releasing granules or a hypochlorite solution (10,000 parts per million of available chlorine) must be available for decontamination of any spillages. Care must be taken as chlorine releasing fumes have occurred when mixed with urine (Safety Action bulletin 1990).

Equipment

This will vary according to the specimen required but must include:

- Disposable gloves (Health and Safety Executive 1998)
- A protective tray
- A sterile container for the specimen
- Appropriate transport medium, if required
- Laboratory specimen form
- A polythene transportation bag
- Biohazard label, if required.

Blood samples

Blood sampling should be performed by a healthcare worker trained and competent in the procedure. As there are many haematological, biochemical, immunological and microbiological blood tests the person should seek information as to the appropriate laboratory containers required for specific tests and the amount of blood required. Protective clothing such as gloves and aprons (and facial protection when appropriate) must be used along with an aseptic non-touch technique.

The 'Broken Needle Technique' (breaking the hub of the needle to obtain blood from small infants) poses an additional risk of injury to the child and user and must **not** be used (Safety Action Notice 2001).

Blood culture

Detection of micro-organisms by culture of blood is essential in the diagnosis of bloodstream infections, including: infective endocarditis; infections presenting as pyrexia of unknown origin; prosthetic material infections; and intravenous catheter infections. Blood culture may also detect bacteraemia associated with primary infections such as pneumonia and septic arthritis. Accurate positive results provide valuable information to guide optimal antibiotic therapy early on, which can improve the outcome from these conditions.

On the other hand, contaminated blood cultures can cause considerable diagnostic confusion and lead to unnecessary or sub-optimal antimicrobial therapy.

Contamination may be prevented by careful collection of the blood using an aseptic non-touch technique (Taking a Blood Culture 2011). If possible, avoid palpating the vein after cleansing the skin. The specimen should also preferably be taken during pyrexial episodes as more bacteria may be present at that time.

Blood cultures should be taken when there is a clinical need to do so in response to any of the following clinical signs suggestive of sepsis and a deteriorating clinical picture including:

- Abnormalities in
  - Heart rate
  - Core temperature
  - Leucocyte count.
- Presence of rigors or chills
- Other focal signs of infection, such as pneumonia, septic arthritis, meningism, urinary tract infection including pyelonephritis and acute abdominal pathology.

Procedure guideline 14.4 Taking a blood culture

Statement	Rationale
1. Use both blood culture bottles and clean the bung with alcohol or with a 2% chlorhexidine in 70% alcohol wipe. Allow to dry.	**1.** To ensure sterility.
2. Soap and water should be used to clean any visibly soiled skin. The skin must then be decontaminated with a 2% chlorhexidine in 70% alcohol wipe and allowed to dry.	**2.** Do not re-palpate the vein (even with a gloved hand) after decontamination as the skin may become contaminated.
3. After withdrawing the blood, insert the blood into the container with a new sterile needle.	**3.** There is a risk of contamination of skin organisms on the needle used to withdraw the blood.
4. The volume of blood is the most critical factor in the detection of blood stream infection. Place as much blood as possible (up to 4 ml in the yellow aerobic bottle (priority) and up to 10 ml in the anaerobic orange bottle. For neonates 1–2 ml of blood is recommended. However, the sensitivity of neonatal blood cultures is increased if more blood is cultured.	**4.** This optimises the identification of the micro-organism if present.
5. Inoculation of the blood into the blood culture bottles should be performed first before inserting blood into other bottles.	**5.** Many other blood bottles are not sterile and accidental contamination may occur.
6a) In children in whom line sepsis is suspected, blood for culture may be taken from a peripheral vein stab and also from the appropriate intravascular lines. **b)** In cases of suspected bacterial endocarditis three blood cultures should be taken from separate venepunctures.	**6a)** If the same micro-organism is identified from both sites this indicates line colonisation or infection. **b)** This optimises recovery of bacteria which may be present in small numbers.

Analysis of antibiotic levels

The relationship between drug dose, drug concentration in biological fluid and the individual child's metabolic process must be understood for interpreting results. The results may be affected by the route of administration, age of the child and disease process such as liver and renal disease. The analysis involves testing levels in blood serum or plasma in direct relationship to drug administration:

- For timing of sampling for antibiotic concentrations see local antibiotic policy.
- Record on the laboratory form/name of the drug, dose and mode of administration, the time the drug is given and whether the sample is a 'peak' or 'trough' level.
- Blood for antibiotic assay must not be taken through the same catheter which has been used to give the antibiotic at any time. Antibiotics bind to plastic and the drug may release intermittently giving false results.

Biopsy material

Specimens such as skin, muscle, kidney, liver, jejunal, tissue or brain biopsies are generally obtained by medical staff either under general or local anaesthetic according to the site. An aseptic non-touch technique is required for all these procedures. All biopsy specimens must be discussed with the relevant laboratory personnel in order that:

- The most appropriate specimen and laboratory tests are undertaken. If the specimen is small it may be necessary to limit the range of tests.
- Check if the specimen is to be fixed in formalin. **Do not** use formalin if the specimen is for microbiological investigation. In many cases both histopathological and microbiological/

virological analysis will be required and it is critical that separate specimens be sent for these purposes so they are processed and transported appropriately.

Cerebro-spinal fluid

Sampling of cerebrospinal fluid is essential for the accurate diagnosis of infective meningitis and may aid in the diagnosis of encephalitis.

Cerebro-spinal fluid (CSF) is most commonly obtained via a lumbar puncture performed by medical staff. An aseptic non-touch technique is required as there is a risk of introducing infection itself causing meningitis. Specimens of CSF should be dispatched to the laboratory immediately. Out of office hours it is essential that the on-call laboratory staff are contacted when the sample is being transported. It is important not to store the specimen in a refrigerator as this may cause the cells to deteriorate or lyse giving rise to misleading results. It is common practice to send three separate collection tubes of CSF when investigating for evidence of sub-arachnoid haemorrhage, as the initial part of the sample may be contaminated with blood from outside the sub-arachnoid space. If this is performed, it is important to label the tubes as such and specifically request counts on the first and third samples. It is also important to remember that a CSF glucose level can only be accurately interpreted in conjunction with a simultaneous plasma glucose level.

Taking swabs

In child health practice there is a range of swabs that may be requested. These are listed below.

Ear swabs

Procedure guideline 14.5 Taking an ear swab

Statement	Rationale
1. No antibiotics or other therapeutic agents should have been in the aural region for about 3 hours prior to sampling the area.	**1.** Local antibiotics may inhibit the growth of micro-organisms.
2. If there is purulent discharge this should be sampled.	**2.** To obtain an adequate specimen.
3. Place a sterile swab into the outer ear and gently rotate to collect the secretions.	**3.** This material is required to identify any micro-organisms.
4. Place swab in transport medium.	**4.** To preserve the growth of any micro-organisms.
5. For deeper ear swabbing a speculum may be used.	**5.** Experienced medical staff only should undertake this procedure as damage to the eardrum may occur.

Eye swabs

Procedure guideline 14.6 Taking an eye swab

Statement	Rationale
1. Where possible ask the child to look upwards and gently pull the lower lid down or gently part the eyelids.	1. To expose the area to be swabbed.
2. Use a sterile cotton wool swab and gently role the swab over the conjunctival sac inside the lower lid. Hold the swab parallel to the cornea.	2. This avoids injury if the child moves.
3. Place the swab in the transport medium.	3. To preserve the growth of the micro-organisms.
4a) For suspected chlamydia infection obtain a chlamydia sampling swab from the laboratory. b) Clean the eye first with sterile normal saline to obtain a clear view of the conjunctiva c) Using the swab, part the eyelids and gently rub the conjunctival sac of the lower lid to obtain epithelial cells. d) Place the swab in the transport medium provided.	4a) To obtain the best specimen. c) Identification of chlamydia is by PCR.

Nose swabs

Procedure guideline 14.7 Collecting nose swabs

Statement	Rationale
1. If the nose is dry, moisten the swab in sterile saline beforehand.	1. This enhances the collection of material.
2. Insert the swab into the anterior nares and direct it up into the tip of the nose and gently rotate.	2. Both nares should be swabbed using the same swab to obtain adequate material.
3. Place in transport medium.	3. To preserve any micro-organisms.
4. For viral investigation same as above and place in viral transport medium.	4. To preserve any viruses.
5. The outside of the nostrils may be rubbed after the procedure to alleviate the unpleasant sensation of swabbing.	5. This procedure may stimulate sneezing.

Pernasal swabs

This investigation is most commonly used to diagnose whooping cough (*Bordetella pertussis*). Specimens for PCR can be taken in patients under 1 year of age; however, in those children over 1 year, requirement for PCR may need to be discussed with the microbiologist. If taking pernasal swabs for PCR, swabs must be placed in transport media that does not contain charcoal as this inhibits PCR.

When obtaining this specimen the nurse must be proficient in the procedure and ensure suction, oxygen and resuscitation equipment is easily available. The child should be held securely and observed carefully as the procedure may produce paroxysmal coughing and/or vomiting.

NB Performing this procedure may generate either droplets or aerosols or both, which can expose healthcare workers to this pathogen. It is therefore essential that appropriate respiratory protection and eyewear is worn when performing this procedure.

Procedure guideline 14.8 Collecting pernasal swabs

Statement	Rationale
1. Place the child in a good light.	**1.** This facilitates better observation of the child.
2. Use a special soft wired sterile swab (pernasal swab).	**2.** This minimises trauma to the nasal tissue.
3. Holding the head upwards, pass the swab along the floor of the nasal cavity to the posterior wall of the naso-pharynx.	**3.** This is where the *Bordetella pertussis* is found.
4. Gently rotate and withdraw the swab and place in its container, dispatch immediately to the laboratory.	**4.** This ensures maximum chance of growth of the organism.
5. For PCR tests the sample should be taken in the same way and delivered immediately to the microbiology laboratory.	**5.** Do not put the sample in charcoal medium as this inhibits PCR.

Throat swabs

Procedure guideline 14.9 Taking throat swabs

Statement	Rationale
1. Place the child in a position with a good light source.	**1.** This will ensure maximum visibility of the tonsillar bed.
2. Either depress the tongue with a spatula or ask the child to say 'aahh'. Quickly but gently rub the swab over the ansilla fossa (tonsillar bed) or area where there is exudate or a lesion.	**2.** The procedure is likely to cause gagging and the tongue will move to the roof of the mouth. This can prevent accurate sampling.
3. Place the sample into transport medium or, if for viral investigation, put into viral transport medium.	**3.** To preserve the micro-organism.

Vaginal swabs

The taking of this specimen in children should be avoided where possible due to its invasive nature.

Procedure guideline 14.10 Taking a vaginal swab

Statement	Rationale
1. In the case of suspected or actual sexual abuse: **a)** Local child protection protocols must be adhered to. **b)** Do not clean the area before obtaining the specimen.	**1.** **a)** To protect the child and healthcare worker. **b)** The identification of semen or sexually transmitted diseases may be required for evidence.
2. If specimens are to be taken in house (rather than by a forensic medical officer or at a genitourinary medicine clinic), contact the laboratory department who will provide the appropriate swab and transport media.	**2.** To ensure the correct specimens are taken.
3. For suspected chlamydia infection: • The first pass urine or low vaginal chlamydia swab samples may be sent.	**3.** To ensure the best material is obtained.
4. For investigation of simple vaginal discharge: **a)** Expose the vaginal area and part the labia. **b)** Use routine charcoal swab. Gently insert the supplied swab into the outer entrance of the vagina. **c)** Place the swab into the supplied transport medium.	**4.** **a)** To prevent contamination of the swab. **b)** Care must be taken not to tear the hymen. **c)** To obtain the specimen.

349

Wound swabs

Interpretation of results must be in conjunction with clinical signs. In the absence of clinical signs of infection wound swabs will provide little, if any, useful information and simply reflects colonisation (Gilchrist 1996).

Procedure guideline 14.11 Taking a wound swab

Statement	Rationale
1. Obtain the specimen prior to any dressing or cleaning procedure of the wound.	**1.** This will maximise the material obtained and prevent killing of the organism by the use of antiseptics.
2a) Use a sterile swab and gently rotate on the area to collect exudate from the wound and place into transport medium. **b)** Where there is pus collect as much as possible in a sterile syringe or sterile container (do not use a swab) and send to the laboratory.	**2a)** To obtain the material for analysis. **b)** Pure pus may contain a concentration of micro-organisms and maximise analysis of the material.
3. For detection of *Mycobacterium tuberculosis*, pus collected neat into a pot or tissue biopsy is preferred, however a calcium alginate swab can be used.	**3.** The alginate swab gradually dissolves, maximising the isolation of the mico-organism as the number of micro-organisms is usually small.

Faeces

Procedure guideline 14.12 Collecting a faecal specimen

Statement	Rationale
1. A faecal specimen is more suitable than a rectal swab.	**1.** More micro-organisms are likely to be in a stool specimen. However, rectal swabs may be taken from neonates before the first stool is passed.
2. A specimen can be obtained from a nappy or clean potty.	**2.** The specimen does not need to be sterile.
3. Using a scoop, place faecal material into a container.	**3.** To prevent contamination of the outside of the container.
4. Where diarrhoea is present, a small piece of non-absorbent material lining the nappy can be used.	**4.** This prevents faeces soaking into the nappy.
5. Examine the sample for consistency, odour or blood and record observations.	**5.** This helps identify any changes.
6. If segments of tapeworm are seen, send to the laboratory.	**6.** Tapeworm segments can vary from the size of rice grains to a ribbon shape, one inch long.
7a) For the identification of *Enterobius vermicularis* (threadworm/pin worm) material should be obtained first thing in the morning on awakening by using a sellotape slide. **b)** Place the sticky side of a strip of sellotape over the anal region to obtain the material and stick the sellotape smoothly onto a glass slide.	**7a)** Thread worm lay their ova on the perianal skin at night and therefore will not be seen in a faecal specimen. **b)** The worm can then be identified under the microscope.
8. Where amoebic dysentery is suspected, the specimen of stool must be freshly dispatched to the laboratory.	**8.** The parasite causing amoebic dysentery exists in a free-living motile form and in the form of non-motile cysts. Both forms are characteristic in their fresh state but the motile form cannot be identified when dead. 'Hot faeces' should be discussed with the laboratory prior to collection to ensure they are processed immediately.

Fungal samples of hair, nail and skin

Procedure guideline 14.13 Collecting fungal samples

Statement	Rationale
1. Special containers may be obtained from the laboratory.	1. This helps to see the material against a dark background under the microscope.
2. Samples of infected hair should be removed by plucking the hair with forceps or gloves.	2. The root of the hair is infected not the shaft.
3. Samples of the whole thickness of the nail or deep scrapings should be obtained.	3. To enable as much infected material to be obtained to increase the chances of identification.
4. The skin should be cleaned with an alcohol swab. Epidermal scales scraped from the active edge of a lesion or the roof of any lesion should be obtained.	4. To prevent secondary infection.

Gastric washings

Swallowed sputum containing *Mycobacterium tuberculosis* may be obtained through gastric washings. Children generally do not produce sufficient sputum therefore gastric washings are obtained for laboratory analysis to aid diagnosis of pulmonary *Mycobacterium tuberculosis*. The detection of alcohol acid fast bacilli (AAFB) is not adequate, alone, for diagnosis of *M. tuberculosis* as other environmental AAFB's may be present. Culture of the organism is always performed and may take between 6–12 weeks to confirm diagnosis. Three consecutive early morning specimens should be obtained. There are usually only small numbers of organisms present so as much material as possible should be obtained. As AAFB are often found in tap water sterile water must be used.

Procedure guideline 14.14 Collecting gastric samples

Statement	Rationale
1. Fast the child for at least six hours overnight or as long as possible.	1. Feeds may not be sterile and environmental AAFB found normally in substances, such as water, will confuse results.
2. Operators must take precautions and use appropriate PPE.	2. The child may cough and infectious material poses a risk to the healthcare worker
3. Pass a naso-gastric tube.	3. To obtain the gastric washings.
4. Aspirate the stomach contents and place in a sterile container.	4. The fasted stomach contents may contain sputum with AAFB.
5a) Instil at least 30 ml of sterile water down the tube to obtain as much stomach content as possible. b) The medical condition and age of the child must be taken into consideration.	5a) To increase the amount of material to be tested. b) If a preterm infant this may be too much to put into the stomach.
6. Aspirate the contents back and place in the same container.	6. To increase the amount of material to be examined.
7. Remove the tube, if appropriate.	

Naso-pharyngeal aspirate

Nasopharyngeal aspiration is required for the diagnosis of viral infections such as influenza, parainfluenza and respiratory syn- citial (RSV) as well as the diagnosis of *Bordetella pertussis* infections by PCR.

Procedure guideline 14.15 Collecting naso-pharyngeal aspirate

Statement	Rationale
1. The healthcare worker must take precautions and wear appropriate PPE.	**1.** The child may cough and infectious material poses a risk to the healthcare worker.
2. Attach a mucus trap to the suction system and the appropriately sized catheter, leaving the wrapper on the suction catheter.	**2.** This maximises the material for analysis and prevents contamination.
3. Turn on the suction and adjust the pressure.	**3.** To obtain the material for analysis.
4. Without applying suction, insert the catheter into the nose, directed posteriorly and towards the opening of the external ear. NB The depth of insertion necessary to reach the posterior pharynx is equivalent to the distance between the anterior naris and external opening of the ear.	**4.** To prevent contamination of the specimen or injury to the naso-pharynx.
5a) Apply suction and slowly withdraw the catheter using a rotating movement. **b)** The catheter should remain in the nasopharynx for no longer than 10 seconds. The trap should be kept upright.	**5a)** To obtain the material. **b)** To minimise discomfort or hypoxia.
6. If necessary rinse the catheter with a small volume of sterile 0.9% sodium chloride to ensure adequate specimen volume.	**6.** To obtain any material left in the tubing.
7. Disconnect suction and seal mucus trap with tubing.	**7.** To be able to send the sputum trap to the laboratory and avoid contamination of the outside of the container.

Sputum

Good quality sputum samples are essential for accurate microbiological diagnosis of pneumonia but also acute tracheitis and bronchitis. Samples contaminated with oro-pharyngeal secretions and saliva are difficult to interpret and can be misleading.

Procedure guideline 14.16 Collecting sputum samples

Statement	Rationale
1. Encourage the child to cough especially after sleep and expectorate into a container. Alternatively, a sample may be obtained from a naso-pharyngeal/tracheal suction using a sputum trap.	**1.** Sitting up and coughing after sleeping encourages sputum production.
2. Chest physiotherapy may be given.	**2.** This may help facilitate expectoration.
3. Ensure the material obtained is sputum and not saliva.	**3.** The cells in the sputum are required for analysis.

Urine

Bedside urine testing for the presence of blood, protein and other analytes is usually undertaken with reagent strips, the results of which indicate that further laboratory investigation is required (Cook 1995).

Most urine samples sent to the microbiology laboratory are for bacteriological investigation. The same collection techniques also apply to samples sent for virological investigation.

Urine samples should be dispatched to the laboratory as soon as possible or no more than 4 hours if kept at room temperature or up to 24 hours if kept at 4°C to avoid overgrowth of organisms and misleading results (Griffiths 1995).

Urine collected from disposable nappies for microscopy and culture analysis has been described (Ahmed *et al* 1991, Roberts and Lucas 1985, Vernon 1995), however this procedure is not used at the GOSH Trust. Practitioners should ensure they are aware of different practices to be able to describe to families why procedures might be different in different hospitals.

Normal social hygiene, such as washing the genitalia with soap and water and drying thoroughly is considered sufficient to minimise contamination from the skin prior to collection of the specimen. Assess the clinical and psychosocial needs of the child as to whether cleaning the genitalia is necessary. The nurse must be sensitive to the cultural issues surrounding touching intimate parts of the body (Department of Health 2001).

Collection of urine by a supra-pubic aspirate should only be considered (this is a painful procedure) when a clean and accurate sample is required. Ultrasound guidance should be used to indicate the presence of urine in the bladder before a supra-pubic aspirate is attempted (NICE Guidelines 2007).

Midstream specimen or clean catch

This is the most reliable non-invasive urine specimen collection method, but it may not be possibleto obtain from the very young child. In the female encourage separation of the labia to prevent perineal contamination whilst passing urine. In the male encourage retraction of the prepuce, if appropriate.

Procedure guideline 14.17 Collecting a midstream specimen

Statement	Rationale
1. The first part of the urine stream is passed into the toilet.	1. This reduces meatal contamination of the specimen.
2. The middle part of the urine stream is collected into a clean container.	2. This is the best sample of the urine for analysis.
3. The remaining urine is passed into the toilet.	3. To empty the bladder.
4. Pour the urine into a sterile container.	4. To avoid leakage or contamination with faeces.

Bag specimen

1. Select the correct size sterile urine bag.	1. To avoid leakage or contamination with faeces.
2. Remove the protective seal: • For the female place the bag over the vulva, starting from the perineum and working upwards, sticking the bag to the skin • For the male, place the bag over the penis and scrotum.	2. To avoid leakage and contamination from faeces.
3. Observe the bag frequently until urine is passed.	3. To avoid leakage.
4. Remove the bag and empty the urine through the relevant port into a sterile container.	4. To obtain the specimen.
5. Wash the genitalia after the procedure.	5. To prevent soreness of the skin.

Catheter specimen

1. This is collected from the self-sealing bung of the urinary drainage tubing in a child who is already catheterised. (For an alternative method of obtaining a urine specimen from a catheter see Chapter 29.)	1. Do not disconnect the closed drainage system as infection may be introduced (Department of Health 2001) nor take the sample from the urinary drainage bag as the specimen maybe contaminated.
2. Using an aseptic non-touch technique, clean the catheter sampling site with 2% chlorhexidine in 70% alcohol wipe and allow to dry.	2. To decontaminate the sampling site.

(Continued)

Procedure guideline 14.17 (*Continued*)

Statement	Rationale
3. Collect the urine using sterile equipment appropriate to access port, i.e. either using a sterile syringe and needle and inserting the needle into the bung at an angle of 45° degrees, or use a needle-less system.	**3.** This will minimise penetration of the wall of the tubing and subsequent needle stick injury.
4. Gently withdraw the urine into the syringe.	**4.** To diminish any pressure on the bladder and obtain the specimen
5. Remove the needle and syringe, wipe the area with the alcohol swab and allow to dry.	**5.** To prevent contamination. The rubber bung will self-seal.
6. Place the urine in a sterile container.	**6.** To obtain the specimen.
7. Discard the needle and syringe into a sharps container.	**7.** To dispose of equipment safely.
Obtaining urine from a Mitrofanoff stoma	
1. The specimen should be obtained by a nurse who is familiar with the Mitrofanoff operation and the specific anatomy of the area on the child.	**1.** This prevents contamination and enhances the collection of the specimen.
2. The specimen should ideally be taken in conjunction with normal bladder emptying.	**2.** This encourages the flow of urine.
3. A new sterile catheter of the child's normal catheter size should be used.	**3.** To prevent contamination.
4. Clean the stoma with soap and water and dry.	**4.** To reduce contamination.
5. Gently insert the lubricated sterile catheter into the stoma and collect the urine into a sterile container. A water-soluble lubricant should be used.	**5.** To prevent irritation.
6. Ensure the bladder is completely empty before withdrawing the catheter.	**6.** To promote comfort.
7. Wipe the area dry with a tissue.	**7.** To prevent soreness.

Vesicular fluid for herpes polymerase chain reaction (PCR)

Procedure guideline 14.18 Taking a vesicular fluid sample

Statement	Rationale
1. Explain to the child and parent/carer that the procedure is usually pain free.	**1.** The needle only penetrates the vesicle not the skin.
2. Obtain a sterile syringe and needle, sterile swab and viral transport medium.	**2.** To obtain the specimen and avoid secondary infection.
3a) Pierce the top of the vesicle with a sterile needle and if there is sufficient fluid draw up the exudate into a syringe. Keep the needle flush to the skin.	**3a)** To prevent accidental stabbing if the child moves.
b) Then draw up some viral transport medium into the syringe and flush the medium plus vesicle fluid back into the bottle of viral transport medium.	**b)** This maximises the material to be analysed.

Procedure guideline 14.18 (*Continued*)

Statement	Rationale
c) If the vesicle is already dry, a positive diagnosis may be reached from a swab which has been vigorously rubbed over the dry base and sent in viral transport medium.	
4. Dispose of the needle in a 'sharps' bin.	**4.** To avoid contaminated material being transmitted and to avoid injury.
5. Send the sample to the laboratory.	**5.** The vesicular fluid should be screened by PCR to confirm the clinical diagnosis such as varicella-zoster (chickenpox or shingles) or herpes simplex type 1 or 2.
6. Place a sterile dressing over the vesicle until dry.	**6.** To avoid leakage of infected material and prevent secondary infection.

References

Advisory Committee on Dangerous Pathogens (2003) Guidance from the Transmissible Spongiform Encephalopathies Risk Management Subgroup. Available at http://www.dh.gov.uk/ab/ACDP/TSEguidance/index.htm (last accessed 19th December 2011)

Ahmed T, Vickers D, Campbell S, Coultard MG, Pedler S. (1991) Urine collection from disposable nappies. Lancet, 338, 674–676

Brent RL. (1989) The effect of embryonic and fetal exposure to X-ray, microwaves, and ultrasound: counselling the pregnant and non-pregnant patient about these risks. Seminars in Oncology, 16(5), 347–368

Bury B, Hufton A, Adams J. (1995) Radiation and women of child bearing potential. British Medical Journal, 310, 1022

Casey A. (1995) Nursing assessment and communication. In: Campbell S, Glaspar EA. (eds) Whaley and Wong's Children's Nursing, pp126–139. London, Times Mirror International

Cook R. (1995) Urinalysis. Nursing Standard, CE Article 343, 9(28), 32–37

Centres for Disease Control and Prevention (2002) http://www.cdc.gov/mmwr/preview/mmwrhtml/rr5110a1.htm

Coptcoat MJ, Reed C, Cumming J, Shah PJR, Worth PHL. (1988) Is antibiotic prophylaxis necessary for routine urodynamic investigations. British Journal of Urology, 61(4), 302–303

Department of Health (2000) The Ionising Radiation (Medical Exposure) Regulations (IR(ME)R2000) 2000 Statutory Instrument 2000/1059. London, Department of Health Available at www.Opsi.gov.uk/si/si/2000/20001059.htm (last accessed 25th August 2007)

Department of Health (2001) Guidelines for preventing infections associated with the insertion and maintenance of short-term indwelling urethral catheters in acute care. The EPIC Project: Developing National Evidence-based Guidelines for Preventing Healthcare Associated Infections. Journal of Hospital Infection, 47(S3–S4), 39–46

Gilchrist B. (1996) Wound infection – sampling bacterial flora: a review of the literature. Journal of Wound Care, 5(8), 386–388

Fegley B. (1988) Preparing children for radiological procedures. Research in Nursing and Health, 11, 3–9

Griffiths C. (1995) Microbiological examination in urinary tract infection. Nursing Times, 91(11), 33–35

Gyll C. (1982) Investigations into and a comparative study of techniques for basic radiography in children's hospitals. Radiography, 48(573), 175–184

Health and Safety Executive (1998) Advisory Committee on Dangerous Pathogens – Protection against bloodborne infections in the workplace: HIV and Hepatitis. Available at http://www.hse.gov.uk/biosafety/diseases/bbv.pdf (last accessed 19th December 2011)

Health and Safety Executive (2003) Safe Working and the Prevention of Infection in clinical Laboratories and Similar Facilities. Available at http://www.hse.gov.uk/pubns/priced/clinical-laboratories.pdf (last accessed 19th December 2011)

Health and Safety Executive (2004) Advisory Committee on Dangerous Pathogens Approved List of Biological Agents. Available at http://www.hse.gov.uk/press/2004/e04078.htm (last accessed 19th December 2011)

Heiney S. (1991) Painful procedures. American Journal of Nursing, Nov, 20–24

Higgins C. (1994) An introduction to the examination of specimens. Nursing Times, 90(47), 29–32

Hindley M. (1997) Reducing exit site infections and the risk of accidental removal of Hickman lines in children within the first month post insertion. Journal of Intravenous Nursing, 15(1), 36–41

Marcoux, C, Fisher S, Wong D. (1990) Central venous access devices in children. Pediatric Nursing, 16(2), 123–133

National Institute for Health and Clinical Excellence (2007) Urinary Tract Infection in children: diagnosis, treatment and long term management. Available at http://guidance.nice.org.uk/CG54/NICEGuidance/pdf/English (last accessed 20th December 2011)

National Institute for Health and Clinical Excellence (2010) Sedation in children and young people: sedation for diagnostic and therapeutic procedures in children and young people. London, NICE

Parker RI, Mahan RA, Giugliano D, Parker MM. (1997) Efficacy and safety of intravenous midazolam and ketamine as sedation for therapeutic and diagnostic procedures in children. Pediatrics, 99(3) 427–431

Roberts SB, Lucas A. (1985) A nappy collection method for measuring urinary constituents and 24 hour urine output in infants. Archives of Diseases in Childhood, 60, 1018–1020

Royal College of Nursing (2005) Perioperative fasting in adults and children: an RCN guideline for the multidisciplinary team. London, RCN

Royal College of Nursing (2008) 'Let's talk about restraint'. Rights, risks and responsibility. London, RCN

Royal College of Nursing (2010) Standards for infusion therapy. The RCN IV Therapy forum. London, RCN

Royal College of Paediatrics and Child Health Ethics Advisory Committee (2000) Guidelines for the ethical conduct of medical research involving children. Archives of Disease in Childhood, 82, 177–182

Royal College of Radiologists (2008) A guide to understanding the implications of the ionising radition (Medical Exposure) regulations in radiotherapy. London, RCR

Royal College of Radiologists (2003) Safe Sedation, Analgesia and Anaesthesia within the Radiology Department. London, RCR

Safety Action Bulletin (1990) Spills of urine: Potential risk of misuse of chlorine-releasing disinfecting agents. SAB, 90, 41

Safety Action Notice (2001) Blood sampling from small infants:improper disposal of needles. SAN (SC)01/31. Available at http://www.hfs.scot.nhs.uk/online-services/incident-reporting-and-investigation-centre-iric/safety-action-notices-sans/sans-issued-in-2001/ (last accessed 19th December 2011)

Scott L, Langton F, O'Donoghue J. (2002) Minimising the use of sedation/anaesthesia in young children receiving radiotherapy through an effective play preparation programme. European Journal of Oncology Nursing, 6(1) 15–22

Singh J, Daftary A. (2008) Iodinated contrast media and their adverse reactions. Journal of Nuclear Medicine Technology 36, 69–74. Available at http://tech.snmjournals.org/content/36/2/69.full.pdf (last accessed 1st November 2011)

Taking a Blood Culture: a summary of Best Practice (2011). Available at http://hcai.dh.gov.uk/files/2011/03/Document_Blood_culture_FINAL_100826.pdf (last accessed 20th December 2011)

Tramer MR, Elm E, Loubeyre P, Hauser C. (2006) Pharmacological prevention of serious anaphylactic reactions due to iodinated contrast media: systematic review. British Medical Journal, 333, 675

Vernon S (1995) Urine collection from infants: a reliable method. Paediatric Nursing, 7(6), 26–27

World Health Organisation (2007) Guidance on Regulations for the Transport of Infectious Substances. Available at http://www.who.int/csr/resources/publications/biosafety/WHO_CDS_EPR_2007_2cc.pdf (last accessed 19th December 2011)

youtube (2011) http://www.youtube.com/watch?v=p9T6m21AZ80 (last accessed 2nd October 2011)

Chapter 15

Administration of medicines

Chapter contents

Procedure guidelines

The Great Ormond Street Hospital Manual of Children's Nursing Practices, First Edition. Edited by Susan Macqueen, Elizabeth Anne Bruce, Faith Gibson.
© 2012 Great Ormond Street Hospital for Children NHS Foundation Trust. Published 2012 by Blackwell Publishing Ltd.

Introduction

Many changes within pharmacology, knowledge and practice management of medication therapies in children have taken place since the early 1990s. Medications now come in multiple forms for administration via multiple routes. The prescribed route is dependent on the availability and cost of forms of medication, the condition being treated, the speed of action of the medication that is required and the child's tolerance to the route of administration. Infants, children and young people are in a constant state of physical, metabolic and psychological change (Kanneh 2002); all this presents a real challenge to the practitioner administering medication to children. This chapter discusses those developmental considerations, the multiple routes of administration, the benefits and contra-indications for using that route, and provides a guide to the safe practice of administering medication to children.

As part of everyday practice nurses administer medication to patients; however, there is a potential for errors and the consequences of this could prove fatal. To protect the public, guidelines for practitioners have been developed based on local policies and government and other agency policies. There are extensive legislation and guidelines on the manufacture, licensing, prescribing, dispensing and administration of medication. The manufacture, supply and administration of medicines are controlled by two acts: The Medicine Act (1968) and The Misuse of Drugs Act (1971).

The Medicines Act (1968) was established as a system for licensing medicine for human use for medicinal purposes. A medicine is classified into three categories, prescription only medicine (POM), general sale medicine (GSL) and pharmacy only medicine (P). This act allows doctors, pharmacists and nurses respectively, to supply and administer medication for their respective professions.

The Misuse of Drug act (1971) was established for the regulation of possession, supply or manufacture of controlled drugs. It is classified into five schedules, each represent a different level of control.

Schedule 1: Cannabis and derivatives but excluding nabilone, LSD (lysergic acid diethylamide)

Schedule 2: Most opioids in common use; cocaine, diamorphine, methodone, pethedine, fentanyl phenoperidine, alfentanyl, amphetamines, morphine papaveretum and codeine, dihydrocodeine and pentazocine (injections only)

Schedule 3: Minor stimulants, barbiturates (excluding hexobarbitone, thiopentone, methohexitone), diethylpropion, buprenorphine and temazepam

Schedule 4: Part 1 anabolic steroids. Part 2 benzodiazepines

Schedule 5: Some preparations containing very low strengths of: cocaine, codeine, morphine, pholcodine and some other opioids.

Schedule 2 and schedule 3 are the two schedules with which practitioners will be more familiar. The purpose of this legislation is to minimise the potential abuse and misuse of the substances concerned. In practice this means that controlled drugs (CDs) must be supplied, stored and administered in accordance with the act.

The effective and safe administration of medication to patients is further clarified by the Nursing and Midwifery Council (2007) stating that the administration of medication is not 'solely a mechanistic task to be performed in strict compliance with the written prescription of a medical practitioner, it involves thought and the exercise of professional judgement'. The NMC expects the nurse to administer medication in a safe manner and to also have a broader knowledge of other influencing factors involved in this process such as a understanding of the pharmacology, i.e. use, action, the normal doses and the side-effects of the drug to be administered, signs of toxicity, as well being competent in numeracy, communication, teaching and knowledge of child development. Further clarification regarding safe and effective drug administration is supplied by the NMC, and states that all practitioners have a professional responsibility to administer medicines safely (NMC 2008a). Therefore, the nurse should be aware of the correct procedure, in order to administer medication safely to children. Administer medication safely and avoid errors by adhering to the following basic principles, the 'five Cs/Rs':

- Correct/right patient/child
- Correct/right medicine
- Correct/right dose
- Correct/right time
- Correct/right route.

Prior to following the five Cs/Rs, the child's prescription chart should be checked to ascertain the medication, the method of administration, the validity and legibility of the prescription and signature of prescriber.

The NMC Code of Professional Conduct (NMC 2008a) supports the single checking of oral medication within strict local policy guidelines and protocols. Please refer to Administration of Medicines Operational Policy (Cope 2009) for GOSH Trust guidelines, but in the first instance refer to local guidelines. Local policies will require a degree of theory and practice training to achieve a level of competency before this practice is undertaken.

As well as the NMC supporting practitioners in the administration of medication, it also welcomes the self-administration of medication and the administration of medication by carer. However, agreed polices and procedures on safety, security and storage arrangements must be in place before it can be implemented. In children's nursing, the majority of parents/carers are encouraged to participate in the administration of medication to their children. In addition, some children are able to self-administer if they have an appropriate level of understanding of their treatment. This is especially common in those children undergoing long-term treatment or those who have chronic conditions requiring the administration of therapeutic interventions. When undertaking this practice, accountability and communication must be defined clearly between child or parent/guardian and practitioner within an established policy. Children are often discharged home on prescribed medication regimens. There are obvious benefits to adjusting the responsibility to self/carer administration while still having professional support prior to the child and family being discharged (NMC 2007). However, although most children/carers are willing to participate in their or their child's treatment, there are occasions when they may wish to take a break from the responsibility. For those children or carers who wish to participate in the self-administration of medication, the responsibility and professional duty of the practitioner does not diminish. The practitioner's responsibility is to educate, train and assess the child or carer's competence in carrying out the task. When the child or carer achieves competence, the practitioner should ensure that the necessary support is provided and that their competence is regularly reviewed (refer to Standard 10, NMC 2007).

The legislation and guidelines are in place to ensure that practitioners are professionally responsible for their own actions and that they act in the best interests of the patient at all times (NMC 2007). Administering medication to children can be a real challenge, as well as having to have the ability to communicate with children of different ages and stages of development, the practitioner must also be familiar with the variety of routes for safe administration of medication.

The traditional role of nurses in drug administration is changing and evolving once again. According to Blatt (1997) nurse prescribing was first recommended by the Royal College of Nursing in 1980, and became part of the government's policy agenda in 1986 with the Cumberlege Report. Pilot sites were established and education provided to enable community nurses to prescribe. Following on from the success of these schemes, and the endorsement of the 1989 Crown Report (Department of Health 1989), meant that most district nurses were able to prescribe from a limited formulary. The 1989 Crown Report (DoH 1989) concluded that only district nurses and health visitors who were seen to have clear responsibility for care and management should be granted prescribing rights. Community psychiatric nurses and nurse specialists were excluded from this at the time because of their dual role within and without the acute setting, however it was suggested that certain specialist nurses might be permitted to prescribe specific items for a named group of patients. The 1999 Crown Report (DoH 1999) expanded upon this stating that new groups of professionals would be able to apply for the authority to prescribe in particular clinical areas but only if this would improve patient care and if patient safety could be assured. Two distinct groups of prescribers were identified at this time in this report:

1. **Independent Prescribers:** professionals who are responsible for the initial assessment of the patient and for devising the broad treatment plan, with the authority to prescribe the medicines required as part of that plan.
2. **Dependent Prescribers:** professionals who are authorised to prescribe certain medicines for patients whose condition has been diagnosed or assessed by an independent prescriber, within an agreed assessment treatment plan.

The preferred term for dependent prescriber is now 'supplementary prescriber' (DoH 2002).

Amendments to Prescription Only Medicines and changes to NHS regulations have been made to enable nurses and pharmacists to take on the role of independent prescriber. This change in role and responsibilities must be supported by appropriate education, accreditation and the maintenance of clinical competence. At the time of writing there are a number of education courses available, but none with a specific remit to educate professionals who specifically care for children. However, the National Prescribing Centre (2001) has produced a document outlining a framework for maintaining competency in prescribing, which could easily be adapted to suit individual needs. Change would seem to have stabilised with a number of practitioners in different specialities now undertaking prescribing courses to be independent prescribers. To keep up to date with the latest news, please refer to the DoH site: http://www.dh.gov.uk/en/Healthcare/Medicinespharmacyandindustry/Prescriptions/TheNon-MedicalPrescribingProgramme/Nurseprescribing/DH_099261.

This was last updated in 2010 with all the relevant documents to inform practice available in one place. In particular, the DoH (2006) document, *Medicines Matters*, is very useful as it presents the history and process of change, in a short concise document. Nurse prescribing must be considered a logical development of the expanded role of nurses. It is an exciting and much awaited change in policy that will see nursing being recognised as an autonomous profession (Jones 1999). As Gibson *et al* (2003) identified in a small local survey, nurses are already making decisions about medications where the need to encompass 'prescribing' in a role that emanated from a desire to improve the care given to children and their families.

Child development considerations

There are some basic principles which will facilitate ease of administration of medication:

- Be confident and firm.
- Approach the procedure, child and family with a positive attitude.
- Be honest and understanding.
- Allow the child to have some control (where appropriate).
- Use appropriate language that the child will understand.
- Explain to the child if appropriate what they will smell, taste, feel, see and hear.
- Listen to all involved.
- Explain the benefits of taking the medication.

Infants (1–12 months)

At this stage of development the infant is usually developing basic trust and a need to have their parents or carer near.

- Use sensory measures, i.e. touching of skin, talking softly.
- Provide comfort, i.e. a cuddle before, during and after administering the medication.
- If the infant has a familiar/favourite blanket or toy, have it nearby for comfort.
- Encourage parental/carer involvement.

Toddlers (1–3 years)

At this stage of development the toddler is developing their use of language slowly and remains very clearly attached to their parents/carer.

- Use a calm and confident approach and encourage the child to express their feelings.

- Use basic language that they will understand to explain what is going to happen, using toys/dolls, etc. and encourage them to role-play with their own toys.
- Give one instruction at a time, e.g. sit down.
- Prepare the child shortly or immediately before the administration.

Pre-schoolers (3–5 years)

By this stage the child has usually further developed the ability to communicate.

- Give simple explanations so the child understands what is going to happen and does not perceive it to be a punishment.
- Use a positive approach and statements/reinforcement, e.g. that they are good *at* taking the medicine not that they are good *for* taking the medicine.
- Allow the child some control by asking them to choose which vesicle they want to use or where and how they would like to position themselves.

School-age (6–12 years)

The child at this stage of development is self-aware and has an awareness of the environment, etc. around them. They have an understanding of illness and treatments.

- Give an explanation of what is going on using teaching dolls, models, diagrams, drawings, etc.
- Involve the child in the decision making and allow time to answer questions.
- Prepare in advance of administration and suggests ways of maintaining control, e.g. counting.

Adolescents

- Adolescents usually value their independence; however, at the same time they like to know someone is there to depend on. Always where appropriate involve them in the discussions about what is about to happen.
- Allow them to share the responsibility and decision making of their own treatment.
- Provide support and reassurance for the adolescent in their decision making as appropriate.

Drug calculations

Dose calculation in child health and adolescent medicine is usually based on either body surface area (mg/m^2) or body weight (mg/kg) of the child. Body weight is most commonly used because of simplicity and ease of calculation. The calcula-

tion of body surface area (BSA) requires both body weight and height, which is then applied to a nomogram (Figure 15.1). In 1998 the UK Chemotherapy Standardisation Group (CCLG) approved the use of the estimation of body surface area in infants and children based on weight alone. This has also been approved by the Drugs and Therapeutics Committee for use in GOSH whenever BSA is required. However, doses need to be modified in infants of **less than 10 kg** body weight.

Guidance for safe practice in paediatric drug calculation:

- Ensure all dosages are reviewed regularly as the child grows.
- Check whether the dose prescribed or stated in a formulary is in terms of a single dose ($mg/kg/dose$, $mg/m^2/dose$) or total daily dose (TDD). If total daily dose is used, then divide by the number of times the drug is to be administered.
- Remember to account for displacement volumes when reconstituting freeze-dried injections. If not, under dosing will be significant for drugs with large displacement volumes or when small doses are administered.
- Remember not to exceed maximum adult doses. For example:

Paracetamol 20 mg/kg/dose four times a day with a maximum of 1 gram/dose
Amikacin 10 mg/kg/dose twice a day with a maximum of 500 mg/dose twice a day for children over 50 kg.

- Discourage the use of decimal points. For example, 100 microgram instead of 0.1 milligram or 10 millimole and not 10.3 millimole. An error would result in a 10-fold difference in dosage, which could be fatal (Figure 15.1).
- Consider the presentation of drug, strength and form to encourage adherence and ease of administration for parents/carers and children.

The drug formula is:

$$\frac{\text{Dose required}}{\text{Present standard quantity of drug}} \times \begin{array}{c}\text{Present quantity of liquid} \\ \text{in which standard quantity} \\ \text{of drug is dissolved}\end{array} = \begin{array}{c}\text{Correct dosage} \\ \text{to be given}\end{array}$$

In other words:

$$\frac{\text{What you want}}{\text{What you have}} \times \text{What it is in (dilution)} = \begin{array}{c}\text{Correct dosage} \\ \text{to be given}\end{array}$$

For example:
A child is prescribed 90 mg of paracetamol and the medication supplied is 120 mg of paracetamol in 5 ml:

$$\frac{90}{120} \times \frac{5}{1} = 3.75\,ml$$

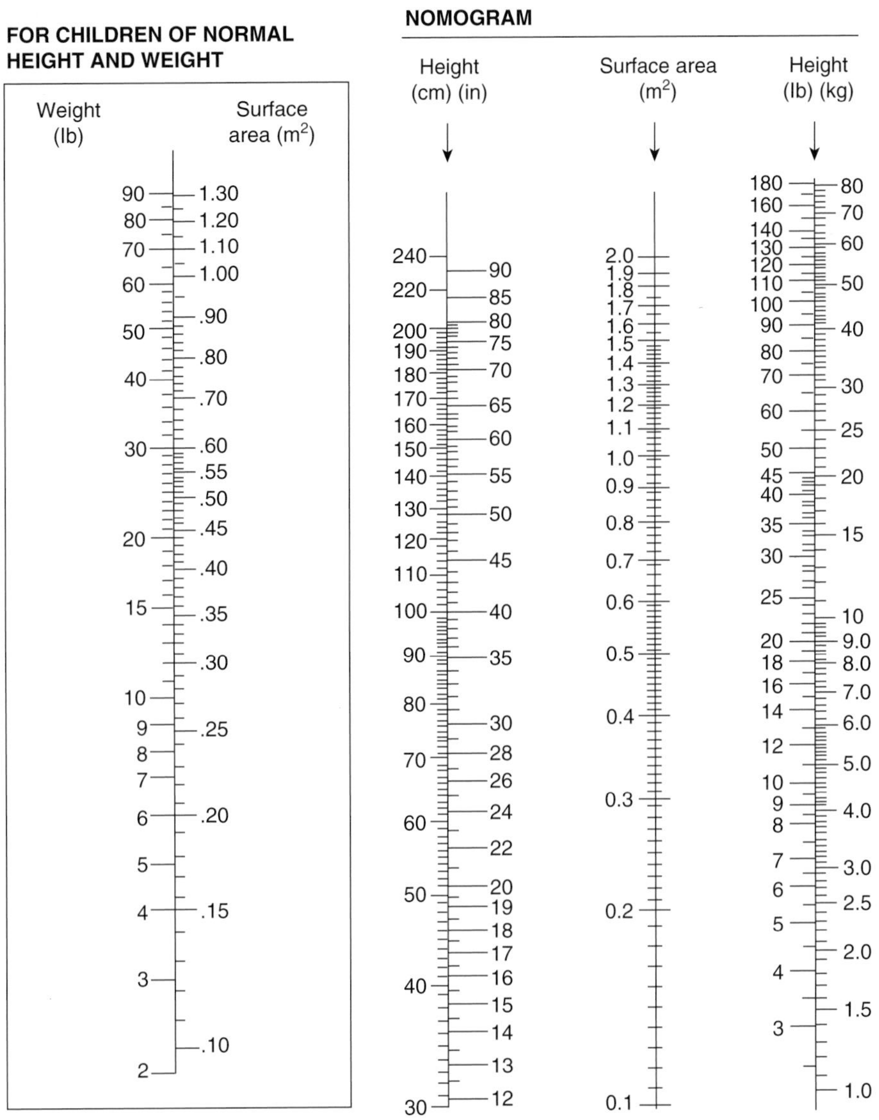
FOR CHILDREN OF NORMAL HEIGHT AND WEIGHT
Weight (lb)
Surface area (m2)
NOMOGRAM
Height (cm) (in)
Surface area (m2)
Height (lb) (kg)

BODY SURFACE AREA FORMULA
(Adult and Pediatric)

$$\text{BSA (m}^2) = \sqrt{\frac{\text{Ht (in)} \times \text{Wt (lb)}}{3131}} \quad \text{or, in metric: BSA (m}^2) = \sqrt{\frac{\text{Ht (cm)} \times \text{Wt (kg)}}{3600}}$$

Figure 15.1 Calculation of body surface area. Lam TK and Leung DT (1988) and Mosteller RD (1987). Reproduced with kind permission from the Massachusetts Medical Society.

Principles table 15.1 General guidelines

The following sections of this chapter provide details for the administration of medications via a number of different routes. For each route there are a number of general principles that need to be followed, the reader is requested to be familiar with the following principles to be applied in each situation.

Principle	Rationale
1. Refer to local policy for administration of medications.	**1.** To adhere to local policy.
2. Do not let yourself be distracted while dispensing and administering medications.	**2.** To reduce the risk of medication error.
3. Never administer medication you have not checked yourself.	**3.** To reduce the risk of medication error. It is unsafe practice.
4. Obtain equipment needed for the procedure.	**4.** To be adequately prepared for dispensing and administering medication.
5. Check the expiry date of all equipment, e.g. syringes.	**5.** To reduce the risk of harm to the child.
6. Refer to local guidelines on writing prescriptions. Check the prescription is clearly and correctly written. It should be written in full in capital letters, with no abbreviations and signed and dated by the practitioner prescribing the medication.	**6.** To adhere to local policy. To ensure the child is given the correct medication at the correct time. To reduce the risk of medication error. To reduce the risk of harm to the child. To adhere to NMC Guidelines for the administration of medication (2002).
7. Check the medication is required and has not already been given.	**7.** To prevent a medication error.
8. Check the child does not have any known allergy or contra-indication to the prescribed medication. If the child does, do not give the medication and inform the responsible prescriber immediately.	**8.** To reduce the risk of medication error. To reduce the risk of harm to the child. To enable the responsible prescriber to make a decision about the child's treatment.
9. Check in an approved medication formulary that the dose, route and frequency of the prescribed medication are accurate.	**9.** To reduce the risk of medication error and to reduce the risk of harm to the child.
10. If more than one medication is prescribed check they are compatible. If they are not compatible, do not give the medications and inform the responsible prescriber immediately.	**10.** To reduce the risk of medication error. To reduce the risk of harm to the child. To enable the responsible prescriber to make a decision about the child's treatment.
11. Remove the medication from the box/holding the canister and check the name, dose and expiry date of the medication's actual container, e.g. ampoule or canister/ inhaler, bottle label.	**11.** To prevent medication error and to ensure the packaging actually containing the medication has not been placed in the incorrect box and that the medication is the correct strength.
12. Wash your hands according to Standard (Universal) Precautions.	**12.** To reduce the risk of cross-infection.
13. Dispense the medication according to the child's prescription and local policy.	**13.** To prevent medication error.
14. Take the medication directly to child for administration.	**14.** To prevent tampering of medication. To prevent misuse of medication by others.

Principles table 15.1 (*Continued*)

Principle	Rationale
15. Do not attempt to administer the medication while the child is asleep or crying.	**15.** To promote the development of a trusting relationship. To reduce the risk of aspiration of medication.
16. Identify if the child has any previous experience of taking medication and if so what the experience was like.	**16.** To facilitate the provision of an appropriate explanation of the administration of the medication.
17a) Explain to the child using age and developmental appropriate language what medication is due and why. Explain this also to the parent/carer. **b)** Negotiate roles for the administration of the medication with the child and parent/carer.	**17a)** To allow time for child and parent/carer to ask questions and discuss any concerns. **b)** To work in partnership with the child and parent/guardian, as well as to obtain informed consent from the child and parent/carer.
18. Check that the name, date of birth and hospital number on the medication chart corresponds with the details on the child's name band. NB There are potential benefits and risks of *also* checking the child's identity with the parent/carer and or child. The nurse should consider this carefully.	**18.** To ensure the correct child receives the correct medication.
19. Where possible allow the child choice and control in the procedure, e.g. the child could choose between administering the medicine themselves or with assistance from their parent/carer or nurse. Be firm but fair with the child.	**19.** Child involvement and participation in decision making can help reduce anxiety and facilitate successful administration of medication.
20. Allow time for the child to take the medication.	**20.** Rushing the child could increase feelings of anxiety, which could result in the child refusing administration of the medication.
21. Provide positive reinforcement as appropriate during and following administration of medication.	**21.** To encourage the child to take the medication.
22. Assist the child in re-positioning (if required) to promote comfort following the administration of the medication.	**22.** To maintain the child's comfort.
23. Inform the responsible prescriber if the child refuses or is unable to take the medication. Document the incident in the appropriate area on the medication chart and in the child's health record.	**23.** To maintain the child's safety. To enable the responsible prescriber to make a decision about the child's treatment. To maintain accurate records.
24. Discard any unused medication according to trust protocol.	**24.** To prevent the misuse of unused medication by others.
25. Dispose of equipment according to trust protocol.	**25.** To reduce the risk of cross-infection.
26. Where appropriate remove gloves and always wash hands according to trust protocol.	**26.** To reduce the risk of cross-infection.
27. Sign for administration of the medication on the child's prescription chart after administration is completed	**27.** To maintain an accurate record of medication administered. To reduce the risk of medication being administered twice. To adhere to NMC guidelines for the administration of medication (2009). To adhere to NMC guidelines for records and record keeping (2009).

363

(Continued)

Principles table 15.1 (*Continued*)

Principle	Rationale
28. Observe, report and document any local reaction or abnormality in the case of injections.	**28.** To enable the responsible doctor to make a decision about the child's treatment, and to maintain accurate records.
29. Observe for and report immediately to the nurse in charge and responsible prescriber any adverse effects of the medication.	**29.** To facilitate early detection and action of any adverse effects of medication.

Oral administration

Medication administered orally passes down the digestive tract for absorption usually from the small intestine to the liver via the portal vein. After the medication has been metabolised by enzymes in the liver it enters the circulatory system, usually for systemic effect. However, some oral medication can have a local effect, e.g. oral antacids reduce the acidity of stomach contents while stimulant laxatives increase intestinal motility (British National Formulary 2010).

The oral route is the most common route of administration in children, this is for several reasons:

- It is generally associated with less pain and anxiety compared to other routes such as intra-muscular injections.
- It is often cheaper than other preparations like intravenous medication.
- Usually, less equipment is required which can make administration less time-consuming.
- Slower absorption of medication compared to other routes e.g. intravenous, allows more time to react should adverse reactions occur.

Considerations

The following should be taken into consideration when administering medicines orally:

- Refer to the responsible practitioner if the child is nil by mouth e.g. pre-operative fasting. In some circumstances the child may still be allowed to take the medication orally, while in others an alternative route of administration may need to be prescribed. NB The dose of medication may differ depending on the route of administration.
- Ensure the child's gag reflex is present and has the ability to maintain their airway in the presence of fluid.
- If the child is critically ill, note that gastric absorption of the medication may be slow and erratic.
- Unless contra-indicated, administer oral medication to a baby prior to a feed, in case of post-feed vomiting.
- Some oral medications such as non-steroidal anti-inflammatories, e.g. diclofenac sodium, can irritate the gastro-intestinal lining. Taking these oral medications during or after food or milk can prevent or partially reduce the irritation (British National Formulary 2010).

- The therapeutic effect of some oral medications can be inhibited by the presence of food/milk, e.g. ampicillin (British National Formulary 2010).
- The therapeutic dose of oral medication may vary depending on its preparation, e.g. 90 mg phenytoin suspension is equivalent to 100 mg tablet (Wright 2002).
- The therapeutic duration of effect of oral medication may also vary depending on its preparation, e.g. morphine suspension has a shorter duration of effect than modified release morphine tablets.
- Protective clothing should be worn when handling some medications, e.g. immunosuppressant and cytotoxic medication, (see Chapter 8 regarding cytotoxic medication).
- Refer to the manufacturer's guidelines and liaise with the ward pharmacist regarding the use of *some* intravenous preparations of medication, which are also suitable for oral administration.
- Some intravenous preparations of medication taste unpleasant, e.g. intravenous midazolam is bitter tasting (Guys, St Thomas' and Lewisham Hospital 2001).
- Child's developmental level and understanding can determine the method of administration, e.g. type of vesicle used such as oral syringe or spoon and form of oral medication such as suspension or tablet.
- Caution should be taken using syringes designed for intravenous use. Cousins and Upton (1998) identified a case where medication intended for oral administration was accidentally given intravenously.
- Some suspensions are very sugary and can cause dental caries with use over a prolonged period of time, consider sugar-free formulations if available.
- Some suspensions can taste extremely unpleasant, e.g. flucloxacillin (Guys, St Thomas' and Lewisham Hospital's Paediatric Formulary 2001).
- Consider alternatives if the volume of suspension is large, e.g. dissolvable tablets.
- Crushing tablets or opening capsules generally makes the mediation unlicensed for use (Wright 2002).
- While written authorisation by the prescriber for the crushing of tablets or opening of capsules is a legal requirement, the nurses administering the medication would share responsibility for any harm caused by this practice (Wright 2002).
- Some tablets are not suitable for crushing, e.g. enteric-coated tablets should **not** be crushed as the coating prevents the

release and absorption of the drug until it reaches the small intestine. Capsules should also not be broken or opened, the medication contained in the gelatin shell may be a slow-release preparation or particularly unpalatable.

- It is good practice to avoid crushing or dissolving tablets or capsules, however if it is necessary, care should be taken in order to deliver as safe and accurate dose as possible. This should include liaising with pharmacy and referring to manufacturer's guidelines.
- Do not break tablets in half in order to administer half the dose unless they are scored.
- Refer to the *BNF for Children* in all prescribing practices (BNF for Children 2010–11).

Contraindications

- Unconscious child
- Absent gag reflex
- Inability to swallow
- Vomiting.

Cautions

- Digestive tract trauma/illness
- Post digestive tract surgery
- Nil by mouth, e.g. pre-operative fasting
- Nausea.

Equipment

The following equipment should be prepared:

- Prescription chart
- Medication formulary
- Manufacturer's drug information (if required)
- Disposable medication tray
- Medication
- Medicine spoon/pot (with measured volumes)
- Oral syringe
- Cup/beaker or teat (if required)
- Tablet divider/mortar and pestle/tablet crusher
- Sterile water (for dissolving medication)
- Non-sterile gloves (if required).

Procedure guideline 15.1 Administration of oral medication

Statement	Rationale
1. Check the medication supplied is suitable for oral administration.	1. To reduce the risk of medical error and to reduce the risk of harm to the child.

2. Negotiate with the parent/carer and child regarding any decision to mix medications with food, e.g. remove the cream filling of a biscuit and mix the medication in the cream and place back between the biscuits.
  NB The potential benefits and risks of covert administration of medication in fluid or food should be considered carefully by the nurse and parent/carer (NMC 2008b).
	2. To promote development of a trusting relationship between the child and nurse.
	  To maintain trusting relationship between child and parent/carer
	  To promote ingestion of medication.
	  To reduce the risk of the child becoming fearful of medication being hidden in food or drinks.

3. If a choice is available, identify the child's preference for the form of oral medication, e.g. suspension or tablet and the type of vesicle to be used for administration.	3. To promote the development of a trusting relationship between the child, parent/carer and nurse. This also facilitates partnership working with the child and parent/carer.
4. Dispense medication into the appropriate vesicle without directly touching the medication with your hands.	4. To reduce the risk of cross-infection.
5. Do not force the medication vesicle into the child's mouth. The oral syringe/spoon can be inserted into the side of the mouth between the cheek and the gum, or alternatively the syringe/spoon placed onto the tip of the tongue.	5. To prevent oral trauma and also promote the development of a trusting relationship.
6a) Ensure the medication is administered slowly.	6a) To promote safe ingestion of medication.

(Continued)

Procedure guideline 15.1 (*Continued*)

Statement	Rationale
b) Gently stroking the cheek or under the chin may encourage the baby's sucking reflex.	**b)** To reduce the risk of the child spitting out the medication and to reduce the risk of aspiration of medication.
c) A medicine spoon can be used to retrieve any medicine spat/spilt on the chin.	**c)** To reduce the risk of spillage of medication.
7. Unless contraindicated, offer the child a flavoured drink or ice cube in-between and after ingestion of medication.	**7.** To promote ingestion of medication.

Enteral tube administration

Enteral tube administration of medication via feeding tubes placed either in the stomach or small intestine can provide systemic or local effect similar to oral administration depending on the position of the tube. There are numerous types of enteral tubes and different reasons why children may require them (see Chapter 19). This section will concentrate only on the general principles of administration of medication by enteral tubes. There is currently limited available research about administration of medication via enteral tubes (Cannaby *et al.* 2002) and therefore there could be potential for variation in nursing practice. The benefits of enteral tube administration of medication include:

- An alternative route of administration for children who are unable to take oral medications, e.g. the unconscious child
- Slower absorption of medication compared to some other routes, e.g. intravenous, allows more time to react should adverse reactions occur.

Considerations

- Oral and enteral tube administration of medication are different and should not be confused.
- Enteral tube administration of medication differs depending on the type and location of the tube.
- The majority of medications are not licensed for enteral administration (Wright 2002).
- Some medications are not suitable for enteral administration, e.g. liquid diazepam, which can be absorbed into the enteral tubing (Thompson *et al* 2000).
- The therapeutic effect of some medications can be inhibited by the presence of enteral feeds, e.g. phenytoin (Bauer 1982).
- Medications should not be added to enteral feeds because of the increased risk of tube blockage and current lack of research into other potential complications (Thompson *et al* 2000).
- Administration of crushed tablets or viscous suspensions should be avoided as they could block enteral tubes.
- If tablets are used, they should be crushed into a fine powder and thoroughly dissolved in water.
- Suspension medication with a high sorbital content or high osmolarity can cause bloating, stomach cramps and diarrhoea (Thompson *et al* 2000).

- Medication should not be administered to children who have enteral tubes on free drainage unless the drainage can be stopped for an appropriate amount of time following administration of the medication.
- Children requiring complete aspiration of stomach contents should not have medication administered prior to the procedure.
- If the child is critically ill, gastric absorption of medication maybe slow and erratic.
- Sterile water is usually used in hospitals for flushing enteral tubes after administration of medication. Cooled boiled water or tap water is sometimes used in the community setting for children over the age of 1 year – refer to local policies.
- The volume of medication and flush administered should be monitored and recorded, especially with children who are fluid restricted or require large amounts of medication.

Contra-indications

- Enteral tube in situ that must remain on continuous free drainage.

Caution

- Nil by mouth e.g pre-operative fasting
- Post-operative digestive tract surgery.

Equipment

The following equipment should be prepared:

- Prescription chart
- Medication formulary
- Manufacturers drug information
- Disposable medication tray
- Medication
- Syringes – appropriate size for dispensing medication plus 50 ml syringes for administration of medication and flush.
- Tablet divider/mortar and pestle/tablet crusher
- Sterile water (for dissolving medication and flush)
- Litmus paper/Universal indicator paper
- Non-sterile gloves
- Apron.

Procedure guideline 15.2 Enteral tube administration

Statement	Rationale
1. Check the medication supplied is suitable for enteral administration.	1. To reduce the risk of medical error and to reduce the risk of harm to the child.
2. Refer to the manufacturer's guidelines and liaise with the ward pharmacist.	2. To promote safe administration of medication. Some medications are not suitable for enteral administration. The dose of enteral administration of medication may be different than other routes of administration.
3. Refer to dietician.	3. To facilitate adequate hydration and nutrition, e.g. the dietician may need to alter the feed regimen to allow for the enteral feeds to be stopped for a specified time for administration of incompatible medication, or in the fluid restricted patient alter the volume/type of feeds to allow for the volume of medication and flush administered.
4. Dispense the medication without directly touching it with your hands.	4. To reduce the risk of cross-infection.
5. If the required volume of a medication is too small to put in a 50 ml syringe, liaise with a pharmacist regarding diluting the required amount of medication further with sterile water. NB Caution should be taken when administering to a child who has fluids restricted.	5. Using smaller syringes causes increased pressure, which could damage the enteral tube (Cannaby et al 2002).
6. If the medication is viscous, liaise with the pharmacist regarding alternative preparations of the medication or dissolving the suspension further with sterile water. Also consider flushing the tube with sterile water half-way through administering the medication. NB Caution should be taken when administering to a child who has fluids restricted.	6. To reduce the risk of enteral tube blockage.
7. Record volume of medication and flush on the child's fluid balance chart.	7. To maintain accurate fluid balance chart.

8. **Orogastric/nasogastric tube:**
   a) Check the tube is in the correct position prior to feeding by testing aspirate with litmus paper (see Chapter 19). If unable to obtain aspirate for testing, use alternative method of testing in accordance with local protocol.
   b) Flush the tube with 5–10 ml of sterile water, depending on the length of the tube and the child's fluid balance.
   c) Administer the medication slowly.
   d) Stop administering the medication if aspiration is suspected and inform the nurse in charge/responsible prescriber.
   e) Flush the tube with 5–10 ml of sterile water between medications, depending on the length of the tube and the child's fluid balance.
   f) Flush the tube with 5–10 ml of sterile water after administration of medications depending on the length of the tube and the child's fluid balance.
	8.
	   a) To promote safe administration of medication.
	
	   b) To ensure the tube is clear for administration of medication and to reduce the risk of tube blockage.
	   c) To reduce the risk of aspiration of medication.
	   d) To promote early detection and prompt action of complications.
	
	   e) To reduce the risk of tube blockage.
	
	   f) To reduce the risk of medication remaining in the tube resulting in the child not receiving an accurate dose of medication at the prescribed time.

367

(Continued)

Procedure guideline 15.2 (*Continued*)

Statement	Rationale
9. Naso-duodenal /naso-jejunal tube: **a)** Liaise with the pharmacist as many medicines are not suitable for naso-duodenal/naso-jejunal administration. **b)** Check the tube is in the correct position prior to feeding by testing aspirate with universal indicator paper. (See Chapter 22.) If unable to obtain aspirate for testing, use alternative method of testing in accordance with hospital protocol. **c)** Flush the tube with 5–10 ml of sterile water depending on the length of the tube and the child's fluid balance. **d)** Administer the medication slowly. **e)** Stop administering the medication if aspiration is suspected and inform the nurse in charge/responsible prescriber. **f)** Flush the tube with 5–10 ml of sterile water between medications, depending on the length of the tube and the child's fluid balance. **g)** Flush the tube with 5–10 ml of sterile water after administration of medications depending on the length of the tube and the child's fluid balance.	**9.** **a)** To promote safe administration of medication. **b)** To reduce the risk of a medical error and to reduce the risk of harm to the child. **c)** To reduce the risk of aspiration of medication and to promote early detection and prompt action of the complications, as well as ensuring the tube is clear for administration of medication. **d)** To reduce the risk of tube blockage and to promote safe administration of medication. **e)** To reduce the risk of aspiration of medication and to promote early detection and prompt action of the complications. **f)** To reduce the risk of tube blockage. **g)** To reduce the risk of medication remaining in the tube resulting in the child not receiving accurate dose of medication at prescribed time and to reduce the risk of tube blockage.
10. Gastrostomy: **a)** Flush the tube with 10–20 ml sterile water depending on the length of the tube and the child's fluid balance. **b)** Administer the medication slowly. **c)** Stop administering the medication if aspiration is suspected and inform the nurse in charge/responsible prescriber. **d)** Flush the tube with 10–20 ml of sterile water between medications depending on the length of the tube and the child's fluid balance. **e)** Flush the tube with 10–20 ml of sterile water after administration of medications depending on the length of the tube and the child's fluid balance.	**10.** **a)** To check the tube is patent and clear for administration of medication, and to promote safe administration of medication. **b)** To reduce the risk of aspiration of medication. **c)** To promote early detection and prompt action of the complications. **d)** To reduce the risk of tube blockage. **e)** To reduce the risk of medication remaining in the tube resulting in the child not receiving accurate dose of medication at prescribed time and to reduce the risk of tube blockage.
11. Jejunostomy: **a)** Liaise with the ward pharmacist as many medicines are *not* suitable for jejunostomy administration. **b)** Flush the tube with 10–20 ml of sterile water depending on the length of the tube and the child's fluid balance. **c)** Administer the medication slowly. **d)** Stop administering the medication if aspiration is suspected and inform the nurse in charge/responsible prescriber. **e)** Flush the tube with 10–20 ml of sterile water between medications, depending on the length of the tube and the child's fluid balance. **f)** Flush the tube with 10–20 ml of sterile water after administration of medications depending on the length of the tube and the child's fluid balance.	**11.** **a)** To promote safe administration of medication and to reduce the risk of a medical error. To reduce the risk of harm to the child. **b)** To ensure the tube is clear for administration of medication and to reduce the risk of tube blockage. **c)** To promote the safe administration of medication and to reduce the risk of aspiration of medication. **d)** To promote early detection and prompt action of the complications. **e)** To reduce the risk of medication remaining in the tube resulting in the child not receiving accurate dose of medication at prescribed time. **f)** To reduce the risk of tube blockage.

Buccal and sublingual administration

The administration of buccal medication can be used for local or systemic effect; it involves administering medication between the facial cheek and upper or lower gum for absorption by the buccal mucous membranes. Sublingual medication is only administered for systemic effect and involves administering medication into the space under the child's tongue for absorption by the sublingual mucous membranes. The onset of action for administration of sublingual medicine is faster than the buccal route but has a shorter duration of effect (Pinnell 1996). Both the buccal and sublingual routes of administration of medication appear to be used less frequently in children. However, they can have a number of benefits including:

- More rapid absorption of medication compared with oral and intra-muscular routes
- An alternative route of administration for some medications when there is no intravenous access
- They are generally associated with less pain and anxiety compared with other routes such as intra-muscular injections
- They are less invasive than some other routes of administration, e.g. rectal
- Usually, less equipment is required which can make administration less time-consuming.

Considerations

- *Buccal and sublingual forms of medication and administration are different and should not be confused.*
- There is currently limited availability of medication suitable for buccal and sublingual administration.
- The therapeutic dose and duration of effect of buccal or sublingual medication may be different than with other routes of administration.
- Tablet form of the buccal and sublingual medication is only suitable for children who understand that the tablet should be allowed to dissolve and not chewed or swallowed.
- Liquid form of buccal or sublingual medication should be carefully administered in small amounts to reduce the risk of

swallowing or aspirating the medication especially in children with an absent gag reflex.
- Large volumes of medication may not suitable for buccal and sublingual administration.
- Refer to manufacturer's guidelines and liaise with the ward pharmacist regarding the use of *some* intravenous preparations of medication, which may be suitable for buccal or sublingual administration. NB Some intravenous preparations of medication taste unpleasant.
- Unpleasant tasting medications may affect the child's adherence with administration of the medication.
- Prolonged or repeated administration could potentially cause deterioration in the buccal/sublingual cavity.

Contra-indications and cautions

There currently does not appear to be any readily available documented contra-indications or cautions for buccal and sublingual administration of medication. However, it could be suggested that the following conditions should be discussed with the responsible prescriber prior to administration of buccal or sublingual medication:

- Oral trauma
- Post-operative maxio-facial surgery
- Buccal or sublingual abrasions or lesions.

Equipment

The following equipment should be prepared:

- Prescription chart
- Medication formulary
- Manufacturer's drug information
- Disposable medication tray
- Medication
- Oral syringe (for liquid form of medication)
- Medicine spoon (for tablet form of medication)
- Non-sterile gloves
- Apron.

Procedure guideline 15.3 Buccal and sublingual administration

Statement	Rationale
1. Check the medication supplied is suitable for buccal or sublingual administration, (depending on the route of administration prescribed and preparation of medication).	1. To reduce the risk of medical error and to reduce the risk of harm to the child.
2. Draw up suspension medication into an appropriate size syringe, e.g. a 1 ml syringe calibrated with 0.1 ml increments for doses less than 1 ml.	2. To facilitate accurate measurement and administration of medication.
3. If the tablet form of medication is being used dispense the tablet into a medicine pot or spoon without touching it.	3. To reduce the risk of cross-infection. In addition, contact with skin could initiate breakdown of the medication.

(Continued)

Procedure guideline 15.3 (*Continued*)

Statement	Rationale
4. Allow time for the child to take the medication.	**4.** Rushing the child could increase feelings of anxiety, which could result in the child refusing administration of the medication.
5. Advise the child not to swallow the medication.	**5.** To promote safe administration and absorption of the medication.
6. Check the condition of the child's buccal or sublingual area (depending on the route of administration prescribed). Refer to the responsible prescriber if abrasions or lesions are observed.	**6.** To reduce the risk of harm to the child. To enable the responsible prescriber to make a decision about the child's treatment.
7. Do not force the syringe containing the liquid preparation of medication into the child's mouth.	**7.** To reduce the risk of oral trauma, as well as to promote a trusting relationship.
8. Buccal administration: **a)** Slowly administer small amounts of liquid medication between the child's facial cheek and upper or lower gum. Administer half of the medication on each side of the mouth. If the tablet form is being used, place the tablet in between the child's facial cheek and lower gum.	**8.** **a)** To reduce the risk of the medication being swallowed. To reduce the risk of aspiration of the medication. To reduce the risk of the child spitting out the medication.
9. Sublingual administration: Place the tablet preparation or slowly administer small amounts of the liquid medication into the space under the child's tongue.	**9.** To reduce the risk of spillage of the medication. To promote safe absorption of the medication.
10. Ensure the child does not have any oral fluid or food until all the medication has been absorbed.	**10.** To promote successful absorption of the medication.

Intranasal administration

Medication absorbed through mucous membranes in the nasal cavities can be used for local and systemic effect. Decongestive, corticosteriods and antibiotic medications are sometimes administered this way for local effect while other medications such as desmospression are administered for systemic effect.

The administration of medication by the intranasal route can have a number of benefits including:

- More rapid absorption of medication compared with the oral and intra-muscular routes
- An alternative route of administration for some medications when there is no intravenous access
- It is generally associated with less pain and anxiety compared with other routes such as intravenous and intra-muscular injections.
- It is less invasive than some other routes of administration, e.g. rectal

- Usually, less equipment is required, which can make administration less time-consuming.

Considerations

- There is currently limited availability of medication suitable for intra-nasal administration.
- The therapeutic dose of intranasal medication may be different from other routes of medication.
- Medication swallowed after intranasal adminstration could result in delayed or neurotoxic complications (Berlin *et al* 1997).

Contra-indications and cautions

- Nasal trauma
- Post-operative nasal surgery
- Nasal infection or discharge
- Epistaxis.

Equipment

The following equipment should be prepared:

- Prescription chart
- Medication formulary
- Manufacturer's drug information

- Disposable medication tray
- Medication
- Syringe (if medication is not in spray/dropper form)
- Gauze/tissue
- Non-sterile gloves
- Apron.

Procedure guideline 15.4 Intranasal administration

Statement	Rationale
1. Check the medication supplied is suitable for nasal administration.	1. To reduce the risk of medical error and to reduce the risk of harm to the child.
2. Check the condition of the child's nostrils. Refer to the responsible prescriber if any abrasions, lesions or other contraindications are observed.	2. To reduce the risk of harm to the child. Also enable the responsible prescriber to make a decision about the child's treatment.
3. If appropriate ask the child to gently blow their nose to clear any congestion.	3. To promote safe administration of the medication.
4. **Intranasal spray** a) Intranasal medication in spray form should be labelled with the child's name and hospital number and for individual use only. b) Ensure the spray nozzle is primed before use. c) Assist the child as necessary in repositioning for administration of medication. Unless contraindicated by their condition or treatment, the child should be assisted to sit or stand upright with their head upright or neck hyperextended. d) Do not force the nozzle into the child's nostrils. Block one nostril and insert the spray nozzle gently into the opposite nostril (just inside at the midline) and administer one spray. If more than one spray is prescribed both nostrils should be used. If appropriate ask the child to gently inhale the medication into the nostril as the spray is squeezed. e) Refer to manufacturer's guidelines regarding cleaning the spray nozzle.	4. a) To reduce the risk of cross-infection and to promote safe administration of the medication. b) To reduce the risk of leakage of the medication. c) To reduce the risk of nasal trauma and to facilitate safe administration of intranasal medication. d) Touching the external nares could stimulate sneezing. e) To reduce the risk of infection
5. **Intranasal dropper** a) Intranasal medication in dropper form should be labelled with the child's name and hospital number and for individual use only. b) Assist the child as necessary in repositioning for administration of medication. Unless contraindicated by their condition or treatment, the child should be assisted to either lie supine with the neck hyper extended or sit with their back tilted backwards and neck hyperextended. A pillow can be placed behind the child's neck to assist with positioning and comfort. c) Do not force the dropper into the child's nostrils. The dropper should be positioned at the midline entry of the nostril and the rubber top of the dropper squeezed to administer one drop into the nostril. If more than one drop is prescribed both nostrils should be used.	5. a) To reduce the risk of cross-infection and to promote safe administration of the medication. b) To reduce the risk of nasal trauma and to promote safe intranasal administration of medication. c) Touching the external nares could stimulate sneezing.

371

(Continued)

Procedure guideline 15.4 (*Continued*)

Statement	Rationale
6. Intranasal medication via syringe **a)** Draw up the suspension medication into an appropriate size syringe.	**6.** **a)** To facilitate accurate measurement and administration of medication and to promote safe administration of the medication.
b) Assist the child as necessary in repositioning for administration of medication. Unless contraindicated by their condition or treatment, the child should be assisted to either lie supine with the neck hyperextended or sit with their back tilted backwards and neck hyperextended. A pillow can be placed behind the child's neck to assist with positioning and comfort.	**b)** To reduce the risk of leakage of the medication.
c) Do not force the syringe into the child's nostrils. **d)** Gently insert the tip of the syringe at the midline of the nostril and administer small amounts of the medication slowly. Administer half of the medication into each nostril.	**c)** To reduce the risk of nasal trauma. **d)** To promote safe intranasal absorption of medication, to reduce the risk of leakage to the medication. Touching the external nares could stimulate sneezing.
7. Encourage the child not to blow their nose until all the medication has been absorbed.	**7.** To promote safe intranasal absorption of medication and to reduce the risk of leakage of the medication
8. Use gauze or tissue to wipe any observed leakage following administration of medication and inform the responsible prescriber. Document the incident in the appropriate area on the medication chart and in the child's health record.	**8.** To maintain the child's safety. To enable the responsible prescriber to make a decision about the child's treatment. To maintain accurate records.

Inhalation administration

The inhalation method of administration of medication is when fine particles of medication are delivered by either nebulisation or aerosolisation. These routes of administration are primarily used for local effects to the respiratory tract, although in some of the medications a systemic response is produced. The aim of inhalation therapy, is to reverse or prevent airway inflammation and constriction in order to control symptoms and maximise respiratory flow (National Institute for Clinical Excellence 2002). Nebulisation is the passing of air or oxygen (if required) through a solution of medication to form a fine spray, e.g. sodium chloride, antibiotics or bronchodilators. These are commonly used in the treatment of respiratory tract conditions, e.g. acute asthma, cystic fibrosis. Aerosolisation means that the medication comes in an inert diluent, either in the form of solution or powder (inhalers), which passes a measured amount of medication through a valve under pressure, delivering the medication to the patient in a controlled measured dose and particle size, in a very fine spray, e.g. bronchodilators or steroids. With this method, although a minimal amount of medication is administered, the concentration at the site is high. This usually achieves effective and rapid control of symptoms without the side effects associated with other systemic routes of administration, e.g. intravenous, of the same medication. This is commonly used for treating acute or chronic asthma.

Benefits

- Delivers the medication directly to where it is required.
- Usually achieves control of symptoms with fewer side effects.

Considerations

- The patient should be assessed prior to, during and post administration of medication to establish the effectiveness of the treatment and the child's tolerance.
- Avoid flexion or hyperextension of the neck, as these positions can cause tracheal compression (Hazinski 1992).
- If a child has severe airway obstruction or a depressed level of consciousness, effective administration can be compromised.

Nebuliser

- The nebuliser solution for administration usually needs to be further diluted according to manufacturer's recommendations and have an air or oxygen (if required) flow of between 8–10 litres per minute in order to produce adequate droplet formation.
- Some nebuliser types are more suitable for specific drugs and there are special connectors available for connecting nebulisers to ventilator tubing.
- The air or oxygen can be delivered via a bottle or piped gas supply or a compressor.
- The use of oxygen instead of air is dependent on the child's condition.
- An appropriate sized mask or mouthpiece attached to the nebuliser pot should be used. If neither of these attachments is used, the dose of medication administered to the child can be significantly reduced as the medication can escape into the surrounding atmosphere.

Aerosoliser (inhalers)

- There are a variety of different inhaler devices on the market that offer different features, each has its own advantages and disadvantages. Selecting a suitable device for the administration of inhalation medication for a child depends on their:
  - age group (their fine and motor skills and understanding)
  - respiratory function
  - complexity of their treatment – including history of condition
  - lifestyle – portability, convenience, stigma
  - adherence to treatment
  - inhaler technique.
- There are three main types of inhalers devices, press and breathe pressurised metered dose inhalers (pMDIs), breathe-actuated pressurised metered dose aerosol inhalers and dry powder inhalers (DPIs) (NICE) 2000)
  - Press and breathe pressurised metered dose inhalers (pMDIs) – this is where the user presses down (actuation) on the metal container (held in a plastic cover) which releases the medication in a pressurised metered dose and breathes in. This requires actuation-inhalation coordination (NICE 2000).
  - Breathe-activated pressurised metered dose inhalers – delivers a pressurised aerosol metered dose of medication which is automatically activated when the user inhales through the mouthpiece. Unlike the press and breathe inhaler, this device does not require the actuation-inhalation coordination.

    However, adherence could be difficult as the sound and sensation of the automatic actuation may differ from other devices (NICE 2002).
  - Dry powder inhalers (DPIs) – this is another breathe-activated inhaler, as the user inhales, a dose of micronised medication in an inert powder is delivered. Like the breathe-activated inhaler, actuation-inhalation coordination is not required. However, some children may find it difficult to exert a high enough inspiration in order to deliver an effective dose and this may also present a problem for children who are in acute respiratory distress. There are a variety of DPI devices available and some children may find one DPI device easier to use than another (NICE 2002).
  - Spacers – There are currently two general types of spacer systems available, which directly attach to the pMDIs, to resolve some of the problems associated with these inhalers. Detachable chambers (small, medium or large volume) – this type is attached to the press and breathe pMDIs mouthpiece when required. The spacer acts as a holding chamber for the aerosol and medication, which allows the child to take in the medication over several breaths. As this system has a valve system, it is imperative that the inhalation technique is taught (NICE 2002).

    Small-volume extended mouthpiece spacers – these provide an increased distance between the point of release of the medication and the oropharyngeal area. This type of spacer can be used with press and breathe and breathe-actuated pMDIs (NICE 2002).

    Detachable plastic chamber spacers are prone to developing a build up of static, which can cause an adhesion of the medication, which could reduce delivery. Following manufacturer's guidelines, careful washing and allowing to dry at appropriate intervals can reduce this problem (NICE 2002)
- For children under 5 years old, a pMDI should be used with a spacer device and facemask. If this is not effective, nebulisation should be considered or if the child is 3–5 year olds, a DPI could also be considered. In this age group, the type of device should be governed by the child's specific need and the child's and/or their parent/carer's adherence to the treatment regimen (NICE 2000)
- NICE (2002) have made the following recommendations on selecting an inhaler device for children aged between 5 and 15 years old with asthma, individual training on the use of a specific inhaler device/devices influences the effective delivery of inhalation therapy. The child should have regular monitoring (once a year) of their inhaler technique, to assess its effectiveness, adherence to therapy and review of their inhaler need, which may change with increasing age or child's condition or preference (NICE 2002). The education and training of the child's parent/carer is also important in this age group, as this can influence the effectiveness of, and the child's adherence to, the inhalation treatment
- A suitable spacer device is recommended for the use of corticosteroids in daily therapy, in order to achieve maximum benefit of the preventive therapy and minimising potential systemic absorption
- Most pMDIs have approximately 200 actuations and each canister should be checked as they come in different strengths. Ensure the inhaler is primed before use
- Establish history of the child's condition and the therapeutic interventions they have undergone, this may influence what type of inhalation therapy to administer, if required
- If a child is using the mouthpiece of inhaler device, the inhaler should be labelled with the child's name and hospital number and for individual use only.

Contra-indications

- Airway obstruction
- A depressed level of consciousness (unless ventilated).

Cautions

- Oral/maxio-facial surgery
- Artificial airways
- Severely compromised airways, i.e. acute inflammation of the airway – croup, epiglottitis
- Flexion and hyperextension of the neck
- History of ingestion or inhalation of a foreign body or volatile chemical
- Congenital malformations or trauma of the head, neck or chest
- Recent history of general anaesthesia or sedation
- Generalised muscle weakness, e.g. Guillain–Barré syndrome.

373

Equipment

The following equipment should be prepared:

- Prescription chart
- Medication formulary
- Manufacturer's drug information
- Disposable medication tray
- Medication and diluent (if required)
- Inhaler with spacer and mask (if required) or nebuliser pot and mask or mouthpiece
- Non-sterile gloves
- Apron.

Procedure guideline 15.5 Inhalation administration

Statement	Rationale
1. Check the medication supplied is suitable for inhalation administration.	**1.** To reduce the risk of medical error and to reduce the risk of harm to the child.
2. Assess the child's respiratory function, e.g. respiratory rate and effort, skin colour etc, prior to the administration of the medication.	**2.** To ensure that the child receives the correct medication if required.
3. Nebuliser	**3.**
a) Dispense the correct amount of nebulise solution into the nebuliser pot. Further dilute to a volume as recommended by the manufacturers. Prepacked nebules may also need to be further diluted to approximately 4 ml.	**a)** To promote the absorption of the medication.
b) Assist the child as necessary in repositioning for administration of medication. Unless contraindicated by their condition or treatment, they should be assisted to sit upright with their head forward.	**b)** To promote the absorption of the medication and increase lung capacity.
c) Connect the nebuliser to either the mask or mouthpiece and then to the tubing. Connect the tubing (connected to the nebuliser pot) to the gas supply or compressor.	**c)** To promote safe administration of the medication.
d) Place the mouthpiece in the child's mouth, ensuring the child seals their mouth around the mouthpiece or place the mask gently over the child's mouth and nose. The nebuliser pot should remain vertical/upright throughout the nebulisation.	**d)** To promote absorption of the medication.
e) Turn the air or oxygen flow to 8–10 litres per minute.	**e)** To promote the safe delivery of the medication.
f) Encourage the child to breathe in and out slowly and gently, if appropriate for their age and development.	**f)** To promote absorption of the medication.
g) Occasionally gently tap the nebuliser pot during the administration until all the solution has evaporated.	**g)** To ensure the large droplets are shaken down and the medication is delivered.
h) Observe and document the child's condition during and after the administration of medication.	**h)** To monitor the effectiveness of the treatment.
i) When administration is complete, the child should rinse their mouth.	**i)** To reduce systemic absorption of the medication.
j) After administration, either discard the nebuliser pot or dismantle and wash it according to manufacturer's guidelines, allow to dry and store for the child's use only.	**j)** To reduce the risk of infection.

Procedure guideline 15.5 *(Continued)*

Statement	Rationale

4. Inhaler with small volume extended mouthpiece spacer (*baby or toddler/under 5 years old*)

a) Position the baby or toddler lying supine.

b) Attach the appropriate size mask to the spacer mouthpiece if required.

c) Remove the protective cap from the inhaler device, shake the inhaler thoroughly and insert into the back of spacer.

d) Place the mouthpiece of the spacer in the child's mouth and ensure they seal their lips around the mouthpiece or position the mask gently over the baby/toddler's nose and mouth and form a seal.

e) Encourage the child to breathe in and out slowly and gently, if appropriate for their age and development. A whistling sound may be heard if the child breathes too quickly. However, this sound may not be heard if using a small volume extended mouthpiece with a mask. When this is established, actuate the medication inhaler once, with your free hand.

f) Hold the spacer in position, whilst the child takes several breaths. Then remove from the child's mouth.

g) Wait for 30 seconds, prior to administering a second dose if required, repeat points d–f.

h) When administration is complete, rinse the child's mouth.

4.

a) To promote the safe delivery of the medication.

b) To promote absorption of the medication.

c) To promote the safe delivery of the medication.

d) To promote absorption of the medication.

e) To promote the safe delivery of the medication, to promote absorption of the medication.

f) To reduce systemic absorption of the medication.

g) To promote the absorption of the medication and increase lung capacity.

h) To promote the safe delivery of the medication.

5. Inhaler with small volume extended mouthpiece spacer (*child/ 5–15 years old*)

a) Assist the child as necessary in repositioning for administration of medication. Unless contraindicated by their condition or treatment, they should be assisted to sit upright or stand upright.

b) Attach the appropriate size mask to the spacer mouthpiece, if required.

c) Remove the protective cap from the inhaler device. Shake the inhaler thoroughly and insert it into the back of the spacer. Place the mouthpiece of the spacer in the child's mouth and ensure they seal their lips around the mouthpiece or position the mask gently over the child's nose and mouth and form a seal. Actuate the medication inhaler once, to release a dose of medication.

d) Encourage the child to take a slow deep breath in. A whistling sound may be heard if the child breathes too quickly. However, this sound may not be heard if using a small volume extended mouthpiece with a mask. Encourage the child to hold their breath for about 10 seconds, then breathe out through the mouthpiece and to breathe in again but not to actuate the inhaler and release another dose of medication. Then remove the mouthpiece from the child's mouth and ask them to breathe out. Wait for a few seconds, before administering a second dose if required, repeat points c and d.

e) When administration is complete, the child should rinse their mouth.

5.

a) To promote the safe delivery of the medication.

b) To promote absorption of the medication.

c) To promote absorption of the medication.

d) To reduce systemic absorption of the medication and promote the absorption of the medication and increase lung capacity.

e) To reduce risk of cross-infection.

375

(Continued)

Procedure guideline 15.5 (Continued)

Statement	Rationale
6. Pressurised metered dose inhaler (pMDIs)	**6.**
a) When not using spacers, inhaler devices should be labelled with the child's name and hospital number and for individual use only.	**a)** To promote the safe delivery of the medication.
b) Assist the child as necessary in repositioning for administration of medication. Unless contraindicated by their condition or treatment, they should be assisted to sit upright or stand upright. Remove protective cap from the inhaler device. Shake the inhaler thoroughly. Ask the child to breathe out. Then place the mouthpiece of the inhaler in their mouth and ensure they seal their lips around the mouthpiece. Encourage them to take a slow deep breath in, simultaneously pressing the inhaler once, on inhalation. To hold their breath for about 5–10 seconds.	**b)** To promote the safe delivery of the medication and promote absorption of the medication.
c) Then remove the device from their mouth and ask them to breathe out.	**c)** To reduce systemic absorption of the medication.
d) Wait for a few seconds, prior to administering a second dose if required, repeat points b and c.	**d)** To reduce risk of cross-infection.
e) When administration is complete, the child should rinse their mouth.	**e)** To promote the absorption of the medication and increase lung capacity.
7. Breathe-actuated pressurised metered dose inhaler or dry powder inhalers (DPIs)	**7.**
a) When not using spacers, inhaler devices should be labelled with the child's name and hospital number and for individual use only. Assist the child as necessary in repositioning for administration of medication. Unless contraindicated by their condition or treatment, they should be assisted to sit upright or stand upright. Remove protective cap from the inhaler device. Shake the inhaler thoroughly or pre-load the dry powder inhaler. Ask the child to breathe out. Place the mouthpiece of the inhaler in their mouth and ensure they seal their lips around the mouthpiece.	**a)** To promote the safe delivery of the medication.
b) Encourage them to take a sharp deep breath in. To hold their breath for about 5–10 seconds. Then remove the device from their mouth and breathe out.	**b)** To promote absorption of the medication.
c) Wait for a few seconds, prior to administering a second dose if required, repeat points a and b.	**c)** To promote absorption of the medication.
d) When administration complete, the child should rinse their mouth.	**d)** To reduce systemic absorption of the medication.

Rectal administration

Rectal medications are available in different forms and can have systemic or local effect. For example, anti-inflammatory medication can provide local effect for ulcerative colitis (Rang *et al* 2003), while other medications such as analgesia, antibiotics and anticonvulsants give a systemic effect.

Suppositories are solid forms of medication, which dissolve through the rectal mucosa at body temperature (Smith-Temple and Johnson 1994). An enema is the term used for rectal admin-

istration of a solution. There are several different types , including medicated enemas, which are also absorbed through the rectal mucosa, and cleansing enemas used for evacuation of the large intestine. This section will focus on the administration of suppositories and medicated enemas.

The benefits of rectal administration of medication include:

- An alternative route of administration for some medications if the child either cannot have the oral form of medication or if there is no intravenous access

- It is generally associated with less pain compared with other routes such as intra-muscular injections.

Considerations

- There is currently a limited variance of medication strength in rectal form. Suppositories should not be cut in half, as there is no guarantee of the dosing accuracy (Pinnell, 1996).
- If a smaller dose of an enema is prescribed the volume should be measured and not estimated.
- Medicated enemas provide more rapid absorption than suppositories.
- The therapeutic dose of rectal medication may be different than other routes of administration. For example, a higher dose of Diazepam is usually prescribed when administered rectally instead of intravenously for the treatment of seizures (British National Formulary 2010).
- The presence of faeces in the large intestine can delay or inhibit absorption of medication.
- Some children do not like to receive medications using the rectal route.
- Some cultural and religious beliefs may oppose rectal administration of medication.
- Rectal administration of medications should be avoided if there is a history of child abuse.
- The child's privacy and dignity should be maintained at all times.
- Consider having a chaperone present during administration of rectal medication.

Contra-indications

- Diarrhoea
- Certain bowel conditions, e.g. imperforate anus
- In the post-operative period of some bowel surgery, e.g. Duhammal Pull Through
- Peri-anal injury, e.g. abrasions and lesions
- Immunosuppressed child (Berlin *et al* 1997)
- Cardiac arrhythmia (Downey and Tortorice 2003).

Caution

Discuss with the responsible doctor administration of rectal medication if the child has:

- A rectal stump
- Any history of bowel, cardiac or haematological disorder
- Constipation. (NB Not a caution for laxative suppositories.)

Equipment

The following equipment should be prepared:

- Prescription chart
- Medication formulary
- Manufacturer's drug information
- Disposable medication tray
- Medication
- Water-soluble lubricant or warm water
- Incontinence pad
- Non-sterile gloves and apron.

377

Procedure guideline 15.6 Rectal administration

Statement	Rationale
1. Check the medication supplied is suitable for rectal administration.	1. To reduce the risk of medical error.
2. Advise the child to open their bowels if necessary and appropriate prior to administration of rectal medication.	2. To reduce the risk of expulsion of rectal medication and to promote absorption of medication.
3. Apply non-sterile gloves and apron.	3. To reduce the risk of cross-infection.
4. Assist the child as necessary in repositioning for administration of the medication. Unless contraindicated by condition or treatment ask the child to lie on their left side with their left leg in a flexed position. Babies can also be positioned supine with their legs elevated and flexed.	4. To promote safe administration of the medication. To propitiate insertion of suppository or enema. To reduce risk of harm to the child.
5. Check the condition of the peri-anal area. Do not administer the medication if abrasions, lesions or any abnormality are observed. Inform the responsible doctor immediately.	5. To reduce the risk of harm to the child.

(Continued)

Procedure guideline 15.6 (*Continued*)

Statement	Rationale
6. Suppositories **a)** Remove the suppository from its plastic cover and unless contraindicated anoint the pointed end of the suppository with a water-soluble lubricant or warm water. Gently lift the child's right buttock and insert suppository pointed end first into the rectum using one finger. NB In a small study by Abd-El-Maeboud *et al* (1991) it was suggested suppositories were more easily inserted and retained when inserted blunt end first. However, many manufacturers' guidelines continue to recommended inserting suppositories pointed end first. **b)** Where possible encourage the child not to have a bowel action for as long as they feel comfortable.	**6.** **a)** To propitiate insertion of the suppository. **b)** To reduce the risk of expulsion of the suppository. To allow time for absorption of the suppository. The onset of action for a suppository depends on the time it takes to dissolve, which can be 3–50 minutes depending on its ingredients.
7. Suppositories via a ileostomy and colostomy • The route of administration is normally into the rectum, but suppositories can be inserted into a colostomy using the same principles as above.	**7.** To use appropriate route of administration.
8. Medicated enemas • Position an incontinence pad underneath the child. • Remove the lid of the enema tube and if necessary anoint the nozzle with either water-soluble lubricant or warm water. NB Refer to manufacturer's guidelines as some enemas are now designed so that the nozzle does not need anointment. • Gently lift the child's right buttock and insert the nozzle of the enema into the child's rectum. • Gently squeeze the contents of the enema into the child's rectum. On completion maintain the squeeze on the enema until it is removed from the rectum. • If appropriate, hold the child's buttocks together for a few minutes. • Where possible encourage the child not to have a bowel action for as long as the child feels comfortable.	**8.** • To minimise the risk of disruption to the child caused by spillage of the enema or leakage of bowel contents onto bed linen. • To propitiate insertion of the enema. • To prevent backflow of the contents of the enema. • To reduce the risk of expulsion of the enema medication. • To reduce the risk of expulsion of the enema. • To allow time for absorption of the enema.
9. Provide positive reinforcement as appropriate during and following administration of the medication.	**9.** To encourage the child to take the medication.
10. Utilise distraction techniques such as asking the child to whistle if the child clenches their buttocks inhibiting administration of rectal medication.	**10.** To facilitate administration of rectal medication.

Injections

Injections are less frequently used in children because of the increased availability of alternative routes of administration of which children are generally less fearful. However, there are some circumstances where injections are unavoidable either because the child is unable to have the medication or it is not available or as effective when administered by another route. (For injection routes and techniques in detail refer to the RCPCH guidelines 2002.)

This section will focus on administration of medication via intradermal, subcutaneous and intramuscular injection; refer to Chapter 13 regarding intravenous administration.

Considerations

- Intradermal, subcutaneous and intramuscular administration of medication are different and should not be confused.
- Medication for injection is usually supplied either as a sterile solution or freeze-dried powder if the medications stability is limited once dissolved (see below).
- Nurses should try to be supportive and understanding of any anxieties the child feels about injections. Fernand and Corey (1981, cited by Smalley 1999) found children aged 3–9 years appeared less anxious when staff were empathetic towards their plight.
- Consider referring to the play specialist for play therapy and/ or distraction therapy.
- Unless contraindicated apply prescribed local anaesthetic cream/spray or consider using an ice cube to numb the site prior to the injection.
- Administration of cold medication may be more painful. Refer to manufacturer's guidelines and pharmacy to see if refrigerated medication can be allowed to warm to room temperature before use.
- Administration of large volumes of medication is more painful. Refer to pharmacy regarding available strengths of medication.

Procedure guideline 15.7 Preparation of medication for injections

Statement	Rationale
1. Medicated solution in a glass vial	**1.**
a) Tap the top of the vial gently to move any medication into the lower part of the vial.	**a)** To facilitate collection of medication.
b) Cover the top of the vial with the inside of a sterile alcohol wipe package and break open the vial on the pre-marked line.	**b)** To reduce the risk of glass injury.
c) Inspect the medicated solution for any glass fragments or signs of contamination. Discard if any signs are observed and start the procedure again.	**c)** To reduce the risk of harm to the child.
d) Insert the filter needle or needle size 23 G attached to the syringe into the vial and withdraw the prescribed amount of medication with the vial held tilted upside down keeping the tip of the needle below the level of the medication.	**d)** To reduce the risk of contamination of medication with shards of glass after opening the vial.
e) Recap the needle after removal from the vial.	**e)** To reduce the risk of needle-stick injury.
f) Hold the syringe in a vertical position and tap the syringe gently to expel the air bubbles.	**f)** To ensure the correct amount of medication is administered.
g) Remove the needle and attach an appropriate size needle depending on the route of administration. Syringes are calibrated to give the correct volume of medication accounting for the medication that remains in the hub of the syringe and needle after administration.	**g)** To reduce the risk of harm to the child and to reduce the risk of accidental tracking of medication.
2. Freeze dried medication in a rubber topped vial	**2.**
a) Remove the metal/plastic cap and clean the rubber bung on the top of the vial using an alcohol wipe.	**a)** To reduce the risk of cross-infection.
b) Do not touch the rubber bung after cleaning it.	**b)** To reduce the risk of cross-infection.
c) Refer to manufacturer's and pharmacy guidelines for the type and volume of diluents suitable for dissolving the freeze-dried medication.	**c)** To account for displacement volumes when reconstituting the medication so that the correct dose is administered.
d) Draw up the appropriate volume of diluent with a filter needle or needle size 23 G and syringe.	**d)** To reduce the risk of contamination with particles of rubber through the rubber bung on the vial.
e) Insert the needle into the rubber top of the vial and inject the required volume of diluent slowly into the vial.	**e)** Fast injection of the diluent can create bubbles in the vial.
f) Allow the freeze-dried medication to disperse completely in the solution.	**f)** To ensure the correct dose of medication is administered.
g) Check the dissolved medication for any signs of contamination, e.g. cloudiness. If any signs of contamination are observed discard and start the procedure again.	**g)** To reduce the risk of harm to the child.

379

(Continued)

Procedure guideline 15.7 (*Continued*)

Statement	Rationale
h) Insert the needle already attached to the syringe into the vial and withdraw all of the medication with the vial held tilted upside down keeping the tip of the needle below the level of the medication.	**h)** To ensure the medication is in the correct volume of solution.
i) Recap the needle after removal from the vial.	**i)** To reduce the risk of needle-stick injury.
j) Hold the syringe in a vertical position and tap the syringe gently to expel the air bubbles.	**j)** To reduce the risk of harm to the child and ensure the correct amount of medication is administered.
k) Discard (according to local protocol), any additional medication from the syringe leaving the prescribed amount of medication in the syringe.	**k)** To ensure the correct amount of medication is administered.
l) Remove the needle and attach an appropriate sized needle depending on the route of administration.	**l)** Syringes are calibrated to give the correct volume of medication accounting for the medication that remains in the hub of the syringe and needle after administration, to reduce the risk of tracking of medication during administration.

Intradermal administration

This is where medication is injected into the dermis, the space just underneath the skin, which is the layer of skin beneath the epidermis, the outermost layer of the skin. This route of administration is usually used for either anaesthetising the skin prior to an invasive procedure, to test for allergies or tuberculosis. Intradermal administration is primarily used for diagnostic purposes, e.g. tuberculin testing, with local rather than systemic effect (Springhouse Corporation 1998). Although not often used with children, there are also intradermal implants which are inserted using a minor surgical procedure into dermal pockets in order to release medication, e.g. hormones over several months or a year.

Benefits

- Provides a local rather than systemic effect
- Lower risk of infection than with intravenous administration
- Lower risk of accidentally injecting a blood vessel compared with intramuscular injection.

Considerations

- More time is required for dispensing and administrating intradermal medication compared with some other routes of administration.
- Care should be taken when reading the syringe, as the measurements are very small.
- Research suggests that only small amounts of fluid can be injected – 0.5 ml or less.
- A small wheal forms where the medication is injected into the skin (Workman 1999).

- Awareness of factors that can influence the rate absorption of medication such as the volume of medication and site of administration.
- The best sites for intradermal injections are highly pigmented, thinly keratinised and hairless skin and the most common site is the median inner forearm area or between the scapulae. However, most subcutaneous injection sites are also suitable for intradermal testing (Workman 1999).
- If testing for allergens, the area should be labelled, in order to monitor the allergic response (Workman 1999).
- When testing for allergens, ensure an anaphylactic shock pack is readily available in case the patient develops a severe allergic reaction.
- The gauge and length of needle should be determined by the child's size and the volume and viscosity of the medication; 25–27 G needles are to be frequently used in practice but again there does not appear to be any evidence base for this.

Contra-indications

- Bleeding disorders, e.g. haemophilia, thrombocytopenia
- Injury or infection at site of injection
- Shock.

Cautions

- Altered tissue perfusion, e.g. critical illness
- Altered skin integrity at site of injection
- Dermatological disease/disorders
- Immunosuppression
- Oedema at site.

Equipment

The following equipment should be prepared:

- Prescription chart
- Medication formulary
- Manufacturer's drug information
- Medication
- Clean plastic medication tray
- Syringe – 1 ml (calibrated in 0.01 ml increments) or pre-filled syringe
- Needle – size 25–27 G ½ – 5/8 inches long
- Sterile alcohol impregnated wipe
- Non-sterile gloves
- Apron.

Procedure guideline 15.8 Intradermal administration

Statement	Rationale
1. Check the medication supplied is suitable for intradermal administration.	**1.** To reduce the risk of medical error.
2. Prepare and administer medication using clean non-touch technique.	**2.** To reduce the risk of cross-infection.
3. Apply non-sterile gloves and apron.	**3.** To reduce the risk of cross-infection.
4. Check the medication supplied is suitable for intradermal administration. Volume 0.5 ml or less is used.	**4.** To reduce the risk of medical error.
5. Draw up medication using a 1 ml syringe calibrated in 0.01 ml increments, if not using a pre-filled syringe.	**5.** To ensure the correct amount of medication is administered, and to reduce the risk of medical error.
6. If air bubbles are present in the syringe, tap the syringe gently with your hand and expel the air bubbles	**6.** To ensure the correct amount of medication is administered, and to reduce the risk of harm to the child.
7. Utilise distraction techniques with the assistance of parent/ carer or play specialist as appropriate.	**7.** Distraction could help reduce any feelings of anxiety the child experiences (Dahlquist et al 2002).
8. Identify an appropriate site for administration of the medication. Do not use an area that feels tender, hard or lumpy if the child is having regular intradermal injections.	**8.** To reduce the risk of a fibrous area developing and to promote effective absorption of the medication.
9. Cleanse the site for administration of medication with a sterile alcohol impregnated wipe using a circular movements moving from inwards out for about 20–30 seconds and allow to dry.	**9.** To reduce risk of cross-infection.
10. Choose the site, ensure injection site is highly pigment, thinly keratinised and hairless, i.e. median inner forearm area or between the scapulae.	**10.** To promote effective absorption of the medication.
11. Stretch the skin taut between thumb and forefinger with the non-dominant hand.	**11.** Stretching the small nerves in the skin reduces pain (Stilwell 1995, cited in Watt 2003).
12. With the other hand insert the short needle with a short bevel into the skin with the bevel up, at a 10–15 degree angle (almost parallel with the surface) to the depth of 2–5 mm just under the epidermis.	**12.** To avoid the risk of accidental subcutaneous administration of medication.
13. When administering the medication a raised blanched bleb (blister or large vesicle) or small wheal may form around the injection site.	**13.** A sign of correct administration of the medication.

381

(Continued)

Procedure guideline 15.8 (*Continued*)

Statement	Rationale
14. Administer the medication according to manufacturer's guidelines.	**14.** To administer the medication correctly and prevent a medication error.
15. Do not massage the site following administration of medication.	**15.** Massaging the site could cause additional discomfort.
16. Do not re-sheath the needle after administration of the medication.	**16.** To reduce the risk of needle-stick injury.
17. Dispose of sharps according to trust protocol.	**17.** To reduce the risk of needle-stick injury.
18. Check injection site and surrounding area.	**18.** To observe site for any signs of inflammatory reaction and taken appropriate action if required.

Subcutaneous administration

Subcutaneous administration of a medication involves injecting a medicated solution into subcutaneous tissue, i.e. the layer of connective and adipose tissue located between the skin dermis and muscle fascia (Tortora and Anagnostakos 1984). Subcutaneous medication can be given as a bolus or as an infusion and is used for both local and systemic effect. The most common sites of administration in children are the lateral upper arm, anterior thigh and lower abdomen. The subcutaneous route is usually used either because the medication is not available in a form suitable for administration by other routes, e.g. insulin or in palliative care management.

The benefit of subcutaneous administration of a medication include:

- Lower risk of infection than with intravenous administration
- Lower risk of accidentally injecting a blood vessel compared with intramuscular injection
- Longer duration of effect than intramuscular and intravenous medication.

There appears to be considerable variation between the research and nursing practice of subcutaneous injections, e.g. cleaning the subcutaneous site with alcohol-impregnated wipes prior to injection. While the available research suggests this is *not* necessary, the majority of this research appears to be based on the care of adults. The limited availability of research specific to children and young people, and in particular high-risk groups such as immunosuppressed children, could be a contributing factor for the variance between current research and nursing practice. Note that if the child is not physically clean, skin cleansing prior to injection may be necessary. Additionally, while much adult based research suggests aspirating with subcutaneous injections is also *not* necessary, Drass (1992, cited in Taylor *et al* 1997) still recommended this procedure in children. This appears to be another area of conflict in current practice.

Considerations

- More time is required for dispensing and administrating subcutaneous medication compared with some other routes of administration.

- There are a range of devices used for administration including standard needle and syringes, pre-filled syringes, pen injections and subcutaneous cannula.
- Some medications, e.g. insulin, are prescribed in units based on international standards of drug potency and so should be dispensed and administered in syringes measured in the same units.
- Sites of administration should be rotated to reduce the risk of fibrosis of subcutaneous tissue occurring, which could influence the absorption of medication.
- Awareness of other factors, which can influence the rate absorption of medication include the volume of medication, site of administration, skin temperature and exercise (Fleming 1999).
- Accidental intramuscular administration of subcutaneous medication could result in faster absorption of medication with a shorter duration of effect.
- The size of syringe should be determined by the volume of medication. There does not appear to be a universal, evidence based recommendation for the maximum volume of bolus subcutaneous injection for children, although Watt (2003) suggested a volume of less than 2 ml.
- The gauge and length of needle should be determined by the child's size and the volume and viscosity of the medication; 25–27 G needles are to be frequently used in practice but again there does not appear to be an evidence base for this.
- If regular subcutaneous injections are required refer to pharmacy and doctors regarding medication being administered via a subcutaneous cannula.

Contra-indications

- Injury or infection at site of injection
- Bleeding disorders, e.g. haemophilia
- Shock.

Cautions

- Altered tissue perfusion, e.g. critical illness
- Altered skin integrity at site of injection
- Oedema at site of injection
- Immunosuppression.

Equipment

The following equipment should be prepared:

- Prescription chart
- Medication formulary
- Manufacturer's drug information
- Medication
- Appropriate diluents

- Clean plastic medication tray
- Syringe 1–2 ml
- Needle 25–27 G
- Subcutaneous cannula if appropriate
- Non-occlusive adhesive dressing for subcutaneous cannula
- Sterile alcohol impregnated wipe
- Gauze
- Non-sterile gloves
- Apron.

Procedure guideline 15.9 Subcutaneous administration

Statement	Rationale
1. Check the medication supplied is suitable for subcutaneous administration.	1. To reduce the risk of medical error.
2. Apply non-sterile gloves and apron.	2. To reduce the risk of cross infection.
3. Prepare and administer medication using aseptic non-touch technique.	3. To reduce the risk of cross infection.
4. Refer to preparation of medications for injections (see above).	4. Safe preparation of medication.
5. Remove the needle used for preparation of medication and attach an appropriate size needle depending on the route of administration.	5. Syringes are calibrated to give the correct volume of medication accounting for the medication that remains in the hub of the syringe and needle after administration. To reduce the risk of accidental tracking of medication.
6. Utilise distraction techniques with the assistance of parent/carer or play specialist as appropriate.	6. Distraction could help reduce any feelings of anxiety the child experiences. A small study by Dahlquist *et al* (2002) found distraction techniques effective in reducing children's distress when having injections.
7. Identify an appropriate site for administration of the medication. Do not use an area that feels tender, hard or lumpy. Ensure injection sites are rotated if the child is having regular subcutaneous injections or cannulas.	7. To reduce the risk of subcutaneous fibrosis. To promote effective absorption of medication.
8. **When using a needle and syringe** a) Gently pinch up a small area of skin and subcutaneous tissue and insert the needle in a dart like motion at a 45° or 90° angle depending on the length of the needle and size of the child. Push the plunger on the syringe slowly and smoothly to administer the medication. b) Wait 10 seconds before releasing the grip on the pinch up of skin and subcutaneous tissue and removing the needle from the site of administration. c) Do not massage the site following administration of medication. d) Use gauze to apply gentle pressure if the injection site bleeds. e) Do not re-sheath the needle after administration of the medication. f) Dispose of sharps according to trust protocol. Dispose of equipment according to trust protocol. Remove gloves and wash hands according to trust protocol. g) Observe, report and document any local reaction or abnormality at the site of administration.	8. a) To reduce the risk of accidental intramuscular administration of medication. b) To reduce the risk of accidental administration of intravenous medication. c) Massaging the site could cause additional discomfort, to reduce the risk of haematoma formation. d) To reduce the risk of leakage of the medication. e) To reduce the risk of needle-stick injury. f) To reduce the risk of cross-infection. g) To facilitate early detection and prompt action of any complications, and maintain accurate records.

(Continued)

Procedure guideline 15.9 (*Continued*)

Statement	Rationale
9. When using a subcutaneous cannula	**9.**
a) Check the medication supplied is suitable for administration via subcutaneous cannula. Check the packaging is intact and expiry date is valid before removing the subcutaneous cannula from its packaging.	**a)** To reduce the risk of medical error.
b) Gently pinch up a small area of skin and subcutaneous tissue with the non-dominant hand. Holding the cannula between the forefinger and thumb of the dominant hand insert the full length of the needle at a 45° angle, bevel upwards.	**b)** To reduce the risk of cross-infection.
c) Holding the subcutaneous cannula in position, release the pinch up of skin and subcutaneous tissue and slowly remove the needle from the cannula.	**c)** To reduce the risk of accidental intramuscular administration of medication.
d) Secure the subcutaneous cannula with a non-occlusive adhesive dressing.	**d)** To reduce the risk of harm to the child and to facilitate observation of cannula site.
e) Insert the needle attached to the syringe of medication into the subcutaneous cannula bung and slowly inject the medication into the cannula.	**e)** To reduce risk of needle-stick injury.
f) Remove the needle and syringe from the cannula bung after the medication has been administered.	**f)** To reduce the risk of cross-infection.
g) Dispose of sharps according to local protocol, dispose of equipment according to trust protocol, remove gloves and wash hands according to trust protocol.	**g)** To reduce the risk of cross-infection.
h) Document date of insertion of subcutaneous cannula and refer to manufacturer's guidelines regarding length of time the subcutaneous cannula can remain in situ.	**h)** To maintain accurate records.
i) See Chapter 13, section 13.26, for guidance on delivering a drug as an infusion.	
10. Observe, report and document any local reaction or abnormality at the site of subcutaneous cannulation.	**10.** Subcutaneous cannula should be removed (and a new one inserted at different site if necessary) if the following are observed at the site of cannulation: • Redness • Pain • Swelling • Fibrosis • Leakage • Cannula dislodged or kinked.
11. Dispose of sharps according to trust protocol.	**11.** To reduce the risk of needle-stick injury.

Intramuscular administration

This is where a medicated solution is injected directly into the muscle fibre underneath the subcutaneous layer (Figure 15.2). The intramuscular route is less frequently used in children because many are fearful of having injections. However, it is sometimes used either because the medication is currently not available in a form suitable for administration by other routes, e.g. Hepatitis B vaccination, or because local reaction occurs with subcutaneous administration.

The benefit of intramuscular administration of medication include:

- Reduced risk of local reaction compared with subcutaneous and intravenous administration

- Faster absorption of medication than subcutaneous administration
- Alternative route for some medications when there is no intravenous access, e.g. administration of intramuscular antibiotics for suspected meningitis by the GP.

Considerations

- More time is required for dispensing and administrating intramuscular medication compared with some other routes of administration.
- Awareness of potential complications such as haemorrhage, abscess, fibrosis or necrosis of the muscle and nerve injury.
- The age, size and condition of the child and the volume and viscosity of medication should determine the choice of muscle.

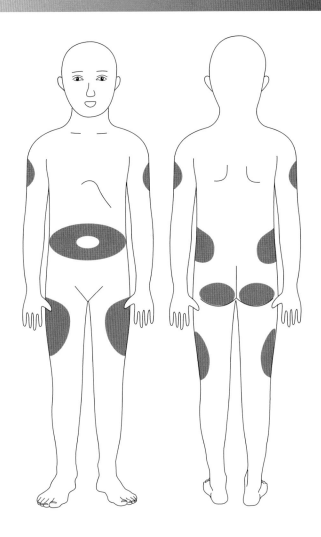

- Awareness of other factors that could influence the rate of absorption of medication such as the volume of medication, site of administration, skin temperature, exercise (Fleming 1999) and obsesity, malnourishment, hypoxia and acidosis (Kanneh 1998).
- Accidental subcutaneous administration of intramuscular medication could result in slower absorption of medication with a longer duration of effect.
- The size of syringe should be determined by the volume of medication. The maximum volume of a intramuscular injection is 1–2 ml depending on the size of the child (Watt 2003).
- Larger volumes could cause more pain and influence the absorption of medication.
- The gauge and length of needle should be determined by the child's size and the volume and viscosity of the medication.

Contra-indications

- Bleeding disorders, e.g. haemophilia
- Children taking anti-coagulant medication (Watt 2003)
- Occlusive peripheral vascular disease (Cahill 1999, cited by Downey and Tortice 2003)
- Shock
- Injury or infection at site of injection.

385

Cautions

- Altered tissue perfusion, e.g. critical illness
- Altered skin integrity at site of injection
- Oedema at site of injection
- Immunosuppression.

Figure 15.2 Sites of subcutaneous administration.

- There does not appear to be a universal agreement for the optimum choice of muscle used for injection but the most commonly used sites in children are the thigh (vastus lateralis and rectus femoris muscle) and buttocks (gluteus minimus and maximus medius muscle). Infants have smaller less developed muscles than older children especially the gluteus minimus muscle (Wong *et al* 1994). The deltoid muscle in the upper arm is generally too small for use in children although it is sometimes used for small volumes of medication such as vaccines in older children.
- Sites of administration should be rotated to reduce the risk of fibrosis of intramuscular tissue developing which could influence the absorption of medication.

Equipment

The following equipment should be prepared:

- Prescription chart
- Medication formulary
- Manufacturer's drug information
- Medication
- Appropriate diluents
- Clean plastic medication tray
- Syringe
- Needles
- Sterile alcohol impregnated wipe
- Gauze
- Non-sterile gloves
- Apron.

Procedure guideline 15.10 Intramuscular administration

Statement	Rationale
1. Check the medication supplied is suitable for intramuscular administration.	1. To reduce the risk of medical error.

(Continued)

Procedure guideline 15.10 (*Continued*)

Statement	Rationale
2. Refer to preparation of medications for injections (see above).	**2.** For safe preparation of medication.
3. Remove the needle used for preparation of medication and attach an appropriate size needle depending on the route of administration.	**3.** Syringes are calibrated to give the correct volume of medication accounting for the medication that remains in the hub of the syringe and needle after administration. To reduce the risk of accidental tracking of medication.
4. Take the medication directly to child for administration.	**4.** To prevent tampering of medication. To prevent use of the medication by others.
5. Utilise distraction techniques with the assistance of parent/carer or play specialist as appropriate.	**5.** Distraction could help reduce any feelings of anxiety the child experiences (Dahlquist *et al* 2002).
6. Identify an appropriate site for administration of the medication (Figure 15.3). Do not use an area that feels tender, hard or lumpy. Ensure injection sites are rotated if the child is having regular intramuscular injections.	**6.** To reduce the risk of muscle fibrosis. To promote effective absorption of medication.
7. Clean the site for administration of medication in circular movements moving outwards for a minimum of 30 s with an alcohol swab and allow time for the site to dry (Taylor *et al* 1997).	**7.** To reduce the risk of cross-infection.
8. Skin stretch technique Stretch the skin between the forefinger and thumb of one hand and using the other hand insert the needle in dart like motion at a 90°angle and then release the stretch on the skin.	**8.** To reduce the risk of accidental subcutaneous administration of medication in obese children. Stretching the small nerves in the skin reduces pain (Stilwell 1995, cited in Watt 2003).
9. Pinch up technique Gently pinch up a small area of skin, subcutaneous tissue and muscle and insert the needle in a dart like motion at a 90° angle and then release the pinch-up.	**9.** To maximise access to muscle and reduce the risk of hitting bone in children with wasted muscle.
10. Z-track technique Push the skin down and then pull the skin taught in one direction. Then insert the needle in a dart like motion at a 90° angle and *keep* the pull on the skin until the needle is ready for removal from the site.	**10.** To reduce the risk of medication leaking into subcutaneous tissue. To reduce the risk of some medications staining the skin, e.g. iron.
11. Aspirate with the syringe for a minimum of 5 seconds and observe for the presence of blood. If no blood is observed administer the medication pushing the plunger slowly and smoothly. NB If blood is observed do *not* administer the medication, remove and dispose of the needle, syringe and medication and start the procedure again.	**11.** To reduce the risk of accidental intravenous administration of medication.
12. Wait 10 seconds following administration of medicine before removing the needle from the site of administration (Taylor *et al* 1997). NB If using the Z-track techniques release the pull on the skin after removal of the needle.	**12.** To allow time for the medication to disperse and reduce the risk of leakage of the medication.
13. Do not massage the site following administration of the medication.	**13.** Massaging the site could cause additional discomfort.
14. Use gauze to apply gentle pressure if the injection site bleeds.	**14.** To reduce the risk of haematoma formation.

386

Insert needle at a 90° angle into the anterolateral thigh muscle

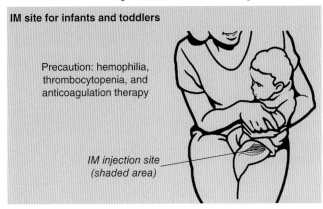

IM site for infants and toddlers

Precaution: hemophilia, thrombocytopenia, and anticoagulation therapy

IM injection site (shaded area)

Insert needle at a 45° angle into the fatty tissue over the triceps muscle. Make sure you pinch up on the SC tissue to prevent injection into the muscle.

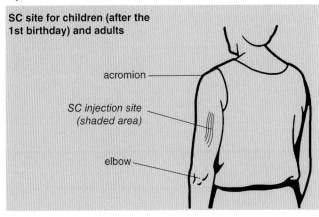

SC site for children (after the 1st birthday) and adults

acromion

SC injection site (shaded area)

elbow

Insert needle at a 90° angle into thickest portion of deltoid muscle - above the level of the axilla and below the acromion.

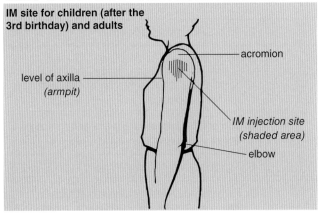

IM site for children (after the 3rd birthday) and adults

acromion

level of axilla (armpit)

IM injection site (shaded area)

elbow

http://www.vhcinfo.org/education.asp?page=administrationtest&title=Test

Figure 15.3 Sites of IM injections. http://www.vhcinfo. orgeducation.asp?page=administrationtest&title=Test © Vaccine Healthcare Centers Network.

Intravenous administration

Intravenous administration of medication involves the administration of medication directly into a vein for systemic action. It can be given by bolus injection, intermittent infusion or continu-ous infusion depending on the type of medication prescribed and the condition of the child. There are different types of intra-vascular access devices including peripheral and central percu-taneous intravenous catheters; non-tunnelled and tunnelled central venous catheters and implanted ports.

The benefits of intravenous medication include:

- Reduced frequency of injection once access is established
- Rapid onset of action of medication in an emergency
- More effective absorption resulting in higher plasma levels compared to other routes, e.g. oral
- Medication can be titrated to achieve the required response, e.g. intravenous insulin in the treatment of diabetes keto-acidosis
- When absorption from the gut is poor or variable
- If a drug is inactivated in the stomach or by the liver before reaching the circulation.

Considerations

- Intravenous medications should only be administered by reg-istered nurses or medical staff who have undertaken a recog-nised period of training and assessment and achieved competence. Refer to local policy for details.
- More time is required for dispensing and administrating intravenous medication compared with some other routes of administration.
- Non-touch techniques should be adhered due to increased risk of infection compared with other routes of administration of medication.
- Awareness of other complications including phlebitis, infiltra-tion, fluid overload, air embolism, and anaphylaxis and action that should be taken.
- Unless an antidote exists it is impossible to reverse the effect or side effects of intravenous medication.
- Concentration levels of medication should be monitored with certain intravenous medications, e.g. gentamicin.
- Some medications are not suitable for administration by peripheral percutaneous catheters, e.g. concentrated potas-sium chloride solutions (40 mmol of potassium chloride in 500 ml of dextrose saline).
- Medication should not be added to blood transfusions, parenteral nutrition or alkaline or strong acidic solutions.
- Liaise with pharmacy and dietician regarding stopping parenteral nutrition for a required time before administration of intravenous medication.
- Refer to local policy about changing intravenous infusion giving sets. The type of medication and length of time it is administered are contributory factors in determining the time frequency.

Intraosseous administration

Intraosseous administration of medications involves delivery via a bone medullary (marrow) cavity for rapid systemic action. It has all the advantages of central venous access in addition to being more rapidly and easily achieved (Resuscitation Council (UK) 2004). In the long bones, the medullary cavity consists of a network of venous sinusoids. These sinusoids drain into large medullary venous channels, which in turn, drain into nutrient or emissary vessels. These vessels exit the bone via the nutrient

387

foramina and empty directly into the systemic venous circulation (Tortora and Grabowski 1993). In the event of circulatory failure (i.e. decompensated clinical shock or cardiac arrest), the peripheral vessels constrict as the child becomes 'shutdown' making it extremely difficult to achieve venous access. The intraosseous route is therefore the preferred route of vascular access when it is urgently required.

Benefits

- The medullary cavity does not collapse in the presence of hypovolaemia or circulatory failure. It acts like a rigid vein making it an ideal site in a situation where vascular access is urgently required (e.g clinical shock or cardiac arrest).
- Rapid onset of medication action.
- Medications can be delivered as a bolus injection or continuous infusion.

Considerations

- This is a vascular route of administration and therefore medications should only be administered via this route, by medical staff or registered nurses who have undergone a recognised period of training. They should have been assessed as having achieved competence in this area of practice as per local policy.
- Non-touch techniques should be adhered to due to the increased potential of infection in comparison with other routes used for administration of medications.

- Knowledge of potential complications and their early detection and management is essential.

Cautions

- Infection
- Extravasation
- Subperiosteal infusion
- Embolism
- Compartment syndrome
- Fracture
- Skin necrosis.

Equipment

The following equipment should be prepared:

- Prescription chart
- Medication formulary
- Manufacturer's drug information
- Medication
- Clean plastic medication tray
- Sterile gloves
- Apron
- Syringes
- Needles
- 0.9% Sodium chloride for injection.

388

Procedure guideline 15.11 Intraosseous administration

Statement	Rationale
1. Check the medication supplied is suitable for intraosseous administration (these are the same medications that are deemed suitable for central intravenous administration).	**1.** To reduce the risk of medical error.
2. Check the medication(s) including dosage as per local policy.	**2.** To prevent medication error.
3. Put on gloves and apron.	**3.** To minimise risk of infection.
4. Prepare the medication(s) as per local policy and manufacturer's guidelines.	**4.** To minimise risk of infection and prevent medication error.
5. Attach the previously primed 3-way tap and flush the cannula with 2–3 ml 0.9% sodium chloride for injection.	**5.** To confirm correct placement and to ensure patency of cannula.
6. Administer appropriate medications/fluids as prescribed.	**6.** To comply with treatment plan.
7. Ensure appropriate volume of 0.9% sodium chloride for injection is used to flush after and/or between each medication.	**7.** To ensure full dosage of medication is delivered. To ensure no drug interactions.
8. Ensure 3-way tap is turned to 'off' position or fluid infusion is continued as prescribed following administration of medication.	**8.** To maintain patient safety, minimise infection risks, to adhere to the prescribed treatment plan.
9. Dispose of sharps and all equipment used as per local policy.	**9.** To minimise risk of injury, to minimise risk of infection.
10. Record medication(s) administered as per local policy.	**10.** To meet local and legal requirements.

Intrathecal administration

Intrathecal medication is administrated directly into the cerebrospinal fluid in either the subdural space or the subarachnoid space between the arachnoid and pia matter, e.g. via a lumbar puncture or directly into the ventricles (intraventricular), e.g. via an reservoir or an external ventricular drainage system. It can only be administered by injection or infusion through a shunt reservoir, an intra-venticular reservoir, a drainage system or a lumbar puncture (Lindsay and Bone 1997). This route is only used for medications such as spinal anaesthesia, antibiotic therapy, specific cytotoxic therapy, X-ray or contrast media containing those substances that do not penetrate the blood-brain barrier.

Benefits

- Allows direct administration of medication to the central nervous system (CNS) of medication that is either normally excluded by the blood–brain barrier or that cross the blood–brain barrier in very limited amounts (Hazinski 1992).

Considerations

- Intrathecal medication must only be administered by medical staff/practitioners who have undergone specific training and been assessed as competent (DoH 2008).
- At present, nurses only support/assist the medical staff who have been suitably trained and assessed as competent to administer intrathecal medication.
- The storage, preparation, dispensing, supply and administration of intrathecal medication should always be separate from medication intended for intravenous administration.
- Check the patient's treatment protocol and determine stage of treatment.

    If administrating intrathecal antibiotics ensure the antibiotic level in the cerebrospinal fluid is checked prior to administration, as this level may directly influence whether the medication dose may need to altered, to maintain therapeutic levels.
- Establish the child's neurological status prior to administration, so any alteration in their neurological condition during and post administration can be detected early.

- Cytotoxic medication must only be administered by medical staff/practitioners who have undergone training, been assessed as competent and registered to administer intrathecal cytotoxic medication. Refer to the specific national and local guidelines that exist in relation to administration of cytotoxic intrathecal medication.
- Intrathecal cytotoxic medication should be prescribed on a specifically designed intrathecal chemotherapy chart.
- Refer to local prescription guidelines, usually the medication and route of administration 'intrathecal' should be clearly written in full on the chart.

Contra-indications and cautions

- Alteration of intracranial pressure
- Infection
- Haemorrhage
- Shock
- Fatality (if incorrect medication is administered).

Equipment

The following equipment should be prepared:

- Prescription chart
- Medication formulary
- Manufacturer's drug information (if required)
- Intrathecal medication
- 0.9% sodium chloride for injection
- Clean plastic medication tray
- Sterile field
- Sterile alcohol impregnated wipes
- 1 × 1 or 2 ml syringe
- 2 × 10–30 ml syringe
- Needles (if required)
- Small non coring bufferfly 25 G needle (if required)
- Three-way tap (if required)
- Sterile gauze and tape (if required)
- Alcohol based skin preparation fluid (if required)
- Sterile gloves
- Apron.

Procedure guideline 15.12 Intrathecal administration

Statement	Rationale
1. Intrathecal medication must only be administered by medical staff who have undergone training and been assessed as competent to administer medication via this route.	1. Enshrined in policy following fatal errors in administration (DoH 2008).
2. Check the medication supplied is suitable for intrathecal administration.	2. To reduce the risk of medical error.
3. Check patient's treatment protocol and determine stage of treatment, e.g. the level of the medication in the cerebrospinal fluid (antibiotic assay, if applicable).	3. The medication level in cerebrospinal fluid directly influences whether the medication dose may need to be altered to maintain therapeutic levels.

(Continued)

Procedure guideline 15.12 (*Continued*)

Statement	Rationale
4. Refer to the manufacturer's guidelines and liaise with the ward pharmacist regarding the administration of the intrathecal medication.	**4.** The effect of some medication is inhibited by the presence of other medication.
5. External ventricular drainage system **a)** Check patient's treatment protocol and determine stage of treatment. **b)** Close clamps on drainage system as near to the injection port as possible. **c)** Put on an apron and perform a surgical hand wash prior to putting on personal protective clothing, i.e. visor according to local policy. **d)** Put on sterile gloves. **e)** Check medication according to local policy. **f)** Prepare the medication using the aseptic non-touch technique. **g)** Clean injection port on the drainage system with an alcohol impregnated wipe and allow to dry. **h)** Then insert the needle and syringe or syringe containing the medication into the injection port. **i)** Inject medication according to manufacturer's guidelines. **j)** Remove the needle and syringe or syringe when the administration is complete. **k)** Insert needle and syringe or syringe containing 0.9% sodium chloride for injection into the injection port and gently flush the line/catheter with 2ml of 0.9% sodium chloride for injection. **l)** Remove the needle and syringe or syringe from the injection port. **m)** Keep drainage system clamped for 1 hour ONLY after administration.	**5.** **a)** To ensure that medication is due according to treatment protocol. **b)** To prevent drug entering drainage system. **c)** To reduce the risk of cross-infection. **d)** To prevent contamination. **e)** To prevent a medication error. **f)** To minimise risk of infection. **g)** To minimise the risk of infection. **h)** To facilitate medication administration. **i)** To promote safe administration of medication. **j)** To facilitate flushing of system and ensure the medication is given. **k)** To ensure safe absorption of medication.
6. Intraventricular access device (reservoir) **a)** To be administered with local anaesthesia, e.g. Emla or Ametop gel, if required. **b)** Check patient's treatment protocol and determine stage of treatment. **c)** Put on an apron and perform a surgical hand wash prior to putting on personal protective clothing, i.e. visor according to local policy and sterile gloves. **d)** Check medication according to local policy. **e)** Position patient comfortably on parent's/carer's lap or lying down. **f)** Open a sterile dressing pack and pour out some alcohol based skin preparation fluid. Assist the doctor to locate the reservoir by slightly depressing the dome several times. Prepare skin and clean the site. **g)** Use a small non-coring butterfly needle 25G connected to a three-way tap, access the reservoir and collect a small amount of CSF (if required). **h)** Connect syringe, containing medication to butterfly needle extension puncture and inject slowly.Compress and release dome after all medication is given.	**6.** **a)** To maintain patient comfort and reduce anxiety. **b)** To ensure that medication is due according to treatment protocol. **c)** To reduce the risk of cross-infection. **d)** To prevent medication error. **e)** To facilitate procedure. **f)** To minimise risk of infection. **g)** To check free flow of CSF and patency of the reservoir, and to send to laboratory for analysis. **h)** To facilitate medication administration and to disperse the drug and promote safe administration of medication.

Procedure guideline 15.12 (*Continued*)

Statement	**Rationale**
i) Remove the needle and syringe or syringe when the administration is complete.	i) To facilitate dispersal of the medication.
j) Spray with Op-site spray and apply pressure with gauze pad. If CSF continues to leak apply a small dressing with gauze and tape.	j) To prevent leakage of CSF and to reduce risk of infection.

7. Administration of intrathecal chemotherapy via a lumbar puncture	**7.**
a) To be administered with general anaesthesia, local anaesthesia or Entonox, in a designated area.	a) To maintain patient comfort and reduce anxiety. In line with the National Guidelines on the Safe Administration of Intrathecal Chemotherapy (DoH 2008).
b) If general anaesthesia or Entonox is to be administered then appropriately trained persons must be present. The child must be starved according to hospital policy.	b) To ensure patient safety and to minimize the risk of aspiration of stomach contents while under anaesthetic.
c) Check patient's treatment protocol and determine stage of treatment.	c) To ensure that medication is due according to treatment protocol.

d) Check patient's full blood count (on pre-op check list)
  i. Minimum platelet count of 50 × 10 9/l
  ii. Ensure coagulation factors are normal. If patient is on aspariginase or has a known clotting abnormality or if there is any doubt. Ensure that a recent coagulation result is also available.
	d) To ensure patient safety and minimise risk of bleeding.

e) Check patient's consent form, prescription chart and name band.	e) To adhere to NMC guidelines for the administration of medication (NMC 2007).
f) Doctor to collect intrathecal chemotherapy from designated fridge and sign book and chart, to confirm that the chemotherapy has been collected from a designated area (Chief Medical Officer 2000, DoH 2001).	f) In line with local policies (DoH 2008).
g) Put on an apron and perform a surgical hand wash prior to putting on personal protective clothing, visor and sleeves.	g) To reduce the risk of cross-infection and to protect from chemotherapy spillage in line with current local policy.
h) Put on sterile gloves.	h) To prevent contamination.
i) The doctor administering the medication must check the intrathecal chemotherapy according to local policy and with a nurse who is chemotherapy competent (Chief Medical Officer 2000, DoH 2001).	i) To adhere to local policy.
j) As soon as the child is anaesthetised they should be monitored according to local policy for children undergoing general anaesthesia.	j) To maintain patient safety and to promote safe administration of medication.
k) Position patient on their side with knees to chest (Foley *et al* 1993, Hollis 2002).	k) To maintain patient safety.
l) Open sterile dressing pack and pour out some alcohol based skin preparation fluid.	l) Monitor effects on cardio-respiratory systems.
m) Open intrathecal chemotherapy drugs by cutting open plastic sealed pack and place on sterile field.	m) To determine need for suction or atropine.
n) Prepare skin and clean site.	n) To determine need for further anaesthetic.
o) Insert a lumbar puncture needle and collect 10 drops of cerebrospinal fluid (Foley *et al* 1993).	o) To facilitate procedure.
p) Connect syringe containing chemotherapy to lumbar puncture needle and inject slowly.	p) To minimise risk of infection.
q) Remove the needle and syringe or syringe when the administration is complete.	q) To minimise the risk of infection, to promote safe administration of medication.

391

(*Continued*)

Procedure guideline 15.12 (*Continued*)

Statement	Rationale
r) Spray with Op-site spray and apply pressure with gauze pad. If CSF continues to leak apply a small dressing with gauze and tape. This dressing must be removed within 24 hours post the procedure or as soon as the leak has stopped.	**r)** To facilitate medication administration, to prevent leakage of CSF and chemotherapy, to reduce risk of infection.
s) To send to laboratory for cytospin to look for leukaemic cells.	**s)** For investigation.

Statement	Rationale
8. Administration of chemotherapy via an intraventricular access device (Ommaya reservoir)	**8.**
a) To be administered with local anaesthesia (Emla or Ametop gel) in a designated area (Chief Medical Officer 2000 and DoH 2001).	**a)** To maintain patient comfort and reduce anxiety. In line with the National Guidelines on the Safe Administration of Intrathecal Chemotherapy (DoH 2008).
b) Check patient's treatment protocol and determine stage of treatment.	**b)** To ensure that medication is due according to treatment protocol.
c) Check patient's full blood count (on pre-op check list): • Minimum platelet count of $50 \times 10\ 9/l$ • Ensure coagulation factors are normal. If patient is on asparaginase or has a known clotting abnormality or if there is any doubt. Ensure that a recent coagulation result is also available.	**c)** To ensure patient safety and minimise risk of bleeding.
d) Check patient's prescription chart and name band.	**d)** To adhere to NMC guidelines for the administration of medication (Keena 2000, NMC 2007).
e) Doctor to collect intrathecal chemotherapy from designated fridge and sign book and chart, to confirm that the chemotherapy has been collected from a designated area (Chief Medical Officer 2000 and DoH 2001).	**e)** To adhere to local policy.
f) Put on apron and perform a surgical hand wash and put on personal protective clothing, visor and sleeves.	**f)** To maintain patient safety and to promote safe administration of medication.
g) Put on sterile gloves.	**g)** To reduce the risk of cross-infection.
h) The doctor administering the medication must check the intrathecal chemotherapy according to local policy and with a nurse who is chemotherapy competent (Chief Medical Officer 2000 and DoH 2001).	**h)** To protect from chemotherapy spillage in line with current local policy, to prevent contamination, too adhere to current policy.
i) Position patient comfortably on parent's lap or lying down.	**i)** To facilitate procedure.
j) Open sterile dressing pack and pour out some alcohol based skin preparation fluid.	**j)** To minimise risk of infection.
k) Open intrathecal chemotherapy drugs by cutting open plastic sealed pack and place on sterile field.	**k)** To minimise the risk of infection.
l) Locate the reservoir by slightly depressing the dome several times. Prepare skin and clean the site.	**l)** To check free flow of CSF and patency of the reservoir.
m) Use a small non-coring butterfly needle 25 G connected to a three-way tap, access the reservoir and collect a small amount of CSF.	**m)** To send to the laboratory for cytospin to look for leukaemic cells.
n) Connect syringe, containing chemotherapy to butterfly needle extension puncture and inject slowly. Compress and release the dome after all medication is given.	**n)** To facilitate medication administration.
o) Remove the needle and syringe or syringe when the administration is complete.	**o)** To disperse the drug and promote safe administration of the medication.
p) Spray with Op-site spray and apply pressure with gauze pad. If CSF continues to leak apply a small dressing with gauze and tape. This dressing must be removed within 24 hours post the procedure or as soon as the leak has stopped.	**p)** To facilitate dispersal of the medication, to prevent leakage of CSF and chemotherapy, to reduce risk of infection.

392

Epidural administration

The epidural route is indicated for use in moderate to severe pain that is likely to be difficult to control via an alternative route. There is a limited range of drugs that can be given into the epidural space. Administration of drugs via the epidural route is an advanced practice and should only be performed by specially trained individuals working within clear local guidelines. Drugs administered via this route have direct access to the brain without having to pass the blood-brain barrier. They should be formulated for epidural use and contain no preservatives, as these can cause neurotoxicity.

Benefits

- Allows direct administration of medication to the central nervous system (CNS) (Rowney and Doyle 1998).
- Can provide more effective analgesia than the intravenous route while minimising the need for opiates, if the block is effective

Considerations

- This route of administration requires verbal consent (written consent is required in the USA).
- Each individual patient should be assessed to ensure that the potential benefits outweigh the risks.
- Insertion of an epidural catheter should be performed by a consultant anaesthetist with experience of caring for children and young people or an anaesthetic registrar under supervision.

Contra-indications

- Local or generalised sepsis
- Coagulation disorders
- Anticoagulation therapy
- Some diseases of the central nervous system
- Spinal deformity.

Epidural drugs can be given as a bolus intra-operatively or continuous infusion. For more information on epidural analgesia administration see Chapter 21 (Pain Management).

Skin patches administration

Skin patches are used as an alternative way of administering medication into the body, providing a systemic effect. Skin patches are thin pads with an adhesive back that are applied to the skin rather like a plaster. Patches contain a reservoir of medicine that passes slowly from the patch through the skin and into the bloodstream. Although the skin is normally impermeable to substances, solutions are used to increase the skin's permeability and allow specific drugs to pass through the skin to the fluid in the tissues and thence to the blood circulation. The use of skin patches in children is often limited because the starting dose of medication contained in the patch is too high (*usually based on an adult starting dose*). However, when used they have a number of benefits including:

- The drug is slowly released and absorbed into the skin continuously so that the effective dose in the blood can be maintained over time.
- They are useful when a child is feeling continuously sick or is unable to take medicines by mouth.
- They provide a pain-free route of administration.
- It is a discreet way of using a medicine.

Considerations

- There is currently limited availability of medication suitable for transdermal administration.
- The therapeutic dose of medication within the skin patch may be different than when administered by other routes (i.e. the oral medication dose is usually higher to allow for the malabsorption and metabolism of the drug).
- For administration in children only small portions of transdermal patches may be needed. Although some patches can be cut for partial administration, cutting others destroys the release of the medication (Lee and Phillips 2002). Furthermore, cutting could also result in an inaccurate dose administration.
- Some patches need to be removed before swimming, showering or bathing, check the manufacturer's drug information before applying.
- Avoid placing the patch under tight clothing or around the area where a child's waistband would be.
- Young children tend to remove patches the same as they do plasters, cover with clothing so that the patch is out of site.
- Ensure the patch applied to children wearing nappies is not placed where a leaking nappy could wet the patch and irritate the skin or dilute the medicine absorption.
- Do not put a patch on a child straight after a bath or shower; allow the skin to cool down first to reduce the possibility of increased absorption through the skin.
- Do not use moisturiser, creams or powder on the skin prior to application as this may stop the patch from sticking properly.
- Do not remove the patch from its protective pouch or remove the protective backing until just before applying it.
- Assess the skin under the patch every time a patch is changed to be certain that the site is not irritated.
- Change the site every time a new patch is applied to decrease the possibility of irritation to the skin.
- Dispose of the used patch carefully as it will still contain some active medicine. Fold the patch so it sticks to itself prior to disposal.

Contra-indications

- Broken, burned, cut or irritated skin
- Epidermolysis bullosa.

Caution

- Sensitive skin
- Children with eczema or other skin conditions.

393

Equipment

The following equipment should be prepared:
- Prescription chart
- Medication formulary
- Manufacturer's drug information
- Medication (skin patch)
- Non-sterile gloves
- Apron.

Procedure guideline 15.13 Skin patches administration

Statement	Rationale
1. Expose the area of skin where the patch will be applied as specified in the manufacturer's drug information instructions. Always apply over the trunk or major muscle, not on distal extremities. Use a non-hairy patch of skin.	1. To prepare for administration and ensure that the patch is applied to the right location on the body. To ensure best absorption.
2. If the skin needs cleaning use **clear water only, no soap or alcohol**. Be sure that the area is completely dry, before applying the patch.	2. Soap or alcohol may affect the absorption of the medication.
3. Put non-sterile gloves on.	3. To reduce risk of absorbing medication.
4. Carefully remove the patch from its pouch, taking care not to tear the patch. Do not use scissors when removing the patch from its pouch.	4. To ensure the patch remains intact and to avoid damaging the patch.
5. Peel off the protective strip exposing the adhesive surface. Do not touch the sticky surface of the patch.	5. To reduce the risk of interfering with the medication dose and possibly absorbing some of the medication oneself.
6. Immediately place the adhesive side against the skin.	6. To reduce the exposure of the medication to the air.
7. Press the patch firmly, for about 10–20 seconds with the palm of your hand. Be sure that the edges adhere to the skin. Run you finger around the edge of the patch once applied to make sure it is sealed properly	7. To ensure that the patch is completely sealed to the skin and that no air or water can get in.
8. Observe for and report immediately to the nurse in charge and responsible prescriber any adverse effects of the medication.	8. To facilitate early detection and action of any adverse effects of medication.

394

Acknowledgements

We wish to thank the following healthcare professionals who were at Great Ormond Street Hospital for Children NHS Foundation Trust, London, as the chapter was conceived and who kindly contributed to this chapter, their knowledge and expertise:

Elizabeth Robinson
Tracey Fisher
Faith Gibson
Paul Griffiths
Helen Johnson
Kuan Ooi
Sheila Simpson
Joseph F. Standing
Carol Walsh

References

Abdi-El-Maeboud K, el-Naggar T, el-Hawi EM, Mahmoud SA, Abd-el-Hay S. (1991) Rectal suppository: Common sense and mode of insertion. Lancet, 338(8770), 798–800

Bauer LA. (1982) Interference of oral phenytoin absorption by continuous nasogastric feedings. Neurology, 32, 570–572

Berlin CM, May-McCarver DG, Nottingham DA, Ward RM, Weisman DN, Wilson GS. (1997) Alternative routes of drug administration – advantages and disadvantages (subject review). Pediatrics, 100(1), July 143–152. Available at www.pediatrics.org (last accessed on 29th May 2003).

Blatt B. (1997) Nurse prescribing: are you ready yet. Practice Nursing, 8(12), 11–13

British National Formulary (2010) Editors. London, British Medical Association and Royal Pharmaceutical Society of Great Britain

British National Formulary (2010–11) BNF for Children. London, British Medical Association and Royal Pharmaceutical Society of Great Britain

Cannaby A, Evans L, Freeman A. (2002) Nursing care of patients with nasogastric feeding tubes. British Journal of Nursing, 11(6), 366–372

Chief Medical Officer Department of Health (2000) An Organisation with a Memory, Report of an Expert Group on Learning from Adverse Events in the NHS. London, Department of Health

Cope J. (2009) Administration of Medicinces Operational Policy. London, Great Ormond Street Hospital

Cousins DH, Upton DR. (1998) Medication errors: inappropriate syringe use leads to fatalities. Pharmacy in Practice, 8, 209–210. Available at www.medication-errors.org.uk (last accessed 6th May 2003)

Dahlquist LM, Busby SM, Slifer KJ, Tucker CL, Eischen S, Hilley L, Sulc W. (2002) Distraction For Children Of Different Ages Who Undergo Repeated Needle Sticks. Journal of Pediatric Oncology Nursing, 19(1), 22–34

Department of Health and Social Security (1986) Neighbourhood Nursing: A Focus For Care. Report of the Community Nursing review (Cumberledge Report). London, HMSO

Department of Health (1989) Report of the Advisory Group on Nurse Prescribing (Crown Report). London, Department of Health

Department of Health (1999) Review of Prescribing, Supply and Administration of Medicines (Crown Report). London, Department of Health

Department of Health (2001) National Guidance on the Safe Administration of Intrathecal Chemotherapy. London, Department of Health

Department of Health (2002) Proposals for supplementary prescribing by nurses and pharmacists and proposed amendments to the prescription only medicines (Human use) order 1997. MLX 284. London, Department of Health. Available at www.mca.gov.uk (last accessed 20th March 2003)

Department of Health (2006) Medicines Matters: A guide to mechanisms for the prescribing, supply and administration of medicines. London, Department of Health

Department of Health (2008) Health Circular: HSC 2008/001 Updated national guidance on the safe administration of intrathecal chemotherapy. Available at http://www.dh.gov.uk/prod_consum_dh/groups/dh_digitalassets/documents/digitalasset/dh_086844.pdf (last accessed January 2010)

Downey P, Tortorice J. (2003) Medication Administration Techniques and Calculation Review. Available at www.ceufast.com/downloads/pdf/82.doc (last accessed 6th May 2003)

Fleming D. (1999) Challenging traditional insulin injection practices. American Journal of Nursing, 99(2), 72–74

Foley GV, Fochtman D, Mooney K (1993) Nursing Care of the Child with Cancer, 2nd edition, pp 76–78. Philadelphia, WB Saunders

Gibson F, Khair K, Pike S. (2003) Nurse prescribing: children's nurses; views. Paediatric Nursing, 15(1), 20–25

Guys, St Thomas' and Lewisham Hospital (2001) Paediatric Formulary, 6th edition. London, Guy's Hospital

Hazinski MF. (1992) Nursing care of the critically ill child, 2nd edition. St Loius, Mosby.

Hollis, R (2002) Accidental Intrathecal administration of Chemotherapy Agents. Cancer Nursing Practice. February, 1 (1) 8–9

Jones M. (1999) The history, the waiting, the battle. In: Jones M. (ed.) Nurse Prescribing: Politics to Practice. Edinburgh, Baillière Tindall

Kanneh A. (1998) Pharmacological principles: Part 2. Paediatric Nursing, 10(4), 24–27

Kanneh A. (2002) Paediatric pharmacological principles: an update. Part 2. Pharmacokinetics: absorption and distribution. Paediatric Nursing, 14(9), 39–43

Keena JB. (2000) Lumbar Puncture. Available at www.nova.edu/~jkeena/lumbarpuncure.htm (last accessed 23rd June 2000)

Lam TK, Leung DT. (1988) More on simplified calculation of body surface area. New England Journal of Medicine, 318(17): 1130 (Letter)

Lee M, Phillips J. (2002) Transdermal patches: High risk for error? Drugs Topic, April 1, 54–55

Lindsay KW, Bone I. (1997) Neurology and Neurosurgery Illustrated. London, Churchill Livingstone

Mosteller RD. (1987) Simplified calculation of body surface area. New England Journal of Medicine, 317(17): 1098 (Letter)

National Institute for Clinical Excellence (2000) Guidance on the use of inhaler systems (devices) for children under the age of 5 years with chronic asthma. London, National Institute for Clinical Excellence

National Institute for Clinical Excellence (2002) Inhaler devices for routine treatment of chronic asthma in older children (aged 5–15 years). London, National Institute for Clinical Excellence, London.

National Prescribing Centre (2001) Maintaining Competency in Prescribing: an outline framework to help nurse prescribers. Liverpool, The National Prescribing Centre

Nursing and Midwifery Council (2008a) Code of Professional Conduct. Nursing and Midwifery Council. London

Nursing and Midwifery Council (2008b) Covert administration of medicines. Available at http://www.nmc-uk.org/Nurses-and-midwives/Advice-by-topic/A/Advice/Covert-administration-of-medicines/ (last accessed January 2010)

Nursing and Midwifery Council (2007) Standards for Medicines Management. London, Nursing and Midwifery Council. Available at http://www.nmc-uk.org/Publications/Standards/

Nursing and Midwifery Council (2009) Record Keeping: guidance for nurses and midwives. London, Nursing and Midwifery Council. Available at http://www.nmc-uk.org/Documents/Guidance/nmcGuidanceRecordKeepingGuidanceforNursesandMidwives.pdf (last accessed 2nd November 2011)

Pinnell NL. (ed.) (1996) Nursing Pharmacology. Philadelphia, W.B. Saunders

Rang HP, Dale MM, Ritter JM, Moore PK. (2003) Pharmacology, 5th Edition. Edinburgh, Churchill Livingstone

Resuscitation Council (UK) (2004) European Paediatric Life Support Course. Provider Manual for use in the UK, 1st edition. London, Resuscitation Council (UK)

Rowney DA, Doyle E. (1998) Review article: Epidural and subarachnoid blockade in children. Anaesthesia, 53, 980–1001

Royal College of Paediatrics and Child Health (2002) Position statement on injection technique. London, RCPCH

Smalley A. (1999) Needle phobia. Paediatric Nursing, 11(2), 17–19

Smith-Temple J, Johnson JY. (1994) Clinical Procedures, 2nd edition. Philadelphia, J. B. Lippincott

Springhouse Corporation (1998) Dosage calculations made incredibly easy! Pennsylvania, Springhouse Corporation

Taylor C, Lillis C, LeMone P. (1997) Fundamentals of Nursing. The Art and Science of Nursing Care. Philadelphia, Lippincott

Thompson FC, Naysmith MR, Lindsay A. (2000) Managing drug therapy in patients receiving enteral and parental nutrition. Hospital Pharmacist, 7(6), 155–164

Tortora GJ, Anagnostakos NP. (1984) Principles of Anatomy and Physiology, 4th edition. Cambridge, Harper and Row

Tortora GJ, Grabowski SJ. (1993) Principles of Anatomy and Physiology, 7th edition. New York, Harper Collins

Watt S. (2003) Safe administration of medicines to children: Part 2. Paediatric Nursing, 15(5), 40–44

Wong DL, Hockenberry EM, Winkelswtein ML, Ahmam E, Divito-Thomas P. (1994) Nursing Care of Infant and Children. St Louis, Mosby

Workman B. (1999) Safe injection techniques. Nursing Standard, 13(39), 47–53; quiz 54

Wright D. (2002) Swallowing difficulties protocol: medication administration. Nursing Standard, 17(14–15), 43–45

Further reading

Bergeson PS, Singer SA, Kaplan AM. (1982) Intramuscular injection in children. Pediatrics, 70(6), 944–947

Bowers S. (2000) All about tubes. Nursing, December, 41–47

Hemsworth S. (2007) Intramuscular injection (IM) technique. Paediatric Nursing, 12(9), 17–20

Hubbard S, Trigg E. (2000) Practices in Children's Nursing: Guidelines for Hospital and Community. London, Churchill Livingstone

Kanneh A. (1998) Pharmacological principles: Part 3. Paediatric Nursing, 14(10), 39–43

Kovisto VA, Feilig P. (1978) Is skin preparation necessary before insulin injection? The Lancet, 20, 1072–1078

Mallett J. Dougherty L. (2000) The Royal Marsden Manual of Clinical Nursing Procedures. Oxford, Blackwell Science

MeReC Bulletin (2000) Prescribing For Children. MeReC Bulletin, 2(11), 5–8

Rowley S. (1997) A Safe and Efficient Handling Technique for IV Therapy. London, Great Ormond Street Hospital NHS Foundation Trust

RCPCH (1999) Medicines for Children. London, RCPCH Publications

Royal College of Paediatrics and Child Health (2002) Position Statement on Injection Technique. London, RCPCH

Vessey JA, Carlson KL, McGill J. (1994) Use of distraction with children during an acute pain experience. Nursing Research, 43(6), 369–372

Watt S. (2003) Safe administration of medicines to children: Part I. Paediatric Nursing, 15(4), 40–43

Winslow E, Jacobson A, Peragallo-Dittko V. (1997) Rethinking subcutaneous injection technique. American Journal of Nursing, 97(5), 71–72

Chapter 16

Moving and handling

Chapter contents

The Great Ormond Street Hospital Manual of Children's Nursing Practices, First Edition. Edited by Susan Macqueen, Elizabeth Anne Bruce, Faith Gibson.
© 2012 Great Ormond Street Hospital for Children NHS Foundation Trust. Published 2012 by Blackwell Publishing Ltd.

This chapter is divided into two parts: (1) moving and handling, which concentrates on the safety and well-being of staff; and (2) an outline on restraint and therapeutic holding of children and young people.

Introduction

Every day healthcare practitioners (HCPs) move and handle a variety of items including equipment and people. This can vary from carrying small pieces of medical equipment, to pushing beds and trolleys or the manual handling of children. Each of these activities presents a unique challenge and has the potential to cause harm to the HCP, child or other carers. The goal of safe moving and handling strategies is to reduce this potential for injury to the lowest reasonably practicable level (HSE 2007). This chapter aims to consolidate knowledge that you will have received from the practical manual handling training that you receive from your employer.

The safe moving and handling of children is a highly skilled activity which requires the healthcare professional to discuss, plan, evaluate, assess and reassess each activity to be undertaken with the child. At the same time, there must be a balance between maintaining staff, equipment and environmental safety and the child's safety, privacy, independence and individuality. This requires a responsive, flexible and knowledgeable HPC who knows their limitations and is fully conversant with current legislation on manual handling practices, protocols and procedures (Manual Handling Operations Regulations (MHOR) 1992, as amended, HSE 2004). They should have a basic understanding of the risks of musculoskeletal injury associated with particular tasks and be able to complete an on-the-spot risk assessment of the task or environment that they are about to engage.

Legislation

Employers have a legal duty to prevent the occurrence of risks of injury or illness in relation to manual handling (HSE 1998). They also have the responsibility of monitoring policy, practice and training of manual handling. Section 2 of the Health and Safety at Work Act 1974 and regulations 10 and 13 of the Management of Health and Safety at Work Regulations 1999 require employers to provide their employees with health and safety information and training (HSE 2010a).

The Health and Safety at Work Act (1974) states:

- That as far as is reasonably practicable, it is the employer's responsibility to ensure health, safety and welfare of all employees.
- Reasonably practical means that the employer must comply with this duty unless the cost (in terms of time, effort and money) of providing it is disproportionate in relation to the likely benefits.
- Employers must ensure that every room where persons work has sufficient floor area, height and unoccupied space for the purposes of health, safety and welfare.
- The employer must maintain handling plans/work systems that are safe and without health risks.

And the employee should adhere to the following:

- Take reasonable care of the health and safety of themselves and others who may be affected by their acts or omissions including reporting to the appropriate line manager any:
  - Medical condition (temporary or permanent) that may develop (including pregnancy) which may affect their ability to carry out moving and handling tasks
  - Problems or unsafe practice that (within their level of competence) they consider to be a risk to health and safety including equipment faults.
- Cooperate with the employer to allow them to comply with their health and safety duties.
- Use equipment appropriately in accordance with training and instructions provided.

Employers and employees are also bound by the Manual Handling Operations Regulations (MHOR) (1992, amended 2002), which provide the minimum health and safety requirement for handling loads where there is a risk, particularly of back injury, to the worker. The employee is required to use the 'safe systems' of work (manual handling procedures) put into place by the employer. The MHOR complements the Health and Safety at Work Act (1974). The regulations encourage safe systems of work based on a hierarchy of measures to reduce the risk of injury from manual handling activities. They include avoiding hazardous handling operations so far as is reasonably practicable; where the hazardous handling cannot be avoided you need to assess, and then reduce, the risks by using an ergonomic risk assessment.

The MHOR has four clear points that should be adhered to in order to maintain health and safety:

1. Avoidance of dangerous manual handling duties
2. Assessment of risk associated with a manual handling task (TILE)
3. Reduce the identified risks associated with the task
4. Document the information and reassess.

Employers should also be familiar with the Management of Health and Safety at Work Regulations (1992) that state that every employer shall make a suitable and sufficient assessment of the risks to their employees, make their employees aware of the risks and aim towards minimal risks and safe systems of work. The regulations states that employees are required to utilise training and equipment provided to them by their employer to ensure the safe handling of loads.

The Royal College of Nursing Manual Handling Assessments in Hospital and the Community (2003) aims to reduce all hazardous manual handling in all but exceptions or life-saving situations. The guidelines encourage patients to assist with their transfers to reduce the risk to the nursing staff.

Additionally in relation to patient handling, Clause 13 in the Nursing and Midwifery Council (2002) document *Practitioner-Client Relationships and the Prevention of Abuse* states:

physical abuse is any physical contact which harms clients or is likely to cause them unnecessary and avoidable pain and distress. Examples include handling the client in a rough manner, giving medication inappropriately, poor application of manual handling techniques or unreasonable physical restraint.

It is important that managers and senior staff are educated in the policies and good practices that have been recommended, and that they regularly encourage the workforce to adopt appropriate techniques and ensure they continue to be used. In the workplace employees must follow their employing organisation's guidelines, policies and procedures, as they should reflect current legislation thus ensuring safe practices and systems of work in the workplace. In general, unfamiliar loads should be treated with caution. If an individual feels that practices are outdated, for whatever reason, they should discuss this with their manager. If an HCP feels there is a need to challenge a particular protocol because of an individual child's need, they must speak to their manager and any other relevant organisational groups, such as health and safety, risk management, legal services or unions for information and support.

Risk assessment

Whether you work in the community or on your employer's premises you need to use a safe protocol of manual handling when working with children whatever their age. This usually begins with the completion and discussion of a risk assessment and leads to you keeping the child as independent as possible by encouraging them to move themselves, using equipment where necessary and avoiding or minimising the need for manually lifting, except in emergencies.

Manual handling risk factor analysis should aim to assess the various individual aspects that lead to the successful completion of the manual handling procedure. These are most commonly the Task, the Individual's capabilities, the Load and the Environment (TILE) (MHOR 1992, amended 2002). Each of these factors will have a bearing on the level of musculoskeletal risk associated with a manual handling procedure and each should be looked at both individually as well as in combination when assessing risk.

Task

One of the main differences between handling adults and children is that children often need supervision and can be constantly demanding on both time and attention. They frequently require repetitive moving and handling from place to place such as from wheelchair to bed or physical support in the bath. The supervised aspect of working with children can often mean the duration of manual handling is longer, and with more urgency of movement, than with adults. Accessing children can make job tasks more difficult as children may be playing on the ground, be situated in cots or lowered beds, therefore increasing the risk associated with completing the task. Children are rarely a 'still weight' and so manually handling can often involve reaching, twisting, awkward postures and stooping. The total weight of the load can often belie the difficulty of the task. If a load requires repetitive lifting this can increase risk. If a load is required to be lifted from an awkward position this can increase risk and if a load has a constantly changing centre of gravity then this also can increase risk of injury (HSE 2010a). Most musculoskeletal and in particular back injuries are not the result of a traumatic 'one off' event but the result of cumulative stress from the strain on the body of small repetitive injuries through twisting, stoop-ing, pulling, pushing and lifting (HSE 2010a). HPCs should be using techniques that prevent or minimise them sustaining such postures.

Many aspects of the task require the same consideration in children's populations as they do with adults. Factors relating to the task that can affect risk include the following (MHOR 1992, amended 2002):

- Static prolonged postures
- The frequency of the task
- The repetition of the task
- Pulling or pushing aspects
- Restrictions of movement for the HCP and the child
- Ensuring safe practice is followed.

Individual

The individual part of the TILE risk assessment pertains to the HCP as the individual and not the child. The HCP should have a keen sense of awareness of their own strengths and limitations when it comes to handling any patient but, in particular, children. Pre-existing musculoskeletal conditions, previous injuries, recent illness, age, strength and fatigue can all have a bearing on the risk presented by a manual handling task. HCP with pre-existing musculoskeletal injuries should alert their manager and seek professional advice and education from their Occupational Health Department. Studies have shown that up to 80% of acute lower back injuries will have a second episode within a year without intervention from a HCP (Hoy *et al* 2010). When assessing a manual handling task for risk, the HCP should be honest about their perceived ability to complete the task and if required use additional equipment or colleague assistance to undertake the task.

When preparing to move a child the HPC must consider their clothing, footwear and whether they need to wear any protective clothing. If the clothing is restricted in any way there is a risk of injury to the staff member or the child (MHOR 1992, amended 2002). The HCP should have adequate training and knowledge of the type of manual handling that they are about to undertake and if not confident then should have support or supervision. Some staff groups are more at risk of injury than others, such as those who are not used to manual work, young staff who are still learning a work procedure or are inexperienced in handling, older staff members, pregnant women, people recovering from an illness or previous manual handling injuries and staff returning after a period of absence such as holiday (Hoy *et al* 2010).

Load

Employees should be trained to recognise loads whose weight, in conjunction with their shape and the circumstances in which they are handled, might cause injury. Simple methods for estimating weight on the basis of volume may be taught but when weight is less important than how the weight behaves, additional considerations need to be made. In general, unfamiliar loads or patients should be treated with caution and employees should be taught to apply force gradually until either too much strain is felt, in which case the task should be reconsidered, or it is apparent that the task is within the handler's capability (MHOR 1992, amended 2002).

When discussing the safer manual handling of children, it is not uncommon to hear people dismiss risks associated with the tasks because of the assumed weight of the child is much less that for an adult. This is a dangerous assumption to make as the load associated with children can vary immensely depending on individual factors.

There are three subgroups that affect load, which are a child's physical state, their psychological state and lastly social aspects (MHOR 1992, amended 2002). Children often present a far more difficult load than adults as they are more likely to be psychologically immature and not forgetting that children can be aged in their late teens and therefore nearing full physical maturity. Additionally, factors affecting adults' mobility can also affect children such as neurological conditions, amputation, and degenerative disorders, and therefore increase the risk of manual handling.

The child's physical state is perhaps the most obvious factor when considering load. The child's perceived weight can be significantly altered by their frailty, balance, pain, sensation and ability to weight bear. Their level of consciousness, ability to speak and the mobility of their upper and lower limbs make up the patient's physical state and all should be assessed when considering manual handling risk.

A child's psychological state may also mean they have a reduced ability or desire to assist a carer in mobilisation. Children can have varying levels of physical and psychological development therefore the child may be prone to making their 'load' more difficult with outbursts or fear. Equally, children are not 'just small adults' they respond both physically and psychologically different to adults and this may have implications for the handling techniques staff may decide to use.

Lastly social aspects such as language and communication barriers, ethical and cultural considerations and family involvement need to be considered as risk factors for the load. It is important in manual handling to work with the patient to have them assist where possible with the task. Children who are unable to communicate present a risk and it is important to engage their family in these cases. Children who require manual handling will be used to being picked up and carried by family or carers, who are likely to have developed techniques and strength through constant manual handling. This often means the expectations of the child on the HCP are sometimes unreasonable.

In all cases, the risk that a child's 'load' presents to an HCP is very real and needs to be assessed with every new manual handling task being considered.

Environment

There are several environmental factors which predispose staff working with children to musculoskeletal injuries. These can include working in awkward, unstable or crouched positioning including bending, forward, sideways or twisting. Children can often require manual handling in static postures near the floor or in cots and low bedding where it is important for the HCP to ensure the surface accessed is at an appropriate height. Where equipment is to be used there needs to be space to use the equipment while still having access to the patient. Manual handing should be planned so that the environment at the beginning and the end (if different) is assessed and prepared in advance. Standard environmental risks also include floor surfaces, temperature, lighting and noise levels (HSE 2010b).

Injury

In any workplace there will be a residual level of musculoskeletal ill health resulting in either absenteeism or presenteeism for the employee (CSP 2010). Absenteeism is where an employee is absent from work while presenteeism is a term used to describe an employee who is at work but not working to their full functional capacity. Musculoskeletal ill-health results in 10 million lost working days per year in the NHS while a survey of 76 NHS trusts found that the average estimated cost of sickness absence was almost £5 million a year (Kendall-Raynor 2008). In addition, the Chartered Society of Physiotherapy (2010) issued a report that estimated that presenteeism could be costing UK companies as much as £15 billion per year (compared to £7.4 billion for absenteeism) due to having staff at work who are not performing to their full potential. The key to reducing these figures lies in preventative and reactive strategies that will be discussed later.

During the risk assessment section above it was suggested that a risk assessment focusing on the TILE principles should be used (HSWA 1974, MHSWR 1999). The task of manual handling with children is often complicated by disability, immaturity of the patient, fear or aggression from the child and the dimensions of the child. The individual HCP may have a pre-existing condition or recent injury that increases their risk of re-aggravation, or there may be a significant size disparity between the HCP and the manual handling task they are expected to achieve. The load, as discussed earlier, with children can be unpredictable and difficult to control. The load can vary in weight and dimensions depending on the requirements of the task. Finally, the environment is important to consider. If the environment does not allow additional manual handling equipment to be used then that presents a risk. Similarly, if the HCP is required to perform the task in an awkward space without the ability to position themselves or their equipment correctly then this presents a risk to the manual handling procedure.

Manual handling injuries are most common in the lumbar spine, the thoracic spine, the cervical spine, the shoulders and the upper limbs (Retsas and Pinikahana 1999).

Anatomy of the spine

The human spine consists of 24 vertebrae that sit on top of each other and are separated by a thin cartilage disc that has a fibrous outer layer and a viscous centre (Figure 16.1). These discs act as shock absorbers and prevent the vertebrae from rubbing against each other when moving. There are seven cervical vertebrae, 12 thoracic vertebrae and five lumbar vertebrae. The vertebrae are held in place by ligaments and muscles that run the length of the spinal column and provide stability and movement throughout. Running inside the vertebral bodies is the spinal cord. This originates at the brain stem and concludes at the cauda equina at the sacral level. Exiting from each vertebral level from the space between the two bones are left and right nerve roots that provide the nerve supply to each part of the body below the head.

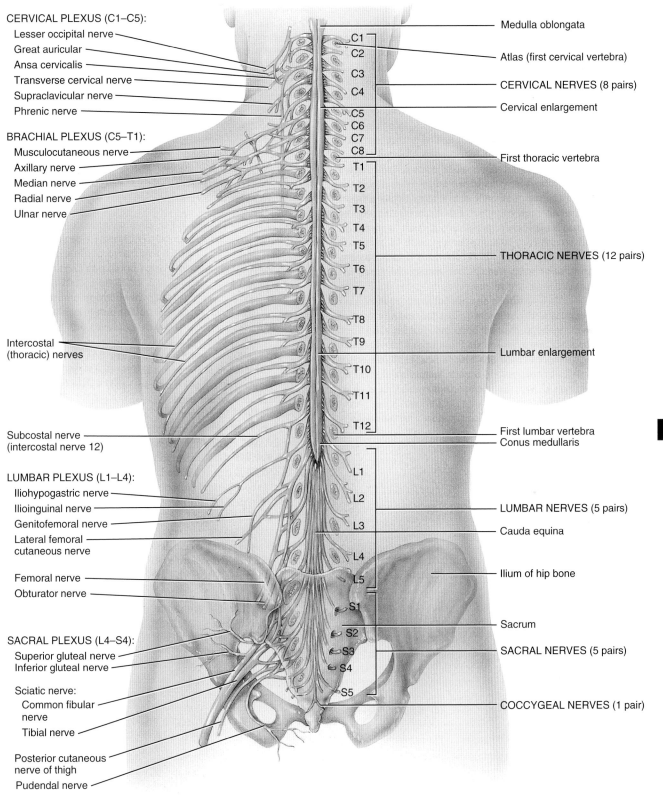

CERVICAL PLEXUS (C1–C5):
Lesser occipital nerve
Great auricular
Ansa cervicalis
Transverse cervical nerve
Supraclavicular nerve
Phrenic nerve

BRACHIAL PLEXUS (C5–T1):
Musculocutaneous nerve
Axillary nerve
Median nerve
Radial nerve
Ulnar nerve

Intercostal
(thoracic) nerves

Subcostal nerve
(intercostal nerve 12)

LUMBAR PLEXUS (L1–L4):
Iliohypogastric nerve
Ilioinguinal nerve
Genitofemoral nerve
Lateral femoral
cutaneous nerve

Femoral nerve
Obturator nerve

SACRAL PLEXUS (L4–S4):
Superior gluteal nerve
Inferior gluteal nerve

Sciatic nerve:
Common fibular
nerve
Tibial nerve

Posterior cutaneous
nerve of thigh
Pudendal nerve

C1
C2
C3
C4
C5
C6
C7
C8
T1
T2
T3
T4
T5
T6
T7
T8
T9
T10
T11
T12
L1
L2
L3
L4
L5
S1
S2
S3
S4
S5

Medulla oblongata

Atlas (first cervical vertebra)

CERVICAL NERVES (8 pairs)

Cervical enlargement

First thoracic vertebra

THORACIC NERVES (12 pairs)

Lumbar enlargement

First lumbar vertebra
Conus medullaris

LUMBAR NERVES (5 pairs)

Cauda equina

Ilium of hip bone

Sacrum

SACRAL NERVES (5 pairs)

COCCYGEAL NERVES (1 pair)

Posterior view of entire spinal cord and portions of spinal nerves

Figure 16.1 External anatomy of the spinal cord and spinal nerves.
From Tortora and Derrickson 2009.

401

Lumbar spine

The lumbar spine is the most common, anatomically the most likely and potentially the most devastating area injured in manual handling (HSE 2011).

The lumbar spine is very stable in its closed packed position of neutral or slightly extended, i.e. standing upright. The lumbar spine has specific muscular support that assists in providing the important stability required in the area and allows the many movements that this area of the back offers. The lumbar spine can flex forward, to the sides and extend backwards as well as performing combinations of these movements. When flexing forwards the bony stability of the lumbar spine is lost and the ligaments and muscles become responsible for its stability. In the first 45° of flexion there is a 'shear' force that acts on the joints of the lumbar spine. This force is magnified if there is increased weight in position forward of the person's centre of gravity. If there is a pre-existing weakness in the joints or if the muscular strength is insufficient to stabilise the movement this force can result in injury to the tissue.

In manual handling, this position of slight to moderate lumbar flexion is common and especially so in children. It is often adopted when tending to children who are lying in bed or are playing on the floor and require feeding or taking blood. HCPs may find they are undertaking tasks in these positions for extended periods of time, under stressful loads and in difficult environments. This is why the lumbar spine is the most commonly injured area in manual handling.

Injury to the lumbar spine can include damage to the muscles, the joints, the discs, the nerves and, commonly, a combination of these. The continuum of lumbar spine injury ranges from a slight strain that can give the individual some discomfort for a few days to a ruptured disc and nerve compression, which can require surgery and month or years of rehabilitation (Burton *et al* 2002).

The neck, thoracic spine and upper limb make up the vast majority of the remaining manual handling injuries (HSE 2010c). Once again posture in relation to the task, individual capabilities, load and environment is the most common risk factor and cause of injury. Injuries can be traumatic, such as a lifting injury resulting in a cervical disc prolapse, or due to repetitive strain as in carpal tunnel syndrome (HSE 2010c).

It is not only the HCP that can be injured due to manual handling. Children for the most part are significantly smaller than adults and therefore require an altered level of force when manual handling to achieve the same results. Correct or incorrect manual handling of a child can result in soft tissue damage to the child. This can be due to difficult handholds, too much pressure application, residual joint and soft tissue tenderness, aggravation of pressure areas or discomfort from poor positioning. Psychologically there can be anger and antagonism towards the HCP due to the lack of communication, depression, withdrawal or non-cooperation due to fear of further mishandling and loss of dignity if the child is left undressed or exposed to onlookers. Occasionally handling equipment may bruise or mark a child, this must also be recorded as there may be a risk of the injury being misconstrued as child abuse and raise unnecessary child protection issues. In either situation, action must be taken to minimise the risk of a repeat incident.

Education and prevention are the keys to reducing the likelihood of these injuries occurring. NHS trusts are required by law to undertake regular manual handling training of employees and additional information should be made available through managers, Occupational Health Departments and other sources (MHOR 1992, amended 2002). Training should have both theoretical and practical elements. The training should be undertaken in an environment similar to the employees' work environment and should analyse and address the various risk factors within the job role (MHOR 1992, amended 2002).

Rehabilitation

The second aspect of musculoskeletal injury that is vitally important in returning the HCP to full health is what occurs once the injury is sustained. Research has shown that early intervention from a physiotherapist or similar HCP and early return to work results in reduced pain levels, improved function and faster return to full duties than would otherwise occur (Boorman 2009). Patients should endeavour to get sound evidence based advice as early as possible and attempt to maintain their mobility throughout the early stages of their injury.

Musculoskeletal injury will typically follow three stages of healing (Brukner and Khan 2000):

1. The first is the inflammatory phase. This stage will typically last 48–72 hours provided there is no further irritation to the area. It is important to remember that if the injured area continues to be aggravated then this inflammatory phase will be prolonged. This phase will respond well to rest from aggravating activities, ice, gentle range of motion exercises and anti-inflammatories as prescribed by a pharmacist or doctor.
2. The next phase produces new tissue to replace the injured tissue. There is a proliferation of this tissue in and around the injury site that responds very well to movement and activity, again within pain free ranges. This stage typically lasts 3–5 weeks.
3. The final stage involves the remodelling of this new tissue and can take anywhere from a few weeks through to months to reach its end.

Lambeek *et al* (2010) found that an integrated approach to rehabilitation in the Occupational Health setting was the most effective and efficient way of returning employees to work and their full duties. The main goal of treatment should be to restore function in the patient's working and personal life and pain should be managed, rather than be the primary focus. The Boorman Report (2009) advocated an integrated biopsychosocial approach to rehabilitation following a work injury that addressed biological, psychological, occupational and compensation factors was again the most effective method. Lambeek *et al* (2010) study utilised the skills of occupational nurses, doctors, physiotherapists to offer a range of support structures to enable the worker to return to work earlier and with less cost to the organisation.

This reinforces the fact that throughout the injury healing process an employee should be in constant contact with their manager and Occupational Health Department. Early return to work is an important part of the rehabilitation process and can be facilitated through phased return to work programmes, utilising light duties and or restricted hours.

Prevention

Training for employees involved in manual handling is mandatory and should be undertaken by a manual handling expert on a regular basis (MHOR 1992, amended 2002). However, information and training need to be coupled with the first objective in reducing the risk of injury, which should be to design the manual handling operations to be as safe as is reasonably practicable in the first place. Training should not be regarded as a substitute for a safe system of work. Analysing and improving the task, the environment, the load and addressing individual employee concerns will result in a more effective training programme and can significantly reduce the risk of manual handling injury.

Employing organisationsl have policies in place to ensure that they provide information and training to comply with MHOR (1992, amended 2002), the HSWA (1974) and MHSWR (1999). These policies state where, when and what training they expect to provide to new employees at induction and the updating of existing employees, which usually takes place annually.

Induction training introduces employees to their new working practices and should make sure that employees understand clearly how manual handling operations have been designed to ensure their safety, while annual updates enable an organisation to communicate and increase awareness of changes in practices, policies and procedures and ensures staff are aware of new equipment in their area and any changes to systems of work. This allows staff to review their handling practices, be exposed to new equipment or changes in environmental conditions or review a child with new or unexpected handling issues. Any training that is given must be recorded with the item, date and content and is usually kept in the personnel files or training department of the organisation.

Employees, their safety representatives and safety committees should be involved in developing and implementing manual handling training, and monitoring its effectiveness. Managers may also wish to monitor sickness absence and near-miss reporting as one way to assess the effectiveness of the training.

The Health and Safety Executive (HSE) states that courses should be suitable for the individual, tasks and environment involved, use relevant examples and last long enough to cover all the relevant information, such information is likely to include advice on:

- Manual handling risk factors and how injuries can occur
- How to implement safe manual handling with good technique
- Appropriate policies of work for the individual's task and environment
- Use of mechanical aids
- A practical component that allows the instructor to correct unsafe habits.

Staff should be taught the basics of load biomechanics and their relationship to paediatric populations. Figure 16.2 shows the different weight for men and women that can be safely lifted at various heights. The guideline weights are reduced if handling is done at high or low levels or with the shoulder flexed as these are the positions that are most likely to result in injury with increased loads. If a weight is lifted through more than one guideline-box then the smallest weight should be used as a guideline. Employees should be given education on lifting anatomy, the muscles and structures involved and the pitfalls of not engaging these areas.

Lifting and handling training should focus on technique above all else. There is no substitute for practise when it comes to lifting and handling techniques, and training should therefore be heavily weighted toward the practical elements of the various job roles that make use of manual lifting and handling.

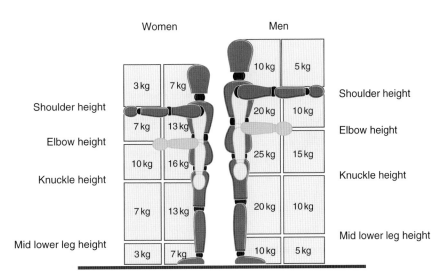

Figure 16.2 Lifting and lowering. HSE (2010). © Crown copyright.

Important principles to consider when lifting or manual handling are the following:

- Is it necessary to move or lift the weight, or can it be made easier?
- The position and shape of the weight to be lifted
- The position of the HCP in relation to that weight
- Are you able to remain close to the weight throughout the lift?
- The actual weight of the patient or object
- Is the patient able to assist with the manual handling procedure?
- The environment around the initial handling procedure and the environment in the area where the procedure will end (if different)
- The ability of the HCP to get into a safe lifting position based on their own health.

Teaching should address the above points and leave employees with the scope to raise additional job specific concerns with the educator. It should aim to promote a thought-pathway that allows the trainees to problem solve, assess risk and make sensible, educated decisions based on the training.

Because of the specific nature of the many job roles (e.g phlebotomy, ICU nursing, physiotherapists, portoring) that are present in the NHS, which require manual handling of different items (children, adults, machinery, equipment, etc.), it is not within the scope of this chapter to give advice on all of them. However, there are some general rules that should be adhered to ensure safe and effective lifting.

General Rules for Manual Handling include the following:

- Stop and think. Assess the risk of the procedure prior to attempting the task (Figure 16.3). Abort and seek assistance if you feel that you may not be able to complete the task safely.
- Patient manual handling instructions must be entered into their care plan or notes.
- Wear appropriate clothing.
- When lifting, moving, pulling or pushing, ensure that the load you are working with is kept as close to your own body as possible. There is a direct relationship between the force required to move a weight and the distance that weight is from your own body.

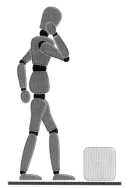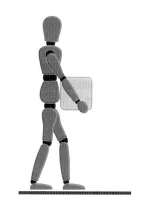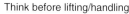

Think before lifting/handling   Keep the load close to the waist

Figure 16.3 Rules for manual handling. HSE (2010). © Crown copyright.

Adopt a stable position with feet apart and one leg slightly forward to maintain balance

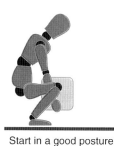

Start in a good posture

Figure 16.4 Lifting an object from the floor. HSE (2010). © Crown copyright.

- When lifting an object from the floor, maintain a neutral (straight) lumbar spine, bend forwards from the hips and bend at your knees to reach the object. Once in your control with a sound grip, reinforce your straight back, push through your legs and extend your hips and knees (Figure 16.4).
- Always move the load within your base of support.
- Your lumbar spine should not flex forward when lifting objects, it should remain straight. Avoid twisting or jerking movements (Figure 16.5).
- Avoid neck holds, bear hugs, pivot transfers to mobilise a patient. HCPs should avoid holding children on their hips to reduce wear and tear.
- When tending to a patient in bed where it is required that you lean over them, attempt to have the patient move as close to you as possible. If they are unable to move then consider using a slide sheet or board to reposition them. Ensure that high-low beds are adjusted so that the area requiring access is within easy reach without leaning. Position yourself against the side of the bed and perform the procedure.
- Babies are often seen as easy to manually handle; however, they may be attached to medical equipment that can make them heavy or difficult to handle. Planning should take this into account.
- When you are required to perform a task over a prolonged period of time attempt to set yourself in a position that is comfortable but also allows repositioning at regular intervals.

Whatever system of handling the HCP chooses for a child based on the risk assessment they must ensure that the child's clear airway can be maintained at all times and, where necessary,

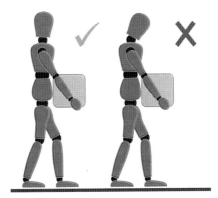

Keep the head up when handling

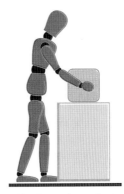

Put down, then adjust

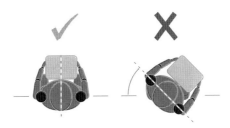

Avoid twisting the back or leaning
sideways, especially while the back is bent

Figure 16.5 Keeping the lumbar spine straight. HSE (2010). © Crown copyright.

405

an HPC has full control of the cervical spine or area of disability or dysfunction.

It is imperative that HCPs who identify handling hazards or risks report them to managers and that managers ensure that the risks are then dealt with along the appropriate channels before reassessing the risk again to ensure the manual handling task is now safe. To comply with the MHOR (1992, amended 2002) this should be documented in the child's notes.

Care of the deceased child

In some health organisations, HCPs handle deceased children (as opposed to porters or undertakers). They may be involved in washing the body after death (depending on religious and cultural beliefs) and transporting the child to the mortuary with the parents/carers.

Everyone, including parents/carers, handling the deceased child should be made aware that deceased children may be cold to touch, 'heavier' than expected when moved, and difficult to position or hold depending on the level of rigour mortis, the age and size of the child. If you are expected to undertake duties in the mortuary area, you should be informed of the handling procedures, risks, equipment used, whether or not duties includes placing bodies in the storage area or dressing children before they are seen in the viewing room by family or friends.

If the child's body should accidentally or inadvertently be injured or marked during handling, an incident form should be completed and the local policy of informing relevant staff and family members be followed. This is particularly important as injuries after death may need to be explained to parents/carers who may be concerned about the pre-death care their child received and/or in certain circumstances at coroner's court.

Documentation

For each child, staff must complete an initial moving and handling risk assessment (as provided by their organisation), which identifies and reflects the child's handling needs, the people required to assist, the equipment and procedures that will be used. This enables staff to maintain consistency in handling, reduce unnecessary handling and ensure nursing records reflect the handling needs of the child while maintaining accurate documentation (NMC 2009). The assessment should be read by all staff before handling the child and updated each time the child's handling needs change. At the end of a patient episode the risk assessment must be filed in the child's notes as it is a record of the care given and received, and may be used for assessing future handling needs or substantiating care given for a complaint or inquiry.

Documentation should reflect the observed effects, both positive and adverse, of each handling episode. Adverse incidents should be reported immediately to the relevant senior staff member and the relevant incident/accident forms completed in line with local policy and the Reporting of Incidents, Diseases and Dangerous Occurrences Regulations (1995). This will

Table 16.1 Type of equipment that can be utilised for manual handling

Aids to be used to assist in sitting to standing	Raised chair, raised toilet seat, tip-up chairs/cushions, grab rails
Aids to be used to encourage independent transfers	Transfer boards, sliding boards, turntables, transfer belts, transfer netting
Aids to be used for bed mobility	Hand block, trapeze, bed ladder, transfer sheets, sliding sheets, hoist
Aids to be used in transfers when manual handling cannot be avoided	Handling slings, transfer sheets, sliding sheets, hoist
Aids for a bathing	Bath seats, bath hoists

facilitate early detection of faulty equipment or user error and ensure the employee or child is treated appropriately.

As noted earlier, injuries can occur even with the best training, technique and advice in place. When injuries occur they must be recorded as per local policy and reported to the relevant manager. Employees who are injured at work may choose to claim some form of compensation but if an accident occurs and the employee is found to have failed in their duty they may find that their entitlement is reduced or compensation is completely withheld. In some circumstances, if an employee's failure to cooperate causes another employee to be injured then that employee could face prosecution and possibly a claim against them for compensation. Many HCPs are also covered by indemnity insurance by their union while workplaces must be covered by public liability insurance. Most staff in healthcare settings are also covered with vicarious liability insurance policy as well. Vicarious liability is where the employer shares responsibility for the acts and omissions of their employees.

Equipment

Manual handling equipment is often used by the HCP in the adult population and the same should be true for children. Table 16.1 details the type of equipment that can be utilised for manual handling.

It is important to remember that equipment or aids should reduce the load on staff, be easy to operate, be able to safely mobilise the patient within the environment it is being used in and it should be in good condition through regular maintenance.

Equipment training

As stated previously, the risk of injury from a manual handling task is increased when workers do not have the information or training necessary to enable them to work safely. It is therefore essential that where equipment for manual handling or mechanical handling aids are available, appropriate training is provided.

Staff must be offered and attend training as required in their local policy (HSWA 1974, MHOR 1992, PUWER 1998 and Lifting Operations and Lifting Equipment Regulations1998). The training should enable staff to identify the advantages and

risks of each piece of equipment, how and when to use it, equipment storage, where to find emergency/replacement equipment, how to buy new equipment and how to identify and report faulty equipment.

Hoists

There are various types of hoist that may be used when moving children. Ceiling track, mobile, standing, bath and walking hoists can assist the HCP with various manual handling tasks. Hoists utilise slings and these should be regularly checked, cleaned and maintained as they hold the load of the patient while being hoisted. Staff must have been trained in the use of the hoist they are using and ensure they use the appropriate sling and have 'sized' the client before applying the sling (LOLER 1998, PUWER 1998).

When using a hoist, staff must ensure the hoist they are using has been serviced annually and load tested every 6 months, the label with date and signature of the tester are usually visible on the hoist. The child and carer should have received an explanation as to why it is being used. Patient hoists should only be used after completion of a risk assessment and are usually used with children who cannot weight bear through their feet (age appropriate). Faulty equipment must be identified, taken out of use and reported as per local procedure.

Ward and specialist equipment

HPCs often move small pieces of equipment such as patient notes, pumps, infusion poles, specialised seating, beds and cots. All of these have handling risks usually associated with their weight and the HPCs ability to handle it. At induction the HPC should be taught the principles of how to move items of equipment safely and how to use them. Risk assessments should be updated when new equipment is introduced in the care environment or if user instructions change.

In the hospital wards height-adjustable beds should be left at their lowest height unless clinical assessment requires otherwise, in which case the bed should be adjusted for the individual HCP. On some electric beds and cots you can lockout the use of the backrest or bed height from the handset ensuring only nursing staff can adjust them. This may help to decrease the risk of injury due to misuse of equipment and especially with children. When leaving the child consider the use of cot sides. In most cases it is acceptable, for children who do not understand the level of risk in falling from a height, that the safety side on a cot, and some beds, may be raised before carers leave the immediate environment. For children outside this category you may have to write a full risk assessment and ensure that your actions are not perceived as restraint.

In the operating theatre there is a predominance of top heavy patterns of movement such as holding a limb for skin prepping, leaning over an abdomen holding a retractor or leaning over a trolley during a patient transfer (Wicker 2000). These actions present considerable risk when performed for prolonged periods or repetitively. To reduce some of the risk, theatres are using pat slide with slide sheets and other equipment and theatre table attachments to reduce the risks from limb holding.

Care of equipment

To maintain a safe working environment for staff, children and carers all moving and handling equipment should be stored clean and dry, away from the children in an easily accessible place for all staff.

All handling equipment must be latex free and stored away from latex containing products to reduce the potential for accidental exposure to latex-containing products during admission, which may induce a reaction in sensitive children, parents/carers or staff.

To prevent and reduce the risk of cross-contamination and infection between equipment, staff and users, HPCs must wash their hands and the equipment, according to local policy, before and after use, when loaning equipment to other areas or sending equipment for repair or servicing (Device Bulletin 2006b (05)).

Fabric equipment such as slide sheets and hoist slings should be labelled with ward/area name to ensure they are returned after laundering or when lent to another area. All fabric equipment should be laundered prior to use, when soiled, or when the child no longer needs it, to reduce the risk or cross-infection both from child to child or from one ward or area to another. Hard surfaced items, such as lateral transfer boards, wheelchairs and handling aids, should be cleaned according to manufacturer's instructions local policy and procedures and this must be documented.

'Single use and single patient use' items must be disposed of according to the local infection control and environmental policies and must not be used on other patients (Devise Bulletin 2006a (04)).All staff must know where replacement items are kept to ensure there is an adequate supply for future patients, how to order further equipment and where to seek advice.

Principles table 16.1 General guidelines

Principle	Rationale
1. Read and understand the local Manual Handling Policy (may be called Moving and Handling, Safer Handling, Minimal Handling Policy).	1. To enable employer and employees to comply with current legislation and local policy. To provide staff with safe systems of work (HSWA 1974, MHOR 1992, amended 2002; MHSWR 1999).
2. Know your limitations and refer to specialist (Back care Adviser, Handling Adviser/Trainer, Ergonomist, Occupational Physiotherapist, Physiotherapist Manager, etc.) where necessary.	2. To protect you own health and safety and that of the child you are handling. To safeguard other healthcare professionals and carers you are assisting or advising.
3. Staff should identify existing or new work or non-work related injuries to their manager at the earliest opportunity and seek advice from the Occupational Health Department.	3. Identified problems can be assessed to minimise the risk of further injury (MHOR 1992). Staff must be physically able to carry out given tasks (MHOR 1992).
4. Staff should attend training relevant to their employment and daily work activities.	4. To provide staff with up-to-date skills and knowledge to undertake activities safety.
5. Wash your hands before and after handling episodes.	5. Hand washing is the single most cost effective method of reducing cross-infection (Trigg and Mohammed 2006).
6. Encourage independent movement where possible.	6. Mobility influences all systems of the body to function to their full potential, in particular skin, digestion, skeleton, cardiovascular and central nervous system (CNS).
7. Where possible, it is essential to prepare the environment with appropriate equipment before the client arrives.	7. To foster the feeling of caring and that you are aware of the person's needs. NB: This may not always be possible in areas such as outpatients and X-ray.
8. Know where the handling equipment is kept and how to use it.	8. To maintain a safe and responsive environment. To minimise the risk of injury to HPCs or others.
9. Gather equipment and check it is clean, complete and working before taking it to the child.	9. To ensure the equipment is both available and usable prior to handling activity and in an emergency.

(Continued)

Principles table 16.1 (*Continued*)

Principle	Rationale
10. Complete/read/update the risk assessment and ensure documentation is completed in conjunction with all relevant parties including the child, carer, and other healthcare professionals where appropriate.	**10.** To maximise adherence and encourage independence and family-centred care. To ensure documentation is reflecting current practice and the child's mobility and abilities. To use the multi-disciplinary team to its full potential for the safety of the child.
11. Plan moving and handling into the child's activities of daily living and seek assistance of other staff where necessary. Use age appropriate language and include an explanation of what the child may feel, see or hear when the equipment or transfer takes place, use play or speech and language therapist if available/necessary.	**11.** To ensure a positive experience, consistency in handling and maintain effective communication. Use as many forms of communication as possible to maximise communication and minimise misunderstandings between child, HPC and carers.
12. Agree and use instructions, such as ready, steady, stand.	**12.** Standardisation of instructions minimises the risk of confusion for the child and staff and therefore minimises the risk of injury.
13. Handling may take place throughout 24 hours. Therefore, the child will need to be assessed for feeding, toileting, and sleeping and social activities. Where necessary this must include psychological state/mood swings.	**13.** To ensure the handling is integrated into the total care package. Handling decisions may be different if the child is for rehabilitation, palliative or long-term care or has fluctuating psychological or verbal responses.
14. Approach the child, parent/carer and other staff with a positive attitude and listen to their concerns. Be honest, understanding and confident. Discuss any concerns openly.	**14.** To maintain honesty and understanding between the child, family and professionals.
15. Take time, especially when using, or changing to, equipment the child/carer has not encountered before.	**15.** To decrease the feeling of anxiety and being 'rushed'.
16. Ensure dignity and privacy (as appropriate) during handling.	**16.** To decrease the risk of feeling 'different' and minimise unwanted attention from others that may not be acceptable to the child.
17. When a child is discharged from your care ensure that other relevant healthcare professionals are aware of the handling needs and any risks associated with this child's care.	**17.** To maintain effective communication and a safe environment for the child, carers and staff.

Principles table 16.2 **Patient assessment**

Principle	Rationale
1. The assessment should be undertaken by a registered healthcare practitioner who has undergone training and is deemed competent (MHOR 1992, amended 2002). In some cases this may be a Health Care Assistant/student who has undergone training and is under the supervision of a registered healthcare practitioner.	**1.** To ensure the safety of the child and other staff during the handling activity and that the assessment is performed thoroughly and systematically.

Principles table 16.2 (*Continued*)

Principle	Rationale
2. The initial Patient Handling Risk Assessment should be explained to the child and family, including why the assessment is necessary and identify when further assessment(s) might take place.	2. To identify an individual child's needs and risks and plan and implement a safe system of work, with or without the use of equipment. To maximise adherence and encourage, where possible, independence and family-centred care.
3. Assess the degree of the child's understanding, mobility and ability to move independently.	3. To determine whether the use of moving and handling equipment is necessary.
4. Weigh and record the child's weight at the earliest opportunity and before placing on weight sensitive equipment such as high/low electric beds/cots. Remember unlike adults, children grow and weight can be under estimated.	4. Take baseline weight to establish if weight sensitive equipment is appropriate. The child's weight may influence the choice of equipment used. To comply with the MHOR (1992, amended 2002), LOLER (1998) and PUWER (1998).
5. Establish what, if any, moving and handling practices and equipment are used at home or other relevant environments such as school.	5. To ensure, where possible, continuity of care within a framework that the child is familiar with. Children with long-term handling issues may have an existing regimen, which may require little or no adaptation for their new environment.
6. Ensure there are no contraindications to continuing an existing handling regimen or proposed new regimen.	6. To reduce the likelihood of confusion for the child and risk of injury to all parties involved in the handling activity.

7. Decisions should be made after full discussion and with the full agreement and involvement of the child, parent/carer, and other healthcare professionals where possible.	7. To obtain cooperation and consent.
	
	  To answer any questions they may have to ease concerns.
	
	  To assist with continuity, safety and partnership in care.

8. Children presenting with a number of risks must have their handling needs discussed with the named nurse, medical team, physiotherapists, occupational therapists, Tissue Viability and Infection Control Nurse Specialists and Moving and Handling Advisers/Trainer as appropriate.	8. To enable the multi-professional team approach.
	
	  To prevent child, parent/carer from receiving conflicting information.
	
	  To negotiate and implement appropriate care.

9. Ascertain from medical record and/or family how the child's medical history has influenced their mobility and current handling practices.	9. To assist in the formulation of a safe system of work.
10. Ascertain from the child/family/notes if an interpreter (sign or language) is required.	10. To enable child, parent/carer to communicate their needs effectively.
11. Speech and language or play therapists may be able to assist with communication issues when staff are having difficulty eliciting the child's wishes because of communication difficulties.	11. To enable the child to communicate their needs/ wishes to staff through the most appropriate medium.
12. Play specialists may assist in communicating information in a child friendly way.	12. To provide distraction therapy or complex information through the medium of play.
13. Where necessary, ensure the child has received appropriate and adequate pain relief prior to handling activity.	13. To provide adequate pain relief to reduce pain and assisting in reducing fear and anxiety.
14. Review handling needs when child's condition changes.	14. To promote high standards of care and to monitor and record changes.

Principles table 16.3 Equipment guidelines

Principle	Rationale
1. Moving and handling activities must only be performed by staff who: **a)** Are conversant with the organisation's policy and procedures. **b)** Are competent in assessment and familiar with the risks and contra-indications of the equipment to be used. **c)** Received induction/update training. **d)** Received extra supervision (if applicable). **e)** Wearing appropriate footwear and clothing which allows freedom of movement and is compatible with the activity to be undertaken. **f)** Have sufficient staff, time and resources to undertake the activity safely. **g)** Aware of the actions to be taken in the event of an incident. **h)** Allow time for debriefing with child/carer other staff, as required.	**1.** **a)** In line with MHOR (1992, amended 2002) Guidelines. **b)** To ensure techniques are appropriately and safely applied to given situation to reduce the likelihood of injury to staff, carer or the child. **c, d)** To establish and maintain the required level of skill and knowledge and comply with current legislation, MHOR (1992, amended 2002) and HSWA (1974). **f)** Ensures time is allowed for all involved to express their views, concerns and feed into an effective action plan. **h)** To facilitate early detection and action of any adverse effects of the handling activity.
2. Use equipment that is: • Clean and usable • Latex free • Serviced and LOLER (1998) tested (where applicable).	**2.** To comply with current hygiene practices. To reduce the risk of sensitisation to all LOLER (1998) and health and safety legislation.

3. Use the equipment on children who have:
a) Been weighed.
b) A signed, updated and completed Risk Assessment.
c) An understanding (age appropriate) of what is about to take place.
d) Where appropriate, been given a choice of handling procedure to be used.
	3. To comply with MHOR 1992 – know the weight of the load being handled and undertake a risk assessment.
	    b) To obtain informed consent, where applicable.
	    c, d) To decrease anxiety and facilitate a successful outcome while working in partnership with the child to promote a trusting relationship and promote independence.

4. Use equipment that is: • Regularly serviced and checked • Bought by the trust and asset marked • Of the appropriate weight and/or has been risk assessed prior to moving it.	**4.** To prevent harm to staff or client.

Principles table 16.4 General positioning

Principle	Rationale
1. Children may have specific positions they favour or meet the specific needs of their mobility problems.	**1.** Risk assessment is necessary as being positioned in the child's position of choice may decrease anxiety but some positions may be detrimental to the child's long-term health and positioning.
2. Ensure child is left in final equipment (bed/chair) in a comfortable position.	**2.** Correct positioning reduces incidence of muscle contractures, pressure sores, physical or psychological stress.
3. Ensure appropriate limbs and joints are supported, seek advice from other healthcare professionals as appropriate.	**3.** For comfort and to maintain spinal alignment. Staff could be accused of abuse if injured due to poor handling (NMC 2002).
4. Ensure correct placement of a child on pressure relieving equipment.	**4.** To prevent pressure ulcers.

Principles table 16.5 Risks when assisting with transfers/using equipment

Principle	Rationale
1. All equipment has risk attached to them. Staff need to establish the risk for each child and situation and ensure everyone is aware of them.	1. Handling aids should be used wherever they can reduce the risk of injury in line with MHOR guidelines.
2. Regular skin assessments should be made to detect skin break down, bruising or marking.	2. Minimise trauma and identify cause of skin marking and to ensure that it is not confused with intentional marking.
3. Examples of equipment: a) Beds/cots – static height/variable height. b) Slide sheets. c) Hoists – various. d) Wheelchairs/commodes.	3. Examples of risks: a) Leaning, reaching, non-adjustable sides, moving around equipment attached to child/bed, prolonged positions over child in poor position. b) Heavy child, difficult child, poorly positioned slide sheet, no additional assistance. c) No assistance, poor positioning of hoist, lack of room to accommodate hoist, awkward positions required to access child/hoist, poor pre-planning of hoist. d) Inadequate space, poorly planned transfer, difficult/sedated/heavy child, poor positioning for HCP to access the child.
4. Individual staff groups may have a greater risk of injury, e.g. pregnant, physiotherapist and other rehabilitation therapist, staff with existing musculoskeletal disorders or illness/injuries work or non-work related.	

Principles table 16.6 Hoisting guidelines

Principle	Rationale
1. Completed risk assessment indicates need for hoisting, all individuals agree.	1. Safety of staff and child.
2. Assistance sought from other healthcare professionals as completed assessment indicates use of hoist.	2. To maintain a safe working environment and safe systems of work for all. To gain a consensus, to allow forum for discussion, debate and resolution.
3. Discussed and informed the child and carer about the procedure and the choice of hoist and sling.	
4. Check, size and apply the appropriate sling, which is compatible with the hoisting system.	4. Failure to do so, may lead to injury and discomfort and there is a risk of 'dropping' the child or causing physical harm.
5. Ensure the hoist can be positioned under the equipment on which the child is placed.	5. Hoisting position may be unsafe if access to the hoist and child is restricted.
6. Wash hands and gather equipment.	6. Reduce the risk of cross-infection.
7. Undertake the hoisting as per local policy and training.	7. All staff using the hoist must be trained in its use and be aware of the risks involved when using the specific hoist.
8. Record untoward incidents as per local policy.	8. As per RIDDOR (1995) and PUWER (1998).
9. Faulty equipment must be reported to the appropriate department, all staff informed and alternative equipment sought, as appropriate.	9. Faulty equipment may cause incidents/accidents to staff and children.

Restraint and therapeutic holding

The NHS Trusts are committed to providing the best quality care from a compassionate, caring and competent workforce. This is best achieved by working in partnership with children and their families to obtain their consent. However, there are times when, in order to provide this care, children may need to be held still or restrained (with or without the explicit consent of their parents/carers) so that care can be delivered safely and effectively. This can raise many complex legal, ethical and practical issues.

This section provides guidance to all staff regarding the restraining and therapeutic holding of children receiving care in hospital. It is designed to be read in conjunction with other local policies including (but not exclusively) those on Consent, Managing the Absconded Child and Holding and Restraint guidelines.

There is currently no precise government guidance specifically on the restraint or therapeutic holding of children in hospital. The following documents have been incorporated into the principles that underpin this policy and may provide additional information to guide good practice:

1. The Children Act 1989
2. Human Rights Act 1998
3. The European Conventions on the rights of the child (ratified 1991)
4. Guidance for Restrictive Physical Interventions (DoH 2002)
5. The Mental Health Act (1983)
6. Restrictive physical intervention and therapeutic holding for children and young people: Guidance for nursing staff (Royal College of Nursing 2010).

Finally, individual practitioners remain accountable for protecting the rights and best interests of their patients while maintaining the standards of practice set out by their own professional body (e.g. General Medical Council, Nursing and Midwifery Council, etc.).

Definitions

Therapeutic holding

Immobilisation, which may be by splinting or by using limited force. It may be a method of helping children, with their permission, to manage a painful procedure quickly and effectively. Holding is distinguished from restraint by the degree of force required and the intention (Royal College of Nursing 2010).

A commonly used and often helpful containing experience for a distressed child (The Children Act 1989).

Restraint

The positive action of force with the intention of over-powering the child.

Physical restraint should be used rarely and only to prevent a child harming himself or others or from damaging property (The Children Act 1989).

Legal considerations

These guidelines have been prepared in the context of The Human Rights Act (1998) and The United Nations Convention on the Rights of the Child (ratified 1991). These policies establish the principle that every child (and adult) is entitled to:

- Respect for their private life
- The right not to be subjected to inhuman or degrading treatment
- The right to liberty and security
- The right not to be discriminated against in their enjoyment of those rights.

Consent

Valid consent should be sought for all forms of healthcare, from providing personal care to undertaking major surgery. This is particularly important if the child or young person has to be held still or restrained for the examination and/or treatment.

Full guidance on issues surrounding children's right to consent to examination or treatment should be followed in local policies (see chapter Introduction). With regard to holding still or restraint, the following principles should be adhered to:

- Patients have a fundamental legal right to determine what happens to their own bodies. Therefore, before examining, treating or caring for a child, you must seek consent.
- If the process of seeking consent is to be a meaningful one, refusal must be one of the child's options.
- Young people aged 16 and 17 are presumed to have the competence to give consent themselves. Younger children who fully understand what is involved in the proposed procedure can also give consent (although ideally their parents/carers will be involved). This can be achieved by ascertaining whether the child has a clear concept of themselves in relation to other people and whether they recognise and understand the decision to be made. Such a child is said to be Gillick (or Fraser) competent after the case in which this principle was established.
- In other cases, someone with parental responsibility must give consent on the child's behalf, except in an emergency.
- If a competent child consents to treatment, this decision cannot be over-ridden by a parent/carer.
- The health professional carrying out the procedure is ultimately responsible for ensuring that the child and parent/carer is genuinely consenting to what is being done.

Refusal of examination or treatment

If a child lacks the competence to consent, the consent of an individual with PR is legally adequate. However, if a child/young person refuses to give consent, serious consideration must be given to the appropriateness of applying to the High Court, even if the parents/carers consent. This should occur if:

- The assessment/treatment is not urgent
- There is any uncertainty as to its being essential
- There are indications that physical force or unusual restraint would have to be used in order to give treatment.

If a competent child refuses life-saving treatment, that refusal is unlikely to be overruled by a Court.

Principles of good practice

General principles

- Restraint or therapeutic holding should be used as the last resort and not the first line of intervention (RCN 2010).
- There should be openness about who decides what is in the child's best interest. Where possible these decisions should be made with the full agreement and involvement of the child and their parent or carer (RCN 2010).
- Staff should not be deterred from normal social contact; however, they should try to ensure that a child does not misinterpret any physical contact. Developmental age and gender should be considerations in deciding the level of appropriate physical contact.
- Staff should ascertain, through discussion with the child, family, professionals, and previous carers, the significance of physical contact. If it is discovered that the child is not comfortable with physical contact, this should be recorded and be borne in mind throughout the child's stay; however, this would not necessarily mean physical contact would be withheld. Cultural factors will be significant in determining unacceptable forms of physical contact.
- Therapeutic holding and restraint should be employed to achieve outcomes that reflect the best interests of the child (i.e. to deliver safe and effective care) and/or others affected by their behaviour (i.e. to prevent the child from causing injury to another person).
- Serious consideration must be given to the appropriateness of applying to the High Court, if there are indications that physical force or unusual restraint would have to be used in order to give treatment, even if the parents/carers consent.
- Therapeutic holding or restraint should not arouse sexual feelings or expectations (RCN 2010) and should cease if the child/young person gives any indication of this.
- Where a member of staff feels it would be inappropriate to respond to a child seeking physical contact, the reasons for denying this should be explained to the child.
- There should be sufficient staff available who are trained and confident in safe and appropriate techniques and in alternatives to restraint and therapeutic holding of children and young people. Staff on the Mildred Creek Unit (Mental Health) and the Clinical Site Practitioners receive specialist training via the GOSH training department and regular updates to maintain skills as appropriate (currently yearly). These staff will act as a resource within the Trust should specialist techniques be required.

Prevention

- Staff should communicate with children and young people in a way that maximises and promotes their understanding of their illness and treatment. Time spent talking and explaining procedures to the child and their family may avoid the need for therapeutic holding or restraint altogether.
- Therapeutic holding and restraint should only be used if other preventative strategies such as dialogue, diversion and distraction techniques have been unsuccessful. Clinical staff should be trained and competent in these preventative strategies and in therapeutic holding children and young people still for clinical procedures.
- Clinical staff working in 'high-risk' specialist areas (as in Mental Health units) may need additional training in de-escalation techniques.

Specific advice regarding infants and young children

- When children are being cared for in hospital, it will not usually seem practicable to seek their parents'/carers' consent on every occasion for every routine intervention such as blood or urine tests or X-rays.
- However, it should be remembered that, in law, such consent is required. Where a child is admitted, you should therefore discuss with the child or their parent/carer what routine procedures will be necessary, and ensure that you have their consent for these interventions in advance.
- If individuals specify that they wish to be asked before particular procedures are initiated, you must do so, unless the delay involved in contacting them would put the child's health at risk.

Therapeutic holding for planned procedures

- For planned procedures (for example, to pass a naso-gastric tube or to take blood) consent should be sought in accordance with the Consent policy summarised above. If staff will have to hold the child to carry out the procedure, the person giving consent should be made aware of this and their consent sought. Consent may be verbal and sought in advance of the procedure (i.e. on admission).
- The involvement of parents/carers may reduce the level of therapeutic holding needed. Consideration should be given to full parental involvement in the examination and/or treatment as this may significantly reduce the child's anxiety. Staff should recognise that the procedure may be as stressful and distressing to the parent/carer as to the child and ensure appropriate support is available.
- Gentle protective containment of the child with bolsters, pads and light straps to gain and maintain the correct positioning for diagnostic imaging or to protect the restless child from self-injury is acceptable. Staff and/or parents/carers may gently restrain their own child, for example to limit movement during cannulation.
- The member of staff should, if at all possible, have an established relationship with the young person and should clearly explain to the child what they are doing and why.

Therapeutic holding in emergency situations

- If consent has not been sought and it is necessary to hold a child/young person to perform an emergency or urgent intervention, there should be careful consideration of whether the procedure is really necessary and whether delay in contacting the parents/carers would put the child's health at risk. If at all possible the procedure should be delayed until consent has been obtained (RCN 2010).
- If immediate initiation of the procedure is deemed to be in the child's best interests, every effort should be made to gain their cooperation.

Restraint

- Physical restraint is permissible in circumstances where staff are attempting to (a) avert an immediate danger or injury to the child or another individual, or (b) avoid immediate damage

to property, when any other course of action would be likely to fail.
- Staff should take steps in advance to avoid the need for physical restraint, e.g. through dialogue and diversion, and the child should be warned verbally that physical restraint will be used unless they desist.
- Restraint is distinguished from therapeutic holding by the degree of force required. At all times the degree of force used must be reasonable and proportionate to both the behaviour of the individual to be controlled and the nature of the harm they may cause. These judgements have to be made at the time, taking due account of all the circumstances, including any known history of other events requiring restraint.
- The minimum necessary force should be used.
- The techniques deployed should be those for which staff are trained and familiar with, and are able to use safely. The team leader should be clearly identified and ensure that all staff are aware of their individual roles during the period of restraint.
- Physical restraint should avert danger by preventing or deflecting a child's action or by removing a physical object. Averting harm by causing or threatening hurt, pain or distress is unacceptable (except in wholly exceptional circumstances such as self-defence).
- Physical restraint should not be used purely to force adherence with staff instruction when there is no immediate risk to people or property.
- Every effort should be made to secure the presence of other staff before applying restraint. The number of staff needed will vary with the situation. If at all possible, a member of staff of the same sex as the child should be present.
- Physical restraint skilfully applied may be disengaged by degrees as the child calms down in response to physical contact. As soon as it is safe, restraint should be gradually relaxed to allow the child to regain self-control.
- Debriefing of the child, and where appropriate, of staff and parents/carers, should take place as soon after the incident as possible (RCN 2010).
- The Senior Nurse (or nominated deputy) and the child's parents/carers must be made aware of all incidents requiring the physical restraint of a child. The Doctor in charge of the ward should be informed of incidents lasting more than 30 minutes. All incidents should be fully documented and the Trust's procedures for reporting incidents should be followed.

Restriction of liberty

- In the ordinary course of maintaining control over a group of children, an adult will limit their liberty by requiring them to do things which may be against their will, including restricting their movements. This is an acceptable part of a child's social education and if the child complies with a reasonable instruction, the question of 'restriction of liberty' does not normally arise.
- However, when instructions require a child to remain in a building or part of a building for an abnormally long time without relief, then this cannot be said to be reasonable and may constitute the use of accommodation to restrict liberty, although no actual 'locking up' occurs.

- The practice of imposing the sanction of 'not being allowed out' is acceptable providing that the child is not physically prevented from so doing.
- A child may insist on leaving a ward or unit in circumstances where there is concern that this may not be in their or other people's best interests. In these circumstances it is reasonable for staff not to let them go without challenge and to stand in their way if they attempt to leave. If the child does not meet the criteria for detention under the Mental Health Act or The Children Act, advice should be sought from the person(s) with parental responsibility and the Trust legal department.
- Under the Children Act (1989) any practice or measure, such as 'time out' or seclusion, which prevents a child from leaving a room or building of his own free will, may be deemed a 'restriction of liberty'. Under this Act, restriction of liberty of children being accommodated by a NHS establishment is only permissible in very specific circumstances (such as under a court order) or when there is no other way to prevent injury or other 'significant harm' (defined in section 31).
- If restriction is used it should be for the minimum time and employing the least force necessary.
- If a child has absconded, the local guidelines should be followed.

The need for repeated restraint or prolonged restriction of liberty

- If the need for restraint is prolonged or required repeatedly, consideration should be given to the need for a specific issue order (via the Courts) or whether the child should be sectioned under the Mental Health Act 1983.
- The maximum period of restriction is 72 hours in 28 days, whether consecutive or not. When this time expires on a Sunday or a public holiday, the time can run to 12 noon on the first day which is not a Sunday or public holiday.
- If restriction is required other than in an emergency (for periods of longer than a few minutes or more frequently than once a week) staff should seek advice from the legal department regarding the use of statutory powers under mental health or childcare legislation (DoH 2002).
- Time is needed to apply for the relevant court order. Advice should be sought through the legal team *at the earliest opportunity*. Out of hours the legal team should be contacted via the manager on call.

Use of medications

- The use of medication to control behaviour would be seen as an extraordinary or unusual step. A decision to use medication should be discussed with those with parental responsibility, and the multidisciplinary team. The consent of the child would be sought if appropriate, bearing in mind the age and understanding of the child.
- If medications are needed to control the child's behaviour, a referral to the psychiatric team should be considered if this has not occurred.

Documentation

- The members of staff involved must keep detailed and accurate records of each occasion where a child is held or restrained.
- An incident report form must be completed and sent to the Modern Matron or equivalent whenever physical restraint is used.

References

Boorman S. (2009) The Boorman Review. Available at http://www. nhshealthandwellbeing.org/ (last accessed 20th November 2011)

Brukner P, Khan K. (2000) Clinical Sports Medicine, 2nd edition. Sydney, McGraw Hill

Burton K, *et al* (2002) The Back Book – UK Edition, 2nd edition. London, TSO

Chartered Society of Physiotherapists (2002) Guidance in Manual Handling for Chartered Physiotherapists. London, CSP

Chartered Society of Physiotherapy (2010) Businesses count the cost of not investing in a healthy workforce. Available at http://www.csp.org.uk/press-releases/2010/10/12/businesses-count-cost-not-investing-healthy-workforce (last accessed 21st November 2011)

The Children Act (1989) London, HMSO

Department of Health (2002) Guidance on Restrictive Physical Interventions. London, HMSO

Devise Bulletin (2006a) (04) Single use Medical Devices: Implications and Consequences of Reuse. Available at http://www.mhra.gov.uk/Publications/Safetyguidance/DeviceBulletins/CON2024995 (last accessed 21st August 2011)

Devise Bulletin (2006b) (05) Managing Medical Devices – guidance for healthcare and social services organisations. Available at http://www.mhra.gov.uk/home/groups/dts-bs/documents/publication/con2025143.pdf (last accessed 9th August 2011)

The European Conventions on the rights of the child (1989 ratified 1991)

Health and Safety Executive (2007) Understanding Ergonomics at Work – Reduce accidents and ill health and increase productivity by fitting the task to the worker. Available at http://www.hse.gov.uk/pubns/indg90.pdf (last accessed 24th August 2011)

Health and Safety at Work Act (1974) Available at http://www.hse.gov.uk/legislation/hswa.htm (last accessed 21st August 2011)

HSE (1998) A Simple Guide to The Provision and Use of Work Equipment Regulations. Available at http://www.hse.gov.uk/pubns/indg291.pdf (last accessed 11th August 2011)

HSE (2004) Manual Handling Operations Regulations 1992. Guidance on Regulations. London, HMSO

HSE (2010a) Health and Safety Regulation. A Short Guide. Available at http://www.hse.gov.uk/pubns/hsc13.pdf (last accessed 11th August 2011)

HSE (2010b) Workplace Health Safety and Welfare. A Short Guide for Managers. Available at http://www.hse.gov.uk/pubns/indg244.pdf (last accessed 11th August 2011)

HSE (2010c) Musculoskeletal Disorders. Available at http://www.hse.gov.uk/msd/uld/index.htm (last accessed 21st August 2011)

HSE (2010d) Getting to Grips with Manual Handling – A short guide for Employers. Available at http://www.hse.gov.uk/pubns/indg143.pdf (last accessed 11th August 2011)

HSE (2011) Back pain. Available at http://www.hse.gov.uk/msd/backpain/index.htm (last accessed 21st August 2011)

Hoy D, Brooks P, Blyth F, Buchbinder R. (2010) Epidemiology of low back pain. Best Practice Research Clinical Rheumatology, 24(6), 769–781

Human Rights Act (1998) London, HMSO

Kendall-Raynor P. (2008) NHS to learn lessons from Royal Mail in cutting sick leave. Nursing Standard, 23(8) 7

Lambeek LC, Van Mechelen W, Knol DL, Loisel P, Anema JR. (2010) Randomised controlled trial of integrated care to reduce disability from chronic low back pain in working and private life. British Medical Journal, 16, 340

Lifting Operations and Lifting Equipment Regulations (LOLER) (1998) Available at http://www.legislation.gov.uk/uksi/1998/2307/contents/made (last accessed 21st August 2011)

Management of Health and Safety Regulations (1999) Available at http://www.legislation.gov.uk/uksi/1999/3242/contents/made (last accessed 21st August 2011)

Manual Handling Operations Regulations (1992, amended 2002) Guidance on Regulations L23, third edition. London, HSE Books

Mental Health Act (1983) Code of Practice, Department of Health and Welsh Office. London, The Stationery Office

Nursing and Midwifery Council (2002) Practitioner-Client Relationships and the Prevention of Abuse. Available at http://www3.shu.ac.uk/hwb/placements/nursing/documents/NMC_PractitionerClientRelationshipsPreventionAbuse.pdf (last accessed 11th August 2011)

Nursing and Midwifery Council (NMC) (2009) Record keeping guidance for nurses and midwives. Available at http://www.nmc-uk.org/Documents/Guidance/nmcGuidanceRecordKeepingGuidanceforNursesandMidwives.pdf (last accessed 9th August 2011)

Provision and Use of Work Equipment Regulations (PUWER) (1998) Available at http://www.legislation.gov.uk/uksi/1998/2306/contents/made (last accessed 21st August 2011)

Retsas A, Pinikahana J. (1999) Manual handling practices and injuries among ICU nurses. Journal of Advanced Nursing, 17(1), 37–42

Reporting of Injuries, Diseases and Dangerous Occurrences Regulations (RIDDOR) (1995) Reporting Incident. Available at http://www.hse.gov.uk/riddor/ (last accessed 31st December 2011)

Royal College of Nursing (2003) Manual Handling Assessments in Hospitals and the Community: An RCN Guide. Available at http://www.rcn.org.uk/__data/assets/pdf_file/0008/78488/000605.pdf (last accessed 11th August 2011)

Royal College of Nursing (2010) Restrictive physical intervention and therapeutic holding for children and young people: Guidance for nursing staff. London, RCN

Tortora G, Derrickson B. (2009) Principles of Anatomy and Physiology, 12th edition. Hoboken, John Wiley & Sons

Trigg E, Mohammed TA. (2006) Practices in Children's Nursing. Guidelines for Hospital and Community. Edinburgh, Churchill Livingstone

Wicker P. (2000) Manual handling in preoperative environment. British Journal Preoperative Nursing, 10(5), 255–259

Chapter 17

Neonatal care

Chapter contents

Procedure guidelines

The Great Ormond Street Hospital Manual of Children's Nursing Practices, First Edition. Edited by Susan Macqueen, Elizabeth Anne Bruce, Faith Gibson.
© 2012 Great Ormond Street Hospital for Children NHS Foundation Trust. Published 2012 by Blackwell Publishing Ltd.

Introduction

The neonatal period is the first 28 days after birth and is not determined by gestational age. Babies who are born prematurely have many additional needs, so will need very careful management and handling. This chapter addresses the needs of all neonates and their families and provides some guiding principles and protocols to assist with their care. In 1907, Pierre Budin (1907), who was known as the 'father of neonatology', working with babies in Paris stated that:

> Unfortunately, a certain number of mothers abandon the babies whose needs they have not had to meet, and in whom they have lost interest. The life of the child has been saved, it is true, but at the cost of the mother.

Society has travelled a long way since this statement was written, but it is still true and very pertinent to the needs of the neonate today, and it should be remembered when caring for the babies and their families. A recent paper, *Toolkit for High Quality Neonatal Services* (DoH 2009), has the following as the first statement in the the executive summary:

> Well organised, effective neonatal sensitive care, can make a life long difference to premature and sick new born babies and their families. Getting this early care right is the responsibility of the NHS at all levels.

The guidelines that follow have been included in this chapter as they are five of the most pertinent areas of neonatal care:

1. Neonatal thermoregulation
2. Vitamin K administration
3. Umbilical care
4. Newborn blood spot screening (formerly known as Guthrie testing)
5. Phototherapy – neonatal jaundice.

Neonatal thermoregulation

Temperature control (thermoregulation) in the neonate is a critical physiological function that is strongly influenced by physical immaturity, extent of illness and environmental factors (Thomas 1994). The neonate's susceptibility to temperature instability needs to be recognised and understood in order to appropriately manage and limit the effects of cold or heat stress. It is essential that neonates are nursed within their 'neutral thermal environment' (NTE). This is defined as 'the environmental air temperature at which an infant with a normal body temperature has a minimal metabolic rate and therefore minimal oxygen consumption' (Merenstein and Gardiner 1993). The maintenance of the NTE, in order to prevent thermal stress is the ultimate aim of neonatal temperature control and management.

Although the term neonate refers to the first 28 days post-delivery, due to the wide range of post-natal ages and gestations seen in neonatal units, this guideline is appropriate for infants up to 6 months of age (post-term). Reference will be made to specific gestational ages. Optimum thermoregulation and related nursing care can be addressed with regard to three interrelated areas:

1. Method of temperature taking
2. Choice of environment
3. Temperature instability and intervention.

Generally, the smaller infants in each weight group will require a temperature in the higher portion of the temperature range. Within each time range, the younger infants require the higher temperature, see Table 17.1 (Klaus and Faranoff 1973).

Principles table 17.1 **Monitoring temperature**

Principle	Rationale
1. The acceptable set-point temperature is an axilla temperature of range 36.7–37.3°C. This range should be maintained at all times.	1. To allow normal physiological function and body metabolism (Thomas 1994).
2. 'Tempadot' (single-use) thermometer is recommended.	2. These are safe, quick and non-invasive to use (Leick-Rude and Bloom 1998) and reduce the risk of cross-infection.
3. A central temperature is obtained by insertion of the thermometer at the axilla site for 3 minutes, placing the dots against the trunk. It must be read 10 seconds following removal.	3. To ensure accurate temperature recording.
4. The axilla temperature should be checked 4–6 hourly and recorded.	4. The axilla is the safest and most accurate site for central temperature readings (Leick-Rude and Bloom 1998, Sheeran 1996, Pontius *et al* 1994). Four hourly is the general recommended interval unless instability occurs.
5. If the temperature falls outside the normal range, readings must be taken more frequently (every 30–60 minutes). This should be continued until the temperature has normalised.	5. To determine whether the temperature is deteriorating or improving.

(Continued)

Principles table 17.1 (*Continued*)

Principle	Rationale
6a) If a neonate undergoes any change of environment or increased exposure (e.g. general cares, procedures, phototherapy, new transfer to an incubator or bassinette), they will require 1–2 hourly temperature checks for the first few hours until the temperature is stable. **b)** The infant should be assessed to determine whether it is able to tolerate more frequent handling.	**6a)** It can take up to 2 hours for a central and peripheral temperature to stabilise following a change to the thermal environment or prolonged exposure in relation to nursing or medical procedures (Mok *et al* 1991). **b)** Continuous monitoring may be required for the at-risk infant or those unable to tolerate increased handling.
7a) For neonates receiving intensive care, peripheral skin temperature is monitored continuously by use of a probe placed on the sole of the foot and covered with a sock. **b)** If an arterial line is in situ, the foot should be left uncovered or covered in a clear plastic glove. **c)** Allow 5 minutes for skin temperature to stabilise once the probe has been applied to the foot. **d)** Peripheral temperature is recorded hourly and the probe site should be changed every 4–6 hours.	**7a)** Peripheral temperature is valuable as one parameter in the assessment of perfusion. The foot is recommended as the most 'peripheral' site (Lyon *et al* 1997). **b)** To ensure arterial line can be visually monitored for disconnection or limb problems. **c)** To ensure an accurate reading is obtained. **d)** To maintain and monitor skin integrity under the probe site.
8a) The 'toe–core' temperature difference is calculated from the difference between the peripheral temperature reading on the monitor and the central readings done at intervals or continuously. **b)** Continuous central monitoring can be done by placing a probe over the abdomen when supine, or the back when prone, preferably over the liver. **c)** The difference should be 1–2°C (Lyon *et al* 1997).	**8a)** Abdominal/liver skin temperature is closest to the body's central temperature and is non-invasive (Sheeran 1996). **b)** Rectal probes are not recommended, due to risk of perforation (Sheeran 1996). **c)** Less than 1°C difference may indicate heat stress while more than 2°C may indicate cold stress, hypovolaemia or infection (Mitchell 1997).
9. Peripheral monitoring can be discontinued when a neonate: • no longer requires cardiovascular support to maintain an adequate blood pressure • is peripherally warm and well perfused. This will require individual assessment.	**9.** The length of time required for optimum perfusion will depend on: • extent of illness • peripheral shutdown • nature and timing of surgery (if applicable).

Principles table 17.2 Environment: incubator

Principle	Rationale
1. Any neonate less than 1.5 kg should be nursed within an enclosed incubator.	**1.** To provide heat by convection within a closed environment (Drager 1997). Neonates have a greater physiological predisposition to heat loss due to a relatively large surface area-to-volume ratio.

2. Any neonate less than 28–30 weeks gestation and in the first 14 days of life should be nursed in a closed incubator with added humidity.
    The optimum level of humidity is determined by gestational age, days of life, skin maturity and underlying pathology.
    Generally a neonate less than 30 weeks' gestation and 1 kg in weight and in the first 7–10 days of life, should be nursed in 50% humidity.
    Sterile water should be used, and humidity levels checked hourly.
	2. The pre-term neonate has high 'trans-epidermal' water loss due to thin, poorly keratinised skin (stratum corneum). This matures by 21 days post-natal age (Blackburn and Loper 1992). Trans-epidermal water loss is a major cause of heat loss in the premature neonate (Marshall 1997).

Principles table 17.2 (*Continued*)

Principle	Rationale
3. Neonates at extremes of prematurity may require up to 85–95% humidity for up to 21 days post delivery.	**3.** The more immature, the greater the predisposition to heat loss by evaporation (Marshall 1997, Merenstein and Gardiner 1993).
4. Set and maintain incubator temperature according to age and gestation by the use of Neutral Thermal Environment (NTE) charts (see Table 17.1). Check and record incubator temperature hourly.	**4.** To minimise oxygen and energy consumption and maintain homeostasis (Merenstein and Gardiner 1993, Sheeran 1996).
5. Alter set temperature according to the neonate's temperature and adjust by 0.5–1°C every 15–30 minutes, depending on the extent of temperature instability.	**5.** To avoid rapid over or under heating or sudden swings in temperature.
6. If a neonate does not require an incubator, they should be transferred to appropriate cot with a suitable warming device.	**6.** To support babies developing thermoregulation ability.
7. Care and interventions, e.g. suction, nappy care, should be carried out via portholes, avoiding opening the side completely.	**7.** To avoid sudden loss of heat from inside the incubator.
8. Where appropriate, the incubator should be changed every 7 days, particularly if humidity is being used.	**8.** To minimise the risk of infection.
9. The date of the incubator change should be recorded, in the nursing documentation.	**9.** For evidence of practice.

Principles table 17.3 Environment: Baby-therm

Principle	Rationale
1. Baby-therms provide heat by a combination of conduction (from below via a gel mattress) and radiation (from above).	**1.** They limit heat loss during exposure and interventions because of easy access and radiant heater responsiveness (Seguin and Vieth 1996).
2a) Any neonate greater than 1.5 kg or who requires ease of access, e.g. for lumbar puncture, central line insertion, particularly surgical and cardiac neonates on admission, is nursed in an open Baby-therm.	**2a)** To allow for easy access to the neonate.
b) If a neonate less than 1.5 kg is admitted into an open cot/ Baby-therm in the first instance, they should be transferred into an incubator as soon as possible.	**b)** To optimise thermoregulation.
3a) When preparing a Baby-therm for use, the mattress is switched to 'on' at a set temperature of 37°C.	**3a)** To meet manufacturer's recommendations.
b) It will take an hour to heat to this set temperature.	**b)** This should be taken into consideration when transferring a baby.

(*Continued*)

Principles table 17.3 (*Continued*)

Principle	Rationale

4. The overhead heater should be turned on and the 'Manual', rather than 'Servo' control should be selected. Servo control is not recommended for 'shocked' neonates who are peripherally vasoconstricted.
    The heater should be switched to level 5 (each level or bar represents a 10% increase or decrease in heat from above).
    It will take 25 minutes to reach the desired temperature from the overhead heater.
	4. The 'Servo' may cause overheating due to the heater responding to the cool skin temperature (Drager 1997).

5. If the neonate is hypothermic, the initial settings are higher. This also applies to a neonate already established in a Baby-therm who needs extra heat. The extended upper range (indicated as >37; i.e. range 37–38.5) is chosen, level or bar 6–10. Above level or bar 6, the heater requires resetting every 15 minutes (press 'reset'), which is indicated by an alarm.	**5.** To avoid the complications associated with cold stress, which include decreased surfactant, increased oxygen consumption, respiratory distress and hypoxia, metabolic acidosis, hypoglycaemia, weight loss and apnoea (Merenstein and Gardiner 1993, Roberton 1995).
6. If the neonate requires cooling, turn the radiant heater off and choose the extended lower range for the mattress, indicated by <37, i.e. 30–35°C). Turn the temperature down by 1°C at 15–30 minute intervals.	**6.** To avoid the complications of heat stress associated with increased fluid losses, hypernatraemia, recurrent apnoeas, convulsions, increased metabolic rate and tachycardia (Merenstein and Gardiner 1993, Roberton 1995).

7. Once established in the Baby-therm, there are two options to determine what the neonate is laid on and covered with:
Option One: Both mattress and radiant heater on:
a) The neonate should lie directly onto a sheet covering the gel mattress.
 	
b) Nesting should be provided around, not under, the neonate.
 	
c) The infant receiving ventilator support then can be covered with bubble wrap, bubbles downwards, or left exposed.
 	
d) In self-ventilating infants bubble wrap should be used with great care or avoided completely.
Option Two: Mattress with no radiant heater.
    As option one but the neonate should be covered with a blanket.
	a) To achieve optimum heat transfer from the heat pad, via the gel mattress, to the neonate (by conduction).
	b) Blankets may block radiant heat transfer from above to the neonate.
	c) Bubble wrap provides an insulation layer to prevent heat loss from convective air currents. The bubbles placed downwards maximise the air trapped between the sheet and neonate.
	d) To minimise the risk of suffocation.
	
	    When there is no radiant heat from above, a blanket can be used.

8. When transferring a neonate on a Baby-therm, e.g. to theatre, X-ray or wards, if possible the transfer should take a maximum of 15 minutes before connecting to mains supply.	**8.** Once switched off, the mattress retains heat for 15 minutes. If transfer is greater than 15 minutes, alternative methods of keeping the baby warm should be used.

Table 17.1 NTE (Klaus and Fanaroff 1973): A guide to recommended environmental temperatures according to age and gestation

Age and weight	At start (°C)	Range
0–6 hours		
Under 1200 g	35.0	34.0–35.4
1200–1500 g	34.1	33.9–34.4
1501–2500 g	33.4	32.8–33.8
Over 2500 g (>36 wks gestation)	32.9	32.0–33.8
6–12 hours		
Under 1200 g	35.0	34.0–35.4
1200–1500 g	34.0	33.5–34.4
1501–2500 g	33.1	32.2–33.8
Over 2500 g (>36 wks gestation)	32.8	31.4–33.8
12–24 hours		
Under 1200 g	34.0	34.0–35.4
1200–1500 g	33.8	33.3–34.3
1501–2500 g	32.8	31.8–33.8
Over 2500 g (>36 wks gestation)	32.4	31.0–33.7
24–36 hours		
Under 1200 g	34.0	34.0–35.0
1200–1500 g	33.6	33.1–34.2
1501–2500 g	32.6	31.6–33.6
Over 2500 g (>36 wks gestation)	32.1	30.7–33.5
36–48 hours		
Under 1200 g	34.0	34.0–35.0
1200–1500 g	33.5	33.0–34.1
1501–2500 g	32.5	31.4–33.5
Over 2500 g (>36 wks gestation)	31.9	30.5–33.3
48–72 hours		
Under 1200 g	34.0	34.0–35.0
1200–1500 g	33.5	33.0–34.0
1501–2500 g	32.3	31.2–33.4
Over 2500 g (>36 wks gestation)	31.7	30.1–33.2
72–96 hours		
Under 1200 g	34.0	34.0–35.0
1200–1500 g	33.5	33.0–34.0
1501–2500 g	32.2	31.1–33.2
Over 2500 g (>36 wks gestation)	31.3	29.8–32.8
4–12 days		
Under 1500 g	33.5	33.0–34.0
1501–2500 g	32.1	31.0–33.2
Over 2500 g (and >36 wks gestation)		
4–6 days	31.0	29.5–32.6
5–6 days	30.9	29.4–32.3
6–8 days	30.6	29.0–32.2
8–10 days	30.3	29.0–31.8
10–12 days	30.1	29.0–31.4
12–14 days		
Under 1500 g	33.5	32.6–34.0
1501–2500 g	32.1	31.0–33.2
Over 2500 g (and >36 wks gestation)	29.8	29.0–30.8
2–3 weeks		
Under 1500 g	33.1	32.2–34.0
1501–2500 g	31.7	30.5–33.0
3–4 weeks		
Under 1500 g	32.6	31.6–33.6
1501–2500 g	31.4	30.0–32.7
4–5 weeks		
Under 1500 g	32.0	31.2–33.0
5–6 weeks		
Under 1500 g	31.4	30.6–32.3
1501–2500 g	30.4	29.0–31.8

Principles table 17.4 Environment: open bassinette

Principle	Rationale
1a) A well neonate, >1.5kg, who no longer requires close monitoring or intensive care and who can maintain a stable central temperature in 26–28°C room temperature, can be transferred to an open bassinette or small cot. **b)** The neonate should be covered or wrapped in blankets and should wear a hat. Advice should be sought by the novice practitioner as to how many blankets an individual infant may require.	**1a)** If well insulated by clothes, blankets and/or swaddling, in the ideal room temperature, a neonate will be able to maintain an adequate central temperature (Medoff-Cooper 1994). **b)** The head has a large surface area for heat loss so should be covered. (Short 1998).
2. Weaning a well neonate from an incubator or Baby-therm should be done according to age and gestation (Table 17.1), turning the incubator or mattress temperature down by 0.5–1°C each day and observing central temperature.	**2.** The environmental temperature must be altered slowly due to the immature heat conserving mechanisms at this age and limited ability to adapt to sudden or extreme changes (Medoff-Cooper 1994, Merenstein and Gardiner 1993).
3. Larger infants, i.e. >4kg, who require warming can be nursed on an open cot with a bear-hugger blanket, heated mattress and/or single overhead heater.	

Principles table 17.5 Interventions: general

Principle	Rationale
1. Maintain a set environmental room temperature of >26°C.	
2. Specific events may precipitate heat loss, the effects of which need to be counteracted (see Table 17.2).	**2.** To prevent heat loss by all means (Altimier et al 1999, Roberton 1995, Sheeran 1996).

Table 17.2 Causes of heat loss

Method of heat loss	Example	Preventative action
Conduction	Cool x-ray plate Theatre table Weighing scales Ttethoscope	Equipment should be pre-warmed and covered
Convection	Draughts Windows	Avoid over-exposure and maintain a 'minimal handling' policy Use portholes for all procedures and close these as soon as possible
Radiation	Cold incubator walls Direct sunlight	Pre-warm incubators, use curtains and covers over the incubator
Evaporation	Cold water Wet skin Nappy Bed	Keep skin and bed dry

Principles table 17.6 Prevention of heat loss

Principle	Rationale
1. Before transferring a neonate to theatre, preparing for procedures or general transportation: • Pack an appropriate sized bonnet, bubble wrap, dry gamgee or blankets, heat pad if available and a clean nappy.	**1.** To provide optimal insulation and prevent heat loss during transfer/change to the NTE (Altimier *et al* 1999).
2. During transfers within the trust, neonates should remain in their incubator or Baby-therm. This should be left switched on, at the same setting, to await their return from the radiological or surgical procedure.	**2.** To maintain a NTE at all times (Merenstein and Gardiner 1993).
3. Temperature must continue to be monitored during transfers and procedures. If this falls outside normal range, recordings must be taken more frequently, i.e. 30–60 minutes, until it has normalised. When it has returned to the normal range it may be done 4 hourly.	**3.** To assess for cold stress due to frequent handling. To evaluate the effectiveness of interventions. Continuous monitoring of temperature may be advocated in the at-risk infant or a baby unable to tolerate increased handling.
4. Any intervention carried out for temperature instability must be recorded in the child's healthcare records.	**4.** To provide an accurate record.

Principles table 17.7 Interventions: cold stress

Principle	Rationale
1. Neonates should be observed for signs and associated problems of cold stress. These are: • central temperature <36.5°C • increase in core–toe gap >2 °C • mottled and pale • increased capillary refill time, i.e. >2 seconds • increased oxygen requirements • metabolic acidosis • tachycardia • hypoglycaemia • apnoeas • bradycardia.	**1.** To enable quick recognition and prevention of adverse consequences (Mitchell 1997).
2. To intervene in this situation: • Place a neonate of <1.5kg in an incubator at the upper range, i.e. >37°C • If using a Baby-therm, set the temperature at the upper range, both above and below, and follow guidelines for Baby-therm use • Increase the set temperature by 1°C every 15 minutes according to the neonate's response • Monitor their temperature every 30–60 minutes until warmed to an acceptable temperature • Identify and eliminate any environmental causes, e.g. wet bed, over exposure, handling • Promote a flexed position • Ensure ventilator gases are adequately warmed to 37°C.	• To avoid the complications of cold stress • To decrease surface area for heat loss.

423

(Continued)

Principles table 17.7 (*Continued*)

Principle	Rationale
3. If the cause of decreased peripheral temperature is not due to cold stress, i.e. central temperature stable but an increase in core–toe gap, the neonate's perfusion status should be assessed.	**3.** Other possible causes include vasoconstriction from shock, hypovolaemia, post-operative stress or handling (Klaus and Fanaroff 1973).
4. The following should be observed (Lyon *et al* 1997): **a)** Capillary refill time. **b)** Colour of mucous membranes and extremities. **c)** Skin. **d)** Heart rate. **e)** Peripheral pulses. **f)** Blood pressure.	**a)** This should be <2 seconds. **b)** To observe for central and peripheral cyanosis. **c)** The baby should be warm to touch. **d)** This should be within normal range. **e)** These should be palpable. **f)** This should be within normal range for age, gestation and condition.

Principles table 17.8 Interventions: heat stress

Principle	Rationale
1. Neonates should be observed for signs and associated problems of heat stress. These are: • Central temperature above 37.3°C and rising • Increased peripheral temperature and decrease in core–toe gap, i.e. <1°C • Tachycardia • Tachypnoea • Restlessness • Dehydration • Stress.	**1.** To enable quick recognition and prevention of adverse consequences (Mitchell 1997).
2. To intervene in this situation: • Check environmental temperature and reduce by 1°C at 15–30 minutes intervals • Remove excess layers and clothing • In a Baby-therm, turn radiant heater off and choose the extended lower range (<35°C) • Turn the temperature down by 1° at 15–30 minute intervals.	**2.** To avoid the complications of heat stress.
3. If the cause is not environmental infection is the most likely cause and should be investigated.	

Vitamin K administration

The Department of Health Circular in May 1998, regarding the administration of vitamin K1 (phytomenadione) to newborn babies, recommended that 'All newborn babies receive an appropriate vitamin K regimen to prevent the rare, but serious disorder of vitamin K deficiency bleeding (VKDB)', also known as haemorrhagic disease of the newborn (DoH 1998, McMillan 1997). The presence of vitamin K (i.e. vitamin K1 itself or substances with vitamin K activity) is essential for the formation within the body of prothrombin, factor VII, factor IX and factor X, and of the coagulation inhibitors, protein C and protein S. Lack of vitamin K leads to increased tendency to haemorrhage (McMillan 1997, Roche 2007). Vitamin K is already added to formula milk (to provide 50 μg daily), but there is insufficient vitamin K in breast milk to prevent VKDB in a minority of babies. Supplemental vitamin K is therefore required to supplement the baby's natural stores during the period of exclusive breast-feeding (DoH 1998, Roche 2007). Studies suggest that VKDB occurs in approximately 1 in 10,000 babies, and that in half of these, bleeding occurs late (i.e. after the first week of life). In babies with late VKDB about 50% suffer intracranial bleeding, which leads to death in about 20 % and brain damage in many of those surviving (DoH 1998). In 1990 and 1992, studies from Bristol raised concern about the possible association between childhood cancer and intramuscular vitamin K1 given to newborn babies. Further research has since been undertaken, and a careful review of data from the UK Children's Cancer Study Group in 2003 found 'no evidence that neonatal vitamin K administration, irrespective of route, influences the risk of children developing leukaemia or any other cancer' (DoH 1998, Fear *et al* 2003). Additional vitamin K should be offered to **all** newborn babies (DoH 1998, Fear *et al* 2003, McMillan 1997). The administration of vitamin K1 is normally discussed with the parents/carers in the ante-natal period to ensure that an informed decision about the route of administration can be made.

Principles table 17.9 **Drug and routes of administration for vitamin K**

Principle	Rationale
1. Vitamin K1 is available as (McMillan 1997, Roche 2005, 2007): • Konakion MM Paediatric 2 mg in 0.2 ml for IV/IM/oral use • Konakion MM 10 mg in 1 ml for IV use.	**1.** Further information on administration can be found in the *British National Formulary for Children* (2011).
2. Konakion ampoules: • Should be protected from light • Should not be allowed to freeze • Should be stored at 25°C or below • Should not be used if turbid (cloudy).	**2.** Following manufacturer's guidelines for optimal storage and use.
3. A single dose of Konakion 1 mg at birth effectively prevents VKBD in virtually all babies (Rennie and Roberton 1999).	

4. Healthy term babies of 36 weeks gestation or older may receive vitamin K in three ways:
1. 1 mg IM single dose at birth (preferred method)
2. 1 mg IV at birth followed by subsequent IV or oral doses as described below (as IV does not provide the prolonged protection of the IM dose)
3. 2 × 2 mg doses orally within the first week of life:
• The first dose is usually given at birth and the second dose at 4–7 days
• A further 2 mg dose orally should be given at 1 month of age for exclusively breast-fed babies (McMillan 1997, Roche 2007).
	4. The recommended dosages to prevent vitamin K bleeding disorder (Rennie and Roberton 1999, Roche 2005).
	  To meet the manufacturer's recommendations (Roche 2005).
	  Vitamin K is already added into formula feeds, so an additional dose is not required in bottle-fed babies (Hey 2003).

5. When the oral preparation is preferred, Konakion MM Paediatric (Roche), 2 mg in 0.2 ml is used.	
6. Pre-term neonates and those at special risk are usually treated with 0.4 mg/kg (up to 1 mg) IM or IV at birth, with subsequent doses depending on coagulation status. Alternatively to address the problem of accurate administration of very small doses and to avoid the risk of errors when drawing up small volumes, a dose of 0.5 mg IM or IV may be used in babies below 1.5 kg.	**6.** To meet the manufacturer's recommendations (BNFC 2011, NHMRC 2000, Roche 2005).
7. If the IV route is used, subsequent IV or oral doses will also be required as stated above.	

Procedure guideline 17.1 **Management of vitamin K**

Statement	Rationale
1. When admitting a baby ascertain: • Has vitamin K1 been given? • What dosage was given? • Which route was been used? • How many doses have been given?	**1.** To enable effective management.

(Continued)

Procedure guideline 17.1 (*Continued*)

Statement	Rationale
2.	
• If IM/IV vitamin K1 has been given, using doses indicated previously, document the details in the child's healthcare records	• To maintain an accurate record
• If child has received IM vitamin K, there is no need for further action.	• The effective dose to prevent VKDB has been already given.
3. If vitamin K1 **has not** been given:	
• Notify the child's doctor	• To initiate appropriate treatment
• Discuss with the child's parents/carers the need for vitamin K	• To obtain consent
• Obtain a prescription for the appropriate medication	• To prevent VKDB
• Administer the medication as prescribed according to the Drug Policy	• To maintain an accurate record.
• Document the administration in the child's healthcare records.	
4. If oral or a smaller IM/IV dose of vitamin K1 has been given inform the child's doctor.	**4.** To enable a decision to be made about further dosage. Inadequate doses of vitamin K could lead to bleeding. Some breast fed babies may have inadequate stores of vitamin K (Hey 2003). Further doses of vitamin K will be required to prevent VKDB.
5. If surgery is indicated:	
• Notify the child's doctor	• Parents/carers should be kept aware of the reason for the administration of vitamin K1
• Whenever possible the issue should be discussed with the parents/carers	• Vitamin K1 is mandatory for all babies undergoing surgery
• As soon as possible, obtain a prescription for IM/IV vitamin K1, using the dosage as indicated previously for the appropriate medication	• To maintain an accurate record.
• Administer the medication as prescribed according to the Drug Policy	
• Document the administration in the child's healthcare records.	
6. If there is uncertainty about the previous administration of vitamin K:	
• Contact the referral hospital	• To clarify the situation.
• Refer to medical staff.	
NB	
Referral hospitals may have different regimens for the administration of this vitamin.	• Regimens vary according to consultant choice.

Umbilical care

The umbilical cord and surrounding area is a potential source of postnatal complication for a newborn baby, requiring regular observation and care. The umbilical cord connects the growing foetus with the maternal placenta, and it normally contains two arteries and one vein (Levene *et al* 2008). Approximately 1% of babies have a single umbilical artery and this is reported to be associated with growth retardation and congenital malformations, especially of the renal tract (Rennie and Roberton 2005). The umbilical cord is normally translucent due to Wharton's jelly, but can be stained green due to meconium or yellow if the baby has hyperbilirubinaemia (Levene *et al* 2008).

Clamping the cord 30–60 seconds post delivery reduces the risk of jaundice requiring phototherapy (Neilson 2008). Two clamps are applied to the umbilical cord 8–10cm from the baby's skin and the cord is then cut between these clamps. When the midwife examines the placenta, she will also examine the umbilical cord and record the number of vessels present in the maternity notes.

The cord stump normally dries and epithelialises within 15 days after birth. Infection can pose a problem during this time and the most common organisms identified are *Staphylococcus aureus*, *Escherichia coli* and other gram-negative organisms. The World Health Organization (WHO 2001) estimates that 460,000 infants die annually in the developing world because of bacterial infections, of which umbilical cord infections are an important precursor. Other conditions associated with umbilical area are umbilical hernia, granuloma, exomphalos, a persistant urachus which discharges urine, and a residual Vitello intestinal duct, where meconium may be passed via the umbilicus (Rennie and Roberton 2005). Surgical repair of the exomphalos, urachus and residual Vitello intestinal duct will be required (Rijhwani *et al* 2005).

Umbilical vessels may be cannulated for arterial or venous access for administration of drugs and intravenous fluids, invasive blood pressure monitoring, blood sampling and exchange transfusion. The associated risks include obstructed blood flow to major vessels, causing ischaemia to a lower limb, infection, thrombosis and necrotising entero-colitis (Rennie and Roberton 2005).

Procedure guideline 17.2 **Preparation of umbilical cord**

Statement	Rationale

1. Inform the family of the following:
  a) That the cord needs to be assessed
  b) The reason for the assessment
  c) What it will entail
  d) The likely duration of the procedure.
	1.
	
	  b) To assess umbilical site for bleeding and infection.
	
	  d) To ensure that parents/carers understand why this is being performed.

2. Co-ordinate procedure to minimise handling baby.	**2.** To conserve energy and minimise oxygen consumption.

3. Collect equipment:
  • Clean nappy
  • Umbilical swab and request form for microbiology if there are signs of infection
  • Alcohol impregnated wipe if there are signs of infection.
	3. To facilitate the efficiency of this procedure.

4. Wash hands immediately prior to and after handling baby.	**4.** To minimise the risk of infection.

5. Observe the umbilicus and surrounding area for:
  • Inflammation or pus
  • A swollen cord
  • Offensive odour from the cord
  • Any abnormality, e.g. granuloma, hernia.
	• Infection in this area can lead to severe complications, including fever, meningitis and septic foci (Zupan *et al* 2004)
	
	• Abnormality may need surgical intervention.

427

Procedure guideline 17.3 **Care of the umbilicus**

Statement	Rationale
1. Perform a clinical hand wash before commencing the procedure.	**1.** To minimise the risk of cross-infection.
2. Standard (universal) precautions must be applied.	**2.** To minimise the risk of cross-infection.

3. To clean the umbilicus:
  a) Remove the nappy.
  b) If there are no signs of infection leave the umbilical area clean and dry.
  c) Using warm tap water clean the umbilical area paying particular attention to the area under the clamp.
 	
  d) If there are signs of infection, take an umbilical swab for microbiology.
  e) The umbilicus should be cleaned with a sterile alcohol impregnated wipe and allowed to dry.
  f) Involve the parents/carers in re-applying the nappy and making the baby comfortable.
	a) To gain access to umbilical area.
	  b) To ensure the umbilical area is clean.
	
	  c) WHO (2001) currently recommends dry cord care and use of soap and water solution to clean the cord if visibly soiled. There is no evidence that applying sprays, creams or powders, are any better than keeping the baby's cord clean and dry at birth (Zupan *et al* 2004).
	  d) To identify micro-organisms.
	
	  e) Bacterial colonisation is significantly reduced by alcohol (Zupan *et al* 2004).
	  f) To minimise discomfort to the baby and ensure they are comfortable.

(Continued)

Procedure guideline 17.3 (*Continued*)

Statement	Rationale
4. Dispose of used equipment according to local waste policy.	**4.** To prevent contamination of area and adhere to hospital policy.
5. Record the completion of the procedure in the child's healthcare records.	**5.** To provide a record of the care given and promote continuity of care.
6. Send any bacterial swabs with a request form to microbiology.	**6.** To ensure that any infection is recognised quickly.
7. If the cord becomes detached it should be disposed of in a waste bag for incineration as per local policy.	**7.** To prevent contamination of the area and adhere to hospital policy.
8. If the parents/carers wish to keep the cord it should be placed in a specimen container.	**8.** The parents/carers may wish to keep the cord as a momento.
9. Inform an experienced nurse or doctor of any abnormalities found.	**9.** To effect treatment of the problem.

Newborn blood spot screening (formerly Guthrie testing)

Neonatal screening for phenylketonuria (PKU) using blood from a heel prick onto a card was first described by Dr R Guthrie in 1962. The screening programme, using drops of blood collected from a heel prick began in Scotland in 1964 and went nationwide in 1969/70. Congenital hypothyroidism was added to the national programme in 1982 (Neonatal Screening Working Group and Family Resource Centre 1999). In London and the surrounding areas, the incidence of PKU is approximately 1:10,000 births and congenital hypothyroidism 1:3–4000 births (Great Ormond Street Hospital for Children NHS Foundation Trust 2002, Neonatal Screening Working Group and Family Resource Centre 1999).

In 1993, the Department of Health recommended routine screening for sickle cell disorders in those districts where births to ethnic minorities at particular risk exceed 15% of all deliveries. As a result of the work of the NHS Sickle Cell and Thalassaemia Screening Programme, all babies in England are now being offered this. Sickle cell disorders occur in frequencies between 1:60 and 1:180 of babies born to parents originating in Africa and the Caribbean, rather less frequently in people from the Mediterranean, India and Pakistan, and occasionally in North Europeans (Neonatal Screening Working Group and Family Resource Centre 1999).

Since March 2004, babies in parts of England have been screened for an additional disorder, medium chain acyl coenzyme A dehydrogenase deficiency (MCADD) (Great Ormond Street Hospital for Children NHS Foundation Trust 2002) as a part of a national pilot project. MCADD affects 1:10,000–20,000 babies and is an autosomal recessive disorder. It is thought that between 1:40 and 1:80 healthy individuals are carriers but have no symptoms. MCADD results from the lack of an enzyme required to metabolise fat into energy (Great Ormond Street Hospital for Children NHS Foundation Trust 2004a, 2004b). Children with MCADD can break down fat to some extent but cannot do so fast enough. If the child needs to break down fats

fast, the accumulated medium chain fats form toxic metabolites, which can lead to serious life-threatening symptoms and even death (Great Ormond Street Hospital for Children NHS Foundation Trust 2004a, 2004b).

Babies and children with MCADD are healthy as long as they are able to avoid low blood sugar levels. The treatment for MCADD is to prevent this happening, especially during illness or fasting (Great Ormond Street Hospital for Children NHS Foundation Trust 2004a, 2004b). A national programme to manage the roll-out of screening for cystic fibrosis started in September 2005. All babies are now screened for cystic fibrosis.

The UK Newborn Screening Programme Centre was set up in October 2003 to 'support the establishment and maintenance of consistent standards in newborn screening throughout the UK for phenylketonuria, congenital hypothyroidism (TSH), cystic fibrosis and sickle cell conditions' (NHS Newborn Bloodspot Screening Programme 2008). These disorders usually cause no obvious problem in the neonatal period, and routine screening is designed to detect affected infants before symptoms develop. It is recommended that treatment be initiated by 21 days, as this is particularly important in improving the outcome for children with PKU and hypothyroidism (Great Ormond Street Hospital for Children NHS Foundation Trust 2002, NHS Newborn Bloodspot Screening Programme 2008, Rennie and Roberton 1999). A firm diagnosis can only be made after further investigation, so when a positive screening test is obtained, the infant is referred to a specialist centre for investigation, counselling and clinical management. In some areas of the country, some screening laboratories also include tests for other conditions such as galactosaemia and other amino acid disorders. These are at present not recommended for universal testing (Neonatal Screening Working Group and Family Resource Centre 1999).

Surveillance can be undertaken for maternal HIV infection based on anonymous testing of spare blood spots. This has been approved by ethics committees and funded by the Department of Health. This does not allow diagnosis to be made in individual cases, but does allow monitoring of disease frequency in a defined population (Neonatal Screening Working Group and Family Resource Centre 1999).

It is preferable to take the blood sample between days 5 and 8 (Neonatal Screening Working Group and Family Resource Centre 1999). In the community, the blood sample is taken by the midwife or health visitor, placed on the special Bloodspot Screening card and send to the local neonatal screening laboratory.

PKU and congenital hypothyroidism are conditions which, if untreated, often lead to severe mental and physical delay (Great Ormond Street Hospital for Children NHS Foundation Trust 2002, Neonatal Screening Working Group and Family Resource Centre 1999). Sickle cell disorders put young children at risk of serious infection (which can be fatal) as well as causing life-threatening anaemia (Rennie and Roberton 1999).

Principles table 17.10 **Assessing the need to test**

Principle	Rationale
1. Newborn Blood Spot tests are done on or after, the 5th day of life, taking the date of birth as day zero. It is essential to do it between days 5 and 8.	1. For local information and national booklets see NHS Newborn Bloodspot Screening Programme (2008)
2. When a baby under 5 days old is admitted to the hospital, a newborn blood spot screening test should therefore be taken between the 5th and 8th day of life.	2. To screen the baby for the abnormalities described.
3. If a baby is over 5 days old and less than 2 months, check that the New Born Blood Spot test has already been done by checking whether this is recorded in the child's notes, parent-held record, or referral letter. If not, contact the local Newborn Blood Spot Screening laboratory for advice.	3. For local information and national booklets see NHS Newborn Bloodspot Screening Programme (2008).
4. If the test has already been done this should be recorded with the date on the child's healthcare records and any other local documentation.	4. To complete documentation of Newborn Blood Spot Screening.
5. If the test has not been done, or if there is any doubt of a sample having been taken, the test should be taken as soon as possible and recorded according to hospital policy.	5. To ensure that Newborn Blood Spot screening is completed preventing long-term developmental delay and potential disability.
6a) If a baby has had a blood transfusion within 5 days, the test should still be automatically done. b) The date of the transfusion must be recorded on the New Born Blood Spot Screening card in the appropriate box.	6a) To ensure that all babies are part of the New Born Blood Spot Screening programme. b) A recent blood transfusion could give an inaccurate result and screening for sickle cell disease cannot be completed.

Procedure guideline 17.4 **Performing the newborn blood spot test**

Statement	Rationale
1. a) The Newborn Blood Spot test is usually done by a capillary blood sample (Liang and Harper 1998). b) The parents/carers should be advised about the reason for the blood test, the procedure explained, and their permission (or refusal) obtained. c) The UK Newborn Blood Spot Screening Centre produces parent/carer information about the test and this should be used to supplement oral information (NHS Newborn Bloodspot Screening Programme 2008).	1. b) This should be clearly documented, to ensure all team members are aware of the parents'/carers' decision.
2. When arterial or venous blood is being taken for another purpose, some of the blood may be used for the test.	2. Co-ordination of blood tests will help to reduce neonatal stress.

(Continued)

429

Procedure guideline 17.4 (*Continued*)

Statement	Rationale

3. To perform a Newborn Blood Spot Screening test:
  a) Take a capillary blood sample according to local practice guidelines (Liang and Harper 1998).
  b) Place blood sample on the provided screening test card using, if possible, one drop of blood in each of the four rings on the card.
  c) Allow the blood to dry.
  d) Complete all parts of the screening card.
  e) Place the card in the special 'waxed paper' envelope for transportation to the laboratory.
  f) Send the card to the local Newborn Blood Spot Screening test centre.
	a) To facilitate testing.
	
	e) The sample must be kept dry so should not be placed directly into a plastic bag.

4a) It is essential that all aspects of the Newborn Blood Spot Screening test card are completed otherwise the test cannot be processed **b)** If the parents/carers refuse to have the Newborn Blood Spot Test, this should be recorded in the child's notes and discharge summary. If the test is declined the Newborn Blood Spot Screening card should be completed with this information and sent to the local screening laboratory.	**4a)** To enable accurate evaluation of blood levels. **b)** To document parental/carer refusal of the screening test.

5. Items which should be recorded on the Newborn Blood Spot Screening card in the 'comments' section include:
  • Antibiotic treatment
  • Any relevant family history
  • If the baby is on Total Parenteral Nutrition.
	5. The neonatal screening laboratory will need this data to facilitate the test.

6. The taking of the Newborn Blood Spot Screening Test should be recorded:
  • In the child's nursing record
  • In the child's healthcare record
  • In the child's parent-held record when available.
	6. To provide accurate information.

Procedure guideline 17.5 **Repeating the newborn blood spot test**

Statement	Rationale

1. Repeat tests will be requested in the following circumstances:
  a) If there is a problem with the blood sample, e.g. inadequate quantity of blood or contamination of the card.
  b) If there is a problem with analysis.
  c) If the results are equivocal or borderline.
 	
  d) If the test has been taken within 72 hours of a blood transfusion. However, the test should be repeated, so that the baby gets into a tracking system.
	1. To ensure that the test is reliable.
	
	c) Each laboratory has a set of values for PKU and TSH and will repeat the screen if these values are exceeded.
	d) Due to mixing with the transfused blood the result may not be considered accurate.

2a) All babies who have had a blood transfusion require a repeat test for sickle disease 3 months after their last transfusion. As most babies will have been discharged by this stage, the local health authority must be informed of the need for a repeat blood test. **b)** All babies born under 36 weeks gestation will need a repeat test for TSH after 36 weeks. **c)** The blood sample gets lost in the post.	**2a)** Sickle cell disease cannot be confirmed or eradicated if the test is done within 3 months of a blood transfusion. **b)** Recent screening results have shown that some preterm babies who have normal TSH levels initially show signs of thyroid deficiency later. **c)** Prepaid envelopes are now being used in some areas to prevent this problem.

Procedure guideline 17.5 (*Continued*)

Statement	Rationale

3. When a repeat sample is requested:
  a) The ward will be informed of the need for a repeat by the Newborn Screening laboratory.
  b) The blood should be taken as soon as possible on another screening card and sent to the laboratory.
  c) The section of the card confirming that it is a repeat sample should be completed.
	a) To ensure that the test is repeated as soon as possible and that the baby is screened correctly.

4. When the test has been taken, it will be recorded in the regional centre.	4. Regional neonatal screening centres are set up throughout the UK (NHS Newborn Bloodspot Screening Programme 2008).

5. If a positive result is found:
  a) Arrangements will be made for the baby to be seen by a paediatric specialist, who is contacted by the regional screening centre, to instigate investigations.
  b) Treatment will be started as soon as possible after the diagnosis is confirmed.
  c) The child's GP will be contacted and informed of the child's investigations and results when available.
	a) To enable urgent specialist referral.
	To inform the family.
	To confirm the diagnosis.
	
	c) To ensure that the primary healthcare team is aware of the potential diagnosis.

6. The family should be advised of the support groups available for babies with PKU, hypothyroidism, sickle cell disease and MCADD, and they should be given a leaflet specific to the condition, from the UK Newborn Screening Programme Centre Website (NHS Newborn Bloodspot Screening Programme 2008).	6. To provide advice and support.

431

Phototherapy – neonatal jaundice

These guidelines are only effective for physiological jaundice, which is a common feature of the newborn baby. Jaundice can result from high levels of conjugated or unconjugated bilirubin. Physiological or neonatal jaundice, results from a high level of circulating unconjugated bilirubin coupled with an immature liver. Most neonates will experience a certain degree of physiological jaundice and have no problems (Totapally and Torbati 2005). In physiological jaundice, the serum bilirubin concentration will be highest around the third day of life. It should then begin to fall rapidly for 2–3 days and then more slowly over a 1–2 week period (Dent 2000). If bilirubin levels rise rapidly above a safe level, and are left untreated, damage to the brain can result. This is known as kernicterus (Juretschke 2005). See Treatment Threshold Graph (NICE http://guidance.nice.org.uk/CG98) for recommended safe levels. Conditions which may increase the risk of hyperbilirubinaemia and kernicterus in the neonate include:

- Prematurity
- Hypoalbuminaemia
- Hypoxia
- Dehydration
- Hypothermia
- Acidaemia
- Polycythaemia
- Haemolytic disease
- Bruising
- Hypoglycaemia
- Hyperlipidaemia
- Sepsis.

Drugs, for example, sulphonamides and heparin, may also increase the risk (Totapally and Torbati 2005). Phototherapy in sick neonates will therefore be commenced earlier. Phototherapy is a safe and effective method of treating the neonate who has high levels of unconjugated bilirubin. It works through the blue part of the spectrum at around 450nm (Dent 2000). The child's doctor must be informed if the phototherapy is unsuccessful and levels of bilirubin have reached a critical level or are rising at a rapid rate. An exchange transfusion may be needed.

NICE clinical guidelines for management of neonatal jaundice (NICE 2011) cover threshold tables, treatment threshold graphs, investigation pathways, phototherapy and transfusion pathways, in addition to providing information for parents/carers and non clinical staff.

Principles table 17.11 **Phototherapy**

Principle	Rationale
1. Most neonates will experience a certain degree of physiological jaundice and have no problems.	1. High bilirubin levels result from a high haemoglobin level and the short lifespan of the neonatal red cell, i.e.: • 40 days in the preterm baby • 60–70 days in the term baby • 120 days in the adult (Roberton 1993).
2. If bilirubin levels rise rapidly above a safe level, and are left untreated, damage to the brain can result.	2. Unconjugated bilirubin is carried in plasma bound to albumin. If dissociated from albumin, it can pass through the blood brain barrier (Fleming *et al* 1991).
3. Phototherapy is a safe and effective method of treating the neonate who has high levels of unconjugated bilirubin (Juretschke 2005, Totapally and Torbati 2005). It works through the blue part of the spectrum at around 450nm (Hart and Hainsworth 1997).	3. Light from the phototherapy lamp isomerises the unconjugated bilirubin passing through the skin into a non-toxic form, which can readily be excreted in stool and urine (Maisels 1996).

Procedure guideline 17.6 **Assessment of neonatal jaundice**

Statement	Rationale
1. Observe for signs and symptoms of jaundice including: • Yellowing of skin colour and sclera of eyes • Lethargy • Poor feeding • Darkened urine • Dark stools.	1. To enable treatment to be initiated.
2. If jaundice is obvious or the neonate has an increased risk of developing jaundice, take a blood sample to check the serum bilirubin level.	2. To ascertain the level of jaundice.
3. Send a capillary sample of venous or arterial blood and request for unconjugated, conjugated and total serum bilirubin levels.	3. Check local blood sampling policy and facilities for these tests.
4. For the jaundiced neonate with a high conjugated bilirubin level, phototherapy should be avoided and further liver function tests will be required. Consult with the medical team.	4. The skin of a neonate with high conjugated bilirubin levels will go deep brown in colour if phototherapy is used (Rubatelli *et al* 1983).
5a) Plot the total bilirubin and unconjugated bilirubin level on the Treatment Threshold Graph (NICE 2011). b) Ensure that the total bilirubin level is charted appropriately against the age and that the appropriate action line is referred to for the term neonate, the neonate less than 37 weeks gestation/less than 2.5kg or for the sick neonate.	5a) The unconjugated bilirubin is responsible for kernicterus and therefore should be monitored used (Rubatelli *et al* 1983). b) Action lines for the initiation of treatment commence at a lower level for the more premature and newborn infant, increasing for the first 6 days of life before it levels off.
6. Once the total bilirubin is plotted on the chart, take the appropriate management indicated by the action lines.	6. To reduce bilirubin levels to within normal limits.
7. If the total bilirubin level is rising or if the neonate is under phototherapy repeat the blood test at least 12 hourly.	7. To evaluate the action taken and the effectiveness of treatment.
8. Consult with the doctor to determine whether phototherapy should be commenced at a lower total bilirubin level in the sick neonate.	8. There is an increased risk of bilirubin toxicity in the sick neonate (Fleming *et al* 1991, Roberton 1993).

Procedure guideline 17.7 Administering phototherapy

Statement	Rationale
1. Commence phototherapy as indicated on the Treatment Threshold Graph (NICE 2011)and inform the child's doctor. Phototherapy units can be obtained from hospital central supplies.	**1.** Check local policy and procedures.
2. More than one set of phototherapy lights may be required if bilirubin levels are very high.	**2.** To maximise the area of skin exposed to phototherapy.
3a) Explain the procedure to the family. **b)** Advise them that phototherapy may be interrupted, i.e. the lights may be turned off, for them to be in contact with their baby and for nursing care. **c)** The baby must still be comforted and their stress minimised as babies do not like being exposed.	**3a)** To minimise stress and keep them informed. **b)** Stopping phototherapy for up to 2 hours for every 6 hours does not decrease effectiveness (Hart and Hainsworth 1997, Maisels 1996).
4. Ensure surfaces of the phototherapy lights and incubator are clean and dust free.	**4.** To optimise the level of irradiance received by the neonate (Totapally and Torbati 2005). Clean equipment as per local policy and reduce infection risks
5. To initiate phototherapy: **a)** Perform a clinical hand wash. **b)** Undress the baby and open their nappy. **c)** Remove any creams or oils from the baby's skin. **d)** Gently cover baby's eyes with 'eye shades'. These can be obtained from hospital supplies. **e)** Place the overhead phototherapy light 40–50cm from the baby's skin and activate the unit. **f)** Perform a clinical hand wash.	**a)** To minimise the risk of cross-infection. **b)** To maximise the effect of the phototherapy. **c)** To prevent skin burns during therapy. **d)** There is the potential for photochemical damage to eyes (Hart and Hainsworth 1997). **e)** To optimise the effectiveness of the treatment without overheating the neonate (Blackburn 1995, Merenstein and Gardiner, 1993). **f)** To minimise the risk of cross-infection.
6. Where possible change the position of the baby after routine nursing care.	**6.** To expose maximum skin area in order to reduce skin bilirubin.
7. Monitor the hydration of the baby and the specific gravity of their urine. Liaise with the child's doctor to ensure adequate hydration. An extra 30ml/kg/day of fluids may be required if urine specific gravity is >1012 or other signs of dehydration exist.	**7.** Insensible losses can occur through the skin, or through loose stools, created by a decrease in gut transit time caused by the osmotic effect of excreted bilirubin (Roberton 1992, 1993).
8. Monitor the baby's temperature: **a)** It must be monitored and recorded every 3 hours following initiation of treatment. **b)** The baby may need to be placed in an incubator during phototherapy treatment. **c)** A thin layer of plastic sheeting may also be used to cover the baby. **d)** It must not be allowed to cover their face.	**a)** Document and report any changes. **b)** To ensure the baby maintains a normal temperature in a neutral thermal environment. **c)** To keep the baby warm. **d)** To prevent suffocation.
9. Document time of commencement and completion of phototherapy in the child's healthcare records and on the Treatment Threshold Graph (NICE 2011).	**9.** To maintain an accurate record.
10. To complete the treatment: Monitor total bilirubin and unconjugated bilirubin levels 6–12 hourly and record on their Treatment Threshold Graph (NICE 2011).	To evaluate the effectiveness of the treatment and assess whether further interventions are required.

433

(Continued)

Procedure guideline 17.7 (*Continued*)

Statement	Rationale
11. Continue phototherapy until the total bilirubin level is below the phototherapy line on the Treatment Threshold Graph (NICE 2011).	**11.** It takes up to 6 days for the liver of a well term neonate, to reach sufficient maturity and be able to metabolise bilirubin (Hart and Hainsworth 1997). It may take longer for the sick or preterm neonate.
12. A prolonged jaundice study may be indicated, if unconjugated bilirubin does not start to fall after 4–5 days, or 5–6 days in the preterm neonate and if it continues to remain high after 14 days. This may be done following liaison with the child's doctor.	**12.** To detect any pathological causes.
13. Once phototherapy is discontinued continue to observe for signs of jaundice and check the bilirubin level 12–24 hours after discontinuation of treatment.	**13.** There is a risk of rebound jaundice, which will require further phototherapy treatment (Roberton 1993).
14. On discontinuation of phototherapy monitor and record the baby's temperature every 3 hours.	**14.** The baby will dramatically cool down and will need their thermal neutral environment re-evaluating.
15. The discontinuation of phototherapy must be recorded on the Treatment Threshold Graph (NICE 2011) and in their healthcare records.	**15.** To maintain an accurate record.
16. On completion of treatment, the phototherapy unit must be sent for cleaning as per hospital policy before being used again.	**16.** For decontamination and to prevent infection. For checking of function.

References

434

Altimier l, Warher B, Amlung S, Kenner C. (1999) Neonatal thermoregulation; Bed Surface Transfers. Neonatal Network, 18(4), 35–37

Blackburn S. (1995) Hyperbilirubinaemia and neonatal jaundice. Neonatal Network, 14(7), 15–25

Blackburn ST, Loper DL. (1992) Thermoregulation. In: Blackburn ST, Loper DL. (eds) Maternal, Fetal and Neonatal Physiology: A Clinical Perspective. London, WB Saunders, pp677–698

British National Formulary for Children (2011) Available at http://bnfc.org/bnfc/bnfc/current

Budin P. (1907) The Feeding and Hygiene of Premature and Full Term Infants. The Nursling, Translated by WJ Maloney. London, Caxton

Department of Health (1993) The Report of the Working Party of the Standing Medical Advisory Committee on Sickle Cell, Thalassaemia and Other Haemoglobinopathies. London, HMSO

Department of Health Circular (1998) PL/ CMO/98/3. PL/CNO/98/4: Vitamin K for Newborn Babies. London, Department of Health

Department of Health (2009) Toolkit for High Quality Neonatal Services, October 2009. London, DoH

Dent J. (2000) Hematological problems. In: Boxwell G. (ed.) Neonatal Intensive Care. Cambridge, Cambridge University Press

Drager Product Information (1997) Closed and Open Incubators. Hemel Hempstead, Drager, pp1–8

Fear NT, Roman E, Ansell P, Simpson J, Day N, Eden OB, United Kingdom Childhood Cancer Study (2003) Vitamin K and childhood cancer: a report from the United Kingdom Childhood Cancer Study. British Journal of Cancer, 89(7), 1228–1231

Fleming P, Spiedel B, Marlow N, Dunn P. (1991) A Neonatal Vade-Mecum. London, Edward Arnold, pp260–271

Great Ormond Street Hospital for Children NHS Foundation Trust (2002) Congenital Hypothyroidism Information for Families. London, Great Ormond Street Hospital

Great Ormond Street Hospital for Children NHS Trust (2004a) Bloodspot Screening for Medium Chain Acyl Coenzyme A Dehydenase Deficiency (MCADD. Information for Midwives/health professionals. London, Great Ormond Street

Great Ormond Street Hospital for London for Children NHS Trust (2004b) Bloodspot Screening for Medium Chain Coenzyme A Dehydrogenase Deficiency (MCADD), Information for Parents/Carers. London, Great Ormond Street

Hart G, Hainsworth A. (1997) Phototherapy for neonates: Step by Step Guide. Journal of Neonatal Nursing, 3(4)

Hey E. (2003) Vitamin K – what, why and when (reviews). Archives of Disease in Childhood, 88(2) 80–83

Juretschke LJ. (2005) Kernicterus: still a concern. Neonatal Network, 24(2), 7–19.

Klaus M, Fanaroff A. (1973) The Physical Environment in Care of the High Risk Neonate. Philadelphia, Saunders

Leick-Rude, Bloom LF (1998) A comparison of temperature-taking methods in neonates. Neonatal Network, 17(5), 21–37

Levene MI, Tudhope SK, Sinha SK. (2008) Essential Neonatal Medicine, 4th edition. Oxford, Blackwell Science

Liang D, Harper M. (1998) Clinical Practice Guideline: Neonatal Capillary Blood Sampling. London, Great Ormond Street Hospital. Available at http://www.gosh.nhs.uk/clinical_information/clinical_guidelines/cpg_guideline_00053 (last accessed 14th May 2011)

Lyon AJ, Pikaar MC, Badger P, McIntosh N. (1997) Temperature control in very low birth-weight infants during the first 5 days of life. Archives of Diseases in Childhood, 76(1), F47–50

Maisels M. (1996) Why we use homeopathic doses of phototherapy. Paediatrics, 98, 283–287

Marshall A. (1997) Humidifying the Environment for the Premature Neonate. Journal of Neonatal Nursing, 3(1), 32–36

McMillan D. (1997) Joint position statement of the Fetus and Newborn Committee, Canadian Pediatric Society (CPS), and the Committee on

Child and Adolescent Health, College of Family Physicians of Canada. Routine administration of vitamin K to newborns. Paediatrics and Child Health, 2(6), 429–431

Medoff-Cooper B. (1994) Transition of the preterm infant to an open crib. Journal of Obstetric Gynecol Neonatal Nursing, 23(4), 329–335

Merenstein GB, Gardiner SI. (1993) Handbook of Neonatal Intensive Care, 3rd edition. St Louis, Mosby

Mitchell A. (1997) Thermal Monitoring of Patients in NICU. Journal of Neonatal Nursing, 2(2), Insert (i–iv)

Mok Q, Bass CA, Ducker DA, McIntosh N. (1991) Temperature instability during nursing procedures in preterm neonates. Archives of Diseases in Childhood, 66(7), 783–786

National Health and Medical Research Council (NHMRC) of the Australian Government (2000) Joint Statement and Recommendations on Vitamin K Administration to Newborn Infants to Prevent Vitamin K Deficiency Bleeding in Infancy (ref CH39). Available at www.nhmrc.gov.au/publications/synopses/_files/ch39.pdf. (last accessed 11th August 2006)

Neilson JP. (2008) Cochrane Update: Effect of timing of umbilical cord clamping at birth of term infants on mother and baby outcomes. Obstetrics & Gynecology, 112(1), 177–178

Neonatal Screening Working Group and Family Resource Centre (1999) Routine blood screening tests on newborn babies. London, Great Ormond Street Hospital for Children NHS Trust

NICE (2011) Clinical Guidelines: Neonatal Jaundice. Available at http://guidance.nice.org.uk/CG98, updated 27th May (last accessed 10th June 2011)

NHS Newborn Bloodspot Screening Programme (2008) Information and national booklets. Available at http://newbornbloodspot.screening.nhs.uk/ (last accessed 14th June2011)

Rennie JM, Roberton NRC, (1999) Textbook of Neonatology, 3rd edition. Edinburgh, Churchill Livingstone

Rennie JM, Roberton NRC. (2005) Textbook of neonatology, 4th edition. Edinburgh, Churchill Livingstone

Rijhwani A, Davenport M, Dawrant M, Dimitriou G, Patel S, Greenough A, Nicholaides K. (2005) Definitive surgical management of antenatally diagnosed exomphalos. Journal of Paediatric Surgery, 40(30),516–522

Roberton N. (1992) Textbook of Neonatology, 2nd edition. Edinburgh, Churchill Livingstone, pp605–624

Roberton N. (1993) A Manual of Intensive Care, 3rd edition. London, Edward Arnold, pp 238–260

Roberton NRC. (1995) A Manual of Neonatal Intensive Care. London, Edward Arnold, pp6–14

Roche Products Ltd (2005) Konakion MM Ampoules (revised December 2005). Welwyn Garden City, Roche Products Ltd

Roche Products Ltd (2007) Konakion MM Paediatric Ampoules (revised July 2007). Welwyn Garden City, Roche Products Ltd

Rubatelli F, Jon G, Reddi E. (1983) Bronze Baby Syndrome : A new porphynn related disorder. Paediatric Research, 17, 327–330

Seguin JH, Vieth R. (1996) Thermal stability of premature infants during routine care under radiant warmers. Archives of Diseases in Childhood (Fetal & Neonatal Edition), 74(2), F137–138

Sheeran MS. (1996) Thermoregulation in Neonates; obtaining an accurate axillary temperature measurement. Journal of Neonatal Nursing, 2(4), 6–9

Short MA. (1998) Comparison of temperature in VLBW infants swaddled verses unswaddled. Neonatal Network, 17(3), 25–31

Thomas K (1994) Thermoregulation in neonate. Neonatal Network, 13(2), 15–21

Totapally BR, Torbati D. (2005) Neonatal jaundice. International Pediatrics, 20(1), 47–54

World Health Organization (WHO) (2001) Estimates in saving newborn lives. State of the Worlds Newborns. Washington DC, Save the Children Federation-US, pp. 1–49

Zupan J, Garner P, Omari AA. (19/07/2004) Topical umbilical cord care at birth. Cochrane Database of Systematic Reviews 2004, 3 (e-pub). Available at http://www.ncbi.nlm.nih.gov/pubmed/15266437 (last accessed 15th December 2010)

Chapter 18

Neurological care

Chapter contents

Procedure guidelines

The Great Ormond Street Hospital Manual of Children's Nursing Practices, First Edition. Edited by Susan Macqueen, Elizabeth Anne Bruce, Faith Gibson.
© 2012 Great Ormond Street Hospital for Children NHS Foundation Trust. Published 2012 by Blackwell Publishing Ltd.

Introduction

This chapter is divided into four sections: neurological care; seizure management; external ventricular drainage (EVD); and lumbar puncture.

Specific investigations utilised within neurology and neurosurgery include scans such as CT (computerised tomography) and MRI (magnetic resonance imaging) and details relating to these investigations can be found in other sections of the book (see Chapter 14).

Neurological observations

Introduction

Formal neurological observations should be undertaken as part of an overall physical assessment of the child and in conjunction with their systemic observations. Appropriate documentation should include the use of a paediatric coma scoring system (Reilly *et al* 1988 and an early warning system (Chapman *et al* 2010). Relevance of the child's surroundings, activities and the presence/absence of their parents/carers must also form part of the assessment. The young child poses challenges when assessing their level of consciousness due to their cognition, limited verbalisation, regression secondary to the illness itself, the effects of hospitalisation, separation from family and home environment, and fear (May and Carter 1995). The parent's/carer's unique knowledge and understanding of their child should be utilised whenever possible in helping to assess the child's behaviour and response.

Consciousness is described as a 'general awareness of oneself and the surrounding environment' (Aucken and Crawford 1999). This 'higher brain function' can be assessed by the subjective observation of arousability and behaviour in response to stimuli (Ellis and Cavanagh 1992). Assessment of consciousness is closely linked to the assessment of pupil reaction:

the reticular activating system (RAS) is situated just above the brainstem and is responsible for arousal; the anatomical proximity of the brainstem to the nuclei of cranial nerves III, IV and VI is also significant as together theses nerves control pupillary responses and eye movement (Disabato and Burkett 2007). The nurse should attempt to first rouse the child and then undertake assessment of pupil reaction to light. Awareness, once the child is roused is controlled in the cerebral cortex. The primary goal for the nurse is to identify changes that may indicate deterioration so that early intervention can be implemented.

A neurological assessment chart known as the Glasgow Coma Scale (GCS) was first introduced by Jennet and Teasdale (1974) and has been adapted worldwide as a standardised assessment for patients with central nervous system dysfunction. The scale is divided into three categories comprising eye opening, best verbal response and best motor response. Each category is further divided and the resulting graph and numerical score is used in conjunction with vital signs, in identifying the patient's clinical status. The lower the numerical score the lower the child's level of consciousness.

Many of the responses required when utilising the GCS involve an adult neurodevelopment response, specifically the development of language and the ability to localise pain; the Adelaide scale was devised for use in children and further adaptations of the scale have since been produced. The Paediatric Neuroscience Benchmarking group in the UK has devised a chart encompassing the developmental and chronological age of the child.

A chart, however, is only as good as the person using it and education in its usage is essential. Neurological assessment of the child on the Intensive Care Unit is outlined by Marcoux (2005), who describes the neurological assessment, pathophysiology, and management of increased intracranial pressure in the critically ill child who has sustained an acute neurological injury.

Principles table 18.1 Neurological observations

Principle	Rationale
1. Neurological observations should be performed on the child as a baseline observation, on those with an altered level of consciousness or those at risk of developing an impaired level of consciousness.	1. Early recognition of changes in conscious level is paramount in the prevention of secondary injury associated with raised intracranial pressure (Norman 2000).
2. Frequency of neurological observations is dictated by the child's condition and can be decided by either medical or nursing staff as appropriate.	2. To enable appropriate, individual assessment to be performed.
3. All staff performing neurological observations should be trained in both the theoretical and practical aspects of these observations.	3. To ensure accurate assessment and recording of the child's condition.

(Continued)

Principles table 18.1 (*Continued*)

Principle	Rationale

4. An appropriate assessment tool is required, taking into account the physical and neurodevelopment age of the child.
    The neurological coma score assessment tool in place at The Great Ormond Street Hospital incorporates an adaptation of the Glasgow Coma Scale (GCS) devised by Jennet and Teasdale (1974) and the Adelaide Paediatric Coma Scale (Simpson and Reilly 1982).
    Incorporated into the charts are a pain score and a record of significant events (see Appendix 18.1).
	4. To ensure accurate assessment and recording of the child's condition.

5. The GCS indicates level of consciousness by assessing a patient's ability to perform three activities: **a)** Eye opening **b)** Verbal response **c)** Motor response. Each activity is given a score and then the three scores are added together to give a score from 3 to 15. A score of 15 indicates a fully alert, orientated patient, while a score of 3 indicates a deep coma.	
6. The GCS is documented in the form of a graph and demonstrated by a series of joined up dots.	**6.** To enable quick and easy evaluation of trends in a child's condition (Aucken and Crawford 1999).
7. When undertaking neurological assessment, it is essential that a baseline be established in relation to the child's individual development.	**7.** To ensure accurate assessment and recording of the child's condition.
8. Any alteration in the child's GCS should be reported to senior nursing/medical staff.	**8.** To enable prompt and appropriate action to be taken as required.
9. A sleeping child should always be woken for neurological assessment.	**9.** To ensure accurate assessment and recording of the child's condition

438

Procedure guideline 18.1 **Neurological observations**

Statement	Rationale
1. Inform the child and family: **a)** That neurological observations are necessary. **b)** Why they are necessary. **c)** What it entails.	**1.** To gain adherence.
2. Encourage the family to participate in the assessment.	**2.** An appropriate fear of strangers may lead some children not to respond to unfamiliar adults.
4. Observe the child from a distance and assess for: **i.** Eye opening **ii.** Appropriateness of vocalisation **iii.** Motor activity. **a)** Determine if the family considers these actions normal for their child. **b)** If the child does not open their eyes or the family considers that actions are abnormal then further assessment is necessary.	**a)** The family knows what normal behaviour is for their child. **b)** Spontaneous eye opening can only be achieved without any stimulation from the nursing staff (Armon *et al* 2003).

Principles table 18.2 Scores for eye opening

Principle	Rationale
Score 4: Spontaneous eye opening.	Demonstrates that arousal mechanisms are intact (reticular activating system) (Appleton and Gibbs 1998).
Score 3: Eye opening to speech. Speak to the child using appropriate language and familiar names. Involve the family to encourage the child to respond to verbal stimuli.	Demonstrates that the cerebral cortex is processing information (Armon *et al* 2003). A child may not open their eyes for unfamiliar adults and this could be behavioural rather than neurological (Barrett-Goode 2000).
Score 2: Eye opening to painful stimuli. If the child is not opening their eye to speech then a central painful stimuli will need to be applied (see Appendix 18.2).	The necessity of painful stimuli to elicit eye opening suggests a decrease in level of consciousness.
Score 1: No eye opening to either speech or painful stimuli. It is essential to note if a child is unable to open their eyes due to orbital swelling or a ptosis, rather than suggestion of a reduced level of consciousness, in which case a '**C**' should be inserted in the appropriate space on the assessment tool.	Indicates that there is a marked depression of the arousal system (Barrett-Goode 2000). To prevent an unnecessary painful stimulus being applied.

Principles table 18.3 Scores for verbal response

Principle	Rationale
This part of the assessment is scored 1–5 and contains a description for the infant/preverbal child and the verbal child.	Verbal response assesses consciousness and cognition (Appleton and Gibbs 1998).
Score 5 • Infant/preverbal child – smiling. • Orientated verbal child. Involve the family to use appropriate familiar words to encourage the child to verbalise.	Orientation in a young child has been defined as an awareness of being in hospital or an ability to give their name (Birdsall and Greif 1990). An appropriate fear of strangers may lead some children not to respond to unfamiliar adults.
Score 4 • Infant not yet able to smile – expected best score. • Infant/preverbal child – crying. • Disorientated verbal child.	
Score 3 • Infant/preverbal child – inappropriate cry. The pitch of the cry is important (Barrett-Goode 2000). A high-pitched cry should be recorded within the significant events. • Verbal child – monosyllabic responses.	It is important to involve the family who will be able to identify if the cry is inappropriate for their child. To ensure accurate recording of the child's condition.
Score 2 • Infant/preverbal child – occasional whimper. • Verbal child – incomprehensible sounds.	At this stage, both verbal and painful stimuli may need to be used to obtain a response (Appleton and Gibbs 1998).

(Continued)

Principles table 18.3 (*Continued*)

Principle	Rationale
Score 1 Infant/preverbal/verbal child – no verbal response to both verbal and painful stimuli. If a child is unable to speak as a result of damage to the speech centres of the brain (dysphasia), then a '**D**' should be placed in the appropriate space on the assessment tool (Appleton and Gibbs 1998).	To ensure accurate assessment and recording of the child's condition.
If a child has a tracheostomy or an endotracheal tube in situ, a '**T**' should be marked in the appropriate space on the assessment tool (Aucken and Crawford 1999).	To ensure accurate assessment and recording of the child's condition.

Principles table 18.4 **Scores for best motor response**

Principle	Rationale
This part of the assessment is scored 1–6.	Upper limbs are used to assess motor response as lower limbs can be inconsistent and there may be a spinal reflex (Appleton and Gibbs 1998).
The motor response of the best arm is recorded (see Appendix 18.3).	If a limb is broken the child may be unable to respond to a painful stimulus.
Limbs with an obvious injury such as a fracture are not assessed (Armon *et al* 2003).	
Score 6 An infant moves the arms spontaneously. A child is able to obey commands.	Demonstrates that the brain is able to receive and interpret sensory information and then coordinate a response (Armon *et al* 2003).
Questions to be avoided when assessing a child's ability to obey commands are: • 'Squeeze my fingers' • 'Open your eyes' (Armon *et al* 2003). Involve the family to encourage the child to obey commands.	The results could be either a reflex grasp or a coincidental action (Armon *et al* 2003). Children may refuse to obey commands from a stranger but may obey commands given by a family member (Barrett-Goode 2000).

Score 5
Central painful stimulus to evoke a localised response will need to be applied and the response observed (Armon *et al* 2003) when:
• An infant does not move limbs spontaneously
• A child does not obey commands.
    Their level of neurological maturity determines the level of best response in a child (Bouffet *et al* 1996).
    Localisation is expected in children between the ages of 6 months and 2 years (Bouffet *et al* 1996).
	If a child is not localising spontaneously then applying a painful stimulus will not be necessary.
	
	Due to neurological immaturity, an infant younger than 6 months is unable to localise to pain (Bouffet *et al* 1996).

440

Principles table 18.4 (*Continued*)

Principle	Rationale

Score 5 continued
The best methods of central painful stimulus to evoke a localised response are:
• Trapezius squeeze
• Supraorbital pressure.
  Localising to pain.
  The arm will move towards the source of the pain in an attempt to remove it.
	Localising to pain indicates that the brain is able to receive sensory information by feeling pain and can coordinate a motor response to attempt to remove the source of the pain (Appleton and Gibbs 1998).

To qualify as localising, the child must bring their hand up beyond the level of the chin (Appleton and Gibbs 1998).	A sternal rub will not show a true localising response, as the child will not have to bring their arm up to chin height (Appleton and Gibbs 1998).
Use of an oxygen mask or nasogastric tube should be avoided as these may cause irritation and the child may localise spontaneously to these sources.	To prevent unnecessary painful stimulus being applied.

Score 4
Normal flexion:
• Infant – best motor response in an infant up to 6 months is flexion (Bouffet *et al* 1996)
• Child – not localising to a central painful stimulus but can bend their arm towards the source of the pain.
  The arm bends at the elbow and the wrist extends rapidly in response to pain but does not attempt to remove the source of the painful stimulus (Appleton and Gibbs 1998).
  Scores below 4 are considered to be abnormal responses.
	Indicates that the brain can receive sensory information by feeling pain and can flex in response, e.g. withdrawal of hand when in contact with a hot object or surface.
	
	Indicates varying degrees of cerebral damage.

Score 3 Abnormal flexion: • The elbow flexes and the wrist rotates in response to a central painful stimulus (Appleton and Gibbs 1998).	Indication of severe cerebral damage and a sign of malfunction in nerve pathways between the brain cortex and the spine (Appleton and Gibbs 1998).
Score 2 Extension to central painful stimulus: • The arm straightens at the elbow and there may be internal rotation of the lower arm (Appleton and Gibbs 1998; Armon *et al* 2003).	Indication of damage to the brain stem by interrupting information being sent to and from the cerebrum. This is a serious sign and may indicate a poor prognosis (Appleton and Gibbs 1998).
Score 1 No response to central painful stimulus.	Indication of extreme depression of brain stem function resulting in no possible sensory input and/or motor output (Armon *et al* 2003).
If a child is paralysed, e.g. as a result of paralysing agents, then a '**P**' should be inserted in the appropriate space on the assessment tool.	To prevent any unnecessary painful central stimulus being applied. To ensure accurate assessment and recording of the child's condition.
When assessing best motor response, it is important to observe for any asymmetry or inability to move a particular limb	An inability to move a particular limb may indicate a hemiplegia.
Add up the total from the three categories to give the Glasgow Coma Score. Record this total on the assessment chart.	To ensure accurate assessment and recording of the child's condition.

441

(*Continued*)

Principles table 18.4 (*Continued*)

Principle	Rationale
Report any alteration to senior nursing staff/medical staff.	To enable prompt and appropriate action to be taken as required.
Assess the child's pain score (see pain assessment guideline) and record total on assessment chart.	To ensure accurate assessment and recording of the child's condition.
Although not part of the Glasgow Coma Scale, vital signs, pupillary reaction and limb movement are an important part of the neurological assessment and should be recorded in addition to the child's conscious level.	To ensure accurate assessment and recording of the child's condition.
Record temperature, pulse rate, respiration rate and blood pressure as condition dictates, together with neurological observations.	A raised blood pressure and a low pulse rate may be an indication of raised intracranial pressure, although this is often a late sign (Bouffet *et al* 1996). Control centres for blood pressure, heart rate and respiration rate are located in the brain stem (Aucken and Crawford 1999).

Procedure guideline 18.2 Pupil reaction

Statement	Rationale
1. The size of both pupils should be observed and noted before applying a light stimulus.	1. This is the pupil size that is recorded on the neurological assessment chart. Unequal pupil size can indicate raised intracranial pressure causing constriction of the occulomotor nerve (Aucken and Crawford 1999) and should be reported to the senior nurse immediately.
2. On the significant events chart, document any medication that may affect pupil size.	2. Some drugs, e.g. atropine, dilate the pupil, while opiates such as morphine cause pupillary constriction (Aucken and Crawford 1999).
3. A pen torch with a bright narrow beam should be used to test both pupils individually. **a)** Both pupils should constrict when light is shone in either eye.	3. Both pupils should react briskly and constrict equally. **a)** If both pupils are not constricting, this may indicate damage to the optic nerve. Fixed dilated pupils indicate a neurosurgical emergency and should be reported immediately.
4. Encourage the family to participate in the recording.	4. Young children may resist having a light shone into their eyes and may respond better to family (Birdsall and Greif 1990).
5. Record pupil reaction in the appropriate space on the chart: • Brisk reaction = + • No reaction = – • Sluggish reaction = **SL**.	5. An absent or sluggish reaction may indicate damage to the oculomotor nerve as a result of raised intracranial pressure.
6. Report any change to senior nursing staff.	6. To enable prompt and appropriate action to be taken as required.
7. Document any known visual problems, e.g. blindness, on the significant events chart.	7. To ensure accurate assessment and recording of the child's condition.

Procedure guideline 18.3 Limb movement

Statement	Rationale

1. The strength of both limbs is measured:
  a) In young babies: observing them moving their limbs will be an indicator of limb strength. Checking the grasp reflex bilaterally is another reliable sign (Birdsall and Greif 1990).
  b) In younger children: limb strength can be assessed through play, e.g. getting them to kick a ball.
  c) In older children: where possible, ask them to respond to commands, e.g. ask the child to push and pull against the assessor.	

2. Document limb strength on the assessment chart. If there is a difference between the two sides, document the right (R) and left (L) sides separately.	2. A developing hemiparesis can be an indication of raised intracranial pressure as a result of damage to the motor cortex (Aucken and Crawford 1999).
3. Report any alteration to senior nursing staff.	3. To enable prompt and appropriate action to be taken as required.
4. If a child is paralysed, for example, as a result of paralysing agents, then a **P** should be inserted in the appropriate space on the assessment tool. If a child has a fracture, then a hash (#) sign should be entered in the appropriate space.	4. To ensure accurate assessment and recording of the child's condition.

Signs of raised intracranial pressure

In infants and young children, some or all of the following signs may be present:

- Tense or bulging anterior fontanelle in infants
- Sun setting pupils in infants
- High pitched cry
- Irritability
- Lethargy
- Vomiting
- Headaches.

If **any** of these signs of raised intracranial pressure occur they should be documented on the significant events chart and the senior nursing staff informed. This will ensure accurate assessment and recording of the child's condition and enable prompt and appropriate action to be taken as required.

Education and training

Staff should receive a theoretical and practical training session from a paediatric nurse with neuroscience experience. Theoretical sessions should include the Trust training video: 'Paediatric Coma Charts – A guide to assessment' (Great Ormond Street Hospital for Children NHS Foundation Trust 1997). This will ensure that the correct assessment is performed with consistent reliability.

In addition, staff should receive supervised practice and assessment.

Seizures

Introduction

This section includes guidelines on the nursing care of children with known seizures (epilepsy) and also those children with first time or new seizures. There are different management approaches for different types of seizures, for example in epilepsy, myoclonic seizures are dealt with differently than tonic-clonic seizures (Castledine 1993). Skilled nursing care, and management of a child having a seizure is of vital importance.

Seizures are of varying classification and are therefore dealt with by differing approaches (see the link at http://www.gosh.nhs.uk/clinical_information/clinical_guidelines/cpg_guideline_00036 for classification of seizures).

Definition of seizures

Seizures are brief malfunctions of the brains' electrical system resulting from cortical neuronal discharge. The manifestations of seizures are determined by the site of origin and may include unconsciousness or altered consciousness, involuntary movements, and changes in perception, behaviours, sensations and postures (Kwong *et al* 2001).

Causes of seizures

When a child has a seizure, it is important to distinguish whether the episode was an epileptic or non-epileptic seizure. Some seizures may result from an acute medical or neurological illness

443

and cease once the illness is treated, e.g. febrile convulsions; electrolyte imbalances such as hypocalcaemia, hypernatraemia; hypoglycaemia, which is typically seen in neonates; infections and drugs (Armon *et al* 2003, Hazinski 1992). On the other hand, the child's seizures may already have been diagnosed as epilepsy (Chin *et al* 2006).

There can be any number of reasons for a seizure to occur. Some examples are:

- Seizure disorders – epilepsy
- Infections (intracranial infections can lead to cerebral oedema, which can be the focus for seizures):
  - Systemic (sepsis), CNS, encephalitis, meningitis, febrile convulsion
  - Focal infection – abscess
- Head injury – especially depressed fractures of the skull and when anoxia has occurred
- Structural lesions – space occupying lesion – tumour (tumours, for example, can act as a focus for seizures.)
- Cerebral infarction, haematoma, intra-ventricular haemorrhage (IVH) – any incident that interferes with normal blood flow can be a focus for seizures
- Hypoxia
- Acidosis
- Metabolic disorders
- Electrolyte imbalances: hypocalcaemia, hypoglycaemia, hyponatraemia, hypernatraemia, dehydration
- Toxic ingestion. Depolarisation is associated with ionic imbalances that alter the chemical environment of the neurons with an intracellular accumulation of sodium, as well as a depletion of intracellular potassium (Hickey 2003). Depolarisation is followed by hyperpolarisation; the cell begins to fire repeatedly producing sustained membrane depolarization and seizure activity (Hickey 2003)
- Hypoxic ischaemic encephalopathy (HIE) (Hazinski 1992).

Physiology of seizures

A prolonged seizure must be treated. There is increasing evidence that the longer the seizures persist, the more difficult it is to terminate them (Holmes 1999). A prolonged seizure is defined as lasting for over 5 minutes (Holmes 1999). Since typical convulsive seizures generally last less than a few minutes in most children, a suggested operational definition of status epilepticus is either continuous seizures lasting at least 5 minutes, or two or more discrete seizures not separated by complete recovery of consciousness (Holmes 1999). If a seizure is continuing after 5 minutes it will commonly continue for at least 30 minutes unless treatment is implemented. Children who have seizures for 5 minutes or longer are likely to be in the early stages of convulsive status and should be treated rapidly (Scott *et al* 1999).

Sustained seizure activity increases adenosine triphosphate (ATP) requirements of neurons, as the constant electrical activity requires an extremely active sodium-potassium pump. This is due to the energy requirements of seizing neurons increasing by up to 250% (Hickey 1997). Systemic physiological changes occur early in a seizure in order to prevent the effects of damage to the brain. These changes include:

- Increased cerebral blood flow with increase in oxygen and glucose delivery to the brain and increased removal of toxic metabolites, with the aim of protecting neurons against damage (Hickey 1997).
- Increased heart rate.
- Increased blood pressure.
- Increased blood glucose levels. At the same time constant muscle contraction and relaxation increases tissue oxygen requirements in the rest of the body leading to an increase in cellular respiration and glycolysis. This can also occur as a result of the metabolic changes from hypoxia leading to acidosis. An example is tonic-clonic seizures where there is prolonged muscular contraction affecting the respiratory muscles. This can also occur as a secondary effect from administration of anti-convulsant medication to terminate seizures.

Respirations can become compromised in certain seizures – therefore oxygenation decreases. After about 30 minutes these physiological mechanisms fail and probably contribute to any neurological damage that may occur. Eventually this can lead to: hypoxaemia or apnoea and hypoglycaemia caused by the increased metabolic activity in skeletal muscles (Hazinski 1992). As a result cellular exhaustion and selected cellular destruction can occur.

Sustained convulsions will increase cerebral blood flow and metabolic requirements and can result in secondary damage to the brain, permanent brain damage or death (Hickey, 1997).

Procedure guideline 18.4 On admission: documentation

Statement	Rationale
1. Information should be clearly documented in the child's healthcare records. The link at http://www.gosh.nhs.uk/clinical_information/clinical_guidelines/cpg_guideline_00036/Appendix_2.doc describes seizure patterns.	1. To ensure good communication between all members of the multi-disciplinary team.
a) An important nursing clinical skill is to accurately observe the seizures and describe their features.	**a)** The more detailed these descriptions, the more valuable they are for assessment and to therefore treat appropriately.

Procedure guideline 18.4 (*Continued*)

Statement	Rationale
2. For a child presenting for the first time with seizures the following should be documented:	**2.**
a) A description of the manifestation of the seizures should be obtained from eyewitnesses, i.e. nurse, doctor, parent, carer, etc.	**a)** This will assist medical staff to classify whether the seizure is focal or generalised.
b) Any impairment or loss of consciousness.	
c) Motor effects, muscular contractions.	
d) Eye movements.	
e) Which parts of the body are affected; whether laterality is present.	**e)** This will assist medical staff to distinguish which side of the brain is affected.
f) Typical duration of seizures and/or occurrence of 'clusters' of seizures.	**f)** As seizures may be treated after a specific duration of time or amount/number.
g) The child's past medical history and any relevant clinical findings should be evaluated.	**g)** This is in order to ascertain and clarify if there is any underlying cause for the seizures.

Predisposing factors

Any significant results of tests and investigations should be taken into account.

Statement	Rationale
3. For a child with a previous history of seizures or epilepsy document the following:	**3.**
a) A full assessment of the types of seizures must be obtained from the parent/carer/child (if appropriate) so that accurate assessment can be obtained. This includes:	**a)** This is in order to treat seizures appropriately when they occur. To work in partnership with the child and parents/carer.
i. The number of different types	
ii. Description of each type	
iii. Child's altered behaviour during the event	
iv. Typical duration of seizures and/or occurrence of 'clusters' of seizures.	**iv.** As seizures may be treated after a specific duration or amount/number.
v. Any aura experienced	
vi. Any impairment or loss of consciousness	
vii. Which parts of the body are affected; whether is laterality present	
viii. Whether cyanosis is present	**viii.** As oxygen occasionally may be required.
ix. Motor or sensory involvement	
x. Muscular contractions	
xi. Eye movements	
xii. Facial expression	
xiii. Triggers or precipitating factors to seizures, i.e. lack of sleep and fatigue, activity, pre-meals, noise, bright flashing lights, loud noises (Couffignal *et al* 2001)	**xiii.** To prevent unnecessary factors that may trigger the child's seizures.
xiv. Time when seizure normally occurs – early morning, nocturnally, during sleep.	
xv. When parents/carers would administer as required medication, i.e. after what time lapse.	**xv.** To ensure continuity of care.
xvi. Post-ictal state.	**xvi.** To ensure that child's seizure has not restarted.
4. Ensure a recent weight is documented on the child's prescription chart.	**4.** To reduce the risk of medication errors.

445

Management and goals

Treatment of a child with seizures requires:

- Maintenance of vital functions, due to the physiological changes that occur in the body as a result of seizure activity
- Termination of seizures – it may not always be possible to abolish seizures completely, but controlling seizures may be a more realistic goal for some children
- Elimination of any precipitating factors

- Reversing correctable causes – management and treatment of correctable reversible underlying causes may terminate seizure activity.

The initial treatment is directed towards:

- Airway – maintaining an airway
- Breathing – supporting breathing and administration of oxygen
- Circulation – support and maintenance of vital functions
- Drugs – administration of drugs (see below)
- Environment – ensure safety of the child and others.

Procedure guideline 18.5 Nursing management during seizures

Statement	Rationale
1. Nurse a child near • Working oxygen • Working suction • Appropriate size bag-valve-mask, e.g. Ambu bag® • Appropriate size airway.	1. Child may need assistance with maintaining a clear airway and breathing, due to the potential of respiratory depression caused by either seizure activity or administration of anti-convulsant medication.
2. Administer oxygen if required. Carry out a risk assessment considering whether portable oxygen and suction may have to be taken to child and utilised if it is not possible to move the child (see local policies for Clinical Service guidelines on Manual Handling: Lifting and Handling Patients).	
3. Nurse the child on their side.	3. This is to assist the maintenance of a clear airway, in cases of vomiting, choking and/or aspiration episodes.
4. Ensure that the environment is safe, i.e. cot sides are in place, that the child is not banging limbs or head on objects. Positioning a blanket or soft object or padding may help prevent injury occurring.	4. To prevent the child from causing injury to themselves.
5. Call for assistance but never leave any child having a seizure.	5. Due to the child potentially losing the airway, or vomiting, or becoming cyanosed.
6. Ensure the seizure is timed.	6. Treatment of the seizure after 4–5 minutes is important to prevent changes in the body's physiological mechanisms (see physiology section).
7. Administer rectal/buccal/intravenous medication according to clinical service guidelines if required, ensuring the correct dosages are administered.	7. To prevent adverse effects of medication errors.
8. Monitor and support child's vital functions.	8. If necessary nurse the child using a saturation monitor to observe oxygen saturations, heart rate and respiration rate. Monitor consciousness level using Glasgow coma scale if deemed necessary.
9. If required administer further doses of rectal/buccal/intravenous medication according to hospital policies continuing to carefully monitor child's vital signs (as stipulated above).	9. If the seizure has not terminated or is not abating then the child may have to progress to having further repeat doses of medication.

446

Procedure guideline 18.5 (*Continued*)

Statement	Rationale
10. Document seizures the child has on the 'seizure events chart'. This chart can be found at http://www.gosh.nhs.uk/ clinical_information/clinical_guidelines/cpg_guideline_00036/ Appendix_3.doc and includes date and time, description of seizure, classification, seizure duration, nursing intervention, medication administered, seizure total and nurse's signature.	

Status epilepticus

Status epilepticus is a **medical emergency**. It requires immediate intervention to prevent possible brain injury or death as sustained convulsions can increase cerebral blood flow and metabolic requirements and result in physiological sequelae. (See section on Physiology of Seizures.)

The currently accepted definition in the International Classification of Epileptic seizures is: 'Any seizure lasting for a duration of at least 30 minutes or repeated seizures lasting for 30 minutes or longer from which the child does not regain consciousness' (Appleton and Gibbs 1998). Seizures that last at least 5–10 minutes are unlikely to spontaneously stop, and will continue for at least 30 minutes unless there is an appropriate intervention (McIntyre *et al* 2005).

Various systems of classification of seizures have been used in the past. The International League Against Epilepsy (ILAE) Task Force (2001) (Fisher *et al* 2005) has revised the previous epilepsy classification and produced a new diagnostic scheme (Engel 2002) See the link at http://www.gosh.nhs.uk/ and search classification of seizures (Panayiotopoulos 2002). See also Figures 18.1 and 18.2.

External ventricular drainage

Introduction

An external ventricular drainage (EVD) is the temporary drainage of cerebrospinal fluid (CSF) from the fluid filled cavities of the brain (lateral ventricles) to a closed collection system outside the body, to relieve raised intracranial pressure (Woodward *et al* 2002). The EVD is inserted in theatre under a general anaesthetic. External ventricular drains should only be cared for by nursing and/or medical staff who have been trained to do so and have achieved competence. For children who move out of the department, e.g. to visit scan or theatres, management guidelines should be adhered to and the transfer checklist completed.

Indications for external ventricular drainage are:

- To relieve raised intracranial pressure (ICP)
- To divert infected CSF in children with hydrocephalus who have a permanent shunt
- To divert bloodstained CSF following neurosurgery/haemorrhage (Neilsen 2007)
- To divert the flow of CSF.

447

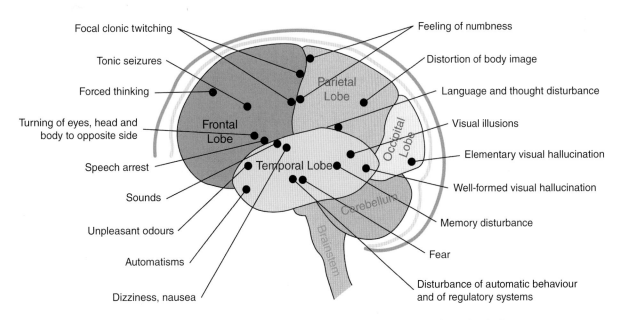

Figure 18.1 The origin of symptoms and signs in focal seizures. A visual display over the dominant hemispheres.

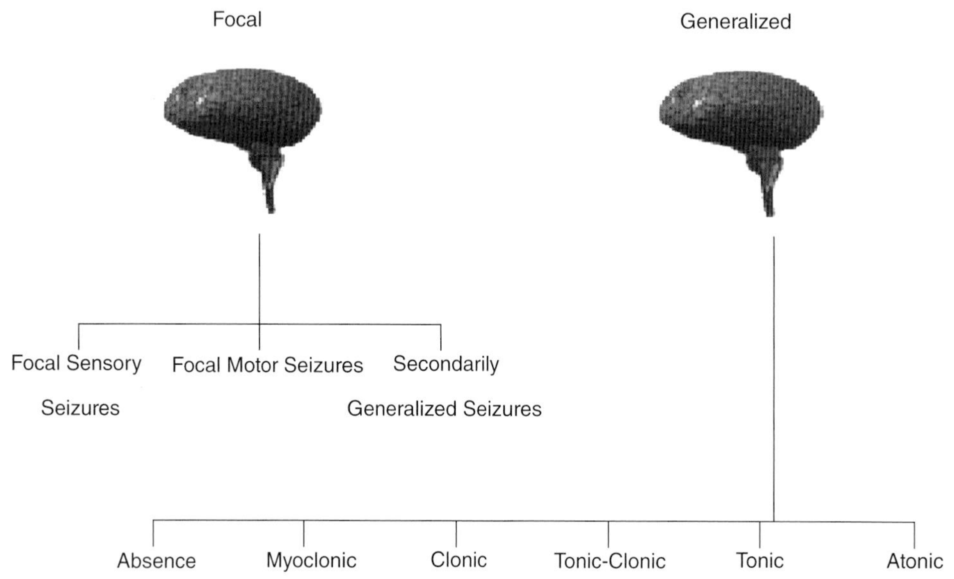

Focal

Generalized

Focal Sensory Seizures

Focal Motor Seizures

Secondarily Generalized Seizures

Absence   Myoclonic   Clonic   Tonic-Clonic   Tonic   Atonic

Figure 18.2 Classification or seizure types.

Principles table 18.5 Treatment for status epilepticus

Principle	Rationale
1. The initial treatment for status epilepticus is directed towards: **a)** Maintaining an airway. **b)** Administration of oxygen.	**1.** **b)** To detect early alterations in vital signs that may indicate impending respiratory depression and respiratory and cardiac arrest.
2. Administration of rectal or buccal or intravenous medication according to clinical service guidelines algorithm.	**2.** (See Appendix 18.4: Algorithm for a convulsing child.)
3. Rectal diazepam and buccal midazolam are safe, simple and effective treatments for pre-hospital management (Alexander and Kendrick 2005). Rectal paraldehyde is still sometimes used and therefore local policies should be adhered to.	**3.** Buccal midazolam is at least as effective as rectal diazepam in the acute treatment of seizures (Scott *et al* 1999). This was first considered to be more advantageous than rectal diazepam for emergency use in 1999 (Scott *et al* 1999). Administration via the mouth is more socially acceptable and convenient than the rectal route especially in older children (Scott *et al* 1999). See the National Centre for Young People with Epilepsy, GOSH Epilepsy Service and GOSH Pharmacy department in collaboration with the Child and Family Information Group, GOSH (2009) for administration of buccal midazolam.
4. Support and maintenance of vital functions.	
5. Followed by intravenous anti-convulsants.	
6. Hydration, e.g. intravenous fluids if required.	

Principles table 18.5 *(Continued)*

Principle	Rationale
7. The child must be closely monitored during administration of intravenous anti-convulsants.	**7.** This is due to the medication potentially causing respiratory depression.
8. Monitor level of consciousness, vital signs of respirations, heart rate, blood pressure and temperature.	
9. If first line drugs are ineffective progress to second line drugs.	
10. Refer to the relevant, appropriate policy and algorithm for the management of a convulsing child (see Appendix 18.4).	
11. The child may need respiratory support of intubation and ventilation on a paediatric intensive care unit.	
12. Outcome is related to aetiology and duration of the status epilepticus.	
13. Always ensure that the drugs are prescribed by the medical staff and that hospital policy and procedures are followed.	**13.** As required by the Nursing and Midwifery (NMC) Council Standards for medicines management (NMC 2002).

There are two types of EVD system:

1. The distal end of the child's existing shunt system is externalised and connected to an external drainage system. This shunt system contains a pressure valve, which controls the amount of drainage from the ventricles (Smith *et al* 2009).
2. The most frequently used system is a new catheter placed into the ventricle through a small hole (burr hole) made in the skull. Once inserted, the scalp incision is sutured and covered with a sterile dressing. The new catheter is tunnelled under the skin, exiting on the abdominal wall and connects to an external drainage system. This system does not have a pressure valve so drainage depends on gravity. The benefits of this system are the prevention of an unsightly scar, the reduction of the risk of infection and the reduction of the risk of accidental removal (Armon *et al* 2003, Smith *et al* 2009, Woodward *et al* 2002).

The ventricular catheter is connected to an external drainage system. The system has several components (see Figure 18.3):

- A sampling/access port – to provide access to the catheter
- An anti reflux collection chamber – to observe CSF drainage
- A drainage bag – to enable on-going collection of CSF
- A pressure scale – to facilitate accurate positioning.

Non-metal clamps, gauze and chlorhexidine impregnated wipes, e.g. Clinell®, **must** be positioned by the child's bed to enable the system to be clamped if the drainage system accidentally becomes disconnected. **The line must be clearly labelled preferably near the injection and sampling port. Ideally a stopcock protection box will be placed over the access point to reduce the risk of accidental administration of intravenous medication.**

The prescribed instructions of the neurosurgeons should be followed for the:

- Position/pressure level of the drain and/or
- Expected hourly amount of CSF drainage.

The external ventricular drainage system should be changed according to specific medical treatment under conditions of strict asepsis, according to microbiological advice/local policy (Wong *et al* 2007). This should minimise the risk of infection/further infection (Armon *et al* 2003). The external ventricular drainage system can then be used for up to 10 days. However, the drainage bag should be changed when three-quarters **full** as overfilling of the drainage bags impairs drainage (Woodward *et al* 2002).

For cases of infected CSF, intrathecal antibiotics are prescribed according to microbiological advice and administered through the injection and sampling port of the external ventricular drain. This should only be undertaken by a healthcare professional who has been trained and achieved competency to ensure safety for the child.

449

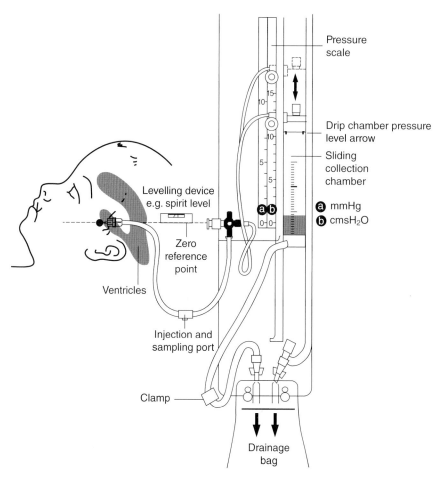

Pressure scale

Drip chamber pressure level arrow

Sliding collection chamber

ⓐ mmHg
ⓑ cmsH₂O

Levelling device e.g. spirit level

Zero reference point

Ventricles

Injection and sampling port

Clamp

Drainage bag

Figure 18.3 External ventricular drainage system.

Procedure guideline 18.6 Inform the child and family

Statement	Rationale
1. Explain the entire procedure and management to the child and family avoiding medical and nursing jargon and complicated language. Information must be given according to the child's age, condition and developmental understanding. Explain the following: **a)** Why the EVD is necessary. **b)** The reason for the EVD. **c)** What it entails. **d)** The likely length of placement of an EVD. **e)** The associated problems of an EVD (Smith *et al* 2009).	**1.** To ensure that the child and family understand the procedure and are psychologically prepared and ensure informed consent is obtained. Parents/carers should be given the *EVD Parents Information Leaflet* to reinforce the verbal information given.
2. If appropriate provide play preparation, involving the play specialist. (Action for Sick Children 2003). Consider involvement of a clinical psychologist if appropriate, particularly if previous procedures have been stressful for the child or if the child is known to have or exhibits signs of anticipatory anxiety or distress (Salmon 2006).	**2.** To give the child the opportunity to express fears in an familiar environment (Bouffet *et al* 1996).

Procedure guideline 18.6 (*Continued*)

Statement	Rationale
3. Ensure a sign is placed above a child's bed or in close proximity to the child to remind healthcare professionals and carers that child has EVD and should not be moved without clamping the drain and following the management guidelines (see http://www.ich.ucl.ac.uk/gosh_families/information sheets/external ventricular drainage).	3. To maintain the child's safety.

Procedure guideline 18.7 **Neurological assessment**

Statement	Rationale

1. The following observations should be carried out on return from theatre.
   The observations must be performed according to the child's condition and hospital policy, but at least 4 hourly.
	1. To establish the baseline for future observations.
	   To monitor change and indentify any necessary changes in treatment, which may include changing the drain height to reduce/increase the volume of CSF draining.

2. Observe for a change in the child's neurological condition by assessing the following: • Level of consciousness • Pupil reaction • Limb movement and strength • Systemic observations: • Heart rate (bradycardia can be a sign of raised intracranial pressure, tachycardia a sign of low intracranial pressure). • Blood pressure (hypertension can be a sign of raised intracranial pressure, hypotension a sign of low intracranial pressure) • Respiratory rate can alter • The fontanelle should be checked in infants. For further information, refer to the previous section on Neurological Observations.	2. To identify changes and act on these findings appropriately. These can indicate a change in intracranial pressure and treatment may need to implemented. A bulging fontanelle indicates raised intracranial pressure; a dipped fontanelle indicates low intracranial pressure.
3. A change in body temperature.	3. Pyrexia could indicate an infection, the source of which should be indentified and treated.
4. The frequency of nausea and vomiting, should be monitored and documented as significant events section of the coma chart.	4. To provide accurate information on which the child's clinical picture can be based.
5. The frequency, duration and severity of any headaches should be monitored and documented significant events section of the coma chart.	5. To provide accurate information on which the child's clinical picture can be based.
6. The family should be included in general observation of child (Action for Sick Children 2003).	6. To use their knowledge of what is 'normal' for the child.

451

Procedure guideline 18.8 Drain management: positioning of drain

Statement	Rationale
1. The system must be positioned accurately according to medical instruction – operation notes or medical notes. **a)** Ensure drain is clamped prior to any repositioning to avoid over draining.	**1.** To ensure desired amount of CSF drainage.
2. Unless otherwise prescribed the drain is measured from the foramen of Monro, which is midway between the outer aspect of the child's eye and the external auditory meatus (Woodward et al 2002). **a)** The midpoint of this line is the zero point for the EVD system (Figures 18.3 and 18.4). **b)** Use a leveling device, e.g. spirit level, to estimate the zero point position against the pressure scale, which is either mounted on an intravenous (IV) pole or on a pressure scale mounting panel (Figure 18.4). **c)** Position and secure the pressure scale, on either the IV pole or the system mounting panel with 0 cm being the estimated zero point (Woodward et al. 2002).	**2.** To calibrate/determine the zero reference point for the drain, i.e. the level of the ventricles for positioning the EVD system (Clar et al 2002). **b)** To ensure accuracy. **c)** For ease of accurate positioning.
3. Position the pressure level arrow at the top of the drip chamber at the prescribed height, e.g. +5, +10 (above) or −2 cm H_2O (below) the zero point (the ventricles) and secure with Velcro straps or the locking bracket. **a)** The position of drain should be documented on either the child's fluid chart and/or the child's neurological observation coma chart. If the height of the drain is changed for any reason, then this must be documented on the neurological observation coma chart and the medical notes.	**3.** To ensure correct CSF drainage. The difference in height between the child's ventricles and the drip chamber creates both a pressure gradient and a safety valve. The height of the drip chamber equates to the pressure inside of the head or intracranial pressure (ICP). This pressure must be reached before any CSF will drain into the collection chamber (Armon et al 2003). **a)** To ensure an accurate record.
4. When moving or repositioning the child: **a)** Clamp both the 3-way tap nearest the child and the external ventricular drain itself. **b)** Re-zero drain. **c)** Unclamp drain immediately.	**4.** The position of the drain always corresponds with the child's ventricles.
5. Parents/carers should be advised of the importance of the following aspects of care when a drain is in situ. **a)** The importance of repositioning the drain. **b)** To clamp the drain if: Moving their child, if their child is crying excessively, or vomiting. **c)** To ask for the assistance of a healthcare professional who has been trained and has achieved competency in EVD management, to rezero/reposition the drain once their child has been moved (Woodward et al 2002). **d)** That the drain should not be clamped for longer than 1 hour unless otherwise specified and prescribed.	**5.** To encourage parental/carer involvement and promote safe management. **a)** To ensure CSF drains as required. **b)** To prevent over drainage of CSF. **c)** For correct CSF drainage. **d)** To minimise risk of blocked catheter and to prevent raised intracranial pressure.
6. This instruction must be documented in the child's healthcare record.	**6.** To provide an accurate record.

452

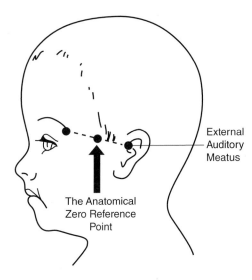

Figure 18.4 Zero reference point.

Procedure guideline 18.9 Drain management: drainage

Statement	Rationale
1. EVD drainage systems should be connected in theatre when first inserted (Smith *et al* 2009).	**1.** To minimise the risk of infection. To prevent blockage of catheter.
2. Once the drain is connected and positioned an initial assessment of CSF drainage should be made.	**2.** To ensure CSF is draining at the correct rate.

3. Subsequently hourly checks should be made of:
a) Amount of drainage.
 	
b) Colour of CSF – should be colourless.
 	
c) Exit site.
	3. To promote safe management of the child.
	a) To ensure CSF drainage rate is as dictated in written medical instructions.
	   A sudden increase in drainage may result from inaccurate zeroing of the drain or could signify a rise in ICP.
	   A decrease in drainage could also indicate inaccurate zeroing of the drain or that the tubing may be kinked, blocked, disconnected or the ports are closed.
	b) Bloodstained CSF could indicate blood in the ventricles
	   Cloudy CSF may indicate the presence of an infection.
	c) To ensure CSF is not leaking.

4. Record the child's fluid balance chart hourly and/or the child's neurological observation coma chart: **a)** The amount of CSF drainage. **b)** The position of the EVD patency of the drain by observing dripping of CSF into the chamber or momentarily lowering the drain.	**4.** **a)** To ensure CSF drainage rate is as prescribed. **b)** To ensure position of drain is correct, to provide an accurate record, and to ensure drain is patent.
5. The neurosurgeon will specify and prescribe a drain height post-operatively and thereafter the drain height is to be: • Maintained • Altered, to drain a certain amount of CSF an hour.	**5.** The child's age and condition and what is prescribed dictates the amount of drainage. **An approximate guide to CSF drainage is:** Infants: 2–5 ml/hour Children: 5–10 ml/hour Adolescents: 10–15 ml/hour.

453

(Continued)

Procedure guideline 18.9 (*Continued*)

Statement	Rationale

6. If the child is crying excessively the drain should be clamped off.
    It **must not** be clamped off for more than 1 hour.
	6. May cause over drainage.
	    To prevent blockage and increase in intracranial pressure.

7. If there is no CSF drainage:
    a) Observe for pulsation movement of CSF in the tubing of the EVD, i.e., this should be a clear rise and fall, not just a flicker.
    b) Ensure system is not clamped or kinked
    c) Lower chamber momentarily below head level.
    d) Advise neurosurgeon immediately if there is no drainage.
	7.
	    a) Drainage may be slow.
	
	    b) This will reduce or stop flow.
	    c) To encourage flow and/or release an air lock.
	    d) The system may need flushing.

8. If a catheter becomes disconnected:
    a) Clamp catheter close to child.
    b) Place end in sterile wrapping/container.
    c) Lie child down.
    d) Thoroughly clean exposed tip using a sterile chlorhexidine impregnated swab and connect a new system aseptically.
    e) Record event in child's healthcare records and inform the child's doctor.
	8. To prevent excess CSF loss.
	    a) To reduce infection risk.
	
	    c) To prevent excess CSF loss.
	    d) To reduce infection risk.
	
	    e) To provide an accurate record.

9. Contact the neurosurgical team immediately if there are concerns about:
    • The amount of drainage
    • The condition of the child.
	9. The position of the drain may need to be re-evaluated.

Procedure guideline 18.10 **Drain management: connecting or changing the system**

Statement	Rationale
1. Newly inserted EVDs will be connected to the drainage system in theatre. (Smith *et al* 2009).	**1.** To minimise the risk of infection.
2. Inform the child and family that the procedure is to be performed.	**2.** To gain understanding and co-operation.
3. The system should be connected by, or under the supervision of a healthcare professional who has been trained and has achieved competency. Two practitioners are required, one to perform the sterile procedure and the other to assist.	

Prepare equipment:
    • Dressing trolley
    • Clamps and gauze
    • A pair of sterile gloves and an apron
    • EVD system
    • Two chlorhexidine impregnated wipes, e.g. Clinell®.
	• To provide a clean work surface.
	
	    • To minimise the risk of infection.
	
	    • To minimise the risk of infection.

4. To change the drainage system:
    a) Clamp catheter close to child using non-sterile gauze and clamps.
    b) Put on apron and perform a ward aseptic procedures handwash.
    c) Open new drainage system and put on sterile gloves.
    d) Assemble drainage set closing clamps.
	4.
	    a) To prevent loss of CSF on disconnection. To protect tubing.
	    b) To prevent contamination.
	    c) To prepare for procedure.
	    d) To prevent CSF drainage until re-positioned.

Procedure guideline 18.10 (*Continued*)

Statement	Rationale
e) Remove last 3-way tap on drainage set.	**e)** It is not required.
f) The assistant cleans the catheter connection with a chlorhexidine impregnated wipe and allows for it to dry.	**f)** To minimise the risk of infection.
g) The 'sterile' practitioner disconnects the old system and cleans the newly exposed catheter end with chlorhexidine impregnated wipe and allows for it to dry.	**g)** To minimise the risk of infection.
h) Connect new system.	**h)** To establish new system.
i) Check connections.	**i)** To prevent CSF loss.
j) Position system as prescribed by the neurosurgeon.	**j)** To establish instructed drainage.
k) Release clamps on new system and those close to the child.	**k)** To commence CSF drainage.
l) Clear away equipment according to waste policy.	**l)** To meet Hospital Policy.
m) Wash hands.	**m)** To minimise the risk of cross infection.
n) Record the procedure in the child's healthcare records.	**n)** To provide an accurate record.

Procedure guideline 18.11 Drain management: repairing a split catheter

Statement	Rationale
1. If a catheter splits: **a)** Clamp catheter close to child using gauze and clamps. **b)** Place end in sterile wrapping/container, e.g. Clinell®. **c)** Lie child down.	**1.** **a)** To prevent excess CSF loss. **b)** To reduce risk of infection. **c)** To prevent excess CSF loss.
2. Catheter should be repaired by, or under the supervision of a healthcare professional who has been trained and has achieved competency. Two practitioners are required, one to perform the sterile procedure and the other to assist.	**2.** To promote asepsis. To minimise the risk of infection.
3. Gather and prepare the following equipment: **a)** Dressing trolley. **b)** A pair of sterile gloves and an apron. **c)** EVD system. **d)** EVD connector. **e)** Sterile scissors. **f)** Alcohol impregnated wipes, e.g. Clinell®.	**3.** **a)** To provide a clean work surface. **b)** To minimise the risk of infection. **c)** To allow CSF drainage. **d)** To connect system safely. **e)** To minimise the risk of infection.
4. To repair a split catheter: **a)** Put on apron and perform a ward aseptic procedures handwash. **b)** Open new drainage system and put on sterile gloves. **c)** Assemble new drainage set closing clamps. **d)** Remove last 3-way tap on drainage set. **e)** The 'sterile' practitioner cleans the exposed catheter end with a sterile chlorhexidine impregnated wipe and allows it to dry. **f)** Using sterile scissors cut just above the split. **g)** Insert EVD connector into the catheter lumen. **h)** Connect new system. **i)** Check connections. **j)** Position system as prescribed by the neurosurgeon. **k)** Release clamps on new system and those close to the child. **l)** Clear away equipment according to Waste Policy. **m)** Wash hands according to local policy. **n)** Record the procedure in the child's healthcare records.	**4.** **a)** To minimise the risk of infection. **b)** To prepare for procedure. **c)** To prevent loss of CSF until repositioned. **d)** It is not required. **e)** To minimise the risk of infection. To create a clean end for connection. **f)** To establish new system. **g)** To prevent CSF loss. **j)** To establish instructed drainage. **k)** To commence CSF drainage. **l)** To meet hospital policy. **m)** To minimise the risk of cross-infection. **n)** To maintain an accurate record.

455

Procedure guideline 18.12 Drain management: unblocking of catheter

Statement	Rationale
1. If a catheter appears to be blocked: **a)** Exclude damage to the EVD system. **b)** Lower drain and observe for CSF movement. **c)** Change EVD.	1. **a)** Connections may be faulty. **b)** Air lock may be present. **c)** Air filter may be wet.
2. If no CSF movement is observed, seek **urgent** advice from a neurosurgeon who may instruct the EVD to be 'milked' or aspirated.	2. The catheter may be blocked resulting in raised intracranial pressure.

3. Catheters **must only** be aspirated by a healthcare professional who has undergone training and has achieved competency. Two practitioners are required, one to perform the sterile procedure and the other to assist.	3. To minimise the potential risks of the procedure.
	   To promote asepsis.
	   To minimise the risk of infection.

4. All EVDs may be aspirated including those with a valve.	4. The valve does not prevent aspiration.
5. Gather and prepare the following equipment: **a)** Dressing trolley. **b)** A pair of sterile gloves and an apron. **c)** EVD system. **d)** Sodium chloride 0.9% for injection. **e)** Alcohol impregnated wipes, e.g. Clinell®. **f)** Blue needle. **g)** 10–30 ml syringes.	5. **a)** To provide a clean work surface. **b)** To minimise the risk of infection. **f)** To draw up sodium chloride 0.9%. **g)** Large syringe sizes reduce pressure exerted on catheter.
6. To aspirate an EVD: **a)** Clamp catheter close to child. **b)** Lie child down. **c)** Put on apron and perform a ward aseptic procedure handwash. **d)** Open new drainage system and put on sterile gloves. **e)** Assemble new drainage set closing clamps. **f)** Remove last 3-way tap on drainage set. **g)** The assistant cleans the catheter connection with an alcohol-impregnated wipe and allows it to dry. **h)** The 'sterile' practitioner disconnects the old system and cleans the exposed catheter end with a chlorhexidine impregnated wipe and allows it to dry. **i)** Insert syringe into end of the catheter. **j)** The assistant should release the clamps close to the child. **k)** Very gently attempt to aspirate CSF. **l)** The assistant should close the clamps close to the child.	6. **a)** To prevent CSF loss on disconnection. **b)** To prevent excess CSF loss. **c)** To prevent contamination. **d)** To prepare for procedure. **e)** To prevent CSF drainage until repositioned. **f)** It is not required. **g)** To minimise the risk of infection. **h)** To minimise the risk of infection. **i)** To enable aspiration of CSF. **j)** To allow aspiration of CSF. **k)** To obtain CSF sample/confirm patency. **l)** To prevent excess CSF loss.
7. If the aspiration has been unsuccessful the EVD should be flushed. This **MUST ONLY** be done by a healthcare professional who has undergone training and has achieved competency. Two practitioners are required, one to perform the sterile procedure and the other to assist.	7. **This is a high-risk procedure.**
8. To flush the EVD: **a)** The competent clinician should draw up 1–2 ml of 0.9% sodium chloride into a syringe. **b)** Insert syringe into the exposed end of catheter.	

Procedure guideline 18.12 (*Continued*)

Statement	Rationale
c) The assistant should release the clamps close to the child.	**c)** To enable catheter to be flushed.
d) Gently attempt to inject the sodium chloride.	**d)** To flush system:

e) If the sodium chloride can be injected the assistant should close the clamps that are close to the child.	**i.** To enable system to be accessed
	   ii. To clear catheter
	   iii. To prevent CSF loss.

9. Continue after aspirating and/or flushing by:
  a) Discard syringe.
  b) Connect new system.
  c) Check connections.
  d) Release clamps on new system and those close to the child.
  e) Gradually lower system to check for drainage.
  f) Position system as instructed by the neurosurgeon.
  g) Clear away equipment according to Waste Policy.
  h) Wash hands.
  i) Record the procedure in the child's healthcare records.
	9.
	
	b) To establish new system.
	c) To prevent CSF loss.
	d) To establish instructed drainage.
	
	e) To check for drainage.
	f) To commence CSF drainage.
	g) To meet hospital policy.
	h) To minimise the risk of cross-infection.
	i) To maintain an accurate record.

10. If the 'flushing' has not been successful the neurosurgeons must be contacted.	**10.** A CT scan will need to be performed.

Procedure guideline 18.13 **Drain management: fluid and electrolyte balance**

Statement	Rationale

1. With younger and sick children, cerebrospinal fluid (CSF) losses should be replaced ml/ml with intravenous 0.9% sodium chloride as prescribed, unless otherwise indicated (Neilsen 2007).
  a) Oral sodium chloride can be used if required.
	1. To maintain fluid and electrolyte balance. Cerebrospinal fluid (CSF) contains sodium.
	
	  a) If the child's oral intake is adequate.

2. Cerebrospinal Fluid (CSF) losses and intravenous fluid replacement should be recorded hourly on a fluid balance chart and reviewed every shift by the nurse in charge.	**2.** To ensure fluid balance is being maintained.
3. Serum electrolytes should be checked according to the child's age, condition and CSF losses, approximately twice weekly.	**3.** To monitor the child's electrolyte balance and treat as appropriate.

457

Procedure guideline 18.14 **Accessing the drain: CSF sampling**

Statement	Rationale

1. Routine CSF sampling is not advised due to the risk of introducing infection to an otherwise sterile circuit.
  However when CSF samples are required they must be taken by either nursing or medical staff who have undertaken training and achieved competency using an aseptic technique.
  a) Infected CSF samples should be taken in line with hospital policy and according to microbiological advice, until the CSF is sterile/infection free.
	1. CSF may be sampled to monitor:
	  • CSF values including antibiotic levels in the CSF
	  • Progress in treatment of a known infection. The following can be utilsed as a marker of infection:
	   i. A raised cell and protein count
	   ii. A lowered glucose count.
	  a) For signs of infection.

(*Continued*)

Procedure guideline 18.14 (*Continued*)

Statement	Rationale
2. CSF samples should be obtained by, or under the supervision of a healthcare professional who has been trained and has achieved competency. Two practitioners are required, one to perform the sterile procedure and the other to assist.	**2.** To promote asepsis and to minimise the risk of infection.
3. Antibiotic levels should be as follows: Vancomycin: less or equivalent to 15 mg/litre Gentamicin: less than 3 mg/litre.	**3.** The levels are checked daily to determine subsequent doses of antibiotics. This must be done in consultation with the microbiologist to avoid overdose of antibiotics.
4. Gather the following equipment: **a)** Sterile paper. **b)** Chlorhexidine impregnated wipe. **c)** Two 10–30 ml syringes. **d)** Two Universal specimen containers. **e)** 1 × container = protein count. **f)** 1 × container = cell count and antibiotic level (if required). **g)** Glucose specimen bottle. **h)** Sterile gloves and an apron. **i)** Computer generated request form.	**4.** **a)** To provide a sterile field. **c)** Large syringe sizes reduce pressure exerted on catheter. **d)** To collect CSF specimen to determine the cell and protein count and the antibiotic level. **g)** To collect CSF specimen for a glucose count. **h)** To minimise the risk of infection.
5. To obtain a CSF specimen: **a)** Close clamps on drainage system close to injection port. **b)** Wash hands and put on apron. **c)** Prepare sterile field. **d)** Perform a ward aseptic procedures handwash and put on gloves. **e)** An assistant should hold the injection port/open and close the 3-way tap. **f)** Clean injection port on EVD system with an alcohol impregnated wipe and allow to dry. **g)** Insert syringe into port. **h)** Slowly withdraw 2 ml of CSF, remove syringe and discard. **i)** Insert second syringe into port. **j)** Slowly withdraw 2 ml of CSF. **k)** Place 1 ml of CSF into the glucose specimen container and 0.5 ml into each universal specimen container. **l)** Open clamps on drainage system close to injection port. **m)** Label samples and send them with completed request forms to the correct laboratory in accordance with local policy. **n)** Dispose of all used equipment according to Waste Policy. **o)** Wash hands according to hospital policy. **p)** Record the procedure in the child's healthcare records.	**5.** **a)** To prevent CSF aspiration from drainage system. **b)** To prevent contamination. **c)** To prevent contamination. **d)** To minimise the risk of infection. **e)** To minimise the risk of infection. **f)** To minimise the risk of infection. **g)** To access system. **h)** To remove contaminated CSF sample. **i)** To access system. **j)** To obtain CSF sample for analysis. **k)** To facilitate analysis. **l)** To continue drainage of CSF. **m)** To facilitate analysis. **n)** To meet hospital policy. **o)** To minimise the risk of cross-infection. **p)** To maintain an accurate record.

Procedure guideline 18.15 Accessing the drain: giving intrathecal drugs

Statement	Rationale
1. Intrathecal drugs, e.g. antibiotics, are administered to enable local treatment of the CSF (Barrett-Goode 2000).	**1.**
a) Antibiotic levels should be checked prior to administering each dose.	**a)** To ensure the correct dosage is administered.
b) Intrathecal antibiotics must only be administered by healthcare professionals who have undergone training and achieved competence.	
2. Gather the following equipment:	**2.**
a) Sterile gloves and an apron.	**a)** To minimise risk of infection.
b) Sterile paper.	**b)** To provide a sterile field.
c) Chlorhexidine impregnated wipe.	**c)** To administer small volumes of drugs.
d) 1 or 2 ml syringe.	**d)** Large syringe sizes reduce pressure exerted on catheter.
e) 2 × 10–30 ml syringes.	**e)** Use to draw up antibiotics.
f) Blue needle.	
g) Prescribed antibiotics.	
h) 0.9% sodium chloride for injection.	**h)** To flush catheter after antibiotics.
i) Child's prescription chart.	**i)** To check drugs prescribed.
3. To administer intrathecal antibiotics:	**3.**
a) Close clamps on drainage system close to injection port.	**a)** To prevent drug entering drainage system.
b) Put on apron and wash hands.	**b)** To prevent contamination.
c) Prepare sterile field.	**c)** To prepare for procedure.
d) Perform a ward aseptic procedures handwash and put on gloves.	**d)** To prevent contamination.
e) Check drugs according to hospital drug policy.	**e)** To maintain hospital policy.
f) Prepare drugs using aseptic non-touch technique.	**f)** To minimise the risk of infection.
g) Check child's identity according to the Drug Policy.	**g)** To maintain hospital policy.
h) Clean injection port on EVD system with an alcohol impregnated wipe and allow to dry.	**h)** To minimise the risk of infection.
i) Slowly withdraw 2 ml of CSF, remove syringe and discard.	**i)** To facilitate drug administration.
j) Insert syringe containing the antibiotic into injection port.	**j)** To meet prescription guidelines.
k) Inject antibiotic according to manufacturer's guidelines.	
l) Remove syringe.	
m) Insert syringe containing 0.9% sodium chloride into port and gently flush catheter with 2 ml 0.9% sodium chloride.	**m)** To facilitate flushing of system. To ensure drug given.
n) Remove syringe.	
o) Keep drainage system clamped for one hour only.	**o)** To ensure absorption of antibiotic.
p) Dispose of all used equipment according to Waste Policy.	**p)** To maintain safe environment.
q) Wash hands according to hospital policy.	**q)** To minimize the risk of cross infection.
r) Record the procedure in the child's healthcare records.	**r)** To provide an accurate record.

Procedure guideline 18.16 Exit site care

Statement	Rationale
1. The child will return from theatre with a dressing over the exit site.	**1.** To keep wound clean and dry.
2. If the exit site is dry it should be dressed with a sterile dressing, e.g. IV3000® or Opsite® to allow observation of the site.	**2.** To reduce the risk of infection. It prevents an excess build up of bacteria.
3. Change the dressing weekly unless contaminated.	**3.** To reduce the risk of infection.
4. The dressing should be changed if it becomes contaminated with CSF or blood (Woodward *et al* 2002).	**4.** To reduce the risk of infection.
5. If the exit site is oozing it should be dressed with sterile gauze pads and surgical tape. **a)** A microbiological swab may need to be taken for culture and sensitivity. **b)** The child's doctor should be kept informed.	**5.** To exert a small amount of pressure to reduce drainage. To soak up any oozing. **a)** To identify any infective organisms.
6. Check exit site dressing hourly for: **a)** Redness. **b)** Inflammation. **c)** Oozing of blood. **d)** Leakage of CSF.	**6.** **a)** An indicator of infection. **b)** An indicator of infection. **d)** The drain may need re-positioning.
7. Loop catheter once at exit site under dressing.	**7.** To reduce the risk of the catheter being accidentally removed.
8. A clear semi-permeable dressing such as IV3000® should be used so the exit site can be observed.	

Procedure guideline 18.17 Removal of the drain

Statement	Rationale
1. The external ventricular catheter should remain in situ for no longer than 10 days unless otherwise specified or according to local policy. After this time the entire system should be removed or changed in theatre.	**1.** To reduce the risk of further infection.
2. Pre-operatively the nurse may be asked to clamp the drain for a specified time prior to surgery.	**2.** To enlarge the ventricles for surgery. To facilitate insertion of catheter.
3. If the child's condition deteriorates due to clamping pre-operatively, unclamp the drain and contact the neurosurgical team.	**3.** The child is likely to have raised ICP.
4. Post operatively assess the child and dress the exit site.	**4.** To ensure recovery form the procedure and anaesthetic and to ensure there is no wound site infection, or CSF leakage.

Procedure guideline 18.18 Transfer management guidelines

Statement	Rationale
1. The drainage chamber is maintained at a level stipulated by the Consultant or the Neurosurgical Registrar. The height of the drain must be specified in the medical notes. If the height of the drain is changed or if the drain is clamped for any reason then this must be documented on the neurological observation chart.	1. To ensure that the correct amount of CSF is drained.
2a) The drain is measured from the foramen of Monro midway between the outer corner of the eye and the external auditory canal unless specified otherwise. b) The drainage system must be put through the cot side and not over the top. c) Blue clamps, gauze and a chlorhexidine swab should be attached to the child's bed at all times in case of disconnection.	2a) To ensure that the drain is set at the correct posisition. b) To ensure that the correct amount of CSF is drained. c) To enable prompt clamping of the drain if it becomes disconnected.
3. Ensure the system is safely and securely attached to the drip stand by the clamp and the pull cord at all times.	3. To ensure that the correct amount of CSF is drained.
4. For good practice when closing the drainage system the drain must be clamped both at the 3-way tap nearest the child and at the drain itself.	4. To prevent incorrect access.
5. The EVD collection system line must be clearly labelled with the EVD sticker, stating date and time of attachment, preferably near to the 3-way tap. A stopcock protection box should be used to cover the access point if available.	5. To maintain child's safety and to reduce the risk of accidental administration of intravenous medication via the EVD.
6. Parents/cares and all non-nursing or medical personnel **must not** clamp the drain under any circumstances, without appropriate training.	6. To maintain child's safety.
7a) Before moving the child for **any** reason, i.e. sitting up or lying down, the drain must be clamped. The drain should be re-measured and then unclamped once the child is in a new position. Parents/carers must only clamp a drain after adequate training from nursing staff. They must **never** unclamp a drain, but must call a nurse for assistance. b) A sign to indicate the child has an EVD must be hung from the pole hanging the drainage system.	7a) To ensure that the correct volume of CSF is drained. b) To maintain child's safety.

461

(Continued)

Procedure guideline 18.18 (*Continued*)

Statement	Rationale
8. The amount of cerebrospinal fluid being lost must be measured and recorded hourly (see above). It is important to also note the colour of the fluid and presence of any debris or pus. With the younger/sick child, the volume of CSF drained, should be replaced with an equal volume ml for ml of 0.9% sodium chloride intravenously, as prescribed. NB Intravenous 0.9% sodium chloride used to dilute intravenous antibiotics should incorporate this replacement.	**8.** To maintain accurate record and ensure correct replacement of losses.
9. If there is no drainage of cerebrospinal fluid, check that: **a)** CSF can be seen pulsating in the tubing (this should be a clear rise and fall and not just a flicker). **b)** The tubing is not clamped off or kinked.	**9.** To identify cause and re-establish patency of drainage system.
10. If the system is found to be patent and still no drainage of cerebrospinal fluid occurs then the Neurosurgical Registrar should be notified immediately.	**10.** To ensure swift action in response to potential blockage of syste, which could result in raised ICP.
11. Observe the child to determine whether the drain is draining too much CSF (child in low pressure) or draining too little (high pressure).	**11.** To ensure swift action in response to potential blockage of syste, which could result in raised ICP.
12. Signs and symptoms include • Headaches • Vomiting. • An open fontanelle that is full/tense indicates high pressure • A dipped fontanelle indicates low pressure. • A change in the child's vital signs is a late sign of intracranial pressure. • Bradycardia, hypertension, altered respiratory rate and a decreased Glasgow Coma Scale (GCS) require immediate attention (raised ICP). • Tachycardia, hypotension, altered respiratory rate and a decreased GCS and pallor (low ICP).	

ANY CHANGES MUST BE REPORTED IMMEDIATELY

Lumbar puncture

A lumbar puncture involves the introduction of a needle into the lumbar subarachnoid space, between L3 and 4, and L4 and 5, avoiding the end of the spinal cord at L1. A lumbar puncture is performed for diagnostic and therapeutic reasons. The main diagnostic indications include the measuring of CSF pressure, and the examination of CSF for blood, protein, sugar, white cells, microscopy cytology and others. The main therapeutic indications include the reduction of intracranial pressure, the introduction of intrathecal drugs (antibiotics and chemotherapeutic) and the introduction of spinal anaesthesia.

Performing a lumbar puncture should be undertaken with caution in those children with raised intracranial pressure, and avoided in children with infratentorial lesions: a sudden pressure decrease in such patients may result in brain stem herniation and ultimately, death. A CT scan should therefore be considered in all children with raised intracranial pressure prior to lumbar puncture.

It is necessary to prepare the child both psychologically and physically for the procedure. Following preparation and explanation, the child must be placed in a lateral recumbent position, with the back arched and knees drawn up, thus allowing maximum separation of the vertebrae for insertion of the needle. The position is uncomfortable and the procedure can be frightening and painful. Although explanation and discussion with the assistance of the play specialist and parents/carers may be adequate in preparing the adolescent for lumbar puncture, the majority of younger children will need sedation or anaesthesia.

Principles table 18.6 CSF

INTRODUCTION

Principle	Rationale
1. All those performing and assisting with the procedure should be trained in the theoretical and practical aspects of the procedure.	1. To achieve a safe and accurate procedure. Staff who are inadequately trained can adversely affect the care of the child.
2. The characteristics of CSF are: a) Normal CSF pressure is 50–180 mm H_2O (depending on age of child). b) Appearance is clear and colourless. c) CSF protein is 15–45 mg/100 ml. d) CSF glucose is 50–80 mg/100 ml. e) CSF cell count is 0–5 WBCs, no RBCs. f) Gammaglobulins 3–12% of the total protein.	2. a) Increased intracranial pressure indicates trauma, infection, obstruction of CSF flow or the presence of a space occupying lesion. b) Cloudy CSF indicates infection; reddish CSF indicates bleeding; brown/orange CSF indicates elevated protein or old blood. c) Increased protein indicates infection, diabetes or inflammatory condition. d) Increased glucose indicates hyperglycaemia; decreased indicates the presence of infection. e) Increased WBC indicates infection, infarction or demyelination; increased RBC indicates bleeding or traumatic lumbar puncture. f) Increased gammaglobulin indicates demyelination, or Guillain–Barré syndrome.

Procedure guideline 18.19 **Preparation for lumbar puncture**

Statement	Rationale
1. Inform the child and family of the following: a) That the lumbar puncture is necessary. b) The reason for the lumbar puncture. c) The implications of the results. d) What it entails. e) The likely duration of the procedure.	1. To obtain informed consent: a) To aid efficiency. b) To aid safety. c) To achieve optimum adherence.
2. An anaesthetic cream should be applied to the site chosen for the lumbar puncture, at the prescribed time.	2. This has been demonstrated to reduce pain during lumbar puncture (Bouffet et al 1996).
3. Administer the chosen method of relaxation, sedation or anaesthesia.	3. To ensure child is safe, comfortable and adherent.
4. The nurse will place and hold the child in the appropriate position: the ideal position is with head flexed down, knees drawn up and spine flexed. a) Occasionally the procedure will be performed with the child sitting up.	4. To allow maximum widening of the laminae, and facilitate placement of needle, while maintaining the child's safety. a) Caution should be exercised when the child is in this position, due to the increased risk of brain herniation.
5. Involve the parent/carer and play specialist as appropriate.	5. To aid with adherence.

Procedure guideline 18.20 Performing a lumbar puncture

Statement	Rationale
1. Aseptic precautions must be undertaken.	**1.** To minimise the risk of cross-infection.
2. The first nurse will continue to hold the child throughout the procedure, providing safety and reassurance.	**2.** To facilitate completion of the lumbar puncture and ensure the child's safety and comfort.
3. The second nurse will assist the doctor with the procedure as requested.	**3.** To facilitate completion of the procedure, while leaving the first nurse to care for the child.
4. Involve the parent/carer and play specialist as appropriate in the psychological care of the child during the procedure.	**4.** To assist with adherence and to minimise psychological trauma. It is considered helpful for a parent/carer to be present during lumbar puncture (Eppich and Arnold 2003).
5. Once the lumbar puncture is completed, allow child to regain comfortable position as desired. **a)** Where possible keep the child flat for a period of time as requested by the clinician.	**5.** To aid comfort. **a)** To reduce risk of post procedural lumbar puncture headache. Although headache following lumbar puncture is considered a lesser risk in children, than in adults (Janssens et al 2003), bedrest, analgesia and adequate fluid intake are recommended (Schwarz et al 1999).
6. Return the child to bed, keeping flat as instructed.	**6.** To indicate to child procedure has finished.
7. Administer further analgesics as required and as prescribed.	**7.** To minimise discomfort to the child.
8. Inform child and family of the result and its implications	**8.** To aid partnership in care.
9. Dispose of used equipment according to Waste Policy.	**9.** To minimise the risk of cross-infection.

464

Training staff

The following list suggests the competencies required of staff caring for a child having a lumbar puncture.

The nurse should be able to:

1. Understand the various reasons why a lumbar puncture may be performed.
2. Understand the potential contraindications and complications.
3. Discuss with child, family and doctor, the appropriate method under which the lumbar puncture is to be performed, i.e. relaxation/sedation/anaesthesia.
4. Provide a safe and calm environment under which the procedure is performed.
5. Ensure the child's safety throughout the procedure.
6. Understand the reasons for holding/ restraining the child during the procedure and be adherent with these.
7. Understand the principles of aseptic technique and assist the doctor is providing these during the procedure.
8. Understand the results provided by the lumbar puncture, and the implications for treatment.

Following the procedure the nurse should provide safety, reassurance, comfort and analgesia as appropriate. A short period of bedrest may alleviate headache associated with a reduction in intracranial pressure after lumbar puncture and nurses should refer to the guidelines provided by their individual hospital regarding mobilisation.

References

Action for Sick Children (2003) Helping children cope with needles. London, Action for Sick children. Available at www.actionforsickchildren.org

Alexander J, Kendrick D. (2005) Pre-hospital seizure management in pediatric patients. Academic Emergency Medicine, 12(5), 165–167

Appleton R, Gibbs J. (1998) Epilepsy in Childhood and Adolescence, 2nd edition. London, Martin Dunitz

Armon K, Stephenson T, Gabri V, MacFaud R. (2003) An evidence and consensus based guideline for the management of a child after seizure. Emergency Medical Journal, 20(1), 13–20

Aucken S, Crawford B. (1999) Neurological assessment. In Guerrero D. (ed.) Neuro Oncology for Nurses. London, Whurr

Barrett-Goode P. (2000) Reliability of the Adelaide Coma Scale. Paediatric Nursing, 12(8), 23–27

Birdsall C, Greif L. (1990) How do you manage external ventricular drainage? American Journal of Nursing, 90, 47–49

Bouffet E, Douard MC, Annequin D, Castaing MC, Pichard-Leandri E. (1996) Pain in lumbar puncture. Results of a two year discussion at the French Society of Pediatric Oncology. Archives of Pediatrics, Jan. 3(1), 22–27

Castledine G. (1993) Neurological emergencies 2: Nurse aid management of fits. British Journal of Nursing, 2(6), 336–337

Chapman CSM, Grocott M and Frank LS (2010) Systematic review of paediatric alert criteria for identifying hospitalised children at risk of critical deterioration. Intensive Care Medicine, 36(4), 600–611

Chin RF, Neville B, Peckham C, et al (2006) Incidence, cause and short term outcome of convulsive status epilepticus in childhood. Lancet 368, 9531, 222–229

Clar R, Walker L, Smith C. (2002) The influence of appraisals in understanding children's experience with medical procedures. Journal of Paediatric Psychology, 27(7), 553–563

Couffignal B, D'Agate B, Bocquet S. (2001) Are epilepsy seizures in patients with medial temporal lobe epilepsy influenced by participating factors. Epilepsies, 13(1), 49–52

Disabato J, Burkett K. (2007) Neurological assessment of the neonate, infant, child, and adolescent. In: Cartwright C, Wallace D. (eds) Nursing Care of the Pediatric Neurosurgery Patient. New York, Springer

Ellis A, Cavanagh S. (1992) Aspects of neurosurgical assessment using the Glasgow Coma Scale. Intensive and Critical Nursing Care, 8(2), 94–99

Engel J. (2002) ILAE (International League Against Epilepsy) Commission Report. A proposed diagnostic scheme for people with epileptic seizures and with epilepsy: Report of the ILAE Task Force on Classification and Terminology. Epilepsia, 42(6), 796–803

Eppich WJ, Arnold LD. (2003) Family member presence in the pediatric emergency department. Current Opinion Pediatrics, June 15(3),294–298

Fisher RS, Van Emede Boas, Blume W, Elger C, Genton P, Lee P, Engel J. (2005) Epileptic seizures and epilepsy: definitions proposed by the international league against epilepsy (ILAE) and the international bureau for epilepsy (IBE). Epilepsia, 46(4), 470–472

Great Ormond Street Hospital for Children NHS Foundation Trust (1997) Paediatric Coma Charts: A guide to assessment. A video teaching guide for the multi-disciplinary team. London, Great Ormond Street Hospital for Children NHS Foundation Trust

Hazinski M. (1992) Nursing Care of the Critically Ill Child, 2nd edition. St Loius, Mosby-Year Book, pp521–628

Hickey J. (1997) The Clinical Practice of Neurological and Neurosurgical Nursing, 4th edition. Philadelphia, Lippincot

Hickey JV. (2003) The Clinical Practice of Neurological and Neurosurgical Nursing, 5th edition. Philadelphia, Lippincott

Holmes G. (1999) Buccal route for benzodiazepines in treatment of seizures? The Lancet, Feb 353(20), 608–609

Janssens E, Aerssens P, Alliet P, Gillis P, Raes M. (2003) Post-dural puncture headaches in Children. European Journal of Paediatrics, 162(3), 117–121

Jennet B, Teasdale G. (1974) Assessment of coma and impaired consciousness. Lancet, July 2(2872), 81–84

Kwong KL, Chak WK, Wong SN, Kwan TS. (2000) Epidemiology of childhood epilepsy in a cohort of 309 Chinese children. Pediatric Neurology, 24(4), 276–282

Marcoux K. (2005) Management of increased intracranial pressure in the critically ill child with an acute neurological injury. AACN Clinical Issues, 16, 212–231

May L, Carter B. (1995) Nursing support and care: meeting the needs of the child and family with altered cerebral function. In: Carter B, Dearman A. (eds) Child Health Care Nursing. Oxford, Blackwell Science, pp 363–391

McIntyre J, Robertson S, Norris E, et al (2005) Safety and efficacy of buccal midazolam versus rectal diazepam for emergency treatment of seizures in children: A randomised controlled trial. The Lancet, July 16 (366), 94

National Centre for Young People with Epilepsy/GOSH (2009) Buccal midazolam. Available at http://www.ich.ucl.ac.uk/gosh_families/information_sheets/medicines_midazolam_buccal/medicines_midazolam_buccal_families.html

Neilsen N, Pearce K, Limbacher E, Wallace DC. (2007) Hydrocephalus. In: Cartwright C, Wallace D. (eds) Nursing Care of the Paediatric Neurosurgery Patient. Berlin, Springer

Norman R. (2000) Controversies in pediatric emergency medicine. Pediatric Emergency Care, 16(4), 229–301

Nursing and Midwifery Council (2002) Guidelines for the administration of medicines. London, NMC

Panayiotopoulos C. (2002) A Clinical Guide to Epileptic Syndromes and their Treatment. Based on the new ILAE diagnostic scheme. Oxfordshire, Bladon Medical Publishing

Reilly PL, Simpson DA, Sprod R, Thomas L. (1988) Assessing the conscious level in infants and young children: a paediatric version of the Glasgow Coma Scale. Child's Nervous System, Feb 4(1), 30–33

Salmon K (2006) Preparing young children for medical procedures: Taking account of memory. Journal of Pediatric Psychology, 1(8), 859–861

Schwarz U, Schwan C, Strumpf M, Witscher K, Zenz M. (1999) Postdural puncture headache: Diagnosis and prevention. Schmerz, Oct 13(5), 332–340

Scott R, Besag FM, Neville BG, et al (1999) Buccal midazolam and rectal diazepam for treatment of prolonged seizures in childhood and adolescence: a randomized trial. The Lancet, 353, 623–626

Simpson D, Reilly P. (1982) Paediatric Coma Scale. Lancet, 2(8295), 450

Smith J, Cheater F, Bekker H. (2009) Parent's involvement in decisions when their child is admitted to hospital with suspected shunt malfunction: study protocol. Journal of Advanced Nursing, 65(10), 198–207

Wong G, Wayne W, Poon W. (2007) External ventricular drain infection. Journal of Neurosurgery, 107(1), 248–250

Woodward S, Addison C, Shah S, Brennan F, MacLeod A, Clements M. (2002) Benchmarking best practice for external ventricular drainage. British Journal of Nursing, 11(1),47–53

Yoong M, Chin R, Scott R. (2009) Management of convulsive status epilepticus in children. Archives of Disease in Childhood, 94, 1–9

465

Bibliography

Appleton R, et al. (2001) Epilepsy, 4th edition. London, Martin Dunitz

Betz C, et al. (1994) Family-centred Nursing Care of Children, 2nd edition. Philadelphia, W.B Saunders, pp 1506–1564

Fuller G, Manford M. (2000) Neurology. An illustrated colour text. London, Harcourt

Lanfear J. (1998) The child/young person with epilepsy. Paediatric Nursing, 10(3), 29–34

Lindsay KW, et al. (1998) Neurology and Neurosurgery Illustrated, 3rd edition. Edinburgh, Churchill Livingstone.

Schwartz R. (1995) The management of epilepsy in childhood. Maternal and Child Health, Dec, 408–411

Taylor M. (2000) Managing Epilepsy. A Clinical Handbook. Oxford, Blackwell Science

Verity C. (1998) Do seizures damage the brain? The epidemiological evidence. Archive of Diseases in Childhood, 78, 78–84

Appendix 18.1 The GOSH Coma Chart

Name		**Coma Scale**	Great Ormond Street **NHS**
Hosp. No			Hospital for Children
DOB	(Affix patient label)		NHS Trust
Ward			

Consultant		Referring Hospital		Weight	Kg

The coma scale is scored on a total of 15 points. A score of less than 12 should give rise for concern. This is a universally accepted tool for measuring coma. A decrease in coma scale will be associated with a decreased level of consciousness. This needs to be considered along with the child's vital signs. Further information about the coma scale can be found in the related clinical procedure guideline.

A.   Eyes Open

If the eyes are closed by swelling, plesse write 'C' in the relevant column, thus indicating the reason for a lower score.

B.   Best Verbal Response

In the left hand margin are two separate scales: on the far left is the scale for babies and infants and on the right is the scale for older children.

The following section gives an explanation of the best verbal response of infants.

a. Smiles

This can be used to describe an alert, contented infant as not all will smile at a stranger. The interaction between parents/carers and the infant should therefore be taken into account.

b. Appropriate Cries

The infant may be unable to settle.

c. Inappropriate Cries

The infant may have periods of being drowsy, but at times is heard to cry out. This is not always associated with being disturbed. The cry may be high pitched.

d. Occasional Whimper

Less frequent than above and may be associated with deep painful stimuli, required to gain a motor response.

e. None

No verbal response.

C.   Best Motor response to Stimuli

The age and cognitive abilities of the child must be taken into account.

D.   Pupils

When recording pupil size in is important to remember the effects of drugs, e.g. morphine will cause pinpoint pupils and atropine drops will dilate pupils for up to 6 hours.

E.   Limb Movements

a. If a child has a permanent hemiparesis please indicate this in the relevant column, e.g. weakness, even though it is normal for the child.
b. A child with a severe developmental delay may score lower on the coma scale, as his motor response may be poor.

Version No: 0.2	Version date: 5th April 2004	Document development lead:	Jacqueline Robinson, Practice Educator, Neurosciences

Name	
Hosp. No	
DOB	(Affix patient label)

Date:
Time:

**Great Ormond Street Hospital for Children NHS Trust
Coma Chart**

Eyes open	Spontaneously	4
	To speech	3
	To pain	2
	None	1

C = Eyes closed by swelling

Best verbal response	Smiles	Orientated	5
	Appropriate cries	Disorientated	4
	Inapproprite cries	Monosylabic response	3
	Occasional whimper	Incomprehensible sounds	2
	None	None	1

T = Endo-tracheal tube

D = Dys-phasia

Best motor response (Record best arm)	Obeys/Spontaneous	6
	Localze pain	5
	Normal flexion	4
	Abnormal flexion	3
	Extension	2
	None	1

P = Para-lysed

Coma scale total

Pain Score	Pain tool in use (see p4)	

Pupil diameter guide

1 mm
2 mm
3 mm
4 mm
5 mm
6 mm
7 mm
8 mm

BP = Blood Pressure
Resp = Respirations

B P & P U l s e

R e s p

240 230 220 210 200 190 180 170 160 150 140 130 120 110 100 90 80 70 60 50 40 30 20 10 0

40.0 39.5 39.0 38.5 38.0 37.5 37.0 36.5 36.0 35.5 35.0 34.5 34.0 33.5 33.0 32.5 32.0

Temperature °C

O₂ Saturation
Air%O₂

Pupils	Right	size (mm)
		Reaction
	Left	size (mm)
		Reaction

+ = reacts
− = no reaction
sl = sluggish

Arms	Normal power
	Mild weakness
	Bevere weakness
	Flexion
	Extension
	No response

Record right (R) and left (L) separately if there is a difference between the two sides

Legs	Normal power
	Mild weakness
	Bevere weakness
	Flexion
	Extension
	No response

P = paralysed
# = fracture

467

Record of Significant Events

Developmental Age:

Coma Scale Prior to Illness:

Date	Time	Description of Significant Event (E.g. post seizure, pain, headache, vomiting etc.)	Signature

Pain Assessment

0	= NO pain
1 – 3	= MILD pain
4 – 7	= MODERATE pain
8 – 10	= SEVERE pain

FLACC   SUGGESTED AGE GROUP: 2 months to 7 years   Behavioural

CATEGORIES	SCORING		
	0	**1**	**2**
Face	No particular expression or smile	Occasional grimace or frown, withdrawn, disinterested	Frequent to constant quivering chin, clenched jaw
Legs	Normal position or relaxed	Uneasy, restless, tense	Kicking, or legs drawn up
Activity	Lying quietly, normal position, moves easily	Squirming, shifting back and forth, tense	Arched, rigid or jerking
Cry	No cry (awake or asleep)	Moans or whimpers, occasional complaint	Crying steadily, screams or sobs, frequent complaints
Consolability	Content, relaxed	Reassured by occasional touching, hugging or being talked to, distractible	Difficult to console or comfort

Each of the five categories: (F) Face; (L) Legs; (A) Activity; (C) Cry; (C) Consolability; is scored from 0 - 2 which results in a total score between 0 and 10   *(Merkel et al, 1997)*

Wong & Baker   SUGGESTED AGE GROUP: 4 years and over   Self-report

Point to each face using the words to describe the pain intensity. Ask the child to choose a face that best describes their own pain and record the appropriate number overleaf.   *(adapted from Wong & Baker, 1988)*

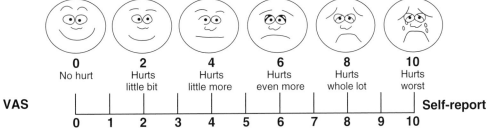

0	2	4	6	8	10
No hurt	Hurts little bit	Hurts little more	Hurts even more	Hurts whole lot	Hurts worst

VAS   **Self-report**

0   1   2   3   4   5   6   7   8   9   10

Analgesic interventions

Analgesic ladder

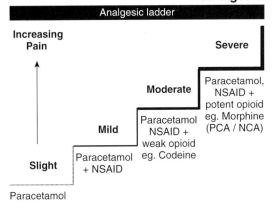

Increasing Pain

- **Severe**
- **Moderate** — Paracetamol, NSAID + potent opioid eg. Morphine (PCA / NCA)
- **Mild** — Paracetamol NSAID + weak opioid eg. Codeine
- **Slight** — Paracetamol + NSAID
- Paracetamol

NB: ■ *Check 'British National Formulary' for contraindications / interactions / precautions etc*

PCA / NCA / Epidural patients

0	No pain *	
1 – 3	**Mild pain ***	
	NCA	- give bolus (10 mins before activity)
	PCA	- encourage bolus (10 mins before activity)
4 – 7	**Moderate pain ***	
	NCA	- give bolus
	PCA	- encourage bolus
	EPIDURAL	- contact Pain Service
8 – 10	**Severe pain ***	
	NCA	
	PCA	⎤ - contact Pain
Service		
	EPIDURAL	⎦

* Ensure supplementary analgesia is given (paracetamol + an NSAID if appropriate)
NB: No codeine

Additional Scales

SEDATION		
	1	Awake
	2	Drowsy
	3	Asleep but moves spontaneously
	4	Asleep responds to stimulation Stop infusion until returns to level 3
	5	Hard to rouse Stop infusion / Contact Pain Service

NAUSEA		
	1	Slight
	2	Moderate
	3	Severe

ITCH		
	1	Slight
	2	Moderate
	3	Severe

469

Appendix 18.2 Types of painful stimuli

The type of painful stimulus used is a controversial issue, although it is generally agreed that a central painful stimulus is required to assess eye opening, and verbal and motor response in children who have a decreased level of consciousness (Appleton *et al* 1998). A central stimulus can be applied in one of three ways:

1. Trapezium squeeze – using a thumb and two fingers, hold and twist the trapezius muscle of the shoulder (Appleton and Gibbs 1998).
2. Supraorbital pressure – using a finger or thumbnail, apply pressure in the supraorbital groove. Applying supraorbital pressure can sometimes make a child grimace and close their eye rather than open it. If this is the case, another form of central stimulus may be required. Supraorbital pressure is also not recommended in children who have facial fractures (Appleton and Gibbs 1998).
3. Sternal rub – using the knuckles of a clenched fist, vertically rub the centre of the sternum (Appleton and Gibbs 1998).

When applying a central painful stimulus, it is important to use caution as pressure on the supraorbital groove or sternum may cause unnecessary injury

Peripheral stimulus can also be used to elicit a response. The most common peripheral stimulus is to apply pressure to the nail beds and observe for a motor response. However, peripheral stimulus may only elicit a spinal reflex, which may not be an accurate assessment of the child's condition.

Appendix 18.3 Examples of motor responses

A. Localising to pain

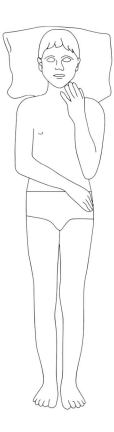

B. Normal flexion

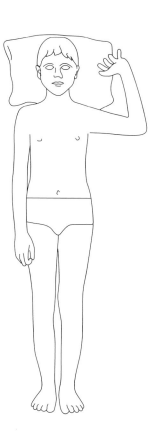

C. Abnormal flexion

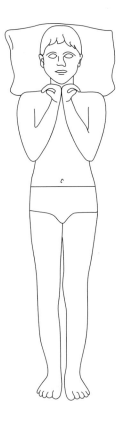

D. Extension

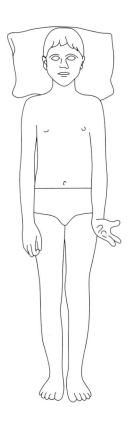

Appendix 18.4 An example of an algorithm for a convulsing child

Disclaimer

No liability can be taken as a result of using this information.

It is strongly suggested that due to the changing and complex nature of seizure management, referring to the latest online algorithm is recommended, examples of which are EPLS, APLS, NICE guidelines.

At the time of going to press the following guideline is currently in use at GOSH (used with permission). Below is an example of the *current* algorithm in use at GOSH, therefore it is advised that the latest version is accessed for use.

North Central London Epilepsy Network Guidelines. Date of Publication: April 2005

The algorithm below can be found on the following website: http://www.ich.ucl.ac.uk/

There are minor differences between these local guidelines and Advanced Paediatric Life Support (APLS) and National Institute for Health and Clinical excellence (NICE) guidelines, for example incorporating pre-hospital care; omission of paraldehyde; addition of buccal midazolam. A recent article by Yoong *et al* (2009) suggests an updated proposal.

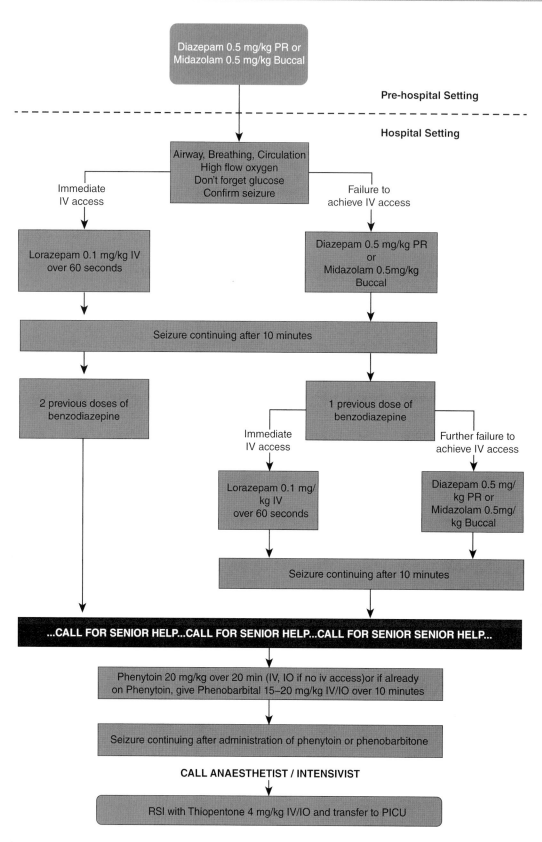

An example of an algorithm for a convulsing child

Chapter 19

Nutrition and feeding

Chapter contents

Procedure guidelines

The Great Ormond Street Hospital Manual of Children's Nursing Practices, First Edition. Edited by Susan Macqueen, Elizabeth Anne Bruce, Faith Gibson.
© 2012 Great Ormond Street Hospital for Children NHS Foundation Trust. Published 2012 by Blackwell Publishing Ltd.

Introduction

Good nutrition is vital for the growth and development of all children in both health and disease. It is important to have a knowledge of the changing nutritional requirements needed throughout childhood in order to assess whether a child's intake is adequate. This chapter describes the nutritional requirements of children from preterm to adolescence and outlines how these can be achieved through normal eating and drinking. Enteral and parenteral feeding are also discussed where children are unable to take adequate nutrition by mouth.

Nutritional requirements

A nutritionally adequate diet is essential for the normal growth and development of children. During illness and recovery, requirements for nutrients are raised. This may be due to factors such as increased losses, e.g. vomiting and diarrhoea, or increased metabolism that expends energy stores, e.g. pyrexia. Sick children are particularly vulnerable to nutritional deficit and there is evidence to suggest that children in UK hospitals often have a poor nutritional status. For this reason, nutritional care should be a priority for all sick children.

A study at Birmingham Children's Hospital to assess the nutritional status of inpatients found that 16% of the total population studied were severely stunted (chronic protein-energy malnutrition); 14% severely wasted (acute protein-energy malnutrition) and a further 20% were at risk of severe malnutrition. Chronic patients were significantly more stunted and wasted than acute/elective patients. Stunting was significantly more common in the cardiac, gastroenterology and respiratory group, but not in oncology or renal patients. This study revealed an alarmingly high prevalence of both acute and chronic malnutrition in a cross-sectional survey of children in hospital (Moy *et al* 1990).

Results from a later study performed at the Royal Hospital for Sick Children in Glasgow revealed: 16% were underweight for age (<5th centile), 15% stunted (<5th centile height-for-age), 8% wasted (<80% weight-for-height); 16% were moderately undernourished or at risk of becoming so. Only one-third of these malnourished children had previously been identified as such. Children with diseases of the digestive system (inflammatory bowel disease, cystic fibrosis and coeliac disease) were most at risk of undernutrition. (Hendrikse *et al* 1997).

A report by the British Association for Parenteral and Enteral Nutrition (BAPEN) looking at hospital food as a medical treatment found that 15% of children in the UK are malnourished on admission to hospital (Allison 1999). Even more worrying, a majority who depend on hospital food for all their nutrition continue to lose weight while in hospital (Allison 1999).

Nutrition screening over a 3-day period in 2007 in 46 Dutch hospitals with a paediatric ward showed that 19% of children were undernourished on admission (Joosten *et al* 2010). The overall prevalence of malnutrition was significantly higher in children with an underlying disease. A further study has shown that the largest proportion of malnourished children are those with multiple diagnoses, mental retardation, infectious diseases and cystic fibrosis (Pawallek 2008). For these reasons it is imperative to monitor the nutritional status of all children in hospital closely to identify any signs of undernutrition. The Care Quality

Box 19.1 Some conditions likely to cause impairment in nutritional status

- Preterm and low birth weight delivery
- Children on inappropriately restrictive diets, e.g. exclusion diets
- Feeding problems: prolonged difficulties with ingesting or swallowing food
- Vomiting, diarrhoea or malabsorption
- Severe or chronic catabolic illness, e.g. recurrent infections or multiple surgery
- Child neglect/abuse
- Eating disorders, e.g. anorexia nervosa
- Diseases/therapies altering the normal pattern of eating, e.g. cancer and chemotherapy

Commission has published essential standards of quality and safety ,which include a requirement for nutritional screening when an individual first starts to use a hospital service, in order to identify where there may be risk of poor nutrition or dehydration (Care Quality Commission 2010). It is also important for all health professionals to be aware that infants and children are not just small adults and that they require both different nutrients and a different balance of nutrients at different stages in their lives.

Nutritional impairment is serious and may:

- Affect long-term health, growth and development in very young infants (Lucas *et al* 1998, 2001).
- Impair health and growth, increase the rate of complications of disease or treatment and, in life-threatening illness, reduce the chances of survival (Hendrikse *et al* 1997).
- Increase length of hospital stay (Joosten *et al* 2010).

Box 19.1 lists some conditions likely to cause impairment in nutritional status.

Energy, protein and micronutrients (vitamins, minerals and trace elements) are required for maintenance as well as growth. It is crucial that requirements are met during infancy, childhood and adolescence. Deficiencies of energy and protein can cause poor growth and development and micronutrient deficiencies can lead to improper functioning of many of the body's systems.

During and following illness and disease, requirements are raised due to hyper-metabolism and anabolism. Total nutritional intake therefore needs to incorporate normal requirements and, in addition, requirements for catch-up growth. In these situations, requirements should be calculated individually for each child to ensure that sufficient nutrition is provided for growth.

Table 19.1 gives a summary of common dietary requirements for healthy children and Table 19.2 shows the dietary requirements for preterm and low birth weight infants. These may change according to the clinical condition of the child.

Nutrition from preterm to adolescence

Breast feeding is the optimum form of nutrition for infants and mothers should be supported in their decision to breast feed. The Department of Health recommends exclusive breast feeding for the first 6 months or 26 weeks of life (Department of Health

Table 19.1 Summary table of selected dietary requirements (Department of Health 1991). © Crown copyright.

Age	Energy*		Protein+	
	kcal/day	kcal/kg/day	g/day	g/kg/day
Males				
0–3 months	545	115–100	12.5	2.1
4–6	690	95	12.7	1.6
7–9	825	95	13.7	1.5
10–12	920	95	14.9	1.5
1–3 years	1230	95	14.5	1.1
4–6	1715	90	19.7	1.1
7–10	1970	–	28.3	–
11–14	2220	–	42.1	–
15–18	2755	–	55.2	–
Females				
0–3 months	515	115–100	12.5	2.1
4–6	645	95	12.7	1.6
7–9	765	95	13.7	1.5
10–12	865	95	14.9	1.5
1–3 years	1165	95	14.5	1.1
4–6	1545	90	19.7	1.1
7–10	1740	–	28.3	–
11–14	1845	–	41.2	–
15–18	2110	–	45.4	–

Age	Sodium+		Potassium+		Vitamin C+	Calcium+	Iron+
	mmol/day	mmol/kg/day	mmol/day	mmol/kg/day	mg/day	mmol/day	μmol/day
Males							
0–3 months	9	1.5	20	3.4	25	13.1	30
4–6	12	1.6	22	2.8	25	13.1	80
7–9	14	1.6	18	2.0	25	13.1	140
10–12	15	1.5	18	1.8	25	13.1	140
1–3 years	22	1.7	20	1.6	30	8.8	120
4–6	30	1.7	28	1.6	30	11.3	110
7–10	50	–	50	–	30	13.8	160
11–14	70	–	80	–	35	25.0	200
15–18	70	–	90	–	40	25.0	200
Females							
0–3 months	9	1.5	20	3.4	25	13.1	30
4–6	12	1.6	22	2.8	25	13.1	80
7–9	14	1.6	18	2.0	25	13.1	140
10–12	15	1.5	18	1.8	25	13.1	140
1–3 years	22	1.7	20	1.6	30	8.8	120
4–6	30	1.7	28	1.6	30	11.3	110
7–10	50	–	50	–	30	13.8	160
11–14	70	–	80	–	35	20.0	260
15–18	70	–	90	–	40	20.0	260

*= EAR, Estimated Average Requirement of a group of people for energy. About half the group will usually need more than the EAR, and half less.
+= RNI, Reference Nutrient Intake for protein or a vitamin or mineral. An amount of the nutrient that is enough, or more than enough, for virtually all people in a group. If the average intake of the group is at RNI, then the risk of deficiency in the group is very small.
It is important to remember that these figures are for populations, not individuals and therefore serve as a guide only.

Table 19.2 Dietary recommendations for growing preterm infants 1000–1500 g birthweight (adapted from Tsang et al 2005)

	Per kg body weight/day
Energy	110–150 kcal
Protein	26–30 weeks PCA 3.8–4.2 g
	30–36 weeks PCA 3.4–3.6 g
Sodium	3.0–5.0 mmol
Calcium	2.5–5.5 mmol
Phosphorus	1.9–4.5 mmol
Iron	2–4 mg from 2 weeks
Vitamin A	210–450 μg
Vitamin C	18–24 mg
Vitamin D	3.75–10 μg (maximum 25 μg/day)
Vitamin E	6–12 mg (maximum 25 mg/day)
Folic acid	25–50 μg

PCA = Post-conceptional age.
See GOSH (2009) for a complete list of nutritional requirements.

Table 19.3a Fortifiers used for preterm infants

		per recommended dose	
		Energy (kcal)	Protein (g)
Breast milk fortifiers	Nutriprem breast milk fortifier (4.3 g/100 ml)	16	0.8
	SMA breast milk fortifier (4 g/100 ml)	15	1.0

Table 19.3b Feeds used for preterm infants

		Average composition per 100 ml	
		Energy (kcal)	Protein (g)
Preterm formulas	Aptamil Preterm, Nutriprem 1, SMA Gold Prem 1	81	2.4
Post-discharge nutrient dense formulas	Nutriprem 2, SMA Gold Prem 2	74	2.0

Table 19.4 Feeds for term infants

		Average composition per 100 ml	
		Energy (kcal)	Protein (g)
Whey-based formulas	Aptamil First, Cow & Gate 1, SMA 1	66	1.3
Casein-based formulas	Aptamil 2 Extra Hungry, Cow & Gate 2, SMA Extra Hungry	66	1.6

2003b). The suck-swallow-breathe sequence that allows the newborn infant to feed is thought to be well developed by 37 weeks gestation. Infants who are not able to coordinate this sequence, whether due to prematurity or clinical disorder, may need to be tube fed. The infants of mothers who are not able to breast feed or where breast feeding is contraindicated, e.g. mothers who are HIV positive, must receive a nutritionally complete infant formula that is appropriate for the age of the infant. Solids should be offered from 6 months of age (Department of Health 2003b). Nutritional requirements for healthy populations have been set by the government (Department of Health 1991) and can be used as a guideline to assess the nutritional adequacy of energy, protein, vitamins, minerals and trace elements in an individual's diet. There are also recommendations concerning the amount of sugars, starch, non-starch polysaccharides (NSP or fibre) and fats that constitute a healthy diet. There is recognition that young children may need a higher fat intake than the rest of the population in order to attain an adequate intake of energy. Recommendations for the population to lower its intake of fat do not apply before 2 years of age, but should be implemented after 5 years of age.

Feeding the premature infant

Up to 220 ml/kg in the well infant feed volumes depend on fluid balance and gut tolerance.

The milk of choice for preterm infants is mother's own breast milk, fed as soon after expression as possible. If the baby cannot take sufficient volumes to provide nutritional adequacy (up to 220 ml/kg may be required to provide adequate energy and nutrients for growth and development) then a breast milk fortifier (BMF) may be added to the expressed breast milk (EBM). Suitable products are given in Table 19.3. Breast milk fortifiers meet the specific needs of preterm infants and should not be used to fortify EBM for babies born at term. If EBM is not available, a preterm infant formula should be used. These are highly specialised milks designed to meet the specific requirements of preterm infants. Nutritional adequacy may be achieved at a feed volume

of 150 ml/kg (Table 19.3). Expressed breast milk with or without BMF and preterm formulas can be fed by tube or by mouth. On discharge from the special care unit, mothers should be encouraged to breast feed on demand. If unable to do so, a nutrient enriched post-discharge formula should be used to aid catch-up growth and bone mineralisation (Table 19.3) (King 2007).

Feeding the term infant

Ideally feed on demand or 150–200 ml/kg until weaning solids established.

If mothers are unable to breast feed then whey-based infant formulas are recommended and can be used from birth (Table 19.4). Some mothers are swayed by advertising and prefer to use casein-based formulas when they perceive their infants to be hungry. The energy and nutrient profile of these two types of formulas are actually very similar and there is no nutritional benefit in changing from one formula to another. Some babies who do not feed well at the breast may be given their mother's expressed breast milk (EBM) by bottle.

Infants who are not breast fed should continue to receive an infant formula as the main milk drink until 12 months of age.

Feed preparation and administration

Ideally infants will receive Ready to Feed (RTF) formulas when in hospital; these are sterile preparations. They need to be stored at cool temperatures, but do not need to be refrigerated. Hands should be thoroughly washed prior to feeding the infant. Warming of formulas for term infants prior to feeding is not necessary, but it is important to continue to provide feeds at the temperature that the baby is used to at home. The bottle may be put under warm running water or placed in an electric warming unit. If warm water baths are used, the bath should be cleaned and fresh water used on a regular basis according to local policy in order to avoid bacterial contamination (American Dietetic Association 2004). The water should not reach the level of the bottle's collar and the lid should not be submersed in the water. If the formula is warmed the process should take less than 15 minutes (American Dietetic Association 2004). Microwave ovens must never be used for warming infant formulas because of the danger of formation of hot spots in the liquid (Department of Health 1994) and overheating can reduce the activity of heat labile vitamins. The bottle cap should only be removed and the teat screwed on immediately prior to feeding the infant. The feed should be shaken to distribute the heat and to ensure that all the components are suspended. The temperature of the feed should be checked by testing a few drops on the inside of the wrist before giving to the baby. The infant formula manufacturers recommend that once opened RTF formulas must be used within 4 hours. In the clinical situation once a bottle has been warmed for feeding and the teat attached it is best practice to discard the feed once it has been at the bedside for 1 hour.

If the infant requires a formula that does not come in a RTF presentation, the formula will need to be reconstituted from powder. In large paediatric hospitals there will be a dedicated special feed unit or milk room where formulas can be made up safely. In smaller paediatric units feeds may be made up at ward level. It is necessary to have a clean room with restricted access to personnel who are trained in the preparation of formulas. Strict protocols for reconstituting feeds must be adhered to, disinfected feed making equipment and bottles must be made available and adequate refrigeration of the prepared feed is necessary to ensure the microbial safety of feeds made at ward level. Guidelines for the requirements of feed making areas are described elsewhere (Paediatric Group British Dietetic Association 2007, Watling 2007). Reconstituted feeds are not sterile and great care must be taken in their storage and handling prior to feeding. The administration of the feed to the baby is the same as described above.

On discharge mothers should be instructed how to make up a bottle of infant formula according to the manufacturer's instructions (1 level scoop of powder to 1 fluid ounce or 30 ml cooled boiled water). All feed making equipment and bottles must be sterilised.

Weaning

In order to comply with the World Health Organization's global recommendation on the duration of exclusive breast

Table 19.5 Weaning foods

	Foods	Milk
First stage Begin by 6 months, but not before 4 months (17 weeks) of age	Smooth pureed or mashed fruit, vegetables, potatoes, baby cereals	Breast feeds or minimum 600 ml infant formula
Second stage 6–9 months	In addition to the above, mashed food with soft lumps: meat, fish, cheese, well-cooked egg, pulses; cereals: rice, pasta, bread, breakfast cereals	Breast feeds or 500–600 ml infant formula or follow-on formula*
Third stage 9–12 months	Minced and chopped 'family foods' incorporating all of the above	Breast feeds or 500–600 ml infant formula or follow-on formula*

*Follow-on formulas should not be used as a sole source of nutrition. They may be used from 6 months of age once a varied weaning diet is taken. Infant and follow-on formulas provide a useful source of iron in the weaning diet.

feeding (WHO 2001) the current Department of Health guidelines suggest that solids should be given around 6 months of age; breast milk (or infant formula) provides all the nutrients that a baby needs until this time. Previous advice, based on the development of the infant's gastrointestinal, immunological and oral motor function, had been that the majority of infants should not be given solid foods before the age of 4 months and that a mixed diet should be offered by the age of 6 months (Department of Health 1994). It will take some time for the new Department of Health guidelines to become common practice and many parents/carers will choose to give solid foods before 6 months. The European Society for Paediatric Gastroenterology, Hepatology and Nutrition recommends that weaning onto solid foods should begin by 6 months, but not before 4 months (Agostoni et al 2008). Table 19.5 provides a guide for weaning. Further information for parents/carers on how to feed their babies, toddlers, older children and teenagers can be found on the Food Standards Agency website (Food Standards Agency 2010a).

Each baby should be assessed on its need for solids individually. Some babies will not need solids until 6 months of age whereas others may benefit from their introduction from 4 months (17 weeks) of age. It is recommended that preterm infants should be given solids some time between 5 and 7 months from birth, i.e. at 5–7 months chronological age (King 2007) provided they have lost the extrusion reflex and are able to eat from a spoon.

Infants must be supervised when eating. Foods should always be given from a spoon and not added to bottle feeds. Salt must not be added to weaning foods. A high salt intake may be associated with hypertension, heart disease and stroke later in life. The Food Standards Agency has made recommendations on the maximum daily salt consumption in children: less than 1 g for infants aged up to 12 months; 2 g for 1–3 year olds; 3 g for 4–6 year olds; 5 g for 7–11 year olds; 6 g for children over 11 years (Food Standards Agency 2010b).

Dental caries is the main dental disease affecting children. Sugar should not be routinely added to weaning foods. Babies should be offered a variety of flavours during weaning and early childhood so that they do not come to expect that all food should taste sweet. Sugar should only be added to foods if the addition will increase their acceptance, e.g. stewed fruits. There is no advantage in replacing sugar with honey – it is also cariogenic and in any case is contraindicated in the under 1s as it may contain *C. botulinum* spores. Babies should not be left with bottles of sugary drinks and any fruit juice given should be well diluted.

In infants at high risk of developing an allergy, i.e. those that have an atopic parent or sibling, it is recommended that they are breast fed throughout the weaning period and that high allergen foods are introduced one at a time so that any reaction to a food can be recognised (Grimshaw 2009). Delaying the introduction of these high allergen foods until after 6 months of age does not reduce the risk of allergy, but some parents/carers may wish to give these foods later (Grimshaw 2009, Muraro *et al* 2004, Venter *et al* 2009). These high allergen foods are: milk, eggs, fish, shellfish, wheat, soya, peanuts, tree nuts, sesame seeds, lupin, celery and mustard.

It is important that mealtimes are introduced when infants are in hospital. It is very easy to forget that giving babies food is part of their treatment. Babies should be placed in high chairs at meal times when able to support themselves and age appropriate spoons, bowls and feeding cups should be used. It may be safer from a microbiological view to give infants in hospital commercial weaning foods because they are sterile. However, there may be paediatric units that can safely provide infants with freshly cooked foods. If the baby is already established on solids it is important to maintain their normal feeding routine as far as possible when in hospital.

A schedule for the introduction of solids is given in Table 19.5.

Other drinks

1. Whole cows milk	1. Pasteurised whole cows milk is low in iron and should not be used as the main milk drink before 1 year of age.
2. Semi-skimmed milk	2. Is lower in fat and energy than whole cows milk; it may be used after 2 years of age if the child has an adequate intake of energy from food.
3. Water	3. Formula-fed infants may need additional water; exclusively breast fed babies rarely need fluids other than breast milk; water given as a drink from a bottle for infants under 6 months must be either sterile or boiled and cooled; drinking water from a cup or beaker does not have to boiled for infants over 6 months of age.
4. 'Baby' juices	4. May be given to quench thirst, but due to their sugar content they should be well diluted and their use confined to mealtimes.
5. Squashes, juices, cordials, fizzy drinks	5. Should not be given to infants; their use in older children should be confined to meal times because of their high sugar content.

From 6 months of age infants should be introduced to drinking from a cup. Bottle feeding should be discouraged from 1 year of age.

Diet throughout childhood

By the time infants have reached their first birthday they should be able to take the family diet, albeit in a mashed up form. Children need to be offered new tastes and textures to enable them to take a wide and varied diet that will provide them with the energy and nutrients needed for continued growth and development. Table 19.6 shows the food groups that meals for children should be selected from. A healthy balanced diet for most children is one rich in starchy carbohydrates, fruits and vegetables with moderate amounts of meat and alternative protein foods, milk and dairy foods. Most children will not be able to meet their energy requirements for the day from the three main meals alone; they will need between meal snacks. Care needs to be taken that these snacks do not rely on foods that are high in fat, sugar and salt, e.g. crisps, biscuits, chocolate though these foods need not be banned and indeed can be useful sources of energy in sick children who have small appetites. The government has given guidance on the menu choices that should be available for children in hospital and acknowledges that children need between-meal snacks (NHS Estates 2003).

It is important that the environment in which meals are served is conducive to eating. Mealtimes should not be a solitary experience; children will be more likely to try new foods and take a wider variety if they are eating with other people who are enjoying their food. Parents/carers friends and family should be encouraged to join the child at mealtimes. Furniture, cutlery and crockery should be appropriate for the age of the child.

Supplementary feeding: Sip feeds

If children have a poor appetite they will get insufficient energy and nutrients from the food that they eat and will experience a faltering in their growth. These children may benefit from a sip feed and a number are available for 1–6 year olds to enhance nutritional intake. The liquid ready-to-drink sip feeds are listed (Table 19.7) and these come in a variety of flavours.

There are no sip feeds specifically designed for the over 6 years age group. The above paediatric sip feeds can be given, or adult sip feeds may be used with caution. It is important to take into account intake of food and drink to make sure that the total diet is nutritionally adequate and that intakes of protein, electrolytes, vitamins and minerals are not excessive. It may be useful to supplement the diet with commercial drinks such as milk shakes to provide a source of energy, protein and calcium, but these are not nutritionally complete.

Supplementary feeding: enteral feeds

Infants and children who are unable to feed adequately by mouth will require supplementary feeding. Enteral feeding may provide total nutritional requirements or be used to supplement a poor oral intake. Enteral nutrition may be delivered via orogastric,

Table 19.6 Foods for children

Food group	Examples	Comment
Cereals and starches	Bread, chapatti, pitta bread, rice, pasta, breakfast cereals, potatoes, sweet potatoes, yams, plantain	Meals should be based on these high-energy nutritious foods. Wholegrain varieties should be included to improve fibre intake
Fruits and vegetables	Apples, bananas, pears, peaches, plums, satsumas, kiwi fruit, mango; broccoli, carrots, cabbage, green beans, sweet corn, peas, tomatoes	Aim for 5 portions a day to provide vitamins, minerals and antioxidants – portion size will depend on the age of the child. Fruit juice can be counted as one of the daily portions of fruit. The vitamin C content will help absorption of iron from breakfast cereals, green leafy vegetables and pulses
Milk and dairy foods	Milk, cheese, fromage frais, yoghurt	Three portions a day will provide adequate calcium. From 5 years of age lower fat varieties should be used
Meat, fish and alternatives	Meat, poultry, fish, eggs, nuts, pulses, e.g. lentils, dhal, chick peas, beans	Two to three portions a day will provide adequate protein and iron. At least two portions of fish per week is recommended, one of which should be oily. Oily fish (mackerel, salmon, sardines) contain beneficial omega 3 fatty acids. Boys may have up to 4 portions of oily fish per week; girls should have no more than 2 portions per week
Drinks	Milk, water, fruit juice	Children need 6–8 drinks a day which should include 350 ml milk. To reduce its cariogenicity fruit juice should be given at mealtimes and diluted for young children to reduce its acidity and sugar content
Fats and sugars	Biscuits, cakes, pastries, chocolate, ice cream, crisps, butter, margarine, oil	Can be offered as extra treats but should not replace the more nutritious foods described above. Children who are overweight should cut down on these high fat, high sugar foods

Table 19.7 Sip feeds for children

		per 100 ml	
		Energy (kcal)	Protein (g)
Standard	PaediaSure	101	2.8
Increased energy/nutrient density	Frebini Energy	150	3.8
	Fortini	150	3.4
	PaediaSure Plus	151	4.2
	PaediSure Plus juce*	150	4.2
	Resource Junior	150	3.0

*Does not contain any fat therefore must not be used as a sole source of nutrition.

Table 19.8 Enteral feeds for infants

		Per 100 ml	
		Energy (kcal)	Protein (g)
Standard	Expressed breast milk	69	1.3
	Infant formula	66	1.3
Increased energy and nutrient density	EBM + 3% infant formula	84	1.6
	15% infant formula	74	1.5
	SMA High Energy	91	2.0
	Infatrini	100	2.6
	Similac High Energy	101	2.6

Table 19.9 Enteral feeds for children

		per 100 ml	
		Energy (kcal)	Protein (g)
Standard	Frebini (8–30 kg)	100	2.5
	Nutrini (8–20 kg)	100	2.8
	PaediaSure (8–30 kg)	101	2.8
	Tentrini (21–45 kg)	100	3.3
Increased energy/nutrient density	Frebini Energy (8–30 kg)	150	3.8
	Nutrini Energy (8–20 kg)	150	4.1
	PaediaSure Plus (8–30 kg)	151	4.2
	Tentrini Energy (21–45 kg)	150	4.9

nasogastric, gastrostomy, nasojejunal or jejunostomy routes and guidelines for administration are given below:

- Infants – feed volume 150–200 ml/kg/day. Infants should be fed either expressed breast milk (EBM) or normal infant formula during the first year of life. If the infant has increased requirements that cannot be satisfied by increasing the feed volume, EBM and infant formula may be fortified to improve the energy and nutrient profile. Alternatively commercial feeds may be used (Table 19.8).
- Children weighing 8–45 kg – feed volume 85–110 ml/kg/day. There are a number of commercial feeds designed for children in this weight range. The feed manufacturers state the age range for which their feed is suitable, but there is some flexibility in which feed to use in a particular clinical situation. Some examples are given (Table 19.9). Some of these feeds are also available with added fibre.
- Children weighing > 45 kg – feed volume 50–70 ml/kg/day. There are no commercial feeds designed for this age group.

Adult enteral formulas may be used but care is needed to regularly check protein, electrolyte, vitamin and mineral status to ensure that intakes are not excessive. Alternatively paediatric enteral feeds can be used and fortified where necessary to improve the energy and protein profile.

Breast feeding

Breast feeding is the most suitable source of nutrition for the newborn baby and the advantages for the baby and the mother are very well recognised. These include the fostering of the mother and baby relationship, the unique 'tailor made' nutrient composition of breast milk, the reduction of infection owing to a range of immune factors in the milk, and the convenience of having the feed available at all times (Henschel and Inch 1996, Shaw and Lawson 2007). The mum too will find that she may lose weight more easily and regain her pre-pregnancy shape more quickly (UNICEF/WHO 1994). Research suggests that there is less risk of pre-menopausal breast and ovarian cancer and hip fractures in women who breast feed (UNICEF/WHO 1994). The World Health Organization now recommends exclusive breastfeeding for the first 6 months of life for most healthy term babies (WHO 2001).

The global UNICEF/WHO Baby Friendly Initiative was launched in June 1991 and in the UK in November 1994. The 'Ten Steps to Successful Breast Feeding' formed the basis of this initiative, and hospitals have to demonstrate that they fully implement the steps and comply with the International Code on the Marketing of Breast Milk Substitutes (WHO 1981). There is no initiative for dedicated paediatric units at present, but the Royal College of Nursing working party on 'Breast Feeding in Paediatric Units, Guidance for Good Practice' (Royal College of Nursing 1998), gives excellent guidelines and a check list to enable the formulation of a policy that will provide a framework for supporting breast feeding. On-going, regular teaching for staff and the assistance for mothers at the bedside are essential (Lang 2002). It is important for staff to know that there are some contra-indications to breast feeding and mothers who are unable to breast feed their baby must also be given support.

The lactation process commences shortly after the placenta separates during the third stage of labour. Where possible, the baby should be encouraged to suckle the breast as soon as possible after delivery. However, in some instances, this may not be possible because of the poor condition of the baby or because of a congenital anomaly.

Colostrum starts to be secreted from the breast once the placenta separates from the uterus. This clear liquid is high in protective immunoglobulins (especially IgA and IgE) and the sugar content helps to prevent hypoglycaemia. It is also a mild laxative so assists the baby to pass meconium.

Milk starts to be produced around the 3–4th day post-partum, but maternal stress and anxiety can delay the process. There are two main hormones involved: prolactin produces the milk in the milk ducts, and oxytocin expels it down the lactiferous sinuses to the nipple. The latter, known as the 'let down' reflex, occurs in response to the stimulation of the areola and the mother seeing and cuddling her baby. When the mother is not able to be present with her baby, this reflex can be replicated by her looking at her baby's photograph, or by her holding a special toy or piece of clothing while she expresses her milk.

The first milk produced by the breast at a feed is the fore milk and this is rather like a sugary drink providing fluid to maintain hydration. Once the baby has settled on the breast and started rhythmic sucking and swallowing (at approximately one suck per second), the milk becomes richer and contains fat and protein – the hind milk. It is essential that the baby suckles long enough at each breast in turn to gain the benefits of both fore and hind milk.

Breast milk contains all the vitamins, minerals and trace elements needed for growth and development in a bio-available form. Together with its anti-infective properties, growth factors, lipase to aid fat digestion and a host of other unique components it has many advantages over infant formula. In addition, it is also warm and always ready for the hungry baby.

Supporting the breast feeding mother

The more the baby is able to suckle at the breast, the greater the volume of milk produced, so regular feeding is essential to establish the lactation process. If the baby cannot suckle then breast milk must be regularly expressed to replicate the stimulation offered by demand breast feeding. The mother will need much support and encouragement during this establishment phase of breast feeding, particularly if she is separated from the baby and/or if her baby is unwell.

Practical assistance includes:

- Arranging for the mother to see a midwife regularly
- Providing privacy when she is breast feeding
- Providing a suitable chair so that her back is supported and that her feet touch the floor
- Providing a pillow for her lap so that the baby can lay more comfortably while feeding
- Ensuring the she has a varied and well-balanced diet and drinks plenty of fluids
- Encouraging her to rest as much as possible.

Demand feeding should be promoted whenever possible.

Leaflets should be available to give advice about breast feeding. Links with the community team are essential, particularly when lactation and breast feeding is not yet fully established. National support agencies, e.g. National Childbirth Trust, La Leche League and the Association of Breast Feeding Mothers are also a great help, and mothers may wish to contact them. Details are given after the reference section.

Expressing breast milk

There are many special circumstances in the paediatric environment which make the establishment of breast feeding more difficult. In some instances the mother cannot be with her baby for 24 hours a day because of her post-partum condition, social, or geographical reasons. Some babies have anatomical anomalies which may prevent the baby sucking at the breast. These include anomalies requiring surgery, e.g. oesophageal atresia, bowel obstruction or bowel motility problems; cranio-facial anomalies like cleft palate or micrognathia; prematurity and the need for on-going respiratory support; cardiac and renal conditions where fluids are restricted and breast milk alone cannot provide adequate nutrition; some rare metabolic disorders may preclude breast feeding.

A number of neonates will need multi-disciplinary input and a long period of hospitalisation making it very difficult for the mother and baby to establish a pattern of feeding.

If the baby is unable to feed at the breast, it is important that lactation is established by the mother expressing her milk. Milk can be expressed either by hand or by using a breast pump. There are several types of pump available, both manual and electric. The mother will need much support with this, and she will need easy access to a pump in a congenial environment. Careful hand washing before expression is essential, and equipment should be sterilised before use.

Principles table 19.1 **Use of breast pumps**

Principle	Rationale
1. The benefits of human milk for preterm infants have been clearly described (Lucas et al 1992). Advantages not only include long-term benefits in developmental indices, blood pressure and lipoprotein profile, but a decreased risk of infection and neonatal necrotising enterocolitis (Lucas and Cole 1990; Lucas *et al* 1992, Singhal *et al* 2001, Singhal *et al* 2004).	
2. An aseptic non-touch technique should be adopted when handling expressed breast milk (EBM) (Rowley *et al* 2010). For further information see Chapter 12 on Infection Prevention and Control.	**2.** To avoid contaminating the EBM.
3. Mothers should be given written and verbal instructions on personal hygiene, and the collection and decanting of EBM (Rathwell and Shaw 2010).	**3.** Information can be confusing to mothers at times of stress. Written information can also help understanding or encourage questions to be asked.
4. A sterile collecting kit and sterile bottle in which to place EBM should be used each time milk is expressed.	**4.** Use of sterile equipment is essential when handling EBM (Balmer *et al* 1997).
5. Milk should be expressed into sterile single use bottles.	**5.** Sterile bottles should be used once only.
6. Ideally milk should be expressed directly into the bottles which are to be used for feeding the baby. If this is not practical because of the small quantity and/or frequency of feeds required, sterile syringes and occlusion caps should be used.	**6.** To prevent contamination of the EBM. To facilitate the safe handling of small volumes of EBM.
7. Breast pumps should be maintained, cleaned and disinfected weekly or when spillage or overflow has occurred.	**7.** To ensure safe and disinfected pumps are in use at all times.

481

Principles table 19.2 **Freshly expressed breast milk**

Principle	Rationale
1. EBM that is to be used within 24 hours should be kept on the ward in a designated milk feed refrigerator.	**1.** To enable fresh EBM to be used as much as possible (Balmer *et al* 1997, Lucas *et al* 1992).
2. The temperature of a refrigerator storing breast milk should be maintained at 2–4°C (Balmer *et al* 1997).	**2.** To ensure safe refrigeration of the EBM.
3. The temperature should be monitored daily.	**3.** To provide an audit trail and ensure safe temperature control.

(Continued)

Principles table 19.2 (*Continued*)

Principle	Rationale
4. Once the milk has been expressed the lid should be replaced and the bottle placed in the refrigerator immediately.	**4.** To prevent contamination of the EBM.
5. All EBM must be handled using an aseptic non-touch technique (Rowley *et al* 2010).	**5.** To prevent contamination of the EBM.
6. The bottle containing EBM should be opened once only and all the milk decanted at that time.	**6.** To reduce the risk of contamination with multiple openings of the bottle.
7. Feeds of 20 ml or less should be placed in a sterile syringe and capped with a sterile occlusion cap.	**7.** Smaller volumes of feed are more easily and accurately decanted if placed in syringes. An occlusion cap will prevent contamination.
8. Babies who are having continuous feeds of EBM should have the feed administered by: **a)** A 60 ml syringe with a maximum of 4 hours of feed. **b)** As soon as the hourly requirement exceeds 5 ml/hour, a feed set and enteral feeding pump should be used. The bottle containing the feed should be agitated 1–2 hourly. **c)** In both instances, the EBM syringe or bottle should be changed 4 hourly.	**8.** **a)** To prevent colonisation of the EBM with bacteria. **b)** To disperse the fat throughout the feed. **c)** To prevent colonisation of the EBM with bacteria.
9. Each feed must be labelled using the patient's identification labels, and the date and time (Balmer *et al* 1997).	**9.** To ensure that the EBM is given to the correct infant.
10. EBM feeds in syringes can be placed in cardboard trays after labelling and placed in the ward milk feed refrigerator.	**10.** To prevent the EBM falling off the shelves of the refrigerator.
11. The EBM in the refrigerator should be used as soon as possible after it has been divided.	**11.** To prevent colonisation of the EBM with bacteria.
12. It must be kept in the main section of the refrigerator until it is required. It should not be placed in the door.	**12.** Temperatures inside the door are higher than in the body of the refrigerator.
13. EBM should be stored at 2–4°C until used.	**13.** To prevent bacterial growth. This temperature is recommended for handling breast milk (Balmer *et al* 1997).
14. Mothers can be taught how to divide their milk. This can be done in the ward milk feed room, ward breast pump room (if available), or at the bedside.	**14.** To prevent contamination of the EBM by other handlers.
15. Written guidelines should be available to assist the mothers. They should be used in conjunction with teaching by nursing staff.	**15.** Written guidelines help to reinforce oral advice and teaching.
16. Hand washing is essential before mothers express and handle their milk (Brekle and Macqueen 2010).	**16.** To prevent contamination of EBM from the hands.
17. Milk that is not used within 24 hours should be frozen in a designated freezer maintained at −18°C until required.	**17.** Frozen milk can be stored safely for 3 months (Balmer *et al* 1997).
18. Occasionally there are instances when breast feeding is contraindicated. These include mothers who are: **a)** Taking some medications. The current *British National Formulary* gives advice about prescribing in breast feeding. **b)** Drug or alcohol abusers. **c)** HIV positive.	**18.** **a)** Some drugs transfer to the baby via EBM. **b)** Transmission of substances may occur. **c)** There is a risk of disease transmission.

Principles table 19.2 (*Continued*)

Principle	Rationale

These include babies who have:
   d) Rare metabolic disorder of long chain fatty acid oxidation.
   e) Galactosaemia.
   f) Glucose-galactose malabsorption.
   g) A chylothorax.
Any of the above situations should be discussed with medical staff before any decision is made.
	d) This can cause developmental damage to the baby.
	e, f, g) Certain nutrients in EBM are contraindicated.

19. Routine bacteriology screening does not need to be carried out (Law *et al* 1989).	**19.** This is not deemed necessary on a regular basis.

Principles table 19.3 **Frozen expressed breast milk**

Principle	Rationale
1. Fresh EBM, which is surplus to requirements for the following 24 hours, should be frozen as soon as possible after expression and stored frozen at −18°C.	**1.** To comply with recommended guidelines (Balmer *et al* 1997).
2. When frozen milk is required it should be left to defrost in the refrigerator.	**2.** To ensure the EBM is defrosted safely. Rapid heating alters the heat labile vitamins.
3. If rapid defrosting is required, the bottle should be placed in cold water taking care to ensure that no water is able to enter it.	**3.** To prevent the EBM being contaminated with the tap water.
4. Once defrosted, the EBM should be used within 24 hours.	
5. An aseptic non-touch technique must be used at all times by staff handling this milk (Rowley *et al* 2010).	**5.** To prevent contamination of the EBM.
6. Milk, which is expressed outside the hospital that arrives frozen, should be placed in a designated freezer.	**6.** To comply with national guidelines (Balmer *et al* 1997).
7. EBM can be stored at −18°C for up to 3 months for sick infants.	

Principles table 19.4 **Dividing and decanting expressed breast milk**

Principle	Rationale
1. The division of the EBM should take place in the breast pump room, in the ward milk feed room or at the bedside.	**1.** To prevent contamination of the EBM.
2. Where possible the mother should be encouraged to handle her own milk. There should be written guidelines for this procedure.	**2.** To minimise the handling of the EBM. Written guidelines complement oral instruction.
3. An aseptic non-touch technique must be used whenever staff handle EBM (Rowley *et al* 2010).	**3.** To prevent contamination of EBM.

(*Continued*)

Principles table 19.4 (*Continued*)

Principle	Rationale
4. To handle milk on behalf of the mother: **a)** An apron should be worn and hands washed thoroughly (Brekle and Macqueen 2010). **b)** Equipment should be assembled as required, e.g. sterile syringes, sterile occlusion caps, sterile quills, sterile EBM bottle, freshly expressed milk, patient name labels. **c)** Surface area should be cleaned, e.g. tray as used for giving IV medications, with an alcohol impregnated wipe. **d)** Hands should be washed thoroughly and non-sterile gloves worn (Brekle and Macqueen 2010). **e)** EBM should be drawn up as required into the syringes or sterile EBM bottles. **f)** Each syringe/bottle should be labelled with the patient name sticker, adding the date and time the milk was expressed. **g)** Feed(s) should be placed in the designated milk feed refrigerator. **h)** Feeds in syringes may be more easily accessed in a cardboard tray. **i)** All the feed should be decanted on one occasion. Half-decanted bottles of EBM should not be left on the wards.	**4.** **a)** To minimise the risk of infection (Rowley *et al* 2010). **b)** To ensure all equipment is available. To minimise the risk of contamination. **c, d)** To minimise the risk of contamination. **e)** To facilitate the use of EBM. **f)** To ensure correct EBM is given to the right baby within 24 hours of being expressed. **g)** To ensure EBM is safely stored. **h)** To facilitate easy use of EBM. **i)** To prevent contamination of open bottles of EBM.
5. Any unused EBM should be placed in a sterile EBM bottle and frozen.	**5.** To prevent wastage.

Fortfication of breast milk for preterm infants

Some preterm babies may not gain weight on raw breast milk if they cannot tolerate the full feeding volumes required for nutritional adequacy. In this situation fortification of expressed breast milk must be considered in order to increase the nutritional value of the milk (Rathwell and Shaw 2009).

484

Principles table 19.5 Qualities of breast milk

Principle	Rationale
1. Breast milk is the preferred source of nutrition for all infants (Sapsford 2000, Shaw and Lawson 2007).	**1.** It is species specific. **a)** It provides the most appropriate balance and concentration of nutrients in a digestible form (Department of Health 1994). **b)** It provides immunity against disease, and possibly protects against necrotising enterocolitis (NEC) and late onset sepsis (Sapsford 2000, Shaw and Lawson 2007). **c)** There is greater enteral feed tolerance (Boyd *et al* 2007) and more rapid weaning from parenteral nutrition (Lucas 1993). **d)** It promotes the maternal–infant relationship (Lang 2002). It is always available, is at the right temperature and at no extra cost. **e)** There is reduced risk of allergy when breast milk is exclusively used (Lucas 1993). **f)** There are possible, but not proven, favourable effects on neuro-cognitive development (Lucas 1993, Sapsford 2000, Shaw and Lawson 2007).

Principles table 19.5 (Continued)

Principle	Rationale
2. However, breast milk may not fully meet the increased nutritional needs of the preterm infant, particularly energy, protein, sodium, calcium, phosphorus and some vitamins (Edmond and Bahl 2007, Lucas 1993, Shaw and Lawson 2007).	
3. Fortification of expressed breast milk (EBM) can minimise these deficiencies in preterm infants (Lucas 1993, Sapsford 2000, Shaw and Lawson 2007).	**3.** Breast feeding is not usually possible in infants <34 weeks gestation, therefore breast milk must be expressed (Lucas 1993).
4. Other babies may benefit from having their EBM fortified but their requirements will be different to those of the preterm infant: • Babies who are fluid restricted, e.g. those with cardiac anomalies • Babies who are failing to thrive due to increased requirements or losses, e.g. in malabsorptive states.	**4.** Preterm and term infants have different nutritional requirements.
5. When fortification is required an aseptic non-touch technique must be used when handling the EBM (Rowley et al 2010, Rathwell and Shaw 2010).	**5.** To prevent contamination of the EBM.

Principles table 19.6 Increasing nutritional intake of preterm infants

Principle	Rationale
1. The first step to improve nutritional intake should be to slowly increase the volume of EBM given.	**1.** Nutritional adequacy can be achieved if sufficient feed volumes are given (Shaw and Lawson 2007).
2. Well preterm babies >1.5 kg can tolerate up to 220 ml/kg (Shaw and Lawson 2007).	**2.** If the maximum volume of EBM tolerated provides inadequate nutrition then fortification should be considered.
3. A commercial breast milk fortifier (BMF) has the advantage over supplementing with a liquid preterm formula.	**3.** It will allow more of the mother's milk to be used (Lucas 1993, Shaw and Lawson 2007).
4. Supplementation with a source of energy alone is not advised (Shaw and Lawson 2007). A multi-nutrient BMF is recommended.	**4.** It will reduce the protein-energy ratio to an unacceptable level (Shaw and Lawson 2007).

Enteral feeding

Enteral feeding is the means of supplying nutrients directly to the gastrointestinal tract. The term is used to describe orogastric, nasogastric, nasojejunal, gastrostomy and jejunostomy tube feeding. It is the preferred method of providing nutritional support to children with a functioning gastrointestinal tract who fulfil the following criteria (Johnson 2007):

• Inability to consume an adequate oral intake due to impaired sucking and swallowing, e.g. neurological handicap and degenerative disorders, ventilated children

• Anorexia associated with chronic illness, e.g. malignancy, congenital heart disease, renal disease
• Increased nutritional requirements, e.g. cystic fibrosis, liver disease, short bowel syndrome
• Congenital anomalies, e.g. oesophageal fistula, orofacial malformations
• Primary disease management, e.g. glycogen storage disease, very long chain fatty acid disorders.

A careful selection of the appropriate feeding route and equipment is essential to ensure optimal nutritional support and patient adherence. Nasogastric tube feeding is most commonly

Procedure guideline 19.1 Adding fortifier to EBM on the ward

Statement	Rationale
1. This procedure should be carried out as an aseptic non-touch technique in a clean area of the ward (Rowley et al 2010, Rathwell and Shaw 2010).	1. To prevent contamination of the feed.
2. The ward milk kitchen or a specific area should be used when available. a) It should be done as close to the feed time as possible.	2. a) To avoid loss of immunological factors. To prevent rise in osmolality of the feed which can begin within 10 minutes of fortification (De Curtis et al 1999).
3. The decision to fortify EBM for a preterm baby must be made by the medical consultant.	3. To ensure that addition of BMF is clinically indicated and safe.
4. The breast milk fortifier (BMF) must be prescribed by the medical staff on the infant's prescription chart.	4. To ensure the correct dose is given.
5. Urea and electrolyte levels must be carefully monitored.	5. Infants receiving BMF have shown raised urea, calcium and phosphate levels.
6. Other vitamin and mineral levels may need to be routinely checked depending on which BMF is used.	6. To obtain baseline levels of these nutrients.
7. Serum levels should be repeated after 2 weeks and then monthly thereafter.	7. To monitor any decline in vitamin and mineral status.
8. Fortification of breast milk should be performed by a trained member of staff. In certain circumstances, this may also be done by the mother under supervision.	8. To ensure that the prescription is accurately implemented.
9. Check if: a) The EBM is for the correct infant. b) The milk is in date. c) It is used in correct rotation. d) Milk, if frozen, is de-frosted correctly (Balmer et al 1997, Rathwell and Shaw 2010).	9. a) To ensure that this is a safe procedure. c) To prevent wastage of EBM. d) To prevent the risk of contamination of EBM.
10. The prescribed fortification is added to the correct amount of feed according to the manufacturer's instructions.	10. To ensure that the nutrient value of the feed is increased as prescribed.
11. The bottle is agitated gently.	11. To ensure an even distribution of fortifier in the breast milk.
12. The bottle is labelled and dated.	12. To ensure that this is a safe procedure.
13. The fortified EBM is fed immediately. Ideally the feed should be given within 10 minutes of fortification. a) If the fortified feed cannot be given immediately, it should be sealed and placed in the milk feed refrigerator on the ward. It must be used within 24 hours. b) Any excess defrosted EBM that has not been fortified must be discarded if not used within 24 hours. c) Any excess fresh EBM should be frozen for later use (Rathwell and Shaw 2010).	13. To minimise bacterial growth and a rise in osmolality (De Curtis et al 1999). a) To ensure that the feed is safely stored at the correct temperature. b) To minimise bacterial growth and prevent contamination. c) To ensure safe storage of the EBM.

employed as a convenient and safe method of feed administration. However, it might not be suitable if long-term feeding is required or for patients with facial/oesophageal structural abnormalities, where gastrostomy tube feeding may be the route of choice. Nasojejunal tube feeding may be necessary if there is a significant risk of aspiration and delayed gastric emptying.

Feeds may be given by bolus or pump-controlled continuous or intermittent feeding. Bolus feeding has considerable advantages as it mimics a physiologically normal feeding pattern and can be adapted to fit in with meal times. However, continuous feeds may be better tolerated in some circumstances and overnight feeding may release the daytime for other activities.

Many of the problems associated with enteral feeding are preventable with a committed multi-disciplinary team. It should consist of the child's dietician, paediatrician and primary nurse.

Nutrition and stoma nurse specialists may help with practical aspects of the child's care.

All health professionals and parents/carers should be aware of the negative aspects of enteral feeding and try to alleviate them. Hygienic storage and handling of both feed and feeding systems are essential in order to prevent microbial contamination and subsequent complications such as diarrhoea, vomiting, malabsorption or pneumonia.

In collaboration with speech and language therapists and occupational therapists an oral stimulation programme should be developed to maintain and improve oromotor skills. The preservation of pleasant associations in connection with food and feeding is essential in order to avoid hypersensitivity to touch and taste and will facilitate the reintroduction of oral feeding.

Principles table 19.7 Handling of enteral feeds

1. Storage

Principle	Rationale
A. Sterile feeds (ready-to-use)	
1. Bottles, cans or containers should be stored in closed, clean cupboards.	**1.** To keep feed container clean, dust free and spoilage free.
2. Stock must be rotated regularly.	**2.** To prevent expiry dates of feed being exceeded.
3. Opened, unused sterile feeds must be discarded.	**3.** To prevent the contamination of opened feed containers.
B. Modular feeds	
4. All modular feeds must be placed in a designated milk refrigerator (or designated area of the refrigerator if at home) immediately after arrival on the ward.	**4.** Ensure that the feed is stored at the recommended temperature as soon as possible.
5. The temperature of a refrigerator storing enteral feeds should be maintained at ≤4°C (Anderton 1995).	**5.** To ensure the safe refrigeration of enteral feeds.
6. The temperature should be monitored daily and recorded in a Temperature Log Book. This should be undertaken by housekeeping/nursing staff (or parent/carer at home) who will alert the nurse in charge to any problems.	**6.** To ensure that the temperature of all milk refrigerators is maintained accurately.
7. Partly decanted bottles of modular feeds must be discarded.	**7.** To prevent the contamination of opened bottles.
2. Infection control issues	
1. Good hygienic practices are essential to ensure that any feed given to a patient is safe.	**1.** To comply with the Food & Safety Act 1990 and to minimise the risk of contamination. Bacterial contamination of enteral feeds may cause diarrhoea and vomiting. Contamination may also contribute to more serious infections including pneumonia and septicaemia (Anderton 1995).
2. Enteral feeds and feed administration systems must not be handled unnecessarily.	**2.** This minimises the risk of contamination.

(Continued)

487

Principles table 19.7 (*Continued*)

Principle	Rationale
3. An aseptic non-touch technique should be adhered to whenever feed administration systems are handled, including the wearing of non-sterile gloves (Rowley *et al* 2010).	**3.** To minimise the risk of contamination. Poor hand hygiene is one of the most frequent causes of enteral feeds being significantly contaminated (Anderton 1995).
4. The feed reservoir used for continuous enteral feeding must not be topped up.	**4.** To prevent contamination of the feed reservoir whilst decanting.
5. Feeds for continuous enteral feeding should be given at room temperature. They must not be heated or given immediately from the refrigerator.	**5.** It is safer to give the feed at room temperature. If the feed is too hot this may damage the mucosal surface and if too cold this may cause the temperature of the baby/child to drop.
6. The integral drug port of feed administration systems must be disinfected with an alcohol-impregnated wipe and allowed to dry before and after giving drugs.	**6.** Each time the connection is touched it increases the risk of introducing bacteria into the system from the hands or the environment.
7. The feed administration set for continuous feeds must be changed every 24 hours (Anderton 1995).	

Principles table 19.8 Preparing the child and family (feeding tube insertion)

Principle	Rationale
1. Adequate psychological preparation for the insertion of a nasogastric, nasojejunal or gastrostomy tube and information on enteral feeding for both the child and the family are essential in order to obtain informed consent, understanding and co-operation.	**1.** Procedures are very distressing to both children and their families (Holden *et al* 1997). Children need to be prepared for painful or uncomfortable procedures sensitively according to their needs. Colouring booklets, training manuals and models, illustrated guides or videos can assist with these preparations (Holden *et al* 1992, Paul *et al* 1993).
2. Nurses or play specialist should explore the child's knowledge and past experience.	**2.** Distraction techniques such as relaxation or guided imagery can help to reduce tension and anxiety during the procedure (Broome *et al* 1992).

Principles table 19.9 Nasogastric tube feeding

Principle	Rationale
1. Nasogastric (NG) feeding is a method of feeding into the stomach and the common route for tube feeding.	**1.** Nasogastric feeding is simple to initiate and manage and is associated with few complications if managed appropriately (Reilly 1998).
2. Wide-bore polyvinyl chloride (PVC) tubes are for short-term use only. They need to be changed at least every 7 days.	**2.** Longer use may cause discomfort and nasal/oesophageal ulceration or irritations. There is a risk of the material of PVC tubes being eroded by gastric juices.
3. Fine-bore (polyurethane or 'Silk') tubes are designed for longer-term use. They need to be changed monthly.	**3.** These tubes are softer and allow the patient to swallow normally. Their use reduces distress as they are changed less frequently.

488

Principles table 19.9 (*Continued*)

Principle	Rationale
4. 6–10 French gauge (Fr) sized tubes are most commonly used in children. The length of the tube (usually 50 or 100 cm depends on the size of the child.	**4.** For feeding purposes the smallest possible tube should be chosen, as a larger size tube predisposes the child to gastroesophageal reflux (Noviski *et al* 1999).
5. Enteral feeds via an NG tube can be administered as either bolus feeds or continuously.	
6. Medication (such as acid inhibitors) alters the pH of the gastric aspirate. This may necessitate radiological confirmation of correct tube placement (Metheny and Titler 2001).	**6.** Bedside confirmation of correct placement relies on a clear pH reading (acid) using Universal Indicator Paper.

Procedure guideline 19.2 **Inserting and managing the nasogastric tube**

Statement	Rationale
1. The following equipment is needed: **a)** Appropriate sized wide-bore or fine-bore tube. **b)** Sterile water to lubricate the tube. **c)** Foil bowl and tissue. **d)** Universal Indicator Paper (pH reading 1–11). **e)** 20 ml syringe for PVC tube/50 ml syringe for polyurethane tube. **f)** Non-sterile gloves and apron. **g)** Tape suitable for the condition of the child's skin. **h)** Glass of water and straw, dummy.	1. **c)** In case of vomiting. **d)** To read the pH level of stomach content. **e)** Larger syringes exert a lower pressure and are less likely to collapse or damage the tube or damage the mucosal surface on suction. **g)** To secure the tube. **h)** If child is able to swallow, this may support tube passage into the stomach.

Insertion

1. The child and family should have been prepared by explaining the procedure.	1. To gain consent and co-operation.
2. Older children should be seated with appropriate support and may hold parent's/carer's hand. Younger children should be lying at angle of >30% or may be sitting on their parent's/carer's lap. A baby might need to be wrapped in a sheet.	2. To prevent the child from pulling the head back on insertion. To prevent the child from pulling the tube out.
3. Choose the most suitable nostril. Ask the child if they have any preferences, where appropriate.	3. To involve the child in the procedure and allow some control.
4. Wash hands thoroughly and dry. Put on an apron and non-sterile gloves.	4. To prevent cross-contamination (Anderton 1995).
5. Check the tube. If a guide wire is used, ensured the guide wire is not bent and is correctly inserted into the tube. The guide wire is lubricated with water by flushing the tube either prior to insertion or just prior to removal.	5. To ensure the tube is patent.
6. The length of the tube is measured from the bridge of the nose to the ear lobe, plus the distance from the ear lobe to the xiphisternum.	6. To estimate the length to which tube should be inserted.

(Continued)

Procedure guideline 19.2 (*Continued*)

Statement	Rationale
7. The end of the tube is lubricated in sterile water.	**7.** Do not use KY-jelly as this may affect the pH measurement of the stomach content.
8. The tip of the tube is gently passed into the child's nostril and guided into the nasopharynx. **a)** If the child can safely swallow offer a sip of water. Babies/toddlers should be offered a dummy. **b)** The tube is slowly advanced until the required length has been passed.	**8.** **a)** This may support the passage of the tube into the stomach and ease the child's discomfort.
9. Should the child show any signs of distress such as coughing or breathlessness, the tube should be removed immediately.	**9.** The tube might have passed into the trachea.
10. Older children should be allowed to have a break to rest at any time during the procedure.	
11. The tube is lightly secured with tape. **a)** Correct placement of the tube must be confirmed. Only Universal Indicator Paper should be used, pH reading 1–11 (Medicines and Healthcare products Regulatory Agency 2004; National Patient Safety Agency 2005a, 2005b). Gastric position pH = 5 Bronchial position pH 6–8 Small bowel position pH 6–8. **b)** Radiography is recommended to check initial placement of tube in patients who are unconscious, intubated or who have absence of swallow reflex.	**11.** **a)** Blue litmus paper is not sensitive enough to confirm placement in the stomach. Bronchial secretions will turn blue litmus paper pink. **b)** NB some medications can elevate gastric pH readings, e.g. proton pump inhibitors.
12. To check the position of the tube, a small amount of stomach content is aspirated using a 20 or 50 ml syringe depending on type of tube.	**12.** Acidity of aspirate is tested using Universal Indicator Paper which should be pH ≤ 5 (Metheny and Titler 2001).
13. If no aspirate can be obtained, the tube should be inserted a further few centimetres or the child's position changed before trying again.	**13.** To ensure the tube is in the fluid in the stomach and to change the fluid level in the stomach.
14. If still unable to aspirate, and it is safe to do so, the child can be offered a drink of water before trying again.	**14.** The stomach may be empty.
15. If it is still not possible to confirm the position of the tube using aspirate, the tube may need to be removed and re-passed.	**15. Air insufflation with abdominal auscultation must not be used as the primary method of checking tube placement as it is not reliable (Metheny and Titler 2001).**
16. In certain circumstances it may be necessary to confirm correct tube placement radiologically.	
17. Following confirmation of correct tube placement, the guide wire can be removed, if present, and the tube gently flushed with 5 ml of water.	**17.** To ensure it is patent.
18. The tube is safely secured to the child's cheek. Depending on the sensitivity of the child's skin a hydrocolloid dressing may be necessary to protect the skin.	**18.** The adhesive tape to secure the tube should not extend beyond the size of the hydrocolloid dressing.

Procedure guideline 19.2 (*Continued*)

Statement	Rationale
19. Record in the patient's notes: all actions, the size of tube, the length of the exposed tube, the appearance of the aspirate and date of passing the tube.	19. To provide accurate record of care and ongoing evaluation. To check the position of the tube.

Tube management

1. The nasal passages should be checked at least twice per day to ensure they are not blocked. Clean with warm water and dry thoroughly.	1. To prevent build-up of dried mucus.
2. The tube must always be tested using Universal Indicator Paper prior to feeding or administration of medicines.	2. Caution: pH reading does not provide useful information during continuous feeding as the feed raises gastric pH. Signs of dislodgement of tube out of stomach: • Sudden decrease in residual volumes • Bile stained feed • Dislodged mark on the tube. Consider the need for a radiological verification of tube placement (Metheny and Titler 2001).
3. The tube should be flushed with 5–10 ml of sterile water depending on the child's fluid balance and size: • Prior to and after each feed • Prior to and after the administration of medicines • 4 hourly if tube is not in use.	3. To prevent blockage of the tube and bacterial contamination due to medicine and feed residues.
4a) A blocked tube must not be manipulated using high pressure. b) Unblocking may be achieved by the use of enzyme preparations, pineapple juice or fizzy drinks (NB check that the child can have these fluids). c) If a tube remains blocked it must be removed and re-passed.	4a) This could damage the tube, lead to gut perforation or the instillation of feeds in the wrong place (Trigg and Mohammed 2006). c) Check there is no medical/surgical reason why the tube should not be removed first.

Principles table 19.10 **Nasojejunal tube feeding**

Principle	Rationale
1. Nasojejunal (or post-pyloric feeding is the method of feeding directly into the small bowel. Jejunal access for feeding may be the preferable method in patients with: • Delayed gastric emptying • Increased risk of aspiration • Persistent vomiting • During the postoperative period, before gastric emptying has resumed.	
2. A long-length, fine-bore tube is passed via the nasogastric route then through the pyloric sphincter and placed in the jejunum.	

(*Continued*)

Principles table 19.10 (*Continued*)

Principle	Rationale
3. Hygienic handling of enteral feeds and feeding systems is paramount when using a jejunal route.	**3.** The stomach's barrier function is bypassed.
4. Jejunal feeds should be delivered continuously rather than as a bolus in order to avoid an overload of the small bowel.	**4.** The reservoir function of the stomach is bypassed.
5. Nasojejunal tubes are made of polyurethane and can remain *in situ* for 1 month. Weighted tubes encourage the tip of the tube to remain in the jejunum once passed.	**5.** Prolonged use affects the condition of the nasal passages.
6. As medication (such as acid inhibitors) alters the pH of the gastric aspirate, the position of the tube may necessitate radiological confirmation of correct tube placement (Metheny and Titler 2001).	**6.** Bedside confirmation of correct placement relies on a clear pH reading using Universal Indicator Paper.

Procedure guideline 19.3 Inserting and managing the nasojejunal tube

Statement	Rationale

1. The following equipment is needed:
   a) An appropriate sized fine-bore tube, (usually 7Fr weighted tip tube with guide wire; 5Fr tube for small infants).
   b) Sterile water to lubricate the tube.
   c) Foil bowl and tissue.
   d) Universal Indicator Paper (pH reading 1–11).
 	
   e) A 50 ml syringe.
 	
   f) Non-sterile gloves and apron.
   g) Tape suitable for the condition of the child's skin.
   h) Glass of water and straw or dummy.
	1.
	
	   c) In case of vomiting.
	   d) To read the changing pH of the aspirate as the tube passes through the stomach into the small bowel.
	   e) Larger syringes exert a lower pressure and are less likely to collapse or damage the tube.
	
	   g) To secure the tube.
	   h) If the child is able to swallow, this may support the tube passage into the stomach.

Insertion

1. The child and family are prepared by explaining the procedure.	**1.** To gain consent and co-operation.
2. Procedures for insertion of NG tube can be followed.	**2.** Prepare equipment on a clean surface, perform a surgical hand wash and wear non-sterile gloves and an apron in order to minimise the risk of infection or any contamination that may occur.
3. The syringe is attached to the tube and stomach contents aspirated and tested using Universal Indicator Paper.	**3.** Gastric indicators: pH $\leq$ 5 and aspirate is grassy green, clear and colourless or brown. Reposition the child if no stomach content can be obtained (Metheny and Titler 2001).
4. If the tube seems to be safely placed in either the stomach or jejunum, the tube is secured to the child's face using an appropriate tape.	**4.** To prevent accidental removal.

Procedure guideline 19.3 (*Continued*)

Statement	Rationale
5. If the tube is sited in the stomach, the tube can be advanced at 1–2 hourly intervals 2–5 cm.	**5.** To assist passage through the pylorus.
6. Retest. This may take a couple of hours. The child should be encouraged to continue with their normal activities while waiting for the tube to pass.	**6.** Intestinal indicators: pH >6 and aspirate is light or dark golden yellow or brownish-green (bile stained) (Metheny and Titler 2001).
7. While the tube is in the stomach it must not be used.	**7.** Consider the nutrition and hydration status of the child while they are not being fed. Consider the use of prokinetic agents.
8. The tube should be flushed after each use.	**8.** To prevent blockage and bacterial contamination.
9. If tube cannot be placed on the ward there should be liaison with medical staff regarding the need for radiological confirmation of placement or radiological placement.	
10. All actions, the size of tube and date of passing must be recorded in the patient's records.	**10.** To provide accurate record of care and ongoing evaluation.

Tube management

1. The tube must always be tested with Universal Indicator Paper prior to feeding or administration of medicines.	**1.** Caution: pH reading does not provide useful information during continuous feeding as the feed slightly lowers intestinal pH. Signs of dislodgement of tube into stomach: • pH ≤ 5 • Sudden increase in residual volumes • Dislodged mark on the tube. Consider the need for a radiological verification of tube placement (Metheny and Titler 2001).
2. It is preferable to avoid using jejunal tubes for the administration of drugs. If there is no alternative, only liquid medication should be used.	**2.** To avoid tube blockage and unnecessary handling of the tube.
3. The compatibility of medicines with the small intestine should be discussed with pharmacy and medical staff.	**3.** To ensure proper absorption of medicine in small intestine.

493

Principles table 19.11 **Gastrostomy tube feeding**

Principle	Rationale
1. A feeding tube is inserted endoscopically or surgically directly into the stomach through the abdominal wall.	
2. Gastrostomy tube feeding is indicated if: • Facial/oesophageal structural abnormalities make NG tube feeding impossible • Prolonged enteral tube feeding needed due to impaired swallow • Longer term need for nutritional support is necessary.	

(Continued)

Principles table 19.11 (*Continued*)

Principle	Rationale
3. Gastrostomy tubes are made of silicone. There are 3 main types: **a)** Temporary balloon device tubes (e.g. G-TUBE).	**3.** **a)** Generally performed in conjunction with a fundoplication procedure requiring a laparotomy or in patients with an obstructive oesophageal lesion. Can be replaced by a skin-level device after 6 weeks, when gastrostomy is well established.
b) Endoscopically placed tubes (percutaneous endoscopic gastrostomy tube, PEG).	**b)** Used in the majority of children, whereby tube is passed via endoscopy. Procedure is relatively safe and associated with low mortality and low complication rate (Broscious 1995). PEG tubes can stay *in situ* for approximately 2 years. They need to be removed endoscopically in order to retrieve the internal fixator (Arrowsmith 1996).
c) Skin-level button devices (e.g. MINI-Button, MicKey-Button).	**c)** Button devices are generally inserted into a pre-formed stoma, mostly for cosmetic and lifestyle reasons. Manufacturer's recommend that they are changed approximately every 6 months as long as both balloon and anti-reflux valve remain intact for this length of time.

Stoma care: newly formed stoma

1. The newly formed stoma should be left undisturbed for 24 hours and then be cleaned aseptically.	
2. For the first 14 days the stoma should be cleaned daily with a sterile saline solution and sterile gauze. At home this can be replaced with cooled boiled water and cotton wool buds.	**2.** To help prevent infection while the wound is healing and to remove exudates.
3. The stoma site needs to be checked regularly for tenderness, irritation and leakage.	
4. An appropriate dry, absorbent dressing may be applied if necessary.	
5. After PEG insertion, the external fixator should not be released for 72 hours.	**5.** To allow the stomach to adhere to the abdominal wall and form the tract.
6. Care has to be taken when handling the tube as it takes 2–3 weeks for a fibrous tract to form (Peters and Westby 1994).	**6.** Before that time a tube will have to be replaced surgically.

Stoma care: established stoma

1. When the stoma has healed it should be cleaned daily with mild soap and water and dried thoroughly.	**1.** To maintain skin integrity.
2. Bathing and showering is allowed as soon as the incision has healed.	
3. The tube and external fixator should be cleaned daily and both should be rotated and pushed in approximately 2.5 cm according to the manufacturer's instructions. This can vary from 360° at least once a week to 180° daily.	**3.** To avoid 'buried bumper' syndrome, where the internal fixator or balloon of the tube is taut against the abdominal wall. This may lead to abdominal discomfort or haemorrhage (Grant and Martin 2000).

Principles table 19.11 (*Continued*)

Principle	Rationale
Tube management and troubleshooting **Checking tube placement**	
1. Correct tube placement needs to be confirmed prior to the administration of the first feed after initial placement with surgically inserted balloon devices and catheters that replace PEG tubes. Gastric acid aspirate must be obtained and balloon volumes checked as per catheter instruction.	1. They can potentially migrate into the small bowel.
Checking balloons	
2. Balloons should be checked weekly as per manufacturer's instruction. A significant loss of water indicates a leakage and the device may need to be changed.	2. A small amount of water may be lost through the semi-permeable membrane of the balloon.
3. A spare device should always be supplied to the patient.	3. To facilitate a quick change of the device.
4. Only syringes indicated for enteral use should be provided.	4. These are recommended to reduce the risk of inadvertent use of content through the intravenous route.
Preventing blockage	
5. The tube should be flushed regularly prior to and after feeding/medicines with 10–20 ml of sterile or cooled, boiled water. Liquid medicines should be used whenever possible.	5. High pressure should not be used while trying to unblock the device.
6. Unblocking may be achieved by the use of enzyme preparations, pineapple juice or fizzy drinks (NB check that the child can have these fluids).	
Replacing the tube	

7. Within the first 2 weeks after initial insertion the device may need to be re-placed either surgically or endoscopically. Gastrostomy devices have to be replaced as quickly as possible in the early days as the tract will start to close within a short period of time. Once the tract is over 6 months old it is stable for 1–2 hours.
    Routine changes of skin-level devices should be carried out as per manufacturer's instruction.
	7. Replacement tubes should not be used for the administration of feeds or medicines until correct placement has been confirmed by medical staff or X-ray.
	    If necessary, a urinary catheter or NG tube could be used to maintain the stoma.
	    If the same size replacement catheter is not available the stoma might need to be dilated under general anaesthesia.

Skin infection	
8. If excoriation of the skin occurs due to leakage of stomach contents from the site a barrier product such as Cavilon (spray or individually wrapped sticks) can be applied.	8. To protect the skin and allow healing to take place.
9. The stoma site should be observed for any signs of infection such as redness, swelling and oozing.	9. If this occurs a swab from the site should be sent to the microbiology laboratory for culture and sensitivity. Bacterial or fungal infections are not uncommon. The device should not be changed because of site infection as this will only lead to a contamination of the new device. The infection should be treated first. For further information see Chapter 14 on Investigations.

495

(Continued)

Principles table 19.11 (Continued)

Principle	Rationale
Over granulation	
10. Over granulation around the stoma site may occur due to a predisposition of the child or friction on the tube. It can cause discomfort and bleeding.	10. Granulation tissue can be treated with silver nitrate sticks, ensuring contact is with the granulation tissue only.

Procedure guideline 19.4 Administration of enteral feeds

Bolus feeds	
Statement	**Rationale**
1. Intermittent bolus feeds are generally delivered by gravity over 15–30 minutes on a schedule of every 2–4 hours.	1. Administration of the feed should take the same length of time as is would take the child to have the same amount orally (Trigg and Mohammed 2006).
2. Bolus feeds are the preferred method of enteral feed administration (Holden *et al* 2000).	2. Bolus feeds mimic a physiologically normal feeding pattern and can be adapted to fit in with meal times. Children on long-term feeding are given greater freedom and mobility (Johnson 2007).

3. Gravity feeding sets are single use only.	3. No attempt should be made to clean/disinfect and re-use any parts of a system that is marked for single use only (Anderton 1999).
	   None of the tested cleaning methods are totally effective in removing bacteria from the lumina of feed administration sets (Anderton and Nwoguh 1991).
	   The remaining bacteria and feed residues may provide an inoculum when the system is refilled with feeds (Anderton 1999).

4. The feed should be warmed to room temperature by placing the bottle in a jug of warm water.	4. Feeds should not be heated in the microwave. Feed bottles may not be suitable and the feed may be too hot to use.
5. A clinical hand wash should be performed according to guidelines and an apron and non-sterile gloves worn.	5. To prevent cross-contamination.
6. The feeding set should be assembled on a clean, dry surface and the reservoir/syringe filled with feed.	6. Air should be removed from the line by flushing the tube with water or feed.
7. The feeding tube is checked, and the patient prepared and positioned.	7. To ensure the child gets the correct feed.
8. The feeding set is connected to the feeding tube. The clamp should be slowly released and the reservoir of the feed system raised to allow feed to flow into the tube.	
9. The child should be encouraged to suck on a dummy or to play with food or feeding utensils.	9. To encourage normal socialisation associated with feeding and to maintain oro-motor skills.
10. Gloves might be removed during feeding for nurturing interactions with the child or when oral stimulation is performed.	

Procedure guideline 19.4 (*Continued*)

Continuous feeds

Statement	Rationale
1. Continuous feeds are administered via an enteral feeding pump.	1. The continuous flow maintained by the pump prevents the blockage of tube/feeding set and avoids back-drainage of stomach/intestine content into the feeding system.
2. Continuous feeds are frequently chosen when enteral feeding is first started.	2. Small amounts of feed continuously infused are usually better tolerated (Holden *et al* 2000).
3. Indications for continuous enteral feeds include: • Severe gastro-oesophageal reflux • Malabsorption syndromes • Crohn's disease • Glycogen storage disease (Johnson 2007).	
4. Sterile feeds are the preferred feeds and should be used whenever possible.	4. To reduce the risk of giving feed to the patient that has already been contaminated during the process of preparation and decanting (Anderton 1999).
5. Sterile feeds in prefilled ready-to-use containers can be hung for up to 24 hours provided that the system remains closed at all times.	5. To prevent the set being accessed frequently and therefore reduce the risk of bacterial contamination. Sterile feed containers remain free of bacterial contamination in closed systems for at least 24 hours (Beattie *et al* 1996).
6. For diluted or decanted sterile feeds and reconstituted modular feeds the hanging time should not exceed 6 hours (Patchell *et al* 1998). For children on home enteral feeding in the community it is recommended that non-sterile reconstituted feeds should hang for a maximum 4-hour period (NICE 2003).	6. To minimise the time for which the feed is exposed to room temperature.

Administering a feed

Statement	Rationale
7. The child is advised that an enteral feed is to be administered.	7. To psychologically prepare the child.
8. The feeding pump is wiped with an all purpose detergent.	8. To decontaminate equipment.
9. Ready-to-use feed container is damp wiped with paper towel.	9. To remove visible dust and dirt.
10. Preparation area is cleaned and allowed to dry.	10. To minimise the risk of cross-infection.
11. Gather equipment as required, e.g. feed containers/bottles, feeding system, alcohol-impregnated wipes, bottle opener/scissors. Type of feed, patient's name and expiry date of feed checked.	11. To ensure the correct feed is administered safely.
12. Wipe the top of the feed container or bottle with a large alcohol-impregnated wipe and allow to dry.	12. To decontaminate the top of the feed container/bottle.
13. Put on a disposable apron. Perform a clinical hand wash and put on non-sterile gloves.	13. To maintain sterility and to avoid contamination.
14. Remove the feeding set from sterile pack and using the inside of the pack as the sterile field, use an aseptic non-touch technique.	

497

(*Continued*)

Procedure guideline 19.4 (*Continued*)

Continuous feeds

Statement	Rationale
15. Decant the sterile (ready-to-use) feed into the feeding set reservoir or sterile bottle.	15. If a sterile bottle is used, the bottle must be attached onto the feeding set taking care not to touch the top of the bottle or the spike set. This reduces the risk of contamination.
16. Prime the line ensuring that all air is expelled.	
17. Insert the feeding set into the feeding pump.	
18. The feeding line should be labelled with a brightly coloured and clearly visible label, especially when simultaneous intravenous (IV) treatment is administered.	18. To prevent any confusion between IV and enteral feeding lines and ensure patient safety.
19. Check the feeding tube is in the correct position, the child is prepared and correctly positioned.	19. To ensure safety and the child is comfortable.
20. Connect the feeding set onto the feeding tube using a non-touch aseptic technique. (Anderton 1995, Anderton 1999, Beattie and Anderton 1998, Trigg and Mohammed 2006).	20. To minimise the risk of contamination.
21. The patient's tube should be aspirated every 4 hours to reconfirm the correct tube location.	
22. The pump rate and alarm settings should be checked and adjusted as required.	22. To ensure that the correct amount of feeds is administered in the correct period of time.
23. Any waste should be discarded according to local waste policy.	
24. Administration of the feed should be documented on the child's fluid balance chart and in their healthcare records.	24. To provide an accurate record.

498

Procedure guideline 19.5 **Monitoring children on enteral feeds**

Statement	Rationale
1. Regular monitoring is a vital part of successful enteral feeding.	1. To prevent potential complications and to ensure that planned progress and improvement in nutritional status is achieved (Reilly 1998).

General observations

1. The child should be observed daily for tube misplacement, nasal or stoma erosion and signs of aspiration.	1. To minimise complications and side effects of tube feeding.

Nutritional observation

1. The child should have their height and weight measured before enteral feeding commences.	1. To monitor the effectiveness of the feeding regimen.

Procedure guideline 19.5 *(Continued)*

Statement	Rationale
2. At the initiation of enteral feeding the weight of infants should be recorded daily (older children weekly) and thereafter plotted frequently on a centile chart.	2. Weight is the best short-term indicator of an improvement in nutritional status (Holden *et al* 2000). The dietician or medical staff can change the nutritional composition of the feed to achieve appropriate weight gain and longer term linear growth.
3. Length and height measurements should be monitored at agreed intervals and plotted on centile charts.	3. To indicate longer term improvements in nutrition and growth.

Monitoring gastrointestinal side-effects

1. As enteral feeding may be an important part of disease management, symptoms such as diarrhoea, nausea, abdominal distension and reflux should be monitored.	1. To assess the improvement/change of symptoms during enteral feeding.
2. Diarrhoea may be caused by the enteral feed through (Johnson 2007, Reilly 1998): • Too fast an infusion rate • Bolus administration • Cold feed straight from the refrigerator • Bacterial contamination • High feed osmolality.	2. Cause should be assessed and treated as quickly as possible.

Oral stimulation

1. Prolonged absence of oral feeding can lead to the loss of oro-motor skills and the build-up of food aversion and anxiety.	1. The loss of normal socialisation associated with feeding and meal times as well as pleasant oral stimulation may cause a hypersensitivity to touch and taste (Trigg and Mohammed 2006).
2. Sucking, swallowing and blowing should be encouraged through oral stimulation and in play, as well as the joyful exploration of food or feeding utensils at meal times.	2. This helps the child to associate food and meal times with pleasure.
3. There needs to be liaison with speech and language therapist, occupational therapist or feeding nurse specialist regarding the implementation of feeding regimens.	3. This ensures the best outcome for the child and prevents complications later.

499

Parenteral nutrition

Parenteral nutrition (PN) is the administration of nutrition directly into the bloodstream, therefore bypassing the gut. It is the method of providing nutrition for children who, for a variety of reasons, cannot absorb enough energy and nutrients to support normal growth and development and maintain health and life (Hill and Long 2001). The need for parenteral nutrition may be on a short- or long-term basis, depending on the underlying medical condition. Parenteral nutrition should only be used when feeding via the oral or enteral route cannot meet nutritional needs, as PN is an invasive treatment and can lead to physiological complications (Pennington 2000). Some children require parenteral nutrition to supplement their nutritional requirements, while others may rely on parenteral nutrition as their sole source of energy and nutrients.

The following are all indications for parenteral nutrition:

• Prematurity
• Autoimmune enteropathy
• Inflammatory bowel disease
• Intestinal failure due to: short gut, hollow visceral myopathy, radiation and/or cytotoxic therapy, post-operative paralytic ileus, protracted diarrhoea
• Liver disease
• Extensive burns
• Severe trauma.

The Nutrition Support Team

A Nutrition Support Team (NST) usually comprises a medical consultant with an interest in nutrition, a clinical nurse specialist, a specialist dietician, a specialist pharmacist and a biochemist. The quality of care for children requiring nutritional support is improved through the involvement of a Nutrition Support Team (Hudson 2000). The NST should monitor the usage and effectiveness of parenteral nutrition in the hospital. There should be assessment by the team members as to the appropriateness of the referral, including nutritional assessment, height and weight measurement with subsequent plotting on a centile chart, other anthropometry as necessary, type of intravenous (IV) access available, gastrointestinal function, accurate fluid balance, diagnosis and history of weight loss.

Regular ward rounds and discussion of the child's overall condition should be carried out in participation with the medical team managing the child's treatment for their underlying illness. As and when the child's condition, oral or enteral intake improves, the NST will recommend how to reduce the PN until it can be discontinued.

Nutrient solutions

For a child requiring parenteral nutrition, it is important to establish a regimen that will provide adequate energy and nutrients to allow for tissue repair, as well as normal growth and development. The solutions are made up of amino acids, glucose, lipids, electrolytes, trace elements and vitamins. The amounts of the various components required are individually calculated for each child.

Provision of PN

Parenteral nutrition must be prescribed by a doctor. The nutritional content should be agreed with NSTs medical consultant and dietician. The prescription for preparing the PN is produced by the pharmacist and is compounded under sterile conditions in a laminar flow unit under supervision of the pharmacist (Hart 1999, Lamb 1999). The conditions in which PN is produced are strictly regulated due to the risks associated with contamination of the solutions by pathogens (Lee and Allwood 2001).

Parenteral nutrition can be administered as a cyclical or continuous infusion. Cyclical PN is an on-going treatment but it is routinely stopped for a set period of time, the length of which depends on the condition of the child. It is used for children of at least 3 months of age who are on a stable PN regimen and who perhaps can tolerate some enteral intake. It is particularly useful when the need for PN is long-term as is the case for children who are receiving PN at home. The time spent off PN (usually during the day) allows the child and family to live as normally as possible, given that the child's activity is not as restricted as it is when the PN infusion is in progress. The infusion rate of cyclical PN must be steadily reduced over the last hour of the infusion to avoid rebound hypoglycaemia once the infusion stops. Depending on the functions of the IV infusion pump, this reduction can be in two stages, i.e. at two successive manually reduced rates at half-hour intervals or perhaps by an automatic gradual reduction in rate throughout the hour.

Continuous PN is a 24 hour continuous treatment. It is used when commencing PN treatment and when warranted by the condition of the child. The amino acid solution is infused over the full 24 hours. The lipid solution, however, is infused for only 20 hours – it is switched off for 4 hours to allow for clearance of the resultant fat emulsion in the plasma. Due to this lipaemia the timing of any necessary blood sampling should be determined by local policy.

Methods of administration

Parenteral nutrition can be administered either peripherally or centrally. It is important to determine how long the child is likely to require parenteral nutrition and consider the most appropriate route of administration. Peripheral lines should only be used for a very short time due to the potential for extravasation injury caused by the components of the PN. The maximum glucose concentration for peripheral use in children is 10–12.5% (Sari and Rollins 1999). The use of peripheral lines therefore reduces the amount of energy, in the form of glucose, which can be given. There is still some debate over the maximum glucose concentration permitted via the peripheral route (some centres will allow 20% glucose), therefore local policy may differ.

Children may receive peripheral PN in certain circumstances, for example when awaiting insertion of a central venous access device (CVAD) or when receiving antibiotic therapy for a CVAD infection. In these circumstances Intralipid (the fat component) may be favoured over Vamin (the amino acid component) for peripheral use as its lower osmolality reduces the risk of extravasation (British Association for Parenteral and Enteral Nutrition 2000, Lamb 1999).

There are a variety of CVADs available and one must select a device suiting short- or long-term use. If it is anticipated that the child is unlikely to require parenteral nutrition for more than 1 month then a peripherally inserted central catheter (PICC) may be useful. Implantable port devices have been used for patients receiving PN but are not recommended for this use.

If it is evident that the child is likely to require long-term PN then a skin tunnelled central venous catheter, such as a Broviac or Hickman line, can be used. If possible a dedicated nutrition line should be established in order to minimise the risk of sepsis. Concurrent administration of IV fluids and medications may necessitate a double or triple lumen central venous catheter (Department of Health 2001). Energy intake can be improved with the placement of a central catheter as a higher concentration glucose solution can be safely used. For further information see Chapter 13 on Intravenous and Intra-arterial Access.

Home parenteral nutrition

When it is established that a child is likely to require PN for at least 2 months, the option of the child going home on parenteral nutrition treatment is considered (Hill and Long 2001). Value rationality underpins discussion surrounding discharging the child on home parenteral nutrition (HPN), with the aim of facilitating the child and family in achieving an improved quality of life at its core (Hill and Long 2001, Wang and Bernhard 2004). A psychosocial assessment is therefore included in the initial steps in this process. The importance of ensuring the child and family receive the support they require from local services at home should not be underestimated. The lifestyle of families with a child who is dependent on PN is altered significantly. Daily life must be organised such that the routine of cyclical PN is sustained and parents/carers need to readily respond to any possible problems consequential to PN treatment, including those associated with the child having an indwelling CVAD.

Prior to the child being discharged home the clinical nurse specialist should carry out a home assessment, which is essential to ascertain that PN treatment can be carried out safely in the home setting. Plans can therefore be put in place for any necessary adaptations to the home. A constant supply of mains electricity to the home is necessary to supply power for a dedicated fridge for storage of PN, and for the IV infusion pumps. There must be sufficient space and suitable washing facilities available such that the Aseptic Non-Touch Technique (ANTT) or similar locally approved aseptic technique can be strictly adhered to.

A home care company can be used to supply the nutrients and equipment required by the child for home parenteral nutrition (HPN) once the pharmacist and the medical consultant have finalised an 'all-in-one' bag PN prescription. The parents/carers need to undergo an intensive training programme with the clini-cal nurse specialist. The HPN training programme must be carefully timed such that on completion of the training programme, all factors in the discharge planning process are in place ready for the child to be discharged straight home. A discharge planning meeting should be held whereby the specific healthcare and social needs of the child and family are made explicit and the commencement of a shared care arrangement is formally marked. Funding needs to be identified and put in place.

The responsibility placed on the parent/carer is onerous and there are a number of very practical issues that need to be addressed. While the PN infusion is running overnight, parents'/carers' sleep can be interrupted by the child needing frequent micturition due to large volume of fluid intake. Parents/carers must also attend to the IV infusion pump when it alarms, to investigate and correct the cause for the alarm. The long-term impact of the responsibility of carrying out highly technical nursing care at home, the emotional stress of the fear of septicaemia and the physical stress placed on the parents/carers necessitates the need for on-going support from local services (Hill and Long 2001).

Procedure guideline 19.6 Delivery of PN in the hospital setting

Statement	Rationale
Inform the child and family	

1. Ensure the child and family are informed of the following:
  a) The reason for commencing PN.
  b) What it will involve.
  c) Likely duration of PN.
  d) Potential side effects of PN.
  e) Likely impact on child and family.
	1. To obtain informed consent (RCN IV Therapy Forum 2003).
	  a) To promote safe delivery of PN.
	
	  c) To maximise effectiveness of PN.

2. The ward play specialist should be informed to enable them to prepare the child.	2. To help to psychologically prepare the child (Bravery 1999).
Refer to nutrition support team	

1. Once the medical team has decided that PN is indicated the child should be referred to a member of the Nutrition Support Team (NST).	1. To determine the child's suitability for PN.
	  To perform a nutritional assessment prior to PN being ordered.
	  To allow the team to determine type of IV access present/required (Burnett 2000).

Baseline parameters	
1. The child's baseline parameters must be measured.	1. To determine effectiveness of PN (Burnham 1999).

2. Prior to starting PN the following observations of the child should be recorded:
  • Temperature
  • Heart rate
  • Respiratory rate
  • Blood pressure. For further information see Chapter 1 on Assessment.
	2. To establish the baseline for subsequent observations.

501

(Continued)

Procedure guideline 19.6 (*Continued*)

Statement	Rationale
3. The weight and height of the child should be recorded on their nursing record and centile chart.	**3.** To allow accuracy of PN formulation and to monitor growth.
4. The child should be weighed according to local policy, ideally unclothed and using the same scales for each weight obtained.	**4.** To obtain an accurate measurement.
5. 'Nutritional' blood and urine samples should be taken according to the monitoring policy.	**5.** To monitor, assess and correct any imbalance of electrolytes, vitamins and trace elements (Puntis 2001). To prevent metabolic complications.

Venous access

1. Long-term PN should be administered via a central venous access device (CVAD). Dextrose concentrations above 10% should be administered via CVAD. Local policy may differ.	**1.** To minimise risk of extravasation injury and phlebitis: a dextrose concentration above 10% is hypertonic and acidic. To ensure the child's nutritional needs are met.
2. The NST must be informed if a CVAD is not available for children for whom PN is prescribed.	**2.** To determine appropriate course of treatment. To allow time to arrange for appropriate IV access.
3. A dedicated nutrition line should be used whenever possible, i.e. a single lumen CVAD.	**3.** To reduce the risk of infection. (Department of Health 2003a). Sometimes a double- or triple-lumen line will be necessary such as when giving cytotoxic therapy or blood products.
4. The intravenous device should be cared for according to the relevant local policy.	**4.** To reduce risks of infection and accidental removal or damage to the device.

Obtaining PN

1. The requesting doctor should ideally liaise with the NST about the nutritional needs of the child. PN must be prescribed by the doctor.	**1.** To ensure the nutritional requirements of the child are met. To comply with legal requirements.
2. When the PN is delivered to the clinical area the following details must be checked: **a)** Name, date of birth, hospital number. **b)** That the bag is intact. **c)** PN has been stored in a fridge. **d)** The temperature of the fridge is recorded daily.	**2.** To avoid delay in treatment. **a)** To ensure correct PN has been delivered. **b)** To minimise risk of infection. **c)** To maintain stability of the PN. **d)** To provide a record for audit and accuracy and to detect equipment failure early.
3. The time to commence the PN should be negotiated with the child and family.	**3.** To promote a partnership in care. To ensure the child is present on the ward when in hospital. To promote effective planning.
4. PN infusion should be prepared in a designated area.	**4.** To minimise the risk of infection. To provide access for resources.
5. Access to the room should be restricted while the PN infusion is being prepared.	**5.** To reduce the risk of error and contamination.
6. PN infusion should be prepared on an individual basis, i.e. immediately prior to connection.	**6.** To reduce the risk of infection and errors.

Procedure guideline 19.6 (*Continued*)

Statement	Rationale
7. PN should be discarded after 24 hours. **a)** A new administration set and filter should always be used. **b)** PN should be administered via an appropriate administration set and a 1.2 micron filter.	**7.** To reduce the risk of infection. **b)** To ensure safe delivery of PN to the child and avoid particulate contamination (Sari and Rollins 1999).
8. PN should be removed from the fridge 1–4 hours before use.	**8.** To ensure stability of PN. To avoid infusing a solution that is too cold causing hypothermia (RCN IV Therapy Forum 2003).
9. PN solution should be checked for leakage and precipitate.	**9.** To avoid infusion of contaminated PN. To avoid risk of infection to the child.
10. Check the following match when comparing the child's intravenous prescription chart against the PN solution and the pharmacy therapy sheet according to local Hospital Drug Policy: **a)** Full name, date of birth, hospital number. **b)** Route of administration. **c)** Dextrose concentration. **d)** Rate of infusion, duration of infusion, volume to be infused.	**10.** To ensure correct product is prepared for correct child (Nicol 1999). **a)** To ensure prescription is correct.
11. If there is a discrepancy between the prescription sheet and the pharmacy therapy sheet: do not commence infusion, contact the relevant pharmacist and medical staff to resolve the problem.	**11.** To ensure appropriate nutrition is maintained. To detect errors and minimise risk to the child. An incident report should be completed.
12. An appropriate intravenous infusion pump must be used.	**12.** To ensure accuracy of infusion.
13. An aseptic non-touch technique (ANTT) (identified in local policy) must be followed when preparing the infusion.	**13.** To minimise the risk of infection (Department of Health 2003a). To comply with local policy.
14. Prime the IV administration set.	**14.** To prevent air embolism. To ensure IV administration set is patent.
15. When lipid is not prescribed water-soluble vitamins should be added in Pharmacy to the amino acid solution. In this case, the bag must be covered and protected from light.	**15.** Some water soluble vitamins are light-sensitive.
16. If the child is having additional IV therapy, the administration set for that should be connected below the filter.	**16.** To minimise the risk of infection by reducing the number of times the CVAD is accessed.
17. Do not add any other drugs or solutions to the PN solution.	**17.** To minimise the risk of infection. To maintain stability of the PN.

Commencement of infusion

1. If possible use the treatment room for connection to PN infusion.	**1.** To minimise number of procedures carried out at the child's bedside.
2. Check identity of child against the PN prescription and solution according to hospital policy.	**2.** To reduce risk of drug error.

503

(*Continued*)

Procedure guideline 19.6 (*Continued*)

Statement	Rationale
3. Use ANTT to access CVAD, to assess patency of CVAD and to connect to PN, according to local policy.	**3.** To minimise risk of infection.
4. The infusion pump should have the following set correctly: rate of infusion, volume to be infused, maximum pressure alarm limit.	**4.** To maintain patient safety. To ensure correct amount of PN is administered.
5. The infusion pump must be secured onto the appropriate infusion stand. The pump must be connected to the mains electricity whenever possible.	**5.** To ensure patient safety. To avoid the rechargable battery from running down.
6. The level of the pump should be positioned correctly and the pressure alarm set according to instructions attached to the infusion device.	**6.** To ensure alarm functions correctly.
7. Ensure all connections are secure in the administration system.	**7.** To prevent accidental disconnection.
8. Ensure all relevant clamps on the administration set and CVAD are open.	**8.** To facilitate flow of PN and avoid unnecessary alarms.
9. All equipment must be disposed of according to hospital waste policy.	**9.** To ensure safety of staff and patients.
10. Ensure prescription charts are signed on commencement of infusion and charted on the child's fluid balance chart.	**10.** To provide record of PN treatment.

Managing the infusion

1. The NST should be contacted if there are any concerns about a child receiving PN.	**1.** To allow issues to be resolved.
2. If there is accidental disconnection of the PN: **a)** Discard PN, flush and lock CVAD as per local policy. **b)** Inform medical staff.	**2.** **a)** To minimise risk of infection. **b)** To ensure safety of the child. The child may need other fluids prescribed.
3. The PN infusion should not be interrupted if possible.	**3.** To ensure the child's nutritional needs are met.
4. If the filter blocks during the administration of the PN infusion: Stop the infusion, inform the child's doctor and pharmacist. **a)** Return the administration set and filter to pharmacy.	**4.** To obtain an appropriate prescription. To obtain a standard PN solution from pharmacy as a replacement. **a)** To enable investigation of the problem.
5. While on PN treatment the child should continue with normal oral hygiene and have oral assessment carried out. Encourage oral-motor stimulation in the patient who is not eating. For further information see Chapter 10 on Personal Hygiene and Pressure Ulcer Prevention.	**5.** To ensure a clean and healthy mouth. To ensure appropriate oral hygiene regimen is used. To prevent feeding problems later on. To prevent problems with speech and language development.

Monitoring

1. Frequency of monitoring and recording observations depends on the clinical condition of the child and any underlying disease process: heart rate, respiratory rate and blood pressure; urinary electrolytes, glucose and ketones; blood glucose; infusion pump pressure, infusion rate, fluid volume infused.	**1.** To meet the needs of the individual child. To assess, monitor and document the response to therapy (Burnham 1999). To observe for fluid overload. To observe for signs of infection. To monitor tolerance of glucose. To ensure accuracy of infusion pump.

Procedure guideline 19.6 (*Continued*)

Statement	Rationale
2. If administering PN peripherally, check cannula site every 30 minutes for redness, pallor, swelling, inflammation, leakage, oozing, tenderness, temperature change. Stop infusion if any of the aforementioned appear. For further information see Chapter 13 on Intravenous and Intra-arterial Access.	2. To detect early signs of extravasation.

3. Weight and height. Calibrate the equipment and use the same weighing scales each time.
    In the case of an infant, head circumference should also be monitored.
	3. To monitor effectiveness of treatment.
	    To enable accuracy of PN formulation.
	    To monitor fluid overload. To enable consistent measurement (Puntis 2001).

Completion of infusion: Continuous PN

Statement	Rationale
1. Record total volume infused on the child's fluid balance chart.	1. To maintain accurate fluid balance.
2. Change administration sets and new solutions without delay.	2. To maintain treatment regimen.
3. Clear the infusion pump settings – these must be re-set when connecting new infusion.	3. To minimise risk of error on re-connection.
4. Follow guidelines for the specific infusion device when disconnecting and when connecting new infusion.	4. To ensure safe and effective use and maintenance of infusion device.
5. Record disconnection and new connection in the child's healthcare records.	5. To maintain accurate records.
6. Dispose of equipment according to Hospital Waste Policy.	6. Maintaining safe practice.

Completion of infusion: cyclical PN

Statement	Rationale
1. If cyclical regimen is new to the child, or if reducing duration of PN infusion, monitor child's blood glucose level.	1. To ensure cyclical regimen is tolerated.
2. Interventions by the multi-professional team should be co-ordinated to suit PN infusion time and child's daily routine.	2. To promote family normality and improve quality of life. To maximise the quality and length of 'free' time available to child and family.
3. During the last hour of the infusion, reduce infusion rate in stages, according to the prescription.	3. To prevent rebound hypoglycaemia.
4. Record total volume infused on the child's fluid balance chart.	4. To maintain accurate fluid balance.
5. Clear the infusion pump settings – these must be re-set when connecting new infusion.	5. To minimise risk of error on re-connection.
6. Follow guidelines for the specific infusion device when disconnecting and when connecting new infusion.	6. Safe and effective use and maintenance of infusion device.
7. Record disconnection and new connection in the child's healthcare records.	7. To maintain accurate records.
8. Dispose of equipment according to Waste Policy.	8. Maintaining safe practice.

(*Continued*)

Procedure guideline 19.6 (*Continued*)

Statement	Rationale
Completion of PN treatment	
1. When PN is coming to an end the volume of PN to be infused should be decreased as the child's enteral intake increases.	**1.** To prevent fluid overload and establish enteral nutrition.
2. The child's doctor should inform the pharmacist when PN is no longer required.	**2.** To reduce wastage and unnecessary costs.
3. The intravenous access device should be removed when it is no longer required.	**3.** To minimise associated risks.
4. The child's height and weight should be recorded at the end of the PN treatment.	**4.** To audit effectiveness of treatment.
5. The child's height, weight and enteral intake should continue to be monitored by the dietician.	**5.** To monitor progress and nutritional adequacy.

Sham feeding

This term is used to describe feeding a baby or young child with a cervical oesophagostomy by mouth while giving nutrition via a gastrostomy at the same time (DeBear 1996). The main indication for forming an oesophagostomy is in the baby with oesophageal atresia where a complete primary repair of the oesophagus is not possible. This is a rare situation today, as every effort is made to correct the defect by connecting the two blind ends of the oesophagus together in the primary repair.

An oesophagostomy is the artificial opening of the oesophagus onto the surface of the neck. It is formed by bringing the upper blind end of the oesophagus out onto the surface of the neck thus forming a stoma. This allows drainage of the nasopharyngeal secretions and sham feeds. The oesophagostomy is closed when the oesophageal atresia repair is done, usually when the baby is aged 6–9 months old.

The advantage of giving sham feeds is that it allows the baby to develop normal oral feeding behaviour. Sham feeds enable the infant to establish feeding by developing and maintaining its sucking reflexes. Infants who need to remain nil by mouth until their corrective surgery is carried out do not experience normal oral feeding and this can lead to difficulties with sucking and swallowing after surgery and the development of oral hypersensitivity and food aversion.

Breast feeding may be established once the oesophagostomy has been fashioned, or formula milk may be given by bottle. The milk will drain out of the oesophagostomy. Wherever possible the sham feed should be given at the same time as the gastrostomy feed so that the baby learns to associate a full stomach with the oral feeds.

The child may be discharged home, depending on their condition and tolerance of feeds, where sham feeding may continue if the parents/carers can cope with this care. The child's Health Visitor, GP and Community Paediatric Nurse must be informed if sham feeds are to be given at home. The parents/carers will need much support and should be able to ring the ward at any time for advice.

Procedure guideline 19.7 Sham feeding

Inform the child and family

Statement	Rationale
1. Inform the child (if appropriate) and family of the following: **a)** The reasons for feeding this way. **b)** The principles of an oesophagostomy and feeding using a gastrostomy. **c)** Why sham feeds are so important. **d)** The likely duration for the need for this procedure.	**1.** To increase understanding so facilitating shared care and family co-operation. **c)** To encourage oral feeding. **d)** To help plan for a later surgical procedure.

506

Procedure guideline 19.7 (*Continued*)

Statement	Rationale
2. The child's parents/carers must be taught all aspects of sham feeding and what to do if the gastrostomy becomes displaced.	**2.** To involve them in their child's care. To ensure the child's safety.
a) This instruction must be documented in the child's healthcare record.	**a)** To provide an accurate record.

Preparing to feed

Statement	Rationale
1. Prepare the following equipment:	**1.** To facilitate feeding.
a) Select appropriate feeding utensils, e.g. bottle and teat or teacher beaker.	
b) Prescribed milk feed (warmed).	
c) Tissues.	
d) Towel.	
e) A new 'oesophagostomy sling'.	**e)** A dressing used to soak up oesophageal secretions.
f) Plastic sheeting.	
g) Barrier cream (if used).	
2. Prepare a clean 'oesophagostomy sling' for use after the procedure has been completed.	**2.** The 'sling' soaks up secretions thus protecting the surrounding skin. This can be made by cutting a length of tubular bandage long enough to cover the stoma and to be able to tie it in a knot underneath the arm. Two pieces of gauze need to be inserted inside the bandage.
3. The gauze is positioned over the stoma site and tied under the opposite arm.	

Feeding the child

Statement	Rationale
1. Before starting the sham feed:	**1.**
a) Remove the infant's upper clothing and 'oesophagostomy sling'.	**a)** To prevent soiling of clothes.
b) Observe the oesophagostomy site and check the stoma is pink and healthy.	**b)** To ensure the blood supply is adequate and no prolapsed has occurred.
c) Check that saliva is draining from it.	**c)** To allow free drainage of the feed.
d) Inform the medical staff if there are signs of infection or thrush.	**d)** Oral thrush may cause thrush at the oesophagostomy site.
e) If there is no saliva draining. **DO NOT** give the feed.	**e)** A lack of drainage may indicate a blockage or an oesophagostomy stricture.
2. An infant who is going to have the sham feed should be wrapped in a blanket allowing room to access the gastrostomy tube.	**2.** To prevent them from becoming cold.
3. Position the plastic sheeting around the baby's shoulders and cover with a towel.	**3.** To protect skin and prevent becoming wet and cold.

(*Continued*)

Procedure guideline 19.7 (*Continued*)

Statement	Rationale
4. Prior to commencing the feed perform a social hand wash and put on a disposable apron.	**4.** To minimise the risk of infection.
5. Where possible, two people should be available to assist with a sham feed.	**5.** To co-ordinate oral 'sham' feeding and gastrostomy feeding.
6. With the aid of the second person, simultaneously give the oral feed and gastrostomy feed.	**6.** The infant will associate a full stomach with oral feeding, To ensure the correct nutritional requirements are given for growth and development.
7. Observe the infant while feeding.	**7.** If the infant becomes upset and distressed stop the oral feed but continue to give the gastrostomy feed slowly. The infant, due to fatigue, may take less orally than via the gastrostomy, especially if this is a new procedure for the infant.
8. The oral volume of feed should be gradually built up as tolerated.	
9. Once the feed is completed the stoma site should be: **a)** Cleaned with warm water and gauze. **b)** Dried. **c)** Protected with an application of soft paraffin.	**9.** To prevent skin excoriation.
10. The new 'oesophagostomy sling' should be placed over the stoma and tied under the opposite arm.	**10.** The 'sling' soaks up secretions thus protecting the surrounding skin. The knot should be checked to ensure it does not cause any pressure.
11. The 'sling' should be changed whenever it becomes wet with saliva.	**11.** To prevent skin excoriation. To maintain comfort.

508

Completing the procedure

Statement	Rationale
1. On completion of the feed a social hand wash should be performed.	**1.** To minimise the risk of cross-infection.
2. The infant should be made comfortable.	
3. Oral feeding equipment should be washed with warm soapy water and decontaminated accordingly, e.g. in a dishwasher. Disposable equipment, e.g. gastrostomy feeding set, should not be re-used.	**3.** To meet local policy.
4. Disposable items and protective clothing should be disposed of according to the local policy.	
5. The quantity of feed taken orally and via the gastrostomy should be recorded on the child's fluid balance chart.	**5.** To be able to assess how much feed the infant takes compared with its total requirements.

Procedure guideline 19.7 *(Continued)*

Statement	Rationale
6. A child receiving sham feeds must be weighed at least twice weekly.	**6.** To determine the effectiveness of the child's feeding regimen.
7. A child receiving sham feeds must have their height/ length measured monthly.	**7.** To determine the effectiveness of the child's feeding regimen.
8. Both recordings must be recorded in the child's healthcare records and plotted on their centile chart.	**8.** To maintain accurate records.

References

Agostoni C, Decsi T, Fewtrell M, Goulet O, Kolacek S, Koletzko B, *et al* (2008) Complementary Feeding: A commentary by the ESPGHAN Committee on Nutrition. Journal of Pediatric Gastroenterology and Nutrition, 46, 99–110

Allison S. (1999) Hospital Food as Treatment. British Association for Parenteral and Enteral Nutrition (BAPEN) report. Redditch, BAPEN

American Dietetic Association (2004) Infant Feedings: Guidelines for Preparation of Formula and Breastmilk in Health Care Facilities. Chicago, The American Dietetic Association

Anderton A. (1995) Reducing bacterial contamination in enteral feeds. British Journal of Nursing, 4(7), 368–375

Anderton A. (1999) Microbial contamination of enteral feeds. How can we reduce the risk? Birmingham, The Parenteral and Enteral Nutrition Group of the British Dietetic Association

Anderton A, Nwoguh CE. (1991) Re-use of enteral feeding tubes – A potential hazard to the patient? A study of the efficiency of a representative range of cleaning and disinfection procedures. Journal of Hospital Infection, 18(2), 131–138

Arrowsmith H. (1996) Nursing management of patients receiving gastrostomy feeding. British Journal of Nursing, 5(5), 268–273

Balmer SE, Nicoll A, Weaver GA, Williams AF. (1997) Guidelines for the collection storage and handling of mother's breast milk to be fed to her own baby on a neonatal unit. London, United Kingdom Association for Milk Banking

Beattie, T.K., Anderton, A. and White, S. (1996) Aspiration of (gastric residuals)-a cause of bacterial contamination of enteral feeding systems? Journal of Human Nutrition and Dietetics, 9(2), pp.105–115.

Beattie TK, Anderton A. (1998) Bacterial contamination of enteral feeding systems due to faulty handling procedures: a comparison of a new system with two established systems, Journal of Human Nutrition and Dietetics, 11(4), 313–321

Boyd CA, Quigley MA, Brocklehurst P. (2007) Formula versus donor breast milk for feeding preterm or low birthweight infants. Archives of the Diseases of Childhood, 92, 169–175

Bravery K. (1999) Paediatric intravenous therapy. In: Dougherty L, Lamb J. (eds.) Intravenous Therapy in Nursing Practice. Edinburgh, Churchill Livingstone

Brekle B, Macqueen S. (2010) Hand Hygiene. Clinical Practice Guidelines Great Ormond Street Hospital for Children NHS Foundation Trust, London. Available at www.gosh.nhs.uk (last accessed 29th June 2010)

British Association for Parenteral and Enteral Nutrition (BAPEN) (2000) Current Perspectives on Paediatric Parenteral Nutrition. Redditch, BAPEN

Broome ME, Lillis PP, McGahee T, Bates T. (1992) The use of distraction and imagery with children during painful procedures. Oncology Nursing Forum, 19(3), 499–502

Broscious SK. (1995) Preventing Complications of PEG Tubes. Dimensions of Critical Care Nursing, 14(1), 37–41

Burnett C. (2000) Patient assessment. In: Hamilton H. (ed.) Total Parenteral Nutrition: a Practical Guide for Nurses. London, Churchill Livingstone

Burnham P. (1999) Parenteral nutrition. In: Dougherty L, Lamb J. (eds.) Intravenous Therapy in Nursing Practice. Edinburgh, Churchill Livingstone

Care Quality Commission (2010) Essential standards of quality and safety. CQC-096-20000-STE-O32010. Available at www.cqc.org.uk (last accessed 10th June 2011).

DeBear K. (1996) Sham feeding: another kind of nourishment. American Journal of Nursing, 86(10), 1142–1143

De Curtis M, Canduso M, Pieltan C, Rigo J. (1999) Effect of fortification on the osmolality of human milk. Archives of Diseases of Childhood Fetal and Neonatal Edition, 81, F141–F143.

Department of Health (1991) Report on Health and Social Subjects 41 Dietary Reference Values for Food Energy and Nutrition for the United Kingdom. London, HMSO

Department of Health (1994) Report on Health and Social Subjects 45 Weaning and the Weaning Diet. London, HMSO

Department of Health (2001) Guidelines for preventing infections associated with the insertion and maintenance of central venous catheters. Journal of Hospital Infection, 47(supplement), S47–S67

Department of Health (2003a) Winning Ways: Working together to reduce healthcare associated infection. London, Department of Health

Department of Health (2003b) Public Health and Clinical Quality > Infant feeding, 9 May 2003. Available at www.doh.gov.uk

Edmond K, Bahl R. (2007) Optimal feeding of low-birth weight infants: Technical Review. Geneva, WHO

Food Standards Agency (2010a) Ages and stages. Available at www.eatwell. gov.uk (last accessed 27th April 2010)

Food Standards Agency (2010b) Salt. Available at www.eatwell.gov.uk (last accessed 27th April 2010)

Grant M, Martin S. (2000) Delivery of enteral nutrition. AACN Clinical Issues, 11(4), 507–516

Great Ormond Street Hospital, Dietetic Department (2009) Nutritional Requirements for Children in Health and Disease, 4th edition. London, GOSH

Grimshaw K. (2009) Infant feeding and allergy prevention: a review of current knowledge and recommendations. A EuroPrevall state of the art paper. Allergy, 64, 1407–1416

509

Hart S. (1999) Infection control in intravenous therapy. In: Dougherty L, Lamb J. (eds) Intravenous Therapy in Nursing Practice. Edinburgh, Churchill Livingstone

Hendrikse WH, Reilly JJ, Weaver LT. (1997) Malnutrition in a children's hospital. Clinical Nutrition, 16, 13–18

Henschel D, Inch S. (1996) Breast Feeding. A Guide for Midwives, 1st edition. Hale, Books for Midwives Press, p 58

Hill S, Long S. (2001) Home enteral and parenteral nutrition for children. In: Nightingale J. (ed.) Intestinal Failure. London, Greenwich Medical Media

Holden C, Fitzpatrick G, MacDonald A, Booth IW, Buick RG. (1992) Gastrostomy Care: A Parent's Guide. Birmingham, Birmingham Children's Hospital NHS Foundation Trust

Holden C, MacDonald A, Ward M, Ford K, Patchell C, Handy D, Chell M, Brown GB, Booth IW. (1997) Psychological preparation for nasogastric feeding in children. British Journal of Nursing, 6(7), 376–385

Holden C, Johnson T, Caney D. (2000) Nutritional support for children in the community. In: Holden C, MacDonald A. (eds) Nutrition and Child Health. Edinburgh, Bailliere Tindall, pp 177–196

Hudson J. (2000) The multidisciplinary team. In: Hamilton H. (ed.) Total Parenteral Nutrition: a Practical Guide for Nurses. London, Churchill Livingstone

Johnson T. (2007) Enteral Nutrition. In: Shaw V, Lawson M. (eds) Clinical Paediatric Dietetics, 3rd edition. Oxford, Blackwell Publishing, pp 33–45

Joosten KF, Zwart H, Hop WC, Hulst JM. (2010) National malnutrition screening days in hospitalised children in The Netherlands. Archives of Diseases of Childhood, 95, 141–145

King C. (2007) Preterm infants. In: Shaw V, Lawson M. (eds) Clinical Paediatric Dietetics, 3rd edition, pp 73–89. Oxford, Blackwell Publishing

Lamb J. (1999) Local and systemic complications of intravenous therapy. In: Dougherty, L, Lamb J. (eds) Intravenous Therapy in Nursing Practice. Edinburgh, Churchill Livingstone

Lang S. (2002) Breast Feeding Special Care Babies, 2nd edition. London, Bailliere Tindall, pp 4–5

Law BJ, Urias BA, Lertzmaan J, Robson D, Romance L. (1989) Is ingestion of milk-associated bacteria by premature infants fed raw human milk controlled by routine bacteriologic screening? Journal of Clinical Microbiology 27, pp 1560–1566.

Lee MJ, Allwood C. (2001) Formulation of parenteral nutrition. In: Nightingale J, (ed.) Intestinal Failure. London, Greenwich Medical Media

Lucas A, Cole TJ. (1990) Breast milk and neonatal necrotising enterocolitis. Lancet, 336, 1519–1523

Lucas A, Morley R, Cole TJ, Lister G, Leeson-Payne C. (1992) Breast milk and subsequent intelligence quotient in children born pre-term. Lancet, 339, 261–264

Lucas A. (1993) Enteral nutrition. In: Tsang RC, Lucas A, Uauy R, Zlotkin S. (eds) Nutritional Needs of the Preterm Infant. New York, Caduceus Medical Publishers Inc, pp 209–216

Lucas A, Morley R, Cole T. (1998) Randomised trial of early diet in preterm babies and later intelligence quotients. British Medical Journal, 317, 1481–1487.

Lucas A, Morley R, Isaacs E. (2001) Nutrition and mental development. Nutrition Reviews 59, S24–32

Medicines and Healthcare products Regulatory Agency (MHRA) (2004) Medical Device Alert Ref: MDA/2004/026. London, MHRA

Metheny NA, Titler MG. (2001) Assessing Placement of Feeding Tubes. American Journal of Nursing, 101(5),36–45

Moy RD, Smallman S, Booth IW. (1990) Malnutrition in a UK children's hospital. Journal of Human Nutrition and Diet, 3, 93–100

Muraro A, Dreborg S, Halken S, Host A, Niggemann B, Aalberse R, et al (2004) Dietary prevention of allergic diseases in infants and young children. Pediatric Allergy and Immunology, 15(4), 291–307

NHS Estates (2003) Better Hospital Food: Catering Services for Children and Young Adults. London, Department of Health

National Patient Safety Agency (NPSA) (2005a) Reducing the harm caused by misplaced nasogastric feeding tubes. London, NPSA

National Patient Safety Agency (NPSA) (2005b) How to confirm the correct position of nasogastric feeding tubes in infants, children and adults. London, NPSA

Nicol M. (1999) Safe administration and management of peripheral intravenous therapy. In: Dougherty L, Lamb J. (eds) Intravenous Therapy in Nursing Practice. Edinburgh, Churchill Livingstone

Noviski N, Yehuda YB, Serour F, Gorenstein A, Mandelberg A. (1999) Does the size of nasogastric tubes affect gastroesophageal reflux in children? Journal of Pediatric Gastroenterology and Nutrition, 29(4), 448–451

Paediatric Group British Dietetic Association (2007) Guidelines for making up special feeds for infants and children in hospital. London, Food Standards Agency

Patchell CJ, Anderton A, Holden C, MacDonald A, George RH, Booth IW. (1998) Reducing bacterial contamination of enteral feeds. Archives of Disease in Childhood, 78, 166–168

Paul L, Holden C, Smith A, Buglass H, Robb TJ, Ford K, Sturny P, Booth IW. (1993) Tube Feeding and You. Birmingham, Nutritional Care Department, Birmingham Children's Hospital NHS Foundation Trust

Pellowe CM, Pratt RJ, Harper P, Loveday HP, Robinson N, Jones S, MacRae ED, and the National Institute for Health and Clinical Excellence (2003) Infection Control: Prevention of healthcare-associated infection in primary and community care. Available at www.nice.org.uk

Pawallek I, Dokoupil K, Koletzko B. (2008) Prevalence of malnutrition in paediatric hospital patients. Clinical Nutrition, 27, 72–76

Pennington C. (2000) What is parenteral nutrition? In: Hamilton H. (ed.) Total Parenteral Nutrition: a Practical Guide for Nurses. London, Churchill Livingstone

Peters RA, Westby D. (1994) Percutaneous endoscopic gastrostomy. British Journal of Intensive Care, 4(3), 88–92

Puntis JWL. (2001) Paediatric Parenteral Nutrition. In Payne-James J, Grimble G, Silk D. (eds) Artificial Nutrition Support in Clinical Practice. London, Churchill Livingstone

Rathwell A, Shaw V. (2009) Clinical Practice Guideline. Expressed breast milk: Fortification. London, Great Ormond Street Hospital for Children NHS Foundation Trust. Available at www.gosh.nhs.uk (last accessed 18th November 2011)

Rathwell A, Shaw V. (2010) Clinical Practice Guideline. Expressing and handling breast milk. London, Great Ormond Street Hospital for Children NHS Foundation Trust. Available at www.gosh.nhs.uk (last accessed 18th November 2011)

Reilly H. (1998) Enteral feeding: an overview of indications and techniques. British Journal of Nursing, 7(9), 510–521

Rowley S, Clare S, Macqueen S, Molyneus R. (2010) ANTT v2: An updated practice framework for aseptic technique. British Journal of Nursing (Intravenous Supplement), 19(5), S5–S11

Royal College of Nursing (1998) Breast Feeding in Paediatric Units. Guidance for good practice. London, RCN

Royal College of Nursing IV Therapy Forum (2003) Standards for Infusion Therapy. London, Royal College of Nursing

Sapsford A L. (2000) Human milk and enteral nutrition products. In Groh-Wargo S, Thompson M, Cox J. (eds) Nutritional Care for the High Risk Infant, rev 3rd edition. Chicago, Precept Press, pp 265–279

Sari A, Rollins C. (1999) Principles and Guidelines for Parenteral Nutrition in Children. Parenteral Nutrition, Paediatric Annals, 28:2/February, 113–122

Shaw V, Lawson M. (eds) (2007) Clinical Paediatric Dietetics, 3rd edition. Oxford, Blackwell Publishing, pp 73–89

Singhal A, Cole TJ, Lucas A. (2001) Early nutrition in preterm infants and later blood pressure: two cohorts after randomised trials. Lancet, 357, 413–419

Singhal A, Cole TJ, Fewtrell M, Lucas A. (2004) Breastmilk feeding and lipoprotein profile in adolescents born preterm: follow-up of a prospective randomised study. Lancet, 363, 1571–1578

510

Trigg E, Mohammed TA. (eds) (2006) Practices in Children's Nursing. Guidelines for Hospital and Community. Edinburgh, Churchill Livingstone

Tsang RC, Uauy R, Koletzko B, Zlotkin SH. (2005) Nutrition of the Preterm Infant: Scientific Basis and Practical Guidelines, 2nd edition. Cincinnati, Digital Educational Publishing

UNICEF/WHO (1994) Mothers Charter: Protecting Breast Feeding Rights. London, UNICEF UK Baby-Friendly Initiative

Venter C, Pereira B, Voigt K, Grundy J, Clayton CB, Higgins B. *et al* (2009) Factors associated with maternal dietary intake, feeding and weaning practices and the development of food hypersensitivity in the infant. Pediatric Allergy and Immunology, 20(4), 320327

Wang KK, Bernhard A. (2004) Technology-dependent children and their families: a review. Journal of Advanced Nursing,45(1), 36

Watling R. (2007) Provision of nutrition in a hospital setting. In: Shaw V, Lawson M. (eds) Clinical Paediatric Dietetics, 3rd edition, pp 21–30. Oxford, Blackwell Publishing

World Health Organization (2001) Fifty-fourth World Health Assembly. WHA54.2 Agenda item 13.1. Infant Feeding and young child nutrition. Geneva, WHO

World Health Organization (1981) International Code of Marketing of Breast Milk Substitutes. Geneva, WHO

World Health Organisation (2001) The optimal duration of exclusive breast feeding – a systematic review. Geneva, WHO

Supporting breast feeding – some useful addresses

Association of Breast Feeding Mothers (ABM)
Maybourne Close
Springfield Road
London SE 26 6HQ
Tel: 020 8676 0965

La Leche League (Great Britain) (LLL)
Breast Feeding Help and Information
BM 3424
London WC1V 6XX
Tel: 0207 242 1278

National Childbirth Trust (NCT)
Breast Feeding Promotion Group
Alexandra House
Oldham Terrace
Acton
London W3 6NH
Tel: 020 8992 8637

Chapter 20

Orthopaedic care

Chapter contents

Procedure guidelines

The Great Ormond Street Hospital Manual of Children's Nursing Practices, First Edition. Edited by Susan Macqueen, Elizabeth Anne Bruce, Faith Gibson.
© 2012 Great Ormond Street Hospital for Children NHS Foundation Trust. Published 2012 by Blackwell Publishing Ltd.

Introduction

Orthopaedic nursing skills are essential for the children's nurse and many have been in use for centuries. Nurses will encounter children undergoing orthopaedic surgery, fractures requiring plaster and children on traction. It is important that all nurses understand how to identify a good plaster cast and be able to take action in case of complications. Any child following a fracture, orthopaedic surgery, or in a cast or bandages is at risk of oedema and neurovascular compromise. It is therefore essential that nurses are aware of the importance of recording and documenting neurovascular observations, and of taking prompt action when compromise is indicated. Early detection and action prevents the long-term damage that can occur in compartment syndrome.

There are 46 compartments in the body, 38 of which are in the extremities (Tucker 1998) Compartments are made up of muscles surrounded by a thick fibrous layer of fascia, within which the nerves and blood vessels that supply the limb traverse (Middleton 2003, Ross 1991, Swain and Ross 1999). Compartment syndrome normally involves skeletal muscles, which contract using nerve stimulation (Edwards 2004, Fort 2003). It occurs when the pressure within the compartment increases, which reduces the capillary blood perfusion, compromising tissue perfusion and oxygenation (Edwards 2004, Love 1998, Middleton 2003, Ross1991). If the pressure outside the capillaries becomes greater than the intravascular pressure (pressure within the capillaries), this will cause the vessels to collapse, which interrupts blood flow. The interruption of blood flow results in tissue ischemia, which creates further swelling and increases the compartment pressure (Altizer 2002, Edwards 2004, Middleton 2003). This progressive and self-perpetuating cycle is known as Volkmann's Ischemia (Altizer 2002, Middleton 2003). Compartment Syndrome occurs from 2 hours to 6 days post injury/surgery but normally within 72 hours (Love 1998, Swain and Ross 1999, Tucker 1998). The blood supply is compromised, creating ischemia. Irreversible muscle damage occurs within 4–6 hours and functional nerve damage within 12–24 hours. Limb contractures can develop as early as 12 hours post insult (Altizer 2002, Booth 1996, Edwards 2004, Footner 1992, Love 1998;).

The use of traction, especially skeletal traction is declining due to improvements in surgical fixation, which allows quicker recovery times and weight bearing, but it is important that nurses maintain the skills to be able care for a child in traction. A child in traction or a plaster cast will have additional hygiene and toileting needs and is at increased risk of developing pressure sores. It is important that the nurse is able to identify these needs and any possible complications.

The care of skeletal pin sites is also an essential skill for the children's nurse. It is important to be able to recognise the difference between the normal healing process and the development of an infection. Skeletal pins have been used for many years but the increase in the use of external fixators has increased the number of pin sites in use. Pin site infections cause discomfort and pain to the child and if not promptly identified can lead to loosening of the pin site, deeper infection and osteomyelitis (Lee Smith *et al* 2001, Patterson 2005). There is, however, little evidence-based consensus in the care of pin sites, including the frequency of cleaning and the best cleaning solution to use, and hence local trusts must review the available literature and agree on a local protocol for pin site cleaning.

Before any orthopaedic procedure, it is essential that the child and family are fully prepared through explanation and that analgesia is given if required. This will reduce anxiety, enable consent to be provided and secure the cooperation of the child and family. All equipment should be prepared in advance to prevent unnecessary delays to the procedure, which can increase anxiety for all those involved.

This chapter covers the following practices:

1. Neurovascular observations.
2. Plaster care.
3. The use of crutches.
4. Traction.

A list of key texts is provided at the end of the chapter.

Neurovascular observations

Monitoring and recording of neurovascular observations is essential to detect early complications in the following situations:

513

Principles table 20.1 Inform child and family (neurovascular observations)

Principle	Rationale
1. The observations that will be carried out and the reason for them must be explained to the child and family.	**1.** To gain informed consent, improve cooperation, reduce fear and provide reassurance.
2. The child should be encouraged to practice the movements shown on the chart regularly (see Figures 20.1 and 20.2). However, the child may be instructed by their physiotherapist to expand the range of movements.	**2.** To reduce fear of movement and the need for passive movement (i.e. physiotherapy). Movement reduces swelling, improves circulation and promotes blood flow, which helps healing.
3. The child should have their pain assessed pre procedure and analgesia given if appropriate.	**3.** To determine whether the procedure is likely to cause pain or discomfort. To minimise pain.

Great Ormond Street **NHS**
Hospital for Children
NHS Trust

Patient Label

Lower Limb Neurovascular Observation Chart

Left / Right (please circle)

Operation Date.................
Operation.......................
....
Consultant......................
Ward..............................

DATE:	
TIME:	
COLOUR:	**PK** = Pink **P** = Pale **D** = Dusky **C** = Cyanotic
WARMTH:	**H** = Hot **W** = Warm **CI** = Cool **Cd** = Cold
SWELLING:	**N** = Nil **S** = Small **M** = Moderate **MK** = Marked
OOZE:	**N** = Nil **S** = Small **M** = Moderate **L** = Large
PULSES: 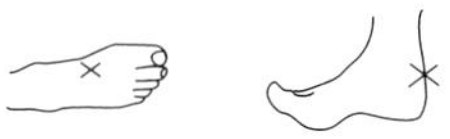	**S** =Strong **W** = Weak **A** = Absent
CAPILLARY: REFILL:	**1** = 1 sec **2** = 2 sec **3** = 3 sec **4+**= 4+ secs
PAIN SCORE:	**0 - 10** (as per pain chart)
MOVEMENT: A⁻ = Active movement without pain A⁺ = Active movement with pain P⁺ = Passive movement without pain P = Passive movement with pain	Peroneal Nerve 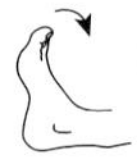 — Dorsiflexion / Tibial Nerve 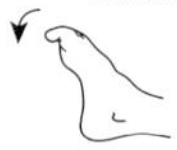 — Plantarflexion
SENSATION: F = Full N = Nil PN = Pins and Needles P = Partial M = Moves to touch	Peroneal Nerve (dorsal surface) 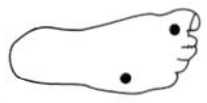 / Tibial Nerve (plantar surface) 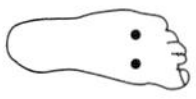
POSITION: **L** = Left side **R** = Right side **S** = Supine **P** = Prone **Sat** = Sat up	
COMMENTS:	
SIGNATURE:	

Adapted from RCH Melbourne

Figure 20.1 Neurovascular observations: lower limb.

Great Ormond Street **NHS**
Hospital for Children
NHS Trust

Patient Label

Upper Limb Neurovascular Observation Chart

Left / Right (please circle)

Operation Date.................
Operation........................
....
Consultant.......................
Ward..............................

	DATE:																	
	TIME:																	
	COLOUR: PK = Pink P = Pale D = Dusky C = Cyanotic																	
	WARMTH: H = Hot W = Warm Cl = Cool Cd = Cold																	
	SWELLING: N = Nil S = Small M = Moderate MK = Marked																	
	OOZE: N = Nil S = Small M = Moderate L = Large																	
	PULSES: S =Strong W = Weak A = Absent																	
	CAPILLARY: 1 = 1 sec 2 = 2 sec REFILL: 3 = 3 sec 4+= 4+ secs																	
	PAIN SCORE: 0 - 10 (as per pain chart)																	
	MOVEMENT: A = Active movement without pain A' = Active movement with pain P' = Passive movement without pain P = Passive movement with pain 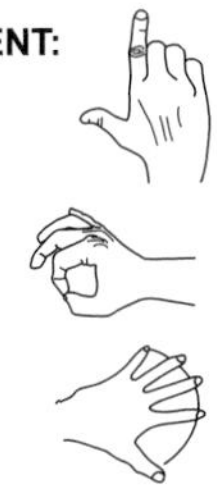	Radial Nerve (into extension)																
		Median nerve																
		Ulnar nerve																
	SENSATION: F = Full N = Nil PN = Pins and Needles P = Partial M = Moves to touch 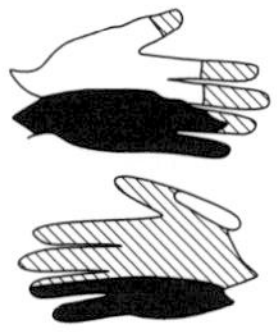	Radial																
		Median																
		Ulnar																
	POSITION: L = Left side R = Right side S = Supine P = Prone Sat = Sat up																	
	VISUAL DISTURBANCE: Y = Yes N = No (c spine patients only)																	
	COMMENTS:																	
	SIGNATURE:																	

Adapted from RCH Melbourne

515

Figure 20.2 Neurovascular observations: upper limb.

Procedure guideline 20.1 How to perform neurovascular observations

Statement	Rationale
1. Colour, warmth, swelling and ooze **a)** Visually assess the naked foot/hand, checking for colour, swelling and ooze. **b)** Check for warmth with superficial touch. **c)** If a chart refers to the colour 'pink', limb perfusion should be checked in children with darker skin. **d)** Ooze requires monitoring for wound care and blood loss. It should be marked on a plaster cast for monitoring and documented.	**1.** **a)** Colour and warmth are provided by a healthy blood supply. A cool pale limb is indicative of a reduced arterial supply, while a dusky, blue or cyanotic limb is likely to be poor venous return. Swelling is an indicator for compartment syndrome and essential to observe. It is especially important if the limb is in any type of cast. Tense refers to a tight shiny limb. (Kunkler 1999, Love 1998). **b)** Increased limb temperature can also be indicative of poor venous return (Altizer 2002, Kunkler 1999). **c)** This is not accurate for all ethnic groups. In these circumstances, assess for a well-perfused limb.
2. Pulse and capillary refill **a)** Check foot/hand for presence and magnitude of pulses distal from the injury/affected area. **b)** Capillary refill should be measured by pressing on the digit for 5 seconds then counting the seconds until the digit returns to its usual colour, normally taking less than 2 seconds.	**2.** **a)** A pulseless limb is a late and unreliable sign of compartment syndrome, as arterial flow may continue while the peripheral perfusion is compromised (Altizer 2002, Edwards 2004, Love 1998, Ross 1991). An absent pulse is significant, however, as it may denote arterial stenosis, whereas an excessively strong pulse can suggest a distal occlusion (Kunkler 1999). **b)** Capillary refill is a significant observation as it is assessing the peripheral perfusion and cardiac output (Kunkler, 1999).
3. Pain score Pain Score should be assessed in conjunction with movement.	**3.** The most reliable and consistent sign of compartment syndrome is pain during movement as ischemic muscles are highly sensitive to stretching (Footner 1992, Kerr 1997, Kunkler 1999, Middleton 2003, Swain and Ross 1999, Tucker 1998). Pain that is disproportionate to the injury and increases with passive extension is indicative of compartment syndrome (Altizer 2002, Dykes 1993, Edwards 2004). However, this can be masked with large doses of opioids (Edwards 2004).
4. Movement when limb is restricted Where movement is restricted by a cast or orthotic, the digits should still be flexed and extended, and the type of cast documented in the comments section.	**4.** This still stretches the muscles and demonstrates nerve function, although to a lesser extent.
5. Movement while child is asleep Where the child is asleep full movement of the limbs should be carried out passively and documented as such.	**5.** Compartment syndrome is as probable in the sleeping child. If the movement is creating significant pain then they require analgesia. If the pain is disproportionate to the injury further assessment is required.

516

Procedure guideline 20.1 (*Continued*)

Statement	Rationale
6. Foot movement **a)** The foot should be actively dorsiflexed as far as mechanically possible (see Figure 20.3a). If active movement is not possible due to language or developmental barriers then full dorsiflexion should be carried out passively (Altizer 2002). **b)** The child should then actively plantarflex the foot as far as mechanically possible (see Figure 20.3b). Where this is not possible due to language or developmental barriers this movement should be carried out passively. See also Figure 20.5. 　It is imperative that the limb is fully flexed and extended in order to assess for compartment syndrome.	**6.** **a)** Active movement demonstrates nerve function (Booth 1996). To assess the function of the peroneal nerve. **b)** To assess the tibial nerve function. 　To detect early signs of compartment syndrome (Dykes 1993, Ross 1991).
7. Hand movement **a)** The thumb and first digit should be made into an L shape and then extended upwards and backwards as far as mechanically possible (Figure 20.4a). **b)** The thumb brought to meet the index finger in an OK sign (Figure 20.4b). **c)** The fingers splayed and mild pressure applied to the external digits to ensure the position can be maintained (Figure 20.4c). 　These tests should be done actively and can easily be made into a game. Where this is not possible, due to language or developmental barriers, these movements should be carried out passively (Altizer 2002).	**7.** **a)** Active movement demonstrates nerve function (Booth 1996). The extended L shape tests the radial nerve function. **b)** To test median nerve function. **c)** To test ulnar nerve function. 　It is imperative that the limb is fully flexed and extended in order to assess for compartment syndrome (Dykes 1993, Ross 1991).
8. Sensation **a)** All touchable/visible surfaces (including in-between digits) should be checked for presence and type of sensation. **b)** If possible, this should be done with the child's eyes closed/not watching.	**8.** **a)** This assesses the peroneal (dorsal) and tibial (plantar) nerves in the foot (Figure 20.5a) and radial, median and ulnar nerves in the hand (Figure 20.5b). Muscles are innervated by nerves and therefore nerve damage can result in permanent loss of function to the whole or part of the limb (Altizer 2002, Edwards 2004). Absence of sensation or complaints of pins and needles/tingling can be indicative of nerve compromise (Booth 1996, Dykes 1993, Love 1998). **b)** It is more effective and accurate if the child is not watching.
9. Position The position of the child should be documented as left, right, supine, prone or sitting.	**9.** To document changes in position as those requiring neurovascular observations commonly have reduced mobility and are therefore at a higher risk of pressure sores. See also Figure 20.1.
10. Visual disturbances If there has been trauma or surgery to the neck (cervical spine) the child should be assessed for any visual abnormalities.	**10.** To check the effect of the cervical spine deformity or damage on the visual field and acuity.
11. Ensure that the child's details, surgical details and the date and time that the observations are carried out have been documented.	**11.** To maintain an accurate record (NMC 2008).

- Bony or muscular trauma
- Burns
- Pre and post orthopaedic/plastic surgery
- Children in traction/plaster
- Application of an orthotic device (Booth 1996, Fort 2003, Love 1998, Tucker 1998).

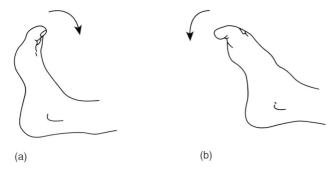

Figure 20.3 (a) Peroneal nerve – dorsiflexion. (b) Tibial nerve – plantarflexion.

Nerves are not renowned for their healing abilities and therefore any damage needs to be diagnosed and assessed promptly in order to reduce the risk of further damage. Neurovascular observations provide information that is essential in the detection of nerve damage or compartment syndrome.

Neurovascular observations must be analysed in conjunction with knowledge of the injury and other observations, as documented complications of compartment syndrome include:

- Loss of limb
- Rhabdomyolysis
- Cardiac arrhythmias
- Hypercalcaemia (Altizer 2002, Edwards 2004, Fort 2003, Love 1998, Middleton 2003, Ross 1991).

The observations should be used in reference to each other and not as individual points of concern. Both limbs should be assessed simultaneously, although it is only required that the injured or affected limb be recorded. It is essential to record a baseline of both/all limbs as a reference point to identify any anomalies such as absent pulses in their feet (Dykes 1993) or altered movement or sensation from a previous injury or condition.

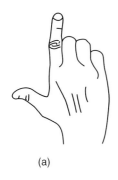 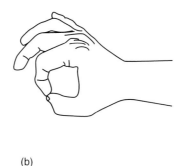 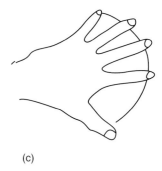

(a)   (b)   (c)

518 **Figure 20.4** Hand movement tests.

Peroneal Nerve
(dorsal surface)

Tibial Nerve
(plantar surface)

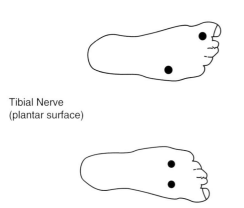

Figure 20.5a Testing sensation in the foot.

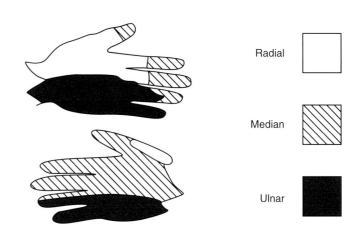

Radial

Median

Ulnar

Figure 20.5b Testing sensation in the hand.

Procedure guideline 20.2 **Management of compartment syndrome**

Statement	Rationale
Actions to take for suspected compartment syndrome	
1. Call child's medical team for an urgent review as time equates to muscle and nerve damage and tissue death.	**1.** To instigate urgent investigation and treatment.
2. If the limb has a bandage or plaster cast in situ, completely split the cast and cut the dressing to skin level.	**2.** To relieve pressure.
3. Elevate the limb to the height of the heart.	**3.** If it is elevated higher, the vascular pressure will continue to increase and exacerbate the condition by increasing the ischemia.
4. Carry out 15–30 minute neurovascular observations.	**4.** To check on the condition of the affected limb.
Action to take for suspected nerve compromise	
1. Refer to child's medical team if condition not previously documented.	**1.** To instigate urgent investigation and treatment.
Treatment	
1. If compartment syndrome has been diagnosed then the child will need to have an emergency fasciotomy in theatre.	**1.** The damage caused by compartment syndrome can occur extremely quickly and urgent surgery is required to reduce the amount of damage caused.
2. If the team is unsure of the diagnosis, a needle will be inserted into the compartment to check the pressure.	**2.** A reading of 0–10 mmHg is considered a normal compartment pressure. Pressure readings are normally taken in conjunction with the child's blood pressure and within 30 mmHg of the diastolic are considered diagnostic (Altizer 2002, Edwards 2004, Love 1998, Swain and Ross 1999).
3. If the pressure is indicative of a compartment syndrome then the child will need emergency surgery.	**3.** To reduce the amount of damage caused.

519

Plaster care

Plaster casts are applied for a number of reasons; to immobilise and support bones and joints following fractures or surgery, reduce pain and to correct deformities by stretching muscles and ligaments. A variety of materials can be used, including plaster of Paris and a range of synthetic materials. Plaster of Paris is used predominantly for fresh fractures, following surgery or where swelling or bleeding is likely (Miles 2001). Synthetic materials are used when the need is for a strong light plaster. A combination of the two materials is useful when the requirement is for a strong light cast that is absorbent and easily moulded (Miles 2001). The nurse caring for a child in a plaster cast must be aware of the reason for the cast and its function, the type of materials used, how to care for it, the duration of the plaster and the mobility limitations it will cause.

Procedure guideline 20.3 **Handling a newly applied plaster cast**

Statement	Rationale
1. Following application of a cast the plastered limb should be elevated if appropriate. This can be achieved by placing the cast on waterproof pillows covered with a towel or by elevating the foot of the bed (Trendelenburg position).	**1.** To aid venous return and prevent oedema to the extremities of the affected limb (Footner 1992).

(Continued)

Procedure guideline 20.3 (*Continued*)

Statement	Rationale
2. When handling a newly applied cast, the carer should use the flat of their hand and extended fingertips ensuring support for the limb at all times.	**2.** To prevent accidental damage and denting to the cast. This could cause pressure sores to develop underneath the plaster. Supporting the cast will also help reduce pain and discomfort associated with the weight of the cast.
3. The newly applied cast should be left uncovered to aid effective drying.	**3.** A plaster of Paris cast can take 1–3 days to dry fully. Covering the cast with clothing or bed linen may inhibit this process (Footner 1992).
4. Artificial means of drying should never be used.	**4.** Plasters dried artificially may become brittle and crack. Artificial methods of drying can also be harmful to the child, as plaster of Paris conducts heat and cold, which may cause burns or blisters.
5. Support and cover unaffected areas of the limb with clothing or bed linen.	**5.** Plaster of Paris casts can be cold and wet until they dry which may cause discomfort.

Management of plaster casts

In addition to removing casts at the end of treatment, it may be necessary for staff to split casts to relieve swelling, or to window casts to allow both the inspection of wound sites or areas of skin where pressure sores are suspected. This task requires the use of a plaster saw and/or plaster shears. Prior to use, all equipment must be checked to ensure it is in working order. Staff carrying out these procedures should have had the relevant training in the correct use of the equipment. Plaster of Paris casts may also require reinforcement with synthetic material.

Procedure guideline 20.4 **Preparation and equipment (cutting a plaster)**

Statement	Rationale
1. Prior to cutting into a cast, perform a clinical hand wash and put on gloves and an apron.	**1.** To prevent cross-infection to the child, for universal precautions against bodily fluids and to protect clothing against plaster.
2. It may be necessary to wear eye or ear protection while splitting the cast.	**2.** To protect the person operating the saw (Miles 1997).
3. Prepare a room/cubicle in which to perform the procedure, ensuring that it is safe and comfortable for the child and carer.	**3.** To allow privacy and to prevent disruption to other patients. Removing a plaster cast can create a lot of dust and noise.

Plaster saw

Statement	Rationale
1. When using the electric saw, hold the blade at 90° to the cast and cut through the plaster using an in and out motion.	**1–3.** The blade will cut the skin or become hot enough to create a burn if used incorrectly (Miles 2001).
2. Avoid sliding the saw up and down the cast and avoid bony prominences.	
3. If the saw becomes hot during the procedure stop and allow the saw to cool before continuing.	
4. Do not use a plaster saw if: a) the plaster cast is not padded. b) the padding has dried blood on it.	**4.** a) To protect the child from harm. b) The padding will be too hard to cut (Bakody 2009).

Procedure guideline 20.4 (*Continued*)

Statement	Rationale
Plaster shears	
1. When using plaster shears, place the blades between the plaster and padding.	1. If the blade of the shear is tilted in either direction the point or the heel of the shears will dig in or nip the skin (Miles 2001).
2. Keeping the shears parallel to the skin, slowly depress the handles in a scissor like motion to cut through the cast (Figure 20.6).	
3. Avoid bony prominences.	
Plaster scissors	
1. Plaster scissors/blunt edged scissors should be used to split padding under plaster (Miles 2001).	1. To reduce the risk of injury to the child's skin.

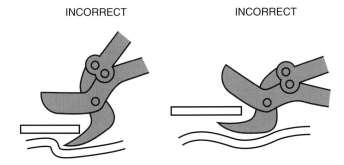

INCORRECT   INCORRECT

Figure 20.6   Using plaster shears.

Procedure guideline 20.5 **Splitting a cast**

Statement	Rationale
1. It may be necessary to split a plaster after application if circulation/neurovascular status is impaired.	1. A plaster cast forms a tight band around a limb and can inhibit circulation.
2. Always seek direction from medical staff prior to splitting the cast.	
3. Splitting of the cast should not be delayed if compartment syndrome is considered.	
4. Splitting a synthetic cast may not relieve swelling, therefore bivalving (when a plaster is cut in two halves back and front) the cast may be necessary.	4. Synthetic material does not have the same level of flexibility as plaster of Paris (RCN and Society of Orthopaedic Nurses 2000).
5. If a limb is expected to swell after surgery/trauma the plaster should be split immediately following application.	5. To protect neurovascular/circulatory status. It is easier to split plaster casts before swelling occurs (RCN and Society of Orthopaedic Nurses 2000).

(*Continued*)

Procedure guideline 20.5 (*Continued*)

Statement	Rationale
6. Plaster should be split by making one continuous cut from the top to the bottom of the cast.	**6.** Constriction will not be relieved unless the whole of the cast is split.
7. This is usually through the centre of the cast following a pencil line.	**7.** To ensure accuracy and to avoid bony prominences (RCN and Society of Orthopaedic Nurses 2000).
8. The surgeon should document in the child's notes where to split the cast if splitting through the centre is contraindicated.	**8.** To prevent unnecessary injury to child and user. To avoid damage to wound sites.
9. The plaster must be split down to the skin. A finger should be run from the top to the bottom of split.	**9.** To ensure that no strands of padding or lining are left intact (Miles 2001). Even one strand of fibre is sufficient to maintain constriction.
10. Plaster spreaders may be required to prise apart the edges of the cast if the limb is very swollen. Extra padding should then be placed in the gap and cast position secured with crepe bandage.	**10.** To prevent tissue swelling into the split edge.
11. After oedema has subsided the plaster can be completed using synthetic cast bandage or a new cast can be applied (RCN 2000).	**11.** To ensure that the plaster cast is secure and not too loose.

Procedure guideline 20.6 **How to window a cast**

Statement	Rationale
1. It may be necessary to cut a window into the plaster cast.	**1.** To observe a small area without removing the integrity of the cast. This may be required to allow the nurse to inspect a wound, remove sutures, or check skin for suspected pressure sores (Miller and Miller 1985).
2. This should be done with direction from medical staff.	
3. A window may be cut using a hand or electric saw.	
4. The area to be windowed should be accurately marked to size prior to cutting.	**4.** To ensure that a whole section is removed, which can be easily replaced (Miles 2001).
5. The removed section should be adequately padded with clean wadding.	**5.** To aid comfort and correct positioning once replaced.
6. Once the wound or skin has been inspected and treated the window section should be replaced and held secure with tape or bandage.	**6.** To prevent tissue swelling into the space made by the window (Miles 2001).

Procedure guideline 20.7 Reinforcing a cast

Statement	Rationale
1. When plaster of Paris is applied following trauma or surgery, the plaster may need to be reinforced using a synthetic material prior to weight bearing.	1. Plaster of Paris may not be durable enough to tolerate weight bearing.
2. The plaster should not be reinforced until neurovascular status is stable.	2. To allow easy splitting of a cast if required. Plaster of Paris can be split more easily than reinforced casts.
3. Synthetic casts usually have to be bivalved.	
4. Use synthetic plaster materials in accordance with manufacturers' guidelines.	4. To ensure effective application.
5. The reinforcement bandages should be applied in a spiral pattern, overlapping by half a bandage width each turn.	5. To ensure even coverage and maintain original form of cast.
6. Take care not to stretch the bandages over the limb. Figure of eight bandaging should be used over heels and other areas of joint flexion.	
7. High impact areas, e.g. heels and base of foot should be doubly reinforced.	7. For added durability and protection.
8. Synthetic bandages should not come into direct contact with the skin.	8. The product will adhere to skin and cause irritation.
9. The reinforced cast should be smooth with no sharp edges (Miles 2001).	9. To prevent damage to skin of affected/adjacent limb.

Procedure guideline 20.8 Removing a cast

Statement	Rationale
1. When removing a plaster cast it should always be cut in to two halves (bivalving) (Miles 2001).	1. To avoid injury to the child, and to use as a splint if required.
2. A guide line should be marked medially and laterally prior to cutting the cast with plaster saw or shears (Miles 2001).	2. To avoid cutting over bony prominences and provide a useful splint.
3. Once the cast is cut on both sides ease the cast open with plaster spreaders, then proceed to cut the padding.	
4. The limb should remain in the cast or the posterior aspect of the cast (back slab) until instructed by medical or physiotherapy notes (Miles 2001).	4. To avoid injury to the child.
5. After cast removal inspect the skin for pressure areas, plaster sores and injuries from foreign bodies. Give skin care as indicated.	5. To identify any complications from the cast.
6. Any pressure sores should be examined by the medical staff and recorded in the case notes (Miles 1997).	
7. Any treatment prescribed and follow-up arrangements must also be documented.	

Observations for a child in a cast

Regular neurovascular observations to all digits of the affected limb must be carried out routinely and regularly following application of a plaster cast (Footner 1992). Swelling is most likely to occur when a plaster is applied following surgery or trauma. For more details regarding neurovascular observations see section one of this chapter.

Regular observation of temperature, pulse and respiration is essential as the child's vital signs may indicate a complication not seen (Footner 1992). Increased temperature or pulse may indicate the beginning of a pressure sore or plaster sore that is undetectable to the eye.

Principles table 20.2 Positioning of a child in a cast

Principle	Rationale
1. Affected limbs should be elevated using pillows or Trendelenburg positioning for lower limbs to no more than 10 cm above the heart.	1. Elevation helps to prevent swelling of the affected limb and also provides support (Miles and Prior 1999a).
2. Slings, collar and cuff or Bradford slings are used to elevate upper limbs.	
3. For children or babies in hip spica plasters, a bed of pillows or a beanbag is a useful way to help provide support.	
4. Areas that are vulnerable to pressure sores, including the heels and sacrum, should never receive direct pressure from the bed (Footner 1992).	4. This may lead to a pressure sore or plaster sore that is undetectable to the eye as they are underneath the cast.
5. Children in large casts should be turned at least 2–4 hourly or repositioned using pillows or beanbags for support.	5. This helps the cast dry and helps to prevent pressure areas developing (Footner 1992).

Procedure guideline 20.9 Performing basic care needs (child in a cast)

Statement	Rationale
1. Cleanse the skin daily in the child's usual way using products of their choice. Pay particular attention to 'hard to reach' areas such as the groin, underarm and back.	1. Plaster crumbs and debris can cause skin irritation and if left may lead to the development of a plaster sore. These areas may be particularly difficult for the child to reach.
2. After washing, ensure that all exposed areas of skin are dried thoroughly and that any powders or creams used are not applied near or under the edges of the cast (Footner 1992).	2. Powders and creams may collect under the cast and encourage skin irritation and breakdown or may even impede the strength of the cast.
3. Throughout the procedure it is imperative that the cast remains dry at all times, and doesn't become wet or damaged in any way.	3. Wet and damaged casts do not provide the support necessary and may cause further complications such as a sore or skin irritation.
4. Ensure clothing is loose and comfortable. Some clothes may need to be altered to accommodate the cast; poppers and Velcro can be placed at the seams to allow for easy dressing (the families will arrange this).	4. Tight clothing may cause restrictions and discomfort and will prevent moisture evaporating away from the surface of the skin.
5. Children who are in hip spica, body casts and bilateral long leg casts may need to use bedpans and urinal bottles for elimination and will most probably need assistance with using these (Footner 1992).	5. These are due to the immobility caused by the cast and rarely are toilets large enough to accommodate a child in a large cast comfortably.

Procedure guideline 20.9 (*Continued*)

Statement	Rationale
6. a) Removable absorbent (not waterproof) tape should be applied to the edges of the cast and around the nappy area for protection. **b)** There should be sufficient padding around the edges of the casts.	**6. a)** Waterproof tape can create a channel, which allows moisture to track further into the cast and can damage the cast. Removable absorbent tape can be changed regularly if it becomes contaminated. **b)** To prevent denting or damage to the cast.
7. Nutrition is an essential component of care for children in casts. Those in hip spicas or body casts should avoid large heavy meals and be advised to eat smaller, more frequent meals to avoid a bloated or overfull feeling in a small space (Footner 1992).	**7.** Hip spicas and body casts are usually quite snug fitting in order to provide support, therefore there is not a lot of room for expansion of the abdomen (Footner 1992).

Principles table 20.3 **Mobilisation in a cast**

Principle	Rationale
1. Mobilising should only be undertaken when the cast is fully dry and reinforced.	**1.** To prevent accidental damage or denting to the cast and injury to the child.
2. Adhere to weight bearing status as directed by medical staff.	
3. Protective plaster boots should be worn at all times (Miles and Prior 1999b).	**3.** Plaster casts need protection even when reinforced, and can be very slippery to walk on.
4. The use of crutches or walking frames may be necessary to aid mobilisation (see above).	**4.** To allow safe mobilisation when no or partial weight bearing is required.
5. Even when mobilising is prohibited the affected limb should be put through a range of exercises above and below the affected area (Footner 1992).	**5.** To prevent joint stiffness and muscle weakness and to help prevent swelling in the extremities.
6. All other limbs should be exercised and used as normal (Footner 1992).	**6.** To help promote independence and to prevent any unnecessary stiffness and weakness.
7. Demonstrate passive exercises whilst giving verbal and written instructions (Footner 1992).	**7.** To reinforce information and use for future reference.

Principles table 20.4 **Complications of a cast**

Principle	Rationale
1. Complications of casts include: • Circulatory and nerve impairment • Excessive ooze or infection of surgical sites • Pressure sores or cast sores • Pain in affected limbs • Skin irritation from the cast • Compartment syndrome (Broughton 1997, Miles 2001).	**1.** These complications can be caused by: • A casts that is too tight • Insufficient padding to allow for swelling, excessive swelling • Uneven tension on application • Local pressure on blood vessels or nerves • Insertion of foreign bodies into the cast • Excessive muscle stretching • Irritation from casting materials.

(Continued)

Principles table 20.4 (*Continued*)

Principle	Rationale
2. Arterial compression Extremities appear white initially then blue and finally black. The beds of the toes and fingernails remain white when blanched and mobility to the digits is severely impaired (Broughton 1997, Miles 2001).	Usual cause of arterial compression would be a constriction caused by the cast being too tight or pressure on an artery from some other source.
3. Venous compression Extremities appear very red, almost purple looking, pain is present and sometimes swelling too (Broughton 1997, Miles 2001).	Usual cause of venous compression would be a constriction caused by the cast being too tight or pressure.
4. Nerve compression The child may complain of pins and needles, followed by numbness, reduced movement and pain (Broughton 1997, Miles 2001).	Nerve compression or impairment is usually due to an injured nerve for example from surgery or the constriction of a plaster cast.
5. Treatment of these conditions is as follows: • Contact a member of the medical team immediately • Spilt the cast through its entire length down to skin (see splitting a cast) • Once the cast is split the edges need to be opened with spreaders and the gap filled with padding to prevent tissue swelling into the gap • The limb must then be elevated and movement encouraged in the extremities • Monitor closely until normal colour and sensation resume and any pain settles (Broughton 1997, Miles 2001) • Document the incident and actions taken in the child's healthcare records.	

Crutches

526

A child may be required to mobilise while non-weight bearing or partial weight bearing. If this is the case, a physiotherapist should assess the child for suitability for a walking aid, then supply and teach the safe use of the appropriate walking aid. Crutches may also be issued by a physiotherapist to improve the gait pattern of a child to increase stability and/or reduce or eliminate weight on the lower limb (Hall and Clarke 1991).

Procedure guideline 20.10 Assessment (walking aid)

Statement	Rationale
1. Read the medical notes, prior to assessing the child.	**1.** To attain the surgeons' plan and the weight bearing status of the child. To determine lifestyle factors impacting on the choice of walking aid. To identify any medical history that would impact choice of walking aid, such as cognitive difficulties, upper limb deformity.
2. Determine the age of the child.	**2.** Children under the age of 6 are unlikely to cope with using crutches (see section on selecting an appropriate aid). Children who use crutches to improve balance or gait may cope at a younger age.

Procedure guideline 20.10 (*Continued*)

Statement	Rationale
3. Where possible, teaching in the use of crutches should be provided prior to surgery. If this is not possible, ensure that oral pain relief is given at least 45–60 minutes before the teaching (15–30 minutes if intravenous analgesia).	3. To ensure that the child is as free as pain as is possible when mobilising for the first time.

Principles table 20.5 **Select appropriate walking aid**

Principle	Rationale
1. If the child is under 6, or is lacking in co-ordination, crutches may not be appropriate. In this situation, a walking frame may be appropriate, or the child's parents/carers may prefer to carry the child or use a wheelchair or buggy.	1. To ensure that the most appropriate and safest method of mobilisation is provided in consultation with the child and family.
2. Elbow crutches are commonly used more often than axillary crutches in the UK. Some hospitals no longer stock axillary crutches. Adapted handles may be required in the presence of upper limb abnormality.	2. Elbow crutches are more likely to be used correctly and have less potential complications if used incorrectly.
3. The decision to use axillary crutches should be based on the stability of the child and the ease with which they use the crutch.	4. Axillary crutches afford more stability to the user than elbow crutches. (Hall and Clarke 1991).
5. A physiotherapist must assess a child who has been prescribed crutches to help them establish a suitable gait pattern.	5. The physiotherapist is the most appropriate person to teach a suitable gait pattern.
6. The person issuing the crutches needs to be aware that they all have weight limits. Although most children are under these limits, if at all unsure the manufacturers should be consulted. Most crutches have limits printed on them.	6. To ensure that the child has been issued with the appropriate crutches for their weight.

Procedure guideline 20.11 **Check safety of crutches**

Statement	Rationale
1. Before issue check that: a) Ferrules (rubber tips) are not worn to the point where no tread is showing. b) Crutches are a matching pair. Do not issue a mismatched pair. c) Crutches are not cracked, warped or damaged. d) Spring clip tips are located into both holes (for axillary crutches make sure the nuts and bolts are tight). e) The adjustment mechanism adjusts freely (elbow crutches). f) The holes on the adjustment legs are round and not worn into an oval shape (elbow crutches).	1. To ensure integrity of the walking aid and thereby insure that the walking aid is in a fit state to be issued for the child's use (Potter and Wallace 1990).
2. Before issuing the crutches, document the batch number of the crutches and record it in the child's healthcare records.	2. To enable recall of all crutches within a batch, in the unlikely event that one is found to be defective.

Procedure guideline 20.12 Education of child and carers (crutches)

Statement	Rationale
1. Explain to the child and their carers: • Why the crutches are needed, • How long they will be required for (if known) • The impact that using crutches will have on the child and family.	1. To gain informed consent for intervention and correct use as instructed.
2. Be sure to explain the risks of improper use of the crutches and how to look for ferrule wear and integrity of the crutches.	2. To ensure that the child remains safe while using the crutches.
3. Make child and carers aware that they should not alter the crutches in any way, e.g. sticking foam onto the handles.	3. Alteration of crutch handles is classed as a customisation and if the crutches fail, the manufacturer will take no responsibility for the failure (European Commission 1994).
4. If the child is having problem with grip, cycling gloves may be recommended.	
5. If sore hands are the problem the physiotherapist should be contacted to determine the availability of crutches with 'Fischer' handles (elbow crutches only).	

Principles table 20.6 Measure the child for crutches

Principle	Rationale
1. If able, measure the child when standing. They should stand with elbows flexed to 15°, with shoes on.	1. To ensure that the child is measured at the height that they will be using the crutches (Potter and Wallace 1990).
2. The height of the crutch handgrips should be measured from the floor to the ulna styloid process using a tape measure.	2. The elbow is flexed to 15° when using the crutches to allow for propulsion.
3. If the child is unable to stand, the crutches should be measured when the child is supine.	3. To ensure that the child is safe and comfortable while being measured for crutches.
4. With the child lying flat, the height of the crutch handle should be measured, using a tape measure, from the ulna styloid process (with elbows as above) to the sole of the shoes the child is going to wear for walking.	4. To ensure that the crutches are the correct height for use with shoes on and that the elbow is flexed to approximately 15°when using the crutches.
5. If the child has a leg length discrepancy, the length of the crutches should normally be measured to the sole of the longest leg when wearing shoes.	5. This allows the long leg to stand with knee in neutral when stationary, and easy toe clearance of the longer leg when walking.
6. Once measured, alter the crutches to the correct height and check them alongside the child to ensure they have been adjusted correctly.	6. Measurement may not be fully accurate; this allows the physiotherapist to correct any error in the measurements.
7. Despite all the above, the crutches may still need to be altered once the child starts using them.	7. The correct height is the height at which the child feels confident and stable and may be slightly longer or shorter than the height measured (Crosbie et al 1992).

Principles table 20.6 (*Continued*)

Principle	Rationale
8. If issuing axillary crutches all the above applies for the handgrips but care must be taken that the axillary pad is two adult finger widths deep from the armpit (with the shoulders relaxed).	8. To avoid potential complications from misuse such as axillary artery aneurysms and radial nerve palsies (Abbott and Darling 1973).
9. If issuing elbow crutches with a height adjustable cuff, they should be adjusted so that they sit just below the elbows but allow the elbows to flex without any impingement.	9. To increase stability.

Principles table 20.7 **Safe use of crutches on the flat**

Principle	Rationale
1. The person issuing the crutches should explain, demonstrate and finally observe the child using the crutches.	1. To ensure that the child and the carers understand how to use the crutches safely.
2. The child should stand up before putting on the crutches and take off the crutches before sitting down.	2. To avoid any injury to the arms from the crutches if the child slips while standing up or sitting down.
3. When standing, the crutches should be between 8–10 cm in front and to the side of the feet, making a triangle shape from the heels and round each crutch.	3. To enhance stability when stationary (Potter and Wallace 1990).
Non weight bearing	
1. Non-weight bearing means keeping the weight off the affected limb. Therefore, the child should be instructed to keep the affected limb off the ground and weight taken through the unaffected limb and the crutches.	1. The crutches should not be in line with the feet because of the instability of this position.
2. Crutches should be placed one step ahead and level with each other.	
3. Putting weight through the crutches, the unaffected limb should be swung to land just in front of the crutches.	
4. Then the cycle should begin again.	
Partial weight bearing	
1. Partial weight bearing means taking some weight through the affected limb.	1. To ensure medical instructions for weight bearing status are adhered to.
2. Therefore the child is instructed to take the appropriate amount of weight through the affected limb, place the crutches one step ahead and level with each other.	
3. The affected limb should be placed between the crutches, weight put through the limb and the crutches then step through with the unaffected limb.	
4. Begin the cycle again.	

529

Safe use of crutches on stairs

Where possible, the child should use a handrail on one side and hold both crutches in the other hand with the spare crutch horizontal, or give spare crutch to someone else. Thus, when they reach the top of the stairs they have both crutches with them.

If the child is non-weight bearing, when going up stairs they should:

- Put weight through handrail and crutch and hop up with the unaffected limb
- Finally bring crutch up to same step as unaffected limb and move hand forward on the handrail
- Start the cycle again.

When going down stairs, they should:

- Put the crutch down one step
- Put weight through the crutch and the handrail
- Keeping the affected limb ahead of the body, hop down onto the same step with the unaffected limb
- Start the cycle again
- If there is no handrail then use both crutches instead of one and the handrail.

If the child is partial weight bearing, to go up stairs they should:

- Putting some weight through the handrail and crutch step up one step with the unaffected limb
- Step up onto the same step with the affected limb
- Finally bring the crutch up onto the same step
- Start the cycle again
- If there is no handrail then use both crutches instead of one and the handrail.

To go down stairs, the partial weight bearing child should:

- Put the crutch down one step
- Putting weight through the crutch and handrail, place the affected limb step onto the same step as the crutch
- Finally, step down onto the same step with the unaffected limb
- Start the cycle again
- If there is no handrail then use both crutches instead of one and the handrail.

Discharge

When the child is safe and independent with the crutches on both the flat and the stairs they may be discharged from hospital. Any earlier discharge from hospital would be unsafe. If a child is unable to go up and downstairs safely using crutches they will need to be supervised at home or taught to go up and down on their bottom to ensure that they can safely negotiate stairs.

Care of a child in traction

Traction is not a new concept. The Italian surgeon Saliceto is considered to have recorded the earliest use of weights and pulleys to reduce fractures over a sustained period of time in the 13th century. Earlier records from Aztec and Egyptian periods describe manual traction being used to reduce dislocations (RCN 2002). In the 18th century, traction use increased, culminating in the development of equipment similar to that we use today. Traction is defined as 'the act of pulling or drawing' (Davis and Barr 1999). Orthopaedic traction is a 'pulling force exerted on a part of the body' (Lucas and Davis 2005). To be able to pull, (or apply traction effectively) there must be something trying to 'pull' in the opposite direction. This is counter traction (Lucas and Davis 2005). Without counter traction, traction is not effective. Counter traction may be provided by body weight (frictional force between the child and the bed) or elevating the foot (where traction is on a lower extremity, or head of the bed (for example in cervical traction), in order to create a greater gravitational pull (Wong *et al* 1995).

There are two mechanisms of traction: **fixed**, which is a pull between two fixed points (e.g. Thomas Splint), and **balanced or sliding**, where the pull is balanced between weights and the child's body (e.g. Pugh's traction). Traction is applied directly to either the skin or skeletal system. **Manual traction** involves pulling a limb by hand and is a simple, temporary method of applying skin traction, which may be used to realign fractured bones (Lucas and Davis 2005). **Skin traction** exerts a force directly on the skin and indirectly on the underlying muscles and bones. Adhesive or non-adhesive strips, with an attached cord, are applied to the limb and secured with a bandage. The cord is either secured to a frame for fixed traction or weights and pulleys are used for balanced traction. Skin traction can be applied to the long bones of the extremities, or using a sling or belt, to the spine or pelvis. **Skeletal traction** directly applies a pulling force to the skeletal structure by pins or wires that have been inserted surgically through the diameter of the bone (Wong and Whaley 1995). The pins are attached to a loop or stirrup, to which cord is attached and weights are then secured to the cord. Skeletal traction can be used for long periods of time, or when a larger amount of weight is required.

Traction may be used:

- To reduce muscle spasm and pain
- To maintain the correct alignment of the limb while ensuring rest and comfort
- To restore and maintain the correct alignment of bone following fractures and/or dislocations, trauma, surgery, or the child's medical condition, while allowing movement of the joints during the healing process
- To prevent or gradually improve contracture deformities to the soft tissues caused by disease or injury
- To allow the child to be moved with ease
- To immobilise the child (Davis and Barr 1999, RCN 2002, Wong and Whaley 1995).

The type of traction applied is determined primarily by the age of the child, the condition of the soft tissue, and the type and degree of displacement of the fracture. Traction is used to immobilise the fracture in the correct position until there is sufficient healing to cast or to splint the limb until fully healed. Splints and casts may be used in conjunction with skeletal traction.

Traction should be used with caution as too much force may damage the nerves and soft tissues and too little force may produce painful muscle spasms and impair healing (RCN 2002). Traction may be used less frequently today due to the developments of orthopaedic fixation devices and techniques that allow children be partial or fully weight bearing, and the expected benefits of reducing the time that children are immobile (Lucas and Davis 2005).

The main forms of traction are described below.

Gallows traction

Gallows, or Bryant's traction, is used to treat a fractured shaft of femur in the very young child (under 2 years or 14 kgs) or to aid hip positioning prior to surgical reduction of development dysplasia of the hip (RCN 2002). Gallows traction can be fixed, with the cord secured to a frame above the cot, or balanced with the use of pulleys and weights. The traction is always applied to both legs to maintain symmetry (RCN 2002). The child lies supine with hips flexed to 90° so that the vertical pull to both legs maintains correct alignment of the bones and the hip joints. The knees are slightly flexed and the buttocks should be just clear of the mattress, with a gap to allow a flat hand to fit underneath. This allows the child's body weight to provide the counter traction (RCN 2002).

Modified gallows traction/abduction traction/hoop traction

Abduction traction is used in some centres pre-operatively in children with developmental dysplasia of the hip prior to a closed reduction. Traction is applied in the same way as gallows traction but after 24 hrs with hips in a neutral position, the child's legs are abducted daily, usually over a week to a maximum of 60° (Figure 20.7). There is some anecdotal evidence that abduction traction prior to closed reduction of the hip may reduce the risk of avascular necrosis of the femoral head. It is also believed to increase the probability of a successful closed reduction by stretching the soft tissues, but this is not proven

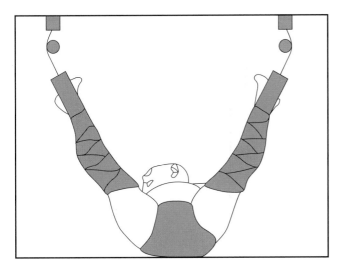

Figure 20.7 Abduction traction (modified Bryant's traction).

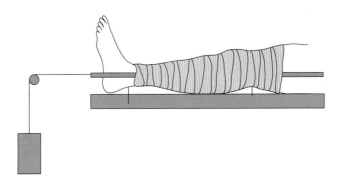

Figure 20.8 Pugh's traction.

(Broughton 1997, Fish *et al* 1991, Hayes 1995, RCN 2002, Weinstein 1997).

To be effective, the traction pull must be maintained continuously throughout the duration of the traction period. However, these types of traction should not be continued for more than 4 weeks due to the potential occurrence of stiffness, porosis and epiphyseal arrest.

Pugh's traction

Pugh's traction (also known as straight leg traction) is applied to either one or both legs using skin extensions and is attached to a bar at the end of the bed or to weights and a pulley (RCN 2002) (Figure 20.8). The foot of the bed is elevated to provide counter traction. A direct pull is applied in a plane that is in line with the body part to be treated. Pugh's traction may be applied pre-operatively for a child with a slipped upper femoral epiphysis, following hip or lower limb surgery, or for developmental dysplasia of the hip, Perthes disease, or irritable hip. Medical staff should document in the notes whether Pugh's traction must be maintained continuously (e.g. following surgery) or can be removed temporarily (e.g. for toileting, washing and physiotherapy).

Slings and springs suspension

Slings and springs are used in the care of children with hip conditions such as Perthes disease or post operatively following hip or lower limb surgery and allow the child to rest the limb/joint while permitting gentle exercise and physiotherapy, maintaining muscle strength and joint mobility. Slings and springs should not be confused with traction as the limb is held in suspension and no counter traction is required. However, the same equipment may be used and slings and springs may also be used in conjunction with traction (Lucas and Davis 2005). The leg is supported by one sling under the thigh and one under the calf, both of which are attached to springs suspended from a traction frame (usually Balkan) frame (Broughton 1997) (Figure 20.9). Padding must be placed under the slings to prevent the edges digging in and causing damage to skin, especially at pressure points. The principles of traction care should be applied to a child on slings and springs, as the child is at risk of the same complications as a child in traction.

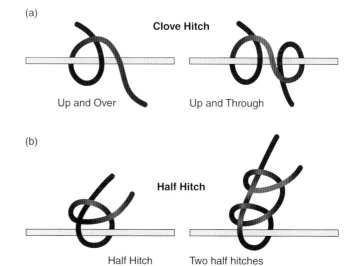

Figure 20.9 Slings and springs suspension.

Figure 20.10 (a) Clove hitch and (b) half hitch knots.

Principles table 20.8 Principles of assembling traction

The type of traction required, including the number of weights and pulleys, must be prescribed and documented by medical staff. All equipment should be checked prior to use to ensure that it is clean and in full working order and the manufacturer's instructions must be followed at all times to ensure safe use. For further detailed information on the use of traction please refer to the RCN Traction Manual (2002).

Principle	Rationale
1. The bed/cot must be compatible with the traction system and have a firm mattress	**1.** To ensure traction is safe and efficient
2. Set up traction with the bed in its lowest position.	**2.** To avoid strain injuries to staff. The weights will hang freely off the floor, once the bed is raised to the required height.
3. Traction cord must be used. The cord is threaded through the track in the pulleys which conveys the traction force.	**3.** To ensure the efficiency of the traction system. Traction cord will not stretch.
4. The correct diameter/strength of cord should be used to fit into the pulley.	
5. The cord must be a continuous single length, with the ends cut short (5 cm) and taped – knots should remain visible.	**5.** To prevent fraying and slipping.
6. The traction cord must not touch the traction frame or the bed.	**6.** To ensure the efficiency of the traction system and prevent cord from fraying.
7. Secure knots should be used to attach and suspend weights at the end of the cord. Knots should be a clove hitch, or two half hitches. See Figure 20.10.	**7.** These are non slip knots.
8. Knots should be positioned away from the pulley.	**8.** To allow free movement of the cord.

532

Principles table 20.8 (Continued)

Principle	Rationale
9. Ensure the prescribed amount of weights are used and hang freely. They should not be in contact with the floor, the traction frame or the bed.	**9.** To ensure the efficiency of the traction system and prevent discomfort to the child.
10. Weights must never hang directly over a child. If there is no option but to do this, then an extra safety cord must be used and checked regularly (RCN 2002).	**10.** To ensure the child's safety.
11. Apply guards (foam balls, squares, soft toys/puppets) over the ends of any protruding traction bars.	**11.** To prevent injury to the child, parents/carers or staff.
12. Use bed cradles to keep heavy covers free from traction cords.	**12.** To maintain the efficiency of the traction system.

Procedure guideline 20.13 **Management of traction**

Statement	Rationale
1. Traction is maintained continuously, unless specified by the orthopaedic surgeon.	**1.** To ensure the treatment programme is effective.
2. Check the traction equipment at the start of each shift, four hourly and after each time the child is repositioned, ensuring the frame, all clamps, and knots are secure, the pulleys are running freely, and the weights are secure, hanging freely and are off the floor.	**2.** To ensure the integrity of the traction apparatus and the efficiency of traction.
3. Ensure correct alignment of the body part in the traction system.	**3.** To maintain traction efficiency.
4. Ensure counter-traction is maintained at all times.	**4.** Without counter-traction, traction is ineffective (Davis and Barr 1999, RCN 2002).
5. Assess the need to elevate the foot or the head of the bed to increase counter-traction, i.e. the balancing force that stops the child being dragged to wards the weight.	**5.** If counter-traction is not present, the child will be pulled in the direction of the traction force and traction will not be effective. To reduce the friction on the sacrum and heels, which may lead to sores.

Procedure guideline 20.14 **Applying skin traction**

Statement	Rationale
1. The area of skin where the traction is to be applied must be clean and dry.	**1.** For hygiene and to aid in the prevention of infection
2. Padding material, routinely integral to the kit, is placed over bony prominences.	**2.** To minimise the risk of a pressure sores.
3. Unroll and stretch the skin extensions prior to removing the backing paper (in adhesive extensions).	**3.** To remove any kinks and to ease handling.
4. The extensions should follow the contours of the limb. This can be facilitated by making nicks in the lengths of the adhesive strips.	

533

(Continued)

Procedure guideline 20.14 (*Continued*)

Statement	Rationale
5. The extensions should be cut to length and the top edges rounded. Ensure the integral protective foam covers any bony prominences, and the adhesive strips are placed in position in accordance with traction prescribed.	**5.** To prevent pressure sores and neurovascular compression.
6. Bandages must be wrapped smoothly and evenly around the limb (maintaining even pressure), in a figure of eight with the limb in internal rotation.	**6.** The 'figure of eight' minimises the risk of slipping. The bandages keep the skin extensions in place, transfer the traction forces to the skin and underlying tissues and encourage neutral rotation.
7. Avoid tight bandaging over pressure areas and vulnerable soft tissue areas (Figure 20.11).	**7.** To prevent neurovascular damage and allow limited movement of the joint.
8. Bandages are secured by a short length of tape.	**8.** The tape must not completely encircle the limb in order to avoid a tourniquet effect.
9. A gap should be left between the child's foot and the end of the skin extension, which allows the foot to touch the footplate when the toes are extended.	**9.** To allow plantar flexion of the foot (RCN 2002).
10. When the skin extensions need to be removed, these should be soaked off in the bath.	**10.** To reduce the risk of skin irritation (RCN 2002).
11. If necessary, gently hold the skin taught and peel back the edges of the skin extensions slowly, using an adhesive solvent.	**11.** This will reduce the risk of damage to the skin.
12. If required, administer analgesia.	**12.** To ensure the child is comfortable and aid adherence.
13. Allow for a gradual pull of traction by removing your hands slowly.	**13.** A sudden onset of traction can cause pain and muscle spasms.

Avoid tight wrapping at these pressure points

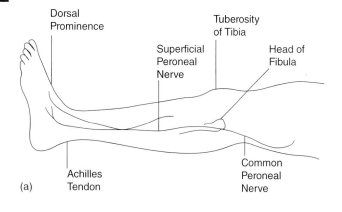

(a)

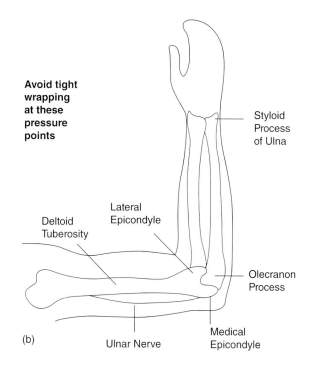

Avoid tight wrapping at these pressure points

(b)

Figure 20.11 Pressure areas (a) Leg. (b) Arm.

Procedure guideline 20.15 Nursing care of the child in traction

For the most part, the nursing care of a child in traction is similar to that for any child on bed rest. The main aims are to meet the child's physical and psychological needs and prevent complications associated with bed rest and immobility, including pressure sores, constipation, chest infection, etc. This section describes the specific nursing care related to traction.

Statement	Rationale
1. The child should be prepared for the application of traction using age appropriate language and pictures or photographs.	1. To obtain consent, aid adherence and facilitate successful treatment.
2. Neurovascular observations must be recorded prior to the application of traction (see section one in this chapter). Always compare the affected limb with the unaffected limb on each occasion.	2. To identify any complications promptly.
3. Report any anomalies to medical staff immediately.	3. Any compromise in neurovascular status is a medical emergency, requiring immediate intervention.
4. Bandages should be removed at least once daily and the skin should be observed for signs of irritation and allergic reaction.	4. To detect and treat complications.
5. When the skin extensions need to be removed, these should be soaked off in the bath.	5. To reduce the risk of skin irritation (RCN 2002).
6. If necessary, gently hold the skin taut and peel back the edges of the skin extensions slowly, using an adhesive solvent.	6. This will reduce the risk of damage to the skin.
7. A pillow underneath a leg in traction relieves pressure on the heel, though it must extend below the popliteal space.	7. A pillow that becomes bunched up underneath the knee keeps the joint flexed and impairs venous flow.
8. Where possible the ankle joint should be left free to allow full plantar flexion and dorsiflexion of the foot.	8. This prevents stiffness and contracture deformity (Mallett and Bailey 1996).
9. Inform the child of any movements to avoid.	
10. A physiotherapy exercise regimen will aim to maintain strength, muscle power, promote good circulation and prevent contractures (RCN 2002).	10. A prolonged period on traction may result in the loss of muscle power. Exercise also prevents muscle weakness in the unaffected limbs.

535

Halo-tibial traction

This section considers the specific care required by a child receiving halo-tibial traction on a Stryker Turning Frame and should be utilised in conjunction with the earlier sections of this chapter. The Stryker Turning Frame is a traction bed designed for total patient care and comfort if traction and/or frequent turning of a child is required during an extended recovery (Stryker UK Ltd 2002a, 2002b). The frame allows a child to be turned prone or supine while maintaining traction by using removable top and bottom canvasses within a turning circle. It is used to treat patients following spinal surgery, trauma, or neurosurgery to aid the straightening of the spine. A general anaesthetic is required to apply Halo-tibial traction and the child remains on a Stryker Turning Frame for the duration of treatment. The manufacturer's guidelines and operating manual must be followed at all times and staff must have appropriate training to ensure they are competent to use the equipment safely and efficiently.

Principles table 20.9 Halo-tibial traction

Principle	Rationale
1. Skeletal traction is applied by the use of a halo frame, secured by two anterior and two posterior pins in the outer skull plates (RCN 2002).	1. To apply the halo traction.
2. A triangular shaped bar attaches to either side of the halo, to which traction cord is secured and threaded through the pulley at the head end of the Stryker turning frame. (See Figures 20.12 and 20.13).	
3. A Steinmann pin is inserted into each tibia and attached to a stirrup. Traction cord is used to attach both stirrups to a spreader bar. Traction cord is attached to the centre of the spreader bar then threaded through the pulley at the foot of the Stryker Turning Frame. Prescribed weights are attached and suspended from the cord.	3. To apply the tibial traction and provide counter traction.

Halo Traction in use

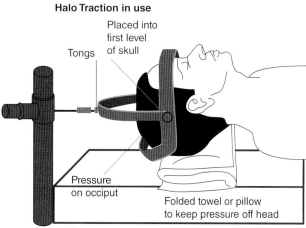

Tongs

Placed into first level of skull

Pressure on occiput

Folded towel or pillow to keep pressure off head

Patient lies flat in bed

Figure 20.12 Halo traction in use.

Stryker Turning Frame

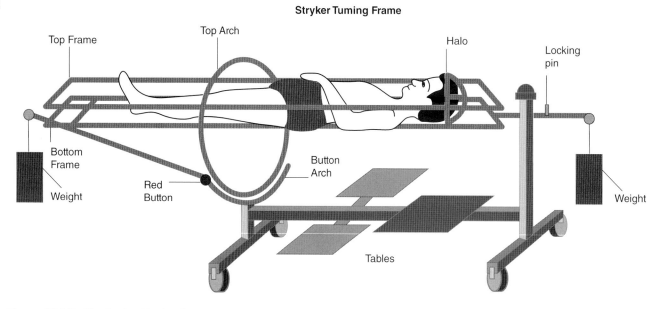

Top Frame

Top Arch

Halo

Locking pin

Bottom Frame

Weight

Red Button

Button Arch

Tables

Weight

Figure 20.13 The Stryker Turning Frame.

Procedure guideline 20.16 Nursing care of the child receiving halo traction

Statement	Rationale
1. Medical staff must torque (tighten) the halo pins to the correct tension using the torque wrench.	1. The initial torque is determined by the spinal surgeon, based on the age and weight of the child.
2. This needs to be rechecked during the course of the treatment.	2. To prevent loosening of the pins, which may lead to a reduction in traction (Fleming *et al* 2000).
3. The traction weight must be prescribed by the spinal surgeon and documented in the child's notes.	3. To ensure the correct traction weight is applied. To maintain accurate documentation.
4. The consultant determines the traction weight by X-rays, neurological function and the absence of pain.	4. To ensure neurovascular status is not compromised.
5. It is likely that different amounts of weight will be prescribed for the halo traction and for the tibial traction.	5. Consider elevating or lowering the foot of the bed accordingly, to ensure sufficient counter traction is provided.
6. Ensure the stirrups are not putting pressure on the skin, superficial nerves, or bony prominences. Pay particular attention to the malleoli, the dorsum of the foot, head of fibula and the popliteal area (back of the knee).	6. To prevent the development of a pressure sore.
7. Ensure both legs are receiving equal traction to ensure there is an equal pull on the spine.	7. To maintain symmetry and prevent pelvic obliquity, which may lead to spinal malalignment.
8. Pin sites should be observed on each shift.	8. To identify problems at an early stage (RCN 2002).
9. If the pin sites are clean and dry they should not be touched.	9. Tampering with pin sites excessively can lead to infection. There is no reliable evidence to support any of the solutions currently used to clean or dress pin sites (Hill and Tucker 1997, RCN 2002).
10. Carry out pin site care, in accordance with local protocol.	10. To ensure the pin sites remain clean and dry and minimise the risk of infection.
11. Check the pins are not becoming loose.	11. Traction will not be effective. A loose pin increases the risk of infection and osteomyelitis.

Turning the frame

1. Read Turning Frame operation instructions (Stryker UK Ltd 2002a, 2002b) before operating the Stryker Turning Frame. Ensure the manual pertains to the model of frame you have.	1–4. To ensure the child's safety.
2. Be aware of the maximum allowable weight for the frame.	
3. The brakes on the Stryker frame must be applied at all times, except when transporting the child.	
4. It is recommended that at least two people are required for the turning of the frame, one to remove the security pin and observe the child, the airway, any tubes/lines and one to do the turning.	
5. The halo and all traction pins are removed in theatre at the end of treatment.	5. To ensure the child's comfort and safety and adherence with the procedure.

Key texts

Kneale JD, Davis PS. (eds) (2005) Orthopaedic and Trauma Nursing, 2nd edition. London, Churchill Livingstone

Royal College of Nursing (RCN)/Society of Orthopaedic and Trauma Nursing (2002) A Traction Manual. London, RCN

Royal College of Nursing (RCN) (2007) Benchmarks for Children's Orthopaedic Nursing Care RCN Guidance. London, RCN

References

Abbott WM, Darling RC. (1973) Axillary artery aneurysms secondary to crutch trauma. American Journal of Surgery, 70(8), 644–646

Altizer L. (2002) Neurovascular assessment. Orthopaedic Nursing, 21(4), 48–50

Bakody E. (2009) Orthopaedic plaster casting: nurse and patient education. Nursing Standard, 23(51), 49–56

Booth Y. (1996) Traction. In Mallett J, Bailey C. (eds) Manual of Clinical Nursing Procedures, 4th edition. Oxford, Blackwell Science

Broughton NS. (1997) A Textbook of Paediatric Orthopaedics. London, WB Saunders

Crosbie J, Armstrong E, Kempson J. (1992) Is walking aid height critical? Australian Physiotherapy, 38(4), 261–266

Davis P, Barr L. (1999) Principles of traction. Journal of Orthopaedic Nursing, 3, 222–227

Dykes PC. (1993) Minding the five Ps of neurovascular assessment. American Journal of Nursing, 93(6), 38–39

Edwards S. (2004) Acute compartment syndrome. Emergency Nurse, 12(3), 32–38

European Commission (1994) Medical Devices: guidance document (meddev 2.1/1), Guidelines relating to the application of: the council directive 90/385/eec on active implantable medical devices the council directive 93/42/eec on medical devices. Available at http://ec.europa.eu/health/medical-devices/files/meddev/2_1_4____03-1994_en.pdf (last accessed 10th August 2011)

Fish DN, Herzenberg JE, Hensinger RN. (1991) Current Practice in the use of prereduction traction for congenital dislocation of the hip. Journal of Pediatric Orthopaedics, 11(2), 149–153

Fleming BC, Krag MH, Huston DR, Sughirara S. (2000) Pin loosening in a halo – vest orthosis: a biomechanical study. Spine, 25(11), 1325–1331

Footner A. (1992) Orthopaedic Nursing, 2nd edition. London, Baillière Tindall

Fort C. (2003) How to combat 3 deadly trauma complications. Nursing, 33(5), 58

Hall J, Clarke AK. (1991) An evaluation of crutches. Physiotherapy, 77(3), 156–160

Hayes MAB. (1995) Traction at home for infants with developmental dysplasia of the hip. Orthopaedic Nursing, 14(1), 33–34

Hill RA, Tucker SK. (1997) Leg lengthening and bone transport in children. Br J Hosp Med, 57(8), 399–404

Kerr GH. (1997) Upper limb trauma. In Broughton N. (ed.) A Textbook of Paediatric Orthopaedics. Philadelphia, WB Saunders

Kunkler CE. (1999) Neurovascular assessment. Orthopaedic Nursing, 18(3), 63–71

Lee Smith J, Santy J, Davis P, Jester R, Kneale J. (2001) Pin site management. Towards a consensus: part 1. Journal of Orthopaedic Nursing, 5, 37–42

Love C. (1998) A discussion and analysis of nurse led assessment for the early detection of compartment syndrome. Journal of Orthopaedic Nursing, 2(3), 160–167

Lucas B, Davis P. (2005) Why restricting movement is important. In: Kneale J, Davis P (eds.) Orthopaedic and Trauma Nursing, 2nd edn. Edinburgh, Churchill Livingstone, pp. 105–139

Mallet J, Bailey C. (1996) The Royal Marsden NHS Trust Manual of Clinical Nursing Procedures, 4th edition. Oxford, Blackwell Science

Middleton C. (2003) Compartment syndrome: the importance of early diagnosis. Nursing Times, 99(21), 30–32

Miles S. (1997) The removal business: safely removing a cast. Journal of Orthopaedic Nursing, 1(4), 195–197

Miles S. (2001) Casting Techniques: application, complications and removal of casts; lecture notes. London, British Orthopaedic Association and Royal College of Nursing

Miles S, Prior M. (1999a) Casting: part one; article 935. Emergency Nurse, 7(2), 33–39

Miles S, Prior M. (1999b) Casting; part two; article 936. Emergency Nurse, 7(3), 32–37.

Miller M, Miller J. (1985) Orthopaedics and Accidents. London, Hodder & Stoughton

Nursing and Midwifery Council (NMC) (2008) The NMC Code: standards for performance, conduct and ethic of professional conduct. London, NMC

Patterson M. (2005) Multicentre pin care study. Orthopaedic Nursing, 24(5), 349–360.

Potter BE, Wallace WA. (1990) Crutches. British Medical Journal, 301, 1037–1039.

Ross D. (1991) Acute compartment syndrome. Orthopaedic Nursing, 10(2), 33–38

Royal College of Nursing (RCN) and Society of Orthopaedic Nurses (2000) A Framework for Casting Standards. London, RCN

Royal College of Nursing (RCN)/Society of Orthopaedic and Trauma Nursing (2002) A Traction Manual. London, RCN

Stryker Medical UK (2002a) Stryker Assembly, Operation Instructions – 124 Wedge Turning Frame and 965 Spinal SurgiBed. Stryker Medical: UK

Stryker Medical UK (2002b) 965 Spinal SurgiBed Operations and Maintenance Manual. Stryker Medical: UK

Swain R, Ross D. (1999) Lower extremity compartment syndrome. When to suspect acute or chronic pressure buildup. Postgraduate Medicine, 105(3), 159–168

Tucker K. (1998) Compartment syndrome: the orthopaedic nurse's vital role. Journal of Orthopaedic Nursing, 2, 33–36

Weinstein SL. (1997) Traction in DDH. Is its use justified? Clinical Orthopaedics, 338, 79–85

Wong DL, Whaley LF (eds) (1997) Whaley and Wong's Essentials of Paediatric Nursing, 5th edn. Michigan, Mosby

Wong DL, Whaley LF, Wilson D. (1995) Whaley and Wong's Nursing Care of Infants and Children, 5th edition. St Louis, CV Mosby

Pain management

Chapter contents

Procedure guidelines

The Great Ormond Street Hospital Manual of Children's Nursing Practices, First Edition. Edited by Susan Macqueen, Elizabeth Anne Bruce, Faith Gibson
© 2012 Great Ormond Street Hospital for Children NHS Foundation Trust. Published 2012 by Blackwell Publishing Ltd.

Introduction

Since the mid-1990s there have been considerable developments in the management of pain in children. An increase in research and education has improved knowledge, changed attitudes towards pain, dispelled myths, and prompted an increase in the use of opiates in children (Clinical Standards Advisory Group 2000, Howard 2003). Pain is an unpleasant sensory and emotional experience, which is unique to individuals and usually associated with tissue damage. If left untreated it can have harmful physical and psychosocial effects and make future painful experiences much more difficult to manage. Children experience a wide range of painful situations and it is unlikely that any admission to hospital will be totally pain-free. Nurses have an ethical and professional responsibility to ensure that pain is prevented and managed as effectively as possible. Numerous guidelines and recommendations have been published, which relate to the provision of healthcare for children and more specifically to the management of pain in children (Box 21.1). Education of staff and audits of practice are essential components of safe, effective pain management (DoH 2004).

Effective pain management involves the use of a combination of pharmacological and non-pharmacological techniques to minimise both the emotional and the sensory components of any potentially painful experiences. Pain in neonates and children with special needs can be particularly difficult to assess and manage. A comprehensive pain management plan should be implemented for all children on admission and continue until discharge. It should be child focused, involving the child and family throughout and various members of the inter-disciplinary team as appropriate (DoH 2004).

This chapter contains the following nursing practice guidelines relating to the assessment and management of pain in children:

- Pain management (general principles)
- Assessment of pain in children
- Entonox administration

> **Box 21.1** UK guidelines and recommendations for the management of pain in children
>
> - Association of Paediatric Anaesthetists of Great Britain and Ireland (2008) Good practice in postoperative and procedural pain management. Pediatric Anesthesia, 18(1), 1–81
> - British Association for Accident and Emergency Medicine (1997), Guidelines for Analgesia in Children in the Accident and Emergency Department. London, BAEM. Revised 2004
> - Clinical Standards Advisory Group (2000) Services for Children with Pain, London, The Stationery Office
> - Commission on the Provision of Surgical Services (1990) Report of the Working Party on Pain after Surgery. Royal College of Surgeons of England and the College of Anaesthetists.
> - Department of Health (2004b) Ill Child Standard, National Service Framework for Children, Young People and Maternity Services. London, Department of Health
> - Royal College of Nursing Institute (2009) The Recognition and Assessment of Acute Pain in Children. London, RCNI
> - Royal College of Paediatrics and Child Health (2001) Guidelines for Good Practice: Recognition and Assessment of Acute Pain in Children. London, RCPCH
> - Royal College of Surgeons of England (2000) Children's Surgery – A First Class Service. London, RCS

- Epidural analgesia
- Patient controlled and nurse controlled analgesia
- Prevention and management of opioid-related complications
- Sucrose.

Further reading is recommended, particularly in relation to the management of chronic pain and pain in palliative care. A number of key texts are suggested at the end of this chapter.

General principles of pain management

This section provides an overview of the main principles of pain management.

Principles table 21.1 General principles of pain management

Principle	Rationale
1a) Pain management guidelines or protocols should be in place in all clinical areas, including ambulance services and accident and emergency departments. The involvement of pharmacists in protocol development is encouraged (DoH 2004a). **b)** Once introduced, regular audit should be carried out to determine whether guidelines or protocols are being followed and they should be reviewed and updated every few years (DoH 2004a).	**1a)** To document the agreed standards for the provision of safe, effective pain management practices locally. To provide support and information for staff. **b)** To ensure that standards of care are met and that the evidence provided is up to date.
2. All staff caring for children should receive education on the assessment and management of pain.	**2.** To ensure that staff are adequately trained to deliver safe, effective pain management for all children (DoH 2004a).
3. Children and their families should be actively involved in decisions regarding the assessment and management of pain (DoH 2004a).	**3.** Pain is subjective. Involvement of children and families increases satisfaction with pain management (Bach 1995, Bookbinder *et al* 1996).

Principles table 21.1 (*Continued*)

Principle	Rationale
4. Information should be given to the child/family, both prior to and on admission, regarding how any potential painful experiences will be prevented and managed. A translator should be used when required. A number of pain related information leaflets can be found at www.gosh.nhs.uk/medical-conditions/procedures-and-treatments/. Where procedures are planned and pain is likely, children should be prepared through play and education.	**4.** To provide adequate information and psychological support (DoH 2004a, RCN 2009). To enable child and family involvement in decision making and facilitate informed consent (DoH 2004a).
5. Pain assessment is an essential part of the pain management process and should be a routine activity (for more information, see next section).	**5.** To treat pain effectively (DoH 2004a). Accurate information regarding the type, location and severity of pain is essential to determine the most appropriate intervention.
6. Pain assessments should be used as a guide to treatment. Intensity scores may be grouped into 'mild', 'moderate' or 'severe' pain to assist decisions regarding the most appropriate intervention.	**6.** To encourage the use of stronger analgesia and a wider range of interventions when pain is more severe (see Figure 21.1).
7. The type of pain, cause and context must also be considered when deciding on the most appropriate intervention.	**7.** To ensure that pain is managed effectively, using the most appropriate intervention(s) for the type and severity of pain experienced.
8a) Pain should be prevented wherever possible. **b)** Treatment should combine drug and non-drug interventions, including psychological therapies such as distraction, coping skills and cognitive-behavioural approaches (DoH 2004a, RCPCH 1997).	**8a)** It is easier to prevent, rather than to treat pain once it occurs. **b)** The experience of pain is both sensory and emotional. For a review of non-drug techniques see key texts (Macintyre *et al* 2010; Twycross *et al* 2009).
9. If there is uncertainty regarding whether pain is present and there is a likelihood of pain, it may be appropriate to treat and reassess.	**9.** Behavioural and physiological responses are not always reliable. If the likelihood of pain is high, analgesia should be pre-emptive (RCPCH 1997).
10. Pain management should be multi-modal where possible and specific to the type of pain experienced. The choice of drug will be determined by a number of factors including the duration of action and side-effect profile of the drug, availability of route of administration and child acceptability.	**10.** Different groups of drugs work in different ways. For a more in-depth review see recommended key texts (Macintyre *et al* 2010, Schechter *et al* 2003, Twycross *et al* 2009). For more information regarding the routes and types of drugs used see points 11–14 below.
11a) The route of administration of analgesia should be safe, effective and acceptable to the child and family. **b)** Verbal consent should be obtained, particularly when using the rectal and epidural routes. Cultural and developmental issues require careful consideration.	**11a)** To provide effective analgesia in partnership with the family. For more information on administration of medicines see Chapter 15. **b)** Many parents/carers have limited knowledge of the rectal route and may be reluctant for drugs to be given this way. Cultural and developmental aspects require careful consideration (Seth *et al* 2000).
12. Simple analgesics (paracetamol and NSAIDs) can be given alone for mild pain, in combination for moderate pain and combined with opiates for moderate to severe pain.	**12.** To provide effective pain relief with minimal complications. Simple analgesics have an opioid 'sparing' effect (Macintyre *et al* 2010).
13. Local anaesthetics are used primarily to prevent procedure-related pain, but are also used to manage chronic pain. These include: **a)** Topical local anaesthetics (e.g. EMLA, Ametop) applied to the skin.	**13.** Local anaesthetics reversibly block conduction along the nerve fibres that they come into contact with (Neal 2002). **a)** To prevent pain during procedures such as suturing, venepuncture, cannulation and local infiltration.

541

(*Continued*)

Principles table 21.1 (*Continued*)

Principle	Rationale
b) Local infiltration, which can be subcutaneous, or target a specific nerve or group of nerves. **c)** Regional anaesthetic (caudal, epidural, spinal).	**b)** To prevent pain during minor surgery (e.g. suturing). **c)** To manage severe pain, usually after surgery.
14. Opioids can be administered for moderate to severe pain. **a)** Morphine is generally considered the 'gold standard'. **b)** Fentanyl and diamorphine are an acceptable alternative to morphine. **c)** Pethidine is generally avoided in children, due to the risk of accumulation of the metabolite norpethidine. **d)** Codeine is a weak opioid with variable efficacy. It is likely to be more effective in combination with paracetamol. If it is ineffective, conversion to an alternative opioid should be considered (e.g. tramadol/oral morphine).	**14.** For more information see key texts (APAGBI 2008, Macintyre *et al* 2010, Twycross *et al* 2009). **a)** The efficacy and side-effect profile are well documented. **b)** They have a different side-effect profile and are quicker and shorter acting, which makes them ideal for short painful procedures. **c)** Accumulation of norpethidine is associated with increased incidence of convulsions. **d)** The main metabolite of codeine that provides analgesia is morphine, but many individuals lack the ability to metabolise the drug (Williams *et al* 2002).
15. Adjuvants or 'co-analgesics' can also provide effective pain relief. These include: **a)** Inhaled anaesthetic agents; primarily nitrous oxide or Entonox. **b)** Ketamine. **c)** Clonidine. **d)** Antimuscarinics, e.g. Buscopan, oxybutynin. **e)** Anxiolytics, e.g. diazepam. **f)** Anticonvulsants, e.g. carbamazepine, gabapentin. **g)** Other drugs such as corticosteroids, chemotherapy and bisphosphonates.	**15.** Co-analgesics either act on the cause of the pain or exert their effect on a specific part of the pain pathway (APAGBI 2008, Macintyre *et al* 2010). **d–e)** For the management of painful spasms. **f)** For the management of chronic pain (Stinson and Bruce 2009). **g)** These treat the cause of the pain: corticosteroids reduce inflammation in conditions such as Crohn's disease, chemotherapy drugs can reduce tumor size and bisphosphonates stimulate bone growth.
16. Sedatives are used to reduce fear of and increase adherence with procedures. The use of sedation alone is not sufficient when a procedure is likely to be painful. However, some sedatives also have analgesic properties.	**16.** For more information, see the NICE sedation guidelines at http://guidance.nice.org.uk/CG112.

Pain assessment

Accurate assessment is an essential part of the pain management process. It enables health professionals to determine the nature and severity of a child's pain; make decisions regarding the most appropriate action to relieve that pain; and to determine whether a specific intervention has relieved pain and if not, what further action is required. There are a wide range of tools available to facilitate accurate pain assessment. Within paediatrics, the range is particularly broad to encompass children of all ages and stages of development, with different types of pain. Research has demonstrated the validity and reliability of these tools and it is recommended that pain should be assessed and documented regularly, using a validated pain assessment tool (Department of Health 2002, 2004a, Royal College of Nursing 2009).

The following pain assessment practices are based on published guidelines and standards and hence do not specify which tools should be used. When choosing pain assessment tools for use with children, healthcare professionals should consider:

- The age and stage of development of child group(s)
- The type of pain to be assessed
- The validity, reliability and ease of use of the chosen tools
- How frequently and where pain assessments will be documented

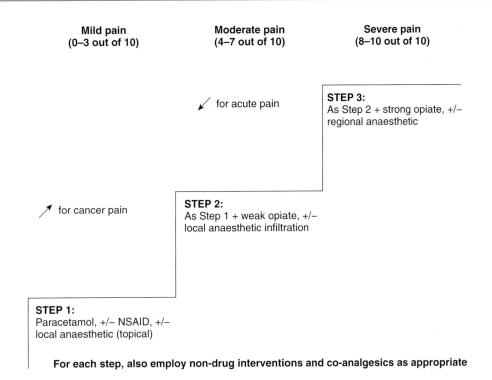

| Mild pain (0–3 out of 10) | Moderate pain (4–7 out of 10) | Severe pain (8–10 out of 10) |

for acute pain

STEP 3:
As Step 2 + strong opiate, +/−
regional anaesthetic

for cancer pain

STEP 2:
As Step 1 + weak opiate, +/−
local anaesthetic infiltration

STEP 1:
Paracetamol, +/− NSAID, +/−
local anaesthetic (topical)

For each step, also employ non-drug interventions and co-analgesics as appropriate

Figure 21.1 Adapted analgesic ladder linking assessment to treatment.
The World Health Organization analgesic ladder (WHO 1986) was originally introduced to recommend a 'step-up' approach to managing cancer pain. However, for surgical or procedural pain, which can be predicted and prevented, the model can be adapted and used to provide a 'step-down' approach.

- How pain assessments will link to treatment
- The amount of education and ongoing support required to implement the tool.

A summary of the available tools and the research evidence regarding those tools can be found on the Royal College of Nursing website, which includes an audit tool for health professionals who wish to audit local practice related to pain assessment. Organisational support, adequate resources and audit activities have been identified as essential for the successful implementation of improved pain assessment practices (Bruce and Franck 2004, 2005). The Department of Health have recently published standards for benchmarking pain (DoH 2010).

Pain assessment tools should be standardised within trusts to provide continuity of care and should include a behavioural tool,

self-report tools for younger and older children and a tool/tools for neonates (term, pre-term and ventilated neonates all require different tools). The assessment of children with cognitive impairment is a particular challenge and tools have been developed for use with this group (Breau et al 2001, Hunt et al 2003, Voepel-Lewis et al 2002). Table 21.1 provides a list of validated pain assessment tools that can be downloaded from the internet (permission may be required before use). This section includes the following practices:

1. General principles of pain assessment.
2. Pain assessment on admission.
3. Pain assessment using a self-report tool.
4. Pain assessment using a behavioural tool.

Table 21.1 Validated pain assessment tools available on the internet

Tool and user group	Website address
Faces Pain Scale – Revised (FPS-R): Self-report tool for verbal children	www.painsourcebook.ca/docs/pps92.html
FLACC: Behavioural tool for children	http://www.wisc.edu/trc/projects/pop/FLACCSCALE.pdf
FLACC revised	http://napnap.dev.vtcus.com/Docs/418_Hellsten(2).pdf
N-PASS: Neonates – pain, agitation and sedation scale	http://www.n-pass.com/index.html
The Oucher: Self-report tool for verbal children	http://www.oucher.org/the_scales.html
Pediatric Pain Profile: Children with severe physical/learning impairment	http://www.ppprofile.org.uk/index.htm
Wong-Baker FACES Pain Rating Scale: Self-report tool	http://www3.us.elsevierhealth.com/WOW/

For a full list of tools, evidence and recommendations go to http://www.rcn.org.uk/development/practice/clinicalguidelines/pain (RCN 2009).

Pain Assessment

Name ....

Hospital No ....

■ **Which pain assessment tool(s) are being used?**

Patient	NRS	☐	Faces	☐	Other
Parent	FLACC	☐			Other
Health professional	FLACC	☐			Other

Instructions *(refer to Clinical Practice Guidelines)*

■ **Always record**   • episodes of pain and interventions   • if patient appears pain free score 0
■ **Frequency**

1. **ALL analgesic infusions**
   (NCA / PCA / Epidural / continuous)

   HOURLY for the total duration of the infusion and for 6 hours after cessation *(then see 3. below)*

2. **Post-op patients** *(if not 1. above)*

   HOURLY for the first 6 hours *(then see 3. below)*

3. **ALL other patients**

   4 HOURLY or AS APPROPRIATE - increase frequency if score is ≥4
   (incl. non-surgical eg. pancreatitis, mucositis, weaning etc, procedural eg. dressing change, venepuncture etc, pre-op & chronic pain)

■ **Any questions?**   Please contact the **Pain Team on bleep 0577**

DATE	TIME	SCORE			INTERVENTIONS / EVALUATIONS	SIGN
	REVIEW AFTER INTERVENTION	patient	parent	health prof	State type of intervention(s) eg. medication, cuddles etc Also note sleep, hunger, complications, etc.	

■	**Assess pain**	Using one of the pain scoring systems on the back of this chart
■	**Plan**	Is an intervention required, if so what?
■	**Implement**	Intervene with appropriate intervention(s)
■	**Evaluate**	Re-score at intervals to evaluate the effectiveness of intervention(s)

Figure 21.2a   GOSH pain assessment Chart (page 1).

Pain Assessment

0	=	**NO PAIN**
1 - 3	=	**MILD** pain
4 - 7	=	**MODERATE** pain
8 - 10	=	**SEVERE** pain

FLACC   SUGGESTED AGE GROUP: 2 months to 7 years   Behavioural

CATEGORIES	SCORING		
	0	**1**	**2**
Face	No particular expression or smile	Occasional grimace or frown, withdrawn, disinterested	Frequent to constant quivering chin, clenched jaw
Legs	Normal position or relaxed	Uneasy, restless, tense	Kicking, or legs drawn up
Activity	Lying quietly, normal position, moves easily	Squirming, shifting back and forth, tense	Arched, rigid or jerking
Cry	No cry (awake or asleep)	Moans or whimpers, occasional complaint	Crying steadily, screams or sobs, frequent complaints
Consolability	Content, relaxed	Reassured by occasional touching, hugging or being talked to, distractible	Difficult to console or comfort

Each of the five categories: **(F)** Face; **(L)** Legs; **(A)** Activity; **(C)** Cry; **(C)** Consolability; is scored from 0 - 2 which results in a total score between 0 and 10
(Merkel et al, 1997)

Wong & Baker   SUGGESTED AGE GROUP: 4 years and over   Self-report

Point to each face using the words to describe the pain intensity. Ask the child to choose a face that best describes their own pain and record the appropriate number overleaf.
(adapted from Wong & Baker, 1988)

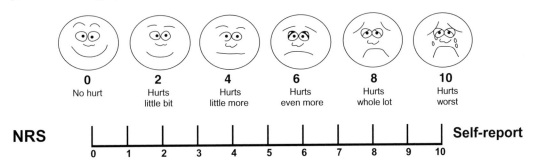

0	**2**	**4**	**6**	**8**	**10**
No hurt	Hurts little bit	Hurts little more	Hurts even more	Hurts whole lot	Hurts worst

NRS   0 1 2 3 4 5 6 7 8 9 10   Self-report

Analgesic interventions

Analgesic ladder

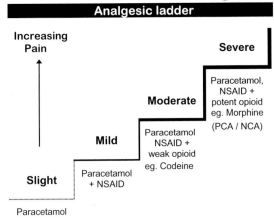

Increasing Pain →

Severe
Paracetamol, NSAID + potent opioid eg. Morphine (PCA / NCA)

Moderate
Paracetamol NSAID + weak opioid eg. Codeine

Mild
Paracetamol + NSAID

Slight
Paracetamol

NB: ■ Check *'British National Formulary'* for contraindications / interactions / precautions etc

PCA / NCA / Epidural patients

0   No pain *

1 - 3   Mild pain *
NCA   - give bolus (10 mins before activity)
PCA   - encourage bolus (10 mins before activity)

4 - 7   Moderate pain *
NCA   - give bolus
PCA   - encourage bolus
EPIDURAL - contact Pain Service

8 - 10   Severe pain *
NCA
PCA   } - contact Pain Service
EPIDURAL

* **Ensure supplementary analgesia is given** (paracetamol + an NSAID if appropriate)
NB: No codeine

© Pain Control Service, GOSH NHS Foundation Trust March 2006

Figure 21.2b   GOSH pain assessment chart (page 2).

Principles table 21.2 **General principles of pain assessment**

Principle	Rationale
1. Involve the family in the assessment and documentation of pain.	**1.** Pain should be assessed in partnership with the family. Parents/carers are able to interpret behavioural cues (DoH 2002, 2004, RCN 2009, RCPCH 2001).
2. Pain should be assessed using validated pain assessment tools wherever possible. These should not be altered unless further reliability and validity testing is planned.	**2.** To ensure that assessments are valid and reliable (DoH 2002, 2004, RCN 2009, RCPCH 2001). Any changes will invalidate the tool and make it unreliable.
3. Assessment should be multidimensional and should include: **a)** The child's self-report of pain wherever possible. **b)** Behavioural indicators. **c)** Physiological measures. **d)** Contextual factors.	**3.** To ensure accurate assessment of pain (RCN 2009, RCPCH 2001). **a)** Pain is a subjective experience. Self-report is considered to be the 'gold standard'. **b)** Many children are unwilling or unable to self-report. Behaviour is a useful indicator of pain in children. **c)** Physiological measures are useful, but are not specific to pain and should not be used in isolation (RCN 2009). **d)** To consider potential causes of pain and prevent painful situations.
4. Accurate documentation of assessments is essential. Space should be provided for documentation of the nature, location and type of pain and any influencing contextual factors.	**4.** Accurate documentation is a legal and professional requirement (DoH 2004, NMC 2004). Most pain assessment tools measure pain intensity, which should not be used in isolation (RCN 2009). For GOSH paperwork see Figure 21.2.
5. Pain assessments should be linked to and used as a guide to treatment (for more information see 'general principles of pain management' section above).	**5.** Scores may be categorised as mild, moderate or severe to enable the use of the WHO analgesic ladder (WHO 1986, 1997).
6. All health professionals caring for children should be trained to recognise and assess pain.	**6.** To enable them to accurately assess and treat pain (DoH 2004, RCN 2009, RCPCH 2001)
7. Pain assessment should be carried out: **a)** On admission. **b)** Whenever pain is suspected. **c)** Prior to and during any interventions that are likely to cause pain. **d)** Following an intervention. **e)** Alongside other cares where possible. **f)** At regular intervals. A sleeping child should not be woken to ask about their pain. The reason for non-assessment should be documented. Assessments should not be done rigidly (e.g on the hour), but should reflect painful and/or pain-free episodes during a period.	**7.** **a)** To provide baseline information with which to compare future assessments. **b)** To confirm whether pain is present. **c)** To determine the most appropriate intervention. **d)** To determine whether an intervention has been effective. **e)** To provide minimal disruption to the child (RCN 2009).
8. The frequency of assessments should be agreed at unit level and determined by: **a)** The type and severity of pain experienced or anticipated. **b)** How long an intervention takes to have an effect.	**8.** To ensure that practice is standardised. **a)** Intense pain and pain related to surgical complications can be harmful and should be treated promptly. **b)** To determine the effectiveness of an intervention as soon as possible.

Procedure guideline 21.1 Pain assessment on admission

Statement	Rationale

1. An accurate pain history should be taken on admission. This should include:
  a) Previous experience of pain and how these were managed.
  b) The words the child uses to describe pain.
  c) Usual behaviour when in pain.
  d) Information regarding comfort measures and analgesia used at home.
  e) A detailed history of any current pain.
	1. To provide information that will assist in the assessment and management of pain during admission (DoH 2002, 2004, RCN 2009, RCPCH 2001).

2. Assessment of any current or illness related pain should include:
  a) Location, intensity and duration of the pain.
  b) The type/nature of the pain (e.g. spasms, burning, etc).
  c) Any factors that exacerbate or alleviate the pain.
	2. To obtain a clear history of the pain and facilitate decision making regarding the most effective way to manage the pain.

3. If the child presents with pain on admission they may require:
  a) A physical examination.
 	
  b) Prompt action to determine the cause of and treat the pain.
	3. a) To determine the underlying condition and/or the cause of the pain. Severe pain can be difficult to manage and may be a sign of underlying pathophysiology (Schechter *et al* 2003).
	b) To manage the pain swiftly and effectively.

4. Pain assessment tools should be explained and the child/family should be taught how to use them wherever possible.	**4.** To familiarise the child/family with the tools and encourage their involvement in pain assessment.

Procedure guideline 21.2 Pain assessment using a self-report tool

Statement	Rationale
1. Children should be encouraged to self-report pain wherever possible. The admitting nurse should assess the individual child's ability, considering factors such as age, language, cognitive ability and willingness to report pain.	**1.** Self-report is considered the 'gold-standard' of pain assessment. Children can self-report from an early age. Validated self-report tools can be used with children as young as 4 (Hicks *et al* 2001).

2. The child should be taught how to use any self-report tool(s) on admission.
  a) The child's ability to use the tool should be tested by asking them to score previous painful experiences.
 	
  b) Younger children should be taught how to use the tool to ensure that they can organise the faces/numbers etc, into the correct order.
  c) If more than one tool is available the child may help choose which tool to use. However, this should be linked to ease and accuracy of use, not just personal preference.
	2. To familiarise the child with the tool and ensure that they are able to use it correctly.
	  a) The child should be able to differentiate on the scale between something that hurt 'a little' and something that hurt 'a lot'.
	  b) Younger children may find more 'concrete' tools easier to use, but if explained correctly, faces scales can be used with children as young as 4 years old (Hicks *et al* 2001).
	  c) To facilitate child choice and familiarity with the tool.

3. The original instructions and wording should be used to explain the tool if available.	**3.** To maintain validity and reliability.
4. The tool should be explained to the child in language that they understand, using the words they use to describe pain.	**4.** To facilitate accurate use. Younger children may not understand the word 'pain' (Jerrett and Evans 1986).
5. It is important that a child is believed if they say that they DO have pain. If a child says that they DO NOT have pain, this should be verified by assessing behaviour and contextual factors.	**5.** Children rarely say that they have pain when they do not. However, they may be reluctant to admit when they do have pain, due to fear of the consequence (e.g. foul tasting medicine or prolonged stay in hospital) (RCNI 1999).

Principles table 21.3 Pain assessment using a behavioural tool

Principle	Rationale
1. Behavioural assessment should be used in combination with verbal reports wherever possible. Physiological and contextual factors should also be considered.	1. To provide the most accurate assessment of pain (RCN 2009).
2. Behavioural indicators of pain are most accurate when assessing acute pain, particularly procedural pain.	2. Behaviour can be modified and pain behaviours are reduced within hours of surgery (Beyer et al 1990).
3. A well researched tool should be used wherever possible. Examples of behavioural tools used at GOSH for different groups include: a) Children aged 3 months and over: FLACC. b) Children with cognitive impairment: FLACC revised. c) Ventilated children and neonates: comfort. d) Neonates: pain assessment tool (PAT).	3. To ensure that assessments are valid and reliable (RCN 2009). For a list of tools available on the internet see Table 21.1. a) (Voepel-Lewis et al 2002). b) (Malviya and Voepel-Lewis 2006). c) (Van Dijk et al 2000). d) (Spence et al 2005).
4. Where possible, observations should be recorded during handling or routine cares.	4. To provide a more accurate assessment. Pain is often greater on movement or handling.

Administration of Entonox

The use of Entonox® has advanced the management of procedural pain in children by providing effective short-term analgesia with minimal risk of adverse effects. Entonox is an inhaled mixture of 50% nitrous oxide and 50% oxygen. It can provide pain relief, sedation and reduce anxiety during painful procedures such as chest drain removal, pin site dressings, physiotherapy and lumbar punctures (Bruce and Franck 2000). Nitrous oxide is both rapidly absorbed and rapidly eliminated through the lungs, although small amounts are eliminated through the skin (Reynolds et al 1996). Because of these properties, the onset of analgesia is extremely fast and once inhalation ceases analgesia and any adverse effects quickly subside. Although the mechanism of action is unclear, the analgesic, sedative and anxiolytic effects of nitrous oxide are thought to be derived from its action at opioid receptors (Mason and Koka 1999). However, this issue remains the subject of debate, and involvement of other receptors has also been suggested (Zacny et al 1999).

Nitrous oxide is an anaesthetic gas and its continuous inhalation can result in moderate to deep sedation (NICE 2010). For this reason, when used in a ward area in the UK, Entonox is usually self-administered. To self-administer the gas a child must be able and willing to cooperate by holding the demand valve and inhaling the gas themselves. If they are unable to do this the use of Entonox should be abandoned and alternative analgesia given. The age at which a child is able to self-administer the gas will vary considerably but is usually around 7–8 years of age. Concordance will depend on the size of the procedure to be performed, the individual child's level of fear and their willingness to inhale the gas. Self-administered nitrous oxide offers several advantages over continuous flow administration, the main one being that it minimises the risk of over-sedation. It also involves the child in their pain management, requires them to focus on regulating their breathing and offers them some control over the situation, which have been shown to have a positive effect on coping with pain (Hodgins and Lander 1997). Entonox should be administered alongside other drugs and non-drug interventions to most effectively manage both the fear and the sensation related to the painful experience. A multimodal approach is particularly important for more painful procedures such as chest drain removal, where Entonox alone may not be effective (Bruce et al 2006a, 2006b).

Healthcare professionals administering Entonox should be trained in its use and familiar with the side-effects and contra-indications (NICE 2010). Online training is also available at http://discover.entonox.co.uk/. Clinical supervision should be provided and level of competence assessed before staff are able to use Entonox on the ward (Box 21.2). A list of staff trained to administer it should be kept on each ward. Entonox is a habit-forming drug and has been subject to abuse. Documented cases are rare, but provide evidence that long-term use can lead to myeloneuropathy and subacute combined degeneration (Reynolds et al 1996). Nitrous oxide is not a controlled substance, but it is good practice to keep a log or audit of use (Figure 21.3) and a weekly check of cylinder levels. This guideline is adapted from the GOSH guideline. The most recent version is available at www.gosh.nhs.uk/health-professionals/clinical-guidelines/.

Training

Entonox must only be administered by staff who:

- Are competent in its administration and in basic life support
- Are familiar with the side-effects of Entonox and its contra-indications
- Are aware of the criteria for child selection (see Box 21.2).

These criteria will ensure that Entonox is administered safely and effectively and the likelihood of side-effects and complications are reduced (NICE 2010).

To establish and maintain the required level of knowledge and skills (NICE 2010), staff should also have received:

- an Entonox training session
- supervised practice
- resuscitation training as per trust policy.

A list of the staff on the ward who have been trained in the use of Entonox should be kept up to date, so that all ward staff know who can administer the gas.

Box 21.2 Suggested competencies for training staff in the use of self-administered Entonox

All staff who use self-administered nitrous oxide with children during painful procedures should be trained and competent to do so. Staff should attend a training session and be familiar with hospital guidelines and protocols

Aim of training: To enable staff to supervise the safe and effective use of self-administered Entonox by children undergoing painful procedures.

Competencies: Staff must be able to:

- Describe the characteristics of nitrous oxide and explain the rational for self-administered versus continuous flow delivery of Entonox
- Give examples of the types of procedures where Entonox might be useful to provide pain relief
- List the selection criteria for the use of Entonox in children
- Describe the contra-indications of nitrous oxide and potential side-effects of its use in children

- Explain why Entonox is not suitable for some children or for prolonged or frequent use
- Describe the nursing care of a child before, during and after Entonox use
- Demonstrate an understanding of the equipment and how it operates, including safety precautions and monitoring
- Demonstrate the ability to instruct a child and family in the use of self-administered nitrous oxide including indications, use, common side-effects and how these are prevented/managed.
- Describe the documentation used within the Trust.

The nurse should be responsible for arranging supervised practice sessions. Training is complete once both supervisor and trainee feel that the required level of competence has been achieved. A record of trained staff should be kept on the ward and regular update sessions made available for staff who need to refresh their skills (i.e. have not used nitrous oxide at least once in the past 6 months).

DATE	CHILD NAME	GAUGE READING		TYPE OF PROCEDURE	DURATION OF USE	COMMENTS: State whether effective, if not why, details of any side-effects, etc.
		AT START	AT END			

Figure 21.3 Audit sheet/log of use.

Procedure guideline 21.3 **Child assessment for use of Entonox**

Statement	Rationale
1. Assess the degree of pain and anxiety likely for the procedure to be carried out.	1. To determine whether Entonox is required.
2. Ensure that Entonox is not contra-indicated for the child.	2. To reduce the likelihood of complications.

(Continued)

Procedure guideline 21.3 (*Continued*)

Statement	Rationale
3. Entonox should not be used if the child has any conditions where air is trapped in the body. These include: • artificial, traumatic or spontaneous pneumothorax • intestinal obstruction • head injuries with impaired consciousness • severe bullous emphysema • maxillofacial injuries • intoxication • following air encephalography • decompression sickness • air embolism • middle ear occlusion • following a recent underwater dive.	3. Nitrous oxide diffuses into air filled cavities, expanding the air to up to three times its original size. It is also thought to cause an increase in intra-cranial pressure (British Oxygen Company 1995).
4. To self-administer Entonox a child must be able to: • Understand and follow simple instructions • Hold the demand valve and inhale the gas through a mask or mouthpiece while breathing normally.	4. To ensure the child is able to use Entonox effectively.
5. Documentation of the assessment should be recorded in the child's healthcare record.	5. To provide information (NICE 2010).

Procedure guideline 21.4 Preparation for Entonox use

Statement	Rationale
1. Ensure the Entonox has been prescribed on the child's prescription chart.	1. To adhere to hospital drug policy.
2a) Liaise with the person carrying out the procedure. b) The person administering the Entonox should not be involved with the procedure.	2a) To agree a suitable time for the procedure. b) To ensure that the child's use of the gas is supervised throughout.
3. If Entonox is to be administered more frequently than every 4 days routine blood cell counts must be performed.	3. To observe for evidence of megaloblastic changes in red cells, reduced production of leucocytes and hypersegmentation of neutrophils (Amos *et al* 1983, Nunn 1987).
4. Staff in the first trimester of pregnancy, or those trying to conceive may wish to avoid the area if Entonox is being administered for long periods in an area with no scavenging.	4. There is some evidence to suggest that exposure to very high levels of nitrous oxide can reduce fertility (Rowland *et al* 1992) and may be harmful to the foetus during pregnancy (Aldridge and Tunstall 1986, Park *et al* 1986).
5. The area should be well ventilated to prevent the accumulation of nitrous oxide.	5. To maintain a safe environment. The occupational exposure standard for long term exposure is 100 parts per million (ppm) (BOC 1995).
6. Gather and prepare the following equipment: a) Entonox cylinder and administration set: • Switch cylinder on and prime the administration set by pressing the test button on the back of the demand valve • Check the cylinder to ensure it is at least one-quarter full.	6. To ensure immediate availability of Entonox once inhalation commences.

Procedure guideline 21.4 (*Continued*)

Statement	Rationale
b) A bacterial/viral filter (e.g. Hydroboy™) and mask or mouth piece: • Attach the filter to the mask or mouthpiece before attaching this to the demand valve.	**b)** To reduce the risk of infection. If no filter is used the whole equipment needs to be cleaned thoroughly between children.
7. Entonox cylinders must be checked carefully before use to ensure they contain the correct mix of 50% nitrous oxide and 50% oxygen.	**7.** To prevent drug errors. Stronger concentrations of nitrous oxide are available for anaesthetic use only.
8. If the child has respiratory or cardiac problems ensure that a saturation monitor is available.	**8.** To observe for post-inhalation hypoxia (BOC 1995).
9. To prepare the child: • Explain the procedure to be carried out and how Entonox will be used, including information about the side-effects • Reassure them that if side-effects occur, these will wear off quickly once they stop inhaling the gas.	**9.** To provide information, relieve anxiety and increase the level of cooperation/concordance.
10. The child should not eat immediately before the procedure. If they have been given sedatives, opioids or already feel nauseous or sedated, a period of fasting is advisable.	**10.** To reduce the likelihood vomiting and associated complications (e.g. aspiration). Vomiting is rare during Entonox use but the risk is increased if more than one sedative has been given (Gall *et al* 2001).
11. Give supplementary analgesia as prescribed: **a)** Oral or rectal drugs should be given about an hour before and intravenous analgesia 20 minutes before starting the procedure. **b)** The child may continue to use their patient controlled analgesia pump (PCA) if one is in use. **c)** A bolus of intravenous opiate may be given if a high degree of pain is anticipated.	**11.** To provide additional pain relief. **a)** to allow adequate time for absorption. **b–c)** It is important to ensure that the child's opiate intake is closely monitored so that they are not too sleepy to inhale the gas.
12. The child should be allowed to practise using the Entonox before the procedure is started.	**12.** To ensure an effective technique is established.

If the child is unable to maintain an effective seal or inhale the gas effectively the use of Entonox should be abandoned and alternative analgesia should be prescribed.

551

Procedure guideline 21.5 **Administration of Entonox**

Statement	Rationale
1. To administer the Entonox: **a)** Calmly explain the procedure; tell the child that they should concentrate on breathing the gas normally. **b)** Offer the demand valve to the child. If they have chosen to use a mask they should hold it over their mouth and nose and, maintaining an airtight seal, breathe normally. **c)** If they have chosen the mouthpiece they should hold it between their teeth and breathe through their mouth only. Some children need considerable encouragement to start inhaling the gas. It is worth persevering as any initial reluctance usually disappears once the child realises that the Entonox is working.	**1.** **a)** To reassure the child and establish an effective inhalation technique. **b)** The mask must only be held in place by the child to minimise the risk of sedation. If they do not maintain a tight seal they will not hear the gas being delivered through the valve. **c)** This technique can be harder for some children. If so they may find the mask easier.

(Continued)

Procedure guideline 21.5 (*Continued*)

Statement	Rationale
2. Inhalation should commence for at least 6–8 breaths before the procedure starts. **a)** Once administration has commenced the child should continue to use the Entonox as required throughout the procedure and should be encouraged to breathe slowly and deeply. **b)** If the child hyperventilates they should be encouraged to exhale slowly and then breathe normally.	**2.** To ensure Entonox has taken effect before introduction of painful stimuli. **a–b)** To provide effective analgesia with minimal side-effects.
3. Observe the child throughout the procedure to determine: • Level of pain • The presence of any side-effects • Whether the child is inhaling the gas effectively. Oxygen saturation level should be monitored during the procedure if the child has an underlying cardiac or respiratory condition.	**3.** To ensure that adequate pain relief is provided with minimal side-effects.

NB If use of Entonox is unsatisfactory at any stage it may be necessary to stop the procedure until alternative analgesia has been prescribed and given.

Procedure guideline 21.6 **Managing side-effects of Entonox**

Statement	Rationale
1. If the child experiences any Entonox related side-effects: **a)** Reassure the child, and remind them that they may stop inhaling the gas until the side-effects wear off. **b)** Negotiate with the child to determine whether the procedure should be halted until they start to inhale the gas again.	**1.** To provide effective analgesia with minimal side-effects.
2. Ear ache: If the child complains of ear ache, inhalation should be stopped and alternative analgesia prescribed.	**2.** Expansion of air trapped in the ear canal could cause perforation of the ear drum (BOC 1995).
3. Dry mouth: This common side-effect is not usually distressing and the child should be encouraged to continue inhaling the Entonox.	**3.** To provide effective analgesia.
4. Dizziness and/or disorientation: If the child starts to feel dizzy or disorientated they may cease inhalation until the sensation starts to wear off. The child may choose to put up with these sensations and continue inhalation to maintain effective pain relief.	**4.** To provide effective analgesia with minimal side-effects.
5. Over sedation: If the child becomes drowsy they will no longer inhale the gas. The child should not be helped to keep the mask in situ. If the child's level of sedation increases: • Monitor the child closely • The procedure may continue if the child's condition is stable. As the gas is self-administered it is unlikely that the child will become over sedated. However, if they are not responding to verbal commands, remove the Entonox and ensure that staff experienced in the management of sedated children are contacted/nearby.	**5.** To prevent the onset of deeper stages of sedation and loss of protection of the laryngeal reflex. Self-administered Entonox should cause only minimal sedation (NICE 2010). For a definition of the levels of sedation see Box 21.3.

Procedure guideline 21.6 (Continued)

Statement	Rationale
6. Nausea and vomiting:	**6.**
a) If the child complains of nausea they may choose to stop inhaling the gas for a while.	**a)** The side-effects of Entonox wear off quickly once inhalation ceases.
b) Less commonly the child may vomit. If so remove the demand valve immediately.	**b)** To prevent inhalation of vomit.
c) Reassure the child and clear any obstruction to breathing.	**c)** To maintain a patent airway.
d) Clean or replace the face mask or mouthpiece.	**d–e)** To ensure the equipment is clean.
e) Clear vomit from the demand valve by vigorously shaking it using a 'flicking' downward action.	
f) Once the equipment has been wiped clean the child may then recommence administration if they wish.	**f)** The side-effects of Entonox wear off quickly once inhalation ceases.
7. Post-administration hypoxia: If the child feels dizzy once they stop inhaling the gas they may benefit from oxygen therapy for 10–15 minutes.	**7.** To prevent post-administration hypoxia (BOC 1995).

Box 21.3 Levels of sedation

- **Minimal sedation**: A drug-induced state during which patients are awake and calm, and respond normally to verbal commands. Although cognitive function and coordination may be impaired, ventilatory and cardiovascular functions are unaffected.
- **Moderate sedation**: Drug-induced depression of consciousness during which patients are sleepy but respond purposefully to verbal commands (known as conscious sedation in dentistry, see below) or light tactile stimulation (reflex withdrawal from a painful stimulus is not a purposeful response). No interventions are required to maintain a patent airway. Spontaneous ventilation is adequate. Cardiovascular function is usually maintained.

- **Conscious sedation**: Drug-induced depression of consciousness, similar to moderate sedation, except that verbal contact is always maintained with the patient. This term is used commonly in dentistry.
- **Deep sedation**: Drug-induced depression of consciousness during which patients are asleep and cannot be easily roused but do respond purposefully to repeated or painful stimulation. The ability to maintain ventilatory function independently may be impaired. Patients may require assistance to maintain a patent airway. Spontaneous ventilation may be inadequate. Cardiovascular function is usually maintained.

(NICE 2010)

Technical problems

It is vital that any faulty equipment is fixed and the safety of children, staff and environment is maintained. If any of the following technical problems occur they should be reported to the hospital's engineering department immediately:

- Equipment not delivering gas
- Leak at joint between regulator and cylinder valve
- Demand valve leaks or does not shut cleanly
- Demand valve does not stop giving flow after test button is released.

Procedure guideline 21.7 **After use**

Statement	Rationale
1. Once the procedure has finished:	**1.**
a) Ensure that the child is comfortable.	
b) Order a new cylinder if required.	**b–c)** To ensure there is an adequate supply for the next child.
c) Check and document the cylinder gauge level.	
d) Turn off the cylinder and depressurise the system fully by operating the test button.	**d)** To prevent misuse and to maintain a safe ward environment.

(Continued)

Procedure guideline 21.7 (*Continued*)

Statement	Rationale
2. Document that Entonox has been given: • On the audit form • In the child's healthcare records.	**2.** To document outcomes of care and promote evidence-based practice.
3. Children should not walk around unaided until any dizziness or disorientation has gone. Monitoring should continue for 30 minutes to ensure that the effects of the Entonox have completely worn off.	**3.** To prevent the child from injury.
4. If the Entonox is used infrequently the cylinder should be checked weekly and its contents recorded. A member of the ward staff should be responsible for ensuring that the equipment is checked regularly.	**4.** To maintain a safe environment and to ensure equipment is in good working order.
5. To clean the equipment: • Depressurise the system • Clean the external surfaces of the demand valve with an alcohol based wipe • If any contamination is suspected between the hose connection into the demand valve it must be sent to HSDU to be autoclaved • Multi-use face masks and mouthpieces should be autoclaved at 121°C by HSDU • Single use face masks and mouthpieces should be discarded • The external surfaces of the administration set should be cleaned with an alcohol based wipe • Filters are for single child use and should be discarded.	**5.** To maintain a safe environment and prevent infection.

Procedure guideline 21.8 **Storage**

Statement	Rationale
1. Entonox cylinders should be kept in a secure environment, attached to a wall or trolley and away from children when not in use.	**1.** To maintain a safe environment.
2. If cylinders are stored outside in cold weather they must be brought inside at least 24 hours before use and stored horizontally.	**2.** The gases will separate if cylinders are stored at temperatures below −6°C. Storing horizontally at 10°C for 24 hours will correct this (BOC 1995).
3. As with all pressurised gases, Entonox should not come into contact with a naked flame.	**3.** Nitrous oxide supports combustion and may produce toxic or corrosive fumes if exposed to fire.

Epidural analgesia

The epidural space is situated between the dura mater (the outer layer of the meninges) and the vertebral canal. It extends from the cranium to the sacrum and contains loose connective tissue, fat, lymph vessels, blood vessels and nerves. Analgesics administered into the epidural space diffuse across the dura and the subarachnoid space and bind to receptors located in the substantia gelatinosa in the dorsal horn of the spinal cord. They also exert an effect on the nerve roots outside the dura mater, are absorbed systemically from epidural blood vessels, and are distributed in the cerebrospinal fluid (CSF). The epidural route is commonly used to manage intra-operative and post-operative pain associated with a variety of procedures. Less commonly, it can be used to control non-surgical or chronic pain. An epidural catheter is inserted into an anaesthetised child by a consultant anaesthetist with experience in paediatrics, or an anaesthetic registrar (SpR) under supervision. In infants under 6 months or 5 kg, the catheter is sometimes inserted via the sacral hiatus (caudal route) and threaded into the epidural space until the appropriate level has been reached.

Local anaesthetics and analgesics can be administered separately or in combination. Intra-operatively these may be given either as a single bolus dose or as an infusion. Post-operative epidural analgesia is usually provided by a continuous infusion via a syringe driver or volumetric pump. The drugs most commonly used to provide analgesia include local anaesthetics and opioids. Each opioid has its advantages and disadvantages and different side effect profiles. Morphine has a slower onset, but longer duration of action than fentanyl and diamorphine (Rowney and Doyle 1998). In neonates, children with sensitivity to opioids, or those at risk of opioid-related complications, local anaesthetic alone may be used. Less commonly, other drugs such as ketamine and clonidine are also administered via the epidural route.

All staff caring for children with an epidural must be trained and competent to do so. Pumps should be standardised and training in their use should be provided (NPSA 2007). Infusion rates, syringe changes and technical problems should be managed by staff who have had additional training and work within written local guidelines (DoH 2004b; Royal College of Anaesthetists (RCOA) 2004).

Principles table 21.4 Assessment and preparation (epidural)

Principle	Rationale
1. Prior to surgery/insertion of the epidural the anaesthetist will consider: **a)** The benefits and risks of an epidural for each individual child. **b)** The effectiveness of epidural analgesia for the type of surgery/pain.	**1.** To ensure that potential risks are balanced against the benefits (Llewellyn and Moriarty 2007).
2a) Parents/carers should be given written and verbal information regarding available methods of pain relief. An anaesthetist will discuss the epidural with the child and family prior to theatre and obtain verbal consent for the procedure. **b)** If verbal consent is not obtained, alternative analgesia will be provided. NB Although only verbal consent is required in the UK, other countries require written consent.	**2a)** To provide information and facilitate informed consent. An information leaflet is available online at www.gosh.nhs.uk/medical-conditions/procedures-and-treatments/pain-relief-after-surgery-using-an-epidural/. **b)** To meet the family's wishes and provide satisfactory analgesia.
3. The anaesthetist may choose not to insert an epidural if the child presents with: **a)** Local or generalised sepsis or a pyrexia of unknown origin. **b)** Coagulation disorders or anticoagulation therapy. **c)** Some diseases of the central nervous system. **d)** Spinal deformity.	**3.** To avoid the risk of epidural-related complications. **a)** To avoid the risk of a centralised infection. **b)** To avoid the risk of a subdural haematoma. **c)** To minimise the risk of exacerbation of the disease. **d)** This may make it impossible to insert the epidural catheter.
4. The child and family should be prepared for the epidural. They should be made aware that: • The epidural will be inserted once the child has been anaesthetised • If the procedure is unsuccessful alternative analgesia will be prescribed.	**4.** To meet information needs and minimise uncertainty and anxiety.
5. Nursing staff should also ensure that: • Any tools that will be used to assess pain are explained to the child/family on admission • Words the child uses for pain and the child's usual pain related behaviours are recorded on their care plan.	**5.** To provide knowledge and obtain information to facilitate accurate assessment of pain (see 'pain assessment' section for further details).
6. The following baseline observations should also be recorded before the child goes to theatre: • Temperature • Heart rate • Respiratory rate • Blood pressure.	**6.** To establish normal parameters with which to compare future observations. Deviation from baseline observations may indicate epidural related side effects or complications.
7. Any neurological abnormality (e.g. altered sensation, limb weakness) should be reported to the anaesthetist and recorded in the child's healthcare records.	**7.** To identify current abnormalities, which if undetected, may be attributed to or exacerbated by the epidural at a later stage.

Principles table 21.5 Drug administration

Principles	Rationale
1. A single bolus of local anaesthetic is usually given initially by the anaesthetist, either through the epidural needle or once the catheter is in position.	**1.** To establish the initial block and provide effective analgesia.
2. Additional boluses may be given intra-operatively or an infusion commenced.	**2.** To provide effective analgesia.
3. A continuous infusion may be administered either via a syringe driver or volumetric pump system according to local policy. See 'Setting up of an Infusion', Chapter 13. In addition, the following principles should be applied: **a)** Only appropriately trained staff working within written hospital guidelines should change epidural infusion rates and syringes or bags. **b)** Pumps and infusion sets should be clearly identifiable as being for epidural use only. **c)** All syringes and equipment should be handled using an aseptic technique. **d)** An epidural filter should always be used.	**3.** To provide effective analgesia with minimal risk of complications. **a–b)** To minimise the risk of drug errors (NPSA 2007, RCOA 2004). **c)** To minimise the risk of infection. **d)** To minimise the risk of infection and nerve damage.
4. By 2013, all epidural infusions and boluses must include connectors that cannot connect with intravenous Luer connectors or intravenous infusion spikes (NPSA 2011).	**4.** To reduce the risk of drugs being given via the wrong route.

Procedure guideline 21.9 Transfer of child (following epidural insertion)

For care of the child during the peri-operative period see Chapter 23.

Statement	Rationale
1. When collecting the child from theatre a verbal report should be obtained from the recovery nurse. This should include details of: • Any intra-operative analgesia and other drugs given • The epidural solution and infusion rate • Any pain or epidural related complications that have been experienced intra-operatively.	**1.** To provide adequate information.
2. The nurse collecting the child should ensure that: **a)** The drug being administered has been prescribed correctly. **b)** The pump's settings have been checked. **c)** The child's pain is being managed effectively. **d)** The child is not excessively sedated. **e)** All documentation has been completed. **f)** **NALOXONE** has been prescribed **BEFORE** the child leaves recovery.	**2.** **a–b)** To prevent drug errors. Any differences between the prescription and the pump settings/syringe label should, ideally, be rectified before the child leaves recovery. **c–d)** To provide effective analgesia with minimal side-effects. **e)** To provide adequate information. **f)** To facilitate immediate treatment of opiate-induced respiratory depression.

Procedure guideline 21.10 **Nursing care of epidural (general)**

Statement	Rationale
1. A care plan/pathway should be available and should be adapted for each individual child.	**1.** To ensure adequate information is recorded.
2. Supplementary analgesia, i.e. paracetamol and an NSAID if possible (e.g. diclofenac or ibruprofen), should be given regularly.	**2.** To provide optimal analgesia. Multi-modal analgesia is more effective than single route analgesia (Macintyre et al 2010).
3. The child should be encouraged to mobilise if their condition allows. Ensure that: **a)** The child is accompanied at all times while mobilising and is accompanied by a staff nurse if leaving the ward. **b)** Older children are warned that they may experience some dizziness initially when mobilising	**3.** Early mobilisation improves circulation, respiratory effort and reduces the risk of complications (NICE 2001). **a)** To prevent falls, complications and inadvertent catheter removal. **b)** Local anaesthetics affect the sympathetic nervous system and can cause hypotension (Gunter 2002).
4. Children with numb or heavy legs, and those on bed rest or reluctant to mobilise should receive regular pressure area care.	**4.** To minimise the risk of pressure sores (for more information on pressure sore prevention see Chapter 10).
5. a) Intravenous access should be available throughout the duration of the epidural and for 6–12 hours after it has been discontinued. **b)** If the cannula has tissued, intramuscular naloxone may be given, but this has a longer onset of action than when given intravenously.	**5. a)** To enable the administration of naloxone by the quickest route if respiratory depression occurs. Morphine remains in the CSF for longer than fentanyl or diamorphine and the risk of respiratory depression is prolonged. **b)** Onset of action is longer if the drug is given via the intramuscular route.

Procedure guideline 21.11 **Nursing care of an epidural (observations)**

Statement	Rationale
1. All observations should be documented in the child's healthcare record. This should include: • Pain scores • Level of sedation • Presence, incidence and severity of any epidural or opioid-related side-effects • Condition of the epidural entry site • The height (dermatome level) and density (e.g. Bromage score) of the block (see point 2 below) • Respiratory rate, pulse and blood pressure • Fluid balance.	**1.** To provide accurate information and early detection of potential complications. See Figure 21.4 for an example of scoring tools and documentation. For the management of epidural and opioid-related side effects and complications see the following sections.

2a) The height of the block is most effectively checked using ice. Touch the ice on the arm or cheek to identify that it is cold. Then work down each side of the body asking the child if they feel hot, warm, cold or no sensation. There is no sensory block in areas where the child can feel cold. The child needs to be able to communicate and willing to cooperate for this test to be effective.
    If the block is at T3 or above the epidural should be suspended.
b) The density of the block is measured by asking the child to bend their knees or move their feet.
c) If the score is 3 the epidural infusion should be suspended or the rate reduced.
d) For thoracic epidurals, ask the child to squeeze your finger, comparing the strength in both hands, then ask them to raise their arms.
e) If the block is too high, STOP the infusion.
	2a) If the block is too low or unilateral (one-sided) the child will feel pain. If the block is too high it may affect the accessory muscles, causing shallow breathing or cause other complications. This test can also help to identify a patchy or unilateral block.
	    For dermatome map, see Figure 21.5.
	    To prevent complications.
	b) The higher the Bromage score, the denser the block (Figure 21.6).
	c) A dense/heavy block (no movement) is unpleasant and greatly increases the risk of pressure sores.
	d) To determine the height of the block.
	e) A high block can affect respiratory function.

557

name _____

hospital no. _____

date _____

Epidural
Observation & Pain Assessment Chart

Instructions – *refer to Clinical Practice Guidelines*

NB: Record ALL observations and assessments AT LEAST HOURLY

Which pain assessment tool(s) are being used?		
	Patient	VAS / Faces / Other
	Parent	FLACC / Other
	Health prof	FLACC / Other

Pain assessment frequency

HOURLY for total duration of infusion +12 hours after cessation

Continue **every 4 hours** on *'Pain Assessment Chart'*

TIME	TOTAL VOL		SYRING: reading	EPIDURAL site	Bromage	Dermatomes Left Right	Pressure Area	N & V	Pruritus	Sedation	PAIN ASSESSMENT patient	parent	health prof	COMMENTS details, interventions and reviews	SIGN
	running	hourly													
00 - 01															
01 - 02															
02 - 03															
03 - 04															
04 - 05															
05 - 06															
06 - 07															
07 - 08															
08 - 09															
09 - 10															
10 - 11															
11 - 12															
12 - 13															
13 - 14															
14 - 15															
15 - 16															
16 - 17															
17 - 18															
18 - 19															
19 - 20															
20 - 21															
21 - 22															
22 - 23															
23 - 24															

SCORES (at least hourly)

© Pain Control Service, GOSH NHS Foundation Trust May 2006

Figure 21.4a Epidural documentation.

Epidural Observations

Sedation Scores

0 Awake / alert
1 Sleepy / responds appropriately
2 Somnolent / rousable (light stimuli)
3 Deep sleep / rousable (deeper physical stimuli)
  Intervene
4 Unrousable to stimuli
  Stop infusion / Bleep 0577

BJA 88(2): 241-5 (2002)

Bromage Score

3 **Stop infusion & contact Pain Team (Bleep 0577)**

2 **Reduce infusion rate by 0.1ml/kg/hr every 12 hours**
  (Extended role for senior nurses)

1 **Observe Hourly**

0 **No intervention required**
  Patient may mobilise with supervision

Bromage 3 (complete)
Unable to move feet or knees

Bromage 2 (almost complete)
Able to move feet only

Bromage 1 (partial)
Just able to move knees

Bromage 0 (none)
Full flexion of knees and feet

Bromage PR (1978) "Epidural Analgesia" WB Saunders (ed), Philadelphia,

Pressure Area Care

S = Sitting   M = Mobilising
R = on Right side F = on Front
L = on Left side   B = on Back

Nausea & Vomiting

1 None
2 Nausea
3 Vomited

Pain Scores

0   No pain
1 - 3 Mild pain
4 - 7 Moderate pain
8 - 10 Severe pain *

Pruritus

1 Slight
2 Moderate
3 Severe

Dermatome Level

Should be documented:
- In recovery
- At the start of each shift
- If the patient is in pain
- 30 minutes after increasing or decreasing epidural infusion

N.B. Level should not be >T3

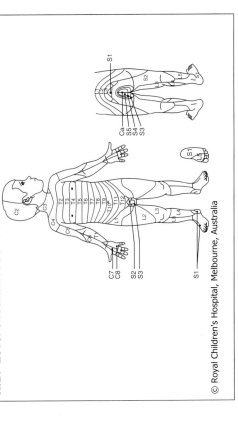

© Royal Children's Hospital, Melbourne, Australia

Epidural Site

R = Red
S = Swelling / Lump
L = Leaking
P = Painful
T = Related Pyrexia

© Pain Control Service, GOSH NHS Foundation Trust May 2006

Figure 21.4b Epidural documentation.

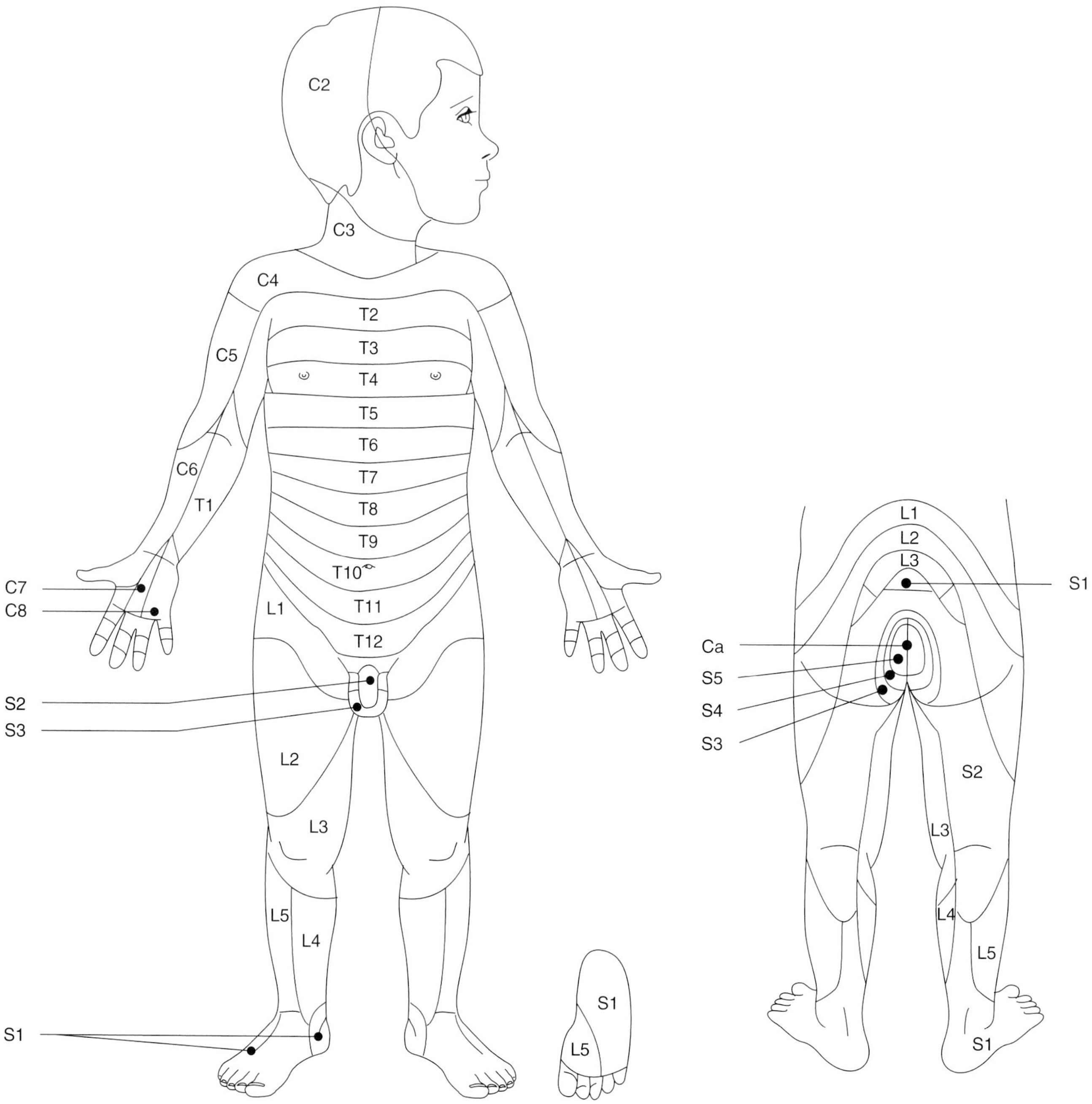

Figure 21.5 Sensory map for dermatome level testing.
© Royal Children's Hospital, Melbourne, Australia – available online at: http://www.rch.org.au/anaes/pain/index.cfm?doc_id=9588.

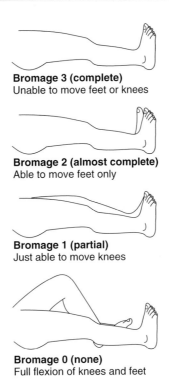

Bromage 3 (complete)
Unable to move feet or knees

Bromage 2 (almost complete)
Able to move feet only

Bromage 1 (partial)
Just able to move knees

Bromage 0 (none)
Full flexion of knees and feet

Figure 21.6 Bromage score (Bromage 1978).

Procedure guideline 21.12 Epidural-related complications

See section on prevention and management of opioid-related complications.

Statement	Rationale
Pain	

1. Assess the level of the block.
   a) If it is too low and the child is not experiencing side effects the infusion rate could be increased.
   b) If it is unilateral or patchy an increase in the rate may also improve the level of pain relief. However, it may be necessary to carefully remove the dressing and pull back the catheter by 0.5–1 cm. This should only be done by an appropriately trained person, usually an anaesthetist.
	1. To establish whether the pain is due to a low, unilateral or patchy block and rectify this if possible.

2. Administer simple analgesics, i.e. paracetamol and an NSAID if appropriate.	**2.** To provide optimal pain relief. Multimodal is more effective than a single mode of analgesia (Macintyre *et al* 2010).
3. It may help to reposition the child.	**3.** To relieve pressure/discomfort.
4. Administer prescribed co-analgesics as appropriate (e.g. anti-spasmodic drugs).	**4.** To treat other causes of pain.
5. Involve parents/carers, play specialist and psychologist if the pain is anxiety related.	**5.** To manage the emotional component of the pain.
6. If the pain is unmanageable or indicative of surgical complications or other cause contact the surgeons, anaesthetist or pain team as appropriate.	**6.** To obtain advice regarding the cause of the pain and the most appropriate intervention.

(Continued)

561

Procedure guideline 21.12 (*Continued*)

Statement	Rationale
7. Some patients may benefit from having a plain epidural (local anaesthetic only) and either oral or intravenous opioids for breakthrough pain.	**7.** To provide effective analgesia.

Urinary retention

Statement	Rationale
1. If the child has no urinary catheter, urine output should be monitored closely.	**1.** Opiates bind to receptors in the bladder, reducing the ability to detect changes in pressure as the bladder fills. Local anaesthetics will also have an effect on bladder sensitivity.
2. The non-verbal child should be observed for signs of increased discomfort. If they have not passed urine recently the bladder should be palpated. Intervention is required if: • The child has a palpable bladder • The verbal child complains of discomfort/inability to pass urine • The length of time since last urine output is excessive and the child is not dehydrated.	**2.** Urinary retention causes abdominal distension, pain and can cause further complications. Increased discomfort or distress in a non-verbal children is sometimes be mistaken for surgical pain.
3. Urinary retention should be treated as follows: **a)** Administer naloxone (0.5 μg/kg) as prescribed. **b)** Four doses can be given at ten-minute intervals. **c)** If not effective, the doses may be repeated after an hour. **d)** A urinary catheter may need to be inserted. This should remain in situ until the epidural infusion is discontinued.	**3.** To maintain adequate urine output. **a)** To reverse opiate-induced retention. **b)** This may reduce the effectiveness of the analgesia. **c)** Naloxone is short acting. **d)** To prevent further complications.
4. If the child has a urinary catheter this should remain in situ until the epidural infusion is discontinued.	**4.** To minimise the risk of retention.

Local anaesthetic toxicity

Statement	Rationale
1. Local anaesthetic toxicity is rare but is most likely in the following situations: **a)** If the drug is accidentally administered intravenously. **b)** In neonates and babies if high rates are infused for long periods. **c)** In children with renal failure.	**1.** **a)** Local anaesthetics should not be given intravenously. **b–c)** Accumulation may occur due to immature or reduced renal function.
2. Observe the child for a reaction to local anaesthetic. Signs include: • Tingling mouth and lips • Increased anxiety • Irritability • Sedation • Nausea • Hypotension • Respiratory distress • Cardiac arrhythmias • Convulsions.	**2.** To ensure prompt detection and prevent worsening of the problem.
3. If any of the above are observed: **a)** Stop the infusion. **b)** Administer basic life support if necessary. **c)** Contact the anaesthetist, surgeon or pain team for advice regarding analgesia.	**3.** **a)** To prevent further accumulation. **b)** To stabilise the child. **c)** To identify an alternative method of analgesia.

The Association of Anaesthetists of Great Britain land Ireland (AAGBI 2010) have provided guidelines for the Management of Severe Local Anaesthetic Toxicity, http://www.aagbi.org/sites/default/files/la_toxicity_2010_0.pdf

Procedure guideline 21.12 (*Continued*)

Statement	Rationale
Epidural entry site	
1. The epidural catheter entry site should be observed when turning the child and at least four hourly.	**1.** To ensure prompt detection of leaking or infection.
2. If leaking occurs:	**2.** This is not uncommon and may not cause any problems, but has the potential to do so.
a) Observe the entry site more frequently, 1–2 hourly if possible.	**a)** To ensure the dressing remains intact and observe for signs of infection.
b) If the dressing starts to peel off, place a new one over the top.	**b)** To minimise the risk of leaking and infection.
c) Removal of the dressing should only be done by a person with advanced training when absolutely necessary.	**c)** To prevent displacement of the catheter.
3. If the dressing falls off:	**3.**
a) Put a new sterile transparent occlusive hypoallergenic dressing on immediately.	**a)** To prevent displacement of the catheter.
b) Contact the pain team/anaesthetist to check the position of the catheter.	**b)** The catheter may have become dislodged and will need to be removed if it is no longer effective.
4. If the child becomes uncomfortable due to the leaking epidural the following actions may be carried out by an appropriately trained individual:	**4.** Excessive leakage may result in ineffective analgesia.
a) Increase the epidural rate if the child is in pain.	**a)** To provide effective analgesia.
b) If the child has no surgical pain reducing the rate may reduce the leaking.	**b)** To prevent further leaking.
c) Redress the entry site.	**c)** If the catheter is kinked under the skin this may relieve the pressure and stop the leaking.
d) Remove the epidural and arrange alternative analgesia.	**d)** Continual leaking increases the risk of epidural site infection. To provide effective analgesia with minimal complications.
Infection	
1. Prompt action should be taken if: • The entry site becomes red or swollen • The catheter has become displaced • The dressing has fallen off • There is excessive leaking of fluid around the entry site • The child has a pyrexia of unknown origin or other signs of unexplained infection.	**1.** To ensure swift action to prevent/treat any potential infection.
2. If an epidural infection is suspected, inform the anaesthetist/pain team/surgeon. The following actions should be taken:	**2.** To ensure prompt, effective treatment and minimise the risk of complications.
a) Remove the epidural catheter.	**a)** To eliminate a potential source of infection.
b) Swab the entry site.	**b)** To identify the micro-organisms that need to be treated.
c) The catheter tip should only be sent to microbiology if a centralised infection is suspected.	**c)** Routine culture of catheter tips is not a good predictor of epidural infection (Seth *et al* 2004).
d) Consider starting antibiotics if the child is clinically unwell.	**d)** To minimise the risks and potential complications of infection.
e) Follow up swab results.	**e, f)** To ensure that the correct antibiotic has been prescribed.
f) Commence antibiotics as appropriate for any micro-organisms isolated.	
g) Document and report the incident as per local policy.	**g)** To ensure effective communication.

(*Continued*)

Procedure guideline 21.12 (*Continued*)

Statement	Rationale
3. Follow up should continue until the infection has cleared. If an epidural abscess is suspected an emergency scan should be arranged and a neurologist involved.	**3.** To minimise the risk of complications.

Neurological complications

Statement	Rationale
1. Neurological complications are rare, but can have serious consequences. Contact the anaesthetist, surgeon or pain team if any of the following are observed: **a)** Headache. **b)** Loss of motor function, sensation or other signs of neurological deterioration.	**1.** Swift action is required to determine the cause (if possible), treat, and to prevent further deterioration. Symptoms may be indicative of: **a)** Dural tap or centralised infection. **b)** Nerve damage/abscess.
2. Record symptoms and any action taken in the child's healthcare records.	**2.** To maintain an accurate record. Long-term follow-up may be required.
3. If neurological damage or an abscess is suspected, the child should be referred to a neurologist for further investigations.	**3.** To obtain specialist advice and ensure prompt detection and appropriate treatment of the problem.

Procedure guideline 21.13 **Technical problems**

Statement	Rationale

Pump occlusion

Statement	Rationale
1. If the pump occludes: **a)** Stop the infusion. **b)** Check that the catheter is not kinked or trapped. **c)** Ensure that the correct administration set is being used. **d)** Check the pump: Pressures may need to be increased or the pump replaced. **e)** Any faulty pumps must be reported.	**1.** **a)** To determine the cause. **b)** Kinked or trapped tubing can cause occlusion. **c–e)** To prevent drug administration errors occurring due to the use of faulty equipment.
2. The following interventions should only be attempted by an anaesthetist or other suitably trained individual: **a)** Check the filter to ensure the connection is not too tight. **b)** Attempt to flush the catheter from the filter with 2 ml of 0.9% sodium chloride for injection in a 5 ml syringe. **c)** Observe and redress the entry site if necessary. If the catheter is kinked under the skin it may be possible to correct this by pulling the catheter back by 0.5–1 cm before redressing.	**2.** To safely determine the cause of the occlusion and attempt to correct it. **a)** A tight connection will increase pressure/resistance. **b)** To determine whether the source of the occlusion is below the filter. Flushing the line may also clear the occlusion. **c)** The catheter may be kinked under the dressing or skin.
3. If these interventions are unsuccessful the epidural may need to be removed and alternative analgesia prescribed.	**3.** To provide effective analgesia.

Catheter disconnection

Statement	Rationale
1. Only appropriately trained staff, working within written hospital/local guidelines should reconnect the filter.	**1.** To minimise the risk of errors and complications (RCOA 2004).

Principles guideline 21.13 *(Continued)*

Statement	Rationale
2. If the catheter becomes disconnected from the filter the following actions may be necessary: **a)** Wrap the filter and catheter in sterile paper. **b)** Do not clamp the epidural catheter. **c)** Stop the infusion.	**2.** These practices should be agreed with at local level with microbiology. **a)** To minimise the risk of infection. **b)** To prevent kinking of the catheter. **c)** To prevent further leakage.
3. The epidural catheter can be reconnected if: • The disconnection occurred less than 2 hours earlier • The fluid level within the catheter does not drop when held at child level • There is less than 2 inches of air the catheter.	**3.** To provide effective analgesia while minimising the risk of infection (Kost-Byerly *et al* 1998, Langevin 1996, McNeely and Trentadue 1997).
4. Reconnect the catheter using an aseptic technique: • Perform a surgical hand wash • Put on a non-sterile apron and sterile gloves • Clean the catheter with an alcohol impregnated swab • With sterile scissors, cut off the section of catheter with air in • Reconnect catheter to the filter • Dispose of used equipment according to local waste policy • Record action in the child's notes.	**4.** To provide effective analgesia while minimising the risk of infection/air in the epidural space.
5. The epidural catheter must be removed if: • It has been disconnected for longer than 2 hours • The catheter is or could have been contaminated • This is a third disconnection.	**5.** To minimise the risk of infection.
6. If the epidural catheter has to be removed, alternative analgesia should be prescribed.	**6.** To provide effective analgesia via an alternative route.

Procedure guideline 21.14 **Discontinuing the epidural**

Statement	Rationale
1. An epidural catheter is usually left in situ for a maximum of 5 days. Local guidelines will vary. Policies should be agreed in liaison with microbiology.	**1.** The risk of infection increases the longer the catheter stays in.
2. If rectal or oral analgesia is not appropriate or sufficient after this period, alternative analgesia (e.g. intravenous patient or nurse controlled analgesia) must be provided.	**2.** To provide effective analgesia with minimal complications. Intravenous opiates may be required.
3. If the epidural catheter is pulled out inadvertently: **a)** Reassure the child. **b)** Put a spot plaster over the entry site. **c)** Check that the catheter is intact.	**3.** **a)** To reduce anxiety. **b)** To minimise the risk of infection. **c)** To ensure that none remains in the epidural space.
4. Prior to the removal of the epidural catheter: **a)** Prepare the child. **b)** Check that the child has no clotting abnormality **c)** If the child has abnormal clotting or is on anticoagulation therapy, discuss with a consultant before removal.	**4.** **a)** To reduce anxiety and minimise the risk of complications. **b–c)** To minimise the risk of bleeding into the epidural space.

(Continued)

Procedure guideline 21.14 (*Continued*)

Statement	Rationale
5. Only suitably trained and competent individuals, working with written local guidelines should remove an epidural catheter.	**5.** To minimise the risk of complications.
6. To remove the epidural catheter: **a)** Gather equipment: • Plastic apron and non-sterile gloves • Spot plaster • Plaster remover • Microbiology swab. **b)** Put on a plastic apron and perform a surgical hand wash. **c)** Position the child comfortably, either on their side or sitting upright. **d)** Remove the dressing using plaster remover. **e)** Put on gloves. **f)** Gently pull the catheter out. **g)** Check that the catheter is intact. **h)** Swab the entry site if red or swollen. **i)** Place a small plaster over the site. **j)** Dispose of used equipment according to local hospital policy. **k)** The plaster should remain in situ for at least 24 hours, after which time the site should have healed.	**6.** **a)** To ensure procedure is carried out with minimal disruption and delay. **b)** To minimise the risk of infection. **c)** For ease of removal. **d)** To cause minimal distress to the child. **e)** To minimise the risk of infection. **f–g)** To ensure that the catheter is removed intact. **h)** To ensure early detection and treatment of infection. **i–k)** To minimise the risk of infection.
7. Any pain, swelling or redness that develops at the entry site after the catheter has been removed should be reported to the pain team or anaesthetist.	**7.** To ensure prompt detection and treatment of infection.
8. If the entry site has been swabbed: **a)** Microbiology results should be checked. **b)** The child's progress reviewed.	**8.** **a)** To ensure that the appropriate antibiotics are/have been prescribed. **b)** To detect and treat complications.

Patient and nurse controlled analgesia (PCA/NCA)

The use of patient controlled (PCA) and nurse controlled analgesia (NCA) has been shown to provide a safe and effective technique for the administration of intravenous or subcutaneous opioids for the relief of pain. (Anderson *et al* 1998, Bray 1983, Doyle *et al* 1993). Patient controlled analgesia refers to a method of pain control that allows the child to press a button to self-administer a pre-programmed amount of an intravenous or subcutaneous opioid (the bolus dose) after a set period of time (the lockout interval). The child may also receive a very small background infusion of the opioid and the pump is programmed with a short lockout interval (5–10 minutes). Nurse controlled analgesia refers to a technique by which the nurse may press a button to give the child a pre-programmed amount of an intravenous or subcutaneous opioid (the bolus dose) after a set period of time (the lockout period). The pump is programmed with a longer lockout interval (20–30 minutes) and the child may be given a larger continuous infusion of the opioid. Neonates, children with renal impairment, or those with sensitivity to mor-

phine may require smaller boluses and no background infusion. Neonates in particular should be closely monitored, as they are at increased risk of sedation and respiratory depression (Howard *et al* 2010).

Patient and nurse controlled analgesia are most commonly used following surgery, but can also be effective for the management of non-surgical pain such as sickle crisis, pancreatitis and cancer related pain and can also be used to manage pain prior to surgery. Staff should be aware that once pain is effectively managed its value as a diagnostic tool is weakened and other indicators of possible deterioration in the child's condition must be observed more closely. Morphine is considered to be the 'gold standard' for intravenous analgesia and is therefore usually the opioid of choice (Lloyd-Thomas 1999). The use of other opioids should only be considered when morphine is contra-indicated.

A child's ability to use patient controlled analgesia depends on their cognitive and motor ability and individual selection is essential, but the technique can be used by some children as young a 4–5 years of age (Llewellyn 1993). The use of PCA and NCA requires a specially designed pump which allows for programming of a continuous infusion rate (if required), bolus dose and lockout interval. Pumps should be standardised and training in their use should be provided (DoH 2004b). All personnel who care for children receiving PCA or NCA must be trained and competent to do so. Additional training should be provided for staff who programme the pumps.

Principles table 21.6 Initial assessment for PCA/NCA

Principle	Rationale
1. Prior to surgery/setting up the infusion the anaesthetist must consider the following: • The suitability of PCA/NCA for each individual child • The effectiveness of PCA/NCA for the type of surgery/pain.	1. To ensure that potential risks are balanced against the benefits.
2. If the child is going to use PCA they must be: • Able to press the button on the handset • Able to understand the technique • Willing to use it.	2. To ensure that the most appropriate technique is used for the child.

Procedure guideline 21.15 Preparation for PCA/NCA use

Statement	Rationale
1. An anaesthetist will discuss the use of PCA/NCA with the child and family prior to surgery/setting up the infusion.	1. To provide information.
2. Written and verbal information should be given to prepare the child and family for the PCA/NCA: **a)** The nursing staff and/or play specialist should explain the technique to the child and family. **b)** The family should be made aware that if the child is unable to use PCA the pump can be changed to NCA programming. NCA may also be changed to PCA at a later date if the child is able and willing to press the button themselves. **c)** The child should be shown the pump and handset before going to theatre.	2. **a)** To meet information needs and reduce anxiety (www.gosh.nhs.uk/medical-conditions/procedures-and-treatments/pain-relief-for-your-child-after-surgery-pca-and-nca/). **b)** To provide the most suitable method of pain relief tailored to the individual child's needs.
3. Nursing staff should also ensure that: • Any tools that will be used to assess pain are explained to the child/family on admission • Words the child uses for pain and the child's usual pain related behaviour are recorded on their care plan.	3. To provide knowledge and obtain information, which will facilitate accurate assessment of pain (see 'pain assessment' section for further details).
4. The following baseline observations should be recorded before the child goes to theatre: • Heart rate • Respiratory rate • Blood pressure.	4. To establish normal parameters with which to compare future observations.
5. Oxygen saturations should also be recorded for: • Neonates • Children with a respiratory condition • Children with a sensitivity to morphine • Any other children with an increased risk of sedation/respiratory compromise.	5. To establish normal parameters with which to compare future observations. These children will require oxygen saturation monitoring during opioid administration.

567

Procedure guideline 21.16 Setting up a PCA/NCA infusion

Statement	Rationale
1. Detailed instructions for setting up infusions are included in Chapter 13. The following principles are specific to setting up a PCA/NCA infusion:	**1.** See Chapter 13 for more information.
a) The PCA/NCA pump must only be programmed by a suitably trained person working within written hospital guidelines. Standardised hospital pump programming and drug concentrations should be used at all times.	**a–b)** To prevent drug errors and to provide effective analgesia with minimal risk of complications.
b) Local procedures for drawing up and administering a controlled drug will apply.	
c) If the intravenous route is not available the subcutaneous route may be used. However, this should be avoided if the child has poor peripheral circulation, infected skin, or clotting problems.	**c)** To avoid the risk of intermittent absorption, infection, or further damage to the skin.
2. Gather and prepare the following equipment:	**2.**
a) 50 ml Luer lock syringe.	
b) 5% glucose solution OR 0.9% saline (saline must be used if the drug is being administered via the subcutaneous route).	
c) Morphine or other opioid – as prescribed.	
d) An administration set with an antisyphon valve for dedicated lines OR	**d)** To prevent free flow of fluid through gravity (Southern and Read 1994).
e) An antisyphon and anti-reflux administration set if running fluids via the same line.	**e)** To prevent the opioid backtracking and accumulating in other lines.
3. To make up the infusion:	**3.**
a) Draw up the glucose or saline in the 50 ml syringe, add the opioid and mix well.	**a)** To ensure an even spread of the drug throughout the syringe.
b) Attach the antisyphon or antisyphon and anti-reflux administration set and prime the line.	**b)** To prevent syphonage and reflux.
c) Ensure that both the syringe and line are labelled.	**c)** To provide accurate information and prevent drug errors.
d) Place 50 ml syringe in pump and purge the solution through the line.	**d)** To prevent administration errors due to mechanical slack.
e) Flush the cannula or line and attach the infusion.	**e)** To ensure that the cannula and line are patent and prevent mixing of drugs.
f) Ensure that the pump programming is checked before starting the infusion.	**f)** To prevent drug errors.
4. When the infusion is commenced an initial 'loading' dose may be given by an appropriately trained person. This is particularly important for children in severe pain, e.g. sickle cell crisis.	**4.** To establish initial pain relief (RCPCH 1997).
5. If the pump is set up on the ward the nurse should ensure that:	**5.**
a) The drug being administered corresponds with the prescription chart.	**a–b)** To adhere to hospital drug policy and prevent drug errors.
b) The pump programming has been checked.	
c) Naloxone has also been prescribed.	**c)** To allow for immediate treatment of opioid induced respiratory depression.
d) These checks should be carried out at the handover of each shift to ensure that the correct drug is being infused at the correct rate, via the correct line.	**d)** To minimise the risk of drug errors.

568

Procedure guideline 21.16 (*Continued*)

Statement	Rationale
6. If the pump has been set up in theatre/recovery, a verbal report should be obtained from the recovery nurse. This should include details of: • Intra-operative analgesia and other drugs given • Drug concentration and pump programming • Any pain-related complications that have been experienced peri-operatively.	**6.** To provide adequate information.
7. Before leaving theatre the nurse should check: • The drug being administered corresponds with the prescription chart • The pump programming is correct • The child's pain is being managed effectively • The child is not excessively sedated • All documentation has been completed.	**7.** To prevent drug errors and minimise the risk of complications.
8. Naloxone should be prescribed **before** the child leaves theatre.	**8.** To enable immediate treatment of opioid induced respiratory depression.
9. Background infusions should usually be reduced or stopped before the NCA/PCA is stopped.	**9.** To ensure that the child is comfortable without a continuous infusion.
10. Syringes and administration sets must be changed every 24–48 hours according to local policy.	**10.** To reduce the risk of infection. This should be agreed locally with pharmacy and microbiology.

Procedure guideline 21.17 Technical problems (PCA/NCA)

Statement	Rationale
1. If the pump alarms: **a)** Stop the infusion. **b)** Check the display panel. **c)** If the line has occluded: • check for kinks or closed clamps • flush the cannula • restart the infusion. **d)** If the syringe is empty a new syringe will need to be made up. **e)** If alarm is due to flat battery plug the pump into the mains. **f)** If the pump is faulty it will need to be replaced and returned to biomedical engineering with a label describing the fault. **g)** If the cause of the alarm is unknown contact the engineer/pain team.	**1.** **a–e)** To determine and correct the cause of the problem. **f, g)** To prevent administration errors due to faulty equipment. The pump will need to be replaced.
2. All faulty pumps must be removed from service and reported to the appropriate department (e.g. risk management, biomedical engineering).	**2.** To prevent administration errors due to faulty equipment.

Procedure guideline 21.18 Care of the child receiving PCA/NCA

Statement	Rationale
1. Record pain scores hourly.	1. To determine effectiveness of analgesia.
2. If child is in pain: a) If using PCA, encourage the child to give a bolus and evaluate its effect after 10–15 minutes. b) If using NCA, administer a bolus and evaluate its effect after 10–15 minutes. c) Administer prescribed simple analgesics, e.g. paracetamol and either diclofenac or ibuprofen, if appropriate. d) Administer prescribed co-analgesics as appropriate, e.g. anti-spasmodic or anti-convulsant drugs. e) Involve parents/carers, play specialist to provide distraction and reassurance, particularly if the child is anxious. f) If pain management is not satisfactory contact the pain service, anaesthetist or surgeon as per hospital policy.	2. To ensure optimal analgesia is provided. c) Regular administration of simple analgesics has an opioid sparing effect (Macintyre 2010). d) To treat a specific cause of pain (e.g. spasms). e) To manage the emotional component of pain (i.e. fear). f) To ensure that swift action is taken to minimise pain.
3. Hourly pump readings should be recorded. This should include: a) Number of demands (tries). b) Number of good demands (good tries). c) Amount infused (hourly and running totals). d) 4 hourly syringe readings if using a syringe driver.	3. To monitor hourly morphine consumption and prevent drug errors. a, b) To ensure that boluses are being used appropriately. c, d) To ensure that the syringe pump is infusing correctly.
4. The PCA/NCA may be discontinued when: • The background infusion has been reduced or stopped • The child is requiring minimal bolus doses • The child is able to take analgesia via an alternative route • Alternative analgesia has been prescribed.	4. To ensure effective analgesia is maintained once the PCA/NCA has been discontinued.

Prevention and management of opioid related complications

The likelihood of opioid related side-effects and complications is affected by a number of factors including the age, genetic makeup and clinical condition of the child, the type of opioid administered, the dose and route of administration and the reason for its use. Prevention and early detection and treatment of unwanted side effects are paramount to ensuring the child's safety. Obtaining a history prior to use will minimise risk related to opioid sensitivity. The use of written guidelines, staff education and competencies for pump programming, plus frequent equipment checks will minimise the risk of an overdose related to pump failures and programming errors. It has been recommended that nurse:child ratios for children with opioid infusions should be a minimum of a 1:4 ratio on a general ward, with a 1:2 or 1:1 ratio following major surgery (RCPCH 1997). This section relates to the prevention and management of complications related to intravenous and epidural opioids.

Box 21.4 GOSH Pain Control Service Sedation Score

0 – Awake/alert
1 – Sleepy/responds appropriately
2 – Somulent/rousable (light stimuli)
3 – Deep sleep/rousable (heavier stimuli)
4 – Unrousable to stimuli (stop infusion).

Procedure guideline 21.19 **Prevention and management of opioid-related complications**

Statement	Rationale

Excessive sedation

---

1. The child's sedation level must be observed and recorded hourly (see Box 21.4):
   a) While a PCA/NCA is in progress and for 4–6 hours after it has been discontinued.
   b) While an epidural infusion is in progress and for 6–12 hours after it has been discontinued.

1. To ensure early detection and treatment of opioid induced sedation.
   a) The risk of excessive sedation continues until the drug has been eliminated (Kart *et al* 1997).
   b) The clearance time of epidural opioids varies. Morphine has a prolonged duration of action, while fentanyl and diamorphine are cleared more quickly (Rowney and Doyle 1998).

---

2. Clear instructions should indicate the action(s) to be taken if the child is over sedated. If the child is difficult to rouse (moderate sedation):
   a) **Stop** the infusion.
   b) Increase frequency of observations and introduce pulse oximetry if not already being recorded.
   c) Contact the pain team, anaesthetist or surgeon if appropriate.
   d) The infusion may be recommenced once the child is rousable to normal stimulation (i.e. touch).
   e) These actions must be recorded in the child's healthcare records.
   f) If the child is unrousable (deep sedation), administer naloxone. This may need to be repeated.

2. To prevent further sedation and an increased risk of respiratory depression.

   a) To prevent further sedation.
   b) To ensure prompt detection of any further deterioration in condition.
   c) The child may require a smaller or no background infusion.
   d) To continue to provide analgesia.

   e) To maintain an accurate record.

   f) To reverse the sedative effects of the opioid. Naloxone is an opiate antagonist. Its half-life is shorter than that of most opioids (Reynolds *et al* 1996).

---

3. Routine oxygen saturation monitoring can be used. It should always be available for the following groups:
   - Children who continue to be excessively sedated (not rousable to touch)
   - Children with respiratory complications, an obstructed airway or a known sensitivity to opioids
   - Infants under one year of age.

3. To ensure early detection and treatment of opioid induced sedation in at-risk groups of children (RCPCH 1997).

Respiratory depression

1. The child's respiratory rate should be recorded hourly:

   a) While a PCA/NCA is in progress and for 4–6 hours after it has been discontinued.
   b) While an epidural infusion is in progress and for 6–12 hours after it has been discontinued.
   c) Increase frequency of observations if the child is excessively sedated or their condition deteriorates.

1. To ensure early detection and treatment of opioid induced sedation.
   a) The risk of respiratory depression continues until the drug has been eliminated (Kart *et al* 1997).
   b) The clearance time of epidural opioids varies. Morphine has a prolonged duration of action, while fentanyl and diamorphine are cleared more quickly (Rowney and Doyle 1998).

---

2. The child's minimum satisfactory respiratory rate should be documented on the prescription chart or in the child's notes or care plan.
   a) This is for guidance only; it does not take into account:
   - Depth of respirations
   - Respiratory pattern and effort
   - Level of sedation
   - Oxygen saturation level.

2. To indicate when it might be appropriate to administer naloxone.

   a) Deterioration in these may also indicate a potential respiratory depression/arrest.

571

(Continued)

Procedure guideline 21.19 (*Continued*)

Statement	Rationale
3. If respiratory depression occurs: 　**a)** **STOP** the infusion. 　**b)** Administer intravenous naloxone as prescribed. This may need to be repeated. 　**c)** Observe the child closely. 　**d)** Contact the anaesthetist, pain team or surgeon. 　**e)** Document actions in the child's healthcare records. 　**f)** The event should be recorded as a critical incident/ near miss, according to local hospital policy.	**3.** 　**a)** To eliminate the possible cause. 　**b)** Naloxone is an opioid antagonist. It has a shorter half-life than most opioids (Reynolds *et al* 1996). 　**c)** To ensure prompt detection of further deterioration. 　**d)** To provide information and to review the child's analgesia. 　**e)** To maintain an accurate record. 　**f)** To learn from potential adverse events and minimise the risk of these reoccurring.
4. If respiratory arrest occurs: 　• Administer basic life support 　• **STOP** the infusion 　• Contact the clinical emergency team 　• Follow steps b–f) as for respiratory depression.	**4.** To ensure that respiratory arrest is treated promptly.

NB Naloxone will only be effective if the respiratory depression/arrest is opiate induced.

5. Once the child's condition has stabilised their analgesic regimen must be reviewed. If the respiratory depression/ arrest was opiate induced: 　• A PCA/NCA can be recommenced with no continuous infusion (i.e. bolus only) and smaller boluses if necessary 　• An epidural infusion can be recommenced with the opioid removed (i.e. local anaesthetic only).	**5.** To provide effective analgesia with minimal risk of complications.

Nausea and vomiting

1. The child should be observed for nausea and/or vomiting at least 4 hourly (1–2 hourly if they feel nauseous or have vomited). This should be recorded on the child's observation chart.	**1.** To ensure early detection of nausea and vomiting.
2. If the child complains of nausea, or has vomited, administer an anti-emetic as prescribed and consider: 　**a)** Aspirating a nasogastric or gastrostomy tube or stopping oral intake. 　**b)** Use of an alternative anti-emetic if nausea/vomiting is not reduced. Dexamethasone may also be effective. 　**c)** Reducing the infusion rate, bolus size or speed of bolus delivery of a PCA/NCA. 　**d)** Reducing the continuous infusion rate of, or removing the opioid from an epidural.	**2.** To ensure effective treatment and prevention of nausea and vomiting. 　**a)** To empty the stomach. 　**b)** Numerous factors are involved in emesis. Each anti-emetic acts on a range of different receptors (Elhakim *et al* 2003, Gan 2003, Litman *et al* 1994). 　**c, d)** To minimise the amount of opioid given. This will only be effective if the nausea and vomiting is opioid induced.

Pruritus (itching)

1. The child should be observed for itching at least 4 hourly (1–2 hourly if itching becomes a problem). 　**a)** Non-verbal children should be observed for an unexplained increase in distress or discomfort.	**1.** To ensure early detection and treatment of opioid-induced pruritus. 　**a)** Non-verbal children may display signs of distress/ discomfort, which can be mistaken for surgical pain.
2. Pruritus should be treated as follows: 　**For epidurals:** 　**a)** Administer naloxone (0.5 μg/kg) as prescribed.	**2.** 　**a)** To reverse opiate-induced pruritus without affecting the quality of analgesia provided (RCPCH 1997).

Procedure guideline 21.19 (*Continued*)

Statement	Rationale
b) Four doses can be given at 10-minute intervals. However, if repeated doses of naloxone are required this may reduce the effectiveness of the analgesia.	**b)** This is equivalent to half the reversal dose and will start to affect analgesia as well as unwanted side effects.
c) The doses may be repeated after an hour if the pruritus returns. If this is effective, the epidural infusion rate should be reduced or the opioid removed from the epidural.	**c)** Naloxone is short acting.
d) If naloxone is not effective an anti-histamine should be prescribed. Other causes of the itching should also be considered.	**d)** Both morphine and persistent itching increase histamine production.

For intravenous opioids:
- **e)** Reduce background rate and/or bolus size.
- **f)** Administer an anti-histamine.
- **g)** If the pruritus is severe and the above is not effective, consider switching to an alternative opioid.

Sucrose

Oral sucrose reduces distress behaviour and physiological response to painful procedures in babies less than 3 months of age (Lefrack *et al* 2006, Morash and Fowler 2004, Stevens *et al* 2010). It is safe and easily administered, but must be prescribed on the drug chart (as required) or administered under a patient group direction. A teaching package and training booklet is available on the Trust website (GOSH 2007). Sucrose should be used in conjunction with other non-pharmacological comfort measures such as non-nutritive sucking, positioning, etc and appropriate analgesia. It is not a substitute for analgesia or comfort measures. A recent study has suggested that sucrose does not affect nociceptive activity in the brain or spinal cord of a neonate and therefore might not provide effective analgesia (Slater *et al* 2010). This article has generated considerable debate (see responses in *The Lancet* in the weeks following the publication of this paper), which will no doubt continue. However, as there is currently no evidence to suggest that sucrose is harmful, its use alongside analgesia is still encouraged at GOSH.

Preparation

24% sucrose solution (sucrose and water) (Sweet-Ease™).

Indications

Sucrose can be given prior to a range of invasive procedures including:

- Heel puncture, venepuncture and cannulation
- Urinary catheterisation
- Eye examination
- Naso-gastric tube insertion
- Intramuscular and subcutaneous injections
- Lumbar puncture.

It can also be used for procedures likely to cause distress such as:

- Colostomy bag change
- Removal of tape and dressing changes
- Scalp electrode placement
- Suturing
- Physiotherapy.

Contra-indications

Sucrose should not be given in the following circumstances:

- Fructose or sucrose intolerance
- Unavailability of oral route (not effective via any other route)
- Paralysed and sedated patients.

Cautions

- Suspected or confirmed necrotising enterocolitis (NEC)
- Intubated patients.

Administration

- Administer 0.1 ml of sucrose solution onto the anterior aspect of the tongue or inside the cheek, or dip the child's dummy into the solution 1–2 minutes prior to procedure
- Offer a dummy if this is part of the baby's normal care (this promotes non-nutritive sucking which will enhance the effect of the sucrose)
- Repeat the dose on commencement of the procedure and every 2 minutes if required
- Maximum dose per administration:

  27–31 weeks: 0.5 ml
  32–36 weeks: 1 ml
  37 weeks: 2 ml
  (no daily maximum has been identified).

573

- The peak action is 2 minutes and duration of action is 5–10 minutes
- Important: discard remaining solution after use (single use only)
- Observe for gagging, choking, coughing and vomiting.

Assessment and documentation

An appropriate pain assessment tool should be used to assess the infant before, during and after the procedure and these scores must be recorded in the child's records. All doses administered must be recorded on the child's prescription chart.

Key texts

Association of Paediatric Anaesthetists of Great Britain and Ireland (APAGBI) (2008) Good practice in postoperative and procedural pain management. Pediatric Anesthesia, 18(1), 1–81

Franck LS, Greenberg CS, Stevens B. (2000) Pain assessment in infants and children. Pediatric Clinics of North America, 47(3), 487–512

Gaffney A, McGrath PJ, Dick B. (2003) Measuring pain in children: Developmental and instrument issues. In: Schechter NL, Berde CB, Yaster M. (eds) Pain in Infants, Children and Adolescents, 2nd edition, pp 128–141 Philadelphia, Lippincott, Williams & Wilkins

Macintyre PE, Schug SA, Scott DA, Visser EJ, Walker SM; APM:SE Working Group of the Australian and New Zealand College of Anaesthetists and Faculty of Pain Medicine (2010) Acute Pain Management: Scientific Evidence, 3rd edition. Melbourne, ANZCA & FPM

Morton NS (1998) Acute Paediatric Pain Management: A practical guide. Philadelphia, Saunders

Royal College of Nursing (RCN) (2009) The Recognition and Assessment of Acute Pain in Children: Update of Full Guideline. London, RCN. Available at http://www.rcn.org.uk/development/practice/clinicalguidelines/pain

Schechter NS, Berde CB, Yaster M (eds) (2003). Pain in Infants, Children and Adolescents, 2nd edition. Philadelphia, Lippincott, Williams & Wilkins

Stinson J. (2009) Pain assessment. In: Twycross T, Dowden SJ, Bruce E. (2009) (eds) Managing Pain in Children – a clinical guide. Oxford, Wiley-Blackwell

Twycross T, Dowden SJ, Bruce E. (eds) (2009) Managing Pain in Children – a clinical guide. Oxford, Wiley-Blackwell

References

Aldridge LM, Tunstall ME. (1986) Nitrous oxide and the fetus: a review and the results of a retrospective study of 175 cases of anaesthesia for insertion of Shirokar suture. British Journal of Anaesthesia, 58, 1348–1356

Amos RJ, Amess JAL, Nancekievill DG, Rees GM. (1983) Prevention of nitrous oxide induced megaloblastic changes in bone marrow using folinic acid. British Journal of Anaesthesia, 56, 103–107

Anderson BJ, McKenzie R, Persson MA, Garden AL. (1998) Safety of postoperative paediatric analgesia. Acute Pain, 1(3), 14–20

Association of Anaesthetists of Great Britain and Ireland (AAGBI) (2010) Guidelines for the Management of Severe Local Anaesthetic Toxicity. Available at http://www.aagbi.org/sites/default/files/la_toxicity_2010_0.pdf (last accessed 12th June 2011)

Association of Paediatric Anaesthetists of Great Britain and Ireland (APAGBI) (2008) Good practice in postoperative and procedural pain management. Pediatric Anesthesia, 18(1), 1–81

Bach DM. (1995) Implementation of the Agency for Health Care Policy and Research postoperative pain management guideline. Nursing Clinics of North America, 30(3), 515–527

Beyer JE, McGrath PJ, Berde CB. (1990) Discordance between self-report and behavioral measures in 3–7 year old children following surgery. Journal of Pain Symptom Management, 5, 350–356

Bookbinder M, Coyle N, Kiss M, Goldstein ML, Holritz K, Thaler H, Gianella A, Derby S, Brown M, Racolin A, Ho MN, Portenoy RK. (1996) Implementing national standards for cancer pain management: program model and evaluation. Journal of Pain & Symptom Management, 12(6),334–347

Bray RJ. (1983) Postoperative analgesia provided by morphine infusion in children. Anaesthesia, 38, 1075–1078

Breau LM, Camfield C, McGrath PJ, Rosmus C, Finley GA. (2001) Measuring pain accurately in children with cognitive impairments: refinement of a caregiver scale. Journal of Pediatrics, 138(5), 721–727

British Association for Accident and Emergency Medicine (1997) Guidelines for Analgesia in Children in the Accident and Emergency Department. London, BAEM

British Oxygen Company (BOC) (1995) Medical Gases Entonox Datasheet. Manchester, BOC Ltd. Updated 2010. Available at http://www.bocsds.com/uk/sds/medical/entonox.pdf (last accessed 11th June 2011)

Bromage PR. (1978) Epidural Analgesia. Philadelphia, WB Saunders

Bruce E, Franck L. (2000) Self-administered nitrous oxide (Entonox) for the management of procedural pain. Paediatric Nursing, 12(7),15–19

Bruce E, Franck L. (2004) Children's pain assessment: Implementing best nursing practices. In: Shaw T, Sanders K. (Eds) Foundation of Nursing studies Dissemination Series, 2(8) London, FoNS

Bruce E, Franck L. (2005) Using the worldwide web to improve children's pain care. International Nursing Review, 52, 204–209

Bruce E, Franck LS, Howard RF. (2006a) The efficacy of morphine and Entonox analgesia during chest drain removal in children. Pediatric Anesthesia, 16, 203–208

Bruce EA, Howard RF, Franck LS. (2006b) Chest drain removal pain and its management: A literature review. Journal of Clinical Nursing, 15, 145–154

Clinical Standards Advisory Group (2000) Services for Children with Pain. London, The Stationery Office

Commission on the Provision of Surgical Services (1990) Report of the Working Party on Pain after Surgery. London, Royal College of Surgeons of England and the College of Anaesthetists.

Department of Health (2002) National Minimum Standards for Independent Health Care. London, HMSO

Department of Health (2004a) Ill Child Standard, National Service Framework for Children, Young People and Maternity Services. London, Department of Health

Department of Health (2004b) National Service Framework for Children, Young People and Maternity Services: Core Standards. London, HMSO

Department of Health (2010) Essence of Care: Benchmarks for the Prevention and Management of Pain. London, The Stationery Office. Available at http://www.dh.gov.uk/en/Publicationsandstatistics/Publications/PublicationsPolicyAndGuidance/DH_119969 (last accessed 9th June 2011)

Doyle E, Harper I, and Morton NS., (1993) Patient controlled analgesia with low dose background infusions after lower abdominal surgery in children. British Journal of Anaesthesia, 6, 121–127

Elhakim M, Ali NM, Rashed I, Riad MK, Refat M. (2003) Dexamethasone reduces postoperative vomiting and pain after pediatric tonsillectomy [La dexaméthasone réduit les vomissements et la douleur postopératoires après une amygdalectomie pédiatrique]. Canadian Journal of Anesthesia, 50, 392–397

Gall O, Annequin D, Benoit G, VanGlabeke E, Vrancea F, Murat I.(2001) Adverse events of premixed nitrous oxide and oxygen for procedural sedation in children. Lancet, 358, 1514–1515

Gan TJ. (2003) Evidence-based management of postoperative nausea and vomiting. Canadian Journal of Anesthesia, 50, R5

GOSH (2007) Protocol for the use of sucrose solution for procedural pain Management. Great Ormond Street Hospital Clinical Practice Guideline.

Available at www.gosh.nhs.uk/health-professionals/clinical-specialties/pain-control-service-information-for-health-professionals/ (last accessed 30th January 2012)

Gunter JB. (2002) Benefit and risks of local anesthetics in infants and children. Paediatric Drugs, 4, 649–672

Hicks C, von Baeyer C, Spafford P, van Korlaar I, Goodenough B. (2001) The Faces Pain Scale – Revised: Towards a common metric in pediatric pain measurement. Pain, 93, 173–183

Hodgins MJ, Lander J. (1997) Children's coping with venepuncture. Journal of Pain and Symptom Management, 13(5), 274–285

Howard RF. (2003) Current status of pain management in children. Journal of American Medical Association, 290(18), 2464–2469

Howard RF, Lloyd-Thomas A, Thomas M, Williams DG, Saul R, Bruce E, Peters J. (2010) Nurse-controlled analgesia (NCA) following major surgery in 10 000 patients in a children's hospital. Pediatric Anesthesia, 20(2), 126–134

Hunt A, Mastroyannopoulou K, Goldman A, Seers K. (2003) Not knowing – the problem of pain in children with severe neurological impairment. International Journal of Nursing Studies, 40(2), 171–183

Jerrett M, Evans K. (1986) Children's pain vocabulary. Journal of Advanced Nursing, 11, 403–40

Kart T, Christupp LL, Rasmussen M. (1997) Recommended use of morphine in neonates, infants & children based on a literature review, part 2: Clinical use. Paediatric Anaesthesia, 7, 93–101

Kost-Byerly S, Tobin JR, Greenberg RS, Billett C, Zahurak M, Yaster M. (1998) Bacterial colonization & infection rate of continuous epidural catheters in children. Anesthesia and Analgesia, 86(4), 712–716

Langevin PB. (1996) Epidural catheter reconnection – safe and unsafe practice. Anesthesiology, 85(4), 883–888

Lefrack L, Burch K, Caravantes R, Knoerlein K, DeNolf, N, Duncan J, Hampton F, Johnston C., Lockey D, Martin-Walters CJ, McLendon D, Porter M, Richardson C, Robinson C, Toczylowski K. (2006) Sucrose analgesia: identifying potentially better practices. Pediatrics, 118, 197–202

Litman RS, Wu CL, Catanzaro FA. (1994) Ondansetron decreases emesis after tonsillectomy in children. Anesthesia and Analgesia, 78, 478–481

Llewellyn N. (1993) The use of PCA for post-operative pain management. Paediatric Nursing, 5(5), 12–15

Llewellyn N, Moriarty A. (2007) The national pediatric epidural audit. Pediatric Anesthesia, 17(6), 520–533

Lloyd-Thomas AR. (1999) Modern concepts of paediatric analgesia. Pharmacology and Therapeutics, 83(1), 1–20

Macintyre PE, Schug SA, Scott DA, Visser EJ, Walker SM; APM:SE Working Group of the Australian and New Zealand College of Anaesthetists and Faculty of Pain Medicine (2010) Acute Pain Management: Scientific Evidence, 3rd edition. Melbourne, ANZCA and FPM. Available at: http://www.anzca.edu.au/resources/books-and-publications/acutepain.pdf (last accessed 11th June 2011)

Malviya S, Voepel-Lewis T. (2006) The revised FLACC observational pain tool: improved reliability and validity for pain assessment in children with cognitive impairment. Paediatric Anaesthesia, 16(3), 258–265

Mason K, Koka B. (1999) Nitrous oxide. In: Krauss B, Brustowicz RM. (eds) Pediatric Procedural Sedation and Analgesia. Baltimore, Lippincott, Williams & Wilkins

McNeely J, Trentadue N. (1997) Comparison of PCA with and without night-time morphine infusion following lower extremity surgery in children. Journal of Pain and Symptom Management, 13(5), 2268–2273

Morash D, Fowler K. (2004) An evidence-based approach to changing practice: Using sucrose for infant analgesia. Journal of Pediatric Nursing, 19(5), 366–370

National Institute for Health and Clinical Excellence (NICE) (2001) Inherited Clinical Guideline B: Pressure ulcer risk assessment and prevention. Available at http://www.nice.org.uk/nicemedia/pdf/clinicalguidelinepressuresoreguidancenice.pdf (last accessed 24th May 2011)

National Institute for Health and Clinical Excellence (2010) Sedation in children and young people Sedation for diagnostic and therapeutic procedures in children and young people. NICE Clinical Guideline 112. National Clinical Guideline Centre. UK. Available at http://guidance.nice.org.uk/CG112 (last accessed 9th June 2011).

National Patient Safety Agency (NPSA) (2007) Patient Alert: Safer practice with epidural injections and infusions. Available at http://www.nrls.npsa.nhs.uk/resources/?entryid45=59807 (last accessed 12th June 2011)

National Patient Safety Agency (NPSA) (2011) Safer spinal (intrathecal), epidural and regional devices. Available at: http://www.nrls.npsa.nhs.uk/resources/?entryid45=94529&p=3 (last accessed 30th January 2012)

Neal MJ (2002) Medical Pharmacology at a Glance, 4th edition. London, Blackwell Publishing, pp16–17

Nursing and Midwifery Council (NMC) (2004) Guidelines for Records and Record Keeping. London, Nursing and Midwifery Council

Nunn JF. (1987) Clinical aspects of the interaction between nitrous oxide and vitamin B12. British Journal of Anaesthesia, 59, 3–13

Park GR, Fulton IC, Shelly MP. (1986) Normal pregnancy following nitrous oxide exposure in the first trimester. British Journal of Anaesthesia, 58(5), 576–577

Reynolds J, Parfitt K, Parsons A, Sweetman S. (eds) (1996) The Extra Pharmacopoeia, 31st edition. London, Royal Pharmaceutical Society of Great Britain

Rowney DA, Doyle E. (1998) Review article: Epidural and subarachnoid blockade in children. Anaesthesia, 53, 980–1001

Rowland AS, Baird DD, Weinberg CR, Shore DL, Shy CM, Wilcox AJ. (1992) Reduced fertility among women employed as dental assistants exposed to high levels of nitrous oxide. New England Journal of Medicine, 327, 993–997

Royal College of Anaesthetists (RCOA) (2004) Good practice in the management of continuous epidural analgesia in the hospital setting. Available at http://www.RCoA.ac.uk/docs/epid-analg.pdf (last accessed 24th May 2011)

Royal College of Nursing Institute (1999) The Recognition and Assessment of Acute Pain in Children: Recommendations. London, RCNI

Royal College of Nursing (RCN) (2009) The Recognition and Assessment of Acute Pain in Children: Update of Full Guideline. London, RCN. Available at http://www.rcn.org.uk/development/practice/clinicalguidelines/pain (last accessed 23rd May 2011

Royal College of Paediatrics and Child Health (RCPCH) (1997) Prevention and Control of Pain in Children: A manual for Health Care Professionals. London, BMJ Publishing

Royal College of Paediatrics and Child Health (2001) Guidelines for Good Practice: Recognition and Assessment of Acute Pain in Children. London, RCPCH

Royal College of Surgeons of England (2000) Children's Surgery – A First Class Service

Schechter NL, Berde C, Yaster M. (eds) (2003) Pain in Infants, Children and Adolescents, 2nd edition. New York, Lippincott Williams & Wilkins

Seth N, Llewellyn NE, Howard RF. (2000) Parental opinions regarding the route of administration of analgesic medication in children. Pediatric Anesthesia, 10(5), 537–544

Seth N, Macqueen S, Howard RF. (2004) Continuous postoperative epidural analgesia in children: the value of catheter tip culture. Paediatric Anaesthesia, 14(12), 996–1000

Slater R, Cornelissen L, Fabrizi L, Patten D, Yoxen J, Worley A, Boyd S, Meek J, Fitzgerald M. (2010) Oral sucrose as an analgesic drug for procedural pain in newborn infants: a randomised controlled trial. Lancet, 376(9748), 1225–1232

Southern DA, Read MS. (1994) Overdosage of opiate from patient controlled analgesia devices. British Medical Journal, 309, 1002

Spence K, Gillies D, Harrison D, Johnston L, Nagy S. (2005) A reliable pain assessment tool for clinical assessment in the neonatal intensive care unit. Journal of Obstetric, Gynecological & Neonatal Nursing, 34(1), 80–86

Stevens B, Yamada J, Ohlsson A. (2010) Sucrose for analgesia in newborn infants undergoing painful procedures. Cochrane Database of Systematic

Reviews, Issue 1. Art. No.: CD001069. DOI: 10.1002/14651858.CD001069. pub3

Stinson J, Bruce E. (2009) Chronic Pain in Children. In: Twycross A, Dowden SJ, Bruce E. (eds) Managing Pain in Children – a clinical guide. Oxford, Wiley-Blackwell

Twycross A. (2009) Nondrug Management of Pain. In: Twycross T, Dowden SJ, Bruce E. (eds) Managing Pain in Children – a clinical guide. Oxford, Wiley-Blackwell

Twycross A, Dowden SJ, Bruce E. (eds) (2009) Managing Pain in Children – a clinical guide. Oxford, Wiley-Blackwell

Van Dijk M, de Boer JB, Koot HM, Tibboel D, Passchier J, Duivenvoorden HJ. (2000) The reliability and validity of the COMFORT scale as a postoperative pain instrument in 0 to 3-year-old infants. Pain, 84(2–3), 367–377

Voepel-Lewis T, Merkel S, Tait AR, Trzcinka A, Malviya S. (2002) The reliability and validity of the face, legs, activity, cry, consolability observational tool as a measure of pain in children with cognitive impairment. Anesthesia and Analgesia, 95, 1224–1229

Williams D, Patel A, Howard R. (2002) Pharmacogenetics of codeine metabolism in an urban population of children and its implications for analgesic reliability. British Journal Anaesthesia, 89, 839–845

World Health Organization (1986) Cancer Pain Relief. Geneva, WHO

World Health Organization (1997) Looking Forward to Cancer Pain Relief for All. International Consensus on the Management of Cancer Pain. Geneva, WHO

Zacny JP, Conran A, Pardo H, Coalson DW, Black M, Klock PA, Klafta JM. (1999) Effects of naloxone on nitrous oxide actions in healthy volunteers. Pain, (83), 411–418

Palliative care

Chapter contents

Procedure guidelines

The Great Ormond Street Hospital Manual of Children's Nursing Practices, First Edition. Edited by Susan Macqueen, Elizabeth Anne Bruce, Faith Gibson.
© 2012 Great Ormond Street Hospital for Children NHS Foundation Trust. Published 2012 by Blackwell Publishing Ltd.

Introduction

The speciality of palliative care evolved during the 1960s with the emergence of the modern hospice movement led by individuals such as Alfred Worcester and Cicely Saunders (Saunders and Sykes 1993). 'Palliative care for children and young people with life limiting conditions is an active and total approach to care, embracing physical, emotional, social and spiritual elements. It focuses on enhancement of quality of life for the child and support for the family and includes the management of distressing symptoms, provision of respite and care through death and bereavement' (The Charter for the Association for Children with Life-Threatening or Terminal Conditions and their Families (ACT) and The Royal College of Paediatrics and Child Health 1997, p.7). Palliative care is thus concerned with maintaining quality of life, not just in the stages of dying, but in the weeks, months and years before a child's death (Department of Health (DoH) 2007). More recently, ACT have offered a refined/refreshed definition: paediatric palliative care is as 'an active and total approach to care, from the point of diagnosis or recognition, throughout the child's life, death and beyond. It embraces physical, emotional, social and spiritual elements and focuses on the enhancement of quality of life for the child/young person and support for the family. It includes the management of distressing symptoms, provision of short breaks (formally known as respite) and care through death and bereavement' (Association for Children with Life-threatening or Terminal Conditions and their Families (ACT) 2011).

Palliative care aims to achieve optimal comfort and quality of life for the child. It can be delivered along with treatments with a curative focus or for some children palliation may be the only treatment option. Palliative care for children can be provided at home or in a hospice or hospital (Vickers *et al* 2007). To enable a family to make an informed choice as to which setting seems to be the most appropriate place for their child to be cared for, they need to be provided with accurate information regarding available services and expected progression of the disease. Expert and effective palliative care requires a holistic approach by the multidisciplinary team (MDT) to the child and family (Liben *et al* 2008, McCulloch *et al* 2008). Nurses involved in palliative care and symptom management need to attend not only to the physical symptoms but also anxieties and expectations of the child within the family: this would include talking with parents/carers and children, dependent on their level of understanding and acknowledging their family culture. The nurse must enable, facilitate and empower families in their care (Davies and Oberle 1990).

Symptoms that occur in the palliative phase may be specific to the disease process, e.g. anaemia and dyspnoea in haematological malignancies; they may be part of the general deterioration of the body as death approaches, e.g. anorexia and cachexia; or they may be the side effects of medication and treatment, e.g. constipation associated with opioid analgesia (Goldman *et al* 2006; Pritchard *et al* 2008, Wolfe *et al* 2000).

Caring for a child in hospital, hospice or at home can pose specific and different problems for the professionals involved. Care of the child at home will be affected by local provision of care and the availability of drugs, equipment and paediatric community services and parent/carer confidence. Palliative care as with all aspects of care for children should be a partnership between family and professionals (Casey 1988). Many families who have provided care for their child with a life-threatening or life-limiting condition will have learnt many technical nursing skills and interventions such as naso-pharyngeal suctioning and nasogastric/gastrostomy feeding, and possibly administration of intravenous (IV) medication. Some families will be happy to continue providing this level of care, and even learn further skills. However, the high levels of stress and anxiety at this time in a child's life may influence parents capacity and desire to learn new procedures. Furthermore, the family may feel that they want to relinquish and 'pass back' responsibility for the more technical aspects of their child's care at this time. For many children cared for at home the children's community nurses or local children's palliative care teams will be able to support families in the practical aspects of care. When a child is cared for in hospital, staff may require support when the focus changes from curative to palliation. This particularly comes to light around issues such as monitoring and recording of vital signs. It may be helpful to remember that routine observations are only useful if they can influence the provision of care and child/family comfort.

It is outside the scope of this book to provide detailed guidelines on all aspects of palliative care for children and the nurse should refer to texts such as (Goldman 1998, The West Midlands Paediatric Macmillan Team 2005) for more comprehensive information. Likewise it is impossible to provide detail on all symptoms that may be encountered, see Twycross and Wilcock (2001). This chapter is intended to be a first point of information, with general guidelines to help the nurse provide care for a child until expert advice is available. It includes the symptoms that are most commonly experienced, i.e. nausea and vomiting, constipation and diarrhoea, and dyspnoea (pain being dealt with in another section). Also included is some information on situations that often cause anxiety, namely haemorrhage, anorexia and dehydration, and signs of impending death. There are other situations, for example spinal cord compression and acutely occurring airway obstruction, which will require rapid medical intervention to maintain quality of life. It is again outside the scope of this chapter to discuss these in detail, but careful assessment of the child will ensure timely identification of these situations.

The vision for services of the future is that they will be commissioned and delivered in line with identified local need and national policy, and driven by best practice (DoH 2008). This chapter presents some of the emerging evidence from practice, evidence that must, despite the challenges, begin to be mapped in terms of research-based practice (Hinds *et al* 2007).

Further information with regard to the development and provision of palliative care services can be found in the Key texts section at the end of this chapter.

What follows, is a series of care practices more frequently associated with palliative care.

Assessment of symptoms

Effective symptom management can only be achieved if a full assessment has first taken place. The age and developmental stage of the child needs to be taken into consideration, as does previous family experiences, which may influence how the family view symptoms. Symptom assessment should be ongoing throughout the palliative phase, and used to plan and implement effective management.

Procedure guideline 22.1 **Symptoms assessment (palliative care)**

Statement	Rationale
1. The multidisciplinary team should work together to obtain a full history of symptoms from the child and family.	1. Effective palliative care is best provided by a multidisciplinary approach as each profession brings its own expertise and individual approach to the problem (Doyle 1995).
2. Ask the child (when appropriate) and the family what they consider are the symptoms, which are causing them most problems and distress.	2. Symptom management in the palliative phase must focus on problems as seen by the child and family (Goldman and Burne 1998).
3. Ask the family to describe problems in as much detail as possible, giving prompts as appropriate to gain an accurate assessment.	3. To ensure that professionals are not acting on their own pre-conceived ideas of what the problems may be.
4. Listen carefully to the words used by the child (when appropriate) to describe the symptoms. Ask the parent/carer how the child describes their symptoms.	4. Children may not use the same words as adults to describe their symptoms (Goldman 1998).
5. Ask if any particular activity or event brings on or exacerbates symptoms.	5. To gain as full a picture as possible and ascertain the most appropriate management (Twycross 2002, Twycross *et al* 2009).
6. Ask the child/family whether any medications or intervention have helped to relieve symptoms in the past.	6. To ensure that previously successful methods can be re-instigated.
7. Ascertain what has been tried but has not proved useful. Ensure that accurate information is taken regarding dosage, frequency and previously used medication.	7. To avoid the use of previously ineffective treatments and to ascertain if medication has been used optimally in the past.
8. Reassess daily (or as negotiated with the family) and adjust management as directed by further assessment.	8. Symptoms may not be fully controlled, a family may wish for less frequent contact with professionals at this palliative stage (Twycross 2002).

Nausea and vomiting

Nausea and vomiting may be caused either by the disease or its treatment (Twycross 2002). Nausea is often experienced as a symptom in constipation, renal or hepatic failure. Early morning nausea and vomiting (usually associated with a headache) is commonly experienced in children with brain tumours or central nervous system disease. Literature from adult-based palliative care widely reports opioids as a common cause of nausea and vomiting (Baines and Sykes 1993, Regnard and Tempest 1998, Twycross 2002). However, Goldman (1998) reports that opioid induced nausea and vomiting is less common in children and young people. An assessment of the child's history, current symptoms and previous management is essential for effective management. Vomiting not associated with nausea may not be distressing for the child and may not require intervention.

579

Procedure guideline 22.2 **Nausea and vomiting**

Statement	Rationale
1. Ask the child/family as appropriate to describe the nature, frequency and timing of the nausea and vomiting. **Early morning vomiting is commonly seen in patients with CNS disease.**	1. In order to determine the likely cause (Regnard and Comiskey 1995).
2. Obtain a history of recent bowel action.	2. Vomiting may be related to constipation (Kaye 1999).

(Continued)

Procedure guideline 22.2 (*Continued*)

Statement	Rationale
3. Discuss with medical staff the possible need for further investigations.	**3.** There may be an underlying cause, which could be treatable (Regnard and Comiskey 1995).
4. Discuss with medical staff the prescribing of appropriate anti-emetics drugs, depending on the cause of the nausea and vomiting.	**4.** Antiemetic choice depends on cause (Regnard and Tempest 1998).
5. For the child with CNS disease it may be helpful for them to sleep with their head raised.	**5.** To reduce increase in pressure, which occurs when the child is lying flat (Lissauer and Clayden 2001).
6. Children with signs of raised intracranial pressure, a short pulsed course of a steroid dose twice daily may be considered.	**6.** Dexamethasone in MRI studies has been shown to reduce water content of oedematous brain tissue (Sinha *et al* 2004).
7. Children receiving enteral feeding may require a reduction of volume or concentration of their feed.	**7.** Gut mobility may be reduced in advanced illness (Regnard and Tempest 1998) and can be slowed by the use of opiates (Baines and Sykes 1993).
8. If the child is vomiting, provide receptacle, which is changed frequently. Change clothes and sponge face as necessary. Offer mouthwash and sips of clear fluid.	**8.** To maintain child comfort.
9. Reassure the family that attempts are being made to control the nausea and vomiting.	**9.** To promote family confidence.
10. Be honest with the family if it is likely to be impossible to completely control the symptoms.	**10.** In certain situations it may be impossible to completely control nausea and vomiting (Mannix 1998).
11. If there is a discernable pattern to vomiting, time medication and food accordingly.	**11.** To facilitate the absorption of medication and maximise nutrition.

Constipation and diarrhoea

Constipation is not just a measure of the frequency of bowel action but also refers to difficulty in defecation. It can be described as the infrequent, difficult and often painful passage of hard stools (Saunders and Sykes 1993). In the palliative phase constipation may be caused by poor food and fluid intake, reduced mobility or as a direct result of the disease process. It is an almost universal and troublesome side effect of opioid medication.

Diarrhoea is the passage of frequent loose stools, but the child may also describe a single loose stool along with frequent normal stools. Possible causes include problems with absorption of feeds or infection.

Procedure guideline 22.3 **Patient assessment (constipation and diarrhoea)**

Statement	Rationale
1. Determine from child/family as appropriate, what is the child's usual bowel habit and whether current bowel action differs from normal.	**1.** To obtain baseline for assessment of current bowel actions and to facilitate decision making as to whether any treatment is necessary.
2. Ascertain whether child is taking any opioid analgesia, and liase with medical staff about commencing a laxative with stimulant and softening action as prophylaxis.	**2.** Opioid analgesia effects gut motility and causes constipation (Baines and Sykes 1993).

Procedure guideline 22.3 (*Continued*)

Statement	Rationale
Management of constipation	
1. If current bowel action is abnormal, discuss with medical staff whether there is a need to investigate any underlying cause, e.g. radiological examination, etc.	1. Abnormal bowel actions may have some underlying treatable pathology which, if corrected, would improve the child's quality of life.
2. If the child has been constipated but has now started to pass small amounts of loose stool, discuss with medical staff whether clinical or radiological examination is necessary.	2. To exclude the possibility of impacted stools with overflow of liquid faecal matter (Regnard and Mannix 1995a).
3. If history indicates that the child is constipated, offer dietary advice where appropriate and liase with medical staff for the prescription of laxatives with a suitable mode of action	3. When a child is receiving palliative care it is often impossible to correct bowel action with dietary adjustments alone (Baines and Sykes 1993).
4. Ensure privacy, time and comfort for child when attempting to defecate.	4. To promote effective bowel action and minimise embarrassment.
5. If the child has not had a bowel action in spite of appropriate laxative, discuss with the family the appropriateness of rectal measures, e.g. suppositories, enema	5. The child may require some rectal stimulant in order to open their bowels (Baines and Sykes 1993).
6. Do not discontinue oral laxatives.	6. It is important to continue to soften the stools and stimulate bowel peristalsis (Baines and Sykes 1993).
7. When appropriate encourage good fluid intake and high fibre diet.	7. To maximise normal gastro-intestinal function.
Management of diarrhoea	
1. Obtain a stool specimen for culture and sensitivity and treat if appropriate (Twycross 2002).	1. Acute onset may indicate infection particularly if other children are affected.
2. Review child's drug regimen with medical staff particularly if they are already undertaking a course of antibiotics or laxatives.	2. Identify possible drug related causes of diarrhoea (Regnard and Mannix 1995a).
3. Review child's feeding regimen, particularly if on supportive feeding.	3. To rule out dietary causes of diarrhoea (Curran and Barnes 2000).
4. Discuss with medical staff appropriate use of fluids and drugs.	4. To reduced peristalsis and number of bowel actions and maintain appropriate hydration (Regnard and Mannix 1995a).
5. Assist family and child in cleaning the anal area and application of barrier cream as necessary.	5. To minimise skin excoriation.
6. Ensure privacy for the child.	6. To minimise embarrassment.

Dyspnoea

Dyspnoea describes the sensation of being short of breath rather than the sign of rapid breathing (tachypnoea).

Dyspnoea in the palliative patient has the potential to be a very frightening experience, and it may have several different causes.

It may be the result of pre-existing conditions, e.g. asthma, cystic fibrosis, cardiac failure or may be the symptom of progressive disease, e.g. anaemia. The causative factors along with the overall condition of the child will influence the multidisciplinary team's decision to treat.

Principles table 22.1 **Dyspnoea**

Principle	Rationale
1. Obtain a detailed history from both child and family.	**1.** In order to ascertain the cause and to decide the most appropriate treatment if any (Ahmedzai and Regnard 1995).
2. Discuss with medical staff the appropriateness of investigations and any active management, i.e. antibiotics, blood transfusion or pleural tap.	**2.** In order to ascertain the cause and to decide the most appropriate treatment if any (Ahmedzai and Regnard 1995).
3. Allow child to position themselves as they prefer (this may not look comfortable to professionals or family).	**3.** To improve ventilatory effort (Ahmedzai and Regnard 1995).
4. Oxygen may improve symptoms (see Chapter 26 on Respiratory care).	
5. Use a fan or sit the child near an open window.	**5.** 'Cold air directed to face…has been shown to relieve dyspnoea probably through stimulation of the vagus nerve' (Heyes-Moore 1993 p87).
6. Consider use of low dose opioids.	**6.** Low dose opioids reduce the sensation of breathlessness (Goldman and Burne 1998).
7. Discuss with medical staff the need for sedation.	**7.** Increasing dyspnoea causes anxiety and agitation (Ahmedzai and Regnard 1995).
8. a) Give explanation and reassurance. **b)** Consider use of distraction.	**8a) and b)** To minimise anxiety of parents/carers and child.

Anorexia and reduced fluid intake

Feeding a child is one of the prime functions of parenting, so reduced appetite and difficulty in feeding is generally a source of great anxiety to parents/carers. However, anorexia and reduced oral intake are common at the end of life as the body's requirement for nutrition decreases. Artificial feeding, i.e. nasogastric or gastrostomy may not always be appropriate in the palliative phase (Regnard 1995) and comfort measures such as sips of fluid or mouth care may be more appropriate. Some symptoms may be exacerbated by enteral feeding or hydration; therefore detailed discussion around such issues should take place between the family and professionals involved. The subject of feeding and hydration in the terminal phase is often a cause of anxiety for families and professionals, therefore discussions around the withdrawal of feeding and fluids needs to be handled with sensitivity.

Principles table 22.2 **Anoerexia and reduced fluid intake**

Principle	Rationale
1. Liaise with the multidisciplinary team (MDT) to obtain a full history.	**1.** To ascertain any physical cause which could be treated (Regnard 1995).
2. Discuss with the family and the MDT the appropriateness of artificial feeding.	**2.** To ensure that the family and staff are involved in the decision making process (Regnard 1995).
3. Provide mouth care (see Chapter 10).	**3.** To keep mucosa moist and minimise anorexia resulting from a painful mouth (Regnard and Mannix 1995).
4. Offer small attractive meals and fluid as desired rather than adhering to strict mealtime regimen.	**4.** To ensure that food and fluid is available when child demands.
5. When appropriate offer high calorie nutritional support; however, be aware that in the terminal phase foods high in fat may not be tolerated.	**5.** To maximise calorific intake.

External haemorrhage

Haemorrhage although unusual in children can be a very frightening experience for the family, child and professionals involved. If this is a likely occurrence it is important that the family have adequate preparation. There are certain conditions, including leukaemia, pulmonary aspergillus infection and solid tumours that may involve major blood vessels, in which haemorrhage is more likely to occur. Any previous experience of bleeding may also increase the family's anxiety about a catastrophic haemorrhage during the palliative phase. Children who are severely thrombocytopaenic may be at risk of intracranial bleeding; this is more likely to cause sudden loss of consciousness or seizures rather than visible bleeding.

Principles table 22.3 External haemorrhage

Principle	Rationale
1. Discuss with medical staff any likely precipitating factors of haemorrhage and appropriate preventative treatment.	1. In order to prepare the family for the possibility of such an event.
2. If haemorrhage is a possibility the provision of dark towels and sheets is appropriate.	2. This makes the appearance of blood less frightening by allowing it to look darker and less red (Regnard and Tempest 1998).
3. Discuss with medical staff the possibility of an acute event and the availability of a prescription for sedation.	3. In order for sedation to be administered quickly (Regnard and Makin 1995).
4. In the case of haemorrhage in the ward situation ensure that someone stays with the family while others go for assistance, retrieves drugs, etc.	4. To support the family during a terrifying experience.
5. A child with reduced platelet count is more likely to experience oozing from the gums or nose rather than a catastrophic haemorrhage. This oozing may be managed by the use of topical or oral tranexamic acid (Regnard and Tempest 1998).	5. To minimise distress to child and family and to promote the child's comfort.

Seizures

Seizures can be a very frightening experience for families, especially if the seizure occurs at home and is unexpected. Where there is the potential for a child to have a seizure it is better if families are warned of this and are prepared with what to do. Children with neurodegenerative diseases may have suffered from seizures throughout their illness or they may be as a result of central nervous system tumours, metastatic disease, electrolyte imbalances (hyponatraemia), a cerebral bleed in the case of leukaemia or a high temperature (febrile convulsion).

Procedure guideline 22.4 Seizures

Statement	Rationale
1. Obtain a detailed history of the type of seizure and any precipitating factors.	1. In order to establish a potential cause, decrease precipitating factors where possible, and decide on the best course of management.
2. Children with known epilepsy or those already taking anti-convulsant medication should, where possible, continue to take their regular anti-convulsants. (You may need to consider the best route for administration.) The burden of taking medication needs to be balanced with the distress of the seizure, the drug side effects, and parental/child's wishes.	2. To control/prevent pre-existing seizures and enable the child to participate in activities, as children are often very tired after seizures. The potential distress of a seizure for families can be prevented.

583

(Continued)

Procedure guideline 22.4 (*Continued*)

Statement	Rationale
3. Educate families about what to do if the child has a seizure, including keeping the child safe and protecting them from further injury. Avoid putting anything in the child's mouth or restraining them. Turn the child onto their side in the recovery position after the seizure to protect their airway.	**3.** Parents/carers will cope better if they are prepared with what to expect even if the chance of a seizure is rare (Goldman 1998). They will need reassurance and support in coping if their child has a seizure. Restraining a child during a seizure may cause further injury.
4. Provide emergency medication if there is a potential risk of seizures, and consider the most acceptable route of administration. Examples include rectal diazepam or buccal midazolam.	**4.** Buccal midazolam maybe easier if the child is large and difficult to manoeuvre, in a wheelchair or at school, where rectal medication is less appropriate.
5a) Discuss with medical staff the appropriateness of checking electrolyte levels and drug levels, e.g. phenytoin and phenbarbitone levels. **b)** Infusions can be used if a child continues to have severe and/or prolonged seizures. Examples include subcutaneous midazolam and phenobarbitone. The advantage of midazolam is that it can be mixed with other drugs including opiates in a syringe driver whereas phenobarbitone is more of an irritant that cannot be mixed.	**5a)** It may be possible to correct electrolyte imbalances or alter drug doses. **b)** These will aim to dampen seizures and control them but may cause sedation. Sedation may be desirable in the terminal phase.

Signs of impending death

Although it can be difficult to predict when death will occur, there are certain signs and symptoms, which may predict its imminence. It can be helpful to the family and staff caring for the child to discuss what these might be. Although at times it may be difficult to broach these subjects with the family it would seem that good preparation empowers the family to care for their child, particularly if they have chosen to be at home.

Procedure guideline 22.5 Dealing with impending death

Statement	Rationale
1. Discuss altered **respiratory rate** or a **change in respiratory pattern**: identify that the respiratory rate may be reduced or there could be the **onset of Cheyne–Stokes respirations**, a form of periodic breathing associated with periods of apnoea (Heyse-Moore 1993).	**1** To prepare the family and reduce anxiety.
2a) Discuss **noisy respirations**: (sometimes known as death rattle), an accumulation of secretions usually in the hypopharynx, which oscillate when the child breathes. Explain that this generally occurs in patients who are too weak to expectorate (Twycross 2002). **b)** This may be improved by changing the position of the child or the use of hyoscine hydrobromide either in the syringe driver or a transdermal patch (Regnard and Tempest 1998).	**2a)** To prepare the family and reduce anxiety. **b)** To facilitate drainage of secretions and reduce production of secretions.
3a) Discuss that the child may become **agitated** or **restless** as death approaches. **b)** Ascertain that there are no physical causes for these, i.e. pain, pruritis, urinary retention (Twycross and Lichter 1998) the side effects of drugs (Breitbart *et al* 1998) or psychosocial issues, i.e. unfinished business (Hodgson 1993).	**3a)** To prepare the family and reduce anxiety. **b)** To facilitate appropriate symptom management.

Procedure guideline 22.5 (*Continued*)

Statement	Rationale
c) Discuss with the family the use of a sedative if all of the above have been excluded (Regnard and Tempest 1998).	**c)** To reduce distress.
4. Explain to the family that in their last few days prior to death many children sleep for longer periods and have a reduced level of consciousness.	**4.** To prepare the family and reduce anxiety.
5. Discuss with the family that the child may also demonstrate reduced peripheral circulation leading to coldness and a discolouration of the extremities.	**5.** To prepare the family and reduce anxiety.

After the child dies

It is essential to ensure that a high standard of care is maintained after a child dies. The following guidelines relate predominantly to the death of a child in hospital. However, much of it, particularly the legal requirements, are also relevant to the death of a child at home. Family involvement at this stage is paramount and the nurse should ascertain by sensitive enquiry how much the parents/carers wish to be involved in the preparation of their child's body and with the legal requirements concerning the death. The family will be distressed and possibly shocked at this time. Sensitivity is required when assisting them. The desire to be of assistance and support to the family can at times lead the nurse to take over actions the parents/carers might prefer to do for themselves. Sensitivity and allowing the parents/carers time to make decisions should avoid this situation. Knowledge of the legal requirements following the death will ensure that families are able to make the necessary arrangements with the minimum of difficulty and distress.

We live in a multi-cultural society and rituals and practices around death may be influenced by families' beliefs. There are numerous texts available describing practices associated with different faiths. These should be used as guidelines only. It is essential to remember that although a family professes a recognised faith their beliefs may be individual. When in doubt ask, it rarely causes offence if done sensitively. The behaviour they exhibit will also be influenced by their culture, previous experiences and coping mechanisms. Cultural expressions of grief vary and should be supported by the nurse, even if the nurse perceives it to be inappropriate.

In the period between death and the funeral the child's body may be cared for at home, in a hospice cool room, a funeral director's premises or a mortuary. These options should be discussed with the family, if not already decided, or stated in a care plan (Fraser *et al* 2010).

Procedure guideline 22.6 Communication and responsibilities (following death of a child)

Statement	Rationale
1. If the child's parents or carers are not present they must be informed immediately.	**1.** To facilitate good communication.
2. The following may need to be advised as soon as possible that the child has died if this has occurred in hospital: • Medical staff • Nursing staff • Site manager • Bed manager • Embassy/sponsoring body • Interpreters • Religious representative.	**2.** To initiate practical help and support. To facilitate good communication.

(*Continued*)

Procedure guideline 22.6 (*Continued*)

Statement	Rationale
3. The following also need to be advised, as appropriate, as soon as possible that the child has died if this has occurred in hospital: • Mortuary staff • Nurse specialists • General practitioner (GP) • Health visitor • School nurse • Community nurse • Referring hospital • Hospice (if involved) • Midwife • Social services.	**3.** To initiate practical help and support. To facilitate good communication.
4a) When a child dies at home there is no urgency for nursing staff to contact anybody. **b)** The following need to be informed at an appropriate time: • GP, including the out-of-hours service, ensuring that the authorities are aware that the death was expected • Funeral director • Religious representative • Health visitor • School nurse • Community nurse • Child's local hospital • Child's tertiary centre (if appropriate) • Hospice (if involved) • Other professionals involved in the care of the child.	**4a)** To empower the family and give them control over the situation. **b)** To prevent unnecessary processes requiring investigation into the death by the Child Death Review Panel, to certify the death, to enable the family to discuss care of their child's body and funeral arrangements, to support the family and facilitate funeral arrangements, and to facilitate good communication.
5. Ensure the death of the child is recorded in all the appropriate documentation and any electronic records.	**5.** To ensure subsequent communications with the family are accurate.
6. If the child has died in hospital fill in the 'Notification of Death' slips and send to: • Hospital chaplain • Histopathology • Medical Audit Department.	**6.** To comply with Hospital Policy. To enhance communication between appropriate personnel.
7. If a child dies in theatre the relevant ward must be informed and arrangements made for transfer of the child to an appropriate area.	**7.** To enhance communication between appropriate personnel and allow parents time to say goodbye in more appropriate surroundings.
8. Local procedure should be followed for the child who is HIV positive.	**8.** To ensure sensitive and appropriate handling.
9. In hospital the medical staff should: **a)** Confirm death and enter into the child's healthcare records. **b)** Discuss organ donation (if not previously discussed). **c)** If appropriate discuss post mortem, post death biopsies and organ or tissue retention. **d)** Request these and obtain consent. **e)** Explain the need for coroner's post mortem. **f)** Arrange a coroner's post mortem if required. **g)** Complete and sign the death certificate.	**9.** **a)** To meet legal requirements. **b) and c)** To obtain consent and to maximise viability of organs for donation. **d)** To ensure good communication.

Procedure guideline 22.6 (*Continued*)

Statement	Rationale
h) Complete a Certificate of Examination for cremation. **i)** Arrange family follow-up and discussion of post mortem results. **j)** Notify GP and referring hospital of death.	**i)** To initiate later support for family.
10. In hospital the nursing staff should: • Arrange for keepsakes • Perform last offices and transfer the child to the mortuary • Provide parents/carers with relevant booklets available from DSS or local NHS Trust • Arrange for parents/carers to view their child at a later date • Advise parents/carers about funeral arrangements • Ensure suitable travel arrangements are in place for the family to go home • Notify the health visitor and relevant social worker of death • Ensure that the GP and referring hospital are informed of death • Ensure that other staff members are informed of the death • Consider informing other families on the ward.	**10.** To ensure good communication, to provide psychological support for the family, and to provide practical advice.
11. If the child dies at home: **a)** It may still be appropriate to discuss organ donation if this has not been done previously. **b)** It may be appropriate to discuss post mortem.	**a)** To obtain consent and to maximise viability of organs for donation. **b)** To ensure good communication and parent's/carer's knowledge of legal and practical requirements.

Procedure guideline 22.7 **Legal issues (following death of a child)**

Statement	Rationale
1. A doctor must examine the child after death.	**1.** To certify death.
2. The child's death must be entered into the child's medical and nursing notes.	**2.** To document that the child has died.
3. The doctor should give their child's Death Certificate to the family before they go to register their child's death. **a)** If the child has died in hospital this should ideally be given to the family before they leave the hospital. **b)** This will not be possible if the death is to be investigated by the Coroner or if a post mortem is to be performed.	**3.** The Death Certificate is required to register a death. **a)** To save the family from returning at a later date. **b)** The cause of death will not yet be established.
4. The details on the Death Certificate should be checked for legibility. It should also be clarified with the family. **a)** An additional 'Certificate of Examination' is required for cremation.	**4.** To avoid difficulties when the death is registered. **a)** It is a legal requirement.

(Continued)

Procedure guideline 22.7 (*Continued*)

Statement	Rationale
5. When the medical staff complete the death certificate of a child with HIV, the cause of death should be written as: **a)** Final illness, e.g. pneumonia, septicaemia. **b)** Immune deficiency may be added but not HIV or AIDS. **c)** On the reverse of the certificate is a box that may be ticked indicating that further information may be available later. The Registrar may then contact the doctor for the underlying cause of death. This should be ticked.	**5.** To ensure confidentiality.
6. Registration of death **must** take place within 5 days. **a)** This is normally done by the child's parents/carers, however after discussion with the family and the Registrar (of deaths), it is sometimes possible for a relative, friend or member of hospital staff to do it on the parents'/carers' behalf as long as they are able to identify the child's body.	**6.** To meet legal requirements. **a)** If a family feel unable to do it themselves.
7. The following is required to register a death: • A certificate stating the cause of death • Date and place of death • The child's full name, home address, place and date of birth • The parents'/carers' full names, home addresses and occupations.	**7.** To meet legal requirements.
8. Parents/carers must be given the details of where to register the death by healthcare personnel, ensuring that opening times are made clear.	**8.** To avoid unnecessary distress and time wasting for family members.
9. It is possible to register the child's death in their home area but paper work may take more than a week to process.	
10. The Registrar will provide: **a)** A certificate for burial or cremation for the undertakers. **b)** Form BD8 (revised) notification of death.	**10.** **a)** To enable the funeral to proceed. **b)** To apply for a funeral grant from the Benefits Agency. This is needed to arrange a funeral abroad or if the child had a savings account.
11. The registration and issue of certificates is free. A certified copy of the Death Certificate is available for a nominal fee.	
12. If a post mortem is required by the coroner, normally the coroner's office, or staff from the hospital mortuary contact the family to advise them when and where they may collect the death certificate and how they may then proceed.	**12.** To enable the funeral to be planned.

Procedure guideline 22.7 (*Continued*)

Statement	Rationale
13. If a newborn baby dies, and their birth has not been registered, a declaration of birth can be made at the same time as registration of death. The birth certificate will be sent at a later date. • Parents can still register the birth locally within the normal 6 weeks if they wish to do so. • If the parents are not married, the mother **must** be present. If they wish for the baby to be registered with the father's surname both parents **must** be present.	**13.** To meet legal requirements.
14. It is the responsibility of the parents/carers to contact Social Services to cancel any benefits that they received for their child.	**14.** To meet legal requirements.
15. Post mortems may be: • Ordered by the Coroner • Requested by medical staff • Requested by the family. A full post mortem is not always required.	**15.** To establish cause of death.
16. The post mortem may be limited to specific areas of the body.	**16.** To further medical knowledge
17. Consent is not a legal requirement for a coroner's post mortem but good practice requires discussion and information to be given. **a)** If the doctors request a post mortem or the child's family written consent MUST be given. This may be faxed. VERBAL CONSENT IS UNACCEPTABLE. **b)** Consent forms are available on the wards or from Histopathology. Completed forms should be kept with the child's case notes.	**17.** To comply with good practice. **a)** To comply with good practice. **b)** For future referral.
18. If a post mortem is to be performed, the medical staff should explain the procedure and obtain family consent.	**18.** To obtain informed consent, to provide any additional information related to their child's death, and to comply with recommended good practice.
19. If a post mortem is to be performed, an appointment for about 6 weeks later must be made to see the family with the results.	
20. When obtaining consent it is important to: **a)** Have a thorough discussion to ensure there are no objections. **b)** To include all appropriate family members. **c)** Be accurate about what needs to be done. **d)** Ensure consent to any tissue samples or organs to be retained. **e)** Advise when and where it is likely to occur.	**20.** **a–e)** To ensure there are no objections, and to comply with recommended good practice and the newly operational consent forms (Department of Health, Social Services and Public Safety 2004).

589

(*Continued*)

Procedure guideline 22.7 (*Continued*)

Statement	Rationale
21. All the same issues of consent apply when a sample of body tissue is to be taken from the body of a dead child while they are still on the ward. **a)** Consent may occasionally be obtained in advance of death.	**21.** To ensure there are no objections. **a)** To enable samples to be taken immediately on death.
22. Once consent has been given the mortuary technician should be informed and arrangements made for them to receive the case notes and consent form.	**22.** To provide background information for investigation. It may enable the post mortem to be limited.
23. If a post mortem is to be done, the child should be taken to the mortuary and placed in the refrigerator as soon as possible.	**23.** To prevent serious degeneration of the tissues rendering the investigation less useful.

Organ donation

Statement	Rationale
24. Permission to use a child's organs after death, for donation or research, **must** be sought sensitively and be fully explained. A refusal **must** be accepted graciously. **a)** A request is often anticipated by the family and it can be a source of satisfaction to the family.	**24.** To respect the wishes of the family and to comply with recommended good practice. **a)** They may feel that they are helping others.
25. The Transplant Coordinator (if available) should be contacted wherever possible in advance to discuss the suitability of the child's organs. Contra-indications are: • Viral hepatitis • Syphilis • Tuberculosis • Herpes • Disseminated infection • Undiagnosed illness • HIV positive.	**25.** To enable sensitive discussion of organ donation.
26. If donation is likely to be suitable, the family should be approached by the medical and nursing staff involved in their child's care.	**26.** To provide continuity of care.
27. Criteria for brain stem death **must** be met before organ donation can be carried out.	**27.** To meet legal requirements.
28. Advice should be sought from histopathology if there are any questions about the circumstances of a child's death, or if there is uncertainty about which medical devices can be removed.	**28.** To ensure correct management of the situation.
29. Donation of tissues, e.g. cornea, heart valves and skin should also be considered.	**29.** To enable families who cannot donate their child's organs to have the satisfaction of an altruistic act. Limited donation may be possible in cases of malignancy.
30. Children who die at home can still potentially donate organs. Advice should be sought from the local transplant co-ordinator	**30.** To ensure that families are aware of limitations and requirements to maintain organ viability.

590

Preparation of the body

When a child dies at home, washing and dressing the child may be performed by the family, the funeral director or nurse. The following guidelines relate to the preparation of the body in hospital. If this is performed at home they should be adapted as appropriate.

Procedure guideline 22.8 Preparation of the body

Statement	Rationale
1. Prepare equipment for washing and dressing the child. a) Universal precautions must be taken as if the child were alive.	1. To ensure availability of equipment. a) To prevent cross-infection.
2. Tidy bed space, switch off all monitoring equipment and wherever possible remove it from the bed area.	2. To normalise the environment
3a) If possible lay the child flat with their limbs straight. b) Their eyes should be gently closed using moist cotton wool. c) Aspirate any secretions. If secretions are copious the child's orifices **must** be packed. Their mouth should be gently closed.	3a) This will not be possible at a later stage. c) To prevent oozing of secretions.
4a) All drains, tubes, cannulae etc. may be removed and disposed of in waste disposal bags for incineration. They can be left in place unless the parents/carers wish to see their child in the chapel. b) If medical devices are to be left in situ, they should be disconnected as close to the skin as possible and securely spigotted. c) If a post mortem is to be performed and they have been removed, they must be placed in bags and accompany the child.	4a) To leave the child in a 'natural' state. To meet hospital policy. b) To prevent leakage of body fluids. c) To comply with legal requirements. To facilitate investigation of cause of death.
3. Renew dressings and secure them using waterproof adhesive tape.	3. To prevent oozing of secretions.
4a) If the child has a high intestinal stoma, a new stoma appliance or a larger than usual nappy may be applied rather than a gauze dressing. b) Express the child's bladder into a foil bowl or nappy.	4a) To avoid later leakage onto clothing. b) To ensure the bladder is empty.
5a) Wash the child as appropriate. b) Brush their hair into their usual style. c) Dress the child in the chosen clothes.	5a) To leave the child in a 'natural' state. c) To comply with the wishes of the family.
6. Clean the bed and remake using clean bed linen.	6. To ensure the bed is aesthetically clean.
7a) Check that the child's identity band displays the following: • Full name • Hospital registration number • Date of birth • The name of the ward. b) A second identity band with the same information must be applied to another limb.	7a) To ensure full accurate information is recorded. b) To facilitate ease of identification.
8. Leave the child as if 'asleep' with any special toys, etc.	8. To leave the child in a 'natural' state.
9. Flowers, if available, may be left by the child's bed.	9. To soften the environment.

(Continued)

Procedure guideline 22.8 (*Continued*)

Statement	Rationale
Keepsakes	
10a) Parents/carers may ask to take photographs or a video during the child's last days or after death. **b)** If families do not have their own camera, medical illustration (if available) may be contacted during office hours and at other times the intensive care areas may be able to help. **c)** Ascertain if a 'Polaroid' or other camera is available in the hospital.	**10.** To provide a source of comfort.
11a) Mementoes of the child should be offered to the family before they leave the hospital, e.g. photographs, lock of hair, palm/foot prints. **b)** This can be done on behalf of the family but only with their consent. **c)** If hand and footprint equipment is not kept in the hospital it may be obtained from: Baby Safe Inkless Imprint System Tricorn Industries PLC Bensan House Lambard Street Digbell Birmingham B12 09R	**11.** To aid grieving and be a source of comfort.
12. If the parents/carers do not wish to take the mementos at this time, staff may offer to retain the items in the child's notes until a later time.	**12.** To provide comfort at a later date.
Special considerations	
13. If the child has died from a potentially highly infectious disease, e.g. HIV, viral hepatitis, open pulmonary tuberculosis, they should be placed in a body bag.	**13.** To meet government recommendations.
14. The mortuary technician **MUST** be informed of the disease.	
15. • The child should be placed in a body bag once they are in the mortuary. • Body bags are kept in the mortuary. • A biohazard sticker should be placed on the outside of the body bag. • The child may be removed from the body bag for viewing but must be put back into the bag afterwards. • If the child is removed from the body bag for viewing or examination, infectious precautions **must** be maintained as when the child was alive, i.e. the wearing of protective clothing. • This clothing must also be offered to family members.	
16. Used linen should be disposed of according to the Waste Policy, i.e. in the infectious linen bag.	

Moving the child who dies in hospital

Procedure guideline 22.9 Moving the child who dies in hospital

Statement	Rationale
To the mortuary 1. The child may be transferred to the mortuary as follows: • On the mortuary trolley covered with a blanket • In the arms of a nurse or carer, wrapped in a blanket, which is replaced with a sheet on arrival to the mortuary • In the mortuary concealment trolley if of appropriate size • An oxygen mask may be placed over the child's face.	**1a)** To facilitate the transfer of the child. This can appear to be more acceptable and can reduce the distress of all involved. **b)** Fully covering the child's face may draw unnecessary attention.
2. A nurse should accompany the child.	2. To complete the caring process.
3. The Portering staff should be asked to help move the child from the ward if necessary.	3. To facilitate the safe and smooth transfer of the child.
4. The child should be placed in the mortuary according to their instructions.	4. To meet hospital policy.
5a) The child should be laid supine in the mortuary refrigerator with any accompanying toys. **b)** Any special blanket may be left with the child.	**5a)** To maintain the child in as optimal condition as possible until they are collected by the undertakers. **b)** It can be used to re-wrap the child if their family visit at a later date.
6a) Special toys and keepsakes can be taken to the mortuary. **b)** Toys and keepsakes left with the child must be in a sealed plastic bag. **c)** These should be clearly labelled with the name of the child.	**6a)** These familiar items can provide comfort to the child's family. **b)** To avoid contamination from body fluids. **c)** To ensure each child has its own possessions.
7a) If parents/carers wish to leave jewellery with their child it is advisable to keep the quantities to a minimum. Rings and bracelets should be secured with tape. **b)** If jewellery or religious artefacts are left, this must be indicated in the 'comments' section of the Mortuary Register along with a full description of the items. **c)** The mortuary staff needs written consent to remove any jewellery.	**7a)** Large quantities of valuables are a security risk. **c)** To provide an audit trail.
8. A 'Notification of Death' slip should be attached to the front of the sheet.	8. To meet hospital policy, comply with legal requirements and facilitate identification.
9. All details, as requested, should be entered into the Mortuary Register or written on the white board by the refrigerators as appropriate.	9. The mortician needs to know the child's diagnosis.
10. If a child is HIV positive, 'retrovirus', should be written in the mortuary register and notification of death slips.	
To home 1. Some families may wish to take their child home from the hospital themselves.	1. Unless a post mortem is required there is no legal reason why they cannot do so.
2. The family must have the child's death certificate before taking their child home.	

593

(Continued)

Procedure guideline 22.9 (*Continued*)

Statement	Rationale
3a) The child may be taken home using undertakers or the parent's/carer's own transport. **b)** It is not advisable for the parent/carer to be the driver of the transport. **c)** The child's details must be entered into the mortuary register with name of the parents/carers/undertaker who has taken them.	**3.** To meet the requirements of the family.
4. If the parents/carers wish to take their child home using their own transport, they should also receive a proforma letter detailing the circumstances of their journey. (See Figure 22.1).	**4.** To provide additional information as required. To avoid distressing enquires, e.g. from the Police.
5. Families should be reminded that they should register their child's death within 5 days.	**5.** To meet legal requirements
6. Advice may be sought from the Child Death Helpline (telephone 0800 282 986) or the local Transport Office.	

After care

Procedure guideline 22.10 **After care**

Statement	Rationale
1a) After the family have spent time with their child, if they do not want to assist with last offices, they should be provided with a quiet room away from the child's bedside. **b)** The family should be given the opportunity to telephone a friend or relative to join them.	**1a)** To ensure privacy. **b)** To obtain support from known people.
2a) If the child has died in hospital the family should be informed of the following before leaving: • What will happen to their child • That they may return to see their child at any time • To contact the ward in advance of this • The phone number for the ward • A name of a specific staff member to ask for (wherever possible) • That they will receive an appointment to return to the hospital to meet their child's consultant and other staff to talk over anything they wish to discuss. **b)** They should be given any relevant booklets produced by either the DSS or the local NHS Trust.	**2a)** To ensure they are kept informed and to enable the visit to be organised. **b)** These contain a summary of the actions that need to be taken after a child has died.
3. The following advice may be offered to lactating mothers: • To wear a firm, well supporting bra • To take regular analgesia • Hormone therapy is no longer considered appropriate • To seek advice from their own midwife or health visitor.	**3.** To offer guidance and support.
4. If a child dies in hospital the family should be accompanied from the ward or mortuary when they are ready to leave.	**4.** To provide support.

Procedure guideline 22.10 (*Continued*)

Statement	Rationale
5a) The nurse should establish how the family are returning home. Transport, e.g. a taxi, may have to be arranged and possibly paid for by the Trust. During office hours advice may be sought from the Transport Office and out of hours from the Site Manager.	**5a)** To ensure their safety.
b) If a child dies at home the nurse should ascertain from the family the level and type of contact and support that they would find appropriate in the time immediately following the child's death.	**b)** To provide support.

Great Ormond Street **NHS**
Hospital for Children
NHS Trust

Great Ormond Street
London WC1N
3JH

To whom it may concern

Date:

This letter is to confirm that (Child's Name) ....

has died at Great Ormond Street Hospital For Children.

The child is being driven to the following location:

....

....

....

....

By: Accompanied by:

....

....

....

....

A medical certificate of cause of death has been issued to (this should be one of the above people):

....

Signature: ....

Print Name: ....

Designation: ....

Ward: ....

Telephone Number: ....

Figure 22.1 Proforma letter.

Acknowledgements

Thank you to Jean Simons (Assistant Director of Family Services) and Sam Howard (Clinical Placement Facilitator) for their permission to reproduce in this section from their clinical practice guideline, *Death: care after*.

Key texts

Association for Children with Life-threatening or Terminal Conditions and their Families (ACT) and Royal College of Paediatrics and Child Health (RCPCH) (1997) A Guide to the Development of Children's Palliative Care Services. London, ACT and RCPCH

Association for Children with Life-threatening or Terminal Conditions and their Families (ACT), National Council for Hospice and Specialist Palliative Care Services and Scottish Partnership Agency for Palliative and Cancer Care (SPAPCC) (2001) Palliative Care for Young People Aged 13–24 Years. Bristol, ACT, National Council for Hospice and Specialist Palliative Care Services and SPAPCC

Association for Children with Life-threatening or Terminal Conditions and their Families (ACT) (2004) Integrated multi-agency care pathways for children with life-threatening and life-limiting conditions. Bristol, ACT

Association for Children with Lif -threatening or Terminal Conditions and their Families (ACT) (2009) A Guide to the Development of Children's Palliative Care Services, 3rd edition. Bristol, ACT

Bristol Royal Infirmary Inquiry (2000) Interim Report: Removal and Retention of Human Material. London, Central Office for Information

Department of Health (2008) Better Care: Better Lives Improving outcomes and experiences for children, young people and their families living with life-limiting and life-threatening conditions. London, COI

Goldman A. (1994) Care of the Dying Child. Oxford, Oxford University

Great Ormond Street Hospital for Children NHS Foundation Trust (2000) When a Child Dies Staff Handbook, 2nd edition. London, Great Ormond Street Hospital for Children NHS Foundation Trust

Great Ormond Street Hospital for Children NHS Foundation Trust (2006) End of Life Care Pathway. London, Great Ormond Street Hospital for Children NHS Foundation Trust

Great Ormond Street Hospital for Children NHS Foundation Trust (2007) End of life care pathway: guidance for practitioners. London, GOSH

Royal College of Paediatrics and Child Health (1997) Withholding or Withdrawing Life-Saving Treatment in Children: A Framework for Practice. London, RCPCH

Stewart A, Dent A. (1994) At a Loss. London, Ballière Tindall

596

References

Ahmedzai S, Regnard C. (1995) Dyspnoea. In Regnard C, Hockley J. (eds) Flow Diagrams in Advanced Cancer and other Diseases. London, Edward Arnold

Association for Children with Life-threatening or Terminal Conditions and their Families (ACT) and Royal College of Paediatrics and Child Health (RCPCH) (1997) A Guide to the Development of Children's Palliative Care Services. London, ACT and RCPCH

Association for Children with Life-threatening or Terminal Conditions and their Families (ACT) (2011) Available at http://www.act.org.uk/page.asp?section=56&search=ACT+Charter (last accessed November 2011)

Baines M, Sykes N. (1993) Gastrointestinal symptoms. In Saunders C, Sykes N. (Eds) The Management of Terminal Malignant Disease, 3rd edition. Boston, Hodder and Stoughton

Breitbart W, Chochino HM, Passick S. (1998) Psychiatric aspects of palliative care. In Doyle D, Hanks GWC, McDonald N. (eds) The Oxford Textbook of Palliative Medicine, 2nd edition. Oxford, Oxford University Press

Casey A. (1988) A partnership with child and family. Senior Nurse, 8(4), 8–9

Curran JS, Barnes LA. (2000) Part IV Nutrition, the feeding of infants and children. In Behrman RE, Kleigman RM, Jenson HB. (eds) Nelson Textbook of Pediatrics, 16th edition. Philadephia, W.B Saunders Company

Davies B, Oberle K. (1990) Dimensions of the supportive role of the nurse in palliative care. Oncology Nurses Forum, 17(1), 87–94

Department of Health, Social Services and Public Safety (2004) Post Mortem Examinations. Good Practice in Consent and the Care of the Bereaved. Available online at: http://www.dhsspsni.gov.uk/postmortem.pdf (last accessed 9th January 2012)

Department of Health (2007) Palliative care services for children and young people in England: an independent review for the Secretary of State for Health. London, DH Publications

Department of Health (2008) Better Care: Better Lives: Improving outcomes and experiences for children, young people and their families living with life-limiting and life-threatening conditions. London, DH Publications

Doyle D. (1995) Forward. In Regnard C, Hockley J. (1995) Flow Diagrams in Advanced Cancer and other Diseases. London, Edward Arnold

Fraser J, Harris N et al (2010) Advanced care planning in children with limiting conditions – the wishes document. Archives of Disease in Childhood, 95(2), 79–80

Goldman A. (ed.) (1998) Care of the Dying Child, 2nd edition. Oxford, Oxford University Press

Goldman A, Burne R. (1998) Symptom management. In Goldman A. (ed.) Care of the Dying Child, 2nd edition. Oxford, Oxford University Press

Goldman A, Hewitt M, Collins GS, Childs M, Hain R (2006) Symptoms in children/young people with progressive malignant disease: United Kingdom Children's Cancer Study Group/Paediatroc Oncology Nurses Forum Survey. Pediatrics, 117(6), 1179–1186

Heyse–Moore L. (1993) Respiratory symptoms. In Saunders C, Syke N. (eds) The Management of Terminal Malignant Disease, 3rd edition. Boston, Hodder and Stoughton

Hinds P, Burghen EA, Pritchard M. (2007) Conducting end-of-life studies in pediatric oncology. Western Journal of Nursing Research, 29(4), 448–465

Hodgson G. (1993) Depression, sadness and anxiety. In Saunders C, Sykes N. (eds) The Management of Terminal Malignant Disease, 3rd edition. Boston, Hodder and Stoughton

Kaye P. (1999) Decision Making in Palliative Care. Northampton, EPL Publications

Liben S, Papadatou D, Wolfe J. (2008) Paediatric palliative care: challenges and emerging ideas. Lancet, 371, 852–864

Lissauer T, Clayden G. (2001) Illustrated Textbook of Paediatrics, 2nd edition. Edinburgh, Mosby International

Mannix K. (1998) Palliation of nausea and vomiting. In Doyle D, Hanks G, Cherny N, Calman K. (eds) The Oxford Textbook of Palliative Medicine, 2nd edition. Oxford, Oxford University Press

McCulloch R, Comac M, Criag F. (2008) Paediatric palliative care: coming of age in oncology? European Journal of Cancer, 44, 1139–1145

Pritchard M, Burghen E, Srivastava DK, Okuma J, Anderson L, Powell B, Furman WL, Hinds PS. (2008) Cancer-related symptoms most concerning to parents during the last week and last days of their child's life. Pediatrics, 121(5), 1301–1309

Regnard C. (1995) Dysphagia. In Regnard C, Hockley J. (eds) Flow Diagrams in Advanced Cancer and other Diseases. London, Edward Arnold

Regnard C, Comiskey M. (1995) Nausea and vomiting. In Regnard C, Hockley J. (eds) Flow Diagrams in Advanced Cancer and other Diseases. London, Edward Arnold

Regnard C, Makin W. (1995) Bleeding. In Regnard C, Hockley J. (eds) Flow Diagrams in Advanced Cancer and other Diseases. London, Edward Arnold.

Regnard C, Mannix K. (1995a) Diarrhoea. In Regnard C, Hockley J. (eds) Flow Diagrams in Advanced Cancer and other Diseases. London, Edward Arnold

Regnard C, Mannix K. (1995b) Reduced hydration or feeding. In Regnard C, Hockley J. (eds) Flow Diagrams in Advanced Cancer and other Diseases. London, Edward Arnold

Regnard C, Tempest S. (1998) A Guide to Symptom Relief in Advanced Disease, 4th edition. Hale, Hochland and Hochland

Saunders C, Sykes N. (eds) (1993) The Management of Terminal Malignant Disease, 3rd edition. Boston, Hodder and Stoughton

Sinha S, Bastin ME, Wardlaw JM, Armitage PA, Whittle IR. (2004) Effects of dexamethasone on peritumour odeamatous brain: a DT-MRI study. Journal of Neurology, Neurosurgery & Psychiatry, 75(11), 1632–1635

The West Midlands Paediatric Macmillan Team (2005) Palliative Care for the Child with Malignant Disease. London, Quay Books, MA Healthcare Limited

Twycross R, Wilcock A. (2001) Symptom Management in Advanced Cancer, 3rd edition. Abingdon, Radcliffe Medical Press

Twycross R. (2002) Introducing Palliative Care, 4th edition London, Radcliffe Publishing

Twycross R, Wilcok A, Stark Toller C. (2009) Symptom management in advanced cancer. Palliativedrugs.com Ltd. http://www.palliativedrugs.com/index.html (last accessed January 2012)

Twycross R, Lichter I. (1998) The terminal phase. In Doyle D, Hanks GWC, McDonald N. (eds) The Oxford Textbook of Palliative Medicine, 2nd edition. Oxford, Oxford University Press

Vickers J, Thompson A, Collins GS, Childs M, Hain R. (2007) Place and provision of palliative care for children with progressive cancer: a study by the Paediatic Oncology Nurses Foprum/United Kingdom Children's Cancer Study Group Palliative Care Working Party. Journal of Clinical Oncology, 25(28), 4472–4476

Wolfe J, Grier HE, Klar N, Levin SB, Ellenbogen JM, Salem-Schatz S, Emanuel EJ, Weeks JC. (2000) Symptoms and suffering at the end of life in children with cancer. The New England Journal of Medicine, 342(5), 326–333

Chapter 23

Peri-operative care

Chapter contents

Procedure guidelines

The Great Ormond Street Hospital Manual of Children's Nursing Practices, First Edition. Edited by Susan Macqueen, Elizabeth Anne Bruce, Faith Gibson.
© 2012 Great Ormond Street Hospital for Children NHS Foundation Trust. Published 2012 by Blackwell Publishing Ltd.

Introduction

This chapter is divided into two sections, the first covering preoperative preparation and the second perioperative care. Preoperative preparation has increasingly been recognised as an important part of perioperative care and, as part of the National Health Service (NHS) Plan (Department of Health 2000), the NHS Modernisation Agency (2003) published recommendations for preoperative assessment to improve preparation and assessment of the patient. These guidelines incorporate both physical and psychological aspects of care and although they are adult focused many of the principles apply to children. They highlight the importance of preparing the child and family, physically and psychologically, for the ordeal of surgery and the need for the child to be in optimum condition for the best postoperative result.

It is the responsibility of the perioperative team – medical, nursing and paramedical – to ensure that the environment is as safe as possible so that the only trauma experienced by the child is the intended surgery and appropriate risk assessments, using a relevant risk assessment tool, are carried out where necessary (Royal College of Nursing 2011). They are dependent on their ward-based colleagues to ensure that all information relevant to the child's condition is communicated to the theatre team. This should be done either at the time of booking the procedure, or before the child is brought to the department, as omissions may compromise the quality of the perioperative care. This can range from something as simple as the identification of loose milk teeth to the discussion and agreements required for a Jehovah's Witness child having major surgery, or those children whose condition is exacerbated, for example, by an underlying latex allergy. Some centres advocate the benefits of preoperative visits by theatre staff to enhance such information exchanges (Harris 2007) but this practice is not universal.

The 1959 Platt Report (Welfare of Children in Hospital) recommended that not only should parents/carers be allowed to stay with their child in hospital but suggested that they should accompany their child to the operating department; this practice has been widely adopted (Alsop-Shields 2000). However, parents/carers should not feel pressurised to do so, as their anxiety is liable to transfer to the child and can aggravate an already stressful situation (Donnelly 2005).

Preoperative preparation

The child should be as fit as possible before undergoing surgery and anaesthesia to minimise the risk of complications. A thorough assessment of their physical condition, medical history and appropriate investigations should be undertaken. Investigations have often been performed routinely as a precaution, however the National Institute for Clinical Excellence (NICE) (2003) issued guidelines about preoperative investigations, which should help streamline the tests required and avoid unnecessary tests that are not only traumatic for the child, but are also time consuming and costly to the health service. Whether investigations are required or not will be dependent

on the type of surgery to be undertaken and the health of the child. For children with complex medical histories investigations and treatment may be required to ensure they are in optimum condition. For example, a child with congenital heart disease may need a preoperative echocardiogram to check cardiac function, together with full blood count and urea and electrolyte measurements. The results of these would indicate whether any action was required to optimise the child's condition prior to surgery. It is a recommendation of the Royal College of Surgeons (2007) that complex paediatric surgery should be centralised in units where this work is carried out routinely in order to provide the best outcomes.

Although there is no consensus on the best way to prepare the child for surgery, most studies agree that some form of preoperative preparation is beneficial (Cassady *et al* 1999, Ho Cheung William Li 2007, Kain *et al* 1998, 2007, Mcgraw 1994, RCN 2011) and may help reduce postoperative sequelae including nightmares, bedwetting and other regressive behaviour (Margolis *et al* 1998) as well as reducing pain (Kain *et al* 2006). The adverse effects vary according to the age and cognition of the child: some understanding of child development is required to enable the best methods of preparation to be undertaken. However, it is not only the child who needs to be prepared for the procedure, but also the parents/carers, as their anxiety can affect the way the child copes with the stress (Kain *et al* 1996). As well as preparing the family for the procedure, preoperative preparation should also prepare the child and family about what to expect on discharge from hospital.

Parents/carers are often well informed about the procedure their child is having through access to the internet and services such as NHS direct. However, these resources, although useful, need to be enhanced by preparation from the people who will be caring for the child to ensure the family has accurate information and has fully understood what will happen.

With shorter hospital stays and increasing levels of day surgery, as well as day of admission surgery, there is less time to prepare the family for procedures and an increased likelihood of cancellation if the child is not adequately prepared. As a result, preoperative assessment clinics have become increasingly popular over recent years. These are often nurse led with anaesthetic input as required. These preadmission visits allow the child to become familiar with the hospital environment and, for the older child and parents/carers, there is more time for questions and time to contemplate information that is given to them, which should help to reduce anxiety. It also enables parents/carers to prepare their child for what to expect if they have a greater knowledge and understanding themselves.

It is well documented that individuals who are anxious and stressed are less able to take in and understand information given to them (Quinn 1996). Therefore, giving information early in a more relaxed environment may help parents/carers understand more, with the result that consent for surgery and anaesthesia really is informed.

The preoperative period is a vital part of perioperative care in which nurses play an important role in ensuring that the child and family are fully prepared both physically and psychologically for the ensuing procedure.

Procedure guideline 23.1 **Pre-admission**

Statement	Rationale
1. Where possible the child and family should be offered a pre-admission visit.	**1.** To prepare child and family in advance of surgery in a relaxed manner and allow them to familiarise themselves with the hospital environment.
2. Where a preadmission service is available the following should be undertaken: **a)** A physical assessment of the child. **b)** Relevant investigations (see NICE 2003). **c)** Psychological preparation of the child and family using age appropriate methods. **d)** Information should include written information about the hospital, the surgery and its associated risks, including the risk of surgical site infection.	**2.** **a)** To ensure the child is fit for surgery. **b)** To ensure test results are available prior to surgery and action can be taken if abnormalities are found. **c)** To reduce anxiety and minimise adverse postoperative sequelae. **d)** To ensure that the family are fully informed of risks and benefits and can give informed consent for the procedure (DoH 2001, NICE 2008).
3. If a preadmission service is not available information leaflets should be sent to the family prior to admission, including hospital details, what the procedure entails and what to expect afterwards, suggestions on how to prepare their child, fasting information and a telephone number to ring if there are any queries.	**3.** To ensure they know what to expect both on admission and for discharge and can adequately prepare for the procedure. A range of information leaflets are available on the GOSH website at http://www.gosh.nhs.uk/medical-conditions/

Procedure guideline 23.2 **Admission to hospital**

Statement	Rationale
1. Introduce yourself to child and family when they arrive on the ward and orientate them to the ward.	**1.** To promote a welcoming environment and to put the child and family at ease.
2. If the child has been pre-admitted check that there has been no change in health status since the pre-admission visit.	**2.** To ensure the child is still fit for surgery.
3. If the child has not been pre-admitted they will need to be examined and a history taken, along with any relevant investigations.	**3.** To ensure the child is fit for surgery and anaesthesia.
4. Check with the parent/carer that the child's details are correct and apply an identity band ensuring correct spelling of child's name, date of birth and NHS number, and check that these details correspond with information on the patient notes. If this is not possible (e.g. nonadherence/allergy) then an alternative method of identification must be followed according to local policy.	**4.** To ensure correct identification of child at all stages during the stay and minimise errors.
5. Check and record vital signs including TPR, BP and where appropriate SpO$_2$ (see Chapter 1).	**5.** To provide baseline observations as a reference point for observations during and after surgery.

Procedure guideline 23.2 (Continued)

Statement	Rationale
6. If the child is pyrexial the anaesthetist must be informed.	**6.** The anaesthetist may decide to cancel the operation if the child has a fever because of the risk of post-operative complications.
7. Check that the child has not had a recent cough or 'cold'.	**7.** Recent or current upper respiratory tract infection (URTI) increases the likelihood of an adverse respiratory event during anaesthesia (Cohen and Cameron 1991) and may increase the incidence of hypoxaemia in the recovery period (Levy *et al* 1992).
8. Check that there has been no contact with infectious diseases in past 2 weeks.	**8.** Incubation period of most childhood infectious diseases is between 12 hours and 21 days (e.g. norovirus and varicella respectively).
9. If the child has been in contact with a childhood infectious disease surgery should be postponed.	**9.** The child is at risk of developing the illness and may be an infection risk to other patients as well as having an increasing risk of anaesthetic complications.
10. Depending on hospital policy, admission nose and throat swabs, skin lesions and stool and urine samples may be taken.	**10.** To screen for antimicrobial resistance such as MRSA infection (DoH 2007a) and for any abnormalities in the urine.
11. Weigh the child.	**11.** Accurate measurement of weight is required to prescribe appropriate drug dosages.
12. Complete relevant documentation including weight, allergies and relevant medical and social history.	**12.** To comply with legal and professional requirements and to ensure that the child's records are comprehensive and to provide information to other clinicians.
13. Discuss with the child, if they are old enough, what they understand about why they have come to hospital.	**13.** To ascertain what their level of comprehension is and to correct any misunderstanding.
14. Where appropriate use play therapy to prepare the child for their procedure.	**14.** To help the child understand what is going to happen and allow them to work through any anxieties.

601

Principles table 23.1 Consent

Principle	Rationale
1. Consent should be obtained by a clinician who is capable of performing the procedure or has had specialist training in giving advice about the procedure (DoH 2001).	1. To comply with legal requirements and to ensure that any queries can be fully answered. Ultimately it is the responsibility of the clinician performing the procedure to ensure that the patient is fully informed and consents to the procedure.
2. The consent form must be signed by a person with parental responsibility (if child is not old enough to give consent).	2. Only individuals with parental responsibility can legally give consent for surgery. For more information on consent and parental responsibility see the Introduction.

Principles table 23.2 **Fasting**

Principle	Rationale
1. The following minimum fasting periods prior to surgery and anaesthesia are recommended by the Association of Anaesthetists of Great Britain and Ireland (2010): • 6 hours for food, infant formula and milk • 4 hours for breast milk • 2 hours for a clear drink (one you can read the paper through).	1. To ensure minimal residual gastric volume and minimise the risk of vomiting and aspirating stomach contents into lungs during induction of anaesthesia.
2a) It is essential that the period of fasting is not extended unnecessarily. Good communication with theatre staff regarding list changes and delays will help to avoid this. b) Premature infants and neonates may need an intravenous infusion prior to theatre.	2a) Prolonged fasting can result in malaise, increased stress and irritability (Schreiner et al 1990). b) Young infants are at greater risk of dehydration and hypoglycaemia with prolonged fasting times.
3. Children with certain metabolic conditions need careful consideration with regard to fasting times and placement on the list.	3. These children are at greater risk of metabolic imbalance if starved for too long.

Principles table 23.3 **Premedication**

Principle	Rationale
1. Premedication, when prescribed, should preferably be administered orally. The intramuscular (IM) route should be avoided where possible. However, it may be used for atropine in certain instances as the effect is more reliable than by the oral route.	1. Oral medications are more acceptable to child and family. IM injections are painful and traumatic for all involved.
2. Sedative premedication, most commonly a benzodiazepine such as midazolam, may be prescribed if the child is anxious. This should be administered 30 minutes prior to going to theatre.	2. Peak effects of midazolam are between 30–45 minutes.
3. Anticholinergic drugs such as atropine are rarely used, as modern inhalational anaesthetics are less irritant to the airways than previous agents, but they may be required in certain conditions or for certain procedures such as prior to ear, nose and throat (ENT) surgery.	3. To prevent reflex bradycardia and to reduce secretions.
4. Gastric motility drugs may be prescribed for those children who are predisposed to gastro-oesophageal reflux.	4. To help reduce likelihood of vomiting and aspiration on induction of anaesthesia.
5. Local anaesthetic cream (EMLA or Ametop), where prescribed, should be applied to appropriate sites (e.g. back of the hands and antecubital fossa) 1 hour prior to theatre.	5. To allow time for cream to take effect to reduce the pain of cannula insertion.
6. Children with underlying conditions such as asthma or epilepsy may need medication prior to theatre.	6. To maintain therapeutic drug levels and prevent symptoms of the condition occurring.

Procedure guideline 23.3 Immediately prior to theatre

Statement	Rationale
1. The child should have had a recent bath/wash and will usually wear a theatre gown to go to theatre, although for some procedures it may be possible for the child to wear their own clothes.	1. To minimise the infection risk and provide easy access to the operation site and easy attachment of monitoring equipment.
2. Any nail varnish should be removed and jewellery should be removed or taped over.	2. Nail varnish prevents a clear view of the colour of the nail bed and may obscure cyanosis; it also interferes with pulse oximetry. Jewellery increases the risk of accidental burns when diathermy is used.
3. Final checks and a preoperative checklist must be completed before the child leaves the ward for theatre. Ensure that: • The child is wearing an identity band and that the information matches that on the medical notes • The consent form is present with notes and has been signed • The child has been fasted for the relevant time period.	3. To ensure the child is identifiable and that all relevant documentation accompanies child to theatre.
4. Child and parents/carers should be escorted to theatre by a nurse.	4. The nurse provides support for the family and will handover the care of the child to the theatre staff.
5. If sedation has been used the child should be transferred to theatre on a trolley with oxygen available.	5. Sedation may cause respiratory depression requiring the administration of oxygen.
6. In the anaesthetic room the parents/carers can usually stay with their child until they are anaesthetised.	6. To provide reassurance for the child.
7. The nurse should also remain with the child and parents/carers and escort the parents/carers back to the ward when the child is anaesthetised.	7. To provide help with distracting the child and to support the parents/carers.

Perioperative care

It is important that all areas of the operating department are as clean and dust-free as possible before and after the operating list as well as between cases. This will reduce the potential for cross-infection.

Procedure guideline 23.4 Care in the anaesthetic room

Statement	Rationale
1. The anaesthetic room should be fully prepared to receive the child and family with all of the necessary and appropriate sized equipment available and the drugs already checked and ready for use.	1. To ensure that the equipment is available and safe, the atmosphere within the room remains calm in order to put the child and family at their ease and minimise delays.
2. There should be some methods of distraction available, such as washable pictures on walls and ceilings or washable toys.	2. To focus the child's attention away from stressful procedures such as venous cannulation.

(Continued)

Procedure guideline 23.4 (*Continued*)

Statement	Rationale
3. The child should be allowed to bring a special toy or comforter with them. This item should either be stored safely during the surgical procedure either on the trolley/bed or by the family so that it is available immediately afterwards.	**3.** To enhance the conscious child's comfort during the perioperative period.
4. This may extend to objects of a religious nature that the child/family may insist remains on or near the child during the surgical procedure.	**4.** To assure the child and family that their spiritual needs are being met without compromising the safety of the child.
5. It is important for the child and parents/carers to be put at ease in order to ensure that the induction goes as smoothly as possible.	**5.** Unlike the ward situation, there is no time for the anaesthetic team to build up a rapport with the child and family in order to gain their trust and the parent/carer need to be confident that the team is able to care for their child (Kristensson-Hallstrom 2000).
6. The anaesthetic team should carry out a full check using the patient records and identity band prior to induction to ensure it is the: • Correct child • Correct procedure • Correct starvation time • Correct side/limb marked (if applicable) • Correct consent form signed and dated.	**6.** To avoid an incorrect procedure being carried out (National Patient Safety Agency (NPSA) 2009).
7. Where possible, the removal of clothing should occur once the child is asleep. This may need to be done beforehand if the access for the anaesthetist is restricted.	**7.** To preserve the child's dignity and safety and to promote safe positioning on the operating table (Donnelly 2005).
8. Glasses and/or hearing aids should not be removed until the child is asleep. These aids should be stored safely in order to be put back on the child once they are conscious.	**8.** To facilitate communication before and after the procedure and to avoid heightening the child's stress.
9. The child should be offered a choice of induction agents, even if they have had a topical anaesthetic cream administered.	**9.** The child may cooperate more if they believe they have been consulted and have some control over pending events.
10. The child should be in a comfortable position for the induction; this may be while sitting on the parent/carer's lap.	**10.** To reassure the child during the procedure and to enhance the effect of the induction agent.
11. The parent/carer should be allowed the opportunity to briefly say farewell to their child before leaving the anaesthetic room.	**11.** To meet the parents'/carers' emotional needs.
12a) Cannulation is mandatory for anaesthetised children. This should be secured firmly, in an aseptic manner, once established (DoH 2007b, Walker and Lockie 2000). **b)** If the child's identity band has had to be removed during the cannulation, a new identity band with the correct patient details should be placed on an unaffected limb as soon as possible. **c)** Equipment used for airway management will depend on the type of surgery to be carried out but must be able to be positioned correctly and securely maintained. **d)** Eyes should be taped shut unless ophthalmic surgery is to be carried out.	**12a)** To ensure there is a secure route for the administration of drugs and/or fluids during the surgical procedure and minimise the risk of cannula site infection in the postoperative period (Harris 2007). **b)** To facilitate safe checking throughout the child's stay in the operating department (Morse 2007, NPSA 2009). **c)** To ensure continued airway maintenance throughout the procedure. **d)** To avoid accidental damage (Harris 2007).

Procedure guideline 23.5 Care in the operating theatre

Statement	Rationale
1. The theatre should be fully prepared to receive the child with all of the necessary, appropriate-sized equipment checked and ready for use, including table attachments, positioning aids, tourniquets and diathermy plates.	1. To provide a safe environment for the child and staff.

Thermoregulation	See also Chapter 17 (Neonatal Care).
2. Room temperatures may need to be increased for neonatal surgery and for children with extensive tissue damage, such as burns/scalds.	2. Neonates have immature thermoregulation systems and require assistance to maintain optimum temperature. Hypothermia in neonates may destabilise blood sugar levels and lead to increased oxygen needs (Brown *et al* 2000, Wilson and da Cunha 2007, Yeo 1998). Excess fluid loss with extensive tissue damage can result in hypoxia due to hypovolaemic shock (Methven *et al* 2007).
3. The operating table may be 'prewarmed' and the use of a warming blanket/mattress should be considered for use throughout the surgical procedure.	3. To maintain the child's temperature.
4. Warm antiseptic skin preparations should be considered and the use of alcohol-based solutions should be avoided for preterm infants.	4. Evaporation can increase the potential for hypothermia (Harris 2007).

Manual handling	
5a) Appropriately sized lifting/transfer aids should be used to move the child to and from the trolley and operating table.	5a) To protect the child and staff from injury.
b) Handling of preterm infants, especially extremely low birth weight babies, should be kept to a minimum.	b) To reduce the effects of prolonged environmental stress (Askin and Wilson 2007). Preterm infants are unable to differentiate different types of stimuli so eliciting a physiological over-response to all stimuli (Yeo 1998).

Positioning	
6. The child should be placed in an optimum position for the surgery to be performed, ensuring that limbs are moved and secured in a 'neutral' state.	6. To facilitate surgical access and avoid potential limb dislocation and nerve damage. To avoid potential pressure damage and to avoid accidental disconnection of anaesthetic medical devices (Smith 2007).
7. Skin should be protected from contact with metal including jewellery, which should either be removed prior to admission to the operating department or taped down.	7. To avoid intraoperative contact burns as a result of using diathermy (Kneedler and Dodge 1991).

Pressure care	
8a) Care should be taken to ensure that all potential pressure points are protected using equipment such as gel pads, 'gamgee', etc.	8a) To avoid the formation of intraoperative pressure injuries.
b) The scrub assistant should ensure that the sterile drapes and surgical equipment should not pose a pressure risk for the child during the surgical procedure.	b) Preterm and low birth weight babies have little subcutaneous fat and fragile skin so are at increased risk of pressure damage (Dimond 1994).

Privacy and dignity	
9. The child should remain covered until the start of the surgical procedure.	9. To maintain the child's dignity and to reduce the potential for hypothermia.

605

(Continued)

Procedure guideline 23.5 (*Continued*)

Statement	Rationale
Surgical 'pause'	
10. The surgical, anaesthetic and theatre team should pause prior to the commencement of surgery in order to confirm: • Correct child • Correct site marked (if applicable) • Correct consented procedure • Available imaging to check correct site (if applicable) • Availability of correct prosthesis (if applicable).	**10.** To avoid an incorrect procedure being carried out (NPSA 2009).
Blood loss	
11. Scrub staff should keep accurate blood loss records due to the small circulating volumes of children.	**11.** To avoid intra- and postoperative hypovolaemia and associated complications.
Electrosurgical diathermy	
12a) The appropriate-sized patient plate should be applied to smooth, dry intact skin as near to the surgical site as possible but avoid placement over bony prominences. **b)** The skin beneath the plate should be checked carefully after removal.	**12a)** To ensure safe placement of electrosurgical equipment and to prevent skin damage (Kneedler and Dodge 1991). **b)** To ensure that the skin is intact and injury-free.
Surgical count	
13. A surgical count of all equipment, swabs and sharps should be performed and documented at the start and end of the procedure and at the closing of each cavity and cavity within a cavity.	**13.** To prevent retention of foreign bodies and harm to the patient (Plumridge and Anderson 2011).
Before transfer to recovery	
14a) After the procedure the child's skin should be cleaned of skin preparation solution and any other soiling. **b)** The child should then be dressed in a clean hospital gown or their own clothing prior to transfer to the trolley/bed. An appropriate-sized clean nappy should be put on (if applicable).	**14a)** To enable a check of skin integrity. **b)** To increase the child's comfort.
15. Trolley sides should be fitted with protective 'bumpers' to prevent the child from injuring themselves.	**15.** The child may become restless as consciousness returns (Harris 2007).
16. All intraoperative care records should be completed and authorised by the appropriate staff prior to the child's transfer to recovery, including the surgical counts.	**16.** To ensure completeness of documentation and surgical equipment prior to the child's transfer from the operating theatre.
17. All used equipment, soiled linens and sharps should be disposed of in compliance with Trust waste regulations.	**17.** To ensure the safe decontamination and disposal of surgical equipment and devices.

Recovery

This section provides a brief overview of the care of the child in recovery. For a more extensive version, which includes many of the assessment procedures covered in Chapter 1, go to http://www.gosh.nhs.uk/health-professionals/clinical-guidelines/recovery-care-of-the-child/.

Procedure guideline 23.6 **Recovery**

Statement

1a) The recovery room should be fully prepared to receive the child and family with all of the necessary, appropriate-sized equipment checked and ready for use. This should include near patient testing devices, such as glucometers, and resuscitation equipment.

b) The area should be child-friendly with washable pictures and toys.

2. The recovery staff should receive a complete handover, including documentation, from the anaesthetist and scrub staff on the following points:
  a) Child's name (checked against the patient notes and the identity band).
  b) Anaesthetic details including
  • Anaesthetic drugs, including any reversal agents
  • Intraoperative analgesia and fluid replacement as well as postoperative maintenance
  • Monitoring required in recovery and on return to the ward.
  c) Surgery performed including:
  • Wound closure and dressings
  • Infiltration of local anaesthetic agent (if applicable) including site and amount
  • Details of any drains, catheters and their losses
  • Any specific postoperative instructions from the surgeon.

3a) The recovery staff will observe and maintain the child's airway until the child is able to safely manage it by themselves.
  b) The following routine observations should be carried out:
  • Heart rate
  • Respiratory rate
  • Oxygen saturation
  • Blood pressure
  • Temperature
  • Wound/wound dressing
  • Drains/catheters.
  c) These should be recorded in the patient notes.

4. Pain management and nausea levels should be assessed on a regular basis and postoperative analgesia and anti-emetics should be administered as required.

5a) Once the child is safely maintaining their own airway, their parents/carers may be invited to the recovery.

  b) The recovery staff should be able to relate appropriate information to the parents/carers but may also ask the surgeon and/or anaesthetist to speak to them.
  c) Unless there is an anaesthetic or surgical reason to be nil by mouth, the child may be given a drink while in recovery. This is particularly important for breast-fed babies.

  d) Very restless children or those with special needs may be nursed on a floor mat instead of the trolley or bed.

6. Once the recovery nurse is satisfied that the child is safe for transfer, the ward staff should be sent for and a complete handover, both verbal and written, is given, including any special postoperative instructions.

Rationale

1a) To ensure the area is safe for the care of children in the immediate postoperative period.

b) To provide distraction and reduce the child's stress.

2.

a) So that recovery staff can positively identify the child.

b) So that recovery staff are aware of any drugs that have been given and any pain management needs the child may have.

c) So that recovery staff are aware of any problems associated with the surgical procedure that may arise during the child's stay in recovery and can handover the correct details regarding the child's surgical procedure and care needs to the family and ward staff once the child is ready to return to the ward.

3a) To prevent the upper airway obstruction (Watcha 2000).

b) To ensure homeostatic levels are maintained and to alert the recovery team if there are physiological changes that may require intervention by the medical team.

c) To ensure completeness of documentation.

4. To maintain the child's comfort. For more information see Chapter 21.

5a) To reduce the child's stress levels as consciousness returns by having their parents/carers present as they wake up.
b) To assure the family that the planned surgery has been completed and to alert them as to any other treatment that has been carried out or may be required.
c) To increase the child's comfort and reduce the starvation time. Breast-feeding mothers are often anxious that the anaesthetic or surgical procedure may interfere with their baby's ability to feed so should be allowed to do so as soon as possible.
d) To reduce the potential for injury.

6. To ensure continuity of care (Donnelly 2005, Harris 2007, RCN 2011).

607

References

Alsop-Shields L. (2000) Perioperative care if children in a transcultural context. AORN Journal, 71(5), 1004–1020

Askin D, Wilson D. (2007) The high-risk newborn and family. In Hockenberry MJ, Wilson D. (eds) Wong's Nursing Care of Infants and Children, 8th edition. St Louis, Mosby Elsevier

Association of Anaesthetists of Great Britain and Ireland (AAGBI) (2010) Pre-operative Assessment and Patient Preparation – The Role of the Anaesthetist. Available at http://www.aagbi.org/sites/default/files/preop2010.pdf (last accessed 6th June 2011)

Brown K, De Lima J, McEwan A, Sumner E. (2000) Development and disease in childhood. In: Sumner E, Hatch DJ. (eds) Paediatric Anaesthesia, 2nd edn. London, Arnold

Cassady J, Wysocki T, Miller K, Cancel D, Izenberg N. (1999) Use of preanaesthetic video for facilitation of parental education and anxiolysis before pediatric ambulatory surgery. Anesthesia and Analgesia, 88(2), 246–250

Cohen MM, Cameron CB. (1991) Should you cancel the operation when a child has an upper respiratory tract infection? Anaesthesia and Analgesia, 72, 282–288

Department of Health (2000) The NHS plan, a plan for investment, a plan for reform. London, DoH

Department of Health (2001) Good practice in consent implementation guide: consent to examination or treatment. Crown Copyright. London. Available online at: http://www.dh.gov.uk/prod_consum_dh/groups/dh_digitalassets/@dh/@en/documents/digitalasset/dh_4019061.pdf – last accessed 14th January 2012

Department of Health (2007a) Saving Lives: reducing infection, delivering clean and safe care High Impact Intervention No 2: Peripheral intravenous cannula care bundle. London, DoH

Department of Health (2007b) Saving Lives: reducing infection, delivering clean and safe care High Impact Intervention No 4: Care bundle to prevent surgical site infection. London, DoH

Dimond B. (1994) Pressure sores: a case to answer. British Journal of Nursing, 3(14), 721–727

Donnelly J. (2005) Care of children and adolescents. In: Woodhead K, Wicker P. (eds) A Textbook of Perioperative Care. Edinburgh, Elsevier Churchill Livingstone

Harris S. (2007) Care of the child in the operating theatre. In Chambers MA, Jones S. (eds) Surgical Nursing Care of Children. Edinburgh, Elsevier Churchill Livingstone

Ho Cheung William Li (2007) Evaluating the effectiveness of preoperative interventions: the appropriateness of using the children's emotional manifestation scale. Journal of Clinical Nursing, 16, 1919–1926

Kain Z, Mayes L, O'Connor T, Cicchetti D. (1996) Preoperative anxiety in children: predictors and outocmes. Archives of Pediatric Adolescent Medicine, 150, 1238–1245

Kain Z, Caramico L, Mayes L, Genvro J, Bornstein M, Hofstadter M. (1998) Preoperative preparation programs in children: a comparative examination. Anesthesia and Analgesia, 87(6), 1249–1255

Kain Z, Mayes L, Caldwell-Andrews A, Karas D, McClain B. (2006) Preoperative anxiety, postoperative pain, and behavioural recovery in young children undergoing surgery. Pediatrics, 118(2), 651–658

Kain Z, Caldwell-Andrews A, Mayes L, Weinberg M, Wang S, MacLaren J, Ronald L. (2007) Family-centered preparation for surgery improves peri-

operative outcomes in children: a randomised controlled trial. Anesthesiology, 106(1), 65–74

Kneedler JA, Dodge GH. (1991) Perioperative Patient Care: The nursing perspective, 2nd edn. Boston, Jones & Bartlett

Kristensson-Hallstrom I. (2000) Parental participation in pediatric surgical care. AORN Journal. 71(5), 1021–1029

Levy L, Pandit UA, Randel GI, Lewis IH, Tait AR. (1992) Upper respiratory tract infections and general anaesthesia in children. Anaesthesia, 47, 678–682

Margolis J, Ginsberg B, De L. Dear G, Ross A, Goral J, Bailey A. (1998) Paediatric preoperative teaching: effects at induction and postoperatively. Paediatric Anaesthesia, 8, 17–23

Mcgraw T. (1994) Preparing children for the operating room: psychological issues. Canadian Journal of Anaesthesia, 41, 1094–1103

Methvan A, Duncan O, Chambers M. (2007) Burns and plastics. In: Chambers MA, Jones S. (eds) Surgical Nursing Care of Children. Edinburgh, Elsevier Churchill Livingstone

Morse T. (2007) Day care surgery. In: Chambers MA, Jones S. (eds) Surgical Nursing Care of Children. Edinburgh, Elsevier Churchill Livingstone

NHS Modernisation Agency (2003) National good practice guidance on pre-operative assessment for inpatient surgery. Available at www.wise.nhs.uk

National Institute for Clinical Excellence (NICE) (2003) Preoperative tests, the use of routine preoperative tests for elective surgery. Available at http://www.nice.org.uk/nicemedia/live/10920/29094/29094.pdf (last accessed 6th June 2011)

NICE (2008) Surgical site infection. Prevention and treatment of surgical site infection. Available at http://www.nice.org.uk/nicemedia/pdf/CG74NICE Guideline.pdf (last accessed 6th June 2011)

National Patient Safety Agency (NPSA) (2009) WHO surgical safety checklist. Available at http://www.nrls.npsa.nhs.uk/resources/?entryid45=59860 (last accessed 6th June 2011)

Plumridge J and Anderson C. (2011) Surgical Count. Great Ormond Street Clinical Nursing Practices. Available online at: http://www.gosh.nhs.uk/health-professionals/clinical-guidelines/surgical-count/ – last accessed 14th January 2012

Quinn A. (1996) Communication, consent and the duty of care. Clinical Risk, 2, 147–148

Royal College of Nursing (2011) Transferring children to and from theatre – RCN position statement and guidance for good practice. London, Royal College of Nursing

Royal College of Surgeons (2007) Surgery for Children – Delivering a First Class Service. London, Royal College of Surgeons

Schreiner MS, Triebwasser A, Keon TP. (1990) Ingestion of liquids compared with preoperative fasting in pediatric outpatients. Anesthesiology, 72, 593–597

Smith C. (2007) Care of the patient undergoing surgery. In: Woodhead K, Wicker P. (eds) A Textbook of Perioperative Care. Edinburgh, Elsevier Churchill Livingstone

Walker I, Lockie J. (2000) Basic techniques for anaesthesia. In: Sumner E, Hatch DJ. (eds) Paediatric Anaesthesia, 2nd edition. London: Arnold

Watcha M. (2000) The immediate recovery period. In: Sumner E, Hatch DJ. (eds) Paediatric Anaesthesia, 2nd edn. London, Arnold

Wilson D, da Cunha MF. (2007) Health problems of the newborn. In: Hockenberry MJ, Wilson D. (eds) Wong's Nursing Care of Infants and Children, 8th edn. St Louis, Mosby Elsevier

Yeo H. (1998) Nursing the Neonate. Oxford, Blackwell Science

Chapter 24

Play as a therapeutic tool

Chapter contents

Introduction

Play is a difficult word to describe. It stands for so many activities and is often seen as frivolous or unimportant. For a child play is work, but to an adult play suggests relaxation. A playing child is not just idling away their time until the next important event organised by an adult arises. A child playing is a child at work and means they are making the very best use of their time, practising and learning vital life skills. Role play for instance is a child's way of re-enacting observed adult behaviour and has an important role in children problem solving and understanding the world around them. Play enhances every aspect of a child's development, helping them to develop control of their body, to perfect physical skills and muscular coordination and to refine their sight, hearing and other senses. Play begins at birth and continues through to adult life. Even adults still love to play. Play is important at every stage of the child's life. At home and at school there should be opportunities to play. There are some alarming trends in childhood that affect children's opportunities to play. For example, society's indifference to play and an overemphasis on academic studies in school. In some areas there is inadequate environmental planning, which results in there being a lack of amenities provided that enable children to play. It is important, therefore, that parents/carers, teachers and all those who have responsibility for children ensure that adequate provision for play is made at home, in schools and in the community.

Play is also very important for the sick child both at home and in the hospital environment.

Play in hospital is now well established in most hospitals throughout the United Kingdom. It contributes part of the multi-professional approach to the care of the child in hospital. The Hospital Play Specialist has unique expertise to contribute within such a team. Gone are the days when children were admitted to hospital, taken from their parents/carers, bathed and dressed in hospital pyjamas by a stranger and then left to languish on a hospital ward, often leaving with an emotional scar for life. Play and the role of the Hospital Play Specialist have been a contributory factor in improving the emotional care of the child in hospital. In recent years the role of the Hospital Play Specialist has changed as our understandings of the needs of children have altered. The Department of Health document, – *Welfare of Children and Young People in Hospital* (1991, preface page I), stated 'Over the last thirty years we have come to a better understanding of the unique qualities of children – no longer can they be perceived as just miniature adults'. More recently, the National Service Framework for Children (NSF) (DoH 2003) comments that hospitals need to be child-friendly and that children are not the same as adults and this means designing hospitals services for children from the child's point of view (Wilson 1992). This knowledge has further underlined the importance of the continuing care and support that children need to help them achieve their full potential as adults. This understanding has had an impact on how we care for sick children and their families. In recent years there has been far more emphasis on the unique needs of adolescents. As this is a period of development of notable physical, social and emotional changes, which often leads to adolescents feeling confused and insecure, it is important to remember that the impact of a hospital admission coupled with a greater understanding of the world and what the future may

hold can lead to heightened anxiety levels within adolescents. The NSF 2003 states 'In particular, the needs of adolescents require careful consideration'. In general, adolescents prefer to be located alongside people their own age who are more likely to meet their need for social interaction and this makes it easier for staff to meet their needs for different forms of entertainment, education and additional privacy. The NSF also calls for more focus on the transition to adult services, and planned transition programmes, stating that if handled badly, there is a risk that the young person will 'drop out' from medical services altogether.

It is important to remember that adolescents are no different from anyone else and benefit from having procedures explained before being carried out. They may try to put on a brave face, hide their distress, anger or anxieties, and try to control what is to take place. They need to be given positive control, as much as possible, by giving them the understanding of what is about to happen, why it is going to happen, and techniques for coping with it. It is useful to explore the child's normal coping mechanisms, to work with these and to practice them beforehand. Some techniques that seem to work well are breathing exercises, listening to music of their choice, watching videos/DVDs, guided imagery, relaxation or being, coached, comforted or massaged by their parents/carers or a chosen friend. Most importantly they need to have privacy and permission to express their emotions.

This chapter will look at the development of play in hospital, its contribution within the multi-professional team, the role of the Hospital Play Specialist and the way in which play can be used as a therapeutic tool with the child in hospital.

This chapter includes the following sections:

1. The development of play in hospital.
2. Normal play for development.
3. The importance of play for children in hospital.
4. Preparation for surgery and procedures.
5. Distraction techniques.
6. Therapeutic play – 1:1 sessions.

The development of play in hospital

'Hospitalisation has long been recognised as being a potentially stressful time for both children and their parents' (Darbyshire 1996, p. 1). Following the work of James and Joyce Robertson in the late 1950s and early 1960s, research began on the child either in the short term or the long term (for a review see Alsop-Shields and Mohay 1991). With the publication of the Ministry of Health's Platt Report in 1959 came attempts to make a stay in hospital for children more human by offering open visiting, living-in facilities for parents/carers and by encouraging parents/carers to participate in the care of their child in hospital.

Hospitals solely for children were comparatively new and emerged in the mid-19th century. Up until this time there were dispensaries who gave advice and medicine to parents. The first of these was opened by Dr George Armstrong in 1769. He believed that children should not be separated from their parents/carers by admission to hospital claiming that parents/carers and nurses would find it difficult to work together in the care of sick children. The primary role of such institutions was to deal with the large number of infections and deficiency diseases that were a result of the social conditions of the time. The struggle to overcome such illnesses was based on asepsis and rigid routine and this affected the relationship between children, parents/carers and hospital staff for over a century and a half.

Some paediatricians, like Sir James Spence in 1927, tried to promote keeping mothers and babies together. He set up a small mother and baby unit in Newcastle upon Tyne (Court 1975). Dermot MacCarthy, paediatrician at Amersham Hospital with ward sister Ivy Morris pioneered liberal practice while awaiting the publication of the Platt report (Davies 2010).

The work of John Bowlby (1953) and James Robertson (1962, 1970) on maternal deprivation highlighted the needs of children in hospital. The Robertsons' films in particular make a dramatic effect on both professional and public opinion. It was around this time that some more humane paediatric nurses began to emerge and so began more family-focused practices such as allowing parents/carers in to visit their child in hospital.

This was followed by an article in *The Lancet* in 1965 entitled 'A Parent's Voice' by Dermot MacCarthy and Ronald MacKeith However, the major breakthrough came in the implementation of the Platt Report, although this was a slow process. In 1976 when the Court Report was published 'Fit for the Future', there was still found to be a misunderstanding of the holistic needs of children in hospital.

In 1961 a group of parents/carers for the National Association for the Welfare of Children in Hospital was established and since then they have monitored how the recommendations of Platt have been implemented and have been a source of support and help to parents/carers to enable them to stay with their sick child in hospital.

Normal play for development

All types of play have importance and serve a purpose in a child's physical, emotional, intellectual or social development. Play provides children with the opportunity to discover themselves. It enlarges a child's horizon, but at the same time helps to reduce the world to manageable proportions, enabling the child to make sense of the flood of impressions pouring in from the outside world. Play is the medium through which the child can express positive emotions and channel negative ones. It provides a safe outlet for emotional stresses. Acting out the jealousy of a brother or sister or anger towards a parent/carer in a dramatic game may help the child to cope with the problem in a safe setting, at the same dispersing some of their aggression.

So what is Play? Play is:

Children's Work – it is what children do and how they in turn make sense of the world.

Central and essential to learning. Playing helps the child to develop control of their body, to perfect physical skills and muscular co-ordination and to refine the use of sight, hearing and the other senses.

Holding the source of all that is good (Jolly 1978, 1979)

Dr Hugh Jolly was a great supporter of play and saw the importance and value of play in the life of a child.

Functions of play

The functions of play are:

1. It aids physical growth and development.
2. It is an opportunity to learn about:

a) Yourself.
b) Your environment.
3. It provides an opportunity to practice potential skills.
4. It can be a useful tool in the assessment of children.

Development of play

Children develop through play and play develops through stages:

1. Solitary.
2. Spectatory.
3. Parallel.
4. Associative.
5. Co-operative.

Please also see Table 24.1.

Types of play

Play can be categorised as follows:

1. Spontaneous and active.
2. Exploratory and manipulative.
3. Imitative play.
4. Constructive play.
5. Imaginative play.
6. Games with rules.
7. Hobbies.

Please also see Table 24.1.

The provision of normal play for development in hospital is as important as the provision of therapeutic activities.

The importance of play for children in hospital

Play is essential to the intellectual, social and emotional development of children. It can help them resolve stressful situations like admission to hospital where they may have to undergo painful treatment procedures and suffer separation from family and friends. Parents who accompany their children on admission may find it difficult to devote all their time to one child without interruptions provided by the daily round of chores. Participation in an organised play scheme may, in such circumstances, be a welcome normalising activity. Research shows that play reduces anxiety, facilitates communication and speeds recovery and rehabilitation. (Department of Health 1991, p. 18)

Play in hospital is important for the following reasons:

- To bring normality to a strange and sometime scary environment
- To lessen the impact of pain and anxiety
- To help children express their fears and feelings
- To aid recovery
- To facilitate normal cognitive development and communication through play.

Play in hospital does much more than just keep children happy and occupied. It is a safety valve for their emotions as well as a way of preparing them for some of the different and difficult experiences they may encounter during their stay in hospital. Play in hospital does not need to be limited to clean,

Table 24.1 Children's developmental progress

1 month

Posture and large movements	Vision and fine movements	**Hearing and speech**	**Social behaviour and play**
Lies on back, head to one side	Turn head and eyes to lights	Loud noises startle	Sucks well
Large jerky movements	Follows light briefly at 30 cm	Responds to soothing voice – but not when screaming or feeding	Sleeps between feeds and changing
Hands closed round thumb when relaxed	Eyes follow slow moving object at 15–20 cm		Expression becoming more alert
Hands open when stretching	Begins to watch face of adult when feeding	Cries loudly when hungry or uncomfortable	Smiles
Turns heads when cheek touched		Grunts when content	Will grasp finger
Cannot support head			Stops crying when picked up
Placed downwards head turns to side			Stops crying when spoken to
Has stepping reflex			

3 months

Posture and large movements	Vision and fine movements	**Hearing and speech**	**Social behaviour and play**
Lies on back, head in mid-line	Is visually alert	Turns eyes to sound	Stares at adult face when feeding
Smooth continuous movements of limbs	Follows adult movements nearby by moving head.	Vocalises when spoken to or pleased	Reacts with cooing when pleased
Kicks vigorously	Follows object 15–25 cm above face	Licks lips in response to sound of feeding in preparation	Holds rattle for few moments
Held sitting, can hold back straight for several seconds	Clasps and unclasps hands	Shows excitement at sound of footsteps, water, etc	
Placed face down supports on forearms	Shows excitement when recognises bottle near face		
Held standing sags at knees	Fixates for 1 or 2 seconds		
Hands loosely open	Eyes comerge as object nears face.		

6 months

Posture and large movements	Vision and fine movements	**Hearing and speech**	**Social behaviour and play**
Lying on back can raise head	Visually insatiable	Turns to known voice across room	Takes everything to mouth
Can lift leg and grasp foot	Moves head and eyes in all directions	Uses single and double syllable	Pats bottle when feeding
Can sit with support	Eyes move in unison	Laughs, chuckles, squeals in play	Shakes rattle deliberately
Turns head side to side to look	Stares at objects 15–30 cm	Screams when annoyed	Looks at toy when making sound
Holds up arms	Uses Palmer grasp	Responds to tones of adult's voice	Friendly with strangers
Pulls himself up when hands held	Stretches both hands to grasp objects		Shows some shyness
Kicks strongly			Shows anxiety when mother out of sight
Can roll over front to back			
Held sitting, bounces up and down			

9 months

Posture and large movements	Vision and fine movements	**Hearing and speech**	**Social behaviour and play**
Can sit alone for 10–15 mins on floor	**Very observant**	Shouts to attract attention	Holds, bites and chews biscuit
Can turn body to look sideways	Passes objects from hand to hand – inspects them	Listens then shouts again	Puts hands round bottle or cup when feeding
Progresses on floor rolling or shuffling	Pokes with index finger	Babbles tunefully repeating syllables	Tries to grasp spoon when being fed
Attempts to crawl	Grasps with finger and thumb – scissor fashion	Tries to imitate adult sounds	Throws body back and stiffens when resisting or annoyed
Can stand holding support for short time	Looks for toys which fall		Is suspicious of strangers
When held steps out on alternate feet	Can release toy by pressing it down		Plays peepbo
	Watches activity at distance for several seconds		Holds out toy but cannot yet give
			Will look for toy hidden in front of him

Table 24.1 (*Continued*)

12 months

Posture and large movements

Can sit unsupported for indefinite time

Can rise to sitting position from lying down

Crawls rapidly on all fours

Pulls up by furniture again

Walks sideways holding furniture

Walks ahead holding one or both hands

Stands alone

Vision and fine movements

Picks up small objects with pincer grasp of thumb and index finger

Points with index finger

Looks in correct place for toys which go out of sight

Recognises people at 6 m distance

Shows slight preference for one hand

Hearing and speech

Responds to own name

Understands simple commands like come, clap hands, etc.

Understands several words in context: 'dinner', 'ball', etc.

Babbles loudly, tunefully and incessantly

Imitates adults' sounds

Will give objects to adult on request

Social behaviour and play

Drinks from cup

Holds spoon

Holds out arm and foot when dressed

Puts things in and out of boxes

Listens to sounds showing pleasure

Repeats action making sounds

Wants constant adult company

Shows affection

15 months

Posture and large movements

Walks unsteadily balancing with arms

Can get to feet alone

Crawls upstairs

Kneels unaided or with slight support

Stoops to pick up toys

Vision and fine movements

Picks up small objects neatly with finger and thumb

Can build tower of 2 cubes

Grasps crayon and imitates scribble

Looks at pictures in books with interest

Points to ask for things they wants

Watches happenings for several minutes

Hearing and speech

Jabbers loudly using wide range of sounds

Uses 2–6 words

Understands more

Asks for food, etc. at table

Points to people and objects when asked

Understands and obeys simple commands like shut the door, etc

Social behaviour and play

Holds cup when given it

Holds spoon and puts in mouth, turned over

Chews well

Helps more when being dressed

Indicates when nappy is wet

Has stopped putting everything in mouth

Very curious

Physically restless

Emotionally changeable

18 months

Posture and large movements

Walks well, stops safely

Runs stiffly upright – eyes on ground ahead

Pushes and pulls large toys

Can carry large toy while walking

Backs into small chair to sit

Climbs into large chair and turns to sit

Can walk upstairs holding hand

Can pick up toy from floor without falling

Vision and fine movements

Picks up small object with delicate pincer grasp

Scribbles

Can build 3 brick tower

Recognises pictures in a book

Turns pages 2 or 3 at once

Is beginning to show preference for one hand

Can point at objects outside if interested

Hearing and speech

Uses 6–20 words. Understands more

Echoes prominent or last word they hear

Demands urgently by pointing and single word

Tries to join in nursery rhymes

Attempts to sing

Points to hair, nose, shoes, etc. if asked

Social behaviour and play

Lifts and holds with both hands Chews well

Puts spoon with food into mouth

Takes of shoes, socks, hats

Indicates needs to use toilet

Has attained bowel control

Does not put things into mouth

Remembers where things belong

Imitates simple action

Explores energetically

Alternates between clinging and resistance

2 years

Posture and large movements

Can run safely on whole foot

Starts easily and avoids objects

Squats to play – rises without using hands

Pulls wheeled toy by cord

Can climb furniture and get down again

Can walk upstairs and down holding side – 2 feet to a step

Can throw small ball when trying to kick it

Vision and fine movements

Can build tower of 6 cubes

Can remove sweet wrapper

Does circular scribble and dots

Can imitate vertical line

Recognises detail in pictures

Can turn single page of book

Recognises familiar people in photograph

Has developed right/left handedness

Hearing and speech

Uses 50 or more words

Puts 2 or more words together

Refers to self by own name

Asks names of objects often

Joins in nursery rhymes and songs

Will say and show words hair, mouth, nose, etc. if asked

Social behaviour and play

Lifts cup and replaces after drinking from it

Can eat from spoon

Asks for food and drink

Can put on hat and shoes

Asks for toilet

Is dry during the day

Can open door and run out

Tantrums when frustrated

Parallel play

Demands adult attention

(*Continued*)

613

Table 24.1 (*Continued*)

3 years

Posture and large movements	Vision and fine movements	Hearing and speech	Social behaviour and play
Walks unaided upstairs with alternate feet	Can build tower of 9 cubes	Has large vocabulary	Eats with fork and spoon
Walks unaided downstairs 2 feet to a step	Can build bridge of 3 when shown	Still has some infantile phonetic substitution	Washes hands – needs supervision drying
Climbs with agility	Can draw circle and cross	Can say full name and sex	Can pull up pants
Can turn wide corners on tricycle	Draws man with head and one other part	Uses plurals and pronouns	Dry through night
Can walk on tiptoe	Matches 2 or 3 primary colours	Talks of present events and past experience	Is affectionate and confiding
Can stand on one foot for a moment	Can cut with scissors	Asks questions 'what, where, who?'	Likes to help adult
		Listens to stories and demands favourites	Plays with other children
		Knows several nursery rhymes	Understands past and present
			Invents make-believe games and people

4 years

Posture and large movements	Vision and fine movements	Hearing and speech	Social behaviour and play
Walks up and down stairs one foot per step	Can build tower of 10 or more cubes	Speech completely intelligible	Uses knife and fork
Can climb ladders and trees	Can build several bridges of 3	Can describe recent events and experiences	Washes and dries hands
Can run on tip toe	Can build 3 steps with 6 cubes when shown	Can give home address and age	Brushes teeth
Can hop on one foot	Draws man with head and legs	Asks questions why? When? How?	Undresses and dresses alone
Can stand on one foot for 3–5 seconds	Draws man with head, legs, trunk and features	Asks meanings of words	Is self-willed
Can bend from waist to pick up toy from floor with knees extended	Draws simple house	Listens to and tells long stories	Uses verbal impertinence when crossed
	Can match and name four primary colours		Likes dramatic play and dressing up
			Confuses fact and fantasy
			Alternately co-operative and aggressive with adults and children
			Understands taking turns
			Can show concern and sympathy

5 Years

Posture and large movements	Vision and fine movements	Hearing and speech	Social behaviour and play
Runs lightly on toes	Can write a few letters	Speech fluent and correct	Uses knife and fork
Active in climbing, sliding, etc	Draws man with head, trunk, legs and some features	Likes stories – acts them out in detail	Washes and dries face and hands
Can skip on alternate feet	Draws house with door, windows, roof, chimney	Can give home address	General behaviour controlled and independent
Dances to music	Can count fingers with index fingers	Can give age and birthday	Domestic and dramatic play carried over to next day
Grips strongly with either hand	Can name four primary colours	Can describe what objects are used for	Chooses own friends
	Can match 10–12 colours	Asks meaning of abstract	Understands need for rules and fair play
			Protective towards younger children
			Comforts playmates in distress

quiet and unexciting activities. For example, bedding can be covered with waterproof sheeting, making it possible to play with water, paint and other messy play materials. The provision of normal play activities gives the Hospital Play Specialist the opportunity to build a trusting relationship with the child/adolescent. This may be a very important factor in enabling the child to accept any future medical treatment they may experi-ence. The Hospital Play Specialist will then be a familiar, safe person that they trust and can help them come to terms with future illness and treatment. When the opportunity for normal play has not taken place and the child requires treatment, the Hospital Play Specialist will be less able to support them and gain their co-operation. Normal play in hospital is therefore therapeutic in its own way.

The role of the hospital play specialist

The role of the Hospital Play Specialist can be summarised as follows:

- To organise play to provide diversionary therapy
- To introduce some normality into the child/adolescents day by relieving boredom through a structured programme of developmental activity
- To contribute to clinical judgements through their observation and communication with children
- To prepare children for diagnostic tests, surgery and other invasive procedures
- To identify children and their family members who are distressed or having difficulty coping
- To put play on the agenda – to have play accepted as a normal part of the routine anywhere in a hospital where children/adolescents attend and are admitted
- To work as part of the multi-professional team and sharing the unique expertise and training of the Hospital Play Specialist
- To help create an environment that makes the hospital friendlier for children and adolescents.

The qualified Hospital Play Specialist can fulfil this role and can provide a unique contribution to the care of the child/adolescent in hospital. Working with the multi-professional team they can share their expertise with the team and participate in case reviews and care planning/pathways.

The functions of play in hospital

Aiding normality

The provision of play in hospital first and foremost provides normality. It also gives opportunities for normal development in an abnormal setting. Menzies Lyth (1982) said, 'That when a child enters hospital there is tendency towards developmental regression as a normal reaction to stress.' However, a number of authors such as Langford (1961) and D'Antionio (1984) noted that play in hospital may help to make the experience of hospitalisation one of growth. Whether this is so or not, it is necessary, if children/adolescents are to avoid falling permanently behind in development. The provision of appropriate play will ensure that children/adolescents' normal development is maintained and that they are not deprived of their developmental life experiences. The current trend is that the emphasis should not be on the treatment of the illness in isolation from the child/adolescent's other needs. Their medical needs should be taken into consideration alongside social and emotional concerns – an important aspect of fostering normality.

Reduction of anxiety

A major function of play in hospital is the reduction of stress and anxiety. If play were not provided children would inevitably become bored. Boredom has long been known to be a contributor to stress for both adults and children alike.

There are a number of detailed accounts in which play is described as reducing anxiety not only for the child/adolescent but also for the parents/carers and staff; for example, Robertson (1958), Billington (1972), Jolly (1977, 1981), Weller (1980), Poster, EC (1983) and D'Antonio, IJ (1984). They report that

through play the child actively learns to deal with an environment that might otherwise be too overwhelming to understand. 'In doing so the child gains self confidence that is often severely reduced on admission to hospital' Newman and Lind (1980). However, play on its own is not enough to reduce a child's anxiety, but it is the expertise and the presence of the Hospital Play Specialist as a stable figure among all the comings and goings of other personnel that provides the reassurance of continuity for the children, which in it itself, can allay fears and anxiety. Several specific forms of play have been reported to reduce anxieties in relation to treatment. For example, some children facing surgery have been seen to experience less trauma when prepared through a structured programme designed to familiarise them with the treatment procedures. This was reported by Jolly (1977). Weller (1980) also said that 'aggressive and creative play have been used to relieve frustration in children restricted by the treatment or the hospital itself. This experience may also be acted out and so perhaps integrating painful, memories and fantasies.'

Speeding recovery

Plank (1964) and Jolly (1975) both reported that play on the hospital ward was seen to speed recovery, partly through an increase in the child's awareness of interest in the environment. A direct link between play and speed of recovery through a reduction in anxiety by the child was noted by Billington (1972) and Garot (1986).

There is evidence that play hastens recovery, as well as reducing the need for interventions to be delivered under general anaesthesia. It has been recommended that all children staying in hospital have daily access to a Play Specialist (DoH 2003).

Facilitating communication

According to Weller (1980), play serves to facilitate communication within the hospital environment. For a child, verbal communication is easier when they are happily engaged in play in the company of a trusted adult. However, it goes further than this. Projected play was introduced by Klein (1929) as a technique whereby the child could project anxieties through an object or toy, a process, which in itself has been noted as serving to reduce the anxiety experienced by a child/adolescent. This enhances a child/adolescent's sense of mastery and self-confidence and in turn affects the extent to which they will interact socially. Projective play can also be an insight into how the child/adolescent is feeling and so acts as a form of communication, regardless of whether the child/adolescent's anxiety has been fully expressed. This kind of communication is very helpful in diagnosis.

The presence of play on the hospital ward has been reported to improve communication between staff themselves and in many instances between staff and parents/carers through its promotion of decreased anxiety levels (Department of Health and Social Security 1976, p. 10, World Health Organization 1966).

Preparation for surgery and procedures

Play in hospital has been reported to have beneficial effects by promoting normality, providing a medium through which the child/adolescent may understand hospital procedures in relation to their often limited experience and in reducing anxiety. (Department of Health 1991, p. 18)

Play preparation should be available to every child/adolescent for any procedure they may undergo during their time in hospital. A qualified Hospital Play Specialist (HPS) who has shown competency in this area should carry out play preparation. In their absence a competent, experienced member of the multi-disciplinary team (MDT) may undertake it.

Play preparation requires good communication and close co-operation between:

- All members of the MDT
- The MDT and the child/parent/carer
- The MDT and the Community.

This will provide a consistent team approach for the child/parent/carer and family.

The parent/carer should be actively encouraged to assist/participate in the preparation of their child. Adolescents should be given the choice as to whether they would like their parents/carers involved and in which role. Sibling needs should be considered in the Play Specialist assessment of the child and may need support or to be involved in the preparation process.

Aims of play preparation

- To help children understand the reason for their admission, their illness, medical procedures and treatments
- To allow the child the opportunity to express their feelings (anxiety/fears) and to correct any misconceptions or fantasies they may have
- To enable the children to develop coping strategies
- To reduce the short-/long-term effects of a hospital admission
- For the child/family to develop a trusting relationship between themselves and Hospital Staff
- To aid recovery, to promote confidence and self-esteem
- To facilitate informed consent.

Role of the Hospital Play Specialist (HPS) within the MDT

The HPS should:

- Be familiar with ward, hospital routines, policies and procedures prior to undertaking any form of play preparation
- Observe medical procedures/treatments prior to carrying out preparation (where appropriate)
- Where possible, work alongside other HPSs observing and discussing preparation methods and resources
- When carrying out play preparation for the first time, have support and supervision available from a qualified HPS
- Discuss each individual aspect of the child's needs with the staff involved in their care and the procedure
- Assess each individual child and family's needs
- Document outcome of play preparation session(s) in child's notes and ensure all members of the MDT involved are aware of any fears/anxieties highlighted in the session, and the coping strategies and/or procedure plan to be used.
- Discuss any problems or concerns regarding preparation with Senior HPS.

Evidenced-based practice and professional development is expected to be an ongoing process for all qualified play staff.

Resources

- A quiet area with no interruptions for the play preparation should be made available
- The HPS should ensure that all preparation materials/resources are suitable for all age groups and needs
- Preparation materials/resources, i.e. booklets, should be regularly reviewed and updated.

Process/action

Pre-admission

Preparation for a hospital admission (booked) should ideally begin at home. Prior to admission, a pre-admission leaflet should be sent out and this should include:

- General information about the hospital, the ward and its routine
- Advice on preparation activities that parent/carer can carry out at home
- A ward contact name and number.

Where possible a visit to the ward should be arranged prior to admission to enable the child and parent/carer to look around and ask any questions they may have.

Admission

On admission, there are two essential key factors that preparation involves: the relationship and the assessment. Where possible the HPS should build a trusting relationship with the child, establishing what their interests are and what toys, games and recreation they enjoy. Time should be allowed for non-directive play before introducing hospital play/ preparation. For the assessment, the HPS should take the following into account prior to carrying out any preparation:

- Age of child/adolescent
- Cultural background and language
- Medical history
- Cognitive development
  - Previous hospital experiences
  - Emotional maturity
  - Individual vulnerability
  - Previous preparation techniques used
  - Child and parental/carer anxieties and coping strategies/abilities
  - Child and parental/carer wishes.

Preparation

- HPS to discuss preparation with parent/carer, ensuring they understand the philosophy behind preparation and to establish their role within it, while at the same time giving them an opportunity to ask questions
- Having assessed the child's individual needs the HPS should select an appropriate method of preparation and materials which will allow them to impart the information to the child and/or parent/carer, thereby enabling them to understand what the procedure entails and allowing them to develop their own coping skills
- The timing of preparation is very important and will depend on all the above factors

- Children who have limited or no concept of time are unable to manage their anxieties about forthcoming procedures if told too far in advance. In these cases the child and/or parent/carer should dictate the timing of preparation
- The majority of children will benefit most from individual preparation (rather than in a group); ideally it should take place in a quiet room/area with no distractions (i.e. TV/computers) and when the child is not tired
- The explanation of the procedure should be honest, using factual information at the child's level of understanding and, where possible, real hospital equipment should be used
- The HPS should use words and phraseology that the child will understand. Clear, concise explanation(s) should be given
- HPS should take care when using substitute words, e.g. 'wiggly' (Hickman line), 'magic cream' (Ametop). Correct names should be used to avoid confusion, unless the child wishes to give a piece of equipment/procedure a particular name
- During the preparation session the HPS will demonstrate the procedure with the appropriate preparation materials
- Using this equipment the child will be given the opportunity to 'act/play out' the procedure and any fears/anxieties under close supervision
- The HPS will give the child the opportunity to process the information and to ask questions. Feelings should be acknowledged and reassurances given that fears/anxieties are a normal reaction
- An anxious child may not be able to take in and understand all the information being given in one session, further sessions may be necessary (stress can limit the ability to absorb information). The HPS also needs to be aware of non-verbal indications that a child is no longer concentrating. This could mean the child has had enough information at this time or the HPS may need to find alternative ways to engage the child.
- On occasions a child may not wish to engage in play preparation. If this is the case, the HPS should direct the session to the parent/carer and allow the child to be a passive participant
- The HPS needs to be aware of the implications of the procedure for the child. A child who is to have a procedure performed on vulnerable parts, i.e. eyes; genital or anal area, may have anxieties about this
- An older child or adolescent may wish not to have their parent/carer present during the session, particularly if it is of the above nature. This is not to be assumed and needs to be explored with the child. It may be more appropriate for the preparation to be carried out by a person of the same sex as the child
- Coping strategies should be discussed. Past strategies to be reviewed. Where the child has no known coping strategies these must be introduced (as with preparation, the information gained at the assessment stage will influence this)
- Offer distraction therapy.

Following the procedure

- Provide praise and rewards where appropriate. Stickers and certificates of achievement can be offered to reinforce this
- An evaluation of coping strategies used and effectiveness of preparation should be discussed with child and parent/carer
- Post-procedural role play should be offered to the young child; the older child/adolescent should be allowed to discuss the procedure.

Outcomes

- Through play preparation the child's fears/anxieties should be greatly reduced
- The child will have a better understanding of what the procedure entails and what will happen during it
- The child and parent/carer will have developed some coping strategies and the child will have a better understanding of the importance of co-operation during a procedure
- The HPS should discuss outcomes and any follow up required with the MDT
- The work undertaken by the HPS and outcomes of the session and procedure should be documented and included in the child's notes for future reference
- As a result of effective preparation, a child's stay in hospital may be reduced
- A positive experience for the child and family
- Effective communication has been carried out between child/parent and the MDT.

The role of parents/carers

Parental involvement in preparation is usually essential as it allows parents/carers to be:

1. More involved in the care of their child.
2. More confident and well informed to reassure their child. Calmer parents/carers can give more emotional support.
3. More considerate of the needs of siblings.

Distraction techniques

During normal growth and development, children strive to be in control of their bodies and the world around them. Illness and the accompanying diagnostic and therapeutic procedures place and additional burden on children's ability to cope. Providing children with cognitive strategies helps to lessen their discomfort and allows then some control in the medical procedure. (Kachoyeanos and Fried 1993).

Hospital staff do not enjoy inflicting pain on children, nor do they like to see children undergoing stress. 'A child who cries during a medical procedure is not only distressed but is distressing' (ARW Paediatric Renal Unit 1993). Distraction is the facilitation of an effective coping strategy for children and young people undergoing treatment or procedures, according to the particular situation and the child/young person's individual needs. Everyone, parents/carers and staff alike are more comfortable if children cope without showing signs of distress. When children are relaxed, they are quicker to treat, happier and are not fearful of further treatment that may be necessary. Consequently staff can relax too.

The use of distraction may help to relieve any fears and anxieties that the child may experience during painful/traumatic procedures. It enables the child to manage those fears and anxieties more effectively, allowing them to have some control over the situation. Distraction should also assist medical and nursing staff to carry out procedures more effectively.

'None of them are magical, although the effects can seem magical' (Lansdown 1987).

617

Table 24.2 Books for use with children in hospital

Title	Author	Publisher
For 2–5 year olds		
If I Were a Crocodile	Rowena Sommerville	Beaver
Billy Grump	Chris Smedley	Simon & Schuster
The Day Teddy Got Very Worried	AM Jungman	Frances Lincoln
For 3–7 year olds		
Bad Mood Bear	John Richardson	Beaver Books
There's an Alligator under my Bed	Mercer Mayer	Macmillan
Today Was a Terrible Day	Patricia Reilly	Picture Puffin
When Emily Woke up Angry	Riana Dancon	Andre Deutsch
The Temper Tantrum book	Edna Mitchell	Picture Puffin
Going to Hospital	C Jessel	Methuen
For 5–9 year olds		
Angry Arthur	Hiawyn Oram and Satoschi Kitunura	Picture Puffins
Feelings	Aliki	Piper Books
Anna's Secret Friend	Yoriko Tsutsui	Picture Puffins
Anna's Special Present	Yoriko Tsutsui	Picture Puffins
The Hairy Book	Babette Cole	Magred
Titch	Pat Hutchins	Picture Puffin
Just Awful	Alma Marshak Whitney	Picture Lions
Emergency Mouse	B Stune	Anderson Press
Crocodile Medicine/Plaster	M Watts	Deutsch
For 7–10 year olds		
Paul in Hospital	C Jessel and H Jolly	Methuen

When is the best time to start?

This should take place preferably before the child is admitted to hospital, for example through the use of books that focus on admission to hospital (Table 24.2). Some hospital web sites also have information about how parents/carers can help their child to cope with painful procedures.

Good preparation for the procedure is absolutely vital. The opportunity for play before the procedure is also a way of helping children to achieve a relaxed state of mind.

Standards for distraction

The use of distraction should be offered to all children undergoing medical treatments/procedures when appropriate/possible. Distraction should be carried out by a qualified play specialist or appropriately trained adult.

Resources

The treatment room should be welcoming, well presented and friendly. Each treatment room should contain a distraction box with a wide variety of equipment suitable for all ages, such as:

- Bubbles
- Musical toys/books (lift the flap/counting/musical)
- Puzzle books such as *Where's Wally* for older children
- Puppets
- Music
- Sensory equipment
- DVDs (where suitable).

Process/action

- Liaise with medical/nursing staff in order to understand the procedure. Where possible a 'platform of trust' with the child and family should be built through play or conversation. Assess the child's understanding of the forthcoming procedure, offering appropriate information, i.e. preparation. Decide on appropriate distraction techniques to be used. Consideration should be given to the child's coping strategies, cognitive development and previous experiences.
- Liaise with the medical/nursing team and the psychologist if involved, for any additional information
- Only the people necessary for the procedure should be in the room and the required equipment should be prepared before the child arrives
- Prior to the procedure, the roles of all those involved should be clearly defined
- The timing of the distraction is crucial. It should commence when the child is relaxed and before the procedure begins, or at the agreed point in the process
- During the procedure, ensure that all others involved with the child are aware that you are providing distraction therapy. Others trying to distract simultaneously will only serve as a distraction from the therapy and will have a negative effect.
- Children assessed as highly anxious before a procedure should only have experienced staff used to carrying out the procedure involved
- If after two attempts it has not been possible to carry out the procedure, the professional should stop and find someone else to continue. This does not have to be someone more senior

but it has been observed that the child and the professional become tenser if left to continue, which is not helpful or healthy for either.

For effective distraction to take place:

- The position of the child and the distraction method must be carefully planned
- Body language and eye contact (taking different cultures into account) can help in the engagement and process of distraction
- The child and parent/carer must be receptive towards the concept of distraction. If the child becomes too distressed it may be necessary to withdraw the distraction and offer comfort and support
- Provide praise and reward where appropriate. Stickers and certificates of achievement can be offered to reinforce this.

Outcomes

- The child is able to allow the procedure to be carried out with little or no distress to them
- The anxious child is able to use their coping strategies through the use of distraction to enable them to manage their anxieties more effectively
- The use of distraction may help to reinforce positive behaviours
- If appropriate, discuss with the child and parent/carer(s) the effectiveness of the distraction during the procedure. It may also be useful to discuss this with colleagues after the procedure has taken place
- The use of distraction enables the multi-disciplinary team to function more effectively in providing a team approach for the child/family. It improves cost and time effectiveness
- The distraction method used and its effectiveness should be documented and included in the child's health record for future reference.

Distraction methods

Below is a list of recommended distraction methods for children of different ages.

- Infants
  - Dummy
  - Cuddling
  - Positive touch
  - Fibre optic lights
  - Music
  - Tactile soothing toys.
- Toddlers
  - Bubbles
  - Pop-up/musical books
  - Cause and effect toys
  - Songs and rhymes.
- Pre-school
  - Short story books/pop-up books/musical books/counting books
  - Bubbles
  - Puppets
  - Songs/rhymes
  - Noisy cause and effect toys.

- School-age children
  - Joke/puzzle books
  - Kaleidoscope
  - Songs/rhymes
  - Guided imagery.
- Adolescents
  - Talking, coaching
  - Breathing techniques
  - Sensory equipment
  - Reading aloud
  - Guided imagery.
- Special Needs
  - Fibre optic lights
  - Music/noisy toys
  - Bubbles
  - Sensory tactile toys and equipment.

It is important that children's cognitive age and culture are taken into consideration when selecting distraction tools to ensure that the most effective measures are employed.

Remember: the success of distraction is dependent on the person supporting the child being continuously engaging and able to adjust their techniques based on observation of how the child is interacting and responding. In some cases children do not respond to distraction and comforting and coaching allows for an alternative successful outcome.

Long waits lead to anxiety. If children have to wait in-between treatments and procedures, keep them occupied or let them have a break to play in the play area.

Ensure all medical equipment required for the procedure is prepared and ready. Children's and parents'/carers' anxieties begin to rise if they have to watch professionals drawing up medications. If a procedure isn't going well, stop, give the child time and space (ideally away from the treatment area) to calm down. Go back over the distraction plans before trying again. Most importantly do not assume you know what is concerning or worrying children and decide how they should cope with a procedure. This often leads to more anxiety, frustration, anger and an unsuccessful procedure.

Relaxation

Relaxation is another technique that can be used in enabling children to cope with painful procedures. It is well established that the more relaxed the muscles are, the less pain is experienced.

One of the most common principles of aiding relaxation is to encourage the tensing of muscles followed by a rapid relaxation of that muscle. For example:

- The child squeezes an adult's hand, takes a breath in, tense their body while an adult counts from one to five. At the same time the adult can squeeze back and tense at the same time
- This position is held for a couple of seconds
- The adult then counts slowly from five to one and gradually relaxes the hand. The whole body is allowed to relax at the same time while the child breathes out and relaxes as well
- This should be practised a few times before the procedure.

Again as with distraction it is important to consider the child's cognitive age and culture for optimum effect when considering specific relaxation techniques for children and adolescents.

Listening to a tape of favourite music or a special relaxation tape or CD may have the desired effect.

Time spent with the child following the procedure is just as important as the distraction. They need to be reassured that their cooperative behaviour has been useful. This will hopefully prepare them for the next time a painful procedure needs to be undertaken. Some children, however, still find the procedure distressing and these children need further help as will be discussed below. These children need to be praised, however, for any little improvement that has been seen. The word brave should be avoided in all situations as it reinforces the message that children must not cry or show any form of distress, which is not the case.

Distraction techniques are in most cases a successful means of helping children to cope. With experience and taking account of the needs of the child suitable distraction techniques can usually be found. The aim is to enable each child to feel confident and secure through the feeling of control. They will then feel relaxed and everyone involved will benefit.

Therapeutic play – 1:1 sessions

Some children, despite developing a good relationship with a play specialist or nurse, do not respond to distraction techniques and continue to find procedures distressing. For this group more one-to-one therapeutic play is necessary.

Play when used as a therapeutic tool can enable children in a non-invasive way to take account of what has happened in the past as well as prepare for the future. This kind of play is concerned with a child's feelings and not just their behaviour. It provides the child with an opportunity to play out their feelings and their problems, in the same way as an adult might talk through their difficulties with a counsellor or friend.

> 'To 'play it out' is the most natural self-healing measure childhood affords' (Erikson 1977).

So how can we help the child who is traumatised by medical procedures or even the whole hospital experience?

First and foremost in any kind of therapeutic play is the development of a relationship with the Hospital Play Specialist or other staff member who will be facilitating this kind of play. For children this will usually be developed through the provision of normal play. Finding out what the child is interested in and providing stimulating activities that engage them will enhance the development of this important relationship. Once a relationship is established then one or more of the following strategies might prove successful.

Desensitisation

This has long been used as an approach to tackle fears for adults, but has also been shown to be very helpful with some children. The first step in desensitisation is to help the child to become relaxed. The next step is then to approach the cause of the fear gradually. The objective is to allow the feared object to become associated with feeling relaxed, rather than one of fear and dread. For example, if the fear you are tackling is one of needles, then perhaps you need to begin by showing the child a picture of the needle. Allow the child to look at it and touch it. Maybe you can

also produce an outline drawing that the child can colour. The important aspect of this work in that the child is free of fear. It is important, therefore, that children are given the time and space to overcome the fear. Desensitisation cannot be rushed. You have to allow the child to decide the pace of the treatment. Once this step is mastered you can begin to show the child the real needle. Maybe safely concealed within the packet to begin with. Then move on to looking at the real needle and then slowly allowing the needle to come nearer and nearer the skin, until the child can bear the needle to touch their skin.

Before embarking on this treatment a full discussion with the child and family needs to take place so that they fully understand what is being suggested. This kind of treatment can be very successful for some children. The disadvantage is that it takes time before the child is ready to accept the blood test or injection. This kind of work should not be undertaken without the support of a psychologist.

Case study 24.1

Some years ago I was working with a 6-year-old child, together with our ward psychologist. He was 'hospital phobic', to the extent that he became anxious when he walked in the road where his GP's surgery was located. This child needed to have an invasive X-ray that required an injection. I was asked to work with this child to see if we could desensitise him to the hospital through play. We talked to his mother about what we wanted to do, as this would involve several visits to the hospital before we felt the child would be ready to cope with the X-ray. The first visit involved coming to the Activity Centre to play. During the second visit we invited him to come to a ward playroom and on the third to the play area in X-ray. Again, on both these occasions, the purpose of the visit was just to play. It was not until the fourth visit that we began to prepare him for the X-ray. Several more visits to the X-ray department were required before this child was able to cope cooperatively with the procedure.

Needle play

Children displaying needle anxiety should be provided with therapeutic needle play session(s) in a controlled environment. A qualified Play Specialist, who has shown competency in this area of play should undertake this type of play. The Play Specialist needs to be aware of their own professional limitations and involve a clinical psychologist if necessary.

Assessment

The Hospital Play Specialist should liaise with medical/nursing staff regarding forthcoming procedures/investigations. They should collate information regarding the child's:

· Previous hospital experiences
· Medical background
· Family history
· Impending procedure (liaise with medical/nursing staff)
· Age, cognitive development and emotional maturity.

Where possible, the HPS should establish a relationship with the child and their family beforehand, through a non-directive activity session. They should consult and liaise with the child/parent/carer(s) on the benefits of this type of play and what it entails. This will provide an opportunity for feelings to be discussed, allowing them to decide whether or not it would be appropriate and helpful.

'Parental anxieties' should be assessed and discussed with the parents/carers in question. It can sometimes be useful if this takes place away from the child, as parental anxiety will affect the child's mood. Parents/carers may choose not to accompany their child during play sessions but should be given the opportunity to unless an older child has requested that they do not or the HPS has assessed their anxiety levels will prevent a positive outcome. This should always be carefully and sensitively explained to parents/carers, with advice and support on how to manage their anxiety offered.

Structure/resources

The HPS should have knowledge of and adhere to **their Trust's policies relating to the use and disposal of sharps** and other relevant policies referring to needle stick injuries. A quiet area with no interruptions for the play session should be made available, where the play session will be on a one-to-one (HPS to one child) basis, unless there is a need for a parent/carer to be available. The HPS should ensure that appropriate play equipment is available for the session(s).

Process/action

The HPS should prepare children for what is going to happen during the needle play session(s), dependant on age and cognitive understanding. For younger children too much information or information they don't understand can raise their anxiety levels. Hence, it is more beneficial for this age group to role play using dolls and medical equipment, and to have good distraction that involves their interaction during a procedure rather than preparation.

For children assessed as appropriate for preparation, discuss with the child the importance of handling needles and other safety issues. Explain to the child the reason why they need to have the proposed procedure, for example, blood test. Explain why the blood is taken, where it goes and that the body makes more blood to replace it.

Using appropriate play equipment/materials demonstrate the procedure, to include all the stages the child will experience. For children who have a deep rooted fear of needles, a programme of desensitisation with a clinical psychologist may be required before undertaking the above.

During the play session(s) the HPS should be honest, using factual information and appropriate language for the age and level of understanding of the child. Care should be taken when using substitute words, for example Hickman line (*wiggly*), or Ametop (magic cream). Where appropriate, using suitable play materials, allow the child the opportunity to 'play-out' any fears or anxieties, under close supervision. In addition, allow the child time to process the information and to ask questions.

The Play Specialist needs to give reassurance that it is acceptable to cry, shout, sing, etc. during the procedure. The setting of boundaries prior to the procedure is very important. Emphasis should be placed on keeping the arm/leg still. This can be achieved through games of balancing or reaching out to collect or touch an imaginary object.

The key to success is negotiation between child and MDT so that the child feels they have some choice and control. Therefore,

a 'Plan of Action' should be made with the child, parent/carer and MDT as to how the procedure is to be carried out, i.e. such as when and if local anaesthetic cream/spray is to be applied.

As much choice as possible should be offered to the child. There does need to be an agreed and safe boundary otherwise children will keep pushing to delay the procedure:

- Would the child like to sit or lie down?
- Who would the child like to accompany them?
- Would the child like to watch the procedure or to be distracted and, if so, with what?

Offering the child certain choices about the procedure helps them to manage their anxieties more effectively. Where possible the HPS should show the child where the procedure will take place. If possible, the child should choose who should accompany them through the procedure and what distraction method will be used.

The HPS should give the child and family feedback following the procedure, emphasising their particular achievements, for example keeping their hand/foot still. This feedback should be reinforced through the use of stickers/certificates as rewards for being good, not brave. Bravery certificates or rewards for being brave enforce the message that crying is bad and not allowed where some children find gentle crying soothing. Under control, crying can also be an affective coping method and assist with breathing and relaxation.

Children assessed as highly anxious before a procedure should only have experienced staff to carry out the procedure involved.

If after two attempts it has not been possible to carry out the procedure, the professional should stop and find someone else to continue. This does not have to be someone more senior but it has been observed that the child and the professional become tenser if left to continue, which is not helpful or healthy for either.

Outcomes

- Through the play session(s), the child's fears/anxieties should be greatly reduced
- The child will have a better understanding of what will happen during the procedure
- The child will be able to develop their own coping strategies and have a better understanding of the importance of cooperation during the procedure
- The HPS will discuss with the child/parent/MDT as to whether further play session(s) are required
- The work undertaken by the HPS and the outcome of the procedure should be documented and included in the child's health record for future reference
- The HPS will carry out reflective practice and discuss the child's progress with the MDT for future reference.

Reinterpretation

Children can learn through this method to see repeated pain in a different light. This is particularly successful with children who have a vivid imagination. The first step in this kind of work is to establish what they are interested in. You then need to find a way of reinterpreting the pain in a positive light in view of this interest.

621

Richard Lansdown in his paper, *Helping children cope with needles* (1987), describes the example of a 7-year-old boy who was keen on boxing. He was encouraged to pretend that he was the schoolboy champion of London but he was prevented from becoming champion of Britain because his arms were not strong enough. The injections he needed were to make his arm strong.

An 11-year-old girl is also described. She pretended that she was hiding from enemy soldiers during a war; if she made a noise they would find her. She developed a way of breathing in and out short breaths, which reduced her tension and prevented her from making a noise.

Lansdown also states 'Very young children can often be helped to reinterpret the pain by identifying with a doll or puppet. Try telling them a story about one of their toys who is sick and has to have an injection and ask the child to help the toy overcome any fears.' It is wise not to use the child's favourite toy or teddy unless the child wants to.

Guided imagery

This is a form of self-hypnotherapy. It is, however, different from hypnosis in that it is used with the child using their vivid imagination. The aim of this kind of approach is to allow children to help themselves by using the power of their imagination to influence their body. Guided imagery can be a powerful tool in helping children cope with painful procedures.

> It is an altered state of awareness in which patients are able to accept suggestions which allow them to use their own mental and physical skills in an optimal fashion. (Olness 1986)

Good preparation for this approach is essential. Finding out what the child is interested in is also a key to its success. The first step is to help the child relax. This can be done by asking the child to close their eyes and then taking them throughout a relaxation sequence by asking them to imagine that every muscle in their body from head to feet is being relaxed. There are then two methods of guided imagery.

One way is effectively through the telling of a story. Imagine the 8-year-old boy who is 'football mad'. A story can be told that it is cup final day at Wembley and this boy is going to be at the match. Ask him to imagine that he has to take 10 steps up to his place in the stand. Take him very slowly up the 10 steps and then ask him to imagine that there is a magic door at the top which he has to open. Once the door is open the match begins. The story then unfolds and at the end the child is guided back through the magic door and slowly down the 10 steps.

The other way is, once the child is in a relaxed state, to involve them in the imagery by asking them questions about where they are and what they can see. The end result is often the same – a relaxed child who is able to cooperate with hospital procedures. Sometimes children are in such a relaxed state that they do not realise that the procedure has actually taken place.

Once this approach is learnt, parents/carers and their children can use imagery whenever they need it.

Combining some of the techniques outlined can also be a therapeutic way of enabling children to cope with pain and medical procedures. The common thread in all approaches is the importance of developing a trusting relationship with children and their families.

Case study 24.1 is an example that highlights a number of techniques that were used to help a traumatised child, but the success of this work is the relationship that developed between the Hospital Play Specialist and the child and family.

Case study 24.2

John was 7 years old. He had a kidney transplant at the age of 3 years and since this time, according to his mother, he had always been anxious about having blood taken. She told me that John had seen a psychologist in the past but to no avail. John was referred to me on his second visit to Great Ormond Street. At the time of the referral he was screaming and kicking and both his mother and younger sibling were both crying. I explained that we needed to take blood today but that this whole experience could be made much easier with the help of some therapeutic play. Mother was rather negative that anything could be done to help her son but agreed that she would try anything! Having the blood test taken on this occasion was traumatic, not only for John but also for those of us who observed. Distraction did not work partly because his fear was too great but partly too because he did not know me.

After the procedure I asked his mother if I might visit them at home as I felt that John was very traumatised. She agreed to this arrangement. The aim of the first visit was really to establish a relationship with the child, to get to know him and his family and to discover what his interests were. When I arrived at his home he appeared surprisingly pleased to see me, and I soon discovered that he loved to draw and particularly liked the *Art Attack* television programme and magazines. He was in the process of making a tube for his pencils as outlined in the *Art Attack* magazine. I also spent time chatting to his mother and establishing a relationship with her and his two siblings. This, I feel, is very important and contributes to the final outcome. When the time came for me to leave, John did not want me to go home but I promised that I would visit again in a few weeks time. On the second visit I went prepared to engage in some therapeutic work – needle play! However, I did begin by asking John what he had made recently, so again building on the relationship that I had established on the first visit.

I then explained that I had brought along 'Bill,' my friend who had to have regular blood tests but always got very anxious. I explained that 'Bill' needed a blood test and I wondered if John would be able to help me with this. John was very keen to be involved. I asked him what equipment we would need and showed him my medical box. He was keen to handle all the equipment with the exception of the butterfly needle. We talked about the importance of the blood test for 'Bill' to establish how well his kidney was functioning. We carried out several blood tests on 'Bill' before he felt confident to carry out the whole procedure and even then was clearly still very anxious about handling the needle. At the end of the visit he asked when I would come again and wanted 'Bill' and the medical box to be brought along. I explained that in fact he would be coming to see me at the hospital the following week and that 'Bill' would be in the hospital on that day. I also asked him to think about what we could do while he was having his blood test done. He said he would like to sing! On arrival at the Out Patients Clinic, John was clearly very anxious and found it difficult to concentrate on any of the art activities offered to him. He also did not want to engage in any play with 'Bill'. The thought of the blood test was just too overwhelming to contemplate engaging in any activities. He needed constant reassurance that I would go with him when he had the blood test procedure. When the time came to have the blood test, he was very distressed and needed reassurance from me that I would stay with him throughout. He also asked if he would be able to have a 'well done' certificate to show his teacher when he returned to school the following day. I reminded him about 'Bill' and how he had coped and that we were all going to sing and as we walked into the treatment room we discussed what we would sing. The blood test was achieved with less distress than on the previous occasion, but there was clearly more work to be done to enable John to be more cooperative. Some of the staff also needed to improve their singing! He was also given his certificate, which was clearly very important to him.

A few weeks later I visited him again at home. Once again he was clearly pleased to see me. The aim of this visit was to try to enable John to talk about his fears. On arrival he asked me if I had brought 'Bill' with me and I said I had but that I had a game I would like us to play first. The game is called 'All About Me'. It is an ordinary board game where each player takes it in turn to throw the dice and move their counter the appropriate number of spaces. However, after this each player has to then answer a question. Some questions are very non-threatening like 'What is your favourite colour?' or 'What is your favourite food?' Others are more revealing like 'What is the worst thing that has happened to you this year?' or 'What makes you feel very anxious?' After one of these questions John talked about the fact that he finds blood tests very scary. I asked about when he first starts to feel anxious? He told me 'It is the minute I get to the waiting room and then you have to wait and wait and wait and the longer I wait the more anxious I become.' I suggested that perhaps it might be better if we could arrange for John to have the blood test as soon as he arrived in the waiting room. As this was the worst part of coming to the hospital if we could get this over and done with quickly, then perhaps he could play and enjoy the rest of the visit. He agreed that this might help and so I told him that I would talk to the clinic staff to see if this was possible. We finished the game and played with 'Bill' again before I needed to return to the hospital. I felt that his session had highlighted that the waiting was provoking John's anxiety to such a degree that he was unable to cope.

On return to the hospital I explained what John had said and they agreed to try to see John as soon as he arrived and see if this did improve John's coping mechanism. John came to the hospital 2 weeks later. As soon as he arrived I suggested that we went to the treatment room. He willingly accompanied me and we talked about what we were going to sing. When he was asked to hold his arm out so that they could look for a vein he compiled with this request. I suggested that we started to sing and the whole procedure was completed without any distress. His mother and the clinic staff were amazed at the way in which John was able to cooperate. I agreed with his mother after the procedure that I would not visit until after his next hospital visit to see if he was still coping. At the next visit we conducted the blood test as soon as he arrived and he was again very compliant although needed reassurance that I would stay with him.

I felt that it was no longer necessary to visit him at home but that he still needed my support at the time of his blood test. Two months later John was diagnosed as a diabetic and now has to cope with daily insulin injections that are carried our without fear or distress.

I think this example highlights the impotence of building relationships with children. It also reveals that something very simple can make all the difference in the world to how a child copes. It also highlights the importance of discovering what it is that is provoking the fear. In John's case it was the waiting time that was the cause of much of his distress. Once this had been noted and the appropriate action taken, his fear and distress was reduced which enabled him to cooperate with clinic staff.

Play is a very powerful therapeutic tool, which used in the right way can help children to cope with hospitalisation, illness and treatment.

Children need to play – it's a fundamental part of every child's nature. Children, who know how to play and have the opportunity, thrive, do well in life and develop into well-rounded individuals. Play is the parent of creativity, co-cooperativeness and leadership. Children whose play is denied or restricted fail to thrive. Their spirit dies, their potential is denied. There is a basic and healthy requirement for every child, to be free to spend time doing what every child knows best – how to play. Play requires opportunity, environment, resources and respect. (Fair Play for Children 2000)

The Millennium Resolution of Fair Play for Children is

A world fit for all children to play in – somewhere near paradise.

Key texts

Baldwin D. (2001) All about Children. Oxford, Oxford University Press

Cook P. (1999) Supporting Sick Children and their families. London, Baillière Tindall

Daniel B, Wassell S, Gilligan R. (2003) Child Development for Child Care and Protection Workers. London, Jessica Kingsley

Darbyshire P. (1996) Living with a Sick Child in Hospital. London, Chapman & Hall

Department of Health and Social Security (1976) Report on the expert group on play for children in hospital. London, DHSS

Department of Health (1991) Welfare of Children and Young People in Hospital. London, HMSO

Department of Health (2003) National Service Framework for Children, Getting the Right Start: National Service Framework for Children Young People and Maternity Service. London, DoH

Jenkinson, S. (2001) The Genius of Play. Stroud, Hawthorn Press

Jolly J. (1981) The Other Side of Paediatrics. Basingstoke, Macmillan

Keenan T. (2002) Introduction to Child Development. London, Sage Publication

Lansdown R. (1996) Children in Hospital. Oxford, Oxford Medical Publications

OMEP Play in Hospital (1966) Report by the World Organization for Early Childhood Education. World Organization for Early Childhood Education, UK National Committee

Petrillo M, Sanger S. (1981) The Emotional Care of the Hospitalised Child. Philadelphia, PA Lippincott

Play in Hospital Liaison Committee (1990) Quality Management for Children – Play In Hospital. London, Save the Children Fund

Santrock JW. (2001) Child Development. Boston, McGraw-Hill Higher Education

Save the Children Fund (1989) Hospital a deprived environment for Children – The case for Hospital Play Schemes. London, Save the Children Fund

Schaefer CE, Di Geronimo TF (2000) Ages and Stages. Chichester, John Wiley & Sons

References

Alsop-Shields L, Mohay H. (1991) John Bowlby and James Robertson: theorists, scientists and crusaders for improvements in the care of children in hospital. Journal of Advanced Nursing, 35(1), 50–58

ARW Paediatric Renal Unit (1993) Painful Procedures: Helping Children to cope. Nottingham, ARW Paediatric Renal Unit

Billington GF. (1972) Play program reducing children's anxiety, speeds recoveries. Modern Hospital, 118(4), 90–92

Bowlby J. (1953) Child Care and the Growth of Love. Baltimore, Pelican Books

Court D. (1975) Sir James Spence. Archives of Diseases of Childhood, 50, 85

D'Antonio IJ. (1984) Therapeutic use of play in hospital. Nursing Clinics of North America, 19(2), 351–359

Davies R. (2010) Marking the 50th anniversary of the Platt Report: from exclusion, to toleration and parental participation in the care of the hospitalized child. Journal of Child Health Care, 14, 6–23

Erikson EH. (1977) Childhood and Society. London, Triad/Granada

Fair Play for Children(2000) Their Millennium Resolution. Journal of Fair Play for Children Association Trust Ltd (Reg. Charity 292134) by Premier Promotions

Garot PA. (1986) Therapeutic play: work of both child and nurse. Journal of Pediatric Nursing, 1(2), 111–116

Jolly H. (1975) How play in hospital helps a child's recovery. The Times, 16 July

Jolly J. (1977) How to be in hospital without being frightened. Nursing Times, 73(48), 1887–1888

Jolly H. (1979) Katies First Year. DVD by Concord Media (Concord Video and Film Council) directed by Nigel Evans. Available at sales@concordmedia.org.uk

Jolly H. (1978) More Common Sense about Babies and Children. London, Pelham

Jolly J. (1981) The Other Side of Paediatrics – a quick guide to the everyday care of the sick child. Basingstoke, Macmillan Press

Kachoyeanos MK, Friedhoff HM. (1993) Cognitive and behavioral strategies to reduce children's pain. MCN, 18, 14–19

Klein M. (1929) Personification the play of children. International Journal of Psycho-analysis, 10, 193–204

Langford WS. (1961) The child in the paediatric hospital: adaptation to illness and hospitalisation. American Journal of Orthopsychiatry, 31, 667–684

Lansdown R, Great Ormond Street Hospital, Department of Psychological Medicine (1987) Helping children cope with needles – a guide for parents and staff. London, Great Ormond Street Hospital

MacCarthy D, MacKeith R. (1965) A parent's voice. Lancet, ii, 1289–1291

Menzies Lyth I. (1982) The psychological welfare of children making long stays in hospital: an experience in the art of the possible. Occasional Paper No3. London, The Tavistock Institute of Human Relations

Ministry of Health (1959) The Platt Report

Newman L & Lind J. (1980) The child in hospital: early stimulation and therapy through play. Paediatrician. Vol 9, pp. 147–150

Olness K. (1986) Hypnotherapy in children. Postgraduate Medicine, 79(4), 95–105

Plank EM. (1964) Working with children in hospital. London, Tavistock Publications

Poster EC. (1983) Stress immunization techniques to help children cope with hospital. Maternal and Child Nursing Journal, 12(2), 119–134

Robertson J. (1958), Going into Hospital with Mother. London, Tavistock Publication

Robertson J. (1962) Hospitals and Children: A review of letters from parents to 'The Observer' and the BBC. London, Victor Gollancz

Robertson J. (1970) Young Children in Hospital. London, Tavistock

Spence JC. (1946) The purpose of the family: A guide to the care of children. National Children's homes, London

Weller BF. (1980) Helping Sick Children Play. London, Baillière Tindall

Wilson L. (1992) The Home Visiting Programme. Paediatric Nursing. July: 10–11

World Health Organization (1966) Report for Early Childhood Education. Geneva, WHO

Further reading

Allen KE, Maroth LR. (2000) By the Ages. Delmar, Thomson Levy

Axline V. (1991) Play Therapy. New York, Pelican

Baldwin D. (2001) All about Children. Oxford, Oxford University Press

Bielby E. (1984) A Childish Concept. Nursing Mirror, 14 November, 26–28

Bowlby J. (1990) Child Care and the Growth of Love. London, Penguin

Bowlby J. (1956) The effects of mother-child separation: a follow-up study. British Journal of Medical Psychology, 29, 211

Carter JH, Hancock J. (1988) Caring for Children. How to ease them through surgery. Nursing Oct, 18(10), 46–50

Cleary J. (1992) Caring for Children in Hospital. London, Scutari Press

Cook P. (1999) Supporting Sick Children and their Families. London, Baillière Tindall

Daniel B, Wassell S, Gilligan R. (2003) Child Development for Child Care and Protection Workers. London, Jessica Kingsley

Davenport GC. (1990) Introduction to Child Development. London, Collins

Edwards M, Davis H. (1997) Counselling Children with Chronic Medical Conditions. London, British Psychological Society

Hart R, Mather P, Slack J, Powell M. (1992) Therapeutic Play Activities for Hospitalised Children. St Louis, Mosby–Year Book, Inc

Jenkinson S. (2001) The Genius of Play. Stroud, Hawthorn Press

Keenan T. (2002) Introduction to Child Development. London, Sage

Lansdown R, Walker M. (1991) Your Child's Development from Birth to Adolescence. London, Frances Lincoln

Linden J. (1993) Child Development from Birth to Eight years. London, National Children's Bureau

McConville B. (1997) Delicate operation. Nursery World 6 March, 16–17

Plank EN. (1964) Working with Children in Hospitals. London, Tavistock

Robertson J. (1970) Young Children in Hospital. London, Tavistock

Rodin R. (1983) Will it hurt? Preparing children for hospital and medical procedures. London, RCN

Santrock JW. (2001) Child Development. New York, McGraw-Hill Higher Education

Schaefer CE, Di Geronimo TF. (2000) Ages and Stages. New York, John Wiley & Sons

Sheridan M. (1997) Birth to Five Years: Children's Developmental Progress (revised and updated by Frost M, Sharma A). London, Routledge

Sylva K, Lunt J. (1982) Child Development – A first course. Oxford, Blackwell

Taylor D. (1991) Prepare for the best. Nursing Times, 87(31), 64–66

Weller B. (1980) Helping Sick Children Play. London, Baillière Tindall

West J. (1996) Child Centred Play Therapy. London, Baillière Tindall

Wilson L. (1990) Storytelling for cwith a chronic illness. Paediatric Nursing, September, 6–7

Poisoning and overdose

Chapter contents

Procedure guidelines

The Great Ormond Street Hospital Manual of Children's Nursing Practices, First Edition. Edited by Susan Macqueen, Elizabeth Anne Bruce, Faith Gibson.
© 2012 Great Ormond Street Hospital for Children NHS Foundation Trust. Published 2012 by Blackwell Publishing Ltd.

Introduction

Poisoning in children falls into three categories, accidental, non-accidental and deliberate in older children. Accidental poisoning is most common in children aged 5 or younger and older children who are developmentally delayed. Over the years, the number of children dying as a consequence of poisoning has fallen significantly. This is associated with better treatment, child resistant container regulations, the impact of the restriction of sales of paracetamol to small packs of 16 and a reduction in the number of prescribed tricyclic antidepressants (Hawton and Townsend 2001). The majority of ingestions taken are relatively non-toxic substances and children are discharged home from A&E or Children's Ambulatory Services (Bates *et al* 1997). However, during 2002, children aged 0–14, spent a total of 30,279 in-patient days as a result of suspected poisoning (Royal Society for the Prevention of Accidents (RoSPA) 2010).

Around 75–99% of accidental poisonings in children under 5 years of age occur in a domestic environment (RoSPA 2010). This is usually the child's own home, but as many as 20% of domestic incidents occur in the home of a relative (often a grandparent) or friend (Bates *et al* 1997). The majority of children who have taken poisons do not have serious symptoms. Medicines may be of low toxicity, e.g. the oral contraceptive pill or antibiotics. Many of the household products children take may be relatively non-toxic, but a few, such as caustic soda and paint stripper, may cause serious harm. Box 25.1 identifies the top 10 enquiries received by the London poison centre. This top 10 varies slightly if grouped into ages as illustrated in Table 25.1.

This chapter will address the following topics:

- Non-accidental ingestion and self-harm
- Health promotion strategies
- Common ingestions (paracetamol and ethanol)
- Initial management following poisoning or overdose
- Treatment of ingested poisons
- Gastric lavage.

Non-accidental ingestion and self-harm

There are two groups of children and young people who need specific consideration: those in whom poisoning may have been non-accidental ingestion and those who self-harm by poisoning. Careful consideration must be given to the possibility of non-accidental poisoning, a serious though relatively rare form of child abuse (Bates *et al* 1997). Suspicion should be raised when the story of the incident is vague, lacking in detail and varies from version to version and from person to person, when unusual behaviour is observed in the carer, if there is a delay or refusal to allow proper treatment, unprovoked aggression, or a

Table 25.1 Top 10 substances ingested by age

Children aged 1–5	Children aged 5–9	Children aged 10–14
Paracetamol	Paracetamol	Paracetamol
Ibuprofen	Multivitamins	Ibuprofen
Oral contraceptives	Ibuprofen	Aspirin
Multivitamins	Laburnum	Ethanol
Aspirin	Pens	Co-proxamol
Pseudoephedrine	Oral contraceptives	Mefenamic acid
Thyroxine	White spirit	Codeine
Chlorphenamine	Inhaled preparations	Carbamazepine
Promethazine	Mercury thermometer	Co-dydramol
Amoxicillin	Bleach	Loratadine

history or evidence of repeated ingestions. Numerous agents have been used to poison children intentionally, including opioids, anticonvulsants, salt and tricyclic antidepressants (McClure *et al* 1996). Children who present 'spaced out' and the child who has had an unexplained fall and is behaving 'oddly' should have urine and bloods taken for toxicology and consideration given to the possibility of non-accidental poisoning.

The second group relates to children and young people who self-harm using poisons. Hawton and Hall (2003) suggest the rate of self-harm is relatively low in early childhood, but increases rapidly with the onset of adolescence, with females being the most vulnerable. Unfortunately, most acts of self-harm in young people never come to the attention of care services (Hawton *et al* 2002). Recent recommendations published by the National Institute for Clinical Excellence (NICE) have attempted to set the gold standard in the care and management of children aged 8 years and over who self-harm (NICE 2004). Figure 25.1 outlines the specific issues for children and young people, further guidance, guidelines and management flow charts highlighted in the document.

Children and young people who attend the emergency department having ingested a poison, all undergo triage, where children are prioritised based on their clinical need/urgency to be seen by a doctor. The triage system most commonly used in the UK is the Manchester Emergency Triage System (Mackway-Jones 1996). This system includes a simple flow chart for overdose and self-poisoning as illustrated in Figure 25.2. Following triage, children and young people who have self-harmed should receive the requisite treatment for their physical condition, undergo a risk and full psychosocial needs assessment and mental state examination, with referral for further treatment and care as necessary (NICE 2004). It is recommended that a member from the Child and Adolescent Mental Health Services (CAMHS) team should undertake this assessment and provide consultation for the young person, their family, the paediatric team and social services (NICE 2004). The consensus is that, for children and young people an admission to a paediatric ward will allow for time to 'cool off', to undertake assessment of the child and family, and to address child protection issues, and this should therefore be the normal course of events (Royal College of Psychiatrists 1998). In the absence of specific adolescent provision, admission to a paediatric ward is far preferable to an adult ward (NICE 2004).

626

Box 25.1 Top 10 enquiries received by UK poison centres

Paracetamol	Aspirin
Ethanol	Temazepam
Ibuprofen	Inhaled preparations
White spirit	Salbutamol
Oral contraceptive pill	Disinfectant
	(TOXBASE (2010)

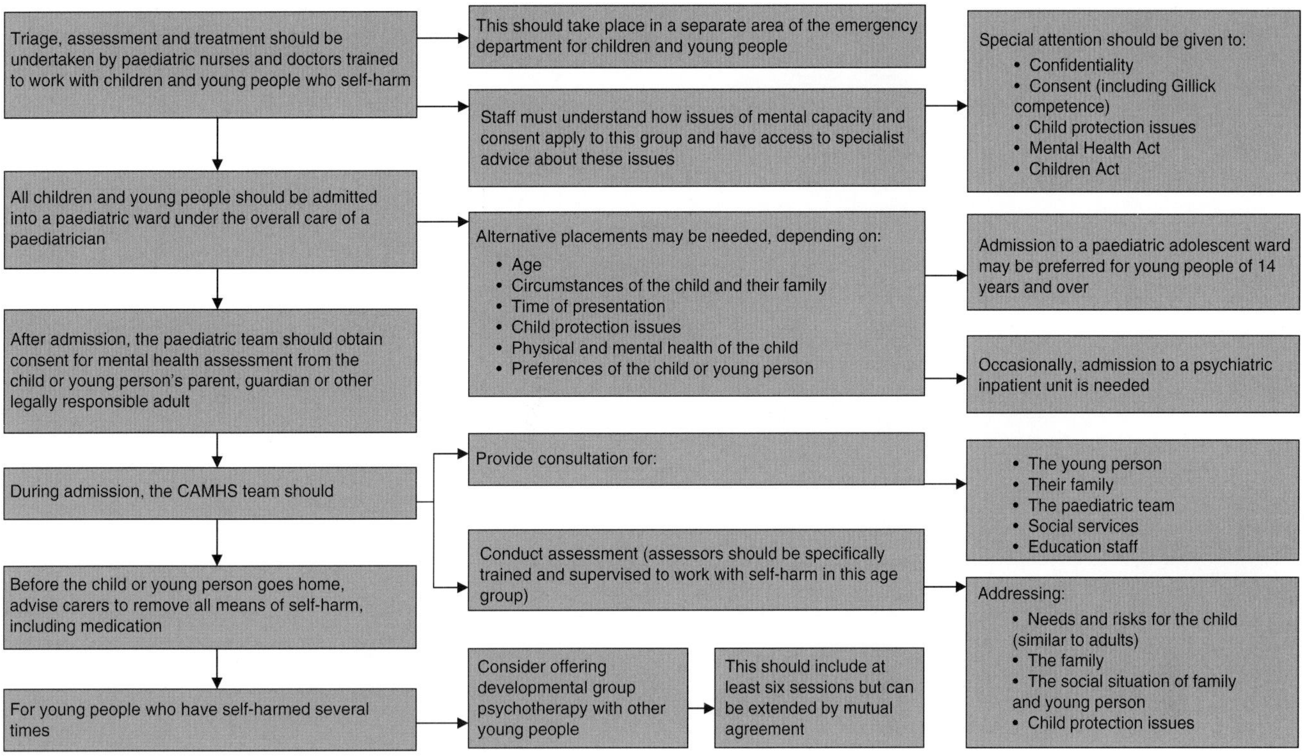

Figure 25.1 Special issues for children and young people (NICE 2004).

Health promotion strategies

Current initiatives to reduce the number of accidental ingestions have focused on restricting access to the container by means of child resistant lids. This has been found to be particularly effective in reducing the number of ingestions in the under-5s age group (Hawton *et al* 2002). However, there is still a need for improvement in the design of containers and packaging. Based on the number of ingestions that occur in the home, the most obvious solution is to keep dangerous products out of the home. This unfortunately is not realistic and therefore parents/carers should be educated in safe practices and encouraged to keep dangerous products out of sight and reach. This change in behaviour can only be brought about by education.

Common ingestions

Paracetamol

Paracetamol is by far the most common ingestion throughout childhood, and unfortunately there are often no initial symptoms, although there may occasionally be nausea and vomiting. The effect on the liver indicated by raised liver function tests and prothrombin time can be detected after 24–48 hours, peaking after 72–96 hours. Gastric decontamination is not necessary in most cases, but should be considered for intentional overdose or where the child has been fed by a sibling. In such cases it is only necessary for ingestions of more than 150mg/kg unless the child falls into a high-risk group, where more than 75mg/kg should be

> **Box 25.2** High-risk groups following ingestion of paracetamol
>
> - Malnourished/anorexic/bulimic children
> - HIV positive children
> - Children with pre-existing liver disease
> - Children taking carbamazepine, phenytoin or rifampicin
> - Children with cystic fibrosis
> - Children with some viral infections e.g. glandular fever
> (Bates *et al* 1997, Paediatric Formulary Committee 2011)

considered potentially toxic (National Poisons Information Service 2008). The high-risk groups are listed in Box 25.2.

Children who have exceeded 150mg/kg need to have bloods taken for paracetamol concentration 4 hours post ingestion. The treatment of choice is either methionine or N-acetylcysteine, but those who fall into one of the high-risk groups should be treated with N-acetylcysteine if their blood paracetamol level is above the highrisk treatment line (National Poisons Information Service 2008). Figure 25.3 illustrates a graph used to estimate the need for acetylcysteine. Activated charcoal may be considered where the dose exceeds 150 mg/kg, but this then prohibits the use of methionine as the charcoal also absorbs this. Oral methionine must be started within 8 hours of ingestion and cannot be used in children who are vomiting, in which case N-acetylcysteine is the treatment of choice. Side effects of this medication, however, include pain along the vein of administration, a rash, nausea, vomiting, pyrexia, headache and tinnitus. In the event of

627

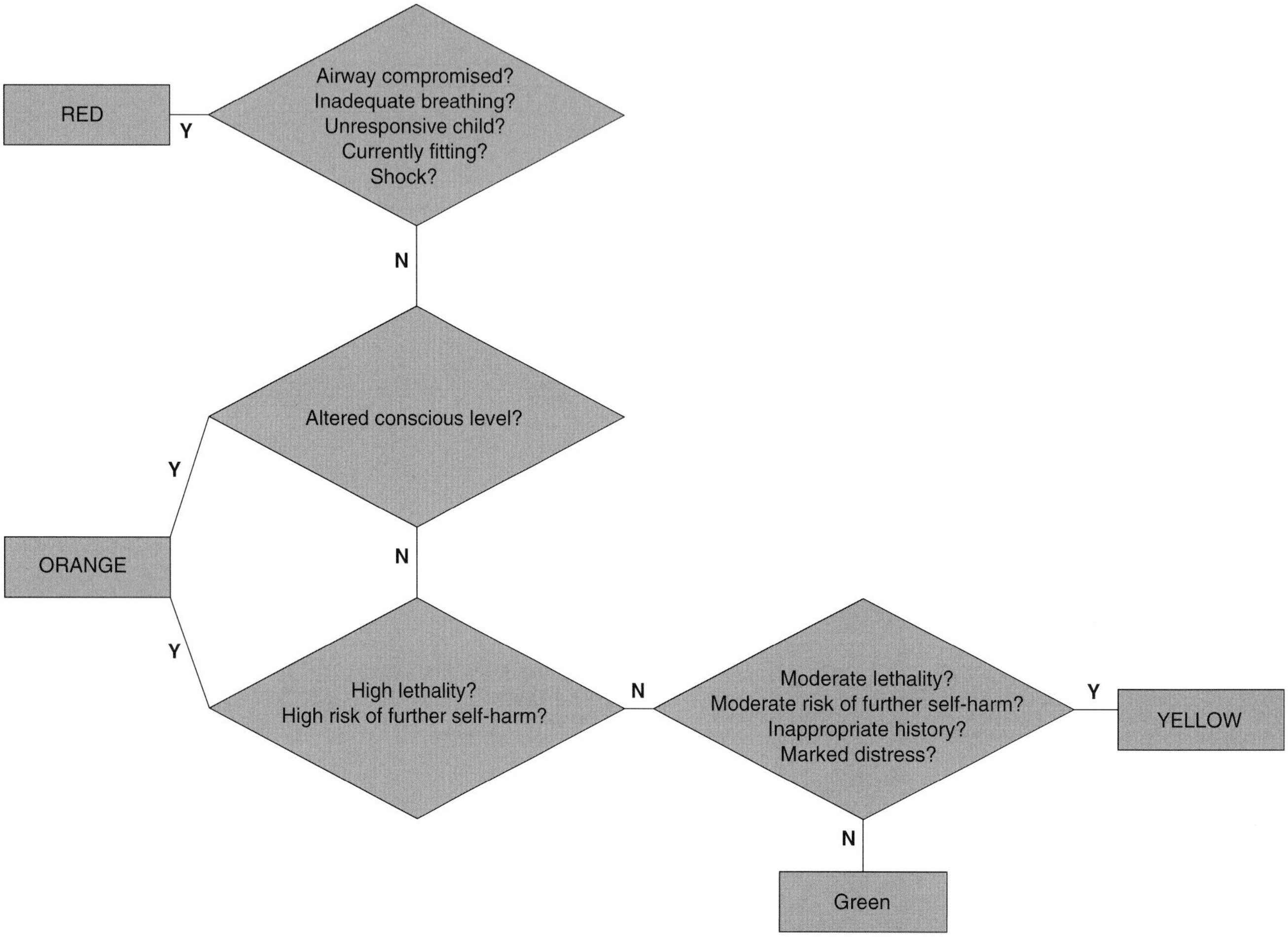

Figure 25.2 Triage flow chart for overdose and self-poisoning (Mackway-Jones 1996).

a severe reaction the infusion must be stopped and medical advice sought.

Ethanol

Ethanol (alcohol) is a poison very commonly ingested in children over the age of 10, but fortunately severe cases are uncommon. Children usually present with in-coordination, slurred speech, ataxia, drowsiness, hypoglycaemia and acidosis (Dolan and Holt 2000). However, care must be taken not to confuse this with symptoms of similar conditions, for example raised intracranial pressure, diabetic hypoglycaemia and drug overdose (Skinner and Driscoll 1996). Severe cases of alcohol ingestion, where the blood alcohol concentration is between 200–400 mg/l, can lead to coma, hypothermia, convulsions, respiratory depression and the risk of aspiration. Due to the risk of rapid central nervous system depression, emesis is not recommended. A period of observation of at least 4 hours is recommend following ingestion equivalent to 0.4 ml/kg (1 ml/kg body weight for 40% spirit, 4 ml/kg body weight for 10% wine, 8 ml/kg body weight for a 5% beer) (Bates *et al* 1997). During this time blood sugar monitoring should be undertaken, and in the event of the blood

sugar dropping below 3 mmol, a bolus dose of 5 ml/kg of 10% glucose should be administered and the blood sugar repeated 30 minutes later (Advanced Paediatric Life Support (APLS) 2005).

Initial management following poisoning or overdose

The initial management of the child is to assess and stabilise their airway, breathing and circulation irrespective of what poison they have ingested. Only after this has been achieved should attention be given to the toxin involved. The airway may be compromised by swelling of the mouth and pharynx and depression of the central nervous system, and can cause reduced respiratory drive and an increased risk of aspiration. Adequacy of breathing should be continually assessed by clinical observation and oxygen saturation monitoring, supplemented by blood gas analysis if appropriate. Inadequate respiratory effort will require intubation and artificial ventilation (APLS 2005). The circulation can be compromised by excessive fluid loss in vomiting and diarrhoea and should be supported with appropriate fluid replacement. Some toxins cause vasodilatation and hypotension, so it is important to obtain intravenous access early in a poten-

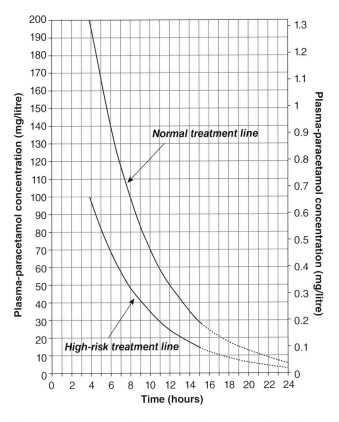

Figure 25.3 Acetylcysteine treatment in paracetamol poisoning. Paediatric Formulary Committee 2011. By permission of Professor P.A. Routledge, All Wales Therapeutics and Toxicology Centre.

tially serious case of poisoning, as this can become more difficult in critically ill children. Appropriate blood samples may be taken at this time. If intravenous access is difficult or unobtainable, using intraosseous access is a useful alternative in the younger child (APLS 2005).

'Shock' is often observed following serious poisoning and poor peripheral perfusion is an early sign, which may be followed by tachycardia and hypotension. It is essential, therefore, that continuous ECG, blood pressure and temperature monitoring be carried out. Mild to moderate shock usually responds to intravenous fluids: initially a 20 ml/kg bolus dose of 0.9% normal saline (isotonic) may be given and repeated as necessary. If fluid replacement is insufficient, the child may need inotropic support, e.g. with a dopamine or dobutamine infusion (McIntosh *et al* 2003).

Arrhythmias are relatively uncommon in paediatric poisoning, and initial management involves adequate resuscitation and correction of any hypoxia, hypercarbia, acid-base or electrolyte imbalances (McIntosh *et al* 2003). Specific therapy need only be considered if supportive measures are inadequate. Metabolic acidosis is frequent but only needs correction with fluids and bicarbonate boluses if severe. Correction of mild acidosis may reduce renal clearance of toxins. Central nervous system depression and convulsions are common features of poisoning. Convulsions induced by toxic agents are usually short-lived, but they may be more refractory to treatment than convulsions due to other causes.

Treatment of ingested poisons

In the past, the removal of poisonous substances from the stomach fell under the broad heading of gastric decontamination and three possible options were available: induced emesis, activated charcoal (which absorbs various toxins or drugs, thus preventing gastrointestinal absorption), and finally gastric lavage. However there has been much debate and a great deal of controversy about the place each of these methods has in the management of ingested poisons (AACT-EAPCCT 1997a, Bates *et al* 1997). They should only be considered in situations, where there are severe ongoing (or predicted) adverse effects as a result of continued exposure to the toxin, for example iron poisoning. However, gastric decontamination should not be considered in cases of hydrocarbon ingestion, such as paraffin or white spirit, or with corrosive substances such as caustic soda, due to the risk of aspiration pneumonia (McIntosh *et al* 2003).

Emesis had long been the favoured method of gastric emptying in children (AACT-EAPCCT 1997b). A number of different emetics have been used in the past, but syrup of ipecacuanha (ipecac) has been the drug of choice for a number of years. The dose is 15ml for children younger than 12 years and 30ml for children aged 12 years and older (Bates *et al* 1997). Despite a good safety record, which may in part account for its long use in the management of acute poisoning, and although is quickly absorbed, there is a delay of up to 20–30 minutes before vomiting occurs, during which time absorption of the agent continues. If vomiting has not occurred after 20 minutes a second dose could be given. However, this method is not without its complications and contra-indications are highlighted in Boxes 25.3 and 25.4. Over time this method has been the subject of many reviews and as a result emesis using ipecacuanha paediatric mixture is no longer used (Bartlett 2003, BNFC 2011, Krenzelok *et al* 1997).

The second method of gut decontamination focuses on the use of activated charcoal, which has been increasingly used in the management of childhood poisoning (AACT-EAPCCT 1997c). Activated charcoal absorbs toxic materials in the gut by offering binding sites and has been used for a variety of drugs including aspirin, carbamazepine and tricyclic antidepressant poisoning. However, it is ineffective in poisons relating to glycol, alcohol, metal and electrolytes. Its routine use is limited by

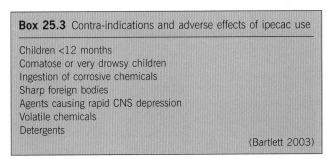

Box 25.3 Contra-indications and adverse effects of ipecac use

Children <12 months
Comatose or very drowsy children
Ingestion of corrosive chemicals
Sharp foreign bodies
Agents causing rapid CNS depression
Volatile chemicals
Detergents

(Bartlett 2003)

Box 25.4 Adverse effects and complications of ipecac

Mallory–Weiss tear of oesophagus
Delay to administration of charcoal
Retropneumoperitoneum gastric rupture

(Bartlett 2003)

its poor acceptance by children and may not be effective more than 1 hour after ingestion (Chyka and Seger 1997). The recommended dose is 1 g/kg for infants, 25–50 g for children (Paediatric Formulary Committee 2011).

Conscious children should be able to drink the charcoal but if they find it impossible to do so, or if vomiting is a problem, it should be given via a nasogastric tube. Palatability of activated charcoal is often a problem and it may be mixed with soft drinks/fruit juices to disguise the taste. Combining activated charcoal with caffeine-free diet cola does not seem to affect the absorptive capacity of charcoal (Rangan *et al* 2001). Its use is not without its complications and adverse effects, which are highlighted in Box 25.5. Contraindications include reduced or absent bowel sounds and use of antidotes that may be absorbed (Brunner and Suddarth 1991).

Gastric lavage

Gastric lavage is the third method of gut decontamination, and its use in children remains poorly studied. Extra care should be taken when performing gastric lavage in children, due to the increased risk of hypothermia if cold fluid is used. Electrolyte imbalance can occur if fluids other than water or isotonic saline are used. Large amounts of water used during the lavage may cause water intoxication, and therefore aliquots of up to 10–20 ml/kg should be used (Bates *et al* 1997). Gastric lavage is

---

Box 25.5 Adverse effects and complications of charcoal

Aspiration
Perforation
Intestinal obstruction
Rectal ulcer

(Brunner and Suddarth 1991)

---

absolutely contraindicated in the comatose child with a depressed gag reflex and an unprotected airway and elective intubation using an appropriate sized endotracheal tube is recommended in these patients. Gastric lavage involves the passage of a large bore orogastric tube with sequential administration and removal of fluid for the purpose of removal of toxins contained in gastric fluids (AACT-EAPCCT 1997a). The orogastric tube should be as large as can be safely tolerated by the child (16F–36Fr) (3.5–8.5 mm) and is dependant on the size of child. This technique of gastric decontamination was used in treating the patient with an acute poisoning ingestion as early as 1812 (Perrone 1994). Until the mid 1980s, the use of gastric lavage up to 4 hours post ingestion followed by the administration of activated charcoal was accepted as the standard of care. However, the types of drug ingestions today are dramatically different and the need and utility of gastric lavage remains controversial. The procedure for undertaking a gastric lavage is outlined below.

Principles table 25.1 Gastric lavage: initial assessment

Principle	Rationale
1. While taking a history it is important to ascertain: • What was ingested and the formulation. (Ideally the parents/carers will have brought the container and remaining tablets with them.) • How much (calculate amounts per kg of body weight).	1. • Parents/carers should be encouraged to bring the remaining tablets or medicines and the container when they attend with the child (Bates *et al* 1997). • It is essential to calculate the maximum possible amount ingested assuming an initial full container and no toxin wasted. If berries or toadstools have been eaten, then they should bring a good sized, un-chewed bit of plant where possible (Bates *et al* 1997).
2. When telephoning a poisons information centre it is helpful to have the following information to hand: • Name, age, sex, weight (in kg) of the child • The time since exposure • The substance(s) to which the child has been exposed • The amount taken or duration of exposure • The constituents and the manufacturer's name of the product if applicable • Packing details and description of product • The clinical condition of the child • Any relevant pre-existing disease • If it is a drug ingestion of a medication the child is taking therapeutically, the child's normal daily dose.	2. The poisons information centre should be contacted if there is any doubt about toxicity of a substance a child has taken or the treatment that is needed (Bates *et al* 1997).
3. Gastric lavage should only be considered if the ingestion has occurred within 1 hour and following recommendation from a poisons information centre.	3. Gastric lavage should not be carried out routinely as there is no evidence to support any improved clinical outcome or reduced mortality (Vale and Kulig 2004).

Principles table 25.2 **Gastric lavage: training**

Principle	Rationale
1. Gastric lavage must only be performed by experienced staff who: a) Are competent in performing the procedure and in basic life-support. b) Are familiar with the indications and contra-indications for the procedure – it should only be considered if the child has ingested a potentially life-threatening amount of poison and the procedure can be undertaken within 60 minutes of ingestion. c) Staff must have received: • Training on how to perform this procedure safely • Supervised practice • Resuscitation training as per trust policy. d) Understand the potential complications of: • aspiration pneumonia • laryngospasm • hypoxia and hypercapnia • mechanical injury to the throat, oesophagus, and stomach • fluid and electrolyte imbalance.	1. To ensure safety and reduce the likelihood of side effects and complications (Bartlett 2003). a) Strong vagal stimulation can induce cardiac dysrhythmias and cardiopulmonary arrest. b) To identify children who are at least at risk from the potential complications of this procedure and would benefit from it. c, d) To establish and maintain the required level of competence.
2) Gastric lavage should not be performed in children who: a) Have a reduced state of consciousness. b) Have ingested a corrosive substance such as a strong acid or alkali solution. c) Have ingested a hydrocarbon (polish, paint stripper/thinner, insecticides, rubber, plastic, etc). d) Are at risk of haemorrhage or gastrointestinal perforation due to recent surgery, or other medical conditions.	2. To ensure safety and reduce the likelihood of side effects and complications. a) Loss of protective reflexes increases the risk of pulmonary aspiration. These patients should be intubated before the procedure. b) To prevent strong acids or alkalis causing further damage to the oesophagus and potential aspiration of a corrosive substance. c) Hydrocarbons have a high aspiration potential. d) To prevent further complications.

Procedure guideline 25.1 **Patient consent and preparation**

Statement	Rationale
1. Obtain consent for the procedure to be carried out. • Ensure the child is awake and cooperative • Explain the procedure to the child (if able to understand) and carer and allow time for any questions.	1. To gain consent from the carer who has parental responsibility and assent from the child (Alderson and Montgomery 1996).
2. To minimise complications. a) Secure airway via orotracheal or nasotracheal intubation in the obtunded or comatose child without a gag reflex. b) Do not attempt to perform a gastric lavage in a completely uncooperative and aggressive child who refuses to swallow a gastric lavage tube.	2. Unconscious children with no cough reflex must be intubated to prevent aspiration while vomiting (Perrone 1994). b) To prevent the risk of pulmonary aspiration and haemorrhage.

631

Procedure guideline 25.2 **Preparation of equipment (gastric lavage)**

Statement	Rationale
1. Assemble the appropriate equipment ensuring the following are available on the trolley prior to performing the gastric lavage: • Incontinence pads • Disposable plastic aprons and gloves, KY jelly • Sterile gastric tube with connector, funnel and connecting tubing • Large jug and bucket for gastric washing • Towel and blankets • Universal container • 50 ml bladder syringe • pH paper <6 • Activated charcoal solution • Warm 0.9% saline (10 ml/kg).	1. To ensure the procedure is conducted as smoothly as possible without unnecessary delays.
2. Ensure the following equipment is available and in good working order: a) Suction, oxygen, child/adult oxygen face mask, appropriate size yanker and a range of suction catheters. b) A bed with the facility to tilt the child head down.	2. To maintain a safe environment and have equipment available which can maintain the child's airway (Perrone 1994). a, b) To minimise the risk of aspiration.
3. Calculate the quantity of liquid required. For children 10 ml/kg body weight of warm normal saline (0.9%) should be given. Water should be avoided in young children because of the risk of inducing hyponatraemia and water intoxication.	3. Small volumes are used to minimise the risk of gastric contents entering the duodenum during lavage. Warm fluids avoid the risk of hypothermia in the very young (Bartlett 2003).

Procedure guideline 25.3 **Procedure (gastric lavage)**

Statement	Rationale
1. In order to undertake the procedure safely and efficiently the following must be adhered to.	1. To ensure the procedure is performed safely and effectively (Perrone 1994).
2. Ensure that there are a minimum of two staff available for the duration of the procedure.	2. One nurse with sole responsibility for managing the airway.
3. Explain procedure to child/relatives if appropriate and ensure they understand the procedure.	3. To gain the child's cooperation and reduce the risks of complications.
4. Ascertain whether a member of the family/carer wishes to be present depending on local/hospital policy.	4. To gain the cooperation of the child and offer reassurance.
5. Throughout the procedure offer reassurance and support.	5. To minimise any complications that may occur should the child become agitated.
6. Lay the child on their left side with the head end of the bed tilted 20 degrees down.	6. Head down tilt will aid the drainage of gastric contents and ensure no secretions/vomit is inhaled.
7. Place disposable sheets under the child's head on a plastic sheet over the floor.	7. To protect the nurse and the child should vomiting occur.

Procedure guideline 25.3 (*Continued*)

Statement	Rationale
8. Turn on suction and place appropriate sized yanker sucker near the child's head.	**8.** To maintain a clear airway should the child vomit.
9. The length of the tube to be inserted is measured and marked before insertion. In children a size 16–36 French gauge with a diameter of 3.5–8.5 mm should be used. The tube should be for single use only.	**9.** To ensure the correct length of tube and minimise trauma while passing the tube.
10. Lubricate the tube and pass a few centimetres at a time while the child swallows.	**10.** To facilitate passage of the tube.
11. Check that the tube is in the stomach by aspirating some of the stomach contents and confirming acidity using pH paper.	**11.** To minimise the risk of aspiration.
12. Place some of the stomach contents in a universal container and send off for toxicology analysis.	**12.** To identify the ingestion of any medications/substances that may be toxic to the body.
13. Slowly pour 0.9% saline solution at 37°C through the funnel to lavage the stomach.	**13.** To prevent sudden lowering of body temperature and possible shock.
14. Fluid is run through the tubing with the funnel held approximately 50 cm above the child's shoulder, taking care not to introduce air into the tube.	**14.** To control the rate at which the fluid is installed.
15. Before the last of the fluid enters the tube, it is compressed and the funnel is lowered into the bucket to allow the lavage fluid to return.	**15.** A siphoning action is needed to recall the contents of the stomach.
16. Observe for tablet debris, which may be seen on the side of the tube or in the bucket. If possible these should be compared to the tablet ingested.	**16.** To confirm ingestion of suspected tablets.
17. As the last of the fluid drains out, care should be taken to compress the tubing to prevent air getting into the system.	**17.** To minimise the risk of the child vomiting and experiencing discomfort.
18. The lavage is repeated until the return is completely clear.	**18.** To maximise clearance of any tablets.
19. Activated charcoal may then be administered down the tube if recommended.	**19.** To absorb any tablets that may be left in the stomach.
20. Disconnect the funnel from the tube and gently but firmly remove the gastric tube and level the head end of the bed.	**20.** Gagging and possible vomiting may occur when the tube is removed. As the tube reaches the pharynx, any fluid left may escape and infiltrate into the lungs.
21. Dispose of all equipment depending on local policy.	**21.** To minimise the risk of infection and adhere to local waste disposal policy.
22. Send sample of gastric contents to toxicology unit for analysis.	**22.** To try and identify the content of the ingested substance.

Procedure guideline 25.4 Post procedure (gastric lavage)

Statement	Rationale
1. Sit the child up and make them comfortable, reassuring the child and carer all the time.	**1.** To minimise the distress to the child and carer.
2. Provide oral hygiene facilities as required.	**2.** To maintain a clean, moist mouth.
3. Document findings and outcome following gastric lavage.	**3.** To ensure effective communication and provide documentary evidence of care provided.

References

Advanced Paediatric Life-support Group (2005) The Practical Approach, 4th edition. London, BMJ

American Academy of Clinical Toxicology: European Association of Poisons Centres and Clinical Toxicologists (AACT-EAPCCT) (1997a) Position Statement: gastric lavage. Journal of Toxicology-Clinical Toxicology, 35(7), 711–719

American Academy of Clinical Toxicology: European Association of Poisons Centres and Clinical Toxicologists (AACT-EAPCCT) (1997b) Position Statement: ipecac syrup. Journal of Toxicology-Clinical Toxicology, 35(7), 699–709

American Academy of Clinical Toxicology: European Association of Poisons Centres and Clinical Toxicologists (AACT-EAPCCT) (1997c) Position Statement: single-dose activated charcoal. Journal of Toxicology-Clinical Toxicology, 35(7), 721–741

Alderson P, Montgomery J. (1996) Health Care Choices: making decisions with children: participation and consent. London, Institute for Public Research

Bartlett D. (2003) The ABC of gastric decontamination. Journal of Emergency Nursing, 29(6), 576–577

Bates N, Edwards N, Roper J, Volans G. (1997) Paediatric Toxicology: handbook of poisoning in children. Exeter: Macmillan

British National Formulary for Children (2011) British National Formulary, 4th edition. London, Royal Pharmaceutical Society of Great Britain

Brunner L, Suddarth D. (1991) The Lippincott Manual of Paediatric Nursing, 3rd edition. London, Harper and Row

Chyka P, Seger D. (1997) Position statement: ipecac syrup. Journal of Toxicology – Clinical Toxicology, 35(7), 721–741

Dolan B, Holt L. (2000). Accident & Emergency: theory into practice. London, Baillière Tindall

Hawton K, Townsend E. (2001) Effects of legislation restricting pack sizes of paracetamol and salicylate on self poisoning in the United Kingdom: before and after study. British Medical Journal, 322(7296), 1203–1207

Hawton K, Hall S. (2003) Deliberate self-harm in adolescents: a study of characteristics and trends in Oxford, 1990–2000. Journal of Child Psychology and Psychiatry, 44(8), 1191–1198

Hawton K, Rodham K, Evans E, Weatherall R. (2002) Deliberate self-harm in adolescents: self report survey in schools in England. British Medical Journal, 325(7374), 1207–1211

Krenzelok E, McGuinan M, Lheur P. (1997) Position statement: ipecac syrup. Journal of Toxicology-Clinical Toxicology, 35(7), 699–709

Mackway-Jones K. (1996) Emergency triage. Plymouth, BMJ Publishing Group

McClure R, Davis PM, Meadow SR, Sibert JR. (1996) Epidemiology of Munchausen syndrome by proxy, non-accidental poisoning. Archives of Disease in Childhood, 75, 57–71

McIntosh N, Helms P, Smyth R. (2003) Forfar & Arneil's Textbook of Pediatrics. London, Churchill Livingstone

National Institute for Clinical Excellence (2004) Self-Harm: the short-term physical and psychological management and secondary prevention of self-harm in primary and secondary care. London, The British Psychological Society

National Poisons Information Service (2008) Paracetamol, Poisons Index. London, National Poisons Information Service

Paediatric Formulary Committee (2011) British National Formulary for Children. London, British Medical Association, the Royal Pharmaceutical Society of Great Britain, the Royal College of Paediatrics and Child Health, and the Neonatal and Paediatric Pharmacists Group

Perrone J. (1994) Gastric lavage. Emergency Medical Clinics of North America, 12, 285–299

Rangan C, Nordt S, Hamilton R, Ingels M. (2001) Treatment of acetaminophen ingestion with a super-activated charcoal-cola mixture. Annual Emergency Medicine, 37, 55–58

Royal College of Psychiatrists (1998) Managing Deliberate Self-harm in Young People. CR64. London, Royal College of Psychiatrists

Royal Society for the Prevention of Accidents (2010) Poisons. Available at: http://www.rospa.com/ (last accessed 18th May 2010)

Skinner D, Driscoll P. (1996) ABC of Major Trauma, 2nd edition. London, BMJ Publishing

TOXBASE (2005) www.spib.axl.co.uk. Available at: www.spib.axl.co.uk. (last accessed 18th May 2010)

Vale JA, Kulig K, American Academy of Clinical Toxicology, European Association of Poisons Centres and Clinical Toxicologists (2004). Position paper: gastric lavage. Journal of Toxicology – Clinical Toxicology, 42(7), 933–943

Chapter 26

Respiratory care

Chapter contents

Procedure guidelines

The Great Ormond Street Hospital Manual of Children's Nursing Practices, First Edition. Edited by Susan Macqueen, Elizabeth Anne Bruce, Faith Gibson.
© 2012 Great Ormond Street Hospital for Children NHS Foundation Trust. Published 2012 by Blackwell Publishing Ltd.

Introduction

Respiratory care is one of the fundamental roles of the nurse, ranging from observation of respiratory rate and effort to the management of long-term ventilation.

Respiratory physiology consists of:

- **Ventilation** – the act of getting air into and out of the lungs
- **Respiration** – the exchange of gases across the alveolar membrane, an essential function of the lungs, providing the body's cells with oxygen.

The lungs are relatively immature at birth but continue to develop into childhood. The anatomy of the respiratory tract is complex, with the lungs surrounded by a double layer of pleural membranes, parietal and visceral layers. To enable efficient ventilation, expansion of the lungs and the parietal pleural spaces is necessary. A small amount of pleural fluid serves as lubrication to the surface of the pleural membranes during respiration. Small spontaneous air leaks that do not cause any symptoms re-seal and air is absorbed back into the body. A moderate collection of fluid can be well tolerated, but large volumes of fluid compress normal lung tissue and therefore interfere with gas exchange.

Appropriate respiratory support in children and young people is critical, as highlighted by the Basic Life Support Guidelines (see Resuscitation, Chapter 27). Infants and small children have small resting volumes and low oxygen reserves. They also have a higher rate of oxygen consumption, which results in a rapid fall in blood oxygen levels when their respiratory state is compromised. All clinical staff, whether they are working in a hospital or community setting, should ensure that they receive regular updates in respiratory assessment skills. Clinical observation and assessment, effective and efficient airway management and support of oxygen delivery are of primary importance to ensure that the child is able to maintain optimal respiratory function, either independently or supported. This is part of the assessment of basic and advanced life support, directing assessment and clinical support strategies. All clinical teams caring for the child need to be competent in clinical observation and assessment of children of all ages using ABCDE (Airway, Breathing, Circulation, Disability, Exposure) (see Resuscitation Chapter).

Early recognition and effective management of respiratory failure or problems will prevent the majority of cardiorespiratory arrests in children, and reduce associated morbidity and mortality. These interventions rely on the relevant skills and knowledge. If clinical staff are in any doubt, they should access immediate help from a more senior member of the clinical team for prompt advice and support, or put out the relevant emergency call.

Standardised assessment using a robust Children's Early Warning System (CEWS) (Pearson and Duncan 2011) and the use of a communication tool such as SBARD (Situation, Background, Assessment, Recommendations, Decision) enable concise communication of problems such as deterioration in the child's respiratory function. This drives patient safety directives and aids assertive, effective communication, reducing the need for repetition in challenging communication situations between all staff levels. These tools also provide a standardised documentation of events (NHS Institute for Innovations and Improvements 2006).

Skills and competence to manage ongoing airway issues are essential for all nurses. Children and young people who have a reduced ability to clear or maintain an airway or need additional oxygen delivery as part of their ongoing care will require the attention of an individual able to provide ongoing assessment. This should be provided by a health professional or, for chronic conditions, another suitably trained person, such a parent or carer, with the relevant skills and competencies to keep the child safe.

The four areas covered in this chapter are:

1. Suction.
2. Oxygen therapy.
3. Chest drains.
4. Long-term ventilation (LTV).

This chapter has close links with the Assessment (Chapter 1) and Resuscitation (Chapter 27) chapters. The reader is also referred to the Tracheostomy chapter (Chapter 28) for guidelines on the suctioning and care of children with a tracheostomy. The use of an inhaler is discussed in Chapters 2 and 15. This chapter does not provide an in-depth account of respiratory physiology or the management of respiratory conditions and the reader is guided to some key texts and websites, which are provided at the end of the chapter.

Airway suction

The aim of airway suction is to clear secretions, thereby maintaining a patent airway and improving ventilation and oxygenation. Removal of such secretions also minimises the risk of atelectasis (Prasad and Hussey 1995). However, suction is not a benign procedure and adverse physiological effects directly attributed to airway suction are well documented. These effects can be both immediate and long-term, and therefore a sound knowledge of the procedure and its effects are a prerequisite for undertaking suction, as is the availability of resuscitation skills and appropriate equipment for the hospital/community setting and any airway adjuncts used. Each case has to be decided on an individual basis, weighing up the benefits against the potentially harmful effects of this invasive procedure.

Airway suctioning is a common practice in the treatment of children with a variety of pathologies. It is most frequently undertaken to remove excessive or retained secretions from a child's respiratory tract, but may also be necessary to obtain specimens for laboratory examination. It may be performed as a single procedure by nursing and medical staff, occasionally by parents/carers, or it may be incorporated into a chest physiotherapy regime.

The principles are the same whether the suction is of the child's pharynx or via an artificial airway (e.g. tracheal tube or tracheostomy). Children may be unable to clear their own tracheobronchial secretions for several reasons, including:

- Respiratory pathology causing an alteration in type or quantity of secretions, or disruption of the normal mucociliary clearance process
- Infants, less than 6 months of age, are preferential nasal breathers and may require assistance to clear the upper airways
- Neurological disorders that inhibit/depress the normal cough reflex
- Presence of an artificial airway or airway adjunct.

Harmful effects of airway suctioning include:

- Tracheobronchial trauma (Brodsky *et al* 1987, Kleiber *et al* 1988, Kuzenski 1978, Sackner *et al* 1973)
- Hypoxia (Boutros 1970, Kerem *et al* 1990, Naigow and Powasser 1977, Rindfleisch and Tyler 1981)
- Atelectasis (Fox *et al* 1977, Nagaraj *et al* 1980)

- Cardiovascular changes (Cordero and Hone 1971, Shim *et al* 1969, Simbruner *et al* 1981, Walsh *et al* 1989, Winston *et al* 1987)
- Intracranial pressure alterations (Durand *et al* 1989; Perlman and Volpe 1983)
- Pneumothorax (Alpan *et al* 1984, Anderson and Chandra 1976, Vaughan *et al* 1978)
- Bacterial infection (Prasad and Hussey 1995).

Procedure guideline 26.1 Assessing the need for suction

Statement	Rationale
1. Assess the need for suction. **a)** Increased work of breathing: • Increased respiratory rate • Alteration in respiratory pattern • Recession • Nasal flaring • Chin tug • Grunting (non-intubated patients) • Altered level of consciousness • Reduced/loss of visible chest movement or unequal movement of the chest on the left and right sides • Suspected aspiration. **b)** Alterations in gas exchange: • Decreased PaO_2 (oxygen levels) and/or increased $PaCO_2$ (carbon dioxide levels) on the blood gas report • Reduced oxygen saturations • Pale and/or mottled appearance • Cyanosis/pallor – colour change due to low oxygen levels and poor gas exchange • Evidence of audible or visible secretions • On auscultation, course breath sounds or lack of chest sounds and/or palpation. • Examination of the chest X-ray • Alteration of respiratory support parameters • Inability to effectively clear secretions independently.	**1.** To ensure that the signs and symptoms exhibited by the child indicate the need for suction thus ensuring that this invasive procedure is not carried out unnecessarily. It is also important that other clinical causes of respiratory distress and possibly an alteration in blood gases that do not require suction are considered, for example a pneumothorax (Alpan *et al* 1984, Anderson and Chandra 1976, Vaughan *et al* 1978).
2. Document the event, assessment of secretions and the child's clinical signs using a children's early warning system (CEWS) (Pearson and Duncan 2011).	**2.** To monitor the safety and comfort of the child, using a standardised assessment score and document accurate records of the event for future care planning.

Procedure guideline 26.2 Preparing the child and family (suction)

Statement	Rationale
1. Provide explanations appropriate to the child's age and condition, even if the child is apparently unconscious.	**1.** To minimise fear, gain co-operation, and provide reassurance and psychological support. An unconscious child may still be able to hear conversations near them.
2. Family members must also receive appropriate explanations.	**2.** To allay their anxieties and reassure them of the benefits of the procedure and to gain their assistance as necessary.

(*Continued*)

Procedure guideline 26.2 (*Continued*)

Statement	Rationale
3. Inform the child and family of the following: • Reason(s) for the suction • What it entails • Potential risks of suction • Duration of the procedure • Expected outcome from suction.	**3.** To gain cooperation, obtain informed consent and minimise anxiety.
4. The child and family must be informed that appropriate holding may be required.	**4.** To obtain informed consent and ensure child safety.
5. The child must be appropriately positioned and securely held using blankets and/or an assistant as appropriate.	**5.** To maximise the child's safety and comfort, minimise the risks of trauma and treatment effectiveness.
6. Any specific considerations/requirements of individual children should be addressed, e.g.: • Nebulised medications administered as prescribed • Pre-oxygenation.	**6.** To comply with the child's treatment plan. To assist or potentiate suction procedure by reducing wheezing and/or loosening secretions. To reduce cardiorespiratory effects.
7. Pre-oxygenation prior to suctioning by an appropriate method will be required for children who, on individual clinical assessment: **a)** Are deemed at risk of desaturation during the procedure. **b)** Require >40% inspired oxygen.	**7.** To prevent complications: **a)** To minimise hypoxia. **b)** To reduce cardiorespiratory effects.
8. Hyperinflation may be required for ventilated children who have reduced lung compliance, e.g. pulmonary oedema.	**8.** To maintain distension of the terminal alveoli and enhance oxygenation during procedure.
9. This **must only** be performed by an experienced nurse or physiotherapist with competency based training.	**9.** To minimse the risk of complications. This procedure has a high risk of cardiac dysrhythmias and reduced cardiac output.
10. Adequate patient hydration and/or efficient humidification of inspired gases must be ensured.	**10.** To reduce the likelihood of thick secretions and therefore maximise airway patency by enhancing the procedure ability to remove secretions.

Principles table 26.1 **Preparation of equipment: negative pressure**

Principle	Rationale
1. The suction unit may be a piped vacuum system or a portable unit. The trust should provide a guide to testing the correct set up of suction units, which should be checked and documented as per unit policy. **a)** This is done by turning on the unit, placing a finger over the end of the suction tubing and then noting the suction manometer reading (Kuzenski 1978). **b)** If necessary, the pressure must be altered appropriately prior to proceeding. **c)** The suction pressure recommendations are: • 60–80 mmHg (8–10 kPa) for neonates • Up to 120 mmHg (<16 kPa) for older children (Young 1984).	**1, 2.** To ensure that equipment is maintained in good working order and ready for use.

Principles table 26.1 (*Continued*)

Principle	Rationale
2. These should be checked daily for function and faults, and prior to use on a new patient admission. Accurate records should be kept of these checks and faulty equipment reported and repaired as per hospital policy. Replacement units must be available.	
3. The negative pressure of the unit must be checked prior to attaching the catheter to the suction tubing.	**3.** To minimise risks of trauma, hypoxia and atelectasis.
4. The vacuum and the suction setting **must be** checked prior to each procedure.	**4.** To ensure the pressure settings have not been altered and are appropriate for the individual child's needs.
5. Catheters must not be 'kinked' prior to insertion in an effort to control the vacuum (Prasad and Hussey 1995).	**5.** To prevent a vacuum build-up which on release causes enormous suction that can result in biopsies of fragile mucosa.

Principles table 26.2 Preparation of equipment: catheter selection

Principle	Rationale
1. Rigid suction catheters (i.e. Yankauer suckers) may be used to clear the mouth of thick and/or particulate matter.	**1.** The relatively wide diameter and rigid design facilitates easier removal of thick secretions/debris.
2. In all other circumstances, catheters must not exceed more than 50% of the internal diameter of the airway (Glass and Grap 1995).	**2.** To enable gas flow between the catheter and the tracheal wall (or tracheal tube) thus minimising the risks of hypoxia and reducing the likelihood of atelectasis.
3. Catheters must have rounded tips.	**3.** To minimise trauma (Link *et al* 1976).
4. Catheters must have two or three small lateral holes. Catheters must not have more than three lateral holes.	**4.** To provide relief if the distal hole becomes occluded.
5. Catheters must not have more than three lateral holes.	**5.** To reduce the risk of the catheter kinking at its tip and damaging the mucosa (Link *et al* 1976). The greater the number of lateral holes the weaker the wall of the suction catheter.
6. Lateral holes of the suction catheters must be smaller than the distal hole (Jung and Gottleib 1976, Link *et al* 1976).	**6.** To ensure that the greatest suction is exerted at the distal end of the catheter, thus minimising the likelihood of lateral invagination of tissue and the potential consequences of tissue trauma.
7. Whenever possible, suction catheters with integrated vacuum controls should be used (Prasad and Hussey 1995). When these are unavailable a 'Y' connector must be incorporated between the suction tubing and catheter.	**7.** To prevent suction being applied to the airway during catheter introduction.

Procedure guideline 26.3 **Performing suction**

Statement	Rationale
1. All individuals performing suction should receive initial training and ongoing assessment in: • Respiratory assessment • Indications for suction • Suction technique • Potential side effects.	**1.** To ensure the child is suctioned appropriately, safely and effectively with minimal side effects and that the individual undertaking the procedure is up to date on the evidence base around this procedure.
2. All staff should have the required level of resuscitation skills and appropriate equipment as agreed for the hospital/ community setting.	**2.** To facilitate rapid clinical emergency interventions if necessary, as appropriate for the child's needs.
3. The frequency of suctioning is determined by the child's clinical condition (including chest auscultation) and not pre-determined time intervals.	**3.** To ensure that care is individualised and appropriate to the child's needs.
4. Before performing suction, gather the following equipment: • Suction unit • Suction catheters of appropriate type and size • Irrigant solution (if considered to be appropriate) • Specimen container (if required) • Non-sterile gloves • Apron • Bowl of clean tap water • Tissues • Blanket (for restraining the child if necessary).	**4.** To enable the procedure to be performed in a timely and safe manner.
5. All the equipment must be checked to ensure it is fully operational prior to procedure.	**5.** To facilitate safe practice and ensure that the procedure is carried out efficiently and effectively.
6. Two people may be required for this procedure, i.e. one to perform suction and the other to restrain the child (Prasad and Hussey 1995).	**6.** To minimise trauma, provide psychological support and facilitate the procedure.
7. The child should be placed on their side if possible.	**7.** To facilitate the procedure and minimise the risk of aspiration.
8. Airway suctioning must be performed as a 'clean' procedure: • A clinical hand wash must be performed. However, in an emergency this may not be practicable. • Gloves should be worn. There should be no contact between the suction catheter and anything other than the practitioner's gloved hand and the child's airway.	**8.** To minimise the risk of infection. National guidelines using 'care bundles' are in place to monitor and reduce infection risks in high-risk procedures (DoH 2011). To minimise the risk of contamination.
9. The person undertaking the procedure should wear the appropriate protective clothing to minimise the risk of exposure to bodily fluids and any associated infective risk. These include: • Gloves • Apron • Mask • Eye protection.	**9.** To protect the staff member undertaking this role and to use appropriate protection as per local and national policies on infection control.
10. The distance a suction catheter is inserted into the airway is determined by measuring the length of the child's airway plus connections.	**10.** To ensure secretions are removed from the child's entire airway.

Procedure guideline 26.3 (*Continued*)

Statement	Rationale
11. Where there is no artificial airway in situ, the appropriate measurement is determined by the distance from the level of central incisors (or where they would be) to the angle of the lower jaw (Advanced Paediatric Life Support Group 2005).	11. To minimise risk of trauma and damage to the airway from the procedure.
12. The aim is then to introduce the catheter just beyond this point. For children who have an artificial airway, the length should be recorded. Catheters are then inserted just beyond this distance, but not as far as the carina (Brodsky *et al* 1987, Runton 1992).	12. To minimise risk of damage to the carina.
13. The child's medical team may occasionally instruct a shorter insertion distance, e.g. post-tracheal surgery.	13. To prevent damage to lesions or surgical sites.
14. Suction catheters must be introduced into the airway gently, ensuring no negative pressure is applied (Jung and Gottleib 1976).	14. To minimise trauma by reducing the direct contact between the catheter and the airway mucosa.
15. Catheters must not be rotated on removal but withdrawn straight out of the airway.	15. To minimise hypoxia which is significantly related to duration of suction attempts
16. The application of continuous versus intermittent suction is contentious (Czarnik *et al* 1991).	16. There is no conclusive evidence as to the efficacy or potential hazards of this practice.
17. The maximum duration of each suction attempt should be determined by the individual child's clinical response, but should be limited to no more than 10–15 seconds (Sumner 1990, Tolles and Stone 1990, Young 1984).	17. To minimise the risk of hypoxia.
18. a) If a child has viscous secretions that are not effectively cleared by suctioning, the use of an irrigant solution may be considered (Prasad and Hussey 1995). b) However irrigants must not be routinely used (Ackerman 1993, Hagler and Traver 1994).	18. a) Inadequately cleared secretions may threaten the patency of the child's airway. b) There is no conclusive evidence as to the efficacy or potential hazards of irrigant use.
19. a) The recommended solution for irrigation is 0.9% sodium chloride. b) Recommended aliquots of irrigants range from 0.5 millilitres in neonates to 2 millilitres for older children. A greater quantity may be required during physiotherapy treatments.	19. a) 0.9% saline solution is an isotonic solution. b) Amounts vary according to the size of the child and their specific requirements. Treatment needs to be applicable to the child's condition.
20. While performing suction, the child must be continuously observed, with particular attention paid to: • Respiratory rate and quality • Colour • Heart rate • SaO_2 (if already being monitored) • Quantity, colour and viscosity of aspirate obtained.	20. To assess the child's tolerance of the procedure and inform future suction practices. To monitor the effectiveness of the procedure and identify any signs of cardiorespiratory compromise.
21. If the child's condition deteriorates, appropriate resuscitation procedures must be initiated immediately.	21. To maximise safety.
22. Disposable suction catheters are designed for single procedure use only. A catheter may be reused only if an immediate further attempt at airway suction is required.	22. To minimise risks of infection and reduce financial costs.
23. Catheters must be changed between suction of an artificial airway and mouth/nostrils.	23. To minimise cross-infection.

641

Procedure guideline 26.4 Completing the suction procedure

Statement	Rationale
1. Suction tubing and flow controls (if appropriate) should be flushed clear with clean tap water. This solution should be discarded and replaced 4 hourly.	1. To ensure that the system is kept clean and to minimise the risk of infection.
2. The child should be made comfortable and feedback given to the child and the family.	2. To meet the comfort and communication needs of the child and family and inform future suction practices.
3. All used equipment must be disposed of according to the local waste policy.	3. To minimise the risk of cross-infection.
4. A clinical hand wash must be performed.	4. To minimise the risk of cross-infection.
5. The suction procedure must be recorded in the child's healthcare records. This should include details of the aspirate obtained, any samples sent, as well as adverse clinical reactions that occurred.	5. To provide accurate records and influence future suction practices.

Oxygen therapy

Oxygen therapy is the administration of oxygen at concentrations greater than that in ambient air with the intent of treating or preventing the symptoms and manifestations of hypoxia and reducing the work of breathing by increasing alveolar oxygen tension (National Guideline Clearing House 2006). It is an essential part of clinical practice, widely utilised in both pulmonary and non-pulmonary conditions. However, some have been critical of its wide use (Downs 2003). Excessive use of oxygen has been demonstrated in several studies, which demonstrate that insufficient attention is shown to pharmacological and physiological principles (Albin *et al* 1992, Gravil *et al* 1997, Jeffrey *et al* 1989, Kor and Lim 2000, Small *et al* 1992). Concentrations required are dependant on condition. Inappropriate concentrations have potentially serious effects, leading to pulmonary epithelial damage (broncho-pulmonary dysplasia), convulsions and, particularly in neonates, retinal damage (Jefferies and Turley 1999). Oxygen is classed as a drug and must be prescribed. Its use should be documented for each child as per national and hospital guidelines (Royal Pharmaceutical Society of Great Britain 2005).

This guideline will including the following:

- Indications for oxygen therapy
- Types of therapy
- Methods and equipment for administration
- Preparation and initial assessment
- Setting up oxygen therapy
- Ongoing assessment
- Discharge planning for children on long-term oxygen.

Indications for oxygen therapy

Oxygen therapy should be considered for any child with one or more of the following:

- Hypoxia – that is, diminished blood oxygen levels (oxygen saturation levels of <92%)
- Acute and chronic hypoxemia (PaO_2 < 65 mmHg, SaO_2 < 92%)
- Signs and symptoms of shock
- Low cardiac output and metabolic acidosis (HCO_3 < 18 mmol/l)
- Cardiac or respiratory arrest
- Chronic type two respiratory failure (hypoxia and hypercapnia) (Balfour-Lynn *et al* 2005a)
  - Hypoxia = blood oxygen levels < 92%
  - Hypercapnia = increased carbon dioxide levels.

Despite a lack of supportive data, oxygen is also administered in the following conditions:

- Dyspnoea without hypoxemia
- Postoperatively, depending on instruction from surgical team (Kbar and Campbell 2006)
- Treatment of pneumothorax (Dinwiddie 1997).

There remains a lack of consensus regarding fundamental issues in oxygen therapy for children, but it differs considerably from adult oxygen therapy and the following issues must be taken into account:

- Assessment can be challenging; it is difficult to obtain arterial/venous blood samples
- Clinical conditions in infancy are exclusive although some overlaps exist in adolescents
- Prognosis in infancy is usually positive – children often require oxygen therapy for limited periods
- Many children who require long-term oxygen therapy only need it overnight
- Low flow equipment is sometimes required
- Supervision from a parent or carer is essential to ensure their ongoing care and safety of therapy
- Oxygen provision maybe necessary within school (Balfour-Lynn *et al* 2005b).

Patient groups within the paediatric population potentially affected by chronic hypoxaemia include children with:

- Chronic lung disease
- Congenital heart disease with pulmonary hypertension
- Pulmonary hypertension secondary to respiratory disease
- Interstitial lung disease
- Obliterative bronchiolitis
- Cystic fibrosis and other causes of severe bronchiectasis
- Obstructive sleep apnoea and other sleep related disorders
- Palliative care for symptom relief (Balfour-Lynn *et al* 2005b).

Types of oxygen therapy

High concentration oxygen therapy – up to 60% of oxygen therapy results in the reduced risk of hypoventilation and retention of carbon dioxide (Joint Formulary Committee 2006). High concentration oxygen therapy can have detrimental effects on the respiratory system, particularly after prolonged usage and can lead to respiratory distress due to absorption atelectasis (collapse of alveoli due to blockage). In the premature infant, retrolental fibroplasias can be a side effect due to vasoconstriction, and could lead to permanent blindness (Jefferies and Turley 1999).

Low concentration oxygen therapy (controlled oxygen therapy) – used to correct hypoxaemia by using an accurate amount of oxygen without depleting existing maintenance of carbon dioxide and respiratory acidosis. Blood gases should be used to measure the precise concentration of oxygen (Joint Formulary Committee 2006).

Long-term oxygen therapy (LTOT) – the provision of continuous oxygen therapy for children with chronic hypoxaemia, requirements vary between 24-hour dependency and dependency during periods of sleep. LTOT principally aims to improve symptoms and prevent harm from chronic hypoxaemia. Any child likely to require LTOT for longer than 3 weeks should be considered for domiciliary oxygen.

Principles table 26.3 **Methods and equipment for administration of oxygen**

Principle	Rationale
1. Consider the most appropriate method of administration (see Table 26.1). Issues such as oxygen requirement and tolerability of the delivery method for the individual child must be considered.	1. To ensure maximum benefit is obtained from treatment.

2. Selection of an appropriate oxygen delivery system must also take into account, clinical condition, the child's size, needs and therapeutic goals (Myers 2002):
• High concentration oxygen is usually delivered via an incubator or humidified head box
• Concentrations below 50%, oxygen can be delivered via nasal cannula
Other methods of delivering oxygen include:
• Face masks
• Re-breathe mask
• Humidified oxygen
• Wafting
• Via nebulisation
• Tracheostomy (see Chapter 28)
   ○ Nasal cannula
   ○ Via a ventilation circuit.
	2. To meet the clinical and age appropriate needs of the child and ensure that the therapeutic goal is reached.

Table 26.1 Selection of the most appropriate method of oxygen delivery

Method	Concentration	Comments
Simple oxygen mask	High concentrations can be delivered safely	Flow below 4 litres could potentially result in carbon dioxide retention (Bell 1995)
High concentration oxygen masks	10–15 litres required	For use in emergency situations
Humidified	26–65% FiO_2	Nasal cannula oxygen should not be humidified. Prolonged periods of high percentage oxygen should be humidified (Chandler 2001)
Wafting	30–40% with 10 litres oxygen per minute	Green oxygen tubing should be used Conventional methods of oxygen delivery recommended if tolerated (Davies *et al* 2002)

Oxygen delivery methods and terms

Face masks

These are supplied in children's sizes but are not always tolerated (Moules and Ramsey 1998). There are two types of face masks dependant on the condition of the child: simple and high-concentration masks (Woodhams 1996):

1. Simple oxygen mask (variable flow masks) – vents in the mask allow for the dilution of oxygen (Chandler 2001). High concentrations of oxygen can be safely administered. If low concentration of oxygen (below 4 litres) required then there is a risk of a carbon dioxide build up (Bell 1995).
2. High-concentration oxygen masks – used for emergency situations (Advanced Life Support Group 1997) due to a large reservoir that allows oxygen only to be breathed in by the child. This prevents the inhalation of mixed gases. The approximate oxygen received is 99% (Bell 1995).

Humidified oxygen

This can be delivered via a face-mask or head box, dependent on the child's age/cooperation. Humidified oxygen should be utilised when high percentages of oxygen are required for prolonged periods and in those with chronic respiratory illness, to prevent drying of the mucosa and secretions. Nasal cannula oxygen does not need to be humidified, as environmental and physiological humidification is sufficient.

Wafting

When conventional delivery methods are not tolerated, wafting of oxygen via a face mask has been shown to deliver concentrations of 30–40%, with 10 litres of oxygen per minute to an area of 35 × 32 cms from top of the mask. Wafting via green oxygen tubing has been assessed as appropriate for short-term use only, for example, while feeding. A standard paediatric oxygen mask placed on the chest can give significant oxygen therapy with minimal distress to the child (Davies 2002).

Other methods

- **Via nebulisation:** If the child is oxygen dependant nebulisers should be delivered via oxygen and not air.
- **Tracheostomy:** Oxygen can be delivered via a tracheostomy mask, Swedish nose or headbox. Consider child's individual need.
- **Nasal cannula:** This can be used for long-term oxygen delivery, allowing the child to vocalise and eat. The concentration is often not controlled, resulting in low inspiratory oxygen concentrations. The use of nasal cannulae can, in the sensitive child, produce dermatitis and mucosal drying (Joint Formulary Committee 2006). Only low flow rates of up to 2 litres per minute can be given comfortably due to inadequate humidification (Jamieson *et al* 1999, Mallet and Bailey 1996). Nasal cannula oxygen does not need to be humidified.
- **Via a ventilation circuit:** Accurate measurement of inspired oxygen is difficult and pulse oximetry must be maintained. Oxygen can be delivered at various points throughout the ventilation circuit (Simonds 2007).
- **Via an Ayres T piece:** An open-ended bag, used by anaesthetists and other experienced practitioners. This administration set gives a reliable impression of the state of the lungs. It also allows manual application of positive end-expiratory pressure (PEEP). It is completely reliant on an effective oxygen source (Advanced Life Support Group 2003).
- **Bag valve mask:** These come in three sizes: 250, 500 and 1500 millilitres. The smallest one is ineffective even at birth. The two smallest bags have a pressure limiting valve set at 4.41 kPa (45 cm H_2O) to protect the lungs from barotrauma (i.e. damage caused to tissues by a change in pressure inside and outside the body). The reservoir bag enables the delivery of oxygen concentrations up to 98%. Without the reservoir bag it is not possible to supply more than 50% oxygen (Advanced Life Support Group 2003).

Principles table 26.4 Education, preparation and initial assessment for oxygen

Principle	Rationale
1. Ensure that adequate education regarding the safe administration safety of oxygen therapy is established.	1. All staff or individuals who deliver oxygen therapy should have up-to-date and ongoing education and competency assessment in its use.
2. Oxygen should not be delivered in the vicinity of any naked flames.	2. Oxygen is an oxidising agent and strongly supports combustion (Ashurst 1995).
3. A thorough assessment should be made in order to determine the reason for the oxygen requirements.	3. To consider if alternative strategies would be appropriate, e.g. suction, repositioning.
4. Age appropriate information must be given to the child and family members must be informed of the following: • Why oxygen therapy is required • The method of delivery • The expected benefits of treatment • Possible side effects • The likely duration of treatment.	4. To gain informed consent and ensure that the child and family are aware and involved in decisions and plans for treatment. To provide reassurance and psychological support.

Principles table 26.4 (*Continued*)

Principle	Rationale
5a) Wherever possible a set of baseline observations should be obtained using a children's early warning system (CEWS) (Pearson and Duncan 2011). **b)** This should be documented appropriately on relevant trust paperwork.	**5.** To ensure that any subsequent changes in the child's condition will be noticed and communicated effectively to the clinical team. **b)** To provide effective communication meet legal requirements and guide future care.
6. A standardised communication tool such as SBARD (NHS Institute for Innovations and Improvements 2006) should be used to report any high scores.	**6.** To aid the prompt detection and concise communication of any deterioration in the child's condition.

7. Baseline observations should include the following:
  a) Respiratory rate.
  b) Use of accessory muscles.
 	
  c) Head bobbing.
 	
  d) Presence of wheeze.
  e) Presence of stridor.
 	
  f) Grunting and/or nasal flaring.
  g) Change in colour (cyanosis).
  h) Capillary refill.
  i) Level of consciousness.
	a) To allow detection of increase work of breathing.
	  b) Intercostal, subcostal or sternal recession show increased effort, particularly in children, resulting from their compliant chest walls.
	  c) Head bobbing demonstrates use of the sternomastoid muscle with each breath.
	  d) Indication of broncho-constriction, usually expiratory.
	  e) Sound during respiration when there is a partial obstruction or collapse of the trachea or larynx.
	  f) Sign of severe respiratory distress.
	  g) Indication of reduced blood oxygen levels.
	  h) To establish peripheral perfusion levels.
	  i) Hypoxia can cause drowsiness and/or agitation.

8. Use a rapid assessment score as part of neurological assessment, e.g. AVPU (Advance Life Support Group 2003): • **A**lert • responds to **V**oice • responds to **P**ain • **U**nresponsive to painful stimuli.	

Procedure guideline 26.5 **Setting up oxygen therapy**

Statement	Rationale
1. Ensure there is an adequate and working oxygen supply.	**1.** To facilitate reliable and effective treatment.
2. If wall a valve supply is being used this must be checked in advance.	**2.** To facilitate effective treatment.
3. If portable oxygen cylinders are being used, these should enable adequate oxygen provision and include back-up cylinders. Litres in cylinders/litres needed per minute = minutes of oxygen available.	**3.** To ensure a continuous and safe delivery of oxygen to the child at all times. All valves on portable oxygen cylinders must be open.
4. Give the oxygen via the approved, or tolerated, method for the child.	**4.** To ensure that the established method for the delivery of oxygen is appropriate for the individual child's needs.
5. Attach tubing from chosen method of delivery to the oxygen supply device.	

645

(*Continued*)

Procedure guideline 26.5 (*Continued*)

Statement	Rationale
6. Set up administration device to enable effective administration as per manufacturer's instructions.	
7. Check the patient's individual prescription. Initiate and maintain oxygen flow rate and concentration as prescribed (Joint Formulary Committee 2006).	**7.** Oxygen is classed as a drug and should be prescribed by law (Bell 1995). Administration of an inappropriate concentration of oxygen can have serious or even lethal consequences.
8. Oxygen should be delivered at the lowest concentration possible and for the shortest possible time (Tucker *et al* 1992).	**8.** Oxygen toxicity can occur with oxygen concentrations of 50% or higher if administered for 24–48 hours or more.
9. Assess whether the delivery system requires humidification (Jamieson *et al* 1999).	**9.** This depends on several factors, especially the method of administration, the length of time of administration and the child's requirements.
10. Determine the reason for the oxygen requirements.	**10.** To ensure that oxygen therapy is the most appropriate management. Is there adequate chest expansion? Does the child need repositioning or suction?
11. Assess the child's level of anxiety and give appropriate explanations. Be aware that the procedure may be frightening for the child.	**11.** To provide appropriate and adequate emotional support.
12. Follow the prescribed protocol for the individual child regarding acceptable oxygen saturations and prescribed oxygen therapy.	**12.** To ensure that individual prescriptions are adhered to and the child's needs are met. Each child has their own acceptable parameters.
13. All oxygen therapy administered must be documented on appropriate chart.	**13.** To provide information and effective communication.

Procedure guideline 26.6 Ongoing assessment of the child (oxygen therapy)

Statement	Rationale
1. Frequent assessment and observation should be an integral part of care, enabling the detection of changes in the child's condition.	**1.** To provide an accurate picture of the child's condition and to assess the effectiveness of the oxygen therapy. Each child will need individual assessment as to their ongoing response to oxygen therapy.
2. Monitor the child's vital signs, level of consciousness and responsiveness during the administration of oxygen.	**2.** To provide an accurate picture of the child's condition and to assess the effectiveness of the oxygen therapy.
3. Monitor the child's colour, respiratory rate and depth and signs of respiratory distress.	**3.** To be alert to early signs of a worsening condition and to enable early detection of the child's respiratory distress.
4. Assess heart rate.	**4.** Hypoxia produces tachycardia. Bradycardia can be caused by severe or prolonged hypoxia.
5. Assess skin tone, taking into account cardiac conditions and possible anaemia.	**5.** Hypoxia initially causes vasoconstriction and skin pallor. Visible cyanosis is a late sign of respiratory distress. Cyanosis could result from cyanotic cardiac disease. Profound cyanosis may not be visible in the severely anaemic child.

Procedure guideline 26.6 (*Continued*)

Statement	Rationale
6. Consider mental status and conscious level, and use a recognised system of assessment such as APVU (alert, responds to voice, responds to pain, unresponsive to stimuli).	**6.** Hypoxia can cause the child to be drowsy and/or agitated.
7. If oxygen requirements increase or the child's condition deteriorates: • Continue to monitor child • Inform the nurse in charge and medical team as necessary • Follow national guidelines for the management of the acutely unwell child (Department of Health 2006).	**7.** To ensure effective detection, reporting and management of any deterioration in the child's condition.

Principles table 26.5 **Discharge planning for children on long-term oxygen**

Principle	Rationale
1. Discharge planning should begin on admission in line with national guidelines.	**1.** To ensure a smooth transition to the home environment (Balfour-Lynn *et al* 2005b).
2. The child's community team should be contacted as soon as discharge planning is commenced.	**2.** Early planning ensures a smoother and increased coordination of the discharge process, ensuring all team members are involved.
3. The child's discharge should be planned in a consistent, systematic and collaborative manner.	**3.** Communication of information between professionals and families is vital in order to ensure the best follow-up care.
4. The clinical decision that a child will receive home oxygen is made by the consultant in charge of the child's care.	
5. Each child's management plan should include the following: • Oxygen prescription (Balfour-Lynn *et al* 2005b) • Amount of oxygen required • Sliding scale of parameters with indications of when to seek advice and from whom • Mode of delivery • Delivery system required (Department of Health 2004).	**5.** To ensure that each child has their own management plan, including guidelines for use and information relating to clinical signs and symptoms.
6. A medical decision will be required regarding whether the use of a pulse oximeter and/or apnoea alarm is appropriate for the home environment (Primhak 2003, RCN 2007).	**6.** There is limited evidence to determine whether the use of an oxygen saturation monitor improves patient care at home. Alarms are often activated by movement and can cause carers to change oxygen flow unnecessarily (RCN 2007). The American Thoracic Society supports the use of oximeters in the home because they feel it reduces the providence of hospital admissions (Myers *et al* 2002).
7. Parents/carers should understand the need for home oxygen therapy and be willing and competent to look after the child in the home environment.	**7.** Parents/carers should be confident in their abilities to care for their child in the home environment.

647

(*Continued*)

Principles table 26.5 (*Continued*)

Principle	Rationale
8. The family must be aware of the risks involved in the child having home oxygen therapy.	**8.** Oxygen is a potential source of combustion and oxygen increases the rate at which fire spreads.
9. Parents/carers must be able to assess their child's respiratory pattern, recognise respiratory distress and be able to take relevant and appropriate action.	**9.** Parents/carers must be aware of early signs of hypoxia and respiratory distress in order to reduce the risk of further deterioration in the child's condition.
10. Ensure the child on home oxygen therapy receives all relevant equipment.	**10.** To maintain quality of life and to ensure that equipment is providing desired outcomes.
11. Parents/carers should have support from the oxygen supplier with regards to equipment.	**11.** To provide ongoing equipment and support.
12. The child may receive oxygen therapy while at school if required.	**12.** To allow the child to access education.
13. The child should have open access to their nearest hospital (Balfour-Lynn *et al* 2005b).	**13.** To ensure swift intervention in an emergency.

Chest drain management

The aims of chest drainage are:

- To remove air or fluid from the pleural space or mediastinum
- To establish normal vacuum pressures within the thoracic cavity
- To enable the lungs to re-expand
- To restore normal respiration.

Conditions requiring chest drain insertion include:

- **Pneumothorax:** Air in the pleural space, which causes a vacuum or increased negative pressure, causing the lung to collapse. The air can come from the lung, trachea or oesophagus, or from external trauma. Tension pneumothorax is a life-threatening condition that develops when air is trapped in the pleural cavity under positive pressure, displacing mediastinal structures and compromising cardiopulmonary function. Promptly recognising this condition saves lives, both inside and outside the hospital. Because tension pneumothorax occurs infrequently and has potentially devastating effects, a high index of suspicion and knowledge of basic emergency thoracic decompression are important for all healthcare personnel.
- **Haemothorax:** An accumulation of blood in the pleural space, which compresses the lung. The bleeding can come from the heart, lungs, vessels or chest wall.
- **Pleural effusion:** A build up of exudate or fluid in the pleural space, often associated with pneumonia. Drainage will allow the re-expansion of the lungs, leading to return of lung function.
- **Chylothorax:** The accumulation of lymph fluid in the pleural space, which occurs after injury to or obstruction of the thoracic duct.
- **Empyema:** The multiplication of bacteria in a pleural effusion secondary to an infection or as a result of trauma (Bourke and Brewis 1998).

- Chest drains are required electively following cardiothoracic surgery to drain blood from the mediastinum to prevent the development of **cardiac tamponade**; compression of the heart, which occurs when blood or fluid builds up in the space between the myocardium (heart muscle) and the pericardium (outer covering sac of the heart).

Insertion of a chest drain should be performed under general anaesthetic or sedation and local anaesthesic infiltration (Association of Paediatric Anaesthetists of Great Britain and Ireland (APAGBI) 2008). There are a variety of chest drainage systems on the market, including a number that allow and promote easy and early mobilisation of the child. Disposable chest drain systems are self-contained, sterile, single patient use and easy to use and change, with the additional aim of optimising safety of the device. The main features include:

- A suction control chamber
- A water seal chamber/one-way valve
- Collecting chambers.

When the chest drain is inserted and connected to the drainage system it maintains a negative pressure, which is lower than the pressure within the pleural space. The pressure gradient created allows air or fluid to move from an area of high to low pressure, i.e. from the pleural or mediastinal space to the chest drainage system. To achieve this, the distal end of the chest drain is placed beneath 2 cms of water, creating a water seal, thereby allowing the movement of air or fluid (Cerfoli *et al* 2001).

The chest drain is removed when:

- The drainage is minimal
- The air leak resolves
- Fluctuations in the water seal chamber stops
- And/or a chest X-ray shows that the lung has re-expanded.

This part of the chapter includes the following sections:

- Assessment of the child pre drain insertion
- Patient preparation and staff competency

- Insertion of a chest drain
- Management of chest drains
- Complications
- Removal of a chest drain.

Procedure guideline 26.7 Assessment of the child pre drain insertion

Statement	Rationale

1. Decision making:
   If the child's airway, breathing or circulation (ABC) are suddenly and severely compromised:
 • Seek prompt medical help
 • Start basic life support
 • Alert the hospital emergency team as per local policy.
	To provide immediate emergency life support (see Chapter 27).
	   A tension pneumothorax should be excluded at this time (see below).

2a) If the child shows no immediate signs of acute deterioration, perform a respiratory assessment for the signs and symptoms of respiratory distress. These include: • Tachypnoea • Use of accessory muscles • Tracheal deviation • Restlessness • Asymmetrical chest movement • Absent or diminished breath sounds on auscultation. **b)** A chest X-ray and/or ultrasound may be performed in a non-urgent situation. **c)** Record observations. Clinical observations include: • Heart rate • Respiratory rate and effort • Blood pressure • Oxygen saturations • Colour/perfusion.	**2a, b)** To measure the extent of respiratory compromise, aid rapid diagnosis and establish appropriate treatment promptly (for more information see Chapter 1). **c)** To monitor and detect changes in the child's clinical condition. All observations should be scored using a children's early warning system (CEWS) (Pearson and Duncan 2011), and reported using a standardised communication tool such as SBARD (Situation, Background, Assessment, Recommendation, Decision), (NHS Institute for Innovations and Improvements 2006).
3. If the child is in respiratory distress consider: **a)** Use of a high flow oxygen mask. **b)** Use of an oxygen saturations monitor. **c)** Repositioning the child in bed or sitting them with their parents/carers.	**3a)** This may ease some of the respiratory distress, depending on how the child tolerates the intervention. **b)** To assist in clinical assessment of effectiveness of oxygen support. **c)** To help ease some of the respiratory distress. Children will naturally assume the position most comfortable for them and which minimises their respiratory distress.

Principles table 26.6 Child preparation and staff competency (chest drainage systems)

Health professionals caring for children with chest drainage systems should be trained and familiar with the management of chest drains and related complications and be able to provide support for the child and family.

Principle	Rationale
1. Children with chest drains must be cared for by staff who have knowledge of respiratory pathophysiology.	**1.** To provide appropriate observation, assessment and evaluation of the child's respiratory effort and cardiovascular status. To reduce the risk of complications and ensure child safety through the swift recognition of any deterioration and when to refer to the medical team.

(Continued)

Principles table 26.6 (*Continued*)

Principle	Rationale
2. Staff should be familiar with the local chest drainage system and have received training in advanced respiratory therapy, including: • Preparing a chest drainage system • Caring for a child with a chest drain and frequent complication • Removal of a chest drain.	2. To establish and maintain the required level of knowledge to care for the child and reduce the risk of complications.
3. Local clinical guidelines and training should be provided for all staff caring for these children and their families.	3. To promote teamwork, reduce the risk of adverse events and provide a framework for the audit of standards and practice.
4. Use evidence based locally agreed guidelines to maintain the patency of the chest drain.	4. The literature related to clamping, milking and stripping of chest drains is inconclusive and does not provide an agreed evidence base in adult or paediatric data sets (Parkin 2002). A Cochrane review (Wallen *et al* 2009) found that 'there are insufficient studies which compare differing methods of chest drain clearance, to support or refute the relative efficacy of the various methods in preventing cardiac tamponade. Nor can the need to manipulate chest drains be supported or refuted by results from RCTs'.
5. Adequate time must be taken to prepare the child and their family. If written information is available, this should be given to the family to read (British Thoracic Society 2008).	5. To reduce the likelihood of complications, relieve anxiety and determine the level of cooperation likely. To ensure that the family have had adequate opportunity to ask questions and understand the procedure.
6. If the child is assessed as competent they should be involved in the consent procedure and ensuing explanations and appropriate written information provided.	6. To ensure the family and child have a clear understanding of the procedure, reasons for the procedure, and the associated risks and complications.
7. A signed consent form must be completed prior to the procedure by the child's legal next of kin or the child if they have been assessed as competent to make this decision.	7. Written consent is required by law, except in an emergency situation.

Procedure guideline 26.8 Insertion of a chest drain

Statement	Rationale
1. The child's chest X-ray should be assessed prior to chest drain insertion. Ultrasound can also be used to locate small or more complex fluid distribution (Laws *et al* 2003).	1. To locate fluid or air and determine the precise site and size, and the need for insertion of chest drain.
2. Risk of haemorrhage: where possible, any coagulopathy or platelet defect should be corrected prior to chest drain insertion (Laws *et al* 2003).	2. Routine measurements of the platelet count and prothrombin time are only recommended in children with known risk factors.
3. Gather and prepare the following equipment: a) Chest drainage system and chest drain insertion pack. b) Sterile water. c) Disposable scalpel blade. d) 10 ml syringe.	3. To ensure immediate availability so that the procedure can be done smoothly and quickly in the safest environment. a) To ensure that the correct equipment is available. b) For the underwater seal drain and suction chamber. c) To make initial incision in the chest wall. d) To aspirate air or fluid to confirm correct drain position.

Procedure guideline 26.8 (*Continued*)

Statement	Rationale
e) 1 × 23G needle (blue) or 1 × 25G needle (orange).	**e)** To draw up and administer local anaesthetic.
f) Lidocaine hydrochloride 1%.	
g) Surgical sutures × 2 (2.0 silk).	**g)** To secure the chest drain in place.
h) Skin preparation as per local policy.	**h)** To cleanse the skin prior to the initial incision.
i) Transparent occlusive dressing.	**i)** To ensure an airtight drainage system that is clearly visible at all times.
j) Y connector.	**j)** For use where two or more drains are connected to the same chest drainage system.
k) Resuscitation trolley in close vicinity.	**k)** To ensure patient safety in the event of an emergency situation or if the child's condition deteriorates.
l) Surgeon's sterile gown and gloves.	**l)** To maintain sterility for the procedure and reduce the risk of infection to the child.
m) Chest clamp, one per drain site.	**m)** To prevent air entering the pleural cavity in an emergency.
n) Appropriate sized catheter drains.	**n)** For further information see below.
4. Ensure that the chest drains are of an adequate size range for the age of the child: A range of sizes of flexible, plastic, intercostal thoracic chest drain catheters exist. • 8–12 Fr for neonates • 12–16 Fr for infants • 16–24 Fr for children • 20–23 Fr for adolescents.	**4.** The actual size of chest drain catheter inserted will depend on the size of the child and what is expected to be drained, e.g. smaller sizes for air and larger sizes for blood/fluid (Laws *et al* 2003).
5. Once the chest drainage system and chest drain insertion pack has been obtained, add sterile water to the water seal to the recommended water level. 　In addition, water must be added to the suction control chamber. The level of suction is usually between 12–15 cm water (Davis *et al* 1994).	**5.** To fill the suction and underwater seal chamber, as per manufacturer's recommendations.
6. Appropriate analgesia and sedation must be given prior to the procedure. National guidelines suggest the use of either general anaesthesia or sedation, in combination with subcutaneous infiltration of buffered lidocaine (APAGBI 2008). Local pain teams or anaesthetic staff can often provide guidance.	**6.** To minimise pain and anxiety.
7. Non-pharmacological techniques such as distraction, play and non-nutritive sucking should also be employed as appropriate for the child's age and stage of development.	**7.** To maximise the use of both pharmacological and non-pharmacological interventions that may help to relieve pain and anxiety as well as the cooperation of the child.
8. Prophylactic antibiotics may be prescribed and given prior to the procedure. This is especially important if there is an underlying infective process (Balfour-Lynn *et al* 2005a).	**8.** To treat any current infective process, using the best evidence base available.
9. Preparation of chest drain site: **a)** The identity of the child should be checked. **b)** The site should be marked by the person undertaking the procedure. **c)** Ultra sound is recommended to confirm the site for chest drain insertion (Laws *et al* 2003), before and during the procedure and to check the site of other organs which could be potentially damaged.	**9.** **a)** To ensure the correct child undergoes the procedure. **b)** To ensure the correct site is used for placement. It also allows for topical local anaesthesia to be applied to the insertion site. **c)** To assess the best site for chest tube placement and to ensure the safety of child. Ultrasound is a ward based, non invasive scan, but needs suitably trained personnel to work the machine effectively.

651

(*Continued*)

Procedure guideline 26.8 (*Continued*)

Statement	Rationale
d) Position the child appropriately for the procedure.	**d)** To ensure ease of chest drain placement, reduce risk of infection and ensure the child is safe during the procedure.
e) Younger children may need assistance from family or staff to maintain the position. Care should be taken to ensure the child remains as still as possible.	**e)** To ensure the chest drain placement is accurate and does not cause the child any additional trauma.
10. Clean and prepare the skin: **a)** Clean the skin with antiseptic solution, covering a wide area at the side of insertion. **b)** The person performing the procedure will administer local anesthetic at the marked site (Laws *et al* 2003).	**10.** **a)** To minimise the risk of infection as per local trust policy. **b)** To minimise pain at the insertion site.

11. Insertion of chest drain:
    A thoracostomy is performed by the doctor inserting the chest drain. See British Thoracic Society Guidelines for details around insertion of chest drains (Laws *et al* 2003).
    Placement of the catheter is dependent on the location of the collection of fluid or air.
• Pneumothorax: the chest drain is usually inserted anterially, near the apex of the lung, in the vicinity of the 3rd or 4th intercostal space
• Haemothorax or pleural effusion; the chest drain is inserted at the level of the 7th or 8th intercostal space. More than one chest drain may be required to drain the air or fluid.
	11.
	To minimise the risk of complications. The procedure should only be performed by a professional trained and competent in chest drain insertion (Laws *et al* 2003).
	
	This is usually because air rises to the top (apex) of the lungs.
	
	This is usually because fluid collects at the base of the lungs.

Initial management of drains post insertion

1. Once the chest drain is inserted, clamp the catheter close to the chest wall until the chest tube is connected to the chest drainage system with either an underwater seal or a one-way valve.	**1.** The effective drainage of air, blood or fluid from the pleural space requires an airtight system to maintain subatmospheric intrapleural pressure. This allows re-expansion of the lung and restores haemodynamic stability by minimising mediastinal shift. The basic requirements are a suitable chest drain with minimal resistance, an underwater seal and a collection chamber. The drainage tube is submerged to a depth of 1–2 cm in a collection chamber of approximately 20 cm diameter. This ensures minimum resistance to drainage of air and maintains the underwater seal even in the face of a large inspiratory effort. The underwater seal acts as a one-way valve through which air is expelled from the pleural space and prevented from re-entering during the next inspiration.

2. Once the person undertaking the procedure is confident that the drain is in the correct position, the sutures will be tied around the tube to secure it and a purse string suture placed for future removal.
    The insertion site is then covered with a sterile dressing.
	2. To reduce the risk of accidental displacement and to assist the process when the chest drain is removed.
	    To reduce the risk of infection at the entry site as per local trust policy.

3. The chest drain system should be kept below the chest insertion site, once connected.	
4. Drainage can be allowed to occur under gravity, or suction may be applied.	**4.** Suction can be used to maintain patency of chest drain tubing or after cardiothoracic surgery (closed chest), where there is a high risk of the drain clotting off.

Procedure guideline 26.8 (*Continued*)

Statement	Rationale
5. Check water suction connection and tubing once every 12 hours.	**5.** To ensure chest tube patency and correct system operation.
6. Check the suction control source and the suction control mechanism are at the set level specified by the medical team. Normally suction control of 10–12 cm H_2O is used. The medical team must specify if a higher level of suction is required.	**6.** To ensure the correct level of suction over time.
7. Check and top up the water chamber to the required level. If it has dropped below the desired level, simply disconnect suction, and top up with sterile water and close again before reapplying suction. This should be checked once every 12 hours.	**7.** The level of the water in the suction chamber, not the suction level dictates suction provided.
8. Regulate the amount of suction at the source or adjust the device to provide for gentle continuous bubbling of the chamber.	**8.** Vigorous bubbling causes rapid evaporation, decreasing the water level and therefore the amount of suction that is exerted on the pleural space.

9. Unclamp the drain once connected to the chest drain system.
    Monitor the immediate effect of unclamping the chest drain on the child's condition.
	9. To maintain patient safety, prevent displacement of chest drain and monitor patient response.
	    To monitor air/fluid loss and observe for air entrainment (see below).

10. Observe and document the output from the chest drain system including: • Bubbling or swinging of the underwater seal • Amount of drainage per hour • Fluid appearance, e.g. blood stained, straw coloured.	**10.** To ensure patient safety and monitor any changes in the output of the chest drainage system.
11. When the child is breathing spontaneously, the water level in the water seal chamber should rise with inspiration and fall with expiration.	**11.** Negative intrapleural pressure becomes greater on inspiration and less negative on expiration.
12. If this is not happening check for the following: • Kinks in the tubing • Tubing still clamped • Child lying on and occluding the tubing • A dependent fluid-filled loop in the tubing • Lung tissue or adhesions blocking the chest drain during expiration • No air leaking from the pleural space.	**12.** To identify and rectify the problem.
13. Order a chest X-ray within 1 hour of insertion, earlier if the child's condition has not improved or deteriorates.	**13.** To confirm the correct radiological position of the chest drain.
14. Settle the child comfortably and conduct and document a full physical assessment, and observations using a children's early warning system (CEWS) (Pearson and Duncan 2011).	**14.** To determine the effect of chest drain insertion on respiratory function and the physical status of the child.
15. Give analgesia as required to ensure the child's comfort.	**15.** If the child is not comfortable it can be difficult to assess the child's condition.
16. The nurse should also be available to answer further questions the child or their family may have at this time and provide additional information as required.	**16.** The child and family will need ongoing support and information.

653

Procedure guideline 26.9 Management of chest drains

Statement	Rationale
1. Perform ongoing respiratory assessments, noting changes in breath sounds and the child's colour/perfusion. The child's chest should be observed and assessed for equal chest movement and equal air entry using auscultation.	**1.** To ensure early detection of the child's improving or worsening respiratory status with the chest drain in situ.
2. Assess ongoing vital signs, rate, regularity, depth and ease of respiration.	**2.** Baseline observations will alert the nurse to changes in the child's condition along with assessment skills with robust documentation.
3. Obtain regular pain assessment scores and administer analgesia regularly for the first 24–48 hours.	**3.** Children with chest drains may be in discomfort or pain, which may impede their respiratory effort.
4. Chest drainage system ongoing assessment Observe: **a)** Swinging in the underwater seal chamber with respiration. **b)** The presence of air bubbling. **c)** Drainage volume and description of fluid type, keep accurate fluid balance charts (see below for effects of fluid loss).	**4.** **a)** Absence of swinging in the underwater seal may indicate obstruction of the drainage system by clots or kinks, loss of sub-atmospheric pressure or complete re-expansion of the lung. **b)** Bubbling should only be seen in the underwater seal drain during expiration, as air and fluid drain from the pleural cavity. Constant bubbling indicates either an air leak in the chest drain system or a persistent broncho-pleural fistula. **c)** To monitor ongoing fluid loss from the chest drain, increase and decrease in volume or changes in type of fluid.
5. Fluid loss Blood/fluid loss greater than 5 millilitres per kilogram will require colloid replacement fluid – inform medical team. Fluid from the chest drain maybe required for: **a)** Analysis of infection. **b)** Haemoglobin levels. **c)** Presence of chyle – a milky fluid comprised of lymph drainage, which carries fat, protein and white blood cells (lymphocytes). It occurs after injury to or obstruction of the thoracic duct.	**5.** Volume of fluid loss may cause the child to become hypovolemic, causing deterioration in the child's condition. **a)** Samples may need to be taken from the drainage system using the manufacturer's directions, to allow analysis of drainage fluid. **b)** Haemoglobin and blood protein levels may need to be monitored if there is no reduction in volume of losses.
6. Do not move the collection chamber above the height of the insertion site, unless it is clamped (see below). Chest drain clamps should be available close to the child at all times, one for each chest drain inserted.	**6.** This is more important as the child becomes more mobile and their clinical condition improves.
7. Clamping a chest drain: **a)** A bubbling chest tube should not be clamped. **b)** Drainage of a large pleural effusion should be controlled with a partial clamp or intermittent unclamping. **c)** In cases of pneumothorax, clamping of the chest tube should usually be avoided.	**7.** **a)** This can result in a life-threatening emergency, tension pneumothorax. **b)** To prevent the potential complication of re-expansion pulmonary oedema. **c)** If a child with a clamped drain becomes breathless or develops subcutaneous emphysema, the drain must be immediately unclamped and medical advice sought.

Procedure guideline 26.9 (*Continued*)

Statement	Rationale
d) If a chest tube for pneumothorax is clamped, this should be under the supervision of a respiratory physician or thoracic surgeon. The child should be managed in a specialist ward with experienced nursing staff, and should not leave the ward environment (Laws *et al* 2003). **e)** Clamping of a chest drain should be avoided except to: • Prevent air entry back into the pleural space in accidental disconnection of any tubing or connections • Replace the drainage system • Locate an air leak in the chest drain system • Lift the chest drain system above the chest insertion site • Prior to chest drain removal.	
8. Check chest drain drainage tubes regularly to ensure patency as per local policy.	**8.** Fluid filled loops or occlusion may cause resistance, back pressure and build up of fluid or air, causing a deterioration in the child's clinical condition or preventing the chest drainage system working effectively. Suction should be considered if drainage tubes continually block.
9. The chest drain site should be checked regularly for security as per local policy. Check that: **a)** The holding sutures are present around chest drain insertion site. **b)** All chest drain connections are secure and air tight. **c)** Occlusive tape secures all connections and the insertion site. **d)** The chest drain tubing is supported at all times. **e)** Two chest drain clamps are available at all times. **f)** Check the chest drain insertion site and surrounding skin. • Subcutaneous emphysema (air leak into the tissues) • Signs of infection, e.g. swelling, redness at the insertion site or clinical signs in the child, e.g. pyrexia.	**9.** To reduce the risk of chest drain complications. **d)** The tubing may cause discomfort if pulled. **e)** For use in an emergency disconnection and at planned removal. **f)** Subcutaneous emphysema may develop, if air leaks into the surrounding tissues. Infection needs to be closely monitored as the chest drain breaks the skin defence barrier. Fluid within the chest maybe infected or become infected over time.
10. In the event of an accidental disconnection: • Immediately reconnect and re secure the site • Assess the child for clinical changes • Order a chest X-ray • Document the incident and report it to the medical team • Inform the family.	**10.** Accidental disconnection can cause additional air to enter the pleural space, causing respiratory compromise and clinical decompensation.
11. Maintain strict aseptic technique when handling, changing drainage system or dressing the insertion site. Document findings and events. Families may wish to be involved with this part of the clinical care.	**11.** To reduce the risk of infection (see complications section below).

655

Procedure guideline 26.9 (*Continued*)

Statement	Rationale
12. Plan and discuss patient activity, including changes in position and mobilising as appropriate. Involve a physiotherapist as early as possible and encourage the child to take deep breaths.	**12.** To encourage drainage, effective respirations and prevent the complications associated with reduced mobility. To reduce the risk of the child developing a chest infection.
13. The child with a long-term chest drain who is well enough to mobilise should be encouraged to do so. Children with chest drains can be encouraged to mobilise away from their bed area by teaching and involving family members about the safety and care aspects of the management of the chest drain. An agreed training sheet should be signed by staff and family members. Ensure chest drain clamps are with the child at all times, at least one per chest drain.	**13.** To ensure the child's safety while encouraging independence. Family members often wish to be involved, as long as they are fully supported and trained in the equipment safety. These would be used in an emergency disconnection of the tubing or chest drain.

Procedure guideline 26.10 Complications associated with chest drains

Statement	Rationale
1. Tension pneumothorax – this is an emergency situation and requires immediate action. It occurs when the intrapleural pressure exceeds atmospheric pressure throughout inspiration and expiration. Symptoms of pleural air under tension include: tachycardia, hypotension, cyanosis, neck vein engorgement, contralateral tracheal deviation. Treatment is high flow oxygen. The medical team will place a large bore cannula via the second intercostal midclavicular space. This should result in a sudden rush of air. Additional air can be aspirated out of the pleural space, until the child has stabilised.	**1.** Clinical diagnosis is usual due to the potential life-threatening nature of this event. Once the child has stabilised, chest X-ray and placement of a permanent chest tube should be considered (Laws *et al* 2003).
2. Bleeding, injured intercostal artery or other internal vessel or organ.	**2.** Bleeding can be from small vessels nicked at the time of insertion. Rarely bleeding may require surgery.
3. Pain in the chest wall, neck or shoulder.	**3.** May be caused by incorrect placement of the chest drain or kinked tubing, injury to the intercostals muscles or perforation of vessels or organs in the chest cavity.
4. Subcutaneous emphysema – this feels like crackling under the child's skin, usually around the insertion site. It can track up and down the body over time, causing the neck and face to swell, and potentially threatening compromise of the child's airway.	**4.** Subcutaneous emphysema is associated with increased morbidity and mortality (Jones *et al* 2001). This can occur if: • Drainage holes of the chest drain are outside the pleural space • The tubing is blocked or kinked • There is a airleak around the insertion site and if the dressing is not secure.
5. Monitor the child for clinical signs of infection.	**5.** Infection can occur at any time from insertion to removal. The longer the chest drain is in situ the higher the risk of infection.
6. Chest drain displacement or accidental removal.	**6.** A displaced drain or accidental chest drain removal can cause pain, internal damage or prevent active resolution of the fluid/air in the pleural space, causing a deterioration or lack of improvement in the child's condition.

Procedure guideline 26.10 (*Continued*)

Statement	Rationale
a) If the chest drain is outside the body, pinch the hole in the skin and alert the medical team.	**a)** To prevent air entering the pleural cavity.
b) Apply clean gauze and non-porous tape, while continuing to pinch.	**b)** To reduce the risk of infection and air entering into the pleural space.
c) Assess the child's respiratory status.	**c)** To note any acute changes in the child's condition.
d) A chest X-ray will be needed.	**d)** To confirm whether the chest drain needs to be replaced or manipulated by the medical team.
e) Document events in the child's notes.	**e)** To maintain good communication.
7. Blockage of the chest drain tubing or the chest catheter. **a)** A chest X-ray may be needed.	**7.** Incorrect position or intermittent blockage by clots, pus or debris can prevent ineffective drainage and be demonstrated by a lack of progress or a deterioration in the child's condition. **a)** To confirm correct chest drain placement.
8a) The medical team may need to flush the chest drain to remove any blockage and aid drainage. **b)** Any entry into the chest drain must be sterile.	**8a)** To remove any blockage preventing the chest drain functioning. **b)** To reduce the risk of introducing infection.

Procedure guideline 26.11 **Removal of a chest drain**

Statement	Rationale
1. Chest drains are assessed for removal when: • The drainage is minimal over a 24 hour period • The air leak has resolved for 24 hours (fluctuations in the water seal chamber stops) • A chest X-ray shows that the lung has re-expanded • Respiratory effort assessment and clinical observations, normal breath sounds are heard over both lungs on auscultation.	**1.** The decision to remove a chest drain is usually made by the medical team responsible for the child. In some areas such as cardiothoracic surgery, clinical pathways and guidelines are used to direct care by other healthcare professionals (e.g. nurses) if certain criteria are met.
2. Perform a clinical assessment of the child's condition.	**2.** To provide a baseline assessment for comparison with post procedure of chest drain removal.
3. Explain the procedure to child and family. The timing of both the explanation and procedure can prevent increased anxiety in the child and family.	**3.** The child will be able to cope better if properly prepared and may be able to assist. Timely preparation and good organisation will mean the child and family are not left waiting, which increases anxiety.
4. Ensure that the ward emergency equipment is available and fully checked.	**4.** To ensure the child's safety should any problems arise from the procedure.
5a) Administer appropriate analgesia as prescribed. Intravenous analgesia should be administered 15–20 minutes, and oral analgesia ¾–1 hour pre procedure. **b)** National guidelines suggest a combination of two or more of the following: • Opioids • Non steroidal anti-inflammatory drugs (NSAIDs) • Nitrous oxide (Entonox) • Sucrose or a dummy (neonates) • Psychological intervention (e.g. play specialist to provide distraction therapy appropriate to the age of the child) (APAGBI 2008).	**5a)** Removal of chest drains can be uncomfortable and a frightening experience (Bruce and Franck 2000, Bruce *et al* 2006b). **b)** Multimodal analgesia is more effective than use of a single analgesic. Even strong analgesia such as morphine and Entonox may not be effective for chest drain removal pain when given alone (Bruce *et al* 2006a).

657

(*Continued*)

Procedure guideline 26.11 (*Continued*)

Statement	Rationale
6. To remove chest drains safely, two people are required to undertake and coordinate the timing of the procedure. **a)** Parental/carer presence is also encouraged to support the child as well as working with the play specialist.	**6.** It is good practice to discuss the procedure with the person you will be undertaking it with to ensure your practice works together for safety of the child and efficiency. **a)** The safety of the child is paramount. A well prepared parent/carer can support the child through the procedure.
7. Prepare a trolley by collecting the following: **a)** Clean gloves. **b)** Skin cleansing solution. **c)** Sterile wound pack. **d)** Sterile gauze. **e)** Sterile stitch cutter. **f)** Metal clamp x1. **g)** Appropriate dressing. **h)** Sterile skin closure strips, e.g. Steristrips. **i)** Occlusive tape.	**7.** Equipment can be collected while analgesia is taking effect, or in advance of analgesia being given. **e)** To cut the anchoring suture of chest drain. **f)** To close off chest drainage tubing. **g)** To reduce infection risk. **i)** To be used if the chest drain site is not fully closed by the suture.
8. The aim is to remove the drains with no air entrapment. If apical and basal drains are to be removed, remove the basal drain first.	**8.** To reduce the risk of residual pneumothorax.
9. Position the child on the side opposite to the insertion site.	**9.** Good positioning enables quick and effective removal. The child may need assistance from family or staff to maintain this position.
10. Drains should remain on suction during removal, unless specific instructions to the contrary are given.	**10.** To promote drainage and any residual air removed at time of chest drain removal.
11. Procedure: If a purse string is present: **a)** Expose and clean the drain site(s) and unwrap the purse string from around the chest drain. **b)** Cut off the knot at the distal end of the purse string. Ask the second nurse to prepare a loose half knot. **c)** Prepare the occlusive dressing. This may be used instead of a purse string suture to close the chest drain site. Check local trust policy. **d)** Clamp any other drains not to be removed. **e)** Cut the anchoring suture and check it is not tethered anywhere else. **f)** Use one hand to withdraw the drain rapidly (within 1 second) and the forefinger and thumb of the other hand to press the skin edges of the drain site together. **g)** If the skin cannot be easily pinched, a finger should be used to press down on the site directly over the hole.	**11.** **a)** To prepare the site and release the purse string suture for use. **c)** The occlusive dressing will be firmly applied over the sterile skin closures, if the purse string is ineffective in sealing the site or the local policy is not to use purse string sutures. **d)** To prevent air entrainment while the first drain is removed. **e)** To release the drain for fast removal. **g)** To prevent air entrainment during drain removal.
12. Timing of drain removal: For spontaneously breathing and cooperative children, ask them to practice taking deep breaths in and hold, then remove the drain at or just at the beginning of expiration. For ventilated children remove on inspiration.	**12.** To increase the intrathoracic pressure, thereby reducing the risk of air from being entrained back into the pleural cavity. If a child is crying, intrathoracic pressure is elevated, which is a good time to remove the drain.

Procedure guideline 26.11 (*Continued*)

Statement	Rationale
13. As soon as the chest drain is out, the second person now ties the purse string securely, taking care to avoid puckering the skin but ensuring closure of the drain site, with a minimum of three knots.	**13.** To ensure good skin closure and future good aesthetic look of the scar site by reducing scaring and enhancing healing.
14. If the wound remains open, the wound site edges should be closed by pushing the edges together to make a seal.	**14.** To allow healing and closure of the entry site and so prevent entrainment of air in the pleural cavity.
15. Assess the drain site and leave exposed if possible.	
16. Observe the site for escaping air or gaping of the wound. If it has not been possible to tie the wound edges together, apply sterile skin closures and nonporous dressing immediately.	
17. Settle the child comfortably and take a full set of observations. See below.	
18. Clinical assessment, vital signs and report signs of: • Increased work of breathing • Tachypnoea • Asymmetrical chest movement • Absent or diminished breath sounds on auscultation • Use of accessory muscles • Tracheal deviation • Restlessness.	**18.** To observe for potential complications take a base line set of observation once the drain is removed and the child has been made comfortable.
19. Obtain chest X-ray within 1 hour, or earlier if there are physical signs of respiratory distress. In some areas such as less complex cardiothoracic surgery, clinical pathways and guidelines are used to direct care by other professionals, e.g. nurses. In some situations children after post chest drain removal will not receive a chest X-ray unless there are clinical reasons. The child will require ongoing clinical assessment to monitor their progress.	**19.** To ensure air leak has resolved and lungs re-expanded. There is a risk of a pneumothorax developing on removal of a chest drain (Pizano *et al* 2002).
20. Dispose of equipment in accordance with hospital infection control standards.	**20.** To minimise the risk of infection and danger to other children and staff.
21. Document the procedure in the child's healthcare records.	**21.** To maintain effective communication.
22. After removal, ensure the child is comfortable and continue with regular observations and respiratory assessment. Administer analgesia to keep the child comfortable after the procedure.	**22.** To minimise pain and to ensure that any clinical deterioration is noted and reported promptly (Pearson and Duncan 2011).
23. If the child is not in hospital 5–7 days after the chest drain removal they must be referred to their local GP for chest suture removal or return to the local hospital if this is the local policy.	**23.** To ensure that the sutures are removed in a safe and timely manner with minimal disruption to the child and family.

Key texts and websites

British Paediatric Respiratory Society, http://www.bprs.co.uk/.

Driver L, Nelson VS, Warschausky SA. (1997) The Ventilator Assisted Child: A practical Resource guide. San Antonio, Communication Skill Builders – a division of the Psychological Corporation

Hall JE. (2011) Text book of Medical Physiology, 12th edition. Philadelphia, Saunders Elsevier

Levein DL, Morriss FC. (1997) Essentials of Pediatric Intensive Care, 2nd edition. London, Churchill, Livingstone

Macnab A, Macrae D, Henning R. (2001) Care of the Critically Ill Child. London, Churchill Livingstone

Madden K, Khemani RG, Newth CJL. (2009) Paediatric applied respiratory physiology – the essentials. Paediatrics and Child Health, 19(6), 249–256

National Institute for Health and Clinical Excellence, NHS, published clinical guidelines. Available at http://guidance.nice.org.uk/CG/Published (last accessed 3rd August 2011)

Noyes J, (1999) Voices and Choices. Young people who use assisted ventilation. Their health and social care, and education. London, The Stationery Office

Robinson C. (1993) Managing Life with a chronic condition: the story of normalisation. Qualitative Health Research, 3(1), 6–28

Simonds AK. (2007) Non-invasive Respiratory Support, A practical handbook, 3rd edition. London, Arnold

References

Ackerman MH. (1993) The effect of saline lavage prior to suctioning. American Journal of Critical Care, 2(4), 326–330

Advanced Life Support Group (1997) Advanced Paediatric Life Support – The Practical Approach. London, BMJ Books

Advanced Life Support Group (2003) Advanced Paediatric Life Support, 3rd edition. London, BMJ Books

Advanced Paediatric Life Support Group (2005) The Practical Approach, 5th edition. London, BMJ Books

Albin RJ, Criner GJ, Thomas S, Abou-Jaoude S. (1992) Pattern of non-ICU inpatient supplemental oxygen utilization in a university hospital. Chest, 102(6), 1672–1675

Alpan G, Glick B, Peleg O, Amit Y, Eyal F. (1984) Pneumothorax due to endotracheal tube suction. American Journal of Perinatology, 1(4), 345–348

Anderson K, Chandra K. (1976) Pneumothorax secondary to perforation of sequential bronchi by suction catheters. Journal of Paediatric Surgery, 11, 687–693

Ashurst S. (1995) Oxygen therapy. British Journal of Nursing, 4(9), 508–515

Association of Paediatric Anaesthetists of Great Britain and Ireland (APAGBI) (2008) Good practice in postoperative and procedural pain management. Pediatric Anesthesia, 18(S1), 1–81

Balfour–Lynn IM, Abrahamson E, Cohen G, Hartley J, King S, Parikh D, Spencer D, Thomson AH, Urquhart D. (2005a) BTS guidelines for the management of pleural infection in children. Thorax, 60, i1–i21. Available at http://thorax.bmj.com/content/60/suppl_1/i1.full.pdf (last accessed 14th December 2011)

Balfour-Lynn IM, Primhak RA, Shaw BN (2005b) Home oxygen for children: who, how and when? Thorax, 60(1), 76–81

Bell C. (1995) Is this what the doctor ordered? Accuracy of oxygen therapy prescribed and delivered in hospital. Profesional Nurse, 10(5), 297–300

Boosfeld B, O'Toole M. 2000) Technology-dependent children: transition from hospital to home. Paediatric Nursing, 12(6), 20–22

Bourke S, Brewis R. (1998) Lecture Notes on Respiratory Medicine, 5th edition. Oxford, Blackwell

Boutros AR. (1970) Arterial blood oxygenation during and after endotracheal suctioning in the apneic patient. Anaesthesiology, 32, 114–118

British Thoracic Society (2008) Chest Drain Insertion. Available at http://www.brit-thoracic.org.uk/delivery-of-respiratory-care/interventional-procedures-chest-drain-insertion.aspx (last accessed 26th July 2011)

Brodsky L, Reidy M, Stanievich J. (1987) The effects of suction techniques on the distal tracheal mucosa in intubated low birth weight infants. International Journal of Paediatric Otorhinolaryngology, 14(1), 1–14

Bruce E, Franck L. (2000) self-administration nitrous oxide (entonox) for the management of procedural pain. Paediatric Nursing, 12(7), 15–19

Bruce E, Franck LS, Howard RF. (2006a) The efficacy of morphine and Entonox analgesia during chest drain removal in children. Pediatric Anesthesia, 16, 203–208

Bruce EA, Howard RF, Franck LS. (2006b) Chest drain removal pain and its management: A literature review. Journal of Clinical Nursing, 15, 145–154

Cerfolio RJ, Bass C, Katholi CR. (2001) Prospective randomised trial compares suction versus water seal for air leaks. Annals of Thoracic Surgery, 71(5), 1613–1617

Chandler T. (2001) Oxygen administration. Paediatric Nursing, 13(8), 37–43

Cordero L, Hone EH. (1971) Neonatal bradycardia following nasopharyngeal stimulation. Journal of Pediatrics, 78, 441–447

Czarnik RE, Stone KS, Everhart CC, Preusser BA. (1991) Differential effects of continuous versus intermittent suction on tracheal tissue. Heart and Lung, 20, 144–151

Davies P, Cheng D, Fox A, Lee L. (2002) The efficacy of noncontact oxygen delivery methods. Pediatrics, 110(5), 964–967

Davis JW, Mackenzie RC, Hoyt DB. (1994) A randomised study of algorithms for discontinuing tube thoracostomy drainage. Journal of American College of Surgery, 179(5), 553–557

Department of Health (2004) Home Oxygen Therapy Service – Service Specification, http://www.dh.gov.uk/en/Publicationsandstatistics/Publications/PublicationsPolicyAndGuidance/DH_4126268 (last accessed 25th July 2011)

Department of Health (2005) Long term ventilation. Available at http://www.dh.gov.uk/prod_consum_dh/groups/dh_digitalassets/@dh/@en/documents/digitalasset/dh_4115102.pdf (last accessed 20th July 2011)

Department of Health (2006) The Acutely Ill or Critically Sick or Injured child in the District General Hospital – A Team Approach. Available at www.dh.gov.uk/en/Publicationsandstatistics/Publications/PublicationsPolicyAndGuidance/DH_062668 (last accessed 25th July 2011)

Department of Health (DoH) (2011) High Impact Intervention Care bundle to reduce ventilation-association pneumonia. Available at http://hcai.dh.gov.uk/files/2011/03/2011-03-14-HII-Ventilator-Associated-Pneumonia-FINAL.pdf (last accessed 7th August 2011)

Dinwiddie R. (1997) Diagnosis and management of paediatric respiratory disease. London, Churchill Livingstone

Downs JB. (2003) Has oxygen administration delayed appropriate respiratory care? Fallacies regarding oxygen therapy. Respiratory Care, 48(6), 611–620

Durand M, Sangha B, Cabal LA, Hoppenbrouwers T, Hodgman JE. (1989) Cardiopulmonary and intracranial pressure changes related to endotracheal suctioning in preterm infants. Critical Care Medicine, 17, 506–510

Fox WW, Berman LS, Dinwiddie R, Shaffer TH. (1977) Tracheal extubation of the neonate at 2 to 3 cm H_2O continuous positive airways pressure. Pediatrics, 59(2), 257–261

Fulmer JD, Snider GL. (1984) American College of Chest Physicians/National Heart, Lung, and Blood Institute National Conference on Oxygen Therapy. Heart Lung, 13(5), 550562

Glass CA, Grap MJ. (1995) Ten tips for safer Suctioning. American Journal of Nursing, 9, 51–53

Gravil JH, O'Neill VJ, Stevenson RD. (1997) Audit of oxygen therapy. International Journal of Clinical Practice, 51(4), 217–218

Gray E (2000) Pain management. Nursing Standard, 14(23) 40–4

Great Ormond Street Clinical Guidelines, www.gosh.nhs.uk/clinical_information/clinical_guidelines/index.html (last accessed 3rd March 2011)

Hagler DA, Traver GA. (1994) Endotracheal saline and suction catheters: Sources of lower airway contamination. American Journal of Critical Care, 3, 444–447

Hall J E (2011) Text book of Medical Physiology (12th Edition), Saunders Elsevier, Philadelphia.

James I. (1996) Centralised paediatric intensive care beds are blocked. British Medical Journal, 312, 1476

Jardine E, O'Toole M, Paton JY, Wallis C. (1999) Current status of long term ventilation of children in the UK: questionnaire survey. British Medical Journal, 318(30), 295–299

Jardine E, Wallis C. (1998) Core guidelines for the discharge home of the child on long term assisted ventilation in the United Kingdom. Thorax, 53(9), 762–767

Jamieson E, McCall JM, Whyte LA. (1999) Clinical Nursing Practices. London, Churchill Livingstone

Jeffrey AA, Ray S, Douglas NJ. (1989) Accuracy of inpatient oxygen administration. Thorax, 44(12), 1036–1037

Jefferies A, Turley A. (1999) Respiratory System. London, Mosby

Joint Formulary Committee (2006) British National Formulary. London, British Medical Association and Royal Pharmaceutical Society of Great Britain

Jones PM, Hewer RD, Wolfenden HD, Thomas PS. (2001) Subcutaneous emphysema associated with chest tube drainage. Respirology, 6(2), 87–89

Jung RC, Gottlieb LS. (1976) Comparison of tracheobronchial suction catheters in humans. Chest, 69, 179–181

Kbar FA, Campbell IA. (2006) Oxygen therapy in hospitalized patients: the impact of local guidelines. Journal of Evaluation and Clinical Practice, 12(1), 31–36

Kerem E, Yatsiv I, Goitein KJ. (1990) Effect of endotracheal suctioning on arterial blood gases in children. Intensive Care Medicine, 16, 95–99

Kleiber C, Krutzfield N, Rose EF. (1988) Acute histological changes in tracheobronchial tree associated with difference suction catheter insertion techniques. Heart and Lung, 17, 10–14

Kor AC, Lim TK. (2000) Audit of oxygen therapy in acute general medical wards following an educational programme. Annals of Academy of Medicine, Singapore, 29(2), 177–181

Levein D L, Morriss F C (1997) Essentials of Pediatric Intensive Care (2nd Edition) Churchill, Livingstone, London.

Kuzenski B. (1978) Effect of negative pressure in tracheobronchial trauma. Nursing Research, 27, 260

Laws D, Neville E, Duffy J. (2003) BTS guidelines for insertion of a chest drain. Thorax, 58(suppl 11), 53–59

Link WJ, Spaeth EE, Wahle WM. et al (1976) The influence of suction catheter tip design on tracheobronchial trauma and fluid aspiration efficiency. Anesthetic Analogues, 55, 290–297

Macnab A, Macrae D, Henning R (2001) Care of the critically ill child, Churchill Livingstone, London.

Madden K, Khemani R G, Newth C J L (2009) Paediatric Applied Respiratory Physiology – the essentials, Paediatrics and Child Health, 19(6): 249–256

Mallet J, Bailey C. (1996) The Royal Marsden NHS Trust Manual of Clinical Nursing Procedures, 4th edition. London, Blackwell Science

Margolan H, Fraser J, Lenton S. (2004) Parental experience of services when their child requires long term ventilation. Implications for commissioning and providing services. Child Care Health and Development, 30(3), 257–264

Moules T, Ramsey J. (1998) The Textbook of Children's Nursing. Cheltenham, Stanley Thornes

Myers TR, American Association for Respiratory Care (AARC) (2002) AARC Clinical Practice Guideline: selection of an oxygen delivery device for neonatal and pediatric patients–2002 revision and update. Respiratory Care, 47(6), 707–716

Nagaraj HS, Shott R, Fellows R, Yacoub U. (1980) Recurrent lobar atelectasis due to acquired bronchial stenosis in neonates. Journal of Pediatric Surgery, 15, 411–415

Naigow D, Powaser MM. (1977) The effect of different endotracheal suction procedures on arterial blood gases in a controlled experimental model. Heart and Lung, 6, 808–816

National Guideline Clearing House (2006) Complete Summary: Oxygen Therapy for adults in an acute care facility: 2002 revision and update. Available at www.guideline.gov/summary/summary.aspx?ss=15anddoc_id=3248andnbr=2474 (last accessed 15th May 2008)

NHS Institute for Innovations and Improvements (2006) www.institute.nhs.uk/safer_care/safer_care/Situation_Background_Assessment_Recommendation.html (last accessed 18th July 2011)

Noyes J. (2000) 'Ventilator-dependent' children who spend prolonged periods of time in intensive care units when they no longer have a medical need of want to be there. Journal of Clinical Nursing, 9(5), 774–783

Parkin C. (2002) A retrospective audit of chest drain practice in a specialist cardiothoracic centre and concurrent review of chest drain literature. Nursing in Critical Care, 7(1), 30–36

Pearson G, Duncan H. (2011) Early warning systems for identifying sick children. Paediatrics and Child Health, 21(5), 230–233

Perlman JM, Volpe JJ. (1983) Suctioning in the preterm infant: effects on cerebral blood flow velocity, intracranial pressure and arterial blood pressure. Pediatrics, 72, 329–334

Pickering E, Bridge HS, Nolan J, Stoddart PA (2002) Double-blind, placebo-controlled analgesia study of ibrufen or refecoxib in combination with paracetamol for tonsillectomy in children. British Journal of Anaesthesia, 88(1) 72–77

Pizano LR, Houghton DE, Cohen SM. (2002) When should a chest radiograph be obtained after chest tube removal in mechanically ventilated patients? A prospective study. Journal of Trauma, 53(6), 1073–1077

Prasad SA, Hussey J. (eds) (1995) Paediatric Respiratory Care. London, Chapman & Hall

Primhak RA. (2003) Discharge and aftercare in chronic lung disease of the newborn. Seminars in Neonatology, 8(2), 117–126

Rindfleisch S, Tyler M. (1981) The effects of duration of endotracheal suctioning on arterial oxygenation in anaesthetised dogs. American Review of Respiratory Disease, 123, 1

Royal College of Nursing (RCN) (2007) Standards for assessing, measuring and monitoring vital signs in infants, children and young people. Available at http://www.rcn.org.uk/__data/assets/pdf_file/0004/114484/003196.pdf (last accessed 3rd August 2011)

Royal Pharmaceutical Society of Great Britain (2005) British National Formulary for Children. London, BNJ

Runton N. (1992) Suctioning artificial airways in children: appropriate technique. Pediatric Nursing, 2, 115–118

Sackner MA, Landa JF, Greeneltch N, Robinson MJ. (1973) Pathogenesis and prevention of tracheobronchial damage with suction procedures. Chest, 64, 284–290

Schmelz J (1999) Effects of position of chest drainage tube on volume drained and pressure. American J Critical Care, 8(5): 319–23

Shim C, Fernandez R, Fine N, Williams H. (1969) Cardiac arrhythmias resulting from tracheal suctioning. American International Medicine, 71, 1149–1153

Simbruner G, Coradello H, Fodor M, Havelec L, Lubec G, Pollak A. (1981) Effect of tracheal suction on oxygenation, circulation and lung mechanics in newborn infants. Archives of Disease in Childhood, 56, 326–330

Simonds AK. (ed.) (2007) Non-invasive Respiratory Support, a practical handbook, 3rd edition. London, Arnold

Small D, Duha A, Wieskopf B, Dajczman E, Laporta D, Kreisman H, Wolkove N, Frank H. (1992) Uses and misuses of oxygen in hospitalized patients. American Journal of Medicine, 92(6), 591–595

661

Staveski SL, Avery S, Rosenthal DN, Roth SJ, Wright GE. (2011) Implementation of a comprehensive interdisciplinary care coordinator of infants and young children on Berlin Heart ventricular assist. Journal of Cardiovascular Nursing, 26(3), 231–238

Sumner E. (1990) Artificial ventilation of children In Dinwiddie R. (ed.) The Diagnosis and Management of Paediatric Respiratory Care. London, Churchill Livingstone

Tolles CL, Stone KS. (1990) National survey of neonatal endotracheal suctioning practices. Neonatal Network, 9, 7–14

Tucker SM, Canobbia MM, Paquette EV, Wells MF. (1992) Patient Care Standards, 5th edition. New York, Mosby Year Book

Vaughan RS, Menke JA, Giacoia GP. (1978) Pneumothorax: a complication of endotracheal tube suction. Journal of Pediatrics, 92, 633–634

Wallen M, Morrison AL, Gillies D, O'Riordan E, Bridge C, Stoddart F. (2009) Mediastinal chest drain clearance for cardiac surgery. Cochrane Database Systematic Review (2) cd003042

Walsh JM, Vanderwarf C, Hoscheit D, Fahey PJ. (1989) Unsuspected hemodynamic alterations during endotracheal suction. Chest, 95(1), 162–165

Winston SJ, Gravelyn TR, Sitrin RG. (1987) Prevention of bradycardic responses to endotracheal suctioning by prior administration of nebulized atropine. Critical Care Medicine, 15, 1009–1011

Woodhams K. (1996) The respiratory system. In McQuaid L, Huband S, Parker E. (eds) Children's Nursing. New York, Churchill Livingstone

Young CS. (1984) Recommended guidelines for suction. Physiotherapy, 70, 106–108

662

Chapter 27

Resuscitation practices

Chapter contents

Procedure guidelines

The Great Ormond Street Hospital Manual of Children's Nursing Practices, First Edition. Edited by Susan Macqueen, Elizabeth Anne Bruce, Faith Gibson.
© 2012 Great Ormond Street Hospital for Children NHS Foundation Trust. Published 2012 by Blackwell Publishing Ltd.

Introduction

Cardiorespiratory resuscitation is a broad concept encompassing many interventions designed to improve or support the respiratory and/or circulatory systems. It is not merely the 'restoration' of a person's vital signs.

The age definitions used in paediatric resuscitation are:

- Newborn – a baby from birth through the first few hours post-delivery (i.e. until the physiological adaptation to extra-uterine life has occurred)
- Neonate – a baby from birth to 28 days old (irrespective of degree of prematurity)
- Infant – a baby from birth until the 1st birthday
- Child – from the 1st birthday until puberty.

The differences between resuscitation of an adult and a child are largely based on differing aetiology. In adults, primary cardiac arrest is more common whereas children usually suffer from secondary cardiac arrest as a result of hypoxia. The onset of puberty (i.e. the physiological end of childhood) would seem the most logical point for the upper age limit to use the paediatric guidelines. It has the advantage of being simple to determine in contrast to an absolute age limit. However, it is clearly both inappropriate and unnecessary to formally establish the onset of puberty; if the rescuer believes the victim to be a child then they should use the paediatric guidelines. If a misjudgement is made, and the victim is actually a young adult, little harm will ensue as studies have shown that the paediatric (i.e. asphyxial) pattern of arrest continues into early adulthood (Biarent *et al* 2010, Resuscitation Council (UK) 2010).

Despite the many advances in medical knowledge and technology, the outcome from paediatric cardiac arrest remains very poor (Eisenberg *et al* 1983, Herlitz *et al* 2005, Lopez-Herce *et al* 2005, O'Rourke 1986, Young and Seidel 1999). Even for those children who do have a return of spontaneous circulation (ROSC), the costs are high, as many will suffer severe neurological sequelae (Ronco *et al* 1995, Schindler *et al* 1996).

A child resuscitated from an out-of-hospital secondary cardiorespiratory arrest has an expected survival of 6–12%, with less than 5% surviving neurologically intact. This is in comparison to a child in secondary cardiorespiratory arrest in hospital, who has a 27% chance of surviving to discharge.

For children who suffer from respiratory arrest but still have cardiac output, there is a much better chance (50–70%) of good quality, long-term survival (Resuscitation Council (UK) 2011a). It is therefore essential that seriously ill children are identified and appropriately managed as early as possible.

However, there will always be a small group of children in whom cardiac arrest cannot be predicted and/or prevented. For them, early Basic Life Support (BLS), rapid activation of appropriate emergency medical services (EMS) and prompt effective advanced life support (ALS) are all vital in order to minimise morbidity and mortality (Hickey *et al* 1995, Kyriacou *et al* 1994).

Aetiology of cardiorespiratory arrest

Unlike adults, the aetiology of paediatric cardiorespiratory arrest is rarely a primary cardiac event, but is secondary to hypoxia (Young and Seidel 1999). In the majority of children, this hypoxia

is the result of respiratory failure. It is generally caused by underlying respiratory pathology (e.g. asthma, infection, foreign bodies) or it may be from a neurological problem (e.g. convulsions, raised intracranial pressure) (Gausche *et al* 1989).

Regardless of the primary cause, the resultant hypoxia and acidosis lead to destruction and death of the cells in every body tissue, and in particular, those of the brain, kidneys and liver. Once the myocardial tissue is also affected, cardiac arrest will ensue.

In some children, the primary problem may be circulatory in origin (e.g. loss or maldistribution of their circulating volume). The resultant inadequate delivery of oxygen and other nutrients to body tissues by the depleted circulating volume causes tissue hypoxia and acidosis, which again ultimately leads to cardiac arrest.

The tried and tested approach to all ill or injured children should be based on ABCDE:

- **A**irway (with cervical spine immobilisation if head/neck trauma is suspected)
- **B**reathing
- **C**irculation
- **D**isability
- **E**xposure

(RCUK 2011b).

Airway management

There are a number of anatomical and physiological features that not only pre-dispose infants and small children to hypoxia, but also necessitate specific management strategies.

The anatomical features include:

- A relatively large tongue
- 'U'-shaped epiglottis (which protrudes into the pharynx)
- Relatively high position of the larynx
- Short and concave vocal cords
- Narrow cricoid ring
- Upper airway easily obstructed by flexion or hyperextension of head and neck
- Preferential nasal breathers until approximately 6 months of age (patent nares and nasopharynx essential for adequate air flow)
- Small narrow airways (easily obstructed by swollen lymph tissue or secretions)
- Poorly developed lower airways (readily occluded by active constriction, e.g. oedema)
- Congenital abnormalities, e.g. vascular ring, tracheomalacia or tumours (resulting in extrinsic obstruction) (Advanced Life Support Group 2011, Resuscitation Council (UK) 2011b).

Airway obstruction results in increased airway resistance. Even a minor reduction in the already small diameter of the paediatric airway, can result in a large loss of the cross-sectional area; just 1 millimetre circumferential oedema at the level of the cricoid ring will produce a 50–75% reduction in the airway's diameter.

The degree of airway resistance is a primary factor in how infants and small children maintain adequate minute ventilation. With limited tidal volumes, sufficient minute ventilation is achieved by higher respiratory rates (Crone 1983):

- Horizontal placement of ribs means that elevation of them does not significantly increase intrathoracic volume.
- Diaphragm placement is also more horizontal and contraction tends to draw the lower ribs inwards.
- Immaturity of intercostal and accessory muscles and rib cartilage results in a very compliant thorax and contributes to the paradoxical movements (sternal and intercostal retractions) seen during active inspiration.

As tidal volume is very dependent on diaphragmatic functioning, any impedance from above (e.g. pulmonary hyperinflation in asthma) or below (e.g. gastric distension) seriously compromises respiration, as the chest wall cannot compensate.

The main physiological features that predispose children to hypoxia are:

- High metabolic rate and oxygen consumption (6–8 ml/kg/min in children: 3–4 ml/kg/min in adults)
- Low resting lung volumes resulting in limited respiratory reserves.

Respiratory function may also be compromised by:

- CNS depression (coma/seizures, cranial trauma, metabolic disturbances, medications)

- Disease process (bronchospasm, atelectasis)
- Artificial airways (accumulated secretions)
- Inflammatory process (anaphylaxis, croup, post-surgery)
- Foreign bodies
- Dehydration (viscous secretions).

Basic airway management techniques

Principles table 27.1 Suction

Principle	Rationale
1. Children with compromised airways frequently require suction to clear their upper airways of secretions and prevent aspiration (for further information see Chapter 26 on Respiratory Care).	1. Reduced conscious level and excessive secretions are common in compromised children.

Procedure guideline 27.1 Head positioning (airway management)

Statement	Rationale
1a) Children who have respiratory distress (increased effort of breathing) but are alert, will usually assume a position of optimal airway patency themselves.	1a) The child will naturally maximise their own airway.
b) They should be supported in this position of choice, e.g. with pillows or in a carer's arms.	b) To provide comfort and keep the child calm, thus minimising oxygen consumption.
c) Placing the child in a supine position should be avoided.	c) This can potentiate airway obstruction (e.g. in epiglottitis).
d) The child should be monitored closely.	d) To rapidly initiate interventions if condition deteriorates.
e) If the child's conscious level is reduced airway patency must be secured.	e) To prevent hypoxia.
2a) There are two basic head positioning manoeuvres that can be used to achieve a patent airway: head tilt/chin lift or jaw thrust.	2a) Head positioning can be safely and rapidly performed with minimal rescuer training.
b) The vast majority of children will require no airway adjuncts to secure a patent airway.	

Head tilt/chin lift

3a) With the child in a supine position, stand at one side of them.
    The rescuer's hand nearest the child's head should be placed on the forehead. Gentle downwards pressure is applied to tilt the head backwards.
	3a) To facilitate manoeuvre.
	    To obtain functional alignment of the airway.

b) The desired head position depends primarily on age, but abnormalities or injury may necessitate modifications.	b) Extension of the head and neck in infants results in airway occlusion due to kinking of their immature tracheal cartilage. As they grow, the cartilage rings mature and the airway lengthens, necessitating varying degrees of extension to achieve airway patency.

665

(Continued)

Procedure guideline 27.1 (*Continued*)

Statement	Rationale
4. In general, infants should be placed in a neutral head position (the nares pointing at the ceiling) and the child should be in a slightly more extended ('sniffing') head position.	
5. The thumb and/or fingers of the other hand should be placed on the chin and if necessary, along the lower jaw. Pressing only on bony parts, the chin should be gently lifted upwards.	**5.** To lift the lower jaw forwards, which displaces the tongue and mandibular block of tissue away from the posterior pharyngeal wall.
6. Care must be taken to avoid pressing on the soft tissues under the chin.	**6.** To prevent airway occlusion from finger pressure on the tracheal rings.

Jaw thrust

Statement	Rationale
7a) This is the manoeuvre of choice if there is any suspicion of cervical spine injury. It is also the recommended method when airway adjuncts or ventilatory devices are to be utilised **b)** With the child in a supine position, stand behind them and place a hand on each side of the child's face. **c)** Depending on the child's size, place one or two fingers from both hands under the angles of the lower jaw and gently lift it upwards.	**7a)** Minimises risk of exacerbating injury. Facilitates easier use of airway and ventilatory equipment and allows for more access to the child by other rescuers. **b)** To facilitate manoeuvre. **c)** To displace the mandibular block of tissue away from the posterior pharyngeal wall.
8. If this manoeuvre is being utilised where there is suspected spinal injury, the rescuer should position themselves with their elbows resting on the surface that the child is laid on.	**8.** To maximise control over immobilising the child's spine should they regain consciousness and attempt to move.
9. Whichever head positioning method is used to open the airway, ABC should be frequently reassessed.	**9.** To rapidly detect changes in condition and initiate appropriate interventions.

Procedure guideline 27.2 Pharyngeal airways

Statement	Rationale
1. If airway patency is difficult to maintain despite optimal head positioning, a pharyngeal airway may be inserted. These are available for oral or nasal insertion.	**1.** To minimise potential for airway obstruction related to the tongue and mandibular block of tissue.

Choice of pharyngeal airway

Statement	Rationale
2a) Oropharyngeal (Guedel) airways should only be used in unconscious children except in very specific situations (e.g. initial management of neonates with bilateral choanal atresia). **b)** Nasopharyngeal airways are generally well tolerated even by conscious children. However, they are contraindicated where basal skull fracture is suspected or in some cases of nasal abnormality.	**2a)** Presence of a gag reflex means that an oral airway is unlikely to be tolerated and may induce vomiting with aspiration risk. **b)** They do not interfere with intact reflexes or activities such as suckling. There is the potential to penetrate cerebral tissue. May cause significant haemorrhage of the vascular nasal bed.

Procedure guideline 27.2 (*Continued*)

Statement	Rationale
Sizing pharyngeal airways	
Select the appropriate size of:	
3. Oral airway, by measuring the length against the side of the child's face. The distance to be determined is from the centre of the incisors (or where they would be) to the angle of the mandible.	**3, 4.** Too small an airway will be ineffective, while one that is too large may cause laryngospasm. Additionally, incorrect sizes can cause trauma and may result in worsened airway obstruction.
4. Nasal airway, by measuring the distance from the tip of the child's nose to the tragus of their ear. An appropriate diameter is one that fits just inside the nostril without causing it sustained blanching.	
Insertion of oropharyngeal airways	
5a) Open the airway using jaw thrust manoeuvre and support the mouth in an open position.	**5a)** To adequately visualise the mouth for placement of the airway.
b) If necessary, use a laryngoscope blade to depress the tongue gently and gently insert the airway as it will sit in situ (i.e. concave side down).	**b)** To prevent tongue being pushed back into pharynx. To prevent trauma to palate and ensure correct placement.
c) In older children, it is appropriate to use the standard 'adult' technique, i.e. the airway is inserted 'upside down' (concave side up) until it passes the soft palate. It is then rotated so that the natural curve follows that of the tongue and pharynx.	**c)** The risk of trauma while still present, is much less than in infants and small children.
Insertion of nasopharyngeal airways	
6a) Lubricate the airway with a water-soluble lubricant.	**6a)** To facilitate insertion. To minimise discomfort for child.
b) If a commercially produced nasopharyngeal airway is to be used, insert a large safety pin through the flange.	**b)** To ensure the airway is not inhaled or inserted too far.
c) If a shortened tracheal tube is to be used, an appropriate connector must be secured to the end of the tube.	**c)** To ensure the airway is not inhaled or inserted too far. This also helps secure it appropriately, and facilitates the application of CPAP (continuous positive airway pressure) if required.
7a) Insert the tip of the airway into the nostril and gently direct it posteriorly (not upwards) along the nasal floor.	**7a)** To minimise potential for trauma.
b) Gently progress the airway past the turbinates with a slight rotating movement until a 'give' is felt. Continue to gently insert the airway until the flange rests at the nostril.	**b)** The loss of resistance indicates that the airway has entered the pharynx. To achieve correct placement.
c) If difficulty is experienced inserting the airway, it should be removed and consideration given to using the other nostril or a smaller diameter of airway.	**c)** To minimise trauma.
8. Whichever pharyngeal airway route is used, observe the child for any signs of trauma to the oral or nasal cavity.	**8.** Difficulty in placement of the airway can lead to significant bleeding from mucous membranes or damage to teeth. Pressure ulceration can develop with improper placement or prolonged usage (McCrory and Downs 1984).
9. Reassess the child's ABC frequently.	**9.** Insertion of a pharyngeal airway should improve the child's condition. If it does not, its use should be reassessed.
10. Continue with clinical assessment and further interventions as appropriate.	**10.** To minimise the risk of morbidity and mortality.

Recovery position

The unresponsive child who is breathing spontaneously with an adequate circulation, should be placed in a safe, side-lying position unless contraindicated (e.g. suspected spinal injury). The purpose of this is to ensure that:

- The tongue does not fall back and obstruct the airway.
- The risk of aspiration of stomach contents is reduced.

There is no universally accepted 'recovery' position, but the general principles are based on ensuring that the child:

- Is in as near a true lateral position as possible
- Has a patent airway maintained
- Can be easily observed and monitored
- Is stable and cannot roll over
- Can freely drain secretions/vomit from their mouth
- Has no pressure on their chest that may impede breathing
- Can be easily turned into a supine position for BLS if indicated.

The following is a description of one method of placing a child in a recovery position.

Procedure guideline 27.3 Placing child in a recovery position

Statement	Rationale
1a) Rescuer should kneel/stand at one side of the child. **b)** Straighten out the child's legs and arms. **c)** Remove any spectacles and sharp/bulky objects (e.g. large hairslides, items in their pockets, etc).	**1a)** To facilitate ease of positioning. **b)** To facilitate turning of child. **c)** To prevent trauma when they are turned on to their side.
2. Loosen any clothing around the child's neck.	**2.** To avoid airway constriction.
3. Extend the child's arm nearest to the rescuer out to their side at an angle of approximately 30°.	**3.** To minimise risk of trauma to child's limb during the manoeuvre.
4. Bring the child's opposite arm across their body towards the rescuer, and hold it against the cheek on the rescuer's side.	**4.** To facilitate turning of child.
5a) With their other hand, the rescuer should bend up the child's farthest leg at the knee. **b)** Pressing against the child's knee, they should be gently rolled over towards the rescuer.	**5a)** To facilitate turning the child safely. **b)** To minimise exertion required by the rescuer while placing child on their side.
6. The hand that was placed against the child's cheek previously (and is now underneath it) should be checked.	**6.** To ensure that it is not causing undue pressure on the face.
7. The child's head can then be positioned slightly backwards if necessary.	**7.** To ensure airway remains patent.
8. A rolled up towel or blanket may need to be placed at the back of a small child or infant.	**8.** To prevent them rolling on to their backs and potentially occluding their airway.
9. The child's breathing and circulation should be reassessed frequently while awaiting further assistance as indicated.	**9.** The child with a decreased conscious level is at increased risk of airway obstruction due to accumulated secretions or aspiration. To rapidly detect any deterioration necessitating turning the child in to a supine position for thorough ABC assessment.
10. If they are to be kept in a recovery position for any longer than 30 minutes, the infant/child should be turned on to their other side.	**10.** To minimise potential for pressure injuries or nerve damage.

Advanced airway and breathing management

In a respiratory or cardiac arrest situation, oxygen should be administered at the highest concentration and as soon as pos-sible; concerns about its potential toxicity should never prevent its use in initial resuscitation.

The equipment usually employed in paediatric resuscitation is a self-inflating bag-mask device with high flow oxygen and a reservoir bag attached. Without a reservoir bag attached, it is almost impossible to provide >50% oxygen concentration (ALSG 2011). With a reservoir in situ and adequate flow of oxygen, up to 98% is achievable.

Ideally the self-inflating bag-mask (B-M) device should have a pressure-limiting (or 'pop off') valve incorporated in its design. This is to prevent inadvertent delivery of excessive inflation pressures, which could cause significant barotrauma to the child's lungs.

Gastric tubes

When children have respiratory distress, they tend to swallow large amounts of air that distends the stomach and makes them prone to vomiting. The use of a B-M device compounds this, as some oxygen tends to be forced into the stomach. This can cause significant vagal stimulation with potential risk of aspiration. Additionally diaphragmatic splinting makes ventilation difficult. It is therefore important that a gastric tube is placed early to deflate the stomach (Berg *et al* 1998).

Laryngeal mask airways

The laryngeal mask airway (LMA) is widely used in adult resuscitation. It has also gained some favour in the field of newborn resuscitation. While LMAs are widely used for paediatric anaesthesia purposes they are not ideal for routine usage in resuscitation of children, as they are supraglottic devices which do not prevent the lower airway from gastric aspiration. However, they should be readily available as someone proficient in their use may find them life saving if dealing with a child with a difficult airway problem in whom adequate ventilation cannot be achieved via B-M or tracheal intubation.

Tracheal tubes

The placement of a tracheal tube is more usually undertaken as a planned urgent procedure rather than an emergency one nowadays. This is because of the improved early recognition of seriously ill children. However, when cardiorespiratory arrest occurs in a non-intubated child, they should ideally be stabilised (or at least as well oxygenated as possible) by other non-invasive means before placement of a tracheal tube is considered. Endotracheal intubation is a technically difficult procedure in children and not without complications (Gausche *et al* 2000). It should therefore be undertaken by someone competent in the procedure and only considered when (Kramer-Johansen 2006):

- B-M ventilation fails to be effective
- The airway is insecure
- Ongoing ventilatory support is anticipated.

When an infant/child is unable to breathe adequately, or is in cardiorespiratory arrest, artificial ventilation must be urgently provided.

Procedure guideline 27.4 **Self-inflating bag-mask ventilation**

Statement	Rationale
Selection of equipment	

1. A correctly sized facemask.
  a) The required properties of the mask include:
    • Transparency
    • Cover the mouth and nose
    • Avoid pressure on the eyes
    • Have a low dead space.
  b) If the mask has an inflatable rim, a check should be made to ensure this is adequately inflated.
	1.
	  a) To facilitate optimal ventilation:
	    • Observation of colour and detection of vomit
	    • Create a good seal
	    • Prevent trauma and vagal stimulation
	    • Avoid CO_2 retention.
	  b) To ensure adequate seal.

2. Appropriate size of self-inflating bag.
  a) These generally come in 3 sizes – 250 ml, 450–500 ml and 1600–2000 ml. The smallest was designed for newborns but is generally considered ineffective as adequate tidal volumes may not be delivered.
  b) Either the middle or largest sizes can be used for children; however, not all manufacturers currently incorporate pressure limiting devices into the large bags, which make them potentially less safe for use in infants and young children. The larger size is generally required in older children (above 20–30 kg) but individual responses need to be considered.
	2.
	  a) This is due to the inability to deliver prolonged inspiratory times required to inflate newborn lungs with it.
	
	  b) This is designed to 'blow off' at a predetermined limit (approximately 30–40 cm H_2O pressure) thus minimising the risk of barotrauma to the lungs.

669

(Continued)

Procedure guideline 27.4 (*Continued*)

Statement	Rationale
3. Reservoir bag.	**3, 4.** To ensure the highest possible concentration of oxygen is administered.
4. Continuous supply of oxygen.	

Checking self-inflating bag-mask device

Statement	Rationale
1. The self-inflating bag should be checked for any visible defects (missing or faulty components).	**1.** To ensure safe functioning.
2. The bag should be squeezed with one hand, with the free hand held near the outlet (inspiratory) valve.	**2.** To ensure that air is felt on the free hand indicating that it has been expelled through the valve.
3. The bag should be squeezed again with one hand while the free hand is held against the inspiratory valve.	**3.** To check that the pressure limiting valve works (i.e. that excess air is vented through it).
4. While squeezing the bag again, the operator should use the thumb of their free hand to ensure that the pressure limiting valve can be depressed.	**4.** There is a metal spring in some of these valves which can rust and become ineffective (e.g. if the bag has been autoclaved).
5. The oxygen flow should be attached and turned on to check that the reservoir bag inflates.	**5.** To detect any leaks or defects in the system that will reduce the oxygen concentration that can be delivered.
6. Attach the appropriate face mask to the bag device.	**6.** To ensure the device is ready for use.
7. Set the oxygen flow meter to an appropriate level (approx 10 litres/minute for 500 ml paediatric bag and 15 litres/minute for large adult bag).	**7a)** It should be turned to as high a flow as possible to maintain a high concentration in the reservoir bag. **b)** The oxygen tubing can blow off the flow meter if set too high.

Self-inflating bag-mask ventilation technique

Statement	Rationale
1. The child's airway should be opened by a jaw thrust manoeuvre (see above).	**1.** To maintain airway patency. This places rescuer in optimal position for using airway adjuncts and ventilatory devices.
2. Place the correctly sized facemask on the child's face.	**2.** In preparation for ventilation.
3. Apply gentle downwards pressure to the mask, while gently lifting the child's mandible upwards into the mask by the continued application of jaw thrust.	**3.** To ensure a good seal and provide an adequate interface between child and ventilation device. To maintain airway patency.
4. In infants this is achieved by using the thumb and forefinger of one hand positioned in a C-shape to depress on the top of the mask. The remaining fingers of that hand perform the jaw thrust. The other hand is then used to gently squeeze the bag.	**4.** Ensures a good seal and prevents pressure on soft tissues under the chin.
5. In small children, the same technique is often possible. However, if there are two rescuers available, or it is an older child, one rescuer maintains the mask seal and jaw thrust with two hands, while the other squeezes the bag.	**5.** This technique is the preferred one for any child over 1 year of age as it can be difficult to maintain airway patency and perform ventilation single-handed.
6. The self-inflating bag should be gently squeezed until chest rise is observed.	**6.** To ensure oxygenation.
7. If no chest rise is seen, the airway position and facemask seal must be rechecked and corrected as necessary.	

Procedure guideline 27.4 (*Continued*)

Statement	Rationale
8. If there is still no chest movement achieved despite appropriate jaw thrust and a good facemask seal the reason why must be sought. If necessary, BLS techniques should be attempted until the problem is rectified.	**8.** To minimise hypoxia.
9. The lack of chest movement may be related to faulty equipment necessitating repair/replacement of the device.	**9.** An undetected defect or a disconnection of device.
10. The child's underlying clinical condition may also be the cause and this must be considered, e.g. **a)** Airway obstruction due to a foreign body (FB) or intense swelling (e.g. in epiglottitis). **b)** 'Stiff' lungs due to underlying respiratory pathology (e.g. prematurity or asthma) may require additional inflation pressure to be administered by over-riding of the pressure-limiting-valve. This should be performed with caution and for short periods only.	**10a and b)** A foreign body may completely obstruct the airway and require other airway and ventilation techniques to be employed. This may also be the same in epiglottitis, however in both of these scenarios, the following technique may also be effective: • Depressing the pressure-limiting valve during delivery of the breath, higher airway pressures are generated and thus may result in chest rise. To minimise the potential for trauma (e.g. pneumothorax).
11. The rate of ventilation is generally 15–30 breaths/minute but is dependent on the age of the child..	**11.** Physiologically, younger children have higher respiratory rates.

Circulation management

When an infant/child is unable to maintain an adequate circulation or is in cardiorespiratory arrest, it is essential that interventions are rapidly initiated. This may include the delivery of chest compressions, management of cardiac arrhythmias, and most likely attaining vascular access.

In a clinical emergency situation, it is imperative to gain access to the circulation for the delivery of medications and possibly fluids. The ideal is access via a central vein to facilitate rapid onset of action of medications. As this can be a relatively time-consuming and skilled procedure, the route of choice in an obtunded or arrested child without existing established central access, is the intraosseous route (McCarthy *et al* 2003).

Intraosseous access

The concept of using the medullary (marrow) cavity of a bone to administer medications and fluids dates from the 1920s when adults suffering from pernicious anaemia were transfused via their sternum (Wheeler 1989).

As intravenous technology and surgical techniques developed, intraosseous cannulation fell from favour and by the 1950s had been largely superseded by other access routes (Rosetti *et al* 1985).

However, as advances in paediatric resuscitation have been made, the need for rapid vascular access in collapsed children was highlighted and the intraosseous route has become the route of choice when the child has no other central access already in situ in a clinical emergency situation (Advanced Life Support Group 2011, Resuscitation Council (UK) 2011a).

Intraosseous administration of medications generally involves delivery via the medullary cavity of a long bone. This not only provides rapid systemic action of medications and fluids (Andropoulos *et al* 1990), but it is also more rapidly and easily achieved than other forms of central venous access (Banerjee *et al* 1994). In the long bones, the medullary cavity consists of a network of venous sinusoids. These sinusoids drain into large medullary venous channels, which in turn, drain into nutrient or emissary vessels. The emissary vessels exit the bone via the nutrient foramina and empty directly into the systemic venous circulation (Tortora and Grabowski 1993).

In the event of circulatory failure (i.e. decompensated clinical shock or cardiac arrest) the peripheral vessels constrict as the child becomes 'shut down', making it extremely difficult to achieve venous access. The intraosseous route is therefore the preferred route of vascular access in a clinical emergency situation where a child urgently requires fluid or medications to be administered.

Although the intraosseous route is often limited to young children because of the physiologic replacement of red bone marrow by the less vascular yellow marrow at around 5–6 years of age (Fiser 1990, Ryder *et al* 1991) it has been demonstrated that although less vascular, yellow marrow still facilitates absorption, and therefore the procedure can also be successfully used in older children and adults.

Benefits of the intraosseous route

Unlike the peripheral vessels, the medullary cavity does not collapse in the presence of hypovolaemia or circulatory failure. It acts like a rigid vein making it an ideal site in a situation where vascular access is urgently required (e.g. clinical shock or cardiac arrest).

The onset of action of medications administered via the intraosseous route is almost as rapid as conventional central venous delivery and considerably quicker than those given via a peripheral vessel. Medications can be delivered as a bolus injection or continuous infusion. The intraosseous route can be used to obtain bone marrow samples for emergency testing (e.g. crossmatch in trauma).

Considerations for using the intraosseous route

In general, any medication or fluid that can be delivered via a central venous route can be delivered via the intraosseous route.

Aseptic non-touch techniques should be adhered to due to the increased potential for infection in comparison with other routes used for administration of medications. Knowledge of potential complications and their early detection and management is essential to minimise risks. For further information see Chapter 12 on Infection Prevention and Control.

Contraindications to using the intraosseous route

1. Osteogenesis imperfecta
2. Osteoporosis
3. Osteopetrosis
4. Fractures (select another site)
5. Loss of skin integrity (select another site).

Potential side-effects

1. Infection
2. Extravasation
3. Subperiosteal infusion
4. Embolism
5. Compartment syndrome
6. Fracture
7. Skin necrosis.

Selection of insertion site

The optimal choice is generally considered to be the anteriomedial aspect of the tibia, with the anteriolateral aspect of the femur being the next most commonly selected site. Both of these permit ease of access to the child's airway and thorax for other life-saving procedures that may be required. The anatomical landmarks for insertion of the intraosseous cannula to these bones are:

1. Tibia – 2–3 cm below the tibial tuberosity
2. Femur – 3 cm above the lateral condyle.

These two sites specifically avoid the epiphyseal (growing) plates of the bone and the joint spaces, though many others may be chosen in particular circumstances (McCarthy and Buss 1998).

In general, infected skin or wounds should not be used as an entry point to minimise infection risks.

Selection of cannula or needle

Commercially prepared, single use designated IO cannulae should ideally be used. These are available in a variety of sizes and a guide to appropriate gauge relative to age is:

1. 0–6 months = 18 G
2. 6–18 months = 16 G
3. >18 months = 14 G.

If a designated intraosseous needle is not available, bone marrow or spinal needles can be used as an alternative in an emergency situation.

There are also powered devices (e.g. EZ-IO drill) which are loaded with the cannula and allow very rapid insertion (Frascone et al 2009). The cannulae for these devices come in several weight-based lengths:

1. 3–39 kg = 15 mm
2. >39 kg = 25 mm
3. >39 kg with excessive amounts of tissue over the chosen insertion site.

Procedure guideline 27.5 Preparation for insertion of an intraosseous cannula

Statement	Rationale
Equipment preparation	
1. In preparation for insertion of an intraosseous needle, the following equipment should be gathered: a) Sterile gloves and apron. b) Alcohol based skin preparation fluid/wipes. c) Syringes. d) Needles. e) Sterile 3-way tap with extension tubing. f) Sodium chloride 0.9% for injection should be drawn up (10 ml) in an appropriately sized syringe and used to prime the 3-way tap with extension tubing. Turn the 3-way tap to the 'off' position. g) Sterile intraosseous needle (appropriate gauge) – either manual insertion type or for powered device as appropriate.	1. To enable the procedure to be performed in a safe and timely manner. a) To minimise infection potential. b) To cleanse skin in a rapid and effective manner. e) To facilitate prompt administration of medication/fluids as per local and manufacturer's policies. f) To facilitate checking of cannula patency and rapid delivery of medications. To prevent introduction of air into the medullary cavity. g) To minimise infection potential.

Procedure guideline 27.5 (*Continued*)

Statement	Rationale
h) Powered device (e.g. EZ-IO drill) if using.	**h)** To insert cannula appropriately.
i) Specimen bottles (as required).	**i)** To collect required specimens in a timely manner.
j) Local anaesthetic agent (if required) – this should be drawn up as prescribed, ready for use.	**j)** To minimise pain if the child is not deeply unconscious.
k) IV fluid administration set (if required).	**k)** To facilitate prompt administration of fluids.
l) Adhesive tape or dressing (if appropriate – see below).	**l)** To secure cannula and prevent accidental dislodgement.
m) If specific medication(s) and/or fluids are to be given, the following should also be prepared: • Child's prescription chart • Medication formulary • Manufacturer's drug information • Relevant medications and/fluids.	**m)** To facilitate prompt administration of medication/fluids as per local policies.

Inform child and family

2. In a clinical emergency scenario, time for explanations may not be appropriate. Where possible, these should be given appropriate to child's age and condition.	**2a)** To minimise fear. **b)** To gain cooperation. **c)** To provide reassurance and psychological support.
3. Family members must also receive appropriate explanations. Information to the family should include: • Reason for intraosseous cannulation • What it entails • Potential risks of intraosseous cannulation • Duration of the procedure • Expected outcome of intraosseous cannulation.	**3.** To allay their anxieties and reassure them of the benefits of the procedure. To obtain informed consent. To minimise anxiety.

Preparation of child

4a) Identify the site of insertion. **b)** Using an appropriately briefed assistant, position the child in a safe position that provides ready access to the chosen insertion site.	**4a)** To ensure appropriate placement. **b)** To facilitate safe and prompt placement of the cannula and minimise trauma to the child.
5. If the insertion site is to be in a limb, it should be supported by placing a towel or nappy behind it.	**5.** To secure the limb and facilitate safe placement of cannula.

Procedure guideline 27.6 **Procedure for manually inserted cannula**

Statement	Rationale
1. Check expiry date and open intraosseous needle packaging.	**1.** To minimise risk of infection.

2. Remove device and check to ensure:
  a) Integrity – no cracks or bends in hub or cannula.
  b) Trocar can be unscrewed and easily withdrawn from cannula.
  c) When trocar is screwed into cannula, that it protrudes past the end of it in readiness for insertion.
	2a) To ensure no damage to device that may hinder safe placement.
	b and c) To facilitate safe and easy placement of device.

673

(Continued)

Procedure guideline 27.6 (*Continued*)

Statement	Rationale
3. Clean the skin around the selected insertion site with the alcohol-based solution/wipe and allow to dry.	**3.** To minimise risk of infection.
4. Infiltrate the skin through to the periosteum with local anaesthetic agent (if appropriate).	**4.** To minimise pain along the intended insertion track of the IO cannula.
5. Immobilise the relevant limb with the non-dominant hand. **a)** Ensure the hand is not placed under the limb being cannulated.	**5.** To secure the limb and facilitate safe placement of cannula. **a)** To prevent injury to practitioner.
6. Holding the cannula in the dominant hand it is positioned at an angle of 90° to the skin at the prepared site.	**6.** To avoid damaging epiphyseal plates.
7. Insertion is achieved by applying firm downwards pressure in a rotating action while maintaining the 90° angle until a loss of resistance ('give') is felt. **a)** Care should be taken to avoid a 'rocking' motion during insertion.	**7.** A 'give' indicates the periosteum has been penetrated and bone cortex accessed. (The cannula should have penetrated the limb approximately 1–2 cm.) **a)** To avoid 'splintering' of the bone.
8. Ensure cannula stands stable in an upright position without support.	**8.** To confirm correct placement.

Procedure guideline 27.7 **Procedure for EZ-IO inserted cannula**

Statement	Rationale
1. Check integrity of packaging and expiry date before opening appropriate size of intraosseous cannula.	**1.** To minimise risk of infection.
2. Clean the skin around the selected insertion site with the alcohol-based solution/wipe and allow to dry.	**2.** To minimise risk of infection.
3. Infiltrate the skin through to the periosteum with local anaesthetic agent (if appropriate).	**3.** To minimise pain along the intended insertion track of the IO cannula.
4. Load the IO cannula on to the end of the drill (they fix together magnetically).	**4.** To prepare the device for use.
5. Hold the loaded drill in the dominant hand and place it on the skin at the selected insertion site at an angle of 90°.	**5.** To avoid damaging epiphyseal plates.
6. Immobilise the relevant limb with the non-dominant hand. **a)** Ensure the hand is not placed under the limb being used.	**6.** To secure the limb and facilitate safe placement of cannula. **a)** To prevent injury to practitioner.
7. Without drilling, push the drill until the cannula penetrates through the child's skin and bone is felt.	**7.** To assist with correct placement of cannula and avoid injury.
8. Apply continuous pressure to the drill button until a loss of resistance ('give') is felt.	**8.** A 'give' indicates the periosteum has been penetrated and bone cortex accessed.
9. Detach the drill from the IO cannula and remove the trocar.	**9.** To prepare the cannula for use.

Procedure guideline 27.8 Using the IO cannulae

Statement	**Rationale**
1. If clinically appropriate, attach a 5 ml syringe and attempt aspiration of bone marrow.	1. To confirm correct placement. To obtain marrow for baseline testing. To rapidly identify misplaced cannulae.
NB It is not always possible to obtain marrow easily due to the narrow lumen of the cannula and the viscosity of marrow.	
2a) If no marrow is obtained, but the practitioner's clinical judgement is that the cannula is correctly placed (i.e. they felt loss of resistance on entering cortex and the cannula is standing in a stable unsupported position) they should assume it is sited correctly and use the cannula accordingly. b) Observations to detect possible extravasation or sub-periosteal placement as described below should be made. c) NB In cardiac arrest, the attempt at aspiration of bone marrow should be omitted.	2. The administration of first-line resuscitation medications must not be delayed. c) To ensure adrenaline administration is not delayed.
3. Attach the previously primed 3-way tap and flush the cannula with 2–3 ml sodium chloride 0.9% for injection.	3. To confirm correct placement. To ensure patency of cannula.
4. Administer appropriate medications/fluids as prescribed.	4. To comply with treatment plan.
5. Observe site and relevant limb for any signs of extravasation, leakage or development of compartment syndrome. If any of these complications are suspected, infusion or injection should be discontinued and advice sought immediately	5. To minimise trauma and initiate appropriate treatments.
6. Ensure appropriate volume of sodium chloride 0.9% for injection is used to flush after and/or between each medication.	6. To ensure full dosage of medication is delivered. To ensure no drug interactions.
7. Ensure 3-way tap is turned to 'off' position or fluid infusion is continued as prescribed following administration of medication.	7. To maintain patient safety. To minimise infection risks. To comply with prescribed treatment plan.
8a) As the intraosseous needle is generally only in situ for a short period (until more permanent vascular access can be secured), it is usually not necessary to secure it in any other way. b) However, if the child's conscious level improves, or they require to be transported to another area, it may be necessary to secure the needle and/or extension tubing. For the manually inserted cannula, this can be easily achieved by placing a gallipot over the top of the cannula (or syringe barrels placed on either side of it under the hilt) and taping them to the child's skin. For the EZ-IO inserted cannula, there is a designated fixation device that should be used.	8a) To minimise potential for infection. b) To minimise risk of accidental displacement. The site must be readily visible at all times.
9. Dispose of all equipment according to local policy.	9. To minimise potential for injury and infection.
10. Record medication(s) administered as per local policy and record procedure in child's clinical records.	10. To meet local and legal requirements.
11. Observe the site frequently (at least hourly) for any side effects such as extravasation, leakage, infection or compartment syndrome.	11. Record and report to senior staff any potential problems so appropriate actions can be initiated.

Basic life support

Basic life support (BLS) is a series of manoeuvres that can be performed to 'buy time' for the collapsed child. It is the basis of all advanced life support (ALS) techniques and without effective BLS techniques, no amount of technological advances will improve patient outcome. Using no more than their hands and expired breath, BLS means that the rescuer(s) can provide a level of oxygenation that affords some protection from hypoxia until more ALS measures are available.

Effectiveness of BLS is increased when the rescuer is proficient in its delivery. However, even sub-optimal BLS is probably better than no BLS if performed safely.

It is recommended that when performing expired air ventilation, a protective barrier device (e.g. plastic face shield) should be used to minimise the potential risks of cross-infection. However, rescue breathing should not be delayed while the rescuer searches for a barrier device (ILCOR 2010).

Expired air ventilation alone will provide no more than 16–17% oxygen, so it is important to maximise this as soon as equipment becomes available. Trained healthcare providers can utilise a self-inflating bag-mask (B-M) device to provide room air (21% oxygen) or better still, attach it to an oxygen flow to supplement this to a high concentration of oxygen.

The sequence of events in paediatric BLS

The order of actions in BLS is important. If one is missed or inadequately performed, the next step may be rendered useless.

If there is more than one rescuer present, one of them should immediately seek further assistance by activating the appropriate EMS team, while the other(s) initiate BLS.

If a child with a known cardiac condition, e.g. cardiomyopathy or congenital cardiac defect, suffers a sudden, witnessed collapse, it is likely that they may have suffered a primary cardiac event. In this instance, they are likely to be in ventricular fibrillation (VF) or pulseless ventricular tachycardia (VT). For these children, optimal outcome will depend on rapid defibrillation and it would be appropriate for a lone rescuer to activate the EMS before commencing BLS and to use an automated external defibrillator (AED) if available.

For the vast majority of children who suffer cardiorespiratory arrest however, it is a secondary event and not of cardiac origin. In the event of only a single rescuer being present, while it is important that ALS is rapidly sought, it must not preclude the delivery of a full minute of BLS. This will provide at least some oxygenation to the already profoundly hypoxic child. Additionally, the most common cardiac arrhythmia encountered in arrests in children is severe bradycardia deteriorating into asystole; effective BLS is therefore, more important than rapid access to a defibrillator.

Paediatric BLS sequence

The sequence of actions in BLS is identical whether in or out of the hospital environment. It can be easily remembered as:

- **S**afety
- **S**timulate
- **S**hout for assistance
- **A**irway
- **B**reathing
- **C**irculation
- **R**eassess.

Procedure guideline 27.9 **BLS provision**

Statement	Rationale
Safety	
1. The first priority is that rescuer(s) are not placed in danger. Second is that the child is in a 'safe' position.	**1.** Rescuer(s) are unable to assist child if they injure themselves. To prevent further injury.
2. Quickly check for potential environmental dangers in immediate vicinity. If necessary, move child to a position of safety before initiating resuscitation. (This applies even if there is suspicion of trauma and movement should ideally be avoided.)	**2.** To avoid endangering child and selves.
3. As all bodily fluids are potentially infectious 'universal precautions' should be followed whenever practical. This includes gloves and barrier devices (e.g. face shields) if readily available. However, initiation of BLS to infants and children should not be delayed for the arrival of any equipment.	**3.** To minimise risks of cross-infection. Any delay in oxygenation will increase the likelihood of morbidity and mortality.
4. On approaching the child, and before touching them, look for any clues as to what may have caused the emergency.	**4.** To modify initial management of the child (e.g. suspicion of head/neck trauma necessitates consideration of C-spine immobilisation).

Procedure guideline 27.9 (*Continued*)

Statement	Rationale
Stimulate	
5a) Establish responsiveness of child through verbal and tactile stimulation. **b)** An appropriate way to do this is to stabilise child's head by placing one hand on their forehead and then use other hand to shake their arm or tug their hair. **c)** At the same time loudly call the child's name or tell them to 'waken up'.	**5a)** To determine whether actually in a critical condition requiring EMS activation. **b)** To immobilise C-spine. To elicit a response through tactile stimulation. **c)** To elicit a response through verbal stimulation.
6a) If the child responds (e.g. moving, crying or talking) their clinical status should be evaluated. **b)** If there is no response to stimulation, the rescuer must proceed with the next step of BLS.	**6a)** To determine whether their condition requires EMS activation. **b)** To minimise delay in oxygenation and accessing EMS.
Shout	
7. While staying with the child, the rescuer must either send someone else to activate an EMS team, or if they are alone, shout out loudly for assistance.	**7.** To facilitate rapid access to EMS.
8. If there is no response to this initial shout for help, the lone rescuer must not leave the child but proceed with the next stages of BLS.	**8.** To avoid delay in ensuring child's airway patency and oxygenation.
9. If there is another person available to alert the EMS, the rescuer must ensure that the individual is capable of providing the following information: **a)** Precise location of the emergency. **b)** Telephone number from which the call is being made. **c)** Number and age of victim(s) – i.e. child(ren) are involved. **d)** Severity and urgency of situation – i.e. that the child requires ALS.	**9.** **a)** To facilitate rapid arrival of EMS. **c)** To ensure appropriate personnel summoned.

10. The individual being sent to activate the EMS must be made aware that they should only hang up after the controller they speak to ends the call. They should also be instructed to return to the scene after they have alerted the EMS.	**10.** To ensure all necessary information has been relayed.
	  To confirm that EMS has been summoned.
	  To provide further assistance.

Airway	
11. To facilitate ventilation and oxygenation, airway patency must be achieved/maintained.	**11.** In the unconscious child, the combination of head flexion/hyper-extension and passive posterior displacement of the tongue is likely to at least partly occlude the airway.
12. If possible, ideally place child in a supine position on a firm, flat surface.	**12.** To facilitate BLS delivery.
13. Open the airway using either head tilt/chin lift or jaw thrust manoeuvres (as described previously).	**13.** To clear tongue away from the posterior pharyngeal wall.
14. While opening the airway, look into the mouth. In infants, the nares should also be checked for patency.	**14.** To ensure no obvious foreign bodies. Blocked nostrils can cause apnoea in small infants who are preferential nasal breathers.
15. Only if there is a visible foreign body in the mouth that the rescuer is confident they can reach, should they consider attempting a single, gentle finger sweep.	**15.** To avoid further impacting a foreign body or risking soft tissue damage.

677

(*Continued*)

Procedure guideline 27.9 (*Continued*)

Statement	Rationale
Blind finger sweeps must not be performed	
16. Once the airway has been opened, the rescuer must proceed with the next step of BLS.	16. To minimise delay in oxygenation.
Breathing	
17. While maintaining the airway open (as above) the rescuer must assess whether or not the child is making adequate spontaneous respiratory effort. To decide this, the rescuer positions their cheek a few centimetres above the child's face. At the same time, they need to look along the child's body towards their feet.	17. To determine the need for rescue breathing by **looking** (for chest/abdominal rise and fall), **listening** (for breath sounds) and **feeling** (for air movement).
18. No more than 10 seconds should be taken to determine respiratory effort.	18. To minimise delay in oxygenation.
19. If there is adequate respiratory effort, the rescuer should continue to monitor the child and summon more assistance as appropriate.	19. To ensure no further deterioration in condition.
20. If there is no suspicion of head or spinal trauma, it would be appropriate to place the child in a safe, side-lying position (see 'Recovery position').	20. To maintain airway patency and minimise potential risk of aspiration.
21. If the child is not making adequate respiratory effort, rescue breaths must be delivered.	21. To deliver oxygen to the child's lungs.
22. While maintaining the airway as described above, five initial rescue breaths should be delivered.	22. It is recognised that the first attempts at rescue breaths are often ineffective.
23. Each breath must be delivered slowly (over approximately 1 to 1.5 seconds).	23. To minimise the potential for gastric distension.
24. Rescuers should remove their mouth from the child's face between each breath.	24. To facilitate child's exhalation and avoid rebreathing of air.
25. Rescuers may wish to take a breath themselves between delivery of each rescue breath.	25. To maximise the amount of oxygen and minimise the amount of carbon dioxide in the expired air that they deliver to the child.
26. Delivery of rescue breaths can be performed by either of these two techniques:	26. Choice is dependent on the size and/or anatomy of the child's face.
27a) **Mouth-to-mouth and nose** is the method generally recommended for use in infants. The rescuer places their mouth over the mouth and nose of the infant and creates a seal around them.	27a) This is more physiologically 'normal' as infants are preferential nasal breathers.
b) **Mouth-to-mouth** is usually used in children, or where a seal cannot be achieved in mouth-to-mouth and nose in infants. The rescuer's mouth is placed directly over the child's creating a seal. With the hand nearest the top of the child's head, the rescuer must occlude the child's nostrils	b) To ensure that there is no air escape from the nostrils during rescue breath delivery.
28a) The probable effectiveness of rescue breaths must be determined by observing for chest rise and fall with each one.	28a) To ensure that air is being delivered to the child's lungs.
b) If chest movement is not observed, the child's head should be repositioned and the breaths repeated.	b) Commonest problem is inappropriate head positioning. An inadequate seal may be causing air to escape.

Procedure guideline 27.9 (*Continued*)

Statement	Rationale
29. If despite repositioning of the head, the rescue breaths continue to fail to achieve chest rise, the likely cause must be sought and remedied.	**29.** The likelihood of a foreign body obstructing the airway should be considered and the rescuer should move straight to chest compression delivery.
30. Once initial rescue breaths have been delivered, the rescuer must proceed with the next step in BLS sequence.	**30.** To minimise delay in oxygenation.

Circulation

Statement	Rationale
31. The rescuer must establish whether the child has an adequate spontaneous circulation.	**31.** To determine further management.
32. No more than 10 seconds should be spent assessing for 'signs of life' (i.e. moving, swallowing or gasping).	**32.** To determine the need for external chest compressions (ECC) to provide a circulation.
33. The presence of a central pulse can be determined by those previously trained to assess for pulses. (Recommended sites are the brachial or femoral in infants and carotid or femoral in children.)	**33.** It is acknowledged that assessing for pulses in collapsed persons is difficult, so determination of 'signs of life' is the priority (Tibballs and Russell 2009).
34. If there are signs of an effective circulation (i.e. pulse > 60/ minute and/or spontaneous movement), the rescuer should reassess the breathing.	**34.** ECC are not indicated. To determine the need for continuing appropriate rescue breathing (12–20 rescue breaths per minute and frequent reassessment of circulation).
35. If there are no signs of an effective circulation (i.e. no signs of life present), or if the rescuer is at all unsure, then ECC must be commenced.	**35.** All pulseless children and those with heart rates too low to adequately perfuse vital organs require ECC.
36. ECC are best delivered with the child in a supine position on a firm, flat surface.	**36.** To facilitate safe and effective delivery.
37. ECC are a series of rhythmic depressions of the anterior chest wall.	**37.** Intended to cause blood to be delivered to the vital organs, in an attempt to keep them viable until the return of adequate spontaneous circulation (ROSC).
38. They should be delivered over the lower half of the sternum, in a smooth, rhythmic fashion. Rate of delivery is approximately 100 times (and no more than 120) per minute.	**38.** To minimise trauma.
39. The depth of compression should be at least approximately one-third of the anterior-posterior diameter of the thorax.	**39.** ECC have previously been noted to be too shallow (Resuscitation Council 2010).
40. Equal time should be spent in the depression and relaxation phases.	**40.** To optimise cardiac filling and emptying.
41. ECC are interspersed with rescue breaths.	**41.** To ensure blood being circulated is oxygenated.

Landmarking for ECC

Statement	Rationale
42a) The area for delivery of ECC for both infants and children is the lower half of the sternum. This can be safely identified by locating the xiphisternum at the angle where the lower ribs meet and compressing approximately one finger's breadth above the xiphisternum.	**42a)** To minimise risk of trauma.
b) However, it is essential to check that the rescuer's fingers are not over the xiphisternum.	**b)** To locate safe position for delivery (Clements and McGowan 2000).

679

(*Continued*)

Procedure guideline 27.9 (*Continued*)

Statement	Rationale
ECC delivery	
43. Method of delivery of ECC is dependent on the: **a)** Size of the child **b)** Number/expertise of rescuers.	
44. Infant ECC can be delivered by either of these techniques: **a)** Two-fingers is the recommended technique for laypersons or the single rescuer. Two fingers from the hand nearest the infant's feet are placed in the correct position (as described above) on the centre of the lower sternum. **b)** Two-thumbs is the technique recommended when two rescuers are present, or when oxygen delivery devices are being utilised. The rescuer's two thumbs are placed side by side (or one on top of the other in a very small infant) in the correct position (as above) on the centre of the lower sternum. **c)** With the other fingers, the rescuer's hands encircle the chest.	**44.** **a)** Considered the easiest method of ECC delivery and can be used for infants of all sizes. **b)** Evidence suggests this method provides greater cardiac output, but it cannot be effectively utilised by single rescuers. **c)** To provide support to the infant's back and optimise output.
45. In children ECC is delivered by placing the heel of one hand along the long axis of the centre of their lower sternum.	**45.** To minimise risk of trauma.
46. The rescuer's fingers should be raised off the chest wall.	**46.** To prevent pressure being exerted over ribs and potentially causing trauma.
47. The rescuer should ideally be positioned close to the side of the child.	**47.** To minimise stress to rescuer's back.
48. Rescuer's shoulders should be directly over the child's chest, with their arm locked straight at the elbow.	**48.** The rescuer's body weight will help to reduce the physical effort required to achieve adequate compression depth.
49. If the rescuer finds it difficult to achieve a depth of at least one-third of the anterior-posterior diameter of the thorax, they should use both hands; the second hand placed on top of the first with the fingers interlocked off the chest wall. **a)** During the relaxation phase of each individual compression, the rescuer must release the pressure, while leaving their fingers/hands in position on the chest wall.	**49.** To allow the heart to refill with blood between compressions and therefore, optimise cardiac output. **a)** To minimise delay in recommencing ECC after ventilations.
50. If a single rescuer is providing both rescue breaths and ECC, they must remove their fingers/hands to perform the chin lift at the end of each series of compressions.	**50.** To ensure airway patency and facilitate effective rescue breath delivery.
51. Where there is more than one rescuer (and they are competent at pulse checks) one should feel for a central pulse whilst ECC is being delivered by another. **a)** In children, ECC should always be interspersed with rescue breaths. **b)** The recommended ratio in infants and children is 5 compressions: 2 breaths. **c)** In newborn babies a compression to ventilation ratio of 3:1 is recommended.	**51.** Adequacy of ECC may be assessed by determining presence of pulsation in a central artery (NB in haemorrhage this may not be possible). **a)** Oxygenated blood is critical to minimise hypoxic tissue damage. **b)** The hypoxic aetiology of children's cardiorespiratory arrests necessitates effective ventilation. **c)** The physiological respiratory rates of newborns are faster than older children and adults, thus greater emphasis is placed on ventilation.

Procedure guideline 27.9 *(Continued)*

Statement	Rationale
Reassessment	
52. Following a full minute of BLS delivery, the rescuer should briefly stop and reassess the situation: a) Firstly, confirmation that the EMS has been summoned must be sought.	**52.** To ensure access to ALS interventions is forthcoming as BLS alone is unlikely to achieve ROSC in cardiorespiratory arrest. a) Any person who has required BLS is likely to need ongoing care in an ALS facility.
53. If EMS has not been summoned or there is any doubt, it must now be done. A mobile telephone should be used if available.	**53.** To minimise delays in ALS availability.
54. If a mobile telephone is not available, and the victim is an infant or small child, the rescuer may be able to carry them safely to activate further assistance and then recommence BLS. If the means of summoning assistance is some distance away, the rescuer should stop en route every minute or so, place the child on the ground and deliver a further minute of BLS before moving on again.	**54.** To provide a basic level of oxygenation in an effort to minimise morbidity and mortality.
55. If the child is too large to carry safely, the rescuer would need to leave them to activate EMS and then return and recommence BLS as rapidly as possible.	**55.** To prevent injury to the child or themselves.
56. If EMS has already been alerted, the rescuer must immediately resume BLS as appropriate, unless there are obvious 'signs of life'.	**56.** To maximise oxygenation and minimise morbidity and mortality.
Continuing BLS	
57. The rescuer should only briefly stop to reassess the situation after the first minute of BLS. Thereafter, BLS should be continued until: a) Child exhibits any signs of response. b) Another person competent in BLS takes over. c) Rescuer is too exhausted to continue. d) Resuscitation attempt is stopped by a medically qualified person.	**57.** To maintain oxygenation. a) ABC should be reassessed and BLS continued as appropriate. b) BLS is a physically demanding procedure. d) It is deemed inappropriate to continue resuscitation attempt.

Choking

When a foreign body (FB) enters their airway, a person will immediately react by coughing – their attempt to expel it. Someone who is choking on an FB but is still able to cough effectively should be actively encouraged to do so. A spontaneous cough is not only safer, but is probably more effective than any manoeuvre that a rescuer might perform.

However, if coughing is absent or ineffective, the choking person is at extreme risk of complete airway obstruction with resultant rapid asphyxiation. Anyone who is unable to effectively cough due to an FB in their airway requires immediate assistance.

Recognition of choking

Choking is characterised by the sudden onset of respiratory distress associated with coughing, gagging and/or stridor.

The majority of choking events in infants and children occur during feeding or playing, and are therefore usually witnessed by a caregiver, who should be able to intervene immediately when necessary. In an adolescent or adult, the FB is usually related to eating and again is frequently witnessed by another person.

However, it is important to be aware that the signs and symptoms of choking can sometimes be confused with those of other airway obstruction causes, e.g. laryngitis or epiglottitis, which require very different management.

General signs of choking in children

- Sudden onset
- Often a witnessed event
- Coughing, gagging, stridor
- History of playing with, or eating small objects immediately preceding event.

Box 27.1 lists effective and ineffective coughing.

Box 27.1 Effective and ineffective coughing	
Effective coughing	**Ineffective coughing**
Crying or verbal response to questions	Inability to vocalise
Able to cough forcefully	Quiet or silent cough
Able to inhale before coughing	Difficulty (or no) breathing
Alert and responsive	Cyanosis
	Decreasing level of consciousness

Procedure guideline 27.10 **Management of choking infant/child**

Statement	Rationale
Safety	
1. Rapidly assess the situation (effectiveness of coughing; age of child) and ensure safety of both rescuer and child.	**1.** To identify the need for, and type of intervention required. To prevent injury to rescuer or child.
Stimulate	
2. The conscious level of the child should be rapidly assessed in a manner appropriate to their age.	**2.** To determine potential degree of hypoxia from airway obstruction.
Shout	
3. Shout for more assistance whether in or out of the healthcare environment. Anyone answering this call for assistance should await further instructions from the rescuer depending on how the event progresses.	**3.** While many episodes of choking can be safely and quickly remedied, they also have the potential for rapidly deteriorating in to a serious clinical emergency.
Back blows in infants	
4. Sit on a chair or kneel on the floor.	**4.** To minimise potential for injury if the infant should fall.
5a) The infant's head should be supported by the rescuer placing the thumb of one of their hands at the angle of the infant's lower jaw, and one or two fingers from this hand at the same point on the other side of the infant's face.	**5a)** To maximise patency of the airway (modified jaw thrust). To support the infant's head and minimise risk of brain trauma.
b) Care must be taken not to compress the soft tissues under the chin.	**b)** To prevent airway occlusion.
6. Hold the infant in a head downwards, prone position down the length of their thigh, or across their lap.	**6.** Gravity will assist with removal of FB.
7. With the heel of their free hand, the rescuer should deliver up to five sharp blows to the middle of the infant's back, between their scapulae.	**7.** The aim is to loosen the object in order that the infant can then expel it and to relieve the obstruction with as few back blows as possible (do not give all five unless necessary).
Back blows in children	
8a) Depending on the size of both the rescuer and the child, they should try to support the child in a head downwards position.	**8a)** Safety of both is utmost priority.
b) If this is not possible, then they should try to support them in a forward-leaning position, with the rescuer standing behind.	**b)** Gravity will help with removal of FB.

Procedure guideline 27.10 (*Continued*)

Statement	Rationale
9. With the heel of their free hand, the rescuer should deliver up to five sharp blows to the middle of the child's back, between their scapulae.	**9.** The aim is to loosen the object in order that the child can then expel it and to relieve the obstruction with as few back blows as possible (do not give all five unless necessary).

Thrusts

Although the ILCOR (2010) guidelines for the delivery of thrusts is that abdominal ones can be used in children (i.e. over 1 year of age), it is important that the rescuer uses their clinical judgement to decide if it is safe to perform these. If the clinical judgement is that the child is too small, then they should deliver chest thrusts as for infants. **Abdominal thrusts (Heimlich manoeuvre) should never be performed in infants due to the very high likelihood of trauma to their internal organs.**

10. If back blows fail, and the infant or child is still conscious, the rescuer must administer thrusts; chest in the infant and abdominal in a child.	**10.** An alternative movement to relieve the airway obstruction.

Chest thrusts in an infant

11. Turn the infant from the head downwards, prone position they were in for back blows, to a head downwards, supine position.	**11.** To facilitate effective delivery of chest thrusts.
a) This can be achieved most easily by placing the free arm down the infant's back and cupping their occiput with the hand, and rolling the baby over in to the supine head downwards position.	**a)** To support the infant's head throughout to minimise risk of injury and to maximise safety.
b) If this is difficult, lay the baby flat on the ground, but avoid lifting their head higher than their trunk.	**b)** To prevent any loosened object falling back down in to the lower airway.
12. Hold the infant in a head downwards, supine position down the length of their thigh, or across their lap.	**12.** Gravity will assist with removal of FB.
13a) The landmark for ECC (i.e. a finger-breadth above the xiphisternum) should be identified and two fingers positioned on the sternum.	**13a)** To minimise trauma.
b) Up to five sharp downward thrusts should be delivered. These thrusts are similar to ECC but are delivered at a slower rate and are sharper in nature.	**b)** The aim is to loosen the object in order that the infant can expel it and to relieve the obstruction with as few chest thrusts as possible (do not give all five unless necessary).

Abdominal thrusts in a child

14a) The rescuer should stand behind the child, place their arms underneath the child's and encircle their torso.	**14a)** To maximise safety.
b) They can then support them in a forward leaning position.	**b)** To have a degree of control over the child if they lose consciousness; can lower their body more safely to the floor.
15. The rescuer should clench one of their fists and place this on the child's abdomen, midway between their umbilicus and the tip of their xiphisternum.	**15.** To minimise risk of trauma to internal organs.
16. The rescuer should grasp this fist with their free hand and by pulling sharply upwards and inwards, they should deliver up to five abdominal thrusts.	**16a)** To cause a change in intrathoracic pressure thus creating an artificial 'cough'.
	b) The aim is to loosen the object in order that the child can expel it.
	c) The aim is to relieve the obstruction with as few abdominal thrusts as possible (do not give all five unless necessary).

683

(*Continued*)

Procedure guideline 27.10 (*Continued*)

Statement	Rationale
Reassessment	
17a) Following delivery of the thrusts (chest or abdominal), the rescuer should briefly stop and reassess the situation.	**17a)** To determine further management required.
b) If the FB has been successfully expelled, the child should be assessed and made comfortable until examined by a medical practitioner.	**b)** Any person who has required back blows and chest/abdominal thrusts needs to be assessed in case of internal trauma or retained FB.
c) If the FB has not been expelled, and the infant/child is still conscious, ensure that EMS is summoned (as in BLS support above) and the sequence of back blows and chest/abdominal thrusts repeated as indicated.	**c)** To minimise delays in ALS availability and to try and relieve the FB while awaiting arrival of EMS.

As with BLS, it is important that rescuers intervene quickly to prevent a manageable situation becoming one of potential cardiorespiratory arrest. The steps for managing a choking infant/child who is conscious but unable to effectively cough are detailed below.

The management of an infant/child who is (or becomes) unconscious as the result of foreign body choking is identical to that of one who shows no 'signs of life', i.e. the procedure for BLS (above) should be followed.

The additional considerations in this scenario are:

1. **Checking the mouth:** The mouth should be checked for the FB each time the airway is opened for rescue breaths. If it is visible, a single finger sweep should be used to try and remove the FB. However, blind or repeated finger sweeps must not be performed as these are likely to impact the FB further into the airway and/or cause trauma.
2. **Initial rescue breaths:** If a rescue breath does not result in chest wall rise, the head should be repositioned before attempting the next breath. If all five initial breaths are ineffective (i.e. no visible chest rise), despite repositioning of the head, and the infant/child demonstrates no 'signs of life' the rescuer should proceed to ECC.
3. **Continued BLS:** The cycle of BLS should be followed with a check for the FB in the child's mouth prior to delivery of each set of two breaths. If the first breath is ineffective, the head should be repositioned prior to the second. If the second is also ineffective, the rescuer should proceed again with ECC.

Should rescue breaths be effective (i.e. there is visible chest rise) full BLS should continue unless/until the child displays 'signs of life'.

If 'signs of life' are displayed, the rescuer should rapidly assess the child's ABC and then continue as appropriate.

Cardiorespiratory arrest management

Cardiac arrest can be defined as the lack of palpable central pulses. It is crucial that effective BLS is continued while specific treatment strategies are incorporated as necessary. ALS measures are designed to re-establish circulation and achieve effective oxygenation. Cardiac arrest management will involve some or all of the following:

- ECG rhythm analysis
- Defibrillation/cardioversion
- Advanced airway management procedures
- Intravascular access
- Fluid and medication delivery
- Ongoing ABCDE assessment.

Body weight estimation

As most treatments in children are weight dependent, it is prudent to determine this as early as possible. If it is not already known, a recognised method of estimation (e.g. Broselow tape measure or centile chart should be utilised). It is essential that whatever method is utilised, practitioners are familiar with it to minimise the potential for calculation errors in an emergency situation.

ECG rhythm analysis

Early identification of the child's ECG rhythm is essential to influence appropriate management. There are essentially two categories of cardiac arrest arrhythmias: shockable and non-shockable.

The shockable arrhythmias are ventricular fibrillation (VF) and pulseless ventricular tachycardia (VT).

The non-shockable rhythms are asystole and pulseless electrical activity (PEA).

Profound bradycardia deteriorating to asystole is the most common ECG presentation of cardiac arrest in children. As with PEA, it should be treated with continued BLS and additional oxygen.

Procedure guideline 27.11 Management of non-shockable rhythms (asystole and PEA)

Statement	Rationale
1a) Perform continuous CPR at 15 ECC:2 ventilations with high-concentration bag-mask ventilation as soon as available. **b)** Deliver ECC at a rate of 100–120/minute.	**1a and b)** To maximise oxygenation to body tissues.
2. If the child's airway is secured with a tracheal tube, continuous ECC should be delivered.	**2.** Minimising interruptions to ECC results in increased coronary perfusion; the tracheal tube allows this as it protects the lower airways from potential aspiration of gastric contents.
3. The ventilation rate once the child is intubated should be 10–12 breaths/minute.	
4. Exhaled CO_2 should be measured.	**4.** To monitor ventilation and ensure correct tracheal tube placement.
5. Adrenaline (10 µg/kg) must be given as soon as venous or IO access is achieved.	**5.** Any delay in administration reduces the likelihood of ROSC.
6. Continue CPR, only pausing briefly every 2 minutes to check for rhythm change (should be coordinated with ventilation delivery if child not intubated).	**6.** To maximise oxygenation to body tissues.
7. Administer adrenaline 10 µg/kg every 4 minutes (i.e. every alternate cycle of CPR) while maintaining uninterrupted effective CPR.	**7.** Adrenaline induces vasoconstriction, increases coronary perfusion pressure, enhances the contractile state of the heart and stimulates spontaneous contractions.

8. Examine the child, their records (e.g. drug chart and blood results) and consider any potentially reversible cause(s) of the arrest:
• Hypoxia
• Hypovolaemia
• Hypo/hyperkalaemia (and other metabolic disturbances)
• Hypothermia
• Tension pneumothorax
• Toxic/therapeutic disturbances
  Tamponade (cardiac)
  Thromboembolism.
  Correct any reversible causes.
	8. It is particularly important to search for the underlying cause of the arrhythmia in children as it is unlikely to be due to coronary artery disease (the usual adult cause).
	  The earlier these are identified and treated, the greater the likelihood of ROSC.
	  Remember there may be more than one reversible cause and that problems can occur during the resuscitation necessitating frequent reassessment.

9a) Consider other medications: Sodium bicarbonate (this is not a first-line medication, but may be useful in a prolonged event).	**9a)** In prolonged events, lactic acid accumulation may have occurred and require treating. NB The best treatment for acidaemia in cardiac arrest is a combination of effective ECC and ventilation.
b) Atropine may be useful in vagal induced bradycardia tone (e.g. after insertion of nasogastric tube). The dose is 20 µg/kg with a minimum dose of 100 µg.	**b)** A dose lower than 100 µg may cause a paradoxical bradycardic effect.

685

Procedure guideline 27.12 Management of shockable rhythms (ventricular fibrillation and pulseless ventricular tachycardia)

This is a much less common situation in paediatric practice, although Mogayzel *et al* (1995) reported an incidence of 19% and Atkins *et al* (2009) up to 27%. It may occur as a secondary event, and is likely when there has been a witnessed and sudden collapse. It is commoner in the paediatric intensive care unit and cardiac wards.

Statement	Rationale
1. Continue with continuous CPR at 15 ECC:2 ventilations with high-concentration bag-mask ventilation as soon as available until defibrillator is ready to use.	1. To maximise oxygenation to body tissues.
2. Establish the energy level required: • 4 J/kg if using manual defibrillator • A paediatric-attenuated dosage if using an AED for a child less than approximately 8 years of age • If using an AED for a child over 8 years, use the standard adult dose.	2. A single 4 J/kg shock strategy improves 1st shock success rate and minimises interruption to ECC (ILCOR 2010).
3. Charge the defibrillator while another rescuer continues chest compressions.	3. To minimise interruptions to ECC.
4. Once the defibrillator is charged, pause the chest compressions and quickly ensure that all rescuers are clear of the patient before promptly delivering the shock.	4. To adhere to best practice safe guidelines. To try and convert the rhythm to a perfusing one.
5. The shock may be delivered by the person doing compressions or by another trained rescuer. This decision should be planned before the ECC are stopped.	5. To minimise interruptions to ECC.
6. Immediately resume CPR without assessing the rhythm or checking for a pulse starting with ECC.	6. To minimise interruptions to ECC.
7a) Examine the child, their records (e.g. drug chart and blood results) and consider any potentially reversible cause(s) of the arrest: • Hypoxia • Hypovolaemia • Hypo/hyperkalaemia(and other metabolic disturbances) • Hypothermia • Tension pneumothorax • Toxic/therapeutic disturbances • Tamponade (cardiac) • Thromboembolism. b) Correct any reversible causes.	7a) It is particularly important to search for the underlying cause of the arrhythmia in children as it is unlikely to be due to coronary artery disease (the usual adult cause). The earlier these are identified and treated, the greater the likelihood of ROSC. b) Remember there may be more than one reversible cause and that problems can occur during the resuscitation necessitating frequent reassessment.
8. Continue uninterrupted CPR for 2 minutes before briefly pausing to check the rhythm.	8. To maximise oxygenation to body tissues.
9. **If still VF/VT:** a) Give a second shock (identical to first). b) Immediately resume CPR without assessing the rhythm or checking for a pulse starting with ECC. c) Continue uninterrupted CPR for 2 minutes before briefly pausing to check the rhythm.	9a) To try and convert the rhythm to a perfusing one. b) To maximise oxygenation to body tissues. c) To maximise oxygenation to body tissues.

Procedure guideline 27.12 (*Continued*)

Statement	Rationale
10. If still VF/VT: a) Give a third shock (identical to first and second) b) Immediately resume CPR without assessing the rhythm or checking for a pulse starting with ECC.	**10a)** To try and convert the rhythm to a perfusing one. b) To maximise oxygenation to body tissues.
11a) Administer adrenaline 10 µg/kg (i.e. after the third shock and once CPR has resumed).	**11a)** Adrenaline induces vasoconstriction, increases coronary perfusion pressure, enhances the contractile state of the heart, stimulates spontaneous contractions and increases the intensity of VF, thereby increasing the likelihood of successful defibrillation.
b) Also administer amiodarone 5 mg/kg. NB Amiodarone can cause thrombophlebitis when administered peripherally, and so should ideally be given via a central vein. If it has to be given peripherally in an emergency then it must be liberally flushed with sodium chloride 0.9% or 5% glucose.	b) Amiodarone is a membrane-stabilising anti-arrhythmic drug that increases the duration of the action potential and refractory period in atrial and ventricular myocardium. Atrioventricular conduction is slowed, and a similar effect is also seen in accessory pathways.
12. Administer adrenaline 10 µg/kg every 4 minutes (i.e. every alternate cycle of CPR) while maintaining uninterrupted effective CPR.	**12.** Higher doses of intravascular adrenaline should not be used routinely in children as it may worsen outcome.
13. Repeat amiodarone 5 mg/kg once more (after the fifth shock) if still in a shockable rhythm.	**13.** To try and convert the rhythm to a perfusing one.
14. Continue delivering shocks every 2 minutes, ensuring ECC are maintained during charging of defibrillator and minimising any interruptions to CPR as much as possible.	**14.** To try and convert the rhythm to a perfusing one.
15. After each 2 minutes of uninterrupted CPR pause briefly to assess the rhythm.	
16. If still VF/VT: a) Continue CPR with the shockable sequence.	**16.** a) To try and convert the rhythm to a perfusing one.
17. If asystole: a) Continue CPR but switch to non-shockable sequence as above.	**17.** a) To manage arrhythmia appropriately.
18. If organised electrical activity is seen: a) Check for 'signs of life' and central pulse. b) If there is ROSC commence post-resuscitation management. c) If there is **no** pulse or it is <60 beats per minute and there are no other 'signs of life' continue CPR as for the non-shockable sequence described above.	**18.** b) To minimise/prevent hypoxic damage. c) To manage arrhythmia appropriately.
19. If defibrillation was successful but VF/VT recurs, resume the shockable CPR sequence with defibrillation. a) Give an amiodarone bolus (unless two doses have already been given) and start a continuous infusion.	**19.** To try and convert the rhythm back to a perfusing one.

NB Uninterrupted, good-quality CPR is vital; ECC and ventilation should be interrupted only for defibrillation. As ECC delivery is tiring for providers, the team leader should continuously assess the quality of the ECC, and change the providers every 2 minutes.

NB Uninterrupted, good-quality CPR is vital; ECC and ventilation should be interrupted only for defibrillation. As ECC delivery is tiring for providers, the team leader should continuously assess the quality of the ECC, and change the providers every 2 minutes.

Defibrillation

Defibrillation is the delivery of electrical energy through the thorax, causing a transient standstill of the heart. The resultant depolarisation of the myocardium, aims to restore organised spontaneous electrical activity and a normal ECG rhythm.

Shockable arrhythmias (VF and pulseless VT) are uncommon in cardiac arrests in children. The children in whom they are most likely to be encountered are those with underlying cardiac pathology, hypothermia or tricyclic antidepressant poisoning.

As with the adult, asynchronous defibrillation should be performed as rapidly as a defibrillator is ready to use. Effective CPR beforehand is likely to enhance a successful outcome, although it is also reported that for every minute delay in defibrillation, there is a 7–10% reduction in the likelihood of successful outcome (Bossaert 1999).

Automated external defibrillators

These machines are now widely available in both hospital and pre-hospital settings. This has led to improvements in survival from VF for adults. Standard AED pads are suitable for use in children older than approximately 8 years. Special paediatric pads (that attenuate the current delivered during defibrillation) should be used in children aged between 1 and 8 years if they are available; if not, the AED should be used as it is. Shockable rhythms are uncommon in children of less than 1 year and the use of an AED is not generally recommended. However, if a shockable rhythm is present and an AED is the only defibrillator available, its use should be considered (Resuscitation Council 2010).

The current recommendation, therefore, is that variable energy defibrillators must still be available in areas where sick children are being cared for.

Pads or paddles

Manual defibrillation can be performed using either self-adhesive pads (i.e. 'hands free') or the rigid paddles on the machine. While the paddles are probably rarely used nowadays, they may still be necessary for a very small infant in whom the paediatric pads (even in anterior-posterior placement) are too large (i.e. they touch one another). If paddles are to be used, then defibrillation gel pads must first be placed on the chest wall to ensure good contact, reduce transthoracic impedance and prevent burning of the skin.

Self-adhesive pads are widely available in adult and paediatric sizes. They are safe, easy and generally preferable to use.

Procedure guideline 27.13 **Manual defibrillation with self-adhesive pads**

Statement	Rationale
1. Confirm presence of shockable rhythm (VF/pulseless VT) via ECG and check for central pulse during brief pause in ECC.	**1.** To ensure correct management.
2. Immediately resume ECC while the necessary equipment for defibrillation is prepared for use.	**2.** To maintain oxygenation.
3. Plan all actions before shock delivery and ensure all rescuers know what is expected of them.	**3.** To minimise interruption to CPR. To ensure shock delivery is safe and coordinated.
4. To facilitate prompt delivery, the child's weight must be determined.	**4.** To calculate the energy levels required.
5. Prompt, effective and safe defibrillation delivery is dependent on:	**5.**
a) Pad size selection – choose largest available that still permits for space between them (infant pads are generally selected for babies <10 kg; manufacturer's guidelines should be followed).	**a)** To maximise contact with chest wall and to prevent arcing of current.
b) Placement of pads – bracket heart.	**b)** To allow for maximum current flow through the heart.
c) Skin-pad interface – ensure smoothed down on chest with no trapped air bubbles.	**c)** To decrease thoracic impedance to current flow.
d) Energy selection – determined by child's body weight.	**d)** To select lowest energy level likely to be effective, thus minimising potential for myocardial damage.
6a) The self-adhesive pads should be positioned on the chest while ECC continues.	**6a)** To minimise interruption to ECC and maintain coronary and cerebral artery perfusion.
b) The standard sites are one over the apex of the heart (left axilla region in small children) and one to the right of the sternum, just below the clavicle. In known dextrocardia, the pads should be applied in reverse position.	**b)** To bracket the heart appropriately for current delivery.

Procedure guideline 27.13 (*Continued*)

Statement	Rationale
c) In a small infant where there are only large pads available, the baby is positioned on it's side and essentially 'sandwiched' between one pad placed on the anterior chest and the other on their back between the scapulae.	**c)** To ensure the pads do not come in to contact with one another and cause arcing of the delivered current.
7. The designated rescuer should select the energy for appropriate level of joules (4 J/kg) and presses the 'charge' button.	**7.** To charge the machine to the previously selected energy level. To inform other rescuers of stage in procedure.
8. While the defibrillator is charging, all rescuers other than the one performing ECC, should be instructed to 'stand clear' and to remove any oxygen delivery devices as appropriate.	**8.** To facilitate prompt delivery of correct energy level. To minimise interruption to ECC and resultant fall in coronary and cerebral artery perfusion. There is a potential for combustion if the atmosphere is enriched with oxygen.
9. Once the machine is charged (change in audible tone) instruct the rescuer performing ECC to 'stand clear' while performing a quick visual check of the child and immediate surrounding area and confirming there is continued VF/pulseless VT.	**9.** To ensure that no one (including self) is in direct or indirect contact with the child or the surface on which they are lying. To confirm that the child is still in a shockable rhythm. To prevent delivery of an inappropriate shock if the child's rhythm has changed to a non-shockable one.
10a) If the child is still in a shockable rhythm, press the discharge button on the machine. **b)** Without reassessing the rhythm or checking for a pulse, resume CPR starting with ECC.	**10a)** To administer the shock effectively. **b)** To comply with current best practice treatment guidelines. **c)** Even if the defibrillation shock restores a rhythm, it is unlikely to be an effectively perfusing one initially.
11. Continue CPR for 2 minutes; consider reversible causes of arrest and prepare for next pause in ECC.	**11.** To rapidly identify and treat reversible causes. To minimise interruptions in CPR.
12. If after 2 minutes of CPR, VF/pulseless VT persists, proceed as before to deliver second shock.	**12.** To comply with current best practice treatment guidelines.
13. Following the resuscitation attempt, ensure that all defibrillation shocks you delivered are accurately documented in the child's healthcare records.	**13.** To record all interventions and maintain accurate records. To influence post-resuscitation observations and management strategies.
14. The interventions should also be documented on clinical emergency audit forms as appropriate.	**14.** To help with data collection which is vital to inform future practice guidelines.

Medications in cardiorespiratory arrest

Administration of medications in a cardiac arrest should ideally be via a central vascular route (intravenous (IV) or intraosseous (IO)). It is important that each medication is followed by a saline flush.

If access to the circulation is not possible and a tracheal tube is in position, this can be used for delivery of some medications, including adrenaline. This route, however, is less effective as absorption of the medication is unpredictable (Kleinman *et al* 1999). It also requires dosages to be increased for endotracheal

(ET) administration. The Resuscitation Council (2010) discourages this route in its latest guidelines.

There are few medications that are routinely used in cardiorespiratory arrest. Adrenaline is given in all cardiac arrests. If the child has a shockable arrhythmia that is resistant to defibrillation, then amiodarone should also be administered.

There is no place for routine administration of alkalysing agents (e.g. sodium bicarbonate) or glucose. Both of these medications may, however, be indicated by the underlying condition or by biochemical results. In those instances, they should be given on an individualised basis.

Adrenaline

Adrenaline is the first line medication in cardiac arrest. The dose is $10 \mu g/kg$ for IV or IO administration. It should be administered as a bolus injection and should be repeated every 3 minutes as necessary.

As there is no conclusive evidence that an increased dose is beneficial to children in cardiac arrest, subsequent dosages of adrenaline remain the same (Carpenter and Stenmark 1997). The possible exception to this is in the event of cardiac arrest caused by a circulatory collapse (e.g. severe sepsis or anaphylaxis). In this scenario, $100 \mu g/kg$ **may** be used for second and subsequent IV or IO dosages.

Amiodarone

Amiodarone is the anti-arrhythmic medication of choice in shock-resistant VF and pulseless VT. The dosage is $5 mg/kg$ via rapid IV or IO bolus. It is given after the third defibrillation shock and may be repeated after the fifth shock.

Glucose

Due to their high glucose requirements and low glycogen stores, sick infants and children can readily become hypoglycaemic. Low blood glucose levels are known to be a common cause of seizures and also to play a part in depressing myocardial contractility. It is therefore important to ensure that glucose levels are monitored carefully. However, there is evidence to show a correlation between raised glucose levels and poor neurological outcome (Ashwal *et al* 1990, Cherian *et al* 1997). Therefore, only proven hypoglycaemia merits the administration of glucose in resuscitation of children, with care being taken not to cause hyperglycaemia. The recommended dosage is $2 ml/kg$ of 10% glucose (Resuscitation Council 2011a, 2011b).

Intravascular fluids

Where circulatory failure has been the cause of the cardiorespiratory arrest (e.g. hypovolaemia or sepsis), the standard recommended volume of fluid is $10–20 ml/kg$ as a bolus via IV or IO routes. Crystalloid (e.g. 0.9% saline) is recommended rather than colloid for routine resuscitation management.

Potentially reversible causes of cardiorespiratory arrest

It is essential to identify any potentially treatable causes of the cardiac arrest in order to treat them as rapidly as possible, and maximise the chances for ROSC. These causes are best remembered as the '4 Hs and 4 Ts':

Hypoxia	Tension pneumothorax
Hypovolaemia	Tamponade
Hypothermia	Toxicity
Hypo/hyperkalaemia	Thrombo-emboli

Rapid and appropriate treatment of these problems may result in ROSC and ultimate survival of the child. This is why ongoing reassessment of the ABCDE is so vital.

Post-resuscitation care

Once ROSC is achieved, the child must be managed in an area capable of providing ongoing ALS measures. Immediate post-resuscitation investigations should include:

- Arterial and central venous blood gases
- Chest X-ray
- 12-lead ECG
- Bloods:
  - glucose
  - haemoglobin, haematocrit and platelet count
  - cross-match
  - urea and electrolytes
  - clotting screen.

Ongoing management may necessitate transfer to another unit with dedicated PICU facilities. Any transfer (whether it is within the same institution or to another hospital) should be undertaken by staff skilled in intensive care.

Close monitoring of the child's vital signs post-resuscitation is essential to rapidly detect any improvement or deterioration in the child's condition, and allow for modification of their treatment accordingly. This monitoring should include:

- Heart rate and rhythm
- BP
- O_2 saturation
- Core and peripheral skin temperature
- Urinary output
- Arterial blood gases
- CO_2 monitoring (capnography).

Consideration should be given to induced hypothermia (Doherty *et al* 2009, Polderman and Herold 2009, Takasu *et al* 2001) and additional invasive monitoring (e.g. central venous pressure).

Ethical considerations

Presence of family members during resuscitation attempts

It has become much more widespread practice to ask parents/carers (and sometimes other close family members) if they wish to be present during the resuscitation attempt. It is important that this is done in a supportive manner, allowing them to make a decision that feels most appropriate for them (Meyers *et al* 1998). While many will choose to be present, some will decline, and many will change their minds, perhaps choosing to be present for some time and leaving at another.

Whether the parents/carers are present or not, an experienced member of the healthcare team should be allocated to remain with them to ensure appropriate support and information is provided (Robinson *et al* 1998). Additionally, the team leader should at some point during the resuscitation attempt ensure that they take time out to speak directly with them. This is particularly important if the resuscitation attempt is prolonged, or if it in some other respect, seems likely to be unsuccessful.

Ending resuscitation attempts

Resuscitation should be stopped when there are signs of established biological death. Additionally, if there has been no ROSC after 30 minutes of full resuscitation efforts, it is extremely unlikely that there will be a positive outcome (Schindler *et al* 1996, Sirbaugh *et al* 1999). The only exceptions are children with a primary hypothermic event or in cases of poisoning, as there are a number of reports of prolonged resuscitation attempts being successful in these situations.

Do not attempt resuscitation (DNAR) orders

A DNAR order is something that requires sensitive and timely discussion. Local policies will dictate the person(s) most appropriate to discuss it with the family and the specific documentation and communication processes necessary. However, the following are some of the necessary considerations included in a joint statement issued in 2007 by the British Medical Association, Royal College of Nursing and Resuscitation Council (UK):

- Prognosis and expected quality of life
- Anticipated cardiorespiratory arrest
- Informed consent
- Accurate documentation
- Specific palliative care measures agreed
- Arrangements for regular review
- Effective communication to all members of child's care team
- DNAR order can be revoked at any time.

The family (and child if appropriate) must be made aware that a DNAR order relates only to active cardiorespiratory resuscitation interventions and that all palliative care measures to maintain the child's dignity and comfort will be continued and increased as appropriate.

References

Advanced Life Support Group (2011) Advanced Paediatric Life Support. The Practical Approach, 5th edition. London, BMJ

Andropoulos DB, Soifer SJ and Schreiber MD (1990) Plasma epinephrine concentrations after intraosseous and central venous injection during cardiopulmonary resuscitation in the lamb. Journal of Pediatrics, 116 (2) 312–315

Ashwal S, Schneider S, Tomasi L, Thompson J. (1990) Prognostic implications of hyperglycaemia and reduced cerebral blood flow in childhood near-drowning. Neurology, 40, 820–823

Atkins DL, et al (2009) Epidemiology and outcomes from out-of-hospital cardiac arrest in children. Circulation, 119, 1484–1491

Banerjee S, Singhi SC, Singh S, Singh M. (1994) The intraosseous route is a suitable alternative to intravenous route for fluid resuscitation in severely dehydrated children. Indian Pediatrics, 31(12), 1511–1520

Bossaert L. (1999) Electrical defibrillation: new technologies. Current Opinion Anaesthesiology, Apr 12(2), 183–193

Berg MD, Idris AH, Berg RA. (1998) Severe ventilatory compromise due to gastric distention during pediatric cardiopulmonary resuscitation. Resuscitation, 36, 71–73

Biarent D, Bingham R, Eich C, et al. (2010) European Resuscitation Council Guidelines for Resuscitation 2010. Section 6. Paediatric Life Support Resuscitation, 81, 1434–1444

Carpenter TC, Stenmark KR. (1997) High-dose epinephrine is not superior to standard-dose epinephrine in pediatric in-hospital cardiopulmonary arrest. Pediatrics, 99, 403–408

Cherian L, Goodman JC, Robertson CS. (1997) Hyperglycaemia increases brain injury in caused by secondary ischaemia after cortical impact injury in rats. Critical Care Medicine, 25, 1378–1383

Clements F, McGowan J. (2000) Finger position for chest compressions in cardiac arrest in infants. Resuscitation, 44, 43–46

Crone RK. (1983) The respiratory system. In Gregory GA. (ed.) Pediatric Anesthesia, vol 1. New York, Churchill Livingstone, pp35–62

Decisions relating to Cardiopulmonary Resuscitation. A Joint Statement from the British Medical Association, the Resuscitation Council (UK) and the Royal College of Nursing (2007) http://www.resus.org.uk/pages/dnar.htm

Doherty DR, Parshuram CS, Gaboury I, et al. (2009) Hypothermia therapy after pediatric cardiac arrest. Circulation, 119, 1492–1500

Eisenberg M, Bergner L, Hallstrom A. (1983) Epidemiology of cardiac arrest and resuscitation in children. Annals of Emergency Medicine, 12, 672–674

Fiser DH. (1990) Intraosseous infusion. New England Journal of Medicine, 322(220), 1579–1581

Frascone RJ, Jensen J, Wewerka SS, Salzman JG. (2009) Use of the EZ-IO needle by Emergency Medical Service Providers. Pediatric Emergency Care, 25, 329–332

Gausche M, Seidel JS, Henderson DP, Ness B, Ward PM, Wayland BW, Almeida B. (1989) Pediatric deaths and emergency medical services (EMS) in urban and rural areas. Pediatric Emergency Care, 5, 158–162

Gausche M, Lewis RJ, Stratton SJ, Haynes BE, Gunter CS, Godrich SM, Poore PD, McCollough MD, Henderson DP, Pratt FD and Seidel JS. (2000) A prospective randomized study of the effect of out-of-hospital pediatric endotracheal intubation on survival and neurological outcome. JAMA, 283, 783–790

Herlitz J, Engdahl J, Svensson L, Young M, Angquist KA, Holmberg S. (2005) Characteristics and outcome among children suffering from out of hospital cardiac arrest in Sweden. Resuscitation, 64(1), 37–40

Hickey RW, Cohen DM, Strausbaugh S, Dietrich AM. (1995) Pediatric patients requiring CPR in the prehospital setting. Annals of Emergency Medicine, 25, 495–501

ILCOR (2010) International Guidelines 2010 for CPR and ECC – A Consensus on Science. Resuscitation, 46, 1–3 (Part 9 Pediatric Basic Life Support p316)

Kleinman ME, Oh W, Stonestreet BS. (1999) Comparison of intravenous and endotracheal epinephrine during cardiopulmonary resuscitation in newborn piglets. Critical Care Medicine, 27, 2748–2754

Kramer-Johansen J, Wik L, Steen PA. (2006) Advanced cardiac life support before and after tracheal intubation–direct measurements of quality. Resuscitation, 68, 61–69

Kyriacou DN, Arcinue EL, Peek C, Kraus JF. (1994) Effect of immediate resuscitation on children with submersion injury. Pediatrics, 137–142

Lopez-Herce J, Garcia C, Rodriguez-Nunez, Dominguez P, Carrillo A, Calvo C, Delgado MA. (2005) Long-term outcome of paediatric cardiorespiratory arrest in Spain. Resuscitation, 64(1), 79–85

McCarthy G, Buss P. (1998) The calcaneum as a site for Intraosseous infusion. Journal of Accident and Emergency Medicine, 15(6), 421–429

McCrory JH, Downs CE. (1984) Cardiopulmonary resuscitation in infants and children. In Hazinski MF. (ed.) Nursing Care of the Critically Ill Child. St Louis, Mosby, pp 39–54

McCarthy G, O'Donnell C, O'Brien M. (2003) Successful Intraosseous infusion in the critically ill patient does not require a medullary cavity. Resuscitation, 56(2), 183–186

Meyers TA, Eichhorn DJ, Guzzetta CE. (1998) Do families want to be present during CPR? A retrospective survey. Journal of Emergency Nursing, 24, 400–405

Mogayzel C, Quan L, Graves JR, Tiedeman D, Fahrenbruch C, Herndon P. (1995) Out-of-hospital VF in children and adolescents: Causes and outcomes. Annals of Emergency Medicine, 25(4), 484–491

O'Rourke PP. (1986) Outcome of children who are apneic and pulseless in the emergency room. Critical Care Medicine, 14, 466

691

Polderman KH, Herold I. (2009) Therapeutic hypothermia and controlled normothermia in the intensive care unit: practical considerations, side effects, and cooling methods. Critical Care Medicine, 37, 1101–1120

Resuscitation Council (UK) (2010) Guidelines 2010. Available at http://www.resus.org.uk/pages/guide.htm (last accessed 20th December 2011)

Resuscitation Council (UK) (2011a) Provider Manual for use in the UK: European Paediatric Life support Course, 3rd edition. London, Resuscitation Council (UK)

Resuscitation Council (UK) (2011b) Provider Manual for use in the UK: Paediatric Immediate Life support Course, 2nd edition. London, Resuscitation Council (UK)

Robinson SM, Mackenzie-Ross S, Campbell-Hewson GL, Egleston CV, Prevost AT. (1998) Psychological effect of witnessed resuscitation on bereaved relatives. Lancet, 352, 614–617

Ronco R, King W, Donley DK, Tilden SJ. (1995) Outcome and cost at a children's hospital following resuscitation for out-of-hospital cardiopulmonary arrest. Archives of Pediatric Adolescent Medicine, 149(2), 210–214

Rosetti VA, et al (1985) Intraosseous nfusion: An alternative route of pediatric intravascular access. Annals of Emergency Medicine, 14(9), 885–888

Ryder IG, Munro HM, Doull IJ.(1991) Intraosseous infusion for resuscitation. Archives of Disease in Childhood, 66, 1442–1443

Schindler MB, Bohn D, Cox PN, McCrindle BW, Jarvis A, Edmonds J, Barker J. (1996) Outcome of out-of-hospital cardiac or respiratory arrest in children. New England Journal of Medicine, 335(20), 1473–1479

Sirbaugh PE, Pepe PE, Shook JE, Kimball KT, Goldman MJ, Ward MA, Mann DM. (1999) A prospective, population-based study of the demographics, epidemiology, management and outcome of out-of-hospital pediatric cardiopulmonary arrest. Annals of Emergency Medicine, 33, 174–184

Takasu A, Saitoh D, Kaneko N, Sakamoto T, Okada Y. (2001) Hyperthermia: is it an ominous sign after cardiac arrest? Resuscitation, 49, 273–277

Tibballs J, Russell P. (2009) Reliability of pulse palpation by healthcare personnel to diagnose pediatric cardiac arrest. Resuscitation, 80, 61–64

Tortora GJ, Grabowski SJ. (1993) Principles of Anatomy and Physiology, 7th edition. New York, Harper Collins

Wheeler CA. (1989) Pediatric intraosseous infusion: An old technique in modern health care technology. Journal of Intravenous Nursing, 12(6), 371–376

Young KD, Seidel JS. (1999) Pediatric cardiopulmonary resuscitation: a collective review. Annals of Emergency Medicine, 33, 195–205

Chapter 28

Tracheostomy: care and management

Chapter contents

Procedure guidelines

The Great Ormond Street Hospital Manual of Children's Nursing Practices, First Edition. Edited by Susan Macqueen, Elizabeth Anne Bruce, Faith Gibson.
© 2012 Great Ormond Street Hospital for Children NHS Foundation Trust. Published 2012 by Blackwell Publishing Ltd.

Introduction

A tracheostomy is one of the oldest surgical procedures and was first successfully performed on children in the late 19th century. Today it is a common procedure and is life saving for many infants and children requiring airway and respiratory support. More children with chronic medical conditions are surviving, largely due to advances in tracheostomy care and technology support. The vast majority of these children are now being cared for in their own homes and at school. However, despite providing a safe and protective airway, tracheostomy in children is often associated with significant morbidity and mortality (Cooke 2009, Midwinter *et al* 2002). A tracheostomy is an artificial opening in the trachea, usually between the 3rd and 4th tracheal rings, into which a tube is inserted (see Figure 28.1). Although a tracheostomy is a life-saving operation, it can also be life-threatening if the airway is not kept clear from secretions and blockages 24 hours a day.

The most common indications for tracheostomy in children are:

- Cystic hygroma
- Haemangioma
- Laryngomalacia
- Papillomatosis
- Sub-glottic stenosis
- Tracheal stenosis
- Tracheomalacia
- Bronchomalacia
- Trauma
- Vocal cord immobility

- Tumour
- Long-term respiratory support.

This chapter has been adapted from the GOSH clinical practice guidelines, the most recent version of which is available on the GOSH website (Cooke 2009). It includes the following sections and guidelines:

1. Caring for a newly formed tracheostomy
2. Management of a stable tracheostomy
3. Resuscitation
4. Discharge planning.

These guidelines are intended to support practitioners looking after children with tracheostomies to improve the care and safety of this group of children. All practitioners should have appropriate clinical experience in dealing with a child with a tracheostomy and should not rely solely on these guidelines for their practice. Children with tracheostomies require constant supervision from those fully trained in their care. Documentation for the assessment of staff and carer competencies are available at www.gosh.nhs.uk/health-professionals/clinical-guidelines/tracheostomy-care-and-management-review/.

Caring for a newly formed tracheostomy

The initial nursing care of a child with a tracheostomy is very different from that for an established stoma. At Great Ormond Street Hospital (GOSH), the first tube change occurs after 1 week. Other units advocate changing the tube after 3 days (Deutsch 1998). The first tube change should be performed by

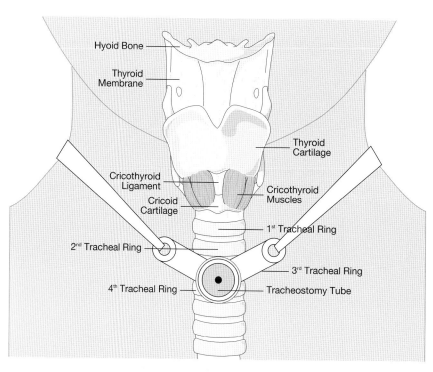

Figure 28.1 Tracheostomy positioning (Cooke 2009).

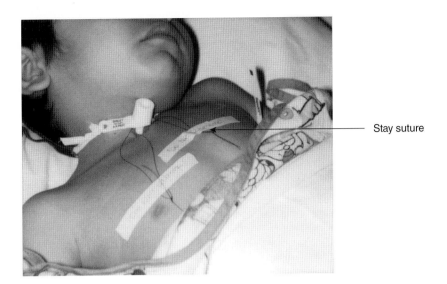

Stay suture

Figure 28.2 Position of stay sutures (Cooke 2009).

a Tracheostomy Nurse Practitioner (TNP) or ENT surgeon. It is essential that the tube stays in situ long enough for the tract to form, so avoiding a difficult and possibly dangerous first tube change. Displacement of the tracheostomy tube in children is a potentially fatal complication. To ensure the safety of the airway, the trachea is sometimes sutured onto the child's skin with tiny interrupted disposable sutures called maturation sutures. These provide an extra safety measure, which facilitates tube replacement (Craig *et al* 2005). In addition, two long looped 'stay' sutures extend from inside the stoma and are taped to the child's chest. These sutures are attached to the tracheal wall on either side of the stoma. These assist with the opening of the stoma during the first week by raising the trachea to the surface of the skin and pulling the stoma apart so that a tube can be inserted. Tape on the child's chest will be labelled '**DO NOT REMOVE**'. Stay sutures are removed after the first tube change when the stoma is more stable (see Figure 28.2).

For information regarding the different types of tracheostomy tubes available and their benefits and disadvantages, see Appendix 28.1.

Principles table 28.1 **Preparation of equipment and environment for tracheostomy**

All equipment must be checked whenever a practitioner takes over the care of a child with a tracheostomy, including breaks and transfers. The child must never be left alone. The accompanying carer (including parents where applicable) must, as a minimum, be able to:
- Recognise the signs of tracheostomy obstruction
- Initiate suctioning of the tracheostomy tube.

Principle	Rationale
1. The child's bed area must be easily accessible from both sides without obstruction for emergency and rapid access. The area should be free from luggage, chairs, etc.	1. To facilitate swift access to the child if required. The child's airway is potentially at risk and they may need immediate attention.
2. Appropriate resuscitation and suction equipment with correct tracheostomy fittings (15mm Smiths Medical (Portex©) swivel connector and a male Smiths Medical (Portex©) adaptor for GOS, Silver and Montgomery tubes) checked and in full working order.	2. To facilitate emergency care quickly.
3. The child should have a dedicated tracheostomy trolley by the bedside containing: a) Oxygen saturation monitoring – if oxygen therapy is required.	3. Specific emergency equipment must be rapidly accessible. a) To enable continual assessment of oxygen requirements.

695

(Continued)

Principles table 28.1 (Continued)

Principle	Rationale
b) Suction catheters – **correct size** – see suctioning section for more details. **c)** Clean gloves. **d)** Clean gauze. **e)** Clean bowl of tap water. **f)** 2 ml syringe. **g)** Ampoule 0.9% sodium chloride. **h)** Waste bag 'for incineration'. **i)** An emergency tracheostomy box containing: • Two spare tracheostomy tubes (one the same size and one a size smaller) • A water based lubricant such as Aqua lube® or KY jelly® • Round ended scissors • Spare tracheostomy tapes • A suction catheter (same internal diameter ID) as the suction catheter used to suction the child).	**b)** To safely suction the tracheostomy tube. **c)** To minimise the risk of cross-contamination. **d)** To clean stoma/secretions. **e)** To flush through suction tubing after use. **f)** To draw up saline for instillation. **g)** For irrigation. **h)** To meet local waste disposal guidelines. **i)** To replace a blocked tube. • If the stomal opening shrinks a smaller tube may need to be inserted • For smoother insertion of the tracheostomy tube • To prevent trauma to the neck when cutting the ties • To secure the tube • To 'railroad' the tube into the stoma (Seldinger technique, refer to resuscitation section).
4. Goggles or protective eye wear should be available.	**4.** To minimise the risk of infection and ensure safety of staff caring for the child.
5. A tube with a 15 mm termination requires a Smiths Medical (Portex©) swivel connector which can be added to the resuscitator and must be available at the child's bedside.	**5.** To enable effective emergency attention if required. This allows a more flexible approach to ventilating the child.
6. A flat-ended tube requires an appropriately sized tracheal tube adapter and a Smiths Medical (Portex©) swivel connector that will 'fit into' the tube as required to create a 15 mm termination that will be compatible with resuscitation equipment.	**6.** To enable effective emergency attention if required. The size must be checked for a 'tight fit'.
7a) At Great Ormond Street, tracheal dilators are kept in the Resuscitation Trolley (not at the child's bedside and must only be used by competent practitioners to assist when reinserting a tube. **b)** Following an audit on dilators, practitioners are now taught the Seldinger technique, which has proven to be effective at replacing tracheosotomy tubes (Lyons et al 2007).	**7a)** Tracheal dilators were removed from the boxes as practitioners were not trained in their use and can 'potentially' cause trauma to the stoma and trachea if used incorrectly. **b)** This is a more non-invasive method of reinserting the tube using a suction catheter.

Procedure guideline 28.1 Caring for a new tracheostomy

Nursing actions and observations during the first 7 days following formation of the tracheostomy centre on observing for possible complications, maintaining the correct positioning and patency of the new tube, stoma maintenance and parental/carer teaching (if appropriate). Replacing tubes in the first week may be problematic, as the stoma may not yet be established.

Statement	Rationale
Initial observations and complications:	
1. The child's vital signs should be recorded in accordance with local policy, with the frequency reducing as the child's condition dictates. Refer to children's early warning scores (CEWS) scoring.	**1.** To ensure the safe recovery from effects of anaesthesia. For more information regarding the CEWS see Chapter 1.

Procedure guideline 28.1 (*Continued*)

Statement	Rationale
2. Practitioners should also carry out routine non-invasive observations:	2. Early detection of potential complications.
a) Check that the tape tension is correct and able to support the tracheostomy tube.	**a)** To prevent accidental decannulation and check for presence of surgical emphysema.
b) Observe any neck swelling (surgical emphysema – see below).	**b)** To observe for surgical emphysema.
c) Check for air entry through tube – place finger above tube opening and feel for a passage of air.	**c–e)** To confirm the position of the tracheostomy tube and rule out complications such as pneumothorax and surgical emphysema.
d) Inspect the chest for bilateral chest movement.	**d–e)** These should be performed by an advanced practitioner or doctor.
e) Auscultate the chest for equal air entry.	

Post-procedural tube check	
1a) For the majority of children a chest X-ray is performed in recovery. If this has not been done a portable chest X-ray must be performed within 1 hour or as soon as possible after the child has returned to the ward.	**1a)** To confirm tube tip position, presence of a pneumothorax or in some cases surgical emphysema (Tarnoff *et al* 1998).
b) If the child is distressed or coughing a flexible endoscopy may be performed post operatively.	**b)** An endoscopy will confirm the tube tip position.

2. Where possible, the child should not leave the ward during the first week unless medically indicated.	2. Their airway is at risk and they must remain in an environment that can cope with any complications.

Procedure guideline 28.2 Detection and management of initial complications

Initial complications include haemorrhage, tube blockage, accidental decannulation, infection and surgical emphysema. These are largely avoidable if the tracheostomy is carefully performed together with dilligent and effective post-operative management.

Statement	Rationale
Haemorrhage	
1. Observe the child and document any bleeding from the tracheostomy.	1. May be primary, reactionary or secondary. A large haemorrhage may be fatal. Secretions may initially be blood stained, but should settle within a few hours.
2. If bleeding continues, contact the Tracheostomy Nurse Practitioner or ENT team.	
3. If any large haemorrhages occur, immediately call the ENT and/or clinical emergency teams as required.	
Tube blockage	
1a) Suction should be performed a minimum of: • ½ – hourly suction for the first 12–24 hours • Then 'as required' until first tube change (Friedman *et al* 2003, Onakoya *et al* 2003, Park *et al* 1999, Seay *et al* 2002, Yaremchuck 2003).	**1a)** To prevent tube occlusion. Although research has shown that children should only be suctioned when required, it is imperative that the tracheostomy tube is kept clear at all times during the first week, so practitioners must be mindful and carry out frequent checks on the tube.

(Continued)

Procedure guideline 28.2 (*Continued*)

Statement	Rationale
2. Children must be nursed in continuous humidity for the first week. This should include warmed humidity for the under 1 year olds and wall humidity for those older, unless requiring oxygen or mechanical support. The humidity may be discontinued for short periods, for bathing or playing.	2. To keep secretions loose and thus easily retrieved from the tube. For more information on humidity, see section below.

Accidental decannulation or tube displacement

Statement	Rationale
1. Care must be taken to ensure that the tube is correctly secured and does not become displaced/dislodged.	1. Early recognition of decannulation or tube displacement is essential as this could be life-threatening. Contact the ENT team/TNP or clinical emergency team for immediate assistance.
2. Check correct tension of the tapes, ensuring that only one finger space can be inserted between the neck and tapes.	2. To minimise the risk of tube displacement.
3. Ensure close observation of respiratory rate, effort, chest movements and air entry on return to the ward.	3. To ensure prompt detection of decannulation or tube displacement.
4. The tube may visibly come out of the stoma or can be pulled out of the trachea and sit in the pre-tracheal tissues. It can be reinserted but **must not be** forced. On reinsertion, tube tip position must be confirmed; ENT team/TNP or clinical emergency team must be contacted immediately to review tube position.	4. Common causes for this include: chubby infant neck, incorrectly chosen tube, loose tracheostomy tapes or the child pulling at the tube.
5. An X-ray or flexible endoscopy may be performed if the position cannot be confirmed with chest auscultation, and/or the child continues to be distressed.	

Infection (chest/stoma site)

Statement	Rationale
1. • The stoma site must be cleaned daily or when soiled using a clean technique and sterile gauze/saline. • The wound must be inspected for signs of inflammation, breakdown/and or infection. • Observe colour and nature of secretions. • Report to medical teams and document all signs of infection.	1. To ensure that any infection or skin breakdown is detected and treated appropriately and as quickly as possible.

Surgical emphysema

Statement	Rationale
2a) Air may leak around the tube into the surrounding tissue – this is particularly problematic if the child has had neck sutures inserted. Contact the ENT team as the stoma sutures may need to be removed.	2a) To allow air to escape from around the neck.
b) Observe for neck/face swelling or if the child complains of discomfort, pain or difficulty with breathing.	b) To detect emphysema.
c) Regularly check tape tension for increased tightness.	c) Checking tape tension not only confirms that the tube is secured correctly but also if they appear tighter may indicate swelling especially if you have never met the child before surgery.

Principles table 28.2 Feeding the child with a tracheostomy

Principle	Rationale
1. If there have been no previous feeding concerns, the child may recommence their normal feeds after a specified time of being 'nil orally'. This is normally 3 hours post-operation, but practitioners must confirm this with the anaesthetic chart.	1. The vocal cords are sprayed during procedure, making them less responsive/effective in protecting the airway from aspiration. The effect of the local anesthetic can continue for up to 3 hours.
2. Water should be offered initially. If the child shows signs of aspiration (e.g. coughing after/during drinking, or visible drink coming out of the tracheostomy), keep child nil orally and contact the ENT team and speech and language therapist.	2. To ensure the child is not put at risk of potential aspiration and that individual feeding issues are addressed.
3. For a child who has had feeding difficulties or has never fed orally, consultation with a speech and language therapist should be sought before commencing oral feeds.	3. To ensure the child is not put at risk of potential aspiration and that individual feeding issues are addressed.
4. It is important that the tracheostomised child remains systemically hydrated and practitioners should consider increasing the child's intake during times of illness such as vomiting, diarrhoea, pyrexia, etc.	4. Good systemic hydration will help keep secretions loose and allow for easy retrieval on suctioning.

Humidification

Maintenance of the humidity and warmth of inspired air is an essential part of tracheostomy management, as the normal functions of the upper respiratory tract have been bypassed (Harkin and Russell 2001). The nose and naso-pharynx normally ensure that inspired air reaches a temperature of 37°C and 100% relative humidity; bypassing these with a tracheostomy dedicates such functions to the lower airways, which are poorly suited to the task. Inspiration of cool and dry air may create many problems for the tracheostomised child. Impairment and destruction of cilia reduces the proximal transportation of mucus (Jackson 1996). Secretions become increasingly thick and tenacious, making their expulsion difficult. This may lead to blockage of the tube. Additionally, cold inspired air increases heat loss from the respiratory tract, a particular danger for the small infant (American Thoracic Society 2000).

Heat and moisture exchangers (HME) consist of multiple layers of water repellent paper or foam membranes, which trap heat and moisture during exhalation. Cold inhaled air is then warmed and moisturised, thus maintaining the optimum respiratory tract environment. Several varieties of HME may be used, but a number of important aspects should be considered. The HME must be lightweight to avoid traction on the tracheostomy tube as this may cause skin irritation or even accidental decannulation. For similar reasons, ventilation attachments should be used with care. Additionally, the internal volume of the HME will add to respiratory dead space, increasing the work of breathing. This may be further increased by the accumulation of secretions within the device; manufacturers therefore recommend changing the HME daily or whenever contaminated. There are several types available and care should be taken to ensure that the correct HME based on the weight of the child is used. In GOSH the Gibeck Mini Vent® is used for infants under 1 year (usually under 10 kgs), which are specially designed for smaller

tidal volumes and cause minimal resistance to breathing. Children over 1 year or 10 kg (whichever comes first) should wear the Thermovent T™ from Smiths Medical, and infants and children requiring additional oxygen should use the Trachphone™ from Platon Medical. These provide the child with an excellent way of providing heat and moisture to inspired air; they are small, easy to use and allow the child to be mobile. They should be worn at all times, where possible. For children who refuse to wear the HME, practitioners should trial the Trachphone as they can be suctioned through. As a last resort, a Buchanan bib could be used, which contains a foam layer that absorbs moisture from the child's expired gases and can easily be tucked into clothing. Some manufacturers' products have securing ties, which may not be suitable for younger children due to the risk of strangulation. An HME should not be used during the first week post tracheostomy formation, as it does not provide enough humidity to prevent tube occlusion in the initial phase.

The ill/hospitalised child with a tracheostomy may require extra humidity and this can be delivered via a nebuliser or by a continuous humidity system. Nebulisers provide aerosol droplets in a saturated vapour. The advantage of using water droplets in the respiratory tract is not well documented or understood and some argue that excessive saturation of the lower airways may cause atelectasis and impair the function of distal cilia (Conway et al 1992, Harris and Riley 1967). For this reason nebulisers should be used as an addition to and not replace a primary method of humidification.

Water humidifiers are particularly useful when there is a higher requirement for humidification, for example, when the child requires a high minute volume during an acute respiratory illness or post anaesthesia (Klein 1974). Care must be taken when assessing the effectiveness of water humidifiers; water droplets must be visible along the whole of the elephant tubing. Warmed humidity must be used for small and vulnerable infants and those receiving oxygen therapy.

Procedure guideline 28.3 Humidification

Statement	Rationale
1. Administer humidity via sterile water and elephant tubing **continuously** for 1 week as far as is practicable. The child may come off for short periods, i.e. to feed, play, bathe, mobilise, etc.	1. Effective humidification will contribute to preventing tube occlusion by keeping secretions loose.
2. Small and vulnerable infants under 1 year must have continuous warmed humidity.	2. To prevent lowering of core temperature.
3. Change humidity apparatus when the bottled water needs changing (usually 24 hrs) or earlier if contaminated with secretions or if the mask comes into contact with the floor. When not in use, the mask should be covered.	3. To reduce infection risk in line with local and national infection control polices.
4. Dating and marking when these should be changed and good documentation will reduce infection risk.	

Procedure guideline 28.4 Other care needs

Statement	Rationale
1. Change the tapes at least daily or when soiled or wet.	1. To minimise bacterial colonisation of the skin/stomal area. Monitor stomal healing.
2. A suitable dressing, such as Trachi-dress®, should be inserted behind the flanges to protect the skin (shiny side to skin). Avoid using bulky substitutes as these may pull the tube away from the neck precipitating accidental decannulation.	2. Use of the correct dressing will enhance skin protection and reduce risks to the child.
3. Never use cotton wool or cut keyhole gauze dressings.	3. Flecks of displaced cotton may enter the respiratory tract.
4. The tracheostomy tube should be changed for the first time 7 days after surgery. The tracheostomy tube should normally be changed for the first time by the ENT surgeon or the Tracheostomy Nurse Practitioner. The stay sutures will be removed at this time.	4. This is potentially the most dangerous of tube changes, as the stoma is still new and not fully formed.
5. Once the stability of the tracheostomy stoma and tract has been verified the child may be allowed off the ward with a person appropriately trained in routine and emergency tracheostomy skills.	5. Continuous risk assessment of the tracheostomy stoma will ensure the appropriate staff care for the child in each environment.

Management of an established tracheostomy

Suctioning

Airway suctioning is a common practice in the care of a child with a tracheostomy, and is undertaken to remove secretions from the child's respiratory tract. A child with a tracheostomy may find it difficult to clear their secretions effectively there-fore suction is an essential aspect of their care. Suctioning is associated with many potential complications and is now only recommended when there are clear indications that the patency or ventilation of the children could be compromised (Ahn and Hwang 2003, Czarnik et al 1991, Dellinger 2001, Fiorentini 1992, Gemma et al 2002, Prasad and Hussey 1995, Pritchard et al 2001, Raymond, 1995, Spence et al 2003);. The GOSH Guideline on Airway Suction is a useful resource (Simpson 2009).

The main complications of suctioning include:

- Hypoxia
- Formation of distal granulation tissue/ulceration
- Cardiovascular changes
- Pneumothorax
- Atelectasis
- Bacterial infection
- Intracranial changes.

Practitioners trained in the skill should perform tracheostomy suctioning to minimise complications and maximise treatment (NMC 2002). The child and family must be informed of the reasons for suctioning, positioning, risks and outcomes as appropriate. A 'clean' technique must be used and the catheter should be discarded if the tip is contaminated with hands, cot sides, etc. Suction equipment must accompany the child at all times, regardless of the nature of the journey or the distance to be travelled.

Practitioners must be aware that some pre-term, vulnerable infants and especially those who are requiring more than 40% inspired oxygen, may require pre-oxygenation prior to suctioning to minimise a potential hypoxic event (Odell *et al* 1993, Pritchard *et al* 2001, Sigler and Willis 1985).

Distal tracheal damage and hypoxia are very real and potential complications especially in the vulnerable paediatric airway. These complications may be reduced by having:

- The correct size catheter: As a guide practitioners should double the size of the tracheostomy tube to obtain the appropriate catheter size, e.g., 4.0 ID tracheostomy tube = size 8Fr catheter. A suction catheter diameter should be less than half of the size of the tracheostomy tube to reduce potential for hypoxia and allow the child to breathe throughout the procedure (Ahn and Hwang 2003, Glass and Grap 1995, Odell et al 1993, Wood 1998).
- One distal and 2 lateral ports with rounded ends: This allows secretions to be collected both distally and from the sides of the tube to minimise tube occlusion; if there were more than three lateral holes then the catheter wall would be too weak. There is no need to 'twist the catheter on withdrawal' (Ahn and Hwang 2003).
- A lateral port that is smaller than the distal port: To prevent mucosal adhesion and biopsy (Fiorentini 1992, Luce *et al* 1998).

- An integrated valve for vacuum control: Suction should only be applied on removal. Catheters should not be kinked prior to insertion in an effort to control the vacuum (Prasad and Hussey 1995).
- Suction catheters with graduations: So that practitioners can measure the exact depth to be suctioned.

Suctioning should not occur distal to the tube tip. Catheters should only be inserted so that the distal hole sits at the end of the tube. This allows collection of secretions but not trauma to the distal tracheal mucosa (Brodsky *et al* 1987, Runton 1992).

Suction pressures should be kept to a minimum; as a general guide, pressures should not exceed 60–80 mmHg (8–10 kPa) for neonates/small infants and up to 120 mmHg <16 kPa for older children (see Table 28.1) (Billau 2004, Dean 1997, Mowery 2002, Simpson 2009, Young 1984). Excessive pressures can cause trauma, hypoxaemia and atelectasis (Czarnik *et al* 1991).

Suctioning is not a painful or distressing procedure if performed correctly; in fact most infants will remain asleep throughout. If the child becomes distressed during suctioning then practitioners should revise their technique. Suctioning a child's tracheostomy is very different from suctioning an adult tube, so adult practitioners will need to adapt their practice. Constant observation of the child during suctioning is essential; practitioners should observe for an improvement or deterioration in respiratory rate and quality, child's colour, and oxygen saturations (if being monitored).

Table 28.1 Tube sizes and suction pressures by age

Age of child	Approximate tube size	Suction Pressures
Pre-term – 1 month	3.0	8–10 kPa 60–75 mmHg
0–3 yrs	3.5–5.0	10–12 kPa 75–90 mmHg
3–10 yrs	5.0–6.0	12–15 kPa 90–112 mmHg
10–16 yrs	6.0–7.0	15–20 kPa 112–150 mmHg

Procedure guideline 28.5 Suctioning

Statement	Rationale
1. Gather the following equipment: • Suction catheters of the correct size (see Table 28.1). • Suction unit with variable vacuum control • Gloves • Apron (if there is time – a child should never wait for suctioning) • Tap water (in clean container) • 2 ml syringe with 0.9% sodium chloride for irrigation (not for routine suctioning) • Waste bag 'for incineration'.	

(Continued)

Procedure guideline 28.5 (*Continued*)

Statement	Rationale
2. Perform a clinical hand wash (if there is time).	**2, 3.** To minimise the risk of infection.
3. Gel squirt and put on gloves as a minimum.	
4. Turn the suction unit on, check the vacuum pressure and set to the appropriate level, according to the child's age.	**4.** To use the correct suction pressure that maximises suction, and minimises complications.
5a) The carer **MUST** know the length and type of the tracheostomy tube. **b)** If the tube is fenestrated then an un-fenestrated inner tube should be inserted prior to suctioning.	**5a)** Accurate knowledge will ensure the child's safety and prevent distal trauma from deep suctioning. **b)** To prevent the catheter going through the fenestration and causing trauma to the posterior tracheal wall.
6a) Insert the catheter gently into the tracheostomy tube, far enough to ensure that the lateral and distal holes just pass through the tip of the tube. Use the graduations on the catheter as a guide. **b)** Do not apply suction on insertion.	**6a)** To prevent distal tracheal damage. Adult literature suggests longer distances (Luce *et al* 1998), however the distance between the tube tip and a child's carina may be a few millimetres. **b)** This may cause mucosal irritation, damage and hypoxia (Czarnik *et al* 1991, Luce *et al* 1998).
7. Handle only the proximal end of the catheter. Catheters should be discarded if the end has been touched before insertion.	**7.** To minimise the risk of infection.
8a) Once the catheter has been inserted, apply suction by placing thumb over the valve, found either on catheter or suction tubing. Do not kink the catheter (Czarnik *et al* 1991). **b)** Do not employ an intermittent suction technique.	**8a)** To prevent a vacuum build-up, which on release may cause high suction pressures, resulting in biopsies of fragile tracheal mucosa. **b)** Iintermittent suctioning is contentious and does not reduce trauma (Luce *et al* 1998).
9. Slowly withdraw the catheter straight out of the tube, maintaining the vacuum. There is no need to rotate the suction catheter on withdrawal.	**9.** Both the distal and lateral holes on the new style of catheter allow for circumferential suctioning.
10. The maximum duration of each suction attempt should be determined by the individual child's clinical response, but should be limited to and should not exceed 5–10 seconds (Sumner 1990, Toils and Stone 1990, Young 1984).	**10.** Limiting the suctioning time minimises hypoxia, which is significantly related to duration of suction attempts. Most of the literature is based on the adult population.
11. Where possible, secretions should be cleared on the first attempt.	**11.** Adult literature suggests that episodes should be limited to three, to limit potential side effects and maximise the recovery period (Luce *et al* 1993).
12. The catheter may be re-used if immediate suction is required, as long as secretions have not occluded the suction ports and the distal end of the catheter has not been contaminated prior to the suctioning episode.	**12.** There is no evidence to suggest that using the same catheter up to three times at the same suctioning episode, increases the risk of infection. In fact with effective re-training on technique, some institutions have repeatedly used the same catheter on the same patient for a 24-hour period and have reported no increase in infection (Scoble *et al* 2001).
13. Wrap the catheter around the gloved hand; remove the glove by inserting it over the used catheter and discard in yellow waste bag according to local waste policy.	**13.** To prevent infection risks and contamination of staff and other patients.
14. Flush suction tubing with tap water and connect a new catheter to the tubing.	**14.** To clear the tubing of secretions.

Procedure guideline 28.5 (*Continued*)

Statement	Rationale
15. Observe for and record secretions that are bloody, purulent, foul smelling or unusually thick in the child's healthcare records. Take samples as required and inform medical team of changes.	**15.** Accurate and early documentation will ensure early alert of infection risks.
16. Deep suctioning may be required in certain circumstances, but this should not be routine practice (Bailey *et al* 1988).	**16.** To provide the most appropriate care for the child's needs.
17. Instillation of saline should not be done routinely (Ackerman and Mick 1998, Blackwood 1999, Hudak and Bond-Domb 1996, Pritchard *et al* 2001, Scoble *et al* 2001).	**17.** Other methods, such as continuous humidity, nebulisers, good systemic hydration are far better ways of keeping secretions loose enough not to occlude the tracheostomy tube.

Procedure guideline 28.6 **Tape changes (cotton)**

A tracheostomy tube is held in place with cotton tapes around the neck. It is essential that the ties are secure and the tension is correct. The tapes are secured with knots tied either side of the tracheostomy tube. Velcro ties are not routinely used at GOSH as they can be easily undone by young children (Cooke 2009). If Velcro ties are used in the trust then a risk assessment must be completed in accordance with Trust policy and documented in the local and trust risk registers.

Statement	Rationale
1. All staff/parents/carers should be taught to tie the tapes in the same way.	**1.** To ensure continuity of training.
2. Parents/carers may prefer to adopt another method of securing the tapes once they have established a routine at home. This method may be continued when the child is re-admitted to hospital but will need individual assessment.	**2.** To ensure the continuity of care for the child and family as an expert carer.
3. Tracheostomy tape changes are normally performed daily.	**3.** To ensure comfort and cleanliness and to assess the stoma site.
4. Only personnel trained and competent in the techniques involved must change tracheostomy tapes (NMC 2002) and two people are required.	**4.** To ensure the child's safety during the procedure.
5. The following equipment should be prepared and readily available: **a)** Appropriate emergency equipment. **b)** Gauze swabs and saline sachets. **c)** Two lengths of 0.6 cm cotton tape with short plastic backing. The backing can be made from appropriately sized available tubing, e.g. 24 hr urine or O_2 tubing. **d)** Cut the ends of the tapes to a point. **e)** Round ended scissors. **f)** A rolled up towel to place under the child's shoulders. **g)** A blanket to swaddle a baby or uncooperative toddler. **h)** Suction equipment available (see suction guidelines). **i)** Non-sterile gloves and an apron. **j)** Goggles/protective eye wear. **k)** Child's own comforter, e.g. dummy, as appropriate.	**5.** **a)** For management of accidental decannulation. **d)** To allow insertion into the tube flanges. **f)** To hyper-extend the neck, making observation and cleaning of the stoma easier. **g)** To minimise the risk of accidental decannulation.

(*Continued*)

Procedure guideline 28.6 (*Continued*)

Statement	Rationale
6. Options for keeping the child still must be discussed with the child and parents/carers, as swaddling the child may cause increased distress. Involve the play specialist where possible. Most children will settle once they get used to the procedure, especially when parents/carers begin to do it. An older child may not require swaddling. Some children assist with the procedure by holding the tracheostomy tube in place and some may even prefer to sit during a change.	**6.** To ensure the child is as comfortable as possible during the procedure and has a say in the procedure as their age and mental capability allows.
7. To change the tracheostomy tapes:	**7.**
a) Perform a clinical hand wash, put on gloves, apron and protective eye wear (parents/carers do not need to wear the protective clothing).	**a)** To reduce the risk of infection.
b) The warmed water should be poured onto the gauze swabs.	
c) Assistant to swaddle baby, exposing shoulders and above.	
d) Place baby/child in supine position, with a rolled up towel under shoulders (as mentioned above, some older children may wish to sit).	**d)** To provide easy access to the tracheostomy.
e) Place clean tapes behind the baby/child's neck.	**e)** To ensure the new tapes are in position for easy use.
f) Assistant should hold tube in position using either their thumb and index finger or index and middle finger (see Figure 28.3). Minimal pressure should be applied.	**f)** To support the tracheostomy tube and preventing an accidental decannulation.
g) Tape changer should cut the tapes between the knot and the flange and remove dirty ties.	**g)** For patient comfort and to prevent any risk to the child.
h) The stoma site (above, below and under each flange and back of the neck should be cleaned and thoroughly dried with the water and gauze using a clean technique.	**h)** For patient comfort and to prevent infection and loss of skin integrity.
i) Thread the new tape through the flange on the side *furthest* away from the tape changer.	
j) Tie the tapes using three knots ensuring the tape is flat to the child's skin.	
k) Thread tape through *near* side flange, tie once and make a bow.	
l) Check tape tension by raising baby/child to a sitting position whilst assistant continues to hold tube in position. With the baby/child's head bent forward it should be possible to slip one finger comfortably between the ties and the baby/child's neck (see Figure 28.4).	**l)** To ensure the tapes are firm enough to hold the tube safely in position.
m) If the ties are too tight or loose lay the baby/child back down, undo the bow and readjust.	
n) If the tension is correct, lie the baby/child down and change the bow into three knots by pulling the loops of the bow through to create a second knot.	**n)** So that the tension is not lost.
o) Tie one further knot to secure the ties.	
p) Cut off excess tape to leave 1 cm remaining.	
q) Assistant may release tube **ONLY** when instructed to do so.	
r) Ensure baby/child is made comfortable.	
s) Clear away equipment according to local waste disposal policy.	**s)** To reduce risk of cross-infection and contamination.
t) Wash hands.	
u) Record the tape change in the baby/child's healthcare records.	**u)** To ensure good communication between colleagues.
v) Check all equipment is replaced and restocked as necessary.	

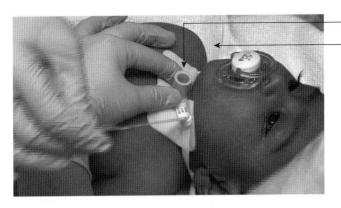

Support tracheostomy tube

Rolled up towel under shoulders

Figure 28.3   Positioning for a tape/tube change (Cooke 2009).

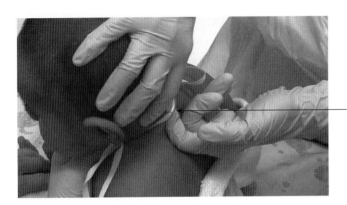

One finger should slip comfortably between the ties and the child's neck

Figure 28.4   Tape tension (Cooke 2009).

Procedure guideline 28.7 Tracheostomy tube changes (planned)

Tracheostomy tubes can be changed weekly or monthly (see Appendix 28.1). Ask the TNP or child's doctor if unsure. Only personnel trained and competent in the technique should perform a tracheostomy tube change (NMC 2002). Two people are required, although a single-handed tube change is taught to parents/carers prior to discharge. An older child should not require swaddling. Some children may assist with the procedure, such as cleaning the stoma site, holding the tracheostomy tube, etc. Some children may need to be swaddled to maintain their safety during the change; assess each child individually.

Statement	Rationale

1. The following equipment should be prepared and readily available:
   - Emergency equipment, oxygen and suction
   - A tracheostomy tube of the same size
   - A tracheostomy tube that is a size smaller
   - A water based lubricant such as Aqualube® or KY jelly®
   - Gauze swabs
   - Saline sachets
   - Two lengths of 0.6 cm cotton tape
   - Round ended scissors
   - A rolled up towel
   - Gloves and an apron
   - Goggles/protective eye wear
   - Two syringes may be required if the child has a cuffed tube.

705

(Continued)

Procedure guideline 28.7 (*Continued*)

Statement	Rationale
To change a tracheostomy tube: **2.** Perform a clinical hand wash. **3.** Put on gloves, apron and protective eye wear.	**2, 3.** To minimise the risk of infection.
4. Assistant to swaddle baby, exposing shoulders and above (baby in supine position if appropriate).	**4.** For patient comfort and safety.
5. Lubricate new tube with a 'dot' of water-based lubricant on the outside bend of the tube.	**5.** For patient safety and to reduce risk of trauma to the stoma.
6. Insert obturator (introducer) into the tube.	**6.** To stiffen the tube.
7. Position the rolled up towel under the child's shoulders, as per tape changes.	**7.** To hyper-extend the neck, exposing the stoma and facilitating an easier change.
8. Place the clean tapes behind the baby/child's neck.	
9. Assistant should hold the tube in position using either their thumb and index finger, or index and middle finger.	**9.** To maximise comfort for the child by not pushing down on the tube.
10. Tube changer should cut the ties between knot and flange.	
11. Remove the dirty ties.	
12. Remove the tube from the stoma with a curved action and dispose.	
13. Quickly insert new tube with a curved action.	
14. Remove obturator.	**14.** This occludes the tube, so the child will not be able to breathe with it in.
15. The assistant should take over and hold the tube in position.	
16. The stomal area and back of the neck should be cleaned and dried with the water and gauze using a clean technique.	
17. The ties are then tied using the method previously described.	

Resuscitation

The basics of cardio-pulmonary resuscitation (CPR) and basic life support (BLS) are universal to all protocols for emergency care: airway management; rescue breathing; circulatory support.

The airway element of BLS will require modification in children with tracheostomies, it is therefore essential that practitioners have received training in both routine and tracheostomy BLS. BLS is similar in the sequence of skills to be performed for those with a tracheostomy: Safety, Stimulate, Shout, Suction, Airway, Breathing, Circulation. When applied to a patient with a tracheostomy, CPR may be more difficult to teach and to learn because additional processes are required to determine and correct the cause of the collapse. Practitioners caring for a child with a tracheostomy must familiarise themselves with the tracheostomy resuscitation algorithm (see Figure 28.6). Patients with a tracheostomy must always have their specific emergency equipment correctly assembled and easily accessible as previously discussed.

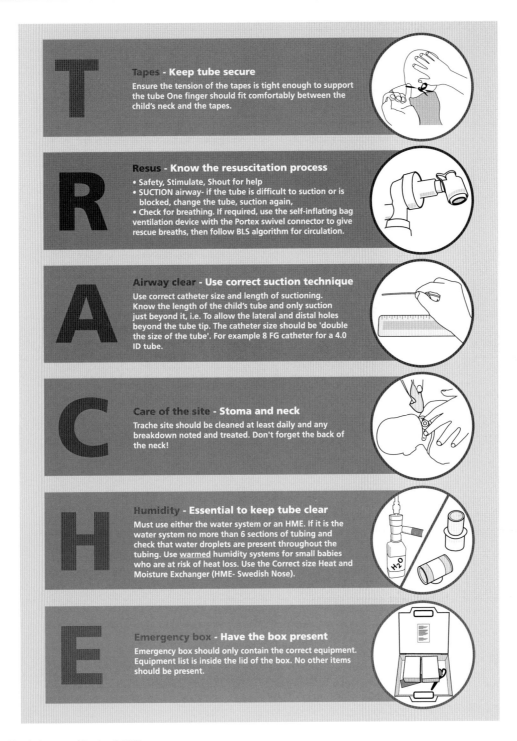

Tapes - Keep tube secure

Ensure the tension of the tapes is tight enough to support the tube One finger should fit comfortably between the child's neck and the tapes.

Resus - Know the resuscitation process

- Safety, Stimulate, Shout for help
- SUCTION airway- if the tube is difficult to suction or is blocked, change the tube, suction again,
- Check for breathing. If required, use the self-inflating bag ventilation device with the Portex swivel connector to give rescue breaths, then follow BLS algorithm for circulation.

Airway clear - Use correct suction technique

Use correct catheter size and length of suctioning. Know the length of the child's tube and only suction just beyond it, i.e. To allow the lateral and distal holes beyond the tube tip. The catheter size should be 'double the size of the tube'. For example 8 FG catheter for a 4.0 ID tube.

Care of the site - Stoma and neck

Trache site should be cleaned at least daily and any breakdown noted and treated. Don't forget the back of the neck!

Humidity - Essential to keep tube clear

Must use either the water system or an HME. If it is the water system no more than 6 sections of tubing and check that water droplets are present throughout the tubing. Use warmed humidity systems for small babies who are at risk of heat loss. Use the Correct size Heat and Moisture Exchanger (HME- Swedish Nose).

Emergency box - Have the box present

Emergency box should only contain the correct equipment. Equipment list is inside the lid of the box. No other items should be present.

Figure 28.5 'Trache' poster (Cooke 2009).

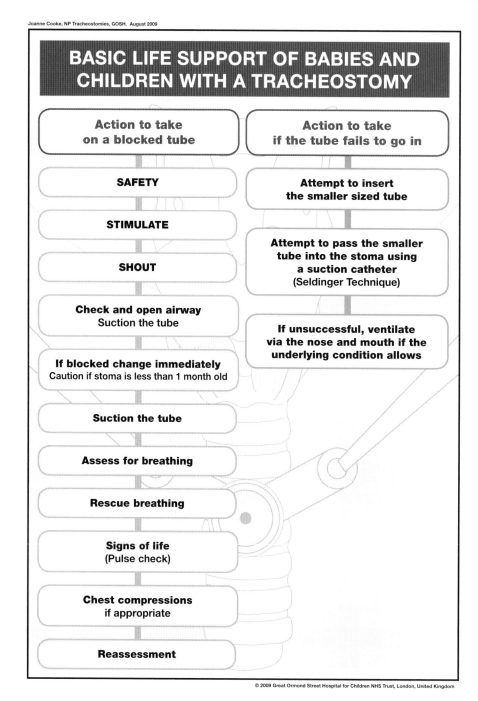

Joanne Cooke, NP Tracheostomies, GOSH. August 2009

BASIC LIFE SUPPORT OF BABIES AND CHILDREN WITH A TRACHEOSTOMY

Action to take on a blocked tube	Action to take if the tube fails to go in
SAFETY	**Attempt to insert the smaller sized tube**
STIMULATE	**Attempt to pass the smaller tube into the stoma using a suction catheter** (Seldinger Technique)
SHOUT	
Check and open airway Suction the tube	**If unsuccessful, ventilate via the nose and mouth if the underlying condition allows**
If blocked change immediately Caution if stoma is less than 1 month old	
Suction the tube	
Assess for breathing	
Rescue breathing	
Signs of life (Pulse check)	
Chest compressions if appropriate	
Reassessment	

© 2009 Great Ormond Street Hospital for Children NHS Trust, London, United Kingdom

Figure 28.6 Tracheostomy resuscitation algorithm (Cooke 2009).

Procedure guideline 28.8 Tracheostomy resuscitation

Statement	Rationale
1. Starting BLS quickly is extremely important.	1. To prevent/minimise hypoxia and subsequent tissue death. Early intervention may prevent progression into full cardio-respiratory arrest.
2. Ensure safety of yourself and the child.	
3. Stimulate the child and call their name, taking care to support their head and body.	3. This may be sufficient to rouse the child.
4. Call for assistance from colleagues.	4. Always summon more help, to assist in tube changes, bringing other equipment, etc.
5. If you are by yourself DO NOT leave the child at this stage.	5. Commencing airway, breathing support is of primary importance as per basic life support policy.
6. Open and check the child's airway by placing them supine on a flat firm surface.	6. To tilt the head and expose the airway.
7. It may be helpful to put a folded towel under the shoulders, only if this is immediately available. Do not waste time by collecting this equipment.	7. To extend the neck and open the airway stoma.
8. Gently tilt the tip of the chin upward, taking care not to press on soft tissue underneath.	8. To ensure the airway is opened.
9. Inspect tube for obvious problems, i.e. signs of blockage: crusts, kinks or dislodgement.	9. Initial assessment of the airway is important for effective future support.
10. **IF IN ANY DOUBT ABOUT CHILD'S CONDITION, SUMMON THE CLINICAL EMERGENCY TEAM IMMEDIATELY.**	
11. Suction the tracheostomy tube.	11. In most circumstances suctioning will clear the obstruction.
12. Change the tracheostomy tube immediately if the tube appears blocked or any resistance is felt and the child is in distress. **Exercise caution if the stoma is less than one week old; if time, contact the TNP/ ENT team/Emergency team first.** However, if the child's condition is unstable, summon the Clinical Emergency Team immediately.	12. If there is a physical airway obstruction changing the tracheotomy tube will improve the child's condition.
13. The same size tube should be inserted. If unable to insert the same size tube try to insert the smaller one.	13. A smaller airway is better than no airway to allow oxygen into the respiratory system.
14. If the stoma closes and the smaller tube cannot be replaced, remove the Obturator from the smaller tube and pass a suction catheter through the tube. Then attempt to insert the end of the catheter through the stoma opening and guide the tracheostomy tube along the catheter and through the stoma (Seldinger technique).	
15. If this is also unsuccessful, ventilation can be attempted via the catheter threaded in to the stoma (as described previously) or by conventional rescue breaths (e.g. mouth-to-mouth or bag and mask over the mouth and nose). These options may not be appropriate for some children due to their underlying airway problem; practitioners must therefore always be aware of the underlying disease/anatomy.	

(Continued)

Procedure guideline 28.8 (*Continued*)

Statement	Rationale
16. The Seldinger technique should be practised as a first line attempt at reinserting a tracheostomy tube. Tracheal dilators should only be used by practitioners familiar and practised in their use. Tracheal dilators are currently kept in the resuscitation trolley for use on request from experienced practitioners (Lyons *et al* 2007).	
17. Assess breathing: Supporting the new tube, place the side of your face over the tracheostomy tube to listen and feel for any breathing. At the same time look at the child's chest to observe any breathing movement. Take up to a maximum of 10 seconds to do this.	**17–20.** To adhere to national life support assessment criteria (Resuscitation Council (UK) 2010).
18. If the child is breathing adequately, give oxygen and keep their airway open by regular suction and await for the clinical emergency team/ENT/TNP and/or CSPs to arrive (practitioners should decide on whom best to call).	
19. If the child is not breathing (or only making agonal gasps), commence artificial respiration with a bag-valve system directly connected to the tracheostomy tube and administer five breaths. This is best achieved with a Smiths Medical (Portex©) 15 mm swivel connector attached to the Ambu bag.	
20. Ensure that the breaths are effective by observing chest movement.	
21. Oxygen should be set at a minimum of 15 litres.	**21.** To ensure adequate oxygen delivery.
22. Parents/carers will be taught mouth to trachy resuscitation by a suitably qualified BLS instructor before discharge. In addition to the other equipment required they must be given a Smiths Medical (Portex©) catheter mount 15 mm female, disconnection wedge and two 'emergency' Velcro tapes.	**22, 23.** To enable parents to secure the airway and perform BLS in an emergency situation at home.
23. Although community teams will supply the equipment for the child's discharge home, the parents/carers should be given two pairs of Velcro tapes, two disconnection wedges, and two tracheostomy extensions from Smiths Medical (Portex©) +/- male to female adapters depending on tube chosen. Practitioners should seek advice from the TNP; these items should be added to their emergency boxes when they get home.	
24. Parents/carers require both theoretical and practical teaching/practice of both emergency algorithms, namely action to take on a blocked tube and action to take if the tracheostomy tube cannot be replaced (Seldinger technique). Practitioners teaching parents/carers must have appropriate knowledge and experience in both areas. At GOSH, a modified 'Resus baby' and 'Little Junior' is used for BLS and a Smiths Medical (Portex©) percutaneous tracheostomy manikin for parents/carers to practise the Seldinger technique.	**24.** Education for the family to assess knowledge and competence is vital to ensure the child's safety.

Further BLS instructions can be found on the Resuscitation Council Guidelines (2010) and in Chapter 27 (Resuscitation) in this book.

Procedure guideline 28.9 Preparation for discharge (see Figure 28.7)

Statement	Rationale
1. The formation of a tracheostomy must be confirmed by telephone with the child's Health Visitor (HV), GP, Paediatric Community Nurse (PCN), School Nurse and local hospital on the day the tracheostomy is inserted. An equipment list and introductory letter must be sent so that equipment can be ordered immediately (New Equipment Form – Figure 28.8). The community team must be contacted after 1 week to confirm tube style/size, which may have had to be changed during the first week.	
2. The progress of supply orders should also be checked. Discussion of respite and carer support should be broached with community team. Most children will be discharged back via their local hospital, which will allow local services and support to be activated. Negotiations to do this should begin as soon as the tracheostomy is formed. However, some children, such as those who have had a planned tracheostomy or who have been in hospital for a long time, may be discharged home straight from hospital. Some equipment may have to be provided to facilitate this; this should be discussed individually with the communities involved. All appropriate documentation and medicines should be ordered/completed.	2, 3. To ensure safe and timely discharge.
3. Ensure that the portable suction unit has been collected from the community team before the day of discharge and bought to the hospital for the transfer home and parents/carers are aware of how it works.	

4. The child's parents, or two main carers, must be taught and be deemed as competent in the following:
• Tracheostomy tube changes (minimum of two)
• Tracheostomy tape changes
• Stoma care
• Suctioning
• Resuscitation skills/emergency care.
  The carer must stay with their child and carry out all care overnight.
  It is important that the carer feels confident in their ability to take the child out of the hospital.
	4, 5. To ensure that parents/carers receive competency based training.

5. Tracheostomy and resuscitation booklets are available to support training. All training provided must be recorded on the child's discharge planner and kept in their health record for future reference. An 8-week ENT outpatient appointment must be arranged prior to discharge (unless indicated otherwise by the medical team).	
6. Confirm discharge of the child with HV and/or PCN and GP as appropriate.	6. To ensure continuity of care.
7. Ensure BLS training and equipment have been provided as described in the previous section.	

Joanne Cooke, NP Tracheostomies, GOSH. August 2009

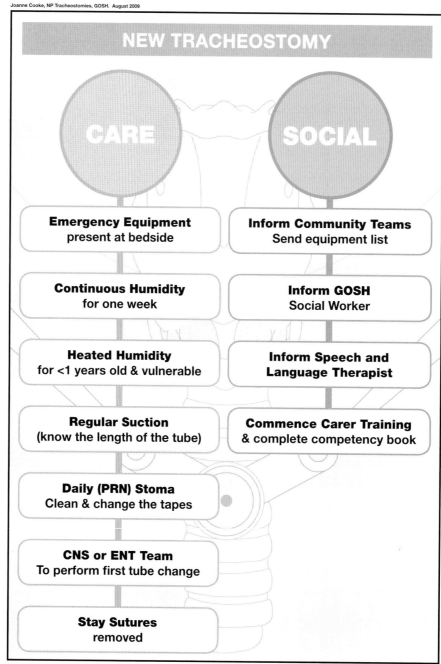

Figure 28.7 Tracheostomy discharge algorithm (Cooke 2009).

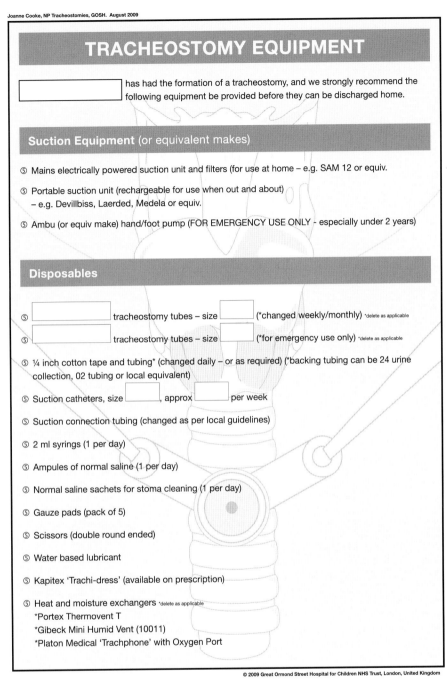

TRACHEOSTOMY EQUIPMENT

[_____] has had the formation of a tracheostomy, and we strongly recommend the following equipment be provided before they can be discharged home.

Suction Equipment (or equivalent makes)

⑤ Mains electrically powered suction unit and filters (for use at home – e.g. SAM 12 or equiv.

⑤ Portable suction unit (rechargeable for use when out and about) – e.g. Devillbiss, Laerded, Medela or equiv.

⑤ Ambu (or equiv make) hand/foot pump (FOR EMERGENCY USE ONLY - especially under 2 years)

Disposables

⑤ [_____] tracheostomy tubes – size [_____] (*changed weekly/monthly) *delete as applicable

⑤ [_____] tracheostomy tubes – size [_____] (*for emergency use only) *delete as applicable

⑤ ¼ inch cotton tape and tubing* (changed daily – or as required) (*backing tubing can be 24 urine collection, 02 tubing or local equivalent)

⑤ Suction catheters, size [_____], approx [_____] per week

⑤ Suction connection tubing (changed as per local guidelines)

⑤ 2 ml syringes (1 per day)

⑤ Ampules of normal saline (1 per day)

⑤ Normal saline sachets for stoma cleaning (1 per day)

⑤ Gauze pads (pack of 5)

⑤ Scissors (double round ended)

⑤ Water based lubricant

⑤ Kapitex 'Trachi-dress' (available on prescription)

⑤ Heat and moisture exchangers *delete as applicable
   *Portex Thermovent T
   *Gibeck Mini Humid Vent (10011)
   *Platon Medical 'Trachphone' with Oxygen Port

Figure 28.8 Equipment list sent to community teams (Cooke 2009).

References

Ackerman MH, Mick DJ (1998) Instillation of normal saline before suctioning in patients with pulmonary infections: a prospective randomized controlled trial. American Journal of Critical Care, 7(4), 261–266

Ahn Y, Hwang T. (2003) The effects of shallow versus deep endotracheal suctioning on the cytological components of respiratory aspirates in high-risk infants. Respiration, 70(2), 172–178

American Thoracic Society (2000) Care of the child with a chronic tracheostomy. American Journal of Respiratory Critical Care Medicine, 161, 297–308

Bailey C, Kattwinkel J, Teja K, Buckley T (1988) Shallow versus deep endotracheal suctioning in young rabbits: pathologic effects on the tracheobronchial wall. Paediatric, 82(5), 746–751

Billau C. (2004) Suctioning. In Russell C, Matta B. (eds) Tracheostomy a multi professional handbook. Cambridge, Cambridge University Press

Blackwood B. (1999) Normal saline instillation with endotracheal suctioning: primum non nocere (first do no harm). Journal Advance Nursing, 29(4), 928–934

Brodsky L, Reidy M, Stanievish JF. (1987) The effects of suctioning techniques on the distal mucosa in intubated low birthweight infants. Journal of Otorhinolaryngology, 14(1), 1–14

Conway JH, Fleming JS, Perring S, Holgate ST. (1992) Humidification as an adjunct to chest physiotherapy in aiding tracho-bronchial clearance in patients with bronchiectasis. Respiratory Medicine, 86, 109–114

Cooke J. (2009) Tracheostomy: Care and Management Review. CPC Guidelines. London, Great Ormond Street Hospital. Available at http://www.gosh.nhs.uk/clinical_information/clinical_guidelines/cpg_guideline_00210 (last accessed 15th July 2011)

Craig D, Bajaj Y, Hartley BE, et al (2005) Maturation sutures for the paediatric tracheostomy an extra safety measure. Journal of Laryngology and Otology, 119, 985–987

Czarnik RE, Stone KS, Everhart CC Jr, Preusser BA. (1991) Differential effects of continuous versus intermittent suction on tracheal tissue. Heart Lung, 20(2), 144–151

Dean B. (1997) Evidence based suction management in accident and emergency: a vital component of airway care. Accident and Emergency Nursing, 5, 92–98

Dellinger K. (2001) Suction injuries: education is the key to prevention. Journal of Pediatric Nursing, 16(3), 147–148

Fiorentini A. (1992) Potential hazards of tracheobronchial suctioning. Intensive Critical Care Nursing, 8(4), 217–226

Friedman E, Kennedy A, Neitzschman HR. (2003) Innominate artery compression of the trachea: an unusual cause of apnea in a 12-year-old boy. South Medical Journal, 96(11), 1161–1164.

Gemma M, Tommasino C, Cerri M, Giannotti A, Piazzi B, Borghi T. (2002) Intracranial effects of endotracheal suctioning in the acute phase of head injury. Journal of Neurosurgical Anesthesiology, 14(1), 50–54

Glass C, Grap MJ. (1995) Ten tips for safe suctioning. American Journal of Nursing, 5(5), 51–53

Harkin H, Russell C. (2001) Preparing the patient for tacheostomy tube removal. Nursing Times, 97(26), 34–36

Harris RL, Riley HD Jr. (1967) Reactions to aerosol medication in infants and children. JAMA, 201(12), 953–955

Hudak M, Bond-Domb A. (1996) Postoperative head and neck cancer patients with artificial airways: the effect of saline lavage on tracheal mucus evacuation and oxygen saturation. ORL Head Neck Nursing, 14(1), 17–21

Jackson C. (1996) Humidification in the upper respiratory tract: a physiological overview. Intensive Critical Care Nursing, 12(1), 27–32

Klein EF Jr, Graves SA. (1974) 'Hot pot' tracheitis. Chest, 65(2), 225–226

Luce JM, Pierson DJ, Tyler ML. (1998) Intensive Respiratory Therapy, 2nd edition. Philadelphia, WB: Saunders Co

Lyons MJ, Cooke J, Cochrane LA, Albert DM. (2007) Safe reliable atraumatic replacement of misplaced paediatric tracheostomy tubes. International Journal of Pediatric Otorhinolaryngology, 71(11), 1743–1746

Midwinter K, Carrie S, Bull P. (2002) Paediatric Tracheostomy: Sheffield experience 1979–1999. Journal of Larynology, 116, 532–535

Mowery BD. (2002) Critical thinking in critial care: tracheostomy troubles. Paediatric Nursing, 28(2), 162

Nursing and Midwifery Council (2002) Code of Professional Conduct for the nurse, midwife and health visitor, 4th edition. London, NMC

Odell A, Allder A, Bayne R, Everett C, Scott S, Still B, West S. (1993) Endotracheal suction for adult, non-head-injured, patients. A review of the literature. Intensive Critical Care Nursing, 9(4), 274–278

Onakoya PA, Nwaorgu OG, Adebusoye LA. (2003) Complications of classical tracheostomy and management. Tropical Doctor, 33(3), 148–150

Park JY, Suskind DL, Prater D, Muntz HR, Lusk RP. (1999) Maturation of the pediatric tracheostomy stoma: effect on complications. Annals of Otology, Rhinology and Laryngology, 108(12), 1115–1119

Prasad SA, Hussey J. (1995) Paediatric Respiratory Care. London, Chapman and Hall

Pritchard M, Flenady V, Woodgate P. (2001) Preoxygenation for tracheal suctioning in intubated, ventilated newborn infants. Cochrane Database of Systems Reviews, 3, CD000427

Raymond SJ. (1995) Normal saline instillation before suctioning: helpful or harmful? A review of the literature. American Journal of Crititcal Care, 4(4), 267–271

Resuscitation Council (UK) (2010) Resuscitation Guidelines. Available at http://www.resus.org.uk/pages/guide.htm (last accessed 15th July 2011)

Runton N. (1992) Suctioning artificial airways in children: Appropriate technique. Pediatric Nursing, 2, 115–118

Scoble MK, Copnell B, Taylor A, Kinney S, Shann F. (2001) Effect of reusing suction catheters on the occurrence of pneumonia in children. Heart Lung, 30(3), 225–233

Seay SJ, Gay SL, Strauss M. (2002) Tracheostomy emergencies. American Journal of Nursing, 102(3), 59, 61, 63

Sigler BA, Willis JM. (1985) Nursing Care of a Patient with a Tracheostomy. London: Churchill Livingstone

Simpson S. (2009) Airway Suctioning, CPC Guidelines. London, Great Ormond Street Hospital. Available at www.gosh.nhs.uk/clinical_information/clinical_guidelines/cpg_guideline_00034 (last accessed 1st July 2011)

Spence K, Gillies D, Waterworth L. (2003) Deep vs shallow suction of endotracheal tubes in ventilated neonates and young infants. Cochrane Database of Systems Review, 3, CD003309

Sumner E. (1990) Artificial ventilation of children. In Dinwiddie R. (ed.) The Diagnosis and Management of Paediatric Respiratory Care. London, Churchill Livingstone

Tarnoff M, Moncure M, Jones F, Ross S, Goodman M. (1998) The value of routine posttracheostomy chest radiography. Chest, 113(6), 1647–1649

Tolles CL, Stone KS. (1990) National survey of neonatal endotracheal suctioning practices. Neonatal Network, 9, 7–14

Tweedie DJ, Skilbeck CJ, Cochrane LA, Cooke J, Wyatt ME. (2008) Choosing a paediatric tracheostomy tube: an update on current practice. Journal of Laryngology Otology, 122(2), 161–169

Wood CJ. (1998) Endotracheal suctioning: a literature review. Intensive Critical Care Nursing, 14(3), 124–136

Yaremchuck K. (2003) Regular tube changes to prevent formation of granulation tissue. Laryngoscope, 113(1), 1–10

Young CS. (1984) Recommendation for suction. Physiotherapy, 70(3), 104–106

Appendix 28.1 Tracheostomy tubes for children

The first types of tracheostomy tubes were made of sterling silver. As other synthetic materials have developed they have improved the flexibility and comfort of paediatric tracheostomy tubes (Tweedie *et al* 2008). See Figure 28.9 for a chart showing the range of tracheostomy tubes.

			Preterm-1 month		1-6 months	6-18 months	18 mths - 3 yrs	3-6 years	6-9 years	9-12 years	12-14 years
	Trachea (Transverse Diameter mm)		5		5-6	6-7	7-8	8-9	9-10	10-13	13
PLASTIC	Great Ormond Street	ID (mm)		3.0	3.5	4.0	4.5	5.0	5.5	6.0	7.0
PLASTIC		OD (mm)		4.5	5.0	6.0	6.7	7.5	8.0	8.7	10.7
PLASTIC	Shiley	Size		3.0	3.5	4.0	4.5	5.0	5.5	6.0	6.5
PLASTIC		ID (mm)		3.0	3.5	4.0	4.5	5.0	5.5	6.0	6.5
PLASTIC		OD (mm)		4.5	5.2	5.9	6.5	7.1	7.7	8.3	9.0
PLASTIC		Length (mm) Neonatal		30	32	34	36				
PLASTIC	*Cuffed Tube Available	Paediatric		39	40	41*	42*	44*	46*		
PLASTIC		Long Paediatric						50*	52*	54*	56*
PLASTIC	Portex (Blue Line)	ID (mm)		3.0	3.5	4.0	4.5	5.0	5.0	6.0	7.0
PLASTIC		OD (mm)		4.2	4.9	5.5	6.2	6.9	6.9	8.3	9.7
PLASTIC	Portex (555)	Size		2.5	3.0	3.5	4.0	4.5	5.0	5.5	
PLASTIC		ID (mm)		2.5	3.0	3.5	4.0	4.5	5.0	5.5	
PLASTIC		OD (mm)		4.5	5.2	5.8	6.5	7.1	7.7	8.3	
PLASTIC		Length Neonatal		30	32	34	36				
PLASTIC		Paediatric		30	36	40	44	48	50	52	
PLASTIC	Bivona	Size	2.5	3.0	3.5	4.0	4.5	5.0	5.5		
PLASTIC		ID (mm)	2.5	3.0	3.5	4.0	4.5	5.0	5.5		
PLASTIC		OD (mm)	4.0	4.7	5.3	6.0	6.7	7.3	8.0		
PLASTIC	All sizes available with Fome Cuff, Aire Cuff & TTS Cuff	Length Neonatal	30	32	34	36					
PLASTIC		Paediatric	38	39	40	41	42	44	46		
PLASTIC	Bivona Hyperflex	ID (mm)	2.5	3.0	3.5	4.0	4.5	5.0	5.5		
PLASTIC		Usable Length (mm)	55	60	65	70	75	80	85		
PLASTIC	Bivona Flextend	ID (mm)	2.5	3.0	3.5	4.0	4.5	5.0	5.5		
PLASTIC		Shaft Length (mm)	38	39	40	41	42	44	46		
PLASTIC		Flextend Length (mm)	10	10	15	15	17.5	20	20		
PLASTIC	TracoeMini	ID (mm)	2.5	3.0	3.5	4.0	4.5	5.0	5.5	6.0	
PLASTIC		OD (mm)	3.6	4.3	5.0	5.6	6.3	7.0	7.6	8.4	
PLASTIC		Length (mm) Neonatal (350)	30	32	3.5	34	36				
PLASTIC		Paediatric (355)	32	36	40	44	48	50	55	62	
SILVER	Alder Hey	FG		12-14	16	18	20	22	24		
SILVER	Negus	FG			16	18	20	22	24	26	28
SILVER	Chevalier Jackson	FG		14	16	18	20	22	24	26	28
SILVER	Sheffield	FG		12-14	16	18	20	22	24	26	
SILVER		ID (mm)		2.9-3.6	4.2	4.9	6.0	6.3	7.0	7.6	
	Cricoid (AP Diameter)	ID (mm)		3.6-4.8	4.8-5.8	5.8-6.5	6.5-7.4	7.4-8.2	8.2-9.0	9.0-10.7	10.7
	Bronchoscope (Storz)	Size		2.5	3.0	3.5	4.0	4.5	5.0	6.0	6.0
		ID (mm)		3.5	4.3	5.0	6.0	6.6	7.1	7.5	7.5
		OD (mm)		4.2	5.0	5.7	6.7	7.3	7.8	8.2	8.2
	Endotracheal Tube (Portex)	ID (mm)	2.5	3.0	3.5	4.0	4.5	5.0	6.0	7.0	8.0
		OD (mm)	3.4	4.2	4.8	5.4	6.2	6.8	8.2	9.6	10.8

Figure 28.9 GOSH chart for paediatric airways. ID, internal diameter; OD, outer diameter.

Tube parts

All tracheostomy tubes have similar parts. In particular, paediatric tubes are designed to accommodate the child's and newborn's neck shape; they provide stability and a means of securing the tube in place.

Ports: A 15 mm termination port is universal 15 mm port providing the means of connecting additional equipment, such as speaking valves and HMEs or ventilatory equipment. It also provides an extension to prevent occlusion from the child's chin (not present on the GOS Rusch®, Silver tubes).

Cannula: Paediatric tubes generally have a single cannula to allow for maximum internal diameter. However, tubes are available with both an inner and outer cannula for older children; the cannula can be fenestrated to allow air to pass upwards through the vocal cords to aid phonation.

Obturator (introducer): This should always be used when inserting the tracheostomy tube, as it provides rigidity to the tube, allowing a smoother insertion.

Tube types

Extensive selections of paediatric tubes are currently available, driven by a variety of specific clinical requirements. Choosing an appropriate tube is just one of the preliminary steps in the management of a child with a tracheostomy. The Consultant and/or Tracheostomy Nurse Practitioner (TNP) will decide the design and size of tube to suit the child. They should be consulted if it is necessary to change the size or style of the tube in the future.

Sizes of tubes are generally measured by the internal diameter (ID). For the majority of children this is the only measurement required. However, some require specifically shorter tubes, for example neonates, whilst others need longer tubes if there is an element of collapse or an obstruction distal to the tube tip. The list below briefly outlines the tubes that are most commonly used at GOSH. Seek advice from the TNP, ENT team, and manufacturer if more information is required.

Bivona®

The Bivona® tube is the most commonly used tube at GOSH, largely replacing other varieties on grounds of comfort and versatility. The range is based around a standard shaft, manufactured from opaque, white siliconised PVC. It is latex free and hydrophobic, hindering protein adhesion and thereby limiting secretion build up and bacterial colonisation. For this reason, these tubes can remain in place for up to 28 days. The silicone is reinforced with wire, producing a tube that is flexible, conforming to the shape of the trachea, but resists kinking. An integrating 15 mm swivelling adapter reduces torque on the shaft and is universally compatible with ventilation appliances. There are two versions: Paediatric (of standard length) and Neonatal (shorter length). The tubes come in a variety of styles, some with independent flexing proximal and distal shafts, which are beneficial for children requiring ventilation (Flextend®); some tubes also have adjustable flanges so that the shaft length can be altered (Hyperflex®). The tubes can be uncuffed or cuffed. The Fome cuff® is a self-inflating tube, providing a high level of protection from aspiration while providing optimal comfort for the child.

Practitioners must ensure that they are familiar with the specifics of this tube when removing and inserting it as it is very different from other tubes. The Tight To Shaft (TTS) is a high-pressure low volume cuff. The cuff is filled with sterile water not air. Care must be taken not to overfill the cuff, and practitioners should only inflate the cuff enough to support artificial ventilation. The cuff can be deflated completely to assume the profile of an uncuffed tube, which makes it very useful when weaning children from the ventilator. This is not a first line tube if ventilatory support is required and other tubes may be appropriate. Bivona® tubes can be sterilised and re-used (maximum of five times or when the integrity of the tube is broken). New 'in hospital and at home' cleaning recommendations are now available from the TNP or the company direct.

The Great Ormond Street Hospital tube

This series is still produced, but no longer commonly used. There are two versions: flat and extended (external fenestrated extension). The extended version is suitable for children whose chin might obstruct the standard flat tube. Both types of tube are made of polyvinyl chloride (PVC) and are clear/brown in colour, with a bevelled tip to facilitate introduction into the stoma and soft, atraumatic flanges. They are available in sizes from 3.0 mm ID to 7.0 mm ID, designed for single use only. More importantly, these tubes are not compatible with ventilator tubing or resuscitation equipment. A Smiths Portex® male/female adapter of appropriate size will be required in such situations but this method is only temporary. If long-term ventilation is required then practitioners should change the tube to one with a 15 mm termination.

Shiley®

The Shiley® range is not commonly used at GOSH. This product range is manufactured from opaque, thermo sensitive, latex-free PVC, with a thin-walled shaft, tapered tip and universal 15 mm connector. Tubes are available in neonatal, standard paediatric and long paediatric varieties, with optional cuffs for the paediatric series. The sizing system used for the Shiley® range was updated several years ago: the internal diameter (mm) is now quoted for reference, in line with other manufacturers' products. From our experiences a weekly tube change is recommended. The Shiley® tube has been superseded by the Bivona® as the product of first choice at GOSH. However, a long paediatric tube (size 5.0–6.5) is not made by other manufacturers, such that the Shiley® remains a unique option for a limited number of children who require a tube that is midway between typical paediatric and adult lengths.

Smiths Portex™

This tube is not commonly used at GOSH. There are two versions available, one without a termination and the other with a 15 mm standard termination. This enables them to be used with anaesthetic and ventilatory equipment. They are made of a clear PVC material with a blue radio-opaque line. Paediatric sizes range from 3.0 mm ID to 7.0 mm ID. Cuffed and fenestrated (to facilitate vocalisation) versions are available.

Silver tubes

A number of silver tubes have been developed. Their designs and general principles remain unchanged for a number of years now. While seldom used by children in GOSH, silver tubes have some important qualities that confer advantages over plastic varieties in certain circumstances. Most significantly, the tubes can be manufactured with very thin walls, permitting the use of an inner tube without compromising airflow. This can be removed and cleaned without taking out the whole tube. Silver tubes may remain in situ for up to one month, a particular advantage for those children requiring long-term tracheostomy. However, silver tubes have certain disadvantages. For example, they are rigid and do not conform to the trachea, which some children find uncomfortable. Additionally, each tube is unique; the unit cost is high (although far fewer tubes are required in the long term) and the components are not interchangeable, creating compatibility problems. Sizes are measured in the French gauge (Fr) and are not comparable to the metric measurements of the plastic tubes. For resuscitation and ventilatory purposes, a Smiths Portex™ male/female adapter of appropriate size will be required. The Sheffield© tube is the only silver product commonly used at Great Ormond Street Hospital. Note that silver tubes are not compatible with MRI scanning and they may distort CT scan pictures of the head, neck and chest. After discussion with the TNP or the child's consultant a suitable alternative must be inserted for the duration of the scan.

Speaking valves

A tracheostomy alters a child's ability to communicate (speak) by affecting the passage of air through the voice box (larynx) and mouth for speech. Air from the lungs passes out of the tracheostomy tube, instead of passing up through the larynx and out of the mouth. A speaking valve is a one-way valve that sits on the end of the tracheostomy tube. The valve opens as the child breathes in and closes as the child breathes out, directing air up through the larynx and out of their mouth. This allows the child to create sounds and words. Not all children will tolerate a speaking valve, as a good air leak around and above the tube is essential. The speaking valve must NOT be used while the child is asleep or when using a cuffed tracheostomy tube. Some variations include the facility for oxygen delivery. Several manufacturers, for example Smiths Portex™, Shiley®, and Rusch® make these. They are designed to facilitate speech in the child with a tracheostomy. A joint decision is made between the ENT Consultant, TNP and the SALT to use a speaking valve, as changes often need to be made to the existing tracheostomy tube to accommodate it. They must not be fitted or used without a full assessment by the child's SALT or TNP. The Rusch® valve is commonly used for initial assessments and then the Passy Muir© is used for long-term use.

Chapter 29

Urinary catheter care

Chapter contents

Procedure guidelines

Introduction

A catheter can be inserted into the urinary bladder via the urethra, via the abdominal wall (suprapubic) or via vesico-ureteric stents which are positioned during bladder surgery.

There are many reasons why a catheter might be inserted, which include:

- Drainage of the bladder when retention occurs
- Accurate recording of fluid output.
- To support an anastomosis
- To promote wound healing
- To prevent obstruction, e.g. after bladder neck surgery
- To minimise pressure and prevent leakage of urine after surgery (Fillingham and Douglas 1997, Robinson 2001)
- For investigations such as urodynamics and micturating cystourethrogram
- End of life care.

Urethral catheterisation is the commonest form of artificial bladder drainage and may be performed by any individual who has been trained and is competent in the procedure for children of either sex (Robinson 2001, RCN 2008).

Clean intermittent catheterisation (CIC) is a procedure that can be taught to children and their families, optimising quality of life by promoting urinary continence. It involves the insertion and removal of a catheter several times a day (Newman and Willson 2011) and has a lower incidence of urinary tract infection than indwelling urethral and suprapubic catheters (Singh et al 2011). It may be necessary to perform CIC for a number of reasons, such as draining post void residuals to prevent infection, or following bladder surgery. CIC may also be performed via a Mitrofanoff, which is a surgically created channel connecting the bladder to the abdominal wall (Mingin and Baskin 2003). As CIC is primarily taught to families, the practice is not included in this chapter.

Suprapubic catheterisation is a procedure that drains the bladder by passing a catheter through the abdominal wall into the bladder (Shah and Shah 1998). The procedure is carried out using an aseptic technique and at GOSH is usually performed under a general anaesthetic.

In life-threatening situations or acute retention of urine, a suprapubic catheter may, however, be inserted under local anaes-thetic. The commonest types of suprapubic catheters at GOSH are Silastic Foley™ and Cystofix™. They are sutured at skin level and secured to the abdomen using a hypoallergenic latex free dressing. They can be clamped to assess the child's ability to void via the urethra.

A vesico-ureteric stent catheter directly drains the kidney and is inserted at the time of surgery. It usually exits the abdomen via the bladder wall and may, in older children, be attached to a drainage bag. In young children who have not been toilet trained it may drain into their nappy. The most commonly used stents at GOSH are the Blue Stent™ and Vygon Ureteric stent™.

All catheters should be inserted for the minimum length of time possible. Duration of catheterisation is strongly associated with risk of infection, i.e. the longer the catheter is in place, the higher the incidence of urinary tract infection (Stamm 1998).

This chapter includes the following sections:

- Catheter care (general principles)
- Catheter insertion
- Catheter care – entry site
- Emptying a catheter
- Maintaining a catheter?
- Flushing a catheter
- Obtaining a specimen
- Catheter removal.

Insertion of indwelling urethral catheters

Despite better products and knowledge regarding care, catheterisation is still the biggest cause of urinary tract infections, and therefore must only be performed when absolutely necessary, for the minimum possible time (Pratt et al 2007). Catheters must always be inserted using an aseptic non-touch technique. Duration of catheterisation is strongly associated with risk of infection, and hence the longer the catheter is in place, the higher the incidence of urinary tract infection (Stamm 1998). The risk of acquiring bacteriuria has been estimated to increase by 5% for each day of catheterisation (Pratt et al 2007). A Silastic Foley™ catheter may remain in situ for up to 6 weeks before it needs to be changed. This section only applies to urethral catheters, as stents and suprapubic catheters are usually placed intra-operatively.

Principles table 29.1 Inform child and family (catheterisation)

Principle	Rationale
1. Inform the child and family: • Why a catheter is necessary • How this will be inserted • The likely duration of the procedure • How long the catheter is likely to remain in situ.	**1.** To provide information enabling informed consent to be given.
2. If the catheter is being inserted in an awake child, the child and family must be informed that restraint may need to be used.	**2.** To fully prepare the child and family.
3. Staff should refer to the local or national holding and restraint guidelines.	**3.** To ensure the safety of the child (RCN 2010).

(Continued)

719

Procedure table 29.1 (*Continued*)

Principle	Rationale
4. The discussion must be recorded in the child's healthcare record.	**4.** To provide an accurate record.
5. Prior to insertion it is essential to consider: • Gender, culture and religious beliefs • Dignity and privacy • Who will be involved in distracting and supporting the child.	**5.** To ensure that insertion of the catheter causes the minimum possible psychological distress.
6. If appropriate a Play Specialist should help to prepare the child.	**6.** To help to psychologically prepare the child.
7. Written information should be available for all children being discharged with a catheter in situ.	**7.** To reinforce verbal explanations (GOSH 2009).

Procedure guideline 29.1 Catheter insertion: preparation

CATHETER INSERTION: PREPARATION

Statement	Rationale
1. Catheterisation must only be performed by or under the supervision of staff who are competent in the procedure: **a)** It normally involves at least two members of staff. **b)** It may be necessary to hold the child. **c)** It may be necessary to sedate the child prior to catheterisation.	**1.** To minimise trauma, discomfort and the potential for catheter-associated infections (Pratt *et al* 2007). **a, b)** To facilitate the procedure and maintain the child's safety. **c)** To minimise distress.
2. When choosing a catheter this should be: **a)** Latex free. **b)** The correct diameter; the smallest diameter catheter that will effectively empty the bladder should be used (Pellowe *et al* 2001). **c)** The correct length; knotting can be prevented by inserting catheters to a minimum distance that is required to obtain urine (Turner 2004). **d)** These issues are particularly important in neonates.	**2.** **a)** To minimise the risk of latex allergy (Woodward 1997). **b)** Smaller gauge catheters minimise trauma and mucosal irritation, which can predispose a child to catheter-associated infection (Pratt *et al* 2007). **c)** Intravesical knotting requiring surgical removal is a well-known hazard of deep catheterisation of the bladder (Carson and Mowery 1997). **d)** For catheter sizes, lengths and models see Tables 29.1 and 29.2 (for neonates).
3. Gather the following equipment: • Catheterisation pack • Catheter of appropriate size and design for intended purpose • Appropriate catheter drainage system • Latex free sterile gloves • Plastic apron • Sachet 0.9% sodium chloride • Sterile lubrication agent • Water based anaesthetic gel (males), e.g. lidocaine 2% • Water based gel (females) e.g. KY gel™ • If Foley catheter: ▪ Prefilled 10 ml syringe of water for injection • Hypoallergenic and latex free adhesive strapping, e.g. Mefix™.	

Procedure guideline 29.1 (Continued)

CATHETER INSERTION: PREPARATION

Statement	Rationale
4. Lay the child in a comfortable position with their head on a pillow: • **Females** should be supine, with their knees bent and flexed outwards. • **Males** should be semi-supine if possible.	4. To provide ease of access for catheterisation.
5. Place an absorbent pad under the child's buttocks.	5. To protect the mattress and bedding.
6. The child's abdomen and lower legs may be covered with a sheet.	6. To maintain dignity and privacy.
7. A parent or carer should remain by the child's head.	7. To provide comfort and restrain hands if necessary.
8. Place a sachet of 0.9% sodium chloride in a bowl of warm water.	8. A cold solution can cause discomfort.
9. Put on an apron. Perform a social hand wash and dry hands thoroughly.	9. To minimise the risk of infection (Pratt *et al* 2007).
10. Open catheter pack and prepare sterile field, adding lubricating agent and catheter.	10–13. To avoid delays and ensure that the necessary equipment is ready for use.
11. Dry sachet of 0.9% sodium chloride and add to sterile field.	
12. Apply alcohol-based gel to hands and put on gloves.	
13. If using a Foley catheter, place prefilled syringe of sterile water on sterile field.	
14. Tear a circular hole in the centre of the sterile sheet and place over the groin area.	14. To give access to groin area.

Table 29.1 An approximate guide to catheter size and models

Weight of child	Model/size of catheter	Rationale
6–29 kg	Foley Silastic size 8 Fr	To prevent urethral trauma when drainage is required for >24 hours
30 kg	Foley Silastic size 10 Fr	To prevent urethral trauma when drainage is required for >24 hours
Attached to:	• A drainable bag with no-return valve	• To facilitate the measurement of output with reduced risk of infection
	• A paediatric urine meter	• To enable very accurate measurement of small volumes with reduced risk of infection

Table 29.2 Catheter size and length for neonates using Self-Cath® urine catheters (Bowden and Greenbers 2003, Carson and Mowery 1997)

Males

Gestation	Weight	Catheter size	Length
LGA	>4 kg	8 Fr	7 cm (+/–2)
Term	3–4 kg	5 or 6 Fr	6 cm (+/–2)
Premature	1–3 kg	5 Fr	5 cm (+/–1)
ELBW	<1 kg	5 Fr	4 cm (+/–1)

Females

Gestation	Weight	Catheter size	Length
LGA	>4 kg	8 Fr	5 cm (+/–2)
Term	3–4 kg	5 or 6 Fr	4 cm (+/–2)
Premature	1–3 kg	5 Fr	3 cm (+/–1)
ELBW	1 kg	5 Fr	2 cm (+/–1)

ELBW, extremely low birth weight; LGA, large for gestational age.

Procedure guideline 29.2 Urethral catheter insertion

Statement	Rationale
To insert a catheter into a female child (see Figure 29.1):	
1. Using non-dominant hand, hold labia open with sterile gauze.	1. To prevent contamination of gloves.
2. Using gauze soaked in 0.9% sodium chloride, clean the vulva using a downward motion.	**2, 3.** To minimise the risk of infection.
3. Clean the outer labia, then the inner labia and then the vulval groove using new gauze for each area.	
4. Position receiver close by.	4. To collect urine.
5. Lubricate tip of catheter with sterile gel.	5. To reduce friction and discomfort from a dry catheter.
6. Ensure child is ready for catheter insertion.	6. To psychologically prepare child.
7. Gently insert catheter tip into urethral meatus.	
8. Insert the catheter using a smooth steady horizontal motion.	
To insert a catheter into a male child (see Figure 29.2):	
1. Gently hold penis with non-dominant hand using sterile gauze and pull it through the hole in the sterile sheet.	1. To give access to penis.
2. Hold the penis vertically and prepare to clean it.	2. To enable effective cleaning.
3. Using gauze soaked in 0.9% sodium chloride, clean prepuce with a singular circular motion. Where possible continue to retract the prepuce.	3. The prepuce is non-retractable in boys under 5 years and excessive force will cause trauma (Thomas *et al* 2002). However, this varies in individuals and some males can never fully retract their foreskin, therefore never force a foreskin to retract.
4. Clean each area of the prepuce/glans with new gauze until prepuce will retract no further or until urethral meatus is visible.	
5. Whilst holding the penis at a 90° angle insert nozzle of lidocaine gel into the urethral meatus/prepuce.	5. Gravity will aid administration of gel.
6. Administer the gel, massaging it downwards into urethra by digital stroking and wait for 4 minutes.	6. Facilitates action of the gel (Addison 2000).
7. Position receiver close by.	7. To collect urine.
8. Ensure the child is ready for catheter insertion.	8. To psychologically prepare the child.
9. Lubricate the tip of the catheter with lidocaine gel.	9. To reduce friction from a dry catheter (Pratt *et al* 2007).
10. Gently insert the catheter tip into the urethral meatus.	
11. Insert the catheter using a smooth steady motion.	
12. On reaching the bladder neck a resistance will be felt.	
13. Encourage the child to take deep breaths.	

Procedure guideline 29.2 (*Continued*)

Statement	Rationale
For both sexes:	
1. Continue to insert the catheter until urine drains freely into the receiver.	

2. If using a Foley catheter:
   a. Insert the catheter to the hilt.
   b. Insert a syringe of 0.9% sodium chloride or sterile water into the one-way valve on side of catheter.
   c. Remove the syringe.
	2.
	   a) To prevent trauma from incorrect balloon position.
	   b) To inflate the balloon at the bladder neck and prevent the catheter from falling out.

3. Secure the catheter to the abdomen or groin using adhesive strapping.	3. To prevent accidental catheter removal (Hanchett 2002).
4. Do not tape it to the child's leg.	4. To minimise trauma to the urethral meatus and bladder neck. This is a greater risk when mobilising with a foley catheter (Hanchett 2002).
5. Attach a sterile drainage bag.	5. To create a closed system (Pratt *et al* 2007).
6. Secure the drainage bag tubing to the abdomen using adhesive strapping.	6. To prevent accidental disconnection of system.
7. Place the bag below the level of bladder using a drainage bag hanger/stand. Do not put it on floor.	7. To promote urine drainage via gravity and minimise the risk of infection (Pratt *et al* 2007).
8. Dispose of equipment according to the trust's waste policy. Perform a social hand wash and dry hands thoroughly.	8. To minimise the risk of cross-infection.
9. Following catheterisation the following must be recorded in the child's healthcare records: • Reasons for catheterisation • Date and time of catheterisation • Type of catheter, including length and size • Volume of sterile water injected into the balloon • Batch number • Manufacturer • Any problems encountered during the procedure • Review date/date to change catheter (Buckley 1999).	9. To provide an accurate record.

Procedure guideline 29.3 Catheter care: general

Statement	Rationale
1. Some children experience bladder spasms or a cramping, burning pain in the lower abdomen. Anti-spasmodic medication, e.g. oxybutynin, may be given as prescribed considering the child's age and underlying condition.	1. To reduce the likelihood of bladder spasms (British Medical Association and Royal Pharmaceutical Society of Great Britain 2003). The tip of the catheter is normally in the trigone of the bladder, which can cause bladder spasm (Fillingham and Douglas 1997).
2. Analgesia should be given as prescribed.	2. The child may experience discomfort from the catheter, even if it is of the correct size and correctly positioned.

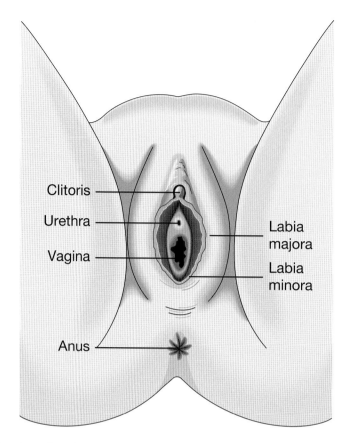

Figure 29.1 Anatomy of the female genito-urinary system. © Great Ormond Street Hospital for Children NHS Foundation Trust.

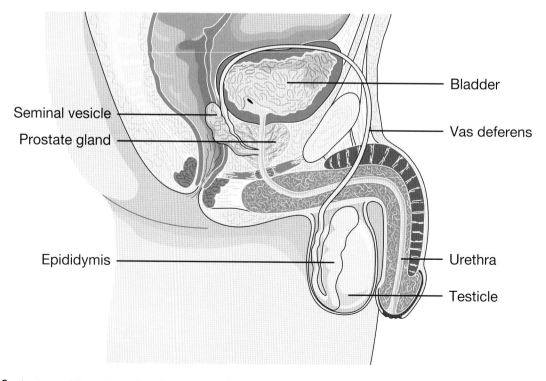

Figure 29.2 Anatomy of the male genito-urinary system. © Great Ormond Street Hospital for Children NHS Foundation Trust.

Procedure guideline 29.4 Catheter care: entry site

Statement	Rationale
1. The catheter must be secured to the abdomen using hypoallergenic adhesive strapping at all times.	1. To prevent accidental removal and trauma to the entry site/ urethral meatus.
2. The strapping – and retention suture for suprapubic catheters and stents – should be checked for security whenever the catheter bag is emptied.	2. To maintain the security of the catheter.

3. Usual hygiene appropriate for the age of the child should be maintained while the catheter is in situ, e.g. nappy care, bathing (Pratt *et al* 2007).
  a) For suprapubic catheters, a shallow bath should be used to avoid soaking the entry site.
  b) Observe the entry site/urethral meatus for trauma and infection.
  c) The child's doctor should be informed of any bleeding, discharge or inflammation. If present this must be recorded in the child's health care records.
	3.
	
	  a) To minimise the risk of infection.
	
	  b) To ensure prevention or early detection and treatment of complications.
	  c) To maintain an accurate record.

4. If an infection is suspected a swab should be taken for microbiological examination.	4. To enable identification of micro-organisms (Higgins 2000).
5. Entry site or meatal cleaning should only be performed if there is bleeding or discharge.	5. Routine entry site/meatal cleansing is not necessary and may increase the risk of infection (Pratt *et al* 2007).

6. Gather the following equipment:
  a) Non-sterile latex free gloves and a plastic apron.
 	
  b) Dressing pack and additional sterile gauze.
  c) Clean non linting gauze.
 	
  d) Foil bowl containing soap and water (urethral catheters).
    OR
    Sachet sterile 0.9% sodium chloride (suprapubic catheters and stents).
  e) Hypoallergenic, latex free adhesive strapping, e.g. Mefix™.
  f) Adhesive remover if necessary.
	6.
	  a) To minimise the risk of cross-infection (National Institute for Clinical Excellence 2003a, 2003b, Sanders 2001).
	  b, c) Cotton wool should not be used as it can deposit fibres around the entry site, which can cause irritation and increase the risk of infection.
	  d) Soap and water provides effective cleansing for urethral catheters. There is no advantage in using antiseptic preparations for cleansing (Sanders 2001).
	
	  e) To replace the strapping if necessary.
	  f) To remove any old tape.

7. To clean a bleeding or infected entry site:
  a) Explain the procedure to the child and family.
 	
  b) Fill a clean foil bowl with warm soap and water. For suprapubic catheters and stents, warm a sachet of 0.9% saline.
  c) Put on plastic apron and perform a social hand wash.
  d) If necessary remove strapping. Dressings for suprapubic catheters should be removed using adhesive remover.
  e) Perform a social handwash.
  f) Apply alcohol-based gel to hands and put on gloves.
  g) With non-dominant hand, hold catheter using sterile gauze.
	7.
	  a) To promote co-operation and involvement and relieve anxiety.
	  b) Warm solution causes less discomfort.
	
	  c) To minimise the risk of infection (Pratt *et al* 2007).
	  d) To enable entry site/meatus to be accessed and to minimise discomfort.
	  e) To minimise the risk of infection.
	  f) To prevent contamination of gloves.
	  g) To minimise the risk of infection.

For urethral catheters (males):
  h) Using gauze soaked in warm soapy water, clean the prepuce/meatus with a circular motion.
  i) Ensure all soap is rinsed off.

(Continued)

Procedure guideline 29.4 (Continued)

Statement	Rationale
For urethral catheters (females):	
j) Using gauze soaked in warm soapy water, clean the outer/inner labia and vulval groove using a vertical downward motion.	**j)** To minimise the risk of spreading infection.
k) Ensure all soap is rinsed off.	
For suprapubic catheters and stents:	
l) Using gauze soaked in 0.9% saline wipe around the entry site once.	
For all catheters:	
m) A new piece of non linting gauze must be used each time until the entry site/meatus is clean.	
n) Ensure the area is dry once the procedure is complete.	
o) Re-secure the catheter.	**o)** To prevent trauma and accidental removal of the catheter.
p) Dispose of equipment according to the trust's waste policy.	**p, q)** To minimise the risk of cross-infection.
q) Remove gloves and apron (dispose of in yellow waste bag). Perform a social hand wash and dry hands thoroughly.	
r) Record procedure in child's healthcare records.	**r)** To provide an accurate record.

Emptying, drainage and flushing

A catheter drainage bag or a child's nappy (if they have a dripping stent in situ) should be emptied/changed 4 hourly to maintain urine flow, prevent reflux and monitor urine output (NICE 2003a, 2003b, Pratt *et al* 2007). Unnecessary emptying of a catheter drainage bag will increase the risk of catheter-related infection and should be avoided (Pratt *et al* 2007, Winn 1996). A dripping stent refers to a catheter that is draining directly into the nappy rather than into a bag. It may be necessary to monitor urine output or to empty the catheter drainage bag more frequently if a child has undergone major surgery, urine output is low due to dehydration, or urine output is high due to overhydration (Methany 2000). If more frequent monitoring is required, the catheter drainage bag could be replaced with an hourly urine output measuring device, e.g. urometer. It is recommended that urine output should equal 1 millilitre per kilogram (ml/kg) of body weight per hour. This is considered the least amount for the kidneys to produce in order to ensure adequate fluid and electrolyte balance. If urine output is lower than this the medical team should be informed. Devices such as urometers enable a child's hourly urine output to be measured without disconnecting the drainage system.

Procedure guideline 29.5 Emptying a catheter drainage bag

Statement	Rationale
1. To empty a catheter drainage bag:	**1.**
a) Inform child and family.	**a)** To promote cooperation and involvement.
b) Put on an apron, perform a social hand wash, dry hands thoroughly and put on clean non-sterile gloves.	**b)** To minimise risk of cross-infection and colonisation of the exit port (NICE 2003a, 2003b, Pratt *et al* 2007).
c) Clean the exit port of the drainage bag using an alcohol impregnated wipe.	**c)** To minimise risk of cross-infection.
d) Empty the urine into a clean jug or foil bowl, taking care not to allow the container to touch the exit port.	**d)** To ensure accurate fluid balance recording and minimise risk of catheter associated infections (NICE 2003a, 2003b, Pratt *et al* 2007).

Procedure guideline 29.5 (Continued)

Statement	Rationale
e) Wipe the exit port again with an alcohol impregnated wipe.	
f) A new receptacle should be used for each catheter.	**f)** To avoid risk of cross-infection (Getliffe 1996, Pratt *et al* 2007).
g) Urine should be measured in a jug or weighed on the sluice scales (i.e. 1 g = 1 ml).	
h) Urine must be discarded in the sluice.	**h)** To avoid cross-infection.
i) The jugs should be decontaminated in the bedpan washer and foil bowls should be discarded as per local waste policy.	**i)** To minimise risk of cross-infection (Getliffe 1996).
j) Remove gloves and apron and dispose of as per local waste policy; perform a social hand wash and dry hands thoroughly.	**j)** To safely dispose of waste and minimise risk of cross-infection (Pratt *et al* 2007, NICE 2003a, 2003b).
k) Urinary output must be recorded on the child's fluid balance chart in millilitres. Children requiring close monitoring of their urine output should also have the amount of urine passed in millilitres per kilogram per hour (ml/kg/hr) calculated and recorded on their fluid balance chart.	**k)** To ensure accurate fluid balance recording.
l) The colour of the child's urine, signs of infection and any debris should also be recorded in the child's nursing notes.	**l)** To monitor for signs of infection.

Procedure guideline 29.6 **Maintaining catheter drainage**

Statement	Rationale
1. If urinary drainage decreases or the child is experiencing increased discomfort:	**1.**
a) Check that the stent or drainage bag tubing is not kinked.	**a)** Kinking will prevent drainage and cause discomfort.
b) Ensure the catheter drainage bag is positioned below the level of the bladder, but is not in contact with the floor.	**b)** To prevent reflux, promote drainage and minimise the risk of infection (NICE 2003a, 2003b, Pratt *et al* 2007).
c) Assess fluid intake in relation to output.	**c)** To assess whether decreased output is related to decreased input (Methany 2000).
d) Look for blockages in the drainage bag tubing caused by debris, blood clots or mucus. If these are present, gently squeeze the catheter above the location of the blockage.	**d)** To break up the blockage and create a vacuum in the tubing, which can mobilise the blockage.
e) Seek medical advice if a blue stent appears blocked. This should only be flushed by the surgeon, or, at their request, by someone with experience of this technique.	**e)** To minimise the risk of complications.
2. It is recommended that urine output should equal at least 1 ml/kg of a child's body weight/hour. If this is not achieved:	**2.** This is considered the least amount for the kidneys to produce in order to ensure adequate fluid and electrolyte balance (Methany 2000).
a) Encourage the child to increase oral intake if the child is tolerating fluid orally.	
b) Consult the surgeons if urine output falls below the required output as an intravenous infusion may need to be commenced or the rate of an existing infusion increased.	**b)** To ensure adequate hydration and increase urine output.
c) It is recommended that all children with an indwelling catheter increase fluids from their normal intake.	**c)** To avoid the colonisation of bacteria in the urine and flush out any micro-organisms or debris in long-term catheterisation.

Procedure guideline 29.7 Flushing supra-pubic, urethral or Mitrofanoff catheters

Statement	Rationale
1. Supra-pubic, urethral and Mitrofanoff catheters may be flushed if the catheter has stopped draining or as part of post-operative/long-term care of an indwelling catheter.	1. To resume catheter drainage by dislodging blockages such as blood and mucus. A blockage can cause a build up of urine, which may cause detrusor spasm, and urine to bypass the catheter (Fillingham and Douglas 1997). An unresolved blockage can also lead to bladder distension, which can compromise the bladder's blood supply and leave the bladder vulnerable to infection (Lowthian 1998).

To flush a urethral, supra-pubic or Mitrofanoff catheter
2. Gather the following equipment:
  a) Large dressing pack.
  b) Plastic apron.
  c) Sterile gloves.
  d) Sachet of sterile water.
  e) Two alcohol impregnated wipes.
  f) New catheter drainage bag.
  g) Hypoallergenic, latex free adhesive strapping, e.g. Mefix™.
  h) A 50 ml bladder syringe.
	2.
	
	h) To reduce the pressure imposed on the bladder mucosa while flushing and minimise the risk of trauma (Fillingham and Douglas 1997).

3.
  a) Explain the procedure to the child and family.
 	
  b) Place a sachet of sterile water in a clean foil bowl, containing warm water.
  c) Put on a plastic apron.
 	
  d) Perform a clinical hand wash and dry hands thoroughly.
  e) Open dressing pack.
  f) Dry the sachet of sterile water and pour into the container provided.
  g) Open alcohol impregnated wipes.
  h) Apply alcohol based gel to hands and put on sterile gloves.
  i) Draw up the prescribed volume of sterile water into the syringe and place it on the sterile field of the dressing pack.
 	
  j) In one circular motion, clean around the join of the catheter and the drainage bag using one alcohol impregnated wipe.
  k) Allow to dry.
  l) Kink the catheter and remove the drainage bag.
  m) Wipe the end of the catheter with a second alcohol impregnated wipe.
  n) Allow to dry.
  o) Insert the syringe into the end of the catheter and unkink the tubing.
  p) If there is **no** resistance push the fluid into the catheter with a smooth and steady motion.
  q) If there is resistance push the catheter a little more firmly.
  r) Do not continue pushing if resistance increases.
 	
  s) If necessary, draw back on the syringe. This should be done gently.
 	
  t) Kink tubing again.
	3.
	  a) To relieve anxiety and promote cooperation and involvement.
	  b) Warm solution reduces discomfort.
	
	  c) To minimise the risk of cross-infection (Pratt et al 2007).
	
	  i) To minimise the risk of transferring micro-organisms to the syringe. The volume used will be related to the underlying condition or nature of the surgery.
	
	  l) To prevent leakage of urine from the catheter.
	  m) To minimise the risk of transferring micro-organisms.
	
	  r) To prevent damage to the bladder mucosa (Fillingham and Douglas 1997).
	  s) To prevent trauma to the urothelium, blockage of the catheter, pain and an increased risk of infection (Fillingham and Douglas 1997).
	  t) To prevent leakage of urine.

Procedure guideline 29.7 (Continued)

Statement	Rationale
u) Remove the syringe. **v)** Unkink the catheter and ensure drainage occurs. **w)** Connect a new drainage bag. **x)** Secure the catheter to the child's abdomen with hypo-allergenic, latex free adhesive strapping. **y)** Dispose of equipment as per local waste disposal policy. **z)** Remove gloves and apron and dispose of as per local policy. Perform a social hand wash and dry hands thoroughly.	**x)** To prevent trauma (Hanchett 2002). **y)** To prevent cross-infection. **z)** To prevent cross-infection (Pratt *et al* 2007).
5. Record procedure and amount drained in child's healthcare records.	**5.** To ensure accurate record keeping and good communication.
6. Inform the medical team if there was resistance to flushing and/or no drainage occurred following the flush.	**6.** Further investigations may be needed to assess reasons for poor drainage.

Obtaining a catheter specimen of urine

A catheter specimen of urine (CSU) may be obtained to determine whether the child has a urinary tract infection or to check urinary electrolytes for children with renal impairment (Postlethwaite and Webb 2002). A clean CSU must be taken to identify the micro-organism causing the infection if a urinary tract infection is suspected, i.e. the urine is smelly, cloudy or has deposits, or the child is pyrexial (Davison *et al* 1997). Urine should never be sampled from the catheter drainage bag as any bacteria present in the urine will quickly multiply and sampling from the bag will provide a false impression of the bacterial content of the bladder (Higgins 2000, NICE 2003a, 2003b, Pratt *et al* 2007). For an alternative method of obtaining a urine specimen from a catheter see Chapter 14, Investigations.

Procedure guideline 29.8 Obtaining a catheter specimen of urine

Statement	Rationale
1. Universal precautions and an aseptic non-touch technique must be employed when obtaining a CSU.	**1.** To minimise the risk of cross-infection and contamination of the specimen (NICE 2003a, 2003b, Pratt *et al* 2007).
2. Prepare the following equipment: • Two alcohol impregnated wipes • Sterile specimen pot • Apron • Non sterile gloves • Eye shields • New catheter drainage bag • Request form.	**2.** To enable CSU to be taken with one break to the closed system thus reducing the risk of introducing further infection to the urinary tract.
3. Check the sample is being collected at the appropriate time.	**3.** An early morning sample may be required for some urinary tests.
4. To take the CSU: **a)** Explain the procedure to the child and family and ensure privacy. **b)** Check the identity of the child against the request form. **c)** Put on an apron and eye shields and perform a social hand wash. Dry hands thoroughly and put on clean non-sterile gloves. **d)** Wipe the join of the catheter with an alcohol impregnated wipe. **e)** Unscrew the lid of the specimen pot and remove.	**4.** **a)** To reduce anxiety and promote cooperation. **b)** To prevent errors. **c)** To avoid cross-contamination of the specimen and cross-infection (NICE 2003a, 2003b, Pratt *et al* 2007).

729

(Continued)

Procedure guideline 29.8 (*Continued*)

Statement	Rationale
f) Kink the catheter to prevent the flow of urine.	**f)** To avoid spillage of urine.
g) Disconnect the catheter from the drainage bag tubing.	
h) Unkink the catheter and allow urine to drip into specimen pot waiting until the appropriate amount of urine is in the specimen pot (as stated on the request card).	**h)** To gain sufficient quantity for urinalysis.
i) Ensure catheter tip does not touch side of specimen pot.	**i)** To prevent contamination of the specimen.
j) Kink the catheter again and wipe the end with the second alcohol impregnated wipe.	**j)** To avoid spillage of urine.
k) Reconnect the catheter to the new drainage bag.	**k)** To reduce introduction of airborne bacteria to the urinary system (Pratt *et al* 2007).
l) Replace and fasten the lid of the specimen pot.	
m) Dispose of used equipment as per local trust policy.	**m, n)** To safely dispose of waste and minimise the risk of infection (Pratt *et al* 2007).
n) Remove apron and gloves. Wash hands and dry thoroughly.	
o) Document the date and time the specimen was taken on the request form and label the specimen clearly.	**o–q)** To maintain an accurate record and link the correct patient to the correct sample.
p) Dispatch for analysis to the appropriate laboratory.	
q) Record the procedure in child's healthcare records.	

Procedure guideline 29.9 Catheter removal

A catheter may only be removed by, or under the supervision of, an experienced nurse or doctor (Pratt *et al* 2007, RCN 2008). Stents should be clamped for several hours prior to removal to ensure the stent is no longer required and the kidney is draining adequately.

Statement	Rationale
1. Gather the following equipment: **a)** An appropriate sized syringe for a Foley catheter. **b)** Non-sterile latex free gloves. **c)** Stitch cutter if required. **d)** Plastic apron. **e)** Adhesive remover.	**1.** To enable the procedure to be performed safely and efficiently.
2. Universal precautions and a non-touch technique must be used.	**2.** To minimise the risk of infection.
3. Give analgesia well in advance of the procedure.	**3.** To relieve any discomfort from catheter removal and first micturition.
4. If the child is prescribed oxybutynin they should not have a dose within 8 hours of a planned catheter removal.	**4.** This reduces bladder tone, which could delay micturition after catheter removal (British Medical Association and Royal Pharmaceutical Society of Great Britain 2003).

To remove the catheter:

Statement	Rationale
1. Prepare the child and family.	**1.** To promote cooperation and involvement and relive anxiety.
2. Put on an apron.	**2–4.** To minimise the risk of cross-infection.
3. Perform a social hand wash and dry hands thoroughly.	
4. Put on gloves.	

Procedure guideline 29.9 (*Continued*)

Statement	Rationale
5. Using adhesive remover, remove adhesive strapping from abdomen, while supporting the weight of the catheter.	**5, 6.** To reduce trauma to the skin.
6. Cut retaining suture if in situ.	
7. Deflate balloon (Foley catheters): **a)** Insert syringe into its one-way valve. **b)** Withdraw the documented volume of sterile water. **c)** If the sterile water cannot be withdrawn consult the child's doctor.	**7.** To avoid trauma to urethra **a)** To enable balloon on catheter to be deflated. **c)** Occasionally the one-way valve fails to release the sterile water.
8. Hold catheter at the entry site.	**8.** To enable catheter to be gently pulled.
9. Encourage the child to take deep breaths.	**9.** To relax abdominal wall and bladder neck.
10. Gently pull on catheter in one steady motion, whilst the child exhales, until the catheter is completely removed.	**10.** To minimise risk of the catheter catching on the bladder neck or urethra, which can cause pain, mucosal damage and bladder spasms.

For suprapubic catheters and stents:

1. Do not use excessive force.	**1.** To prevent the stent from breaking.
2. Contact the child's doctor if the catheter cannot be removed.	**2.** The internal suture may still be intact or it may be caught in oedematous tissue.
3. Following removal, apply pressure using sterile gauze to the entry site for one minute to promote closure of the bladder and abdominal wall.	**3, 4.** To prevent bleeding and leakage of urine.
4. Leave gauze in situ and apply strapping to secure.	
5. If site is bleeding/leaking urine inform the child's doctor.	**5.** The entry site may not have sealed following the application of initial pressure.

For all catheters

1. Dispose of urine and equipment according to the Trust's Waste Policy.	**1, 2.** To minimise the risk of cross-infection.
2. Remove gloves and apron, perform a social hand wash and dry hands thoroughly.	
3. Record volume of urine in drainage bag on fluid balance chart.	**3, 4.** To maintain an accurate record.
4. Record procedure in the child's healthcare records.	

Care after catheter removal

1. Observe the child to ensure that they are able to pass urine urethrally.	**1.** To ensure the child is not retaining urine.
2. The time limit to first micturition should be determined by the child's doctor.	**2.** If the child has had bladder or urethral surgery there is a risk of urine leakage due to excess pressure.
3. The child and family must be informed that the first micturition may be painful.	

(*Continued*)

Procedure guideline 29.9 (*Continued*)

Statement	Rationale
4. The first micturition must be documented on the fluid balance chart and in the child's healthcare record.	**4.** To maintain an accurate record.
5. The child's doctor must be informed if the child: **a)** Is unable to pass urine. **b)** Has dysuria.	**5.** **a, b)** The bladder neck or urethra may be oedematous, which can cause pain and/or obstruction.

In addition, for suprapubic catheters and stents

Statement	Rationale
1. The doctor should be informed if the entry site leaks on first micturition.	**1.** Increased bladder pressure may cause a leak.
2a) The entry site must be observed for haemorrhage and urine leakage. **b)** If either occurs, pressure must be applied and the child's doctor informed.	**2a)** If the bladder bleeds or leaks urine a haematoma or urinoma may form, creating a risk of infection (Fillingham and Douglas 1997). **b)** To ensure that the complication is treated swiftly.
3. The dressing should be removed after 24 hours.	**3.** To promote healing. Once the site is healed a dressing will no longer be required.
4. Inform the Children's Community Nursing (CCN) team prior to discharge.	**4, 5.** To provide support in the community and care after discharge.
5. The child's parents/carers should be advised to contact the CCN team or the ward if they have concerns about the wound site after discharge.	

References

Addison R. (2000) Catheterisation using lignocaine gel. Nursing Times, 96(41), 43–44

Bowden VR, Greenbers CS. (2003) Pediatric Nursing Procedures. London, Lippincott Williams and Wilkins

British Medical Association and Royal Pharmaceutical Society of Great Britain (2003) British National Formulary 46. London, BMA

Buckley R. (1999) Keep it legal. Nursing Times, 95(6), 75–79

Carlson D, Mowery B. (1997) Standards to prevent complications of urinary catheterisation in children: should and should-knots. Journal of the Society of Pediatric Nursing, 2, 37–41

Davison AM, Cameron JS, Grunfeld JP, Kerr DNS, Ritz E, Winearls CQ. (eds) (1997) Oxford Textbook of Clinical Nephrology. Oxford, Oxford University Press

Fillingham S, Douglas J. (eds) (1997) Urological Nursing. London, Baillière Tindall

Getliffe K. (1996) Care of urinary catheters. Nursing Standard, 11(11), 47–54

GOSH (2009) Looking after your child's urethral catheter. www.gosh.nhs.uk/medical-conditions/procedures-and-treatments/looking-after-your-childs-urethral-catheter/ (last accessed 22nd January 2012)

Hanchett M. (2002) Techniques for stabilizing urinary catheters: tape may be the oldest method, but it's not the only one. American Journal of Nursing, 102(3), 44–48

Higgins C. (2000) Understanding Laboratory Investigations: A text for nurses and healthcare professionals. Oxford, Blackwell Science

Lowthian P. (1998) The dangers of long-term catheter drainage. British Journal of Nursing, 7(7), 366–379

Methany NM. (2000) Fluid and Electrolyte Balance: Nursing Considerations. Philadelphia, Lippincott

Mingin GC, Baskin LS. (2003) Surgical management of the neurogenic bladder and bowel. International Brazilian Journal of Urology, 29(1), 53–61. Available at http://www.brazjurol.com.br/january_february_2003/Baskin_ing_53_61.htm (last accessed 13th July 2011)

National Institute for Clinical Excellence (2003a) Clinical Guideline 2 Infection Control: Prevention of healthcare-associated infection in primary and community care; (No 1) Standard Principles. London, NICE

National Institute for Clinical Excellence (2003b) Clinical Guideline 2 Infection Control: Prevention of healthcare-associated infection in primary and community care; (No. 2) Care of Patients with Long-Term Urinary Catheters. London, NICE

Newman DK, Willson MM. (2011) Review of intermittent catheterization and current best practices. Urology Nursing, 31(1), 12–28

Pellowe C, Loveday H, Harper P, Robinson N, Pratt R (2001) Preventing infections from short-term indwelling catheters. Nursing Times, 97, 34–35

Postlethwaite R, Webb N. (eds) (2002) Clinical Paediatric Nephrology, 3rd edition. Oxford, Oxford University Press

Pratt RJ, Pellowe CM, Wilson JA, Loveday HP, Harper PJ, Jones SR, McDougall C, Wilcox M. (2007) Epic2: National evidence-based guidelines for preventing healthcare associated infections in NHS hospitals in England. Journal of Hospital Infection, 65(suppl 1), 1–64

Robinson J. (2001) Urethral catheter selection. Nursing Standard, 15(25), 39–42

Royal College of Nursing (RCN) (2008) Catheter Care. RCN Guidance for Nurses. London, RCN. Available at www.rcn.org.uk/_data/assets/pdf_file/0018/157410/003237.pdf (last accessed 4th July 2011)

Royal College of Nursing (2010) Restrictive physical intervention and therapeutic holding for children and young people guidance for nursing staff. London, RCN. Available at www.rcn.org.uk/_data/assets/pdf_file/0016/312613/003573.pdf (last accessed 4th July 2011)

Sanders C. (2001) Suprapubic catheterisation: Risk management. Paediatric Nursing, 13(10), 14–18

Shah N, Shah J. (1998) Percutaneous suprapubic catheterisation. Urology News, 2(5), 11–12

Singh R, Rohilla RK, Sangwan K, Siwach R, Magu NK, Sangwan SS. (2011) Bladder management methods and urological complications in spinal cord injury patients. Indian Journal of Orthopaedics, 45(2), 141–147

Stamm WE. (1998) Urinary tract infections. In Bennett JV, Brachman PS. (eds) Hospital Infection, 4th edition. Philadelphia, Lippincott-Raven, pp 477–485

Thomas DFM, Rickwood AMK, Duffy PG. (eds) (2002) Essentials of Paediatric Urology. London, Martin Dunitz

Turner TW. (2004) Intravesical Catheter Knotting: An uncommon complication of urinary catheterisation. Paediatric Emergency Care, 2(2), 115–117

Winn C. (1996) Basing catheter care on research principles. Nursing Standard, 10(18), 38–40

Woodward A. (1997) Complications of allergies to latex urinary catheters. British Journal of Nursing, 6(14), 786–790

Chapter 30

Drug withdrawal – prevention and management

Chapter contents

Procedure guidelines

The Great Ormond Street Hospital Manual of Children's Nursing Practices, First Edition. Edited by Susan Macqueen, Elizabeth Anne Bruce, Faith Gibson.
© 2012 Great Ormond Street Hospital for Children NHS Foundation Trust. Published 2012 by Blackwell Publishing Ltd.

Introduction

The prolonged use of opioids (e.g. morphine or fentanyl) and benzodiazepines (e.g. midazolam) for pain management and sedation of children in intensive care are well-established practices that reduce the physiological and biochemical response to critical illness and extensive surgery (Anand and Arnold 1994, Cho et al 2007, Eddlestone et al 1997, Franck and Vilardi 1995, Ista et al 2007). However, the use of any opioid or benzodiazepine has inherent consequences, which may include drug tolerance, physical dependence, cross tolerance with similar pharmacological agents and drug withdrawal. Strategies and treatment regimens are required to manage these effectively (Carr and Todres 1994, Grehn 1998, Tobias 2000, Yaster et al 1996).

Clinical studies have identified the incidence of withdrawal in critically ill children. Playfor et al (2006) found that the incidence ranged from 17–35% in patients receiving midazolam, while Ista et al (2007) found that it may be as high as 57% in patients receiving potent opioids such as fentanyl. However, despite this, there is a lack of research into the causes of iatrogenic withdrawal and limited advice regarding standardised weaning regimens or tools to assess withdrawal in children and young people (Franck et al 2004). Misconceptions related to the nature of withdrawal are common; therefore it is vital that the healthcare professional is familiar with some standard definitions (see Box 30.1).

The mechanisms of tolerance and dependence are not clearly understood (Franck and Vilardi 1995, Puntillo et al 1997, Playfor 2008, Franck et al 2012). It has been hypothesised that when opioids and benzodiazepines are continuously administered to a patient, adaptation occurs in the central nervous system in response to prolonged receptor site occupancy (Yaster et al 1996). Continuous blockage of the neural pathways by opioids or benzodiazepines may cause them to become unusually hypersensitive (Puntillo et al 1997). In addition, other minor neural pathways not normally involved may become active to compensate for other routes being blocked (Franck and Vilardi 1995). Slow reduction of the drugs causing this change allows the neural pathway to return to normal. Abrupt discontinuation exposes the patient's hypersensitive neural pathway to immediate bombardment by messages formally blocked, causing the child or young person to exhibit symptoms resulting from amplified neural responses (Franck and Vilardi 1995). Other suggested mechanisms include interactions between receptors, intracellular enzyme systems and involvement of the noradrenergic system (Playfor et al 2006).

The health professional's role in the treatment of patients on long-term opioids or benzodiazepines includes: the slow reduction of these drugs to prevent the onset of withdrawal symptoms (Franck et al 2004, Ista et al 2007, 2009, Playfor 2008, Tobias 2000, 2003), close monitoring for symptoms (Eddlestone et al 1997, Franck et al 2008, 2012) and the complimentary use of non-pharmacological therapies (Anand and Ingraham 1996, Katz 1994). In addition, the goals of treatment aim to prevent excessive sedation, maintain the child or young person's normal sleep-wake pattern (Puntillo et al 1997), and ensure that the patient's medical condition is not compromised, in order to ultimately avoid unnecessary hospitalisation (Osborn et al 2003).

Box 30.1 Definitions

Tolerance	Reduction in a drug's efficacy over a period of time, requiring steady increase of the drug dose to produce the same initial response (Franck and Vilardi 1995, Jage 2005, Tobias 2000).
Physical dependence	Requirement for ongoing administration of a drug to prevent the occurrence of withdrawal symptoms (Anand and Ingraham 1996, Franck and Vilardi 1995, Jage 2005).
Cross tolerance	A patient who is tolerant to one drug may also exhibit some tolerance to other similar drugs, e.g. a child who is tolerant to morphine may also show signs of tolerance to other opioids (Franck and Vilardi 1995, Jage 2005).
Withdrawal (abstinence) syndrome	A response to sudden discontinuation of long-term sedative or analgesic drug treatment, characterised by a wide range of symptoms. This condition may affect the child's physical well-being and ultimately delay their recovery (Cunliffe et al 2004, Franck and Vilardi 1995, Franck et al 2004, Tobias 2000).
Addiction	Describes a multifaceted pattern of behaviours, which includes psychological, as well as a physiological dependence, due to habitual administration of a drug for its non-medicinal qualities (Anand and Ingraham 1996). The use of this term can be confusing to patients and parents/carers and is not appropriate in describing iatrogenic withdrawal (i.e. withdrawal induced by medical treatment).
Pseudo-addiction	Behaviours that may seem inappropriately drug-seeking but are the result of under-treatment of pain and resolve when pain relief is adequate (Weissman and Haddox 1989).

Healthcare professionals may be concerned that slow reduction of opioids or benzodiazepines as part of the weaning process may prolong the duration of mechanical ventilation (Ducharme et al 2005). However, others suggest that, on the contrary, tolerance to the respiratory depressive effects of opioids occurs rapidly (Franck et al 2004), and a rapid reduction in sedatives may be associated with increased episodes of agitation and distress and other physical symptoms, which can obstruct the process of weaning mechanical ventilation (Alexander et al 2002). Extubation or early discharge from the intensive care unit should not necessitate an excessively rapid withdrawal of opioids or benzodiazepines, as it is unlikely that appropriate weaning will disrupt patient treatment (Carr and Todres 1994, Tobias 2003). In many cases, patients may be effectively weaned from the ventilator before opioid or benzodiazepine drugs are discontinued, even when the patient is receiving relatively high-dose therapy (Tobias 2003).

Withdrawal prevention

Principles table 30.1 Prevention of withdrawal

Principle	Rationale
1a) All patients receiving analgesic or sedative infusions should have regular pain and sedation assessment (Eddlestone *et al* 1997, Playfor *et al* 2006).	**1a)** To inform decisions regarding weaning of opioids and benzodiazepines. Frequent pain and sedation scores allow for reductions in opioid and benzodiazepine rates to be made confidently and accurately (Playfor *et al* 2006, Tobias 2000).
b) This enables the amount of analgesic or sedative drug to be kept to the minimum required for efficacy.	**b)** To minimise the risk of tolerance.
2. Adjunct therapy and non-pharmacological techniques should be considered for all patients.	**2.** To provide adjuncts that will help keep opioid and benzodiazepine therapy to a minimum (Playfor *et al* 2006). Opioid sparing adjuncts (e.g. multi-modal analgesia) enhance the effect of more potent analgesics and can potentially reduce the occurrence of unwanted side-effects.
3. Strategies that can limit the impact of prolonged sedative and analgesic therapy should be employed. These include: • Opioid rotation • 'Wake up' protocols/drug holidays (where muscle relaxants are temporarily suspended to assess patient response to sedation).	**3.** To minimise the incidence and severity of withdrawal and inform decisions regarding weaning. Various strategies have been proposed to reduce the incidence and severity of physical dependence and drug tolerance in patients in the intensive care setting. However, the physiological basis and clinical effectiveness of such techniques has not been established (Du Pen *et al* 2007).

Principles table 30.2 Preparation for weaning opioid or benzodiazepine therapy

Principle	Rationale
1. A weaning and withdrawal plan should be written as soon as opioid or benzodiazepines are commenced. The weaning plan should be reassessed daily by the multi-disciplinary team, who should be aware of the adverse effects of prolonged sedation therapy.	**1.** To ensure continuous monitoring of the child or young person, so that treatment plans can be tailored to the patient's individual needs (Grehn 1998) and any signs of withdrawal are treated in the early stages (Franck *et al* 1998).
2. The plan must take into account the child or young person's: • Age • Cognitive status • Physical condition or disease process • Current or previous drug regimens.	**2.** Management of withdrawal varies from patient to patient and there is no one formula for drug management that applies to all patients (Tobias 2000, 2003, Yaster *et al* 1996).
3. Prior to weaning, a history of the patient's drug usage should be taken, including: **a)** Analgesic and sedative drug dosages, including the highest (peak) dose administered during treatment. **b)** Duration of analgesic and sedative therapy. **c)** Any weaning already undertaken (as a percentage of the peak dose).	**3.** The likelihood of withdrawal is related to the drug the patient has been receiving, the dose and the duration of therapy (Eddlestone *et al* 1997, Tobias 2000). **a)** The percentage of the drug weaned per day is calculated from the highest dose administered, unless this was only maintained for a few hours. **b)** The longer the duration, the higher the risk of withdrawal (see section on weaning protocols). **c)** To determine the effect of the wean and assist decisions regarding the appropriate rate for future weaning.

Principles table 30.2 (*Continued*)

Principle	Rationale
d) The use of any muscle relaxants.	**d)** Neuro-muscular blocking agents increase the risk of withdrawal and masks the signs normally displayed by patients, which would otherwise prompt weaning of sedation. Patients receiving these drugs have been found to also receive higher doses of opioids and benzodiazepines (Birchley 2009, Tobias 2000).
e) Any previous history of opioid or benzodiazepine use or withdrawal problems.	**e)** This information assists the health care professional to identify 'at risk' patients and tailor care to the individual (Tobias 2003).
4. A diagnosis of withdrawal syndrome should only be made if there has been a recent reduction or abrupt discontinuation of opioids or benzodiazepines and all other possible causes of the symptoms have been excluded (see Box 30.2).	**4.** To correctly identify and treat the underlying cause. Ongoing or associated conditions may have similar symptoms and these should be considered and discounted before a diagnosis of withdrawal is made (Ista *et al* 2007, 2009, Playfor *et al* 2006, Tobias 2000, 2003).
5. It is important to note that due to delayed metabolism or excretion of an analgesic or sedative agent, withdrawal symptoms may not be observed for 8–48 hours after discontinuation of drug therapy (Ista *et al* 2007, Wong *et al* 2003).	**5.** A number of factors may cause differences in the individual's response to the sedative or analgesic agent, which may delay the expression of withdrawal symptoms. These include: • Changes in hepatic blood flow • Interactions between drugs • Variations in the plasma protein-binding properties of a drug • The reduced efficacy over time of a drug given continuously (common in drugs that effect the nervous system) (Eddlestone *et al* 1997).

Box 30.2 Other potential causes of withdrawal-like symptoms

• Central nervous system insults or infections
• Intensive care unit psychosis
• Metabolic abnormalities/conditions
• Hypoxia
• Hypercarbia
• Cerebral hypoperfusion from alterations in cardiac output
• Cerebrovascular disease
• Sepsis
• Hypoglycaemia (neonates)
• Insufficient sedation
• Pain
• Ventilator distress
• Noisy environment
    (Berlin 1998, Ista *et al* 2007, Playfor 2006, Tobias 2003)

Withdrawal assessment

Symptoms of withdrawal from either opioids or benzodiazepines are often similar, but may also vary from one individual to another (Ista *et al* 2007, 2009). Thus, patient assessment should form the basis of any weaning plan, with treatment changes made in relation to the child or young person's individual response to treatment (Puntillo *et al* 1997).

The signs and symptoms of withdrawal (Franck *et al* 2004, Ista *et al* 2007, 2008, 2009) are illustrated in Box 30.3 and may be grouped under the following headings:

• Dysregulation of the autonomic nervous system (evident as physiological changes).

• Hyper-irritability of the nervous system and abnormal motor movements (more pronounced in withdrawal from benzodiazepines).
• Gastrointestinal disturbances (not seen in benzodiazepine withdrawal).

Box 30.3 Clinical symptoms of withdrawal

Dysregulation of the autonomic nervous system

• Pupil dilation
• Tachycardia
• Sweating
• Sneezing
• Hypertension
• Tachypnoea
• Mottling
• Increased secretions (suctioning)
• Pyrexia
• Yawning

Hyper-irritability and abnormal motor movements

• Increased muscle tension
• Jittering, tremors
• Behavioural changes
• Repetitive movements
• High pitched/insolable crying
• Grimacing
• Agitation
• Visual/auditory hallucinations
• Anxiety

Continued

Box 30.3 continued

- Insomnia/sleep disturbance
- Seizures, particularly in some infants (Katz 1994)
- Motor disturbances.

Gastrointestinal disturbances

- Poor feeding
- Vomiting
- Diarrhoea

(Anand and Ingram 1996, Franck and Vilardi 1995,
Franck et al 2004, 2008, 2012, Ista et al 2007, 2008, 2009,
Playfor et al 2006, Puntillo et al 1997, Yaster et al 1996)

Withdrawal assessment tools

The 'Sedation Withdrawal Score' (Cunliffe et al 2004) has been found to be clinically sensitive in detecting withdrawal symptoms in children and young people discharged from an intensive care unit to the ward (see Box 30.4). The *Withdrawal Assessment Tool-1* (WAT-1) has been tested for validity and reliability in the intensive care setting (Franck et al 2008, 2012) (Figure 30.1).

Additional resources for the assessment of withdrawal may be found at: www.gosh.nhs.uk/health-professionals/clinical-guidelines/.

Box 30.4 Sedation withdrawal score (Cunliffe *et al* 2004)

Tremor	Sneezing
Irritability	Respiratory distress
Hypertonicity	Fever
Hyperactivity	Diarrhoea
Vomiting	Sweating
High-pitched cry	Convulsions

For each parameter score 0 = absent, 1 = mild, 2 = severe.
Maximum possible score = 24.

Instructions

Score (six hourly)
<6 Current regimen to remain
6–12 Do not reduce regimen further
12–18 Revert to former regimen
>18 Seek advice

Principles table 30.3 Withdrawal assessment

Principle	Rationale
1. At the point when weaning is deemed suitable, withdrawal assessment should be observed and recorded (Anand and Ingraham 1996, Franck et al 1998).	1. To check for any existing symptoms and to determine the effectiveness of any weaning programme implemented.
2. A reliable assessment tool should be used to guide the weaning process.	2. To objectively ascertain whether the child's drug regimen needs to be increased or decreased (Berlin et al 1998, Eddlestone et al 1997).
3. The interval between assessments is dependent on the specific withdrawal assessment tool chosen (Cunliffe et al 2004, Franck et al 2008).	
4. No 'gold standard' assessment of withdrawal currently exists (Franck et al 2008) and there are a limited number of tools that may be used for assessing withdrawal in children and young people who have been exposed to opioid or benzodiazepines (Ista et al 2009). Nevertheless, when choosing a withdrawal assessment tool, the following should be considered (Easley and Nichols 2008): • Ease of application • Willingness of all members of the multidisciplinary team to use the tool • A strategy for staff education in the use and interpretation of the tool • The availability of a flexible weaning protocol.	4. Some promising research has been undertaken to validate tools for use in the paediatric setting (Easley and Nichols 2008, Franck et al 2008, 2012, Ista et al 2007, 2009). However, further study is required to determine: • Cut-off scores that help to diagnose withdrawal in order to guide treatment intervention or changes • The most appropriate interval between assessments • The reliability of assessment tools in a variety of ages and settings • The sensitivity of tools to differentiate between opioid and benzodiazepine withdrawal (Franck et al 2008).
5. Scoring tools should be modified on an individual basis to exclude symptoms of underlying conditions that may influence the withdrawal score and result in unnecessary treatment. For example, the occurrence of loose stools in a child with an ileostomy should be discounted as a symptom of withdrawal, as this is a normal event for this child (Franck et al 1998).	5. In order to make an objective assessment it is important that any assessment tool is modified on an individual basis to ensure that any underlying condition does not skew the withdrawal score and delay the weaning process unnecessarily (Franck and Vilardi 1995).

WITHDRAWAL ASSESSMENT TOOL VERSION 1 (WAT – 1)

Patient Identifier													
	Date:												
	Time:												
Information from patient record, previous 12 hours													
Any loose /watery stools	No = 0 / Yes = 1												
Any vomiting/wretching/gagging	No = 0 / Yes = 1												
Temperature > 37.8°C	No = 0 / Yes = 1												
2 minute pre-stimulus observation													
State	SBS[1] ≤ 0 or asleep/awake/calm = 0 / SBS[1] ≥ +1 or awake/distressed = 1												
Tremor	None/mild = 0 / Moderate/severe = 1												
Any sweating	No = 0 / Yes = 1												
Uncoordinated/repetitive movement	None/mild = 0 / Moderate/severe = 1												
Yawning or sneezing	None or 1 = 0 / ≥2 = 1												
1 minute stimulus observation													
Startle to touch	None/mild = 0 / Moderate/severe = 1												
Muscle tone	Normal = 0 / Increased = 1												
Post-stimulus recovery													
Time to gain calm state (SBS[1] ≤ 0)	< 2min = 0 / 2 - 5min = 1 / > 5 min = 2												
Total Score (0-12)													

WITHDRAWAL ASSESSMENT TOOL (WAT – 1) INSTRUCTIONS

- Start WAT-1 scoring from the **first day of weaning** in patients who have received opioids +/or benzodiazepines by infusion or regular dosing for prolonged periods (e.g., > 5 days). Continue twice daily scoring until 72 hours after the last dose.
- The Withdrawal Assessment Tool (WAT-1) should be completed along with the SBS[1] at least once per 12 hour shift (e.g., at 08:00 and 20:00 ± 2 hours). The progressive stimulus used in the SBS[1] assessment provides a standard stimulus for observing signs of withdrawal.

Obtain information from patient record (this can be done before or after the stimulus):
✓ **Loose/watery stools**: Score 1 if any loose or watery stools were documented in the past 12 hours; score 0 if none were noted.
✓ **Vomiting/wretching/gagging**: Score 1 if any vomiting or spontaneous wretching or gagging were documented in the past 12 hours; score 0 if none were noted
✓ **Temperature > 37.8°C**: Score 1 if the modal (most frequently occurring) temperature documented was greater than 37.8 °C in the past 12 hours; score 0 if this was not the case.

2 minute pre-stimulus observation:
✓ **State**: Score 1 if awake and distress (SBS[1]: ≥ +1) observed during the 2 minutes prior to the stimulus; score 0 if asleep or awake and calm/cooperative (SBS[1] ≤ 0).
✓ **Tremor**: Score 1 if moderate to severe tremor observed during the 2 minutes prior to the stimulus; score 0 if no tremor (or only minor, intermittent tremor).
✓ **Sweating**: Score 1 if any sweating during the 2 minutes prior to the stimulus; score 0 if no sweating noted.
✓ **Uncoordinated/repetitive movements**: Score 1 if moderate to severe uncoordinated or repetitive movements such as head turning, leg or arm flailing or torso arching observed during the 2 minutes prior to the stimulus; score 0 if no (or only mild) uncoordinated or repetitive movements.
✓ **Yawning or sneezing** > 1: Score 1 if more than 1 yawn or sneeze observed during the 2 minutes prior to the stimulus; score 0 if 0 to 1 yawn or sneeze.

1 minute stimulus observation:
✓ **Startle to touch**: Score 1 if moderate to severe startle occurs when touched during the stimulus; score 0 if none (or mild).
✓ **Muscle tone**: Score 1 if tone increased during the stimulus; score 0 if normal.

Post-stimulus recovery:
✓ **Time to gain calm state** (SBS[1] ≤ 0): Score 2 if it takes greater than 5 minutes following stimulus; score 1 if achieved within 2 to 5 minutes; score 0 if achieved in less than 2 minutes.

Sum the 11 numbers in the column for the total WAT-1 score (0-12).

[1]Curley et al. State behavioral scale: A sedation assessment instrument for infants and young children supported on mechanical ventilation. Pediatr Crit Care Med 2006;7(2):107-114.

Figure 30.1 The Withdrawal Assessment Tool-1 (Franck *et al* 2008). Reproduced with permission from Lippincott Williams & Wilkins.

Management of withdrawal

Procedure guideline 30.1 Non-pharmacological management

Statement	Rationale
1. Ensure all children receive appropriate non-pharmacological interventions to prevent or minimise the occurrence of withdrawal symptoms, even if they are also receiving drug therapy.	1. Non-pharmacological methods are effective in reducing the severity of withdrawal symptoms (Anand and Ingraham 1996) and can enhance the effectiveness of drug therapy.
2. Reduce environmental stimulation by: • Nursing the child or young person in a quiet area of the ward, if possible and appropriate • Sequencing nursing procedures to promote minimal disturbance to the child • Liaising with family or carer to limit visitors • Removing mobiles, balloons and noisy toys. Keep a few familiar and comforting toys nearby • Turning off televisions and ensuring that music is kept at a low level • Dimming lights, if possible and appropriate for patient observation • Keeping bed sheets plain. Brightly coloured bedside curtains should be covered or removed if they are exacerbating distress in a child or young person suffering from hallucinations.	2. To reduce over stimulation and hallucinations in a hyperirritable child and promote rest (Anand and Arnold 1994, Anand and Ingraham 1996, Franck and Vilardi 1995, Playfor *et al* 2006, Yaster *et al* 1996).
3a) For small children, comfort measures can be helpful. These include: • Swaddling (Anand and Arnold 1994, Franck and Vilardi 1995, Osborn *et al* 2003, Wong *et al* 2003, Yaster *et al* 1996) • Holding or rocking (Anand and Arnold 1994, Anand and Ingraham 1996, Franck and Vilardi 1995, Wong *et al* 2003) • Bathing and massage (Osborn *et al* 2003) • Non-nutritive sucking, e.g. dummies (Osborn *et al* 2003). b) For older children, comfort measures include: • Massage (Osborn *et al* 2003) • Relaxation (Osborn *et al* 2003, Playfor *et al* 2006) • Promotion of sleep (Playfor *et al* 2006).	

Nutritional concerns

1. Monitor and adjust nutritional intake according to energy expenditure and feeding tolerance in consultation with the multidisciplinary team.	1. Withdrawal increases the use of energy and calories, which are vital to the recovery of a critically ill child (French and Nocera 1994). Increasing activity in the withdrawing child such as irritability, tremors, persistent crying, or sleep disturbance may lead to feeding difficulties, calorie deficiency and weight loss; particularly in neonates (Berlin *et al* 1998, Katz 1994). In addition, the effects of gastrointestinal disturbances such as diarrhoea, vomiting, persistent gastric residuals following enteral feeding and uncoordinated suck and swallow reflexes may also lead to nutritional concerns (Tobias 2000).

Procedure guideline 30.1 (Continued)

Statement

2. Intravenous management of electrolyte imbalance may be necessary in extreme cases. Small frequent feeds of high calorie formula or supplements are usually sufficient to meet the child's additional calorific requirements. Advice should be sought form the dietician whenever necessary.

Maintenance of skin integrity

1. Close attention should be paid to pressure area care, particularly the skin integrity of the heels and toes and nappy area. Consult the Tissue Viability Nurse for advice regarding pressure-relieving mattresses (Osborn et al 2003) if necessary.

Rationale

2. Calories and electrolytes may be lost through vomiting, drooling and diarrhoea (Berlin et al 1998).

1. Repetitive movements in an irritable child may cause redness or skin abrasions. Diarrhoea may also result in skin breakdown (Franck and Vilardi 1995). For more information regarding pressure area care, see Chapter 10.

Weaning protocols

The dose and duration of therapy are key indicators in predicting the risk of withdrawal symptoms (Ista et al 2007). Continuous therapy over a number of days increases the risk of withdrawal. In one study where neonates received continuous infusions of more than 1.6 mg/kg fentanyl for longer than 5 days, the incidence of withdrawal was significantly increased (Arnold et al 1990). Katz et al (1994) found that, neonates and infants who received more than 2.5mg/kg fentanyl or had an infusion duration of more than 9 days had a 100% incidence of withdrawal, despite the drug having been weaned over 2 days. Similarly, the occurrence of withdrawal symptoms may be observed when high dose midazolam is administered over a period of >7 days (Ista et al 2007, Sury et al 1989). Withdrawal syndrome is generally seen after two weeks of morphine administration, but may occur after a few days of therapy (Yaster et al 1996). In some infants and children, tolerance has developed in a matter of hours following initial administration of opioids (Anand and Ingraham 1996, Eddlestone et al 1997).

Children on low dose opioids for less than a week may require a shorter period of weaning than those receiving high-dose opioid infusions (Anand and Arnold 1994), while children on short-term therapy (less than 3–5 days) can be weaned as rapidly as 10–15% every 6–8 hours (Ducharme et al 2005, Tobias 2000).

There is currently no standardised weaning regimen universally utilised in paediatric units in the UK (Birchley 2009, Easley and Nichols 2008, Playfor et al 2006). Dose reduction is based on a percentage decrease (or 'wean') of a peak dose of an opioid or benzodiazepine (Easley and Nichols 2008). This may vary, depending on the unit/hospital, from 10–50% within a 24-hour period (Franck et al 2008). Recommendations in the literature relating to management of opioid weaning in children identify that those on short-term therapy (less than 3–5 days) may be weaned as rapidly as 10–15% every 6–8 hours (Tobias 2000, Ducharme et al 2005). Weaning of longer term therapy should begin with dose reductions of 20% of the peak dose per day

(Anand and Arnold 1994, Carr and Todres 1994, Franck and Vilardi 1995, Ista et al 2007, Yaster et al 1996). Dose reductions of 10% of the peak dose should be employed if the child is particularly sensitive to small decreases (Ducharme et al 2005, Franck and Vilardi 1995, Ista et al 2007). Weaning guidance relating to the reduction of benzodiazepine therapy (midazolam) is less apparent in the literature, with daily dose reductions of between 5% and 25% of the peak dose being suggested (Cho et al 2007).

Table 30.1 Categorising patients' risk of developing withdrawal

Risk category	Duration of opioid/benzodiazepine
Category 1 (low risk)	Less than 5 days
Category 2 (medium risk)	5–14 days
Category 3 (high risk)	More than 14 days

(Great Ormond Street Hospital for Children's NHS Foundation Trust 2008)

Box 30.5 Treatment regimens

Category 1 Patients (low risk)
- No formalised weaning necessary unless symptoms occur
- Observe patient condition using a suitable withdrawal score.

Category 2 Patients (medium risk)
- Wean by 20% of the peak dose (i.e. highest continuous prescribed dose of opioid or benzodiazepine prior to wean) every 24 hours.
- Observe efficacy of treatment using a suitable withdrawal score.

Category 3 Patients (high risk)
- Wean by 5–10% of the peak dose every 24 hours
- Observe efficacy of treatment using a suitable withdrawal score.

(Great Ormond Street Hospital for Children's NHS Foundation Trust 2008) (Cunliffe et al 2004)

Principles table 30.4 Weaning protocols

Principle	Rationale
1. Whatever the weaning protocol adopted, it should be based on the premise of a regular delivery of a decreasing amount of the drug responsible for the actual, or likely cause of withdrawal.	1. Drug tolerance and withdrawal are thought to be related to the length of exposure to the drug and the number of days that it occupies a receptor site (Ducharme *et al* 2005, Yaster *et al* 1996). The administration of the drug dose in progressively smaller amounts maintains a degree of receptor occupancy that prevents susceptible neurones becoming abnormally excited, until the sedative or analgesic agent can be tapered off and stopped completely (Anand and Ingraham 1996). Other suggested mechanisms include interactions between receptors, intracellular enzyme systems and involvement of the nor-adrenergic system (Playfor *et al* 2006).
2. The child should be categorised in relation to the length of time they have received a continuous opioid or benzodiazepine infusion (see Table 30.1).	2. To identify the likelihood of them developing withdrawal symptoms if the analgesic or sedative agents are stopped abruptly (Ducharme *et al* 2005, Franck *et al* 1998).
3. The percentage wean can then be agreed and its effect monitored (see Box 30.5).	3. To minimise the risk of withdrawal.

Procedure guideline 30.2 Conversion from intravenous to oral medication

Statement	Rationale
1. Intravenous opioids and benzodiazepines should be converted to an oral equivalent as soon as possible (Birchley 2009). Criteria for conversion include: a) The child must be tolerating enteral feeds. b) Withdrawal scores should be consistently low. If these criteria are not met, weaning management should continue on intravenous therapy. c) The intravenous dose, when converted to the oral equivalent, should not exceed the dose recommended in the Trust's paediatric formulary.	1. Converting from an intravenous to an oral drug simplifies the weaning process and may allow for earlier patient discharge (Anand and Ingraham 1996, Tobias 2003, Yaster *et al* 1996). a) Inability to tolerate or absorb the oral drug may lead to increase in withdrawal symptoms. b) The efficacy of the oral dose cannot be accurately ascertained if the child is already showing signs of withdrawal.
2. The choice of agent used in the conversion to an oral dose should match the drug that has the potential to cause withdrawal. Practical considerations such as ease of administration, dose reduction and drug half-life should also be considered (Berlin *et al* 1998, Yaster *et al* 1996).	2. A plan of progressive dose reduction often involves the substitution of similar drugs with longer half-lives, while maintaining analgesic potency where necessary. Each drug may be converted at a separate time of the day or on alternate days.
3. As opioids and benzodiazepines are often co-administered both agents may need to be included in the weaning regimen.	3. It may be difficult to identify which drug is causing the withdrawal symptoms (Birchley 2009).

Conversion to oral

1. Approximate conversion factors can form the basis of a weaning strategy. However, the change from intravenous drugs to the oral equivalent should be made with caution, using conversion factors as a guide only.	1. When converting from intravenous to oral drugs, the substitute drug must be calculated to deliver an equipotent dose (Anand and Ingraham 1996).

Procedure guideline 30.2 (*Continued*)

Statement	Rationale
2. In some cases, the dose calculated should be reduced to ensure patient safety.	2. The risk of over or under dosing is significant, as drugs are not necessarily equal in their effect when given via a different route (Anand and Arnold 1994, Anand and Ingraham 1996, Indelicato and Portnoy 2002).
3. Particular caution is required when converting to a different drug in the same group (e.g. from intravenous midazolam to oral diazepam).	3. Changing from one drug to another may require a reduction in the total dose administered, as cross-tolerance may vary (Indelicato and Portnoy 2002, Tobias 2003).

For suggested conversion factors used at GOSH, go to:
www.gosh.nhs.uk/health-professionals/clinical-specialties/pain-control-service-information-for-health-professionals/

Statement	Rationale
4. When a converted dose is prescribed, the oral dose may be given initially and the corresponding infusion stopped an hour later.	4. To keep drug levels as constant as possible and thus avoid triggering further withdrawal symptoms (Franck and Vilardi 1995).
5. The following observations should be documented regularly: • Withdrawal scoring • Pulse • Respiratory rate • Sedation score • Blood pressure.	5. To detect for early signs of respiratory depression, hypotension and withdrawal. The risk of over or under dosing is significant during the conversion phase and careful monitoring of the patient's cardio-respiratory condition is essential (Tobias 2000).
6a) The initial converted dose may need to be given for 24–48 hours before any further weaning is attempted. b) This is particularly important in a child converting to oral opioids and benzodiazepines at the same time.	6a) To avoid triggering further withdrawal symptoms (Anand and Arnold 1994, Anand and Ingraham 1996, Yaster *et al* 1996). b) The drugs may have a synergistic effect when given together (Anand and Arnold 1994, Anand and Ingraham 1996).
7. Throughout the weaning process the child should have regular pain assessment and appropriate analgesia.	7. To provide effective analgesia in addition to any opioids being given as part of a weaning regimen (Franck and Vilardi 1995).
8. It is important to remain vigilant regarding the practicality of any dose reduction made. It may be sensible to stop dose reduction and start to omit doses once small volumes are being administered.	8. Small volumes are difficult to draw-up and administer, and increase the risk of drug errors.
9. When omitting doses as part of the weaning regimen, ensure the remaining doses are re-prescribed, keeping the drug intervals evenly spaced.	9. Drugs should be given on a 'round the clock' basis, at staggered time intervals (Yaster *et al* 1996).
10. If more than one drug is being given, both drugs should be uniformly spread over a 24-hour period.	
11. If two drugs are being weaned on the same day, it may be helpful to reduce the doses alternately (i.e. 12 hours apart).	11. To identify if one or other drug is being reduced too quickly.
12. If the child develops withdrawal during weaning, stop and return to the last dose on which the child was stable.	12. To prevent worsening of the withdrawal. For example, an increase in gastro-intestinal signs may be an indication to return to the previous/a higher opioid dose for 24 hours to see if symptoms improve (Wong *et al* 2003).

Principles table 30.5 Education

Principle	Rationale
1. Families should be given clear information including explanations relating to: • The reversible neurological adaptation that takes place during the development of tolerance, and physical dependence • The symptoms of withdrawal • Misconceptions related to addiction.	1. In some cases families may mistakenly believe that the symptoms they are witnessing are the result of a neurological assault, psychological damage or worsening of their child's disease process or clinical condition.
2. Members of the multidisciplinary team should involve families and carers in all stages of the weaning process, offering support and reassurance, advocating for the child, and communicating any concerns to the multi-disciplinary team (Alexander et al 2002, Osborn et al 2003).	2. Ongoing education for parents/carers and children is essential (Tobias 2000). Infants who suffer withdrawal may be exposed to additional problems such as risk of poor parental/carer bonding (Katz 1994).
3. All members of the multidisciplinary team should be educated in the practical aspects of the weaning process (Easley and Nichols 2008).	3. The management of analgesic and sedative reduction should be based on shared goals and effective communication between members of the multidisciplinary team (Cho et al 2007).
4. Whenever possible a named healthcare professional should lead on the formulation and implementation of an individual child's weaning regimen.	4. To ensure continuity of care and adherence to the principles of the weaning protocol adopted by the unit (Cho et al 2007). Inappropriate attitudes and beliefs, or lack of attention to the implementation of weaning plans should be avoided (Ducharme et al 2005, Franck et al 2004, Puntillo et al 1997).
5. Decisions regarding the weaning of analgesic or sedatives should be made on the basis of practicality (Franck et al 2004), the most current research evidence available and in the best interests of the individual child (Puntillo et al 1997).	5. To use the best available evidence to provide safe, effective care which is tailored to the individual needs of the child.
6. Multidisciplinary review of difficult cases should be held.	6. To ensure that the rationale for weaning guidance is based on best available evidence (Easley and Nichols 2008).
7. The management of children on continuous opioids or benzodiazepines should be audited in line with local policies.	7. To ensure that local guidelines are being followed and to monitor the incidence of withdrawal. Regular audit ensures that best evidence care is being implemented and can identify trends in patient response that may influence changes in practice.

References

Alexander E, Carnevale F, Razack S. (2002) Evaluation of a sedation protocol for intubated critically ill children. Intensive and Critical Care Nursing, 18, 292–301

Anand KJS, Arnold JH. (1994) Opioid tolerance and dependence in infants and children. Critical Care Medicine, 22(2), 174–342

Anand KJS, Ingraham J. (1996) Tolerance, dependence and strategies for compassionate withdrawal of analgesics and anxiolytics in the pediatric ICU. Critical Care Nursing, 16(6), 87–93

Arnold JH, Troug RD, Orav EJ, Scarvone M, Hershenson MB. (1990) Tollerence and dependence in neonates sedated with fentanyl during extracorporeal membrane oxygenation. Anaesthesiology, 73, 1136–1140

Berlin CM, McCarver DG, Notterman DA, Ward RM, et al (1998) American Academy of Pediatrics Committee on Drugs. Neonatal Drug Withdrawal. Pediatrics, 101(6), 1079–1088

Birchley G. (2009) Opioid and benzodiazepine withdrawal syndromes in the paediatric intensive care unit: a review of recent literature. Nursing in Critical Care, 14(1), 26–37

Carr DB, Todres ID. (1994) Fentanyl infusion and weaning in the pediatric intensive care unit: Towards science based practice. Critical Care Medicine, 22(5), 15–17

Cho HH, O'Connell JP, Cooney MF, Inchiosa MA. (2007) Minimising tolerance and withdrawal to prolonged pediatric sedation: Case report and review of the literature. Journal of Intensive Care Medicine, 22(3), 173–179

Cunliffe M, McArthur L, Dooley F. (2004) Managing sedation withdrawal in children who undergo prolonged PICU admission after discharge to the ward. Pediatric Anesthesia, 14, 293–298

Ducharme C, Carnevale FA, Clermont M, Shea S. (2005) A prospective study of adverse reactions to the weaning of opioids and benzodiazepines among critically ill children. Intensive and Critical Care Nursing, 21, 179–186

Du Pen A, Shen D, Ersek M. (2007) Mechanisms of opioid and induced tolerance and hyperalgesia. Pain Management Nursing, 8(3), 113–121

Easley RB, Nichols DG. (2008) Withdrawal assessment in the pediatric intensive care unit: Quantifying a morbidity of pain and sedation management in the critically ill child. Critical Care Medicine, 36(8), 2479–2480

Eddlestone J, MacDonald I, Littler C. (1997) Withdrawal of sedation in critically ill patients. British Journal of Intensive Care, November/December, 210–222

Franck L, Vilardi J. (1995) Assessment and management of opioid withdrawal in ill neonates. Neonatal Network, 14(2), 39–49

Franck L, Vilardi J, Durand D, Powers R. (1998) Opioid withdrawal in neonates after continuous infusions of morphine or fentanyl during extracopporeal membrane oxygenation. American Journal of Critical Care, 7(5), 364–369

Franck L, Naughton I, Winter I. (2004) Opioid and benzodiazepine withdrawal symptoms in paediatric intensive care patients. Intensive Critical Care Nursing, Dec 20, 344–351

Franck L, Harris S, Soetenga D, Amling J, Curley M. (2008) The Withdrawal Assessment Tool–1 (WAT–1): An assessment instrument for monitoring opioid and benzodiazepine withdrawal symptoms in pediatric patients. Pediatric Critical Care Medicine, 9(6), 573–580

Franck L, Scoppettuolo LA, Wypij D, Curley MAQ. (2012) Validity and generalizability of the Withdrawal Assessment Tool–1 (WAT–1) for monitoring iatrogenic withdrawal syndrome in pediatric patients. Pain, 153, 142–148

French JP, Nocera M. (1994) Drug withdrawal symptoms in children after continuous infusion of fentanyl. Journal of Paediatric Nursing, 9(2), 107–113

Grehn L. (1998) Adverse responses to analgesia, sedation, and neuromuscular blocking agents in infants and children. American Association of Critical Care Nurses, Clinical I, 9(1), 36–48

Great Ormond Street Hospital for Children's NHS Foundation Trust (2008) Clinical Procedure Guidelines. Opioid and Benzodiazepine Withdrawal Management. London, GOSH. Available online at: http://www.gosh.nhs.uk/health-professionals/clinical-specialties/pain-control-service-information-for-health-professionals/

Indelicato R, Portnoy RK. (2002) Opioid rotation in the management of refractory cancer pain. Journal of Clinical Oncology, 20(1), 348–352

Ista E, van Dijk M, Gamel C, Tibboel D, de Hoog M. (2007) Withdrawal symptoms in children after long term administration of sedatives and/or analgesics: a literature review. 'Assessment remains troublesome'. Intensive Care Medicine, 33, 1396–1406

Ista E, van Dijk M, Gamel C, Tibboel D, Hoog M. (2008) Withdrawal symptoms in critically ill children after long-term administration of sedatives and/or analgesics: A first evaluation. Critical Care Medicine, 36(8), 2427–2432

Ista E, van Dijk M, de Hoog M, Tibboel D, Duivenvoorden HJ. (2009) Construction of the Sophia Observation withdrawal Symptom Scale (SOS) for critically ill children. Intensive Care Medicine, 35, 1075–1081

Jage J. (2005) Opioid tolerance and dependence – do they matter? European Journal of Pain, 9, 157–162

Katz R, Kelly HW, His A. (1994) Prospective study on the occurrence of withdrawal in critically ill children who receive fentanyl by continuous infusion. Critical Care Medicine, 22(5), 763–767

Osborn DA, Jeffery HE, Cole MJ. (2003) Sedatives for opiate withdrawal in newborn infants (Corchrane Review). The Cochrane Library, Issue 4

Playfor SD. (2008) Pharmacy update: Analgesia and sedation in critically ill children. Archives of Disease in Childhood Education and Practice, 93, 87–92

Playfor S, Jenkins I, Boyles C, et al (2006) Consensus Guidelines on sedation and analgesia in critically ill children. Intensive Care Medicine, 32, 1125–1136

Puntillo K, Casella V, Reid M. (1997) Opioid and benzodiazepine tolerance and dependence: Application of theory to critical care practice. Heart and Lung, 26(4), 310–44

Sury M, Russell G, Hopkins C, Thornington R, Vivori E. (1989) Acute benzodiazepine withdrawal syndrome after midazolam infusions in children. Critical Care Medicine, 17, 301–302

Tobias JD. (2000) Tolerance withdrawal and physical dependency after long term sedation and analgesia of children in the pediatric intensive care unit. Critical Care Medicine, 3(6), 2122–2132

Tobias DJ. (2003) Pain management for the critically ill child in the pediatric intensive care unit. In Schecter N, Berde C, Yaster M. (eds) Pain in Infants and Children, 2nd edition. Philidelphia, Lippincott Williams and Wilkins

Weissman DE, Haddox JD. (1989) Opioid pseudoaddiction – an iatrogenic syndrome. Pain, 36, 363–366

Wong MC, McIntosh N, Menon G, Frank L. (2003) Chapter 37: Pain (and Stress) in Infants in a Neonatal Intensive Care Unit In Schecter, N. Berde, C. Yaster, M (2003) Pain in Infants and Children 2nd ed. Philidelphia; Lippincott Williams and Wilkins

Yaster M, Kost-Byerly S, Berde C, Billet C. (1996) The management of opioid and benzodiazepine dependence in infants, children and adolescents. Pediatrics, 98(1), 135–140

Index

30° tilt, 212, 213–14

A&E, procedures for children attending, 128–9
AAFB, 351
ABCDE, 636, 664, 690
abdominal thrusts, 683
abduction traction, 531
absenteeism, 400
abstinence syndrome *see* withdrawal syndrome
abuse *see* child abuse
ACE procedure, 90, 97–8
acetylcysteine, in paracetamol poisoning treatment, 627–8, 629
acid mantle, 168
acidosis
    and cardiac arrest, 664
    and seizures, 444
    treatment, 148
ACT, 154
activated charcoal, 627, 629, 630, 633
activated clotting time (ACT), 154
activity level, 13
acute kidney injury (AKI)
    causes, 147
    dialysis sessions, 149
    IV fluid and electrolytes requirements, 146
acute laryngotracheobronchitis (croup), isolation precautions, 250
acute protein-energy malnutrition, 474
acute renal failure *see* acute kidney injury
addiction, definition, 735
Adelaide Paediatric Coma Scale, 437, 438
adenovirus, isolation precautions, 250
adipose tissue, 63, 104
adjunct therapy, 736
adjuvants, in pain management *see* co-analgesics
administration of medication, 357–94
    by carer, 358–9
    by self, 358

child development considerations, 359–60
    adolescents, 360
    infants, 359
    pre-schoolers, 360
    school-age, 360
    toddlers, 359–60
drug calculations, 360–4
general guidelines, 362–4
nurse's role, 359
see also buccal and sublingual administration; enteral tube administration; epidural administration; inhalation administration; injections; intradermal administration; intramuscular administration; intranasal administration; intraosseous administration; intrathecal administration; intravenous administration; oral administration; rectal administration; skin patches administration; subcutaneous administration
adolescents, needs, 610
Adoption and Children Act (2002), 121
adrenaline
    in anaphylaxis management, 42, 43
    in cardiorespiratory arrest management, 685, 687, 689, 690
    in circulation management, 675
adrenaline auto-injector devices (AAD), 42–3
Advanced Level Nursing, 292
advanced life support (ALS), 664, 676, 684, 690
adverse events following immunisation (AEFIs), 50, 226
AEDs, 676, 688
aerosolisation, 372
aerosolisers, 373
agitation, near death, 585

air enema, 336–7
airborne transmission, 240
airway management, 664–7
    advanced, 668–71
        in gastric tubes, 669
        laryngeal mask airways (LMAs), 669
        self-inflating bag-mask (B-M) ventilation, 669–71
        tracheal tubes, 669
    basic techniques, 665–7
        head positioning, 665–6
        pharyngeal airways, 666–7
        suction, 665
airway stenosis, 337
airway suction, 636–42
    assessment, 637
    completing procedure, 642
    continuous vs. intermittent, 641
    harmful effects, 637
    irrigation in, 641
    performing suction, 640–1
    preparation of child and family, 637–8
    preparation of equipment
        catheter selection, 639
        negative pressure, 638–9
    uses, 636
AKI *see* acute kidney injury
albumin
    administration, 81–2
        infusion of component, 81
        observations and recordings, 82
    strengths, 80
alcohol acid fast bacilli (AAFB), 351
alcohol misuse, in parent, 121
alcohol poisoning, 628
Allen's test, 312
allergens, 39
    common, 42
    in healthcare setting, 48–51, 246
    high allergen foods, 478
    testing for, 380
allergic dermatitis, 184
allergic march, 40